The Natural Pharmacy

The Natural Pharmacy

REVISED AND UPDATED 3RD EDITION

Complete A–Z Reference to
Natural Treatments for Common Health Conditions

Alan R. Gaby, M.D., Chief Science Editor

Jonathan V. Wright, M.D.

Forrest Batz, Pharm.D.

Rick Chester, R.Ph., N.D., Dipl.Ac.

George Constantine, R.Ph., Ph.D.

Linnea D. Thompson, Pharm.D., N.D.

With contributions by
Amber Ackerson, N.D. • Jeremy Appleton, N.D. • Steve Austin, N.D. • Deah Baird, N.D. • Kimberly Beauchamp, N.D.
Matthew Brignall, N.D. • Donald J. Brown, N.D. • Regina Dehen, N.D., MAcOM, LAc
Tori Hudson, N.D. • Darin Ingels, N.D., M.T. (A.S.C.P.) • James Gerber, D.C. • Ronald LeFebvre, D.C.
Michael Murray, N.D. • Ronald Reichert, N.D. • Trina Seligman, N.D.
Maureen Williams, N.D. • Eric Yarnell, N.D.

Schuyler W. Lininger, Jr., Healthnotes Publisher

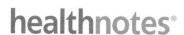

 THREE RIVERS PRESS • NEW YORK

Published in the United States by Three Rivers Press, an imprint of the Crown Publishing Group, a division of Random House, Inc., New York.
www.crownpublishing.com

THREE RIVERS PRESS and the Tugboat design are registered trademarks of Random House, Inc.

Library of Congress Cataloging-in-Publication Data

The natural pharmacy : a complete A-Z reference to natural treatments for common health conditions / edited by Alan R. Gaby; with contributions by Amber Ackerson . . . [et al.].—Rev. and updated 3rd ed. Includes index.
  1. Naturopathy. 2. Homeopathy. 3. Herbs—Therapeutic use. 4. Vitamin therapy.
5. Minerals—Therapeutic use. I. Gaby, Alan. II. Ackerson, Amber. [DNLM: 1. Naturopathy.
2. Homeopathy. 3. Minerals—therapeutic use. 4. Phytotherapy. 5. Vitamins—therapeutic use.
WB 935 N2852 2006]
  RZ440.N354 2006
  615.5'35—dc22   2005022263

ISBN-13: 978-0-307-33665-1
ISBN-10: 0-307-33665-4

Printed in the United States of America

10 9 8 7 6 5 4 3 2 1

Third Edition

For my wife, Beth, who has shared my journey in pursuing the truth regarding natural medicine.—ARG

For the Healthnotes team.—SWL

Acknowledgments

THIS BOOK IS the result of the work of many dedicated healthcare professionals who believe in the power of evidence-based natural medicine. They receive well-deserved credit on the title page, but special recognition goes to Chief Science Editor Alan R. Gaby, M.D. His hard work, sense of humor, and dedication to excellence and quality are an inspiration to all of us.

The "hidden" work is done by the hardworking, talented, and dedicated members of the Product Development and Marketing teams at Healthnotes, Inc. Although many people were involved, Jenefer Angell, Kurt Kremer, Loren Jenkins, and Jeannette Shupp deserve special mention for their efforts on this book.

Thanks are also due our publisher, Three Rivers Press. Our editor, Kathryn McHugh, has been a strong advocate for this new and greatly expanded edition. Her efforts are really appreciated.

Finally, thanks to our families, friends, and customers who continue to strongly support our company and our work.

—*Dr. Skye Lininger, Healthnotes Publisher*

Contents

PART ONE:

Health Concerns

PART TWO:

Nutritional Supplements

PART THREE:

Herbs

Note: Herbs are listed by their most common names. To look up an herb by other common names or by their Latin (scientific) name, look in the index.

Foreword

As PEOPLE INCREASINGLY explore their power to improve their own lives and an aging baby boomer population reaches out for alternatives to traditional therapies, attention has turned to integrative medicine. The rising cost of healthcare has encouraged consumers to take more responsibility for their own physical well-being, from prevention to treatment. In particular, the emergence of new public health issues, such as the epidemic increases in childhood obesity and diabetes, urges us to find complementary and alternative solutions to these problems.

When one is taking a more active role in self-care, the importance of education cannot be overstated, particularly as it relates to the different forms of nutritional supplements, the potencies of different extracts, and how specific intake amounts may benefit particular health concerns. *The Natural Pharmacy* provides numerous examples of how supplementing one's diet with a vitamin, mineral, or herb can provide significant preventative or therapeutic effects.

The primary authors of *The Natural Pharmacy* are respected for their expertise and knowledge in a form of medicine that relies on nature rather than drugs or surgery. Their contributions to this field go beyond their expertise, as they are true visionaries and pioneers, dedicated to making a difference in the lives of others by educating physicians, patients, and the public at large on the value of natural products. Consumers need objective, reliable sources of health information. Accessible science, such as readers will find here, helps them come to safe conclusions about healthcare and natural treatments. *The Natural Pharmacy* is grounded in the mission of providing comprehensive, scientifically based information from leading natural medicine experts to empower individuals to make informed decisions about their health. As a physician, I can't emphasize strongly enough how important it is to review the supplements you're considering with your physician, especially any potential interactions you've uncovered in this very useful guide.

— *Dr. Bob Arnot, NBC news correspondent, expert health and fitness author and columnist*

Preface

THE LAST TWO decades have seen an explosion of interest in natural medicine. The public has an ever-increasing appetite for information on diet and nutrition, and sales of natural remedies such as nutritional supplements and medicinal herbs continue to grow. The number of natural health practitioners now exceeds the number of medical doctors, which bears testament to the fact that individuals all over the globe are being drawn to holistic approaches as an adjunct to or even replacement for conventional medicine.

Driving this change is growing skepticism about the principles and practice of orthodox medicine. In my experience, many individuals are simply not comfortable with the largely symptom-suppressive approach and are increasingly concerned about both the safety and effectiveness of pharmaceutical drugs. Questions are also being asked about the scrupulousness and integrity of the companies that make these agents, and there has even been some erosion in the trust that the public has traditionally had in doctors who prescribe them. With these factors in the background, it is perhaps no surprise that individuals are seeking alternatives.

Another important force in the move toward natural medicine has been the growing recognition that it can so often promote healing in a way that is safer, less expensive, and even more effective than conventional medical practices. More and more, it seems, individuals are feeling motivated to take their health issues into their own hands and are finding that natural medicine often provides them with the tools they need. As the demand for more holistic healthcare increases, people are seeking increasingly sophisticated information and advice about what options are available to them for regaining and maintaining their health.

With this in mind, I regard *The Natural Pharmacy* as a truly unique source of natural healthcare information. Within these pages you will find comprehensive advice on a wide range of health conditions and how they may be approached and healed using natural remedies. One of the most useful features of this book is its detail. The authors have, for instance, included important information on the multiple forms of specific nutrients, such as vitamin E, and the different ways these affect the body. The book also includes guidance on the specific amounts of nutrients that have been found to benefit particular health concerns, and specifies the needed potencies of herbal extracts. Another critical feature of *The Natural Pharmacy* is that it is fully scientifically referenced—which means we can all be confident that the material it contains is validated, trustworthy, and reliable.

The Natural Pharmacy is a valuable source of information people need to take natural approaches in a truly educated way. I heartily recommend it to all who feel empowered to take control of their own health.

—*Dr. John Briffa, leading British natural medicine specialist, award-winning journalist, author, and columnist*

Introduction

OVER THE LAST several decades, the line between conventional and alternative medicines has blurred as more people explore the benefits of vitamins, minerals, and herbs for the treatment of a range of health concerns. Widespread use has made many remedies familiar to the general public, and many people have adopted them as part of their regular self-care practices. At the same time, these natural remedies have gotten more attention from the medical community as a complement to conventional medicine, as evidenced by the explosion of research in recent years.

Despite all the new attention on natural medicine, however, it is still almost as hard to sort out the fact from folklore as it was thirty years ago. The millions of people taking vitamins and herbs are bombarded with anecdotes, fragmented information, and conflicting media messages. Strict regulations restrict supplement manufacturers from advising people on what health conditions an herb or supplement may be used for and on the intake amounts appropriate for a particular condition, so consumers are often left guessing. *The Natural Pharmacy* was conceived to fill this gap and to give people a credible resource for science-based information about herbs and nutritional supplements, with specific information on what, when, and how much to take, in an easy-to-use format.

Over the years, the steady stream of scientific articles has formed a solid foundation for nutritional therapies. When we began working on our electronic knowledge base, Healthnotes, which is the foundation for this book, the number of useful scientific articles on the role of vitamins and herbs in human health exceeded 25,000. Since then, our team of researchers has continued to comb through thousands of articles in over 600 medical journals to keep up to date on breaking research. Those who contributed to this book are among the most knowledgeable natural medicine physicians in the world. Our expert scientific and evidence-based medical team consists of medical doctors, pharmacists, naturopaths, and doctor of chiropractic.

This newest edition of our best-selling book *The Natural Pharmacy* is greatly expanded, with 150 new articles featuring 64 new health concerns, 44 new herbs, and 41 new nutritional supplements. In addition, every article has been updated with the latest scientific research. We have added an informative new article, "Vitamins and Minerals for Healthy People," and provided a thorough evaluation of hot topics, such as the safety of supplementing with vitamin E, and the strengthened evidence for many natural remedies, such as St. John's wort for treating depression and echinacea for preventing the common cold.

Otherwise, this revised third edition shares the same characteristics as the original:

- All statements that might be controversial have been documented with a reference from the scientific literature. Thousands of citations are referenced and available online, so the serious reader can retrieve the article and review the source material.

- We have used primarily human studies, although animal or test tube studies are sometimes used to support the human research.

- A section on contraindications and side effects includes information on possible areas of concern when taking a specific supplement or herb. Millions of people who have never before taken vitamins or herbs are now doing so, and people who use natural medicines are legitimately concerned about the safety (and efficacy) of these products. The information we provide gives you a way to make sensible choices for yourself and your family. For a complete look at drug-nutrient depletions and interactions, see our companion volume, the *A–Z Guide to Drug-Herb-Vitamin Interactions*.

• All of our key contributors have actually been in practice with patients and are also trained to recog-

nize the difference between reliable and questionable scientific evidence.

In short, we have done our best to create the most useful, comprehensive, and balanced book available on this topic, knowing it will be the first place many people turn as they take charge of their health.

All of the Healthnotes team joins me in wishing you good health.

—Alan R. Gaby, Chief Medical Editor,
Healthnotes, Inc.

How to Use This Book

Design Features

The Natural Pharmacy's unique design allows you to access information in several ways.

- **Look Up by Health Condition**—You can look up a specific health concern to learn what nutritional supplements or herbs might be helpful treatments.

- **Look Up by Nutritional Supplement or Herb**—You can look up a nutritional supplement or herb on its own to see the full list of health concerns for which it has been found useful, known side effects and interactions, and other information specific to that nutrient or herb.

- **Find Your Section**—The book is divided into three parts, Health Concerns, Nutritional Supplements, and Herbs, which can be easily found by looking at the gray tabs at the edge of the pages. Once in the right part, flip through the alphabetized listings to find your health concern, nutritional supplement, or herb of interest.

- **Follow Cross-References**—For easy navigation, health concerns, nutritional supplements, and herbs are in boldface and followed by a page number that will take you to information on that topic, much the way hyperlinks work online. If a health concern topic mentions vitamin C, for example, then "**vitamin C**" will appear in bold type, followed by a page number that takes you to the entry on vitamin C.

- **Use the Table of Contents and Index**—The table of contents lists health concerns, nutritional supple-

ments, and the common names of herbs. Try the index for alternative names and the botanical names of herbs.

- **Find References**—We have tried not to make any statements without referring to scientific documentation. We rely most heavily on human studies published in major medical and scientific journals, which can be found using reference numbers. If you or your doctor wants to see the original study, the full references for each entry can be easily accessed online at www.healthnotes.com/naturalpharmacy.

What You'll Find

The following explains what information is covered in each section of the book:

- **Part One: Health Concerns**—Look here for information about specific health concerns ranging from A to Z. Each entry includes a section that describes the concern, makes appropriate dietary and lifestyle recommendations, and suggests which nutrients and herbs might be of help. Special features:

  - *What Do I Need to Know?*—Popular health concerns open with "Where Do I Focus?" sections that help you quickly see doctor-recommended self-care options.

  - *3-Star Checklist Ranking System*—At the end of each condition is the Checklist of the nutritional supplements and herbs discussed in the text, ranked as either 3-star, 2-star, or

1-star, according to the strength of the scientific documentation. See "About the Checklist" (below) for full definitions.

- **Part Two: Nutritional Supplements**—Look here for information about specific vitamins, minerals, amino acids, and other nutrients (such as CoQ_{10}). Each nutrient entry includes information about where it is found, health concerns for which the nutrient might be supportive, suggested dosage ranges, and possible side effects or interactions.

- **Part Three: Herbs**—Look here for information about specific herbs. Each herb includes information about where it is found, what part is used, concerns for which the herb might be supportive, information about historical and traditional use (which may or may not be supported by scientific studies), data on the active compounds (if known), suggested dosage ranges, and possible side effects or interactions.

Many herbs are available in multiple forms: dried (usually in capsules, tablets, poultice, or tea), liquid (as tinctures or extracts), or standardized (where a particular compound is measured and quantified). We have tried to give you dosages for all the various forms when that information is available.

When and How Much to Take

Each health condition covered in this book includes specific, useful information about nutritional and herbal support for the condition. Keep in mind that unless the text specifies differently, the suggested amounts of vitamins, minerals, amino acids, or herbs apply only to an average-size male or female adult.

Children's doses should be determined in consultation with your physician.

Unless otherwise specified in the text, nutritional supplements and herbs should be taken with meals.

Important Disclaimer

It is important to realize that this book is provided for information or educational purposes only and should be used in consultation with a healthcare professional knowledgeable in natural medicine. Information in this book is not meant to replace any medical information supplied by a doctor or pharmacist.

About the Checklist

Information about the effects of a particular supplement or herb on a particular condition has been qualified in terms of the methodology or source of supporting data (for example, clinical, double-blind, meta-analysis, or traditional use). For the convenience of the reader, the information in the table listing the supplements for particular conditions is also categorized. The criteria for the categorizations are:

★★★ Reliable and relatively consistent scientific data showing a substantial health benefit.

★★☆ Contradictory, insufficient, or preliminary studies suggesting a health benefit or minimal health benefit.

★☆☆ For an herb, supported by traditional use but minimal or no scientific evidence. For a supplement, little scientific support and/or minimal health benefit.

Vitamin and Mineral Supplements for Healthy People

Why take vitamin and mineral supplements?

For healthy people, supplements may help prevent vitamin and mineral deficiencies when the diet does not provide adequate quantities of all necessary nutrients. They can also supply amounts of nutrients larger than the diet can provide. Larger amounts of some nutrients may help to protect against future disease. Many of these nutrients will be briefly discussed here. However, for more information, refer to individual nutrient articles.

People may consume diets that are deficient in one or more nutrients for a variety of reasons. The typical Western diet often supplies less than adequate amounts of several essential vitamins and minerals.[1] Recent nutrition surveys in the United States have found that large numbers of people consume too little calcium, magnesium, iron, zinc, and possibly copper and manganese.[2, 3]

Weight-loss, pure vegetarian, macrobiotic, and several other diets can also place some people at risk of deficiencies that vary with the type of diet. Certain groups of people are at especially high risk of dietary deficiencies. Studies have found that elderly people living in their own homes often have dietary deficiencies of vitamin D, vitamin A, vitamin E, calcium, and zinc,[4] and occasionally of vitamin B_1 and vitamin B_2.[5] Premenopausal women have been found often to consume low amounts of calcium, iron, vitamin A, and vitamin C.[6]

What is the potential importance of taking vitamin A?

Dietary deficiency of vitamin A is uncommon in healthy people except in older age groups.[7] Although vitamin A is important for the function of the immune system, vitamin A supplementation did not help prevent infections in elderly people living in nursing homes, in one study.[8] Due to concerns about birth defects[9] and bone loss,[10] people should not take more than 10,000 IU of supplemental vitamin A in the form of retinol without consulting a doctor.

What is the potential importance of taking beta-carotene?

Beta-carotene is a precursor to vitamin A but may have a separate role in human health. Controlled research has shown that beta-carotene supplements can increase the numbers of some white blood cells and enhance cancer-fighting immune functions in healthy people who take 25,000 to 100,000 IU per day.[11, 12] However, some studies of smokers have reported that supplements of *synthetic* beta-carotene *increased* the risk of both heart disease[13, 14] and lung cancer.[15, 16] Other trials found no positive or negative effect of synthetic beta-carotene on the risk of many other diseases, including several types of cancer,[17, 18, 19, 20, 21, 22, 23, 24] angina pectoris,[25] diabetes,[26] age-related eye disease,[27, 28] or intermittent claudication.[29] Natural beta-carotene, though similar to synthetic, was found in one preliminary study to reverse precancerous changes, while synthetic beta-carotene did not.[30] No other studies have investigated whether natural beta-carotene could be more effective than the synthetic form in preventing other diseases, but the potential harm from taking synthetic beta-carotene suggests it should be avoided by smokers.

What is the potential importance of taking B vitamins?

Some of the B vitamins, including thiamine (vitamin B_1), riboflavin (vitamin B_2), and niacin (vitamin B_3), may be adequately supplied by the typical Western diet, because they are added to white flour products and other foods that have been depleted of those vitamins. Another vitamin, biotin, is produced by intestinal bacteria in amounts that, along with typical dietary biotin intake, provide enough of this vitamin to prevent deficiency in healthy people. Pantothenic acid (vitamin B_5), on the other hand, appears to be in short supply in the typical diet. In one study, 49% of a group of male and female adolescents were consuming less than adequate amounts of pantothenic acid in their diet.[31] No research has investigated whether supplements of these B vitamins prevent disease.

Vitamin B_6 (pyridoxine) deficiency, at least in a mild form, may exist in 10 to 25% of people living in Western societies,[32] and may be most common in the elderly.[33, 34, 35] The possible role of vitamin B_6 in the prevention of heart disease by helping to regulate blood homocysteine levels is discussed below. No other research on preventive effects of vitamin B_6 supplementation has been done.

What is the potential importance of taking folic acid?

Folic acid deficiency has been considered somewhat common in the United States. It affects about 11% of healthy people,[36] with a higher prevalence among African-Americans and Mexican-Americans.[37] Recently, however, the U.S. Food and Drug Administration (FDA) mandated that some grain products provide supplemental folic acid. This appears to be causing a reduction in the prevalence of folic acid deficiency in the general population.[38] Nonetheless, some authorities believe the recent increases in folic acid content of the food supply are not enough to optimally prevent diseases such as heart disease and birth defects (see discussions below).[39]

The requirement for folic acid doubles during pregnancy,[40] and insufficient intake of folic acid has been linked to low birth weight and an increased incidence of neural tube defects in newborns. Supplementation with 400 mcg per day of folic acid prior to and shortly after conception is effective in preventing neural tube defects.[41]

What is the potential importance of taking vitamin B_{12}?

Vitamin B_{12} deficiency is not common among healthy young people,[42] except for vegans (vegetarians who also avoid dairy and eggs).[43] However, about 12 to 15% of the elderly in the U.S. have been found deficient in this vitamin.[44, 45] Vitamin B_{12} deficiency may also occur in people who take acid-blocking drugs or antacids for long periods of time.[46] Although vitamin B_{12} deficiency in the elderly is often due to age-related declines in absorption of vitamin B_{12} from food, vitamin B_{12} supplements can be absorbed sufficiently in members of this age group if they do not have pernicious anemia or significant gastrointestinal disorders.[47] Supplementation with 100 mcg per day of vitamin B_{12} was adequate to reverse vitamin B_{12} deficiency in healthy elderly people, according to one recent report.[48]

The B vitamins folic acid, B_{12}, and pyridoxine (vitamin B_6) are important for the control of homocysteine levels in the blood.[49] Elevated homocysteine levels are associated with several diseases, including heart disease,[50] stroke,[51] Alzheimer's disease,[52] and osteoporosis,[53] and some, though not all, research suggests that homocysteine has a direct role in causing these diseases. Daily supplementation with these B vitamins, typically at least 400 mcg of folic acid, 10 mg of vitamin B_6, and 50 mcg of vitamin B_{12}, lowers elevated homocysteine levels in most people.[54, 55, 56] Some studies have shown that supplementing with one or more of these vitamins helps prevent or reverse hardening of the arteries (atherosclerosis) and may also reduce the risk of bone fractures.[57, 58]

What is the potential importance of taking vitamin C?

Severe vitamin C deficiency is uncommon in people who consume Western diets, but mild insufficiency is found in 6% of healthy adults[59] and larger numbers of college students[60] and smokers.[61] On the basis of extensive analyses of published vitamin C studies, some authorities have suggested that optimal intake for disease prevention may be at least 90 to 100 mg per day.[62, 63] However, supplementation with over 200 mg per day of vitamin C by healthy people does not result in higher vitamin C concentrations in the body[64] and may be no more helpful for preventing disease than smaller amounts.

What is the potential importance of taking vitamin D?

Vitamin D can be obtained either from the diet or from sunlight exposure, but these sources can be insufficient, especially in older people and vegans during the winter months.[65, 66] Six to 14% of healthy adult Western European populations have been reported to be vitamin D deficient,[67] but good data are not available for the United States. Vitamin D insufficiency is associated with bone loss and fractures in older people.[68, 69] Reduced bone loss from vitamin D supplements has been reported in some,[70, 71] though not all,[72] studies. In one double-blind study, supplementation with 800 IU per day of vitamin D prevented bone loss more effectively than 200 IU per day in postmenopausal women.[73] In addition, vitamin D supplementation has been shown to reduce the risk of falls in older people.[74] While vitamin D is known to be toxic in very high amounts, up to 2,000 IU per day is considered safe.[75]

What is the potential importance of taking vitamin E?

A nationwide study recently reported that 27% of the U.S. population had low blood levels of vitamin E.[76] Supplementing with at least 100 IU per day of vitamin E is associated with lowered risk of heart disease,[77, 78] and a double-blind study found that 400 to 800 IU of vitamin E per day reduced the risk of nonfatal heart attacks, but not fatal ones.[79] However, another double-blind trial found no beneficial effect from 400 IU per day of vitamin E supplementation on the risk of nonfatal heart attacks,[80] while another study found that 50 IU per day had no effect on heart attack risk.[81] A more recent study found that taking large amounts of vitamin E (400 IU per day or more) may result in a small increase in all-cause mortality,[82] while another study found that 400 IU per day increased the risk of heart failure.[83] Because of these studies, some doctors are advising people not to take large amounts of vitamin E. On the other hand, circumstantial evidence suggests that mixed tocopherols, as opposed to the more widely used alpha-tocopherol, may be safer and more beneficial with respect to heart-disease prevention.[84, 85]

A reduced risk of prostate cancer in smokers was reported in a double-blind trial with 50 IU per day of vitamin E.[86] However, similar studies have not found vitamin E supplements to protect against other cancers.[87, 88, 89, 90]

What is the potential importance of taking vitamin K?

Vitamin K deficiency severe enough to cause bleeding problems is rare in healthy people. However, low vitamin K in the blood[91, 92] and in the diet[93] has been associated with osteoporosis. Preliminary research has suggested that supplements of at least 1 mg per day of vitamin K reduce indicators of bone loss in some women.[94, 95, 96, 97]

What is the potential importance of taking calcium?

Compared with recent calcium intake recommendations, most people have calcium-deficient diets, and less than 10% of women in the United States have adequate dietary intakes.[98] Good calcium nutrition throughout life is essential for achieving peak bone mass and preventing deficiency-related bone loss.[99] Calcium supplements are effective in increasing bone mass in children[100, 101, 102] and slowing bone loss in adults, according to most,[103, 104, 105, 106, 107, 108] though not all,[109] double-blind studies. Calcium supplements have also been shown to reduce the risk of bone fractures in some elderly adults.[110, 111, 112, 113] The protective effect of calcium on bone is one of very few health claims permitted by the FDA. In order to achieve the 1,500 mg per day calcium intake deemed optimal by many researchers for postmenopausal women, 800 to 1,000 mg of supplemental calcium is generally added to diets that commonly contain between 500 and 700 mg of calcium per day.

What is the potential importance of taking phosphorus?

Phosphorus is a necessary nutrient, but diets are almost always adequate in this mineral.[114] Some authorities have suggested that excess intake of phosphorus is hazardous to normal calcium and bone metabolism.[115] However, this idea has been challanged.[116] In any case, for most people there does not seem to be a need for phosphorus supplementation. For this reason, many multivitamin-mineral supplements do not contain phosphorus. The only exception is for elderly people, whose diets tend to be lower in phosphorus. Calcium interferes with phosphorus absorption, so older people who are taking a calcium supplement might benefit from taking additional phosphorus.[117]

What is the potential importance of taking magnesium?

Dietary magnesium deficiency may occur in up to 25% of adult women in the United States and in even higher numbers of elderly people of both sexes.[118] Magnesium supplements of at least 250 mg per day may help prevent bone loss.[119, 120]

What is the potential importance of taking potassium?

While potassium is lower in modern diets compared with so-called primitive diets, true deficiencies are uncommon.[121] Some,[122] though not all,[123] research suggests that raising potassium intake may help prevent high blood pressure. Other research suggests that higher potassium intake may help prevent stroke.[124] However, the maximum amount of supplemental potassium allowed in one pill (99 mg) is far below the recommended amounts (at least 2,400 mg per day). Multiple potassium pills should not be taken in an attempt to get a higher amount, since they can irritate the stomach. The best way to get extra potassium is to eat several servings per day of fruits, vegetables, or their juices.

What is the potential importance of taking iron?

Iron deficiency is not uncommon among some groups of healthy people, including some vegetarians,[125] menstruating girls and women,[126] pregnant women,[127] and female and adolescent athletes.[128] Nonetheless, many people in these groups are not iron deficient [129] and excessive iron intake has been associated in some studies with heart disease,[130] some cancers,[131] diabetes,[132] increased risk of infection,[133] and exacerbation of rheumatoid arthritis.[134] While none of these links has yet been proven, people should avoid iron supplements unless they have been diagnosed with having, or being at high risk of, iron deficiency.

What is the potential importance of taking iodine?

Iodine deficiency is a concern in many developing countries.[135] Until recently this mineral was considered abundant in Western diets, due to the introduction of iodized salt and the iodine added to many foods.[136] However, iodine intake has decreased considerably in recent years and may be low in as much as 12% of the total U.S. population and 15% of women of childbearing age.[137] These numbers may be greater in countries where iodized salt is not available. Still, most people have adequate iodine intake unless they avoid iodized salt, seafood, and sea vegetables. People with thyroid diseases should check with their doctor before using iodine supplements.

What is the potential importance of taking zinc?

Zinc deficiency is not common in Western countries, except in people with low incomes.[138, 139] Zinc supplements (10 mg per day) have prevented growth impairment in deficient American and Canadian children.[140] Supplementation with 25 to 150 mg of zinc per day has been shown to increase immune function, in healthy people.[141, 142, 143, 144] However, too much zinc has been reported to impair immune function and some healthcare practitioners recommend no more than 30 to 50 mg per day.[145] It is unknown whether these immune system changes are sufficient to cause or prevent infections or other diseases in people taking zinc supplements. Regular supplementation with zinc should be accompanied by copper supplements to prevent zinc-induced copper deficiency.

What is the potential importance of taking copper?

The average dietary copper intake in the United States has been found to be below accepted standards.[146] However, the significance of this is unclear, since symptomatic copper deficiency is quite rare.[147] Supplementation with 3 mg per day of copper may help prevent bone loss.[148] Since zinc can interfere with copper absorption, copper should be taken whenever zinc supplements are used for more than a few weeks.[149]

What is the potential importance of taking manganese?

Dietary intake of manganese is adequate for most people, according to recent studies in the United States.[150] However, manganese, along with other trace minerals, is often low in refined and processed foods.[151, 152] People whose diets consist primarily of these types of foods may have low manganese intake. Manganese deficiency has been associated with osteoporosis in an unpublished study.[153] A double-blind trial found that a combination of mineral supplements including manganese prevented bone loss in postmenopausal women.[154] No other studies have investigated the health effects of manganese supplementation. Manganese may be especially important to include when iron is supplemented, since iron can reduce manganese absorption and cause lower body levels of manganese.[155]

What is the potential importance of taking chromium?

Chromium nutrition has been difficult to study because of technical problems in analyzing foods and human body fluids for chromium content. Partly for this reason, there is disagreement about the extent of chromium deficiency in Western societies. Many studies have found suboptimal levels of chromium in the diet, compared to published recommendations.[156, 157, 158] However, some authorities question the validity of the recommended minimum requirements.[159] Chromium deficiency has been associated with blood sugar and cholesterol abnormalities.[160] Also, chromium levels in the body decline as people get older, which is when these problems often appear.[161] Therefore, while chromium supplements have not been tested for their ability to prevent diabetes or heart disease, many health-care practitioners recommend them as a reasonable precaution. A few single case reports have described possible serious side effects in people taking large amounts of chromium, from 600 to 2,400 mcg per day,[162, 163, 164] although it is not clear whether chromium was responsible for these reactions.

What is the potential importance of taking selenium?

Dietary intake of selenium appears to be adequate in most people. This is according to recent studies in the United States based on the Recommended Dietary Allowance of 70 mcg per day of selenium.[165] However, a double-blind study found that people given a supplement of 200 mcg of yeast-based selenium per day for four and a half years had a 50% drop in the cancer death rate over seven years compared with the placebo group.[166] Higher amounts of selenium than are available in the diet may be necessary for this protective effect. The upper end of safe long-term selenium intake has been estimated to be 350 to 400 mcg per day.[167]

What is the potential importance of taking molybdenum?

Molybdenum is an essential trace element with low potential for toxicity.[168] Since little is known about human needs and deficiencies are quite rare, estimated requirements are based on what people typically receive in their diets.[169] Cancer and cardiovascular disease prevention studies in China found no benefit from a supplement containing molybdenum and vitamin C.[170, 171] No other research has investigated disease prevention with molybdenum supplements.

PART ONE
Health Concerns

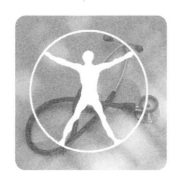

ABNORMAL PAP SMEAR

Sexually active teenagers and women 20 to 65 years old are advised to have periodic Pap smears, where a small amount of tissue is swabbed from the cervix and examined for evidence of precancerous or cancerous changes. A pap smear is considered abnormal when abnormal cervical cells are found. Cervical dysplasia is a term used to describe abnormal cervical cells taken during the pap smear. Cervical dysplasia is usually graded according to its severity, which can range from mild inflammation to precancerous changes to localized cancer.

If an abnormality is detected early, the doctor can prescribe effective treatment before the problem becomes more serious. Cervical **cancer** (page 87) is a common, sometimes fatal disease. It is now known that human papilloma virus (HPV), also the cause of genital **warts** (page 445), is the major cause of cervical dysplasia.

What are the symptoms of an abnormal pap smear?

There are no symptoms of cervical dysplasia until the disease has progressed into advanced cancer. Therefore, it is crucial that sexually active women, or women over age 20, have yearly Pap smears until the age of 65. Women who experience bleeding between menstrual periods, bleeding after intercourse, abnormal vaginal discharge, abdominal pain or swelling, urinary symptoms, or pelvic pain should be evaluated by a healthcare provider, even if it is not the regular time for a Pap test.

Medical treatments

If the Pap smear is normal, no further tests are necessary until the next yearly Pap test. If the cells collected on the Pap smear are abnormal, a repeat test and a pelvic exam where the doctor looks at the cervix with a special magnifying lens (colposcope) may be recommended. Sometimes a small piece of tissue is removed from the cervix (biopsy) and examined under a microscope to see if there are any precancerous changes or cancer present. If these additional tests find an early stage of cervical cancer, it is either treated by removing the affected portion of the cervix (cone biopsy) or by removing the entire cervix and uterus (abdominal hysterectomy).

CHECKLIST FOR ABNORMAL PAP SMEAR

Rating	Nutritional Supplements	Herbs
★★★	**Folic acid** (page 520) (for women using oral contraceptives)	
★★☆		**Green tea extracts** (page 686) (poly E or (-)-epigallocatechin-3-gallate)
★☆☆	**Selenium** (page 584) **Vitamin A** (page 595) **Vitamin E** (page 609)	**Echinacea** (page 669), **Goldenseal** (page 683), **Marsh-mallow** (page 708), **Myrrh** (page 713), **Usnea** (page 754), **Yarrow** (page 763) (suppository; in various combinations)

Dietary changes that may be helpful

Most dietary studies have found that women consuming high amounts of nutrients from fruits and vegetables have less risk of cervical dysplasia.[1, 2] Protective effects may be especially strong from diets high in dark yellow/orange vegetables (carrots, winter squash, etc.)[3] and tomatoes.[4, 5]

Lifestyle changes that may be helpful

Cigarette smoking increases the risk of cervical dysplasia,[6, 7, 8] and increases the likelihood that mild forms of dysplasia will progress to more severe forms.[9, 10] Quitting smoking and avoiding exposure to secondhand smoke are essential for this and many other health reasons.

Certain sexual behaviors are consistently associated with cervical dysplasia, such as becoming sexually active at an early age and having multiple sexual partners.[11, 12] Avoiding these behaviors may reduce the risk of cervical dysplasia. For those who are sexually active, using barrier methods of contraception, such as a condom or diaphragm, is associated with reduced risk of cervical dysplasia.[13, 14, 15]

Nutritional supplements that may be helpful

Large amounts of **folic acid** (page 520)—10 mg per day—have been shown to improve the abnormal Pap smears of women who are taking birth control pills.[16] Folic acid does not improve the Pap smears of women who are not taking oral contraceptives.[17, 18] High blood levels of folate (the food form of folic acid) have been linked to protection against the development of cervical dysplasia[19] but these folate levels may only be a marker for eating more fruit and vegetables.

Women with cervical dysplasia may have lower blood levels of **beta-carotene** (page 469) and **vitamin E** (page 609)[20, 21] compared to healthy women. Low levels of **selenium** (page 584)[22] and low dietary intake of **vitamin C** (page 604)[23, 24] have also been observed in women with cervical dysplasia. Women with a low intake of **vitamin A** (page 595) have an increased risk of cervical dysplasia.[25] However, there is little research on the use of vitamin A as a treatment for cervical dysplasia.

In a double-blind trial, when women with cervical abnormalities were given either 500 mg of vitamin C or 50,000 IU beta-carotene per day for two years, no significant evidence of improvement was seen in either group, and those assigned to both supplements experienced a statistically insignificant worsening of their condition.[26] Given that the apparent association between these supplements and deterioration of the condition of the cervix appears to have been due to chance, there is currently no sound evidence supporting the use of vitamin C or beta-carotene supplements for women with cervical dysplasia.

Are there any side effects or interactions?
Refer to the individual supplement for information about any side effects or interactions.

Herbs that may be helpful

In a preliminary study, women with cervical dysplasia were randomly assigned to receive either (1) 200 mg per day of (-)-epigallocatechin-3-gallate (a flavonoid found in **green tea** [page 686]), (2) 200 mg per day of poly E (a green tea extract), or (3) no treatment (control group) for 8 to 12 weeks. Approximately two-thirds of the women receiving (-)-epigallocatechin-3-gallate or poly E had an improvement in their Pap smear, compared with only 10% of the women in the control group.[27]

Several other herbs have been used as part of an approach for women with mild cervical dysplasia, including **myrrh** (page 713), **echinacea** (page 669), **usnea** (page 754), **goldenseal** (page 683), **marshmallow** (page 708), and **yarrow** (page 763).[28] These herbs are used for their antiviral actions as well as to stimulate tissue healing; they are generally administered in a suppository preparation. No clinical trials have proven their effectiveness in treating cervical dysplasia. A doctor should be consulted to discuss the use and availability of these herbs.

Are there any side effects or interactions?
Refer to the individual herb for information about any side effects or interactions.

ACNE ROSACEA

Acne rosacea, now more accurately know just as rosacea, is a chronic skin condition of the forehead, cheeks, nose, and chin. It consists of flushing, which turns into red coloration from the dilation of the capillaries and can lead to pustules that resemble acne.

Rosacea occurs mostly in middle-aged adults with fair skin. The cause of rosacea is unknown, but there is likely a genetic component. Severe, untreated rosacea can be disfiguring to the face.

What are the symptoms of acne rosacea?

The skin of the center of the face—typically on or surrounding the nose—is red and swollen, with acne-like blemishes. As the condition progresses, parts of the eye can become inflamed and the nose may enlarge.

CHECKLIST FOR ACNE ROSACEA		
Rating	Nutritional Supplements	Herbs
★☆☆	Betaine hydrochloride (page 473) Digestive enzymes (page 506) Vitamin B-complex (page 603)	Burdock (page 648)

Medical treatments

Prescription medications used to treat rosacea include topical and oral antibiotics. The main topical drug, metronidazole (Metrogel), is thought to have antibacterial and anti-inflammatory effects. The vitamin A-related medication tretinoin (Retin A), which is used for acne vulgaris, may also be prescribed. The most commonly used oral antibiotic is tetracycline (Sumycin).

Dietary changes that may be helpful

Alcohol may increase the reddening of the skin affected by rosacea, but alcohol is not the cause of this disease.[1] Spicy foods and hot drinks have been reported anecdotally by rosacea sufferers to cause flare-ups,[2] but no controlled research has evaluated these claims. One small, preliminary report suggested that fasting followed by a vegan diet (allowing no animal flesh foods, dairy products, or eggs) had only small and inconsistent effects on rosacea.[3]

Lifestyle changes that may be helpful

Sun exposure, stress, excessive exercise, and extreme temperatures (hot or cold) of weather or bathing water may trigger flare-ups of rosacea, so avoiding these conditions is recommended.[4]

Nutritional supplements that may be helpful

Azelaic acid is found naturally in wheat, rye, and barley and is used topically in a 20% strength cream. Controlled clinical trials have found this cream effective for mild to moderate acne, including rosacea.[5, 6] Azelaic acid cream is available by prescription only and should be used only under the supervision of the prescribing physician.

Preliminary reports in the 1940s claimed that rosacea improved with oral supplements or injections of **B vitamins** (pages 597–604)[7, 8, 9] On the other hand, one report exists of rosacea-like symptoms in a patient taking 100 mg per day of **vitamin B6** (page 600) and 100 mcg per day of **vitamin B12** (page 601); these symptoms subsided when the supplements were discontinued.[10] More research is needed to evaluate the potential benefits or hazards of B vitamins for rosacea.

Some people with rosacea have been reported to produce inadequate **stomach acid** (page 260).[11] In a preliminary trial, supplemental hydrochloric acid, along with vitamin B complex, improved some cases of rosacea in people with low stomach-acid production.[12] Similarly, improvement in rosacea has been reported anecdotally after supplementation with **pancreatic digestive enzymes** (page 506), and a controlled study found that rosacea patients produced less pancreatic **lipase** (page 547) than healthy people.[13] Controlled trials are needed to evaluate the effects of hydrochloric acid and digestive enzyme supplements in rosacea. Hydrochloric acid supplements should not be taken without the supervision of a healthcare practitioner.

A topical preparation of retinaldehyde (a prescription form of **vitamin A** [page 595]) may be effective in treating people with mild rosacea. In a small, preliminary trial, women with rosacea used a retinaldehyde cream (0.05%) once daily for six months.[14] Inflammation was improved in most participants, and blood vessel abnormalities responded in about half the people after six months. Controlled research is needed to confirm these effects. Retinaldehyde cream is available by prescription only and should be used only under the supervision of the prescribing physician.

Are there any side effects or interactions?
Refer to the individual supplement for information about any side effects or interactions.

Herbs that may be helpful

Historically, tonic herbs, such as **burdock** (page 648), have been used in the treatment of skin conditions. These herbs are believed to have a cleansing action when taken internally.[15] Burdock root tincture may be taken in 2 to 4 ml amounts per day. Dried root preparations in a capsule or tablet can be used at 1 to 2 grams three times per day. Many herbal preparations combine burdock root with other alterative herbs, such as **yellow dock** (page 763), **red clover** (page 735), or **cleavers** (page 660). In the treatment of acne rosacea, none of these herbs has been studied in scientific research.

Are there any side effects or interactions?
Refer to the individual herb for information about any side effects or interactions.

ACNE VULGARIS

What do I need to know?

Self-care for acne vulgaris can be approached in a number of ways—but it can be hard to know just where to start. To make it easier, our doctors recommend trying these simple steps first:

Clean your skin
> Washing with cleaning lotions, oil-removing pads, and medicated bar soaps can help control acne

Try zinc
> 60 to 90 mg each day improves some people's acne

Add copper
> If taking extra zinc, your body will need 1 to 2 mg each day of copper to avoid deficiency

About acne vulgaris

Acne vulgaris, also known as common acne, is an inflammatory condition of the sebaceous glands of the skin. It consists of red, elevated areas on the skin that may develop into pustules and even further into cysts that can cause scarring.

Acne vulgaris occurs mostly on the face, neck, and back of most commonly teenagers and to a lesser extent of young adults. The condition results in part from excessive stimulation of the skin by androgens (male hormones). Bacterial infection of the skin also appears to play a role.

CHECKLIST FOR ACNE VULGARIS

Rating	Nutritional Supplements	Herbs
★★★	**Niacinamide** (page 598) (topical) **Zinc** (page 614)	**Tea tree oil** (page 751) (topical)
★★☆		**Guggul** (page 688)
★☆☆	**Pantothenic acid** (page 568) **Vitamin A** (page 595) **Vitamin B₆** (page 600)	**Burdock** (page 648) **Vitex** (page 757) (associated with menstrual cycle)

What are the symptoms of acne?

Acne is a skin condition characterized by pimples, which may be closed (sometimes called pustules or "whiteheads") or open (blackheads), on the face, neck, chest, back, and shoulders. Most acne is mild, although some people experience inflammation with larger cysts, which may result in scarring.

Medical treatments

Over the counter products such as astringent lotions, oil-removing pads, and medicated bar soaps are used to keep the skin clean. Non-prescription topical agents containing salicylic acid (Clearasil Acne-Fighting Pads, Stri-Dex Pads) and benzoyl peroxide (Oxy 10 Maximum Strength Advanced Formula, Fostex 10% Wash, Clear By Design) are often recommended to prevent the formation of pimples and to treat preexisting cysts.

Topical prescription medications include benzoyl peroxide (Benzac, Desquam, Triaz); antibiotics such as erythromycin (Akne-mycin, Erygel), clindamycin (Cleocin T), and azelaic acid (Azelex); and tretinoin (Retin-A). Oral antibiotics such as erythromycin (Ery-Tab, E-Mycin) or tetracycline (Sumycin) are often prescribed. Women with severe acne are sometimes treated with birth control pills. People with the most severe acne are usually prescribed isotretinoin (Accutane).

Dietary changes that may be helpful

Many people assume certain aspects of diet are linked to acne, but there is not much evidence to support this idea. Preliminary research found, for example, that chocolate was not implicated.[1] Similarly, though a diet high in **iodine** (page 538) can create an acne-like rash in a few people, this is rarely the cause of acne. In a preliminary study, foods that patients believed triggered their acne failed to cause problems when tested in a clinical setting.[2] Some doctors of natural medicine have observed that **food allergy** (page 14) plays a role in some cases of acne, particularly adult acne.[3] However, that observation has not been supported by scientific studies.

Nutritional supplements that may be helpful

In a double-blind trial, topical application of a 4% **niacinamide** (page 598) gel twice daily for two months resulted in significant improvement in people with acne.[4] However, there is little reason to believe this vitamin would have similar actions if taken orally.

Several double-blind trials indicate that **zinc** (page 614) supplements reduce the severity of acne.[5, 6, 7, 8] In one double-blind trial,[9] though not in another,[10] zinc was found to be as effective as oral antibiotic therapy. Doctors sometimes suggest that people with acne take 30 mg of zinc two or three times per day for a few months, then 30 mg per day thereafter. It often takes 12 weeks before any improvement is seen. Long-term zinc supplementation requires 1–2 mg of copper per day to prevent copper deficiency.

Large quantities of **vitamin A** (page 595)—such as 300,000 IU per day for females and 400,000–500,000 IU per day for males—have been used successfully to treat severe acne.[11] However, unlike the long-lasting benefits of the synthetic prescription version of vitamin A (isotretinoin as Accutane), the acne typically returns several months after natural vitamin A is discontinued. In addition, the large amounts of vitamin A needed to control acne can be toxic and should be used only under careful medical supervision.

In a preliminary trial, people with acne were given 2.5 grams of **pantothenic acid** (page 568) orally four times per day, for a total of 10 grams per day—a remarkably high amount.[12] A cream containing 20% pantothenic acid was also applied topically four to six times per day. With moderate acne, near-complete relief was seen within two months, while severe conditions took at least six months to respond. Eventually, the intake of pantothenic acid was reduced to 1 to 5 grams per day—still a very high amount.

A preliminary report suggested that **vitamin B$_6$** (page 600) at 50 mg per day may alleviate premenstrual flare-ups of acne experienced by some women.[13] While no controlled research has evaluated this possibility, an older controlled trial of resistant adolescent acne found that 50–250 mg per day decreased skin oiliness and improved acne in 75% of the participants.[14] However, another preliminary report suggested that vitamin B$_6$ supplements might exacerbate acne vulgaris.[15]

Are there any side effects or interactions?
Refer to the individual supplement for information about any side effects or interactions.

Herbs that may be helpful

A clinical trial compared the topical use of 5% **tea tree oil** (page 751) to 5% benzoyl peroxide for common acne. Although the tea tree oil was slower and less potent in its action, it had far fewer side effects and was thus considered more effective overall.[16]

One controlled trial found that **guggul** (page 688) *(Commiphora mukul)* compared favorably to tetracycline in the treatment of cystic acne.[17] The amount of guggul extract taken in the trial was 500 mg twice per day.

Historically, tonic herbs, such as **burdock** (page 648), have been used in the treatment of skin conditions. These herbs are believed to have a cleansing action when taken internally.[18] Burdock root tincture may be taken in the amount of 2 to 4 ml per day. Dried root preparations in a capsule or tablet can be used at 1 to 2 grams three times per day. Many herbal preparations combine burdock root with other alterative herbs, such as **yellow dock** (page 763), **red clover** (page 735), or **cleavers** (page 660). In the treatment of acne, none of these herbs has been studied in scientific research.

Some older, preliminary German research suggests that **vitex** (page 757) might contribute to clearing of premenstrual acne, possibly by regulating hormonal influences on acne.[19] Women in these studies used 40 drops of a concentrated liquid product once daily.[20]

Are there any side effects or interactions?
Refer to the individual herb for information about any side effects or interactions.

Holistic approaches that may be helpful

Acupuncture may be helpful in the treatment of acne. Several preliminary studies have reported that a series of acupuncture treatments (8 to 15) is markedly effective or curative in 90 to 98% of patients.[21, 22, 23] Besides traditional Chinese acupuncture using needles alone, a technique called "cupping" is frequently used in the treatment of acne. Cupping refers to the use of cup-shaped instruments to apply suction to the area being needled. Two preliminary trials of cupping treatment for acne reported marked improvement in 91 to 96% of the study participants.[24, 25] Controlled trials are necessary to determine the true efficacy of acupuncture and other traditional Chinese therapies in the treatment of acne.

Some hypnotherapists believe that hypnosis might help prevent facial scarring associated with acne. In one case study, a patient was instructed to say the word "scar" in place of picking her face, and the scratch marks resolved. The underlying acne was unaffected.[26]

ACRODERMATITIS ENTEROPATHICA

Acrodermatitis enteropathica is a rare inherited childhood disorder that results in the inability to absorb adequate amounts of zinc from the diet. Anyone who is severely **zinc** (page 614) deficient can develop the same symptoms that occur in the inherited form of this disorder.

Symptoms of acrodermatitis enteropathica include skin lesions, hair loss, and diarrhea. If untreated, the condition can result in death during infancy or early childhood.

CHECKLIST FOR ACRODERMATITIS ENTEROPATHICA		
Rating	**Nutritional Supplements**	**Herbs**
★★★	Zinc (page 614)	

What are the symptoms of acrodermatitis enteropathica?

Symptoms of this condition include growth retardation, **diarrhea** (page 163), hair loss, and a red skin rash. Skin around the fingernails may be red and swollen.

Medical treatments

Individuals with acrodermatitis are usually given over the counter **zinc** (page 614) supplements.

Dietary changes that may be helpful

Oysters, beef, liver, pumpkin seeds, pecans, and Brazil nuts are all high in zinc.[1] However, people with acrodermatitis enteropathica also need to take zinc supplements.

Nutritional supplements that may be helpful

Supplementation with **zinc** (page 614) brings about complete remission in hereditary acrodermatitis enteropathica. Zinc supplements in the amount of 30 to 150 mg per day are used by people with this condition.[2] People with acrodermatitis enteropathica need to be monitored by a healthcare professional to ensure that their level of zinc supplementation is adequate and that the zinc supplements are not inducing a copper deficiency.

Are there any side effects or interactions?
Refer to the individual supplement for information about any side effects or interactions.

AGE-RELATED COGNITIVE DECLINE

A decline in memory and cognitive (thinking) function is considered by many authorities to be a normal conse-

quence of aging.[1, 2] While age-related cognitive decline (ARCD) is therefore not considered a disease, authorities differ on whether ARCD is in part related to **Alzheimer's disease** (page 19) and other forms of dementia[3] or whether it is a distinct entity.[4, 5] People with ARCD experience deterioration in memory and learning, attention and concentration, thinking, use of language, and other mental functions.[6, 7]

ARCD usually occurs gradually. Sudden cognitive decline is not a part of normal aging. When people develop an illness such as Alzheimer's disease, mental deterioration usually happens quickly. In contrast, cognitive performance in elderly adults normally remains stable over many years, with only slight declines in short-term memory and reaction times.[8]

People sometimes believe they are having memory problems when there are no actual decreases in memory performance.[9] Therefore, assessment of cognitive function requires specialized professional evaluation. Psychologists and psychiatrists employ sophisticated cognitive testing methods to detect and accurately measure the severity of cognitive decline.[10, 11, 12, 13] A qualified health professional should be consulted if memory impairment is suspected.

Some older people have greater memory and cognitive difficulties than do those undergoing normal aging, but their symptoms are not so severe as to justify a diagnosis of Alzheimer's disease. Some of these people go on to develop Alzheimer's disease; others do not. Authorities have suggested several terms for this middle category, including "mild cognitive impairment"[14] and "mild neurocognitive disorder."[15] Risk factors for ARCD include advancing age, female gender, prior **heart attack** (page 212), and **heart failure** (page 212).

What are the symptoms of age-related cognitive decline?

People with ARCD experience deterioration in memory and learning, attention and concentration, thinking, use of language, and other mental functions.

Medical treatments

Though there is no standard drug therapy for ARCD, several experimental "nootropic" agents may provide improvements in cognitive function. Nootropic drugs are used specifically to facilitate learning and memory and might prevent the cognitive deficits associated with dementias. Nootropic drugs that are currently being investigated include ergoloid mesylates (Hydergine, Gerimal), idebenone (a synthetic analogue of CoQ_{10}

marketed as a "smart drug"), and derivatives of an inhibitory brain chemical called GABA (vinpocetine and bifemelane, which are also known by the investigational drug names piracetam [Nootropil], oxiracetam, and nebracetam).

CHECKLIST FOR AGE-RELATED COGNITIVE DECLINE

Rating	Nutritional Supplements	Herbs
★★★	Acetyl-L-carnitine (page 461) Phosphatidylserine (page 569) (bovine brain PS only; soy-derived PS does not appear to be effective) Vinpocetine (page 594)	Ginkgo biloba (page 681)
★★☆	Vitamin B₁₂ (page 601) (for treating people with B₁₂ deficiency only) Vitamin B₆ (page 600)	Huperzine A (page 694)
★☆☆	Melatonin (page 555) Vitamin C (page 604) Vitamin E (page 609)	Bacopa (page 632)

Dietary changes that may be helpful

In the elderly population of southern Italy, which eats a typical Mediterranean diet, high intake of monounsaturated fatty acids (e.g., olive oil) has been associated with protection against ARCD in preliminary research.[16] However, the monounsaturated fatty acid content of this diet might only be a marker for some other dietary or lifestyle component responsible for a low risk of ARCD.

Caffeine may improve cognitive performance. Higher levels of coffee consumption were associated with improved cognitive performance in elderly British people in a preliminary study.[17] Older people appeared to be more susceptible to the performance-improving effects of caffeine than were younger people. Similar but weaker associations were found for tea consumption. These associations have not yet been studied in clinical trials.

Animal studies suggest that diets high in **antioxidant** (page 467)-rich foods, such as spinach and strawberries, may be beneficial in slowing ARCD.[18] Among people aged 65 and older, higher **vitamin C** (page 604) and **beta-carotene** (page 469) levels in the blood have been associated with better memory performance,[19] though

these nutrients may only be markers for other dietary factors responsible for protection against cognitive disorders.

One preliminary study found that, among middle-aged men, those who ate more tofu had a *higher* rate of cognitive decline compared with men who ate less tofu.[20] Since tofu and other soy products have consistently demonstrated important health benefits in this age group (e.g., as cholesterol-lowering foods), middle-aged men should not limit their consumption of these foods until the results of this isolated study are independently confirmed.

Lifestyle changes that may be helpful

Cigarette smokers and people with high levels of education appear to have some protection against ARCD.[21] The reason for each of these associations remains unknown. However, as cigarette smoking generally is not associated with other health benefits and results in serious health risks, doctors recommend abstinence from smoking, even by people at risk of ARCD.

A large, preliminary study in 1998 found associations between **hypertension** (page 246) and deterioration in mental function.[22] Research is needed to determine if lowering blood pressure is effective for preventing ARCD.

A randomized, controlled trial determined that group exercise has beneficial effects on physiological and cognitive functioning, and well-being in older people. At the end of the trial, the exercisers showed significant improvements in reaction time, memory span, and measures of well-being when compared with controls.[23] Going for walks may be enough to modify the usual age-related decline in reaction time. Faster reaction times were associated with walking exercise in a British study.[24] The results of these two studies suggest a possible role for exercise in preventing ARCD. However, controlled trials in people with ARCD are needed to confirm these observations.

Psychological counseling and training to improve memory have produced improvements in cognitive function in persons with ARCD.[25, 26, 27]

Nutritional supplements that may be helpful

Several clinical trials suggest that **acetyl-L-carnitine** (page 461) delays onset of ARCD and improves overall cognitive function in the elderly. In a controlled clinical trial, acetyl-L-carnitine was given to elderly people with mild cognitive impairment. After 45 days of acetyl-L-carnitine supplementation at 1,500 mg per day, significant improvements in cognitive function (especially memory) were observed.[28] Another large trial of acetyl-L-carnitine for mild cognitive impairment in the elderly found that 1,500 mg per day for 90 days significantly improved memory, mood, and responses to stress. The favorable effects persisted at least 30 days after treatment was discontinued.[29] Controlled[30, 31, 32] and uncontrolled[33] clinical trials on acetyl-L-carnitine corroborate these findings.

Phosphatidylserine (page 569) (PS) derived from bovine brain phospholipids has been shown to improve memory, cognition, and mood in the elderly in at least two placebo-controlled trials. In both trials, geriatric patients received 300 mg per day of PS or placebo. In an unblinded trial of ten elderly women with depressive disorders, supplementation with PS produced consistent improvement in depressive symptoms, memory, and behavior after 30 days of treatment.[34] A double-blind trial of 494 geriatric patients with cognitive impairment found that 300 mg per day of PS produced significant improvements in behavioral and cognitive parameters after three months and again after six months.[35]

Most research has been conducted with PS derived from bovine (cow) brain tissue. Due to concerns about the possibility of humans contracting infectious diseases (such as Creutzfeld-Jakob or "mad cow" disease), bovine PS is not available in the United States. The soy- and bovine-derived PS, however, are not structurally identical.[36] Doctors and researchers have debated whether the structural differences could be important,[37, 38] but so far only a few trials have studied the effects of soy-based PS.

Preliminary animal research shows that the soy-derived PS does have effects on brain function similar to effects from the bovine source.[39, 40, 41] An isolated, unpublished double-blind human study used soy-derived PS in an evaluation of memory and mood benefits in nondemented, nondepressed elderly people with impaired memories and accompanying **depression** (page 145).[42] In this three-month study, 300 mg per day of PS was not significantly more effective than a placebo. In a double-blind study, soy-derived PS was administered in the amount of 300 or 600 mg per day for 12 weeks to people with age-related memory impairment. Compared with the placebo, soy-derived PS had no effect on memory or on other measures of cognitive function.[43] While additional research needs to be done, currently available evidence suggests that soy-derived

PS is not an effective treatment for age-related cognitive decline.

A double-blind trial found both 30 mg and 60 mg per day of **vinpocetine** (page 594) improved symptoms of dementia in patients with various brain diseases.[44] Another double-blind trial gave 30 mg per day of vinpocetine for one month, followed by 15 mg per day for an additional two months, to people with dementia associated with hardening of the arteries of the brain, and significant improvement in several measures of memory and other cognitive functions was reported.[45] Other double-blind trials have reported similar effects of vinpocetine in people with some types of dementia or age-related cognitive decline.[46, 47] However, a study of Alzheimer patients in the United States found vinpocetine given in increasing amounts from 30 mg to 60 mg per day over the course of a year neither reversed nor slowed the decline in brain function measured by a number of different tests.[48]

Vincamine, the unmodified compound found naturally in *Vinca minor*, has also been tested in people with dementia. A large double-blind trial found 60 mg per day of vincamine was more effective than placebo for improving several measures of cognitive function in patients with either Alzheimer's disease or dementia associated with vascular brain disease.[49] A small double-blind study of vascular dementia also reported benefits using 80 mg per day of vincamine.

Vitamin B₆ (page 600) (pyridoxine) deficiency is common among people over age 65.[50] A Finnish study demonstrated that approximately 25% of Finnish and Dutch elderly people are deficient in vitamin B₆ as compared to younger adults. In a double-blind trial, correcting this deficiency with 2 mg of pyridoxine per day resulted in small psychological improvements in the elderly group. However, the study found no direct correlation between amounts of vitamin B₆ in the cells or blood and psychological parameters.[51] A more recent double-blind trial of 38 healthy men, aged 70 to 79 years, showed that 20 mg pyridoxine per day improved memory performance, especially long-term memory.[52]

Supplementation with **vitamin B₁₂** (page 601) may improve cognitive function in elderly people who have been diagnosed with a B₁₂ deficiency. Such a deficiency in older people is not uncommon. In a preliminary trial, intramuscular injections of 1,000 mcg of vitamin B₁₂ were given once per day for a week, then weekly for a month, then monthly thereafter for 6 to 12 months. Researchers noted "striking" improvements in cognitive function among 22 elderly people with vitamin B_{12} deficiency and cognitive decline.[53] Cognitive disorders due to vitamin B_{12} deficiency may also occur in people who do not exhibit the anemia that often accompanies vitamin B_{12} deficiency. For example, in a study of 141 elderly people with cognitive abnormalities due to B_{12} deficiency, 28% had no anemia. All participants were given intramuscular injections of vitamin B_{12}, and all showed subsequent improvement in cognitive function.[54]

Vitamin B_{12} injections put more B_{12} into the body than is achievable with absorption from oral supplementation. Therefore, it is unclear whether the improvements in cognitive function described above were due simply to correcting the B_{12} deficiency or to a therapeutic effect of the higher levels of vitamin B_{12} obtained through injection. Elderly people with ARCD should be evaluated by a healthcare professional to see if they have a B_{12} deficiency. If a deficiency is present, the best way to proceed would be initially to receive vitamin B_{12} injections. If the injections result in cognitive improvement, some doctors would then recommend an experimental trial with high amounts of oral B_{12}, despite a current lack of scientific evidence. If oral vitamin B_{12} is found to be less effective than B_{12} shots, the appropriate treatment would be to revert to injectable B_{12}. At present, no research trials support the use of any vitamin B_{12} supplementation in people who suffer from ARCD but are not specifically deficient in vitamin B_{12}.

Melatonin (page 555) is a hormone secreted by the pineal gland in the brain. It is partially responsible for regulating sleep-wake cycles. Cognitive function is linked to adequate sleep and normal sleep-wake cycles. Cognitive benefits from melatonin supplementation have been suggested by preliminary research in a variety of situations and may derive from the ability of melatonin to prevent sleep disruptions.[55, 56, 57, 58] A double-blind trial of ten elderly patients with mild cognitive impairment showed that 6 mg of melatonin taken two hours before bedtime significantly improved sleep, mood, and memory, including the ability to remember previously learned items.[59] However, in a double-blind case study of one healthy person, 1.6 mg of melatonin had no immediate effect on cognitive performance.[60]

The long-term effects of regularly taking melatonin supplements remain unknown, and many healthcare practitioners recommend that people take no more than 3 mg per evening. A doctor familiar with the use of melatonin should supervise people who wish to take it regularly.

Use of **vitamin C** (page 604) or **vitamin E** (page 609) supplements, or both, has been associated with better cognitive function and a reduced risk of certain forms of dementia (not including Alzheimer's disease).[61] Clinical trials of these antioxidants are needed to confirm the possible benefits suggested by this study.

Are there any side effects or interactions?
Refer to the individual supplement for information about any side effects or interactions.

Herbs that may be helpful
Most[62, 63, 64, 65, 66, 67, 68] but not all[69] clinical trials, many of them double-blind, have found **ginkgo** (page 681) supplementation to be a safe and effective treatment for ARCD.

Huperzine A, an isolated alkaloid from the Chinese medicinal herb **huperzia** (page 694) *(Huperzia serrata)*, has been found to improve cognitive function in elderly people with memory disorders. One double-blind trial found that huperzine A (100 to 150 mcg two to three times per day for four to six weeks) was more effective for improving minor memory loss associated with ARCD than the drug piracetam.[70] More research is needed before the usefulness of huperzine A is confirmed for mild memory loss associated with ARCD.

Animal studies have found the Ayurvedic herb **bacopa** (page 632) has constituents that enhance several aspects of mental function and learning ability.[71, 72, 73] A controlled study found that a syrup containing an extract of dried bacopa herb given to children improved several measures of mental performance.[74] A double-blind trial in adults found that a standardized extract of bacopa (300 mg per day for people weighing under 200 lbs and 450 per day for people over 200 lbs) improved only one out of several measures of memory function after three months.[75] Another double-blind trial lasting twelve weeks found 300 mg per day of bacopa improved four out of fifteen measures of learning, memory, and other mental functions in adults.[76] A third double-blind study found no effects on mental function in a group of healthy adults given 300 mg of standardized bacopa and tested two hours later. Bacopa has not been tested on people with memory problems.[77]

Are there any side effects or interactions?
Refer to the individual herb for information about any side effects or interactions.

ALCOHOL WITHDRAWAL

Alcohol withdrawal is a set of symptoms that occur with the elimination of alcohol when a person is psychologically and/or physiologically addicted to it.

A majority of people who have been drinking alcohol and decide to stop (often for health-related reasons) are able to do so without much trouble. Alcohol withdrawal typically becomes difficult only when problem drinkers—alcoholics—attempt to quit. Almost inevitably, alcoholics need help in achieving this goal. Sometimes, this help requires medical intervention in detoxification centers.

Finding doctors who work with alcohol detoxification is often as easy as calling the local chapter of Alcoholics Anonymous (AA) and asking for referral information. Most programs successful in getting alcoholics to quit drinking are either part of the AA network or employ AA techniques. Natural approaches to alcohol withdrawal should not be a substitute for detox centers or for AA or AA-related programs.

CHECKLIST FOR ALCOHOL WITHDRAWAL

Rating	Nutritional Supplements	Herbs
★★★		Milk thistle (page 710)
★☆☆	Beta-carotene (page 469) D,L-phenylalanine (page 568) (DLPA) Evening primrose oil (page 511) Glutamine (page 530) L-tyrosine (page 544) Magnesium (page 551) Multiple vitamin-mineral (page 559) Vitamin A (page 594) Vitamin B-complex (page 603) Vitamin B$_3$ (page 598) Vitamin B$_6$ (page 600) Vitamin C (page 604) Vitamin D (page 607) Vitamin E (page 609)	Kudzu (page 700)

What are the symptoms of alcohol withdrawal?

A person typically has a mild to severe hangover that lasts several days. Symptoms may include **stomach upset** (page 260); headache; shakes or jitters; feelings of generalized **anxiety** (page 30) or panic attacks; and **insomnia** (page 270) that may be accompanied by bad dreams. There may also be increases in heart rate, breathing rate, and body temperature. In a small proportion of alcoholics, withdrawal may result in severe symptoms, such as hallucinations, delirium tremens (DTs), or generalized seizures.

Medical treatments

Over the counter treatment involves supplementing with multiple **B vitamins** (pages 597–604), including **thiamine** (page 597).

Prescription treatments in detoxification centers may begin with an injection of **vitamin B$_1$** (page 597) in cases that involve malnutrition. In treating severe acute withdrawal symptoms, a nervous system depressant, such as the benzodiazepines such as diazepam (Valium) and lorazepam (Ativan), is prescribed with a dosage that is tapered down over three to five days. The beta-adrenergic blocking drugs atenolol (Tenormin) and propranolol (Inderal) are also occasionally used.

Further treatment includes adequate nutrition, fluid intake, and rest.

Dietary changes that may be helpful

Some of the nutritional deficiencies associated with alcoholism can be caused by a poor diet—a factor that needs correction on an individual basis. Improving the overall diet should be done in conjunction with a doctor. Sometimes **liver** (page 290) or pancreatic disease associated with alcoholism also contributes to nutritional deficiencies. These problems require medical assessment and intervention.

In one trial, a hospital diet was compared with a special diet including fruit and wheat germ and excluding caffeinated coffee, junk food, dairy products, and peanut butter.[1] After six months, fewer than 38% of those on the hospital diet remained sober, compared with over 81% of those eating the special diet. A review of the research shows that diets loaded with junk food increase alcohol intake in animals.[2] In a human trial, restricting sugar, increasing complex carbohydrates, and eliminating caffeine also led to a reduction in alcohol craving.[3] While the support for dietary intervention remains somewhat unclear, some doctors suggest that alcoholics reduce sugar and junk food intake and avoid caffeine.

Lifestyle changes that may be helpful

Most experts agree that alcoholics must stop drinking completely in order to overcome the addiction. Moreover, before nutritional supplements can be used, effective treatment of the **malabsorption** (page 304) problems requires a complete avoidance of alcohol.

Nutritional supplements that may be helpful

Many alcoholics are deficient in B vitamins, including **vitamin B$_3$** (page 599). John Cleary, M.D., observed that some alcoholics spontaneously stopped drinking in association with taking niacin supplements (niacin is a form of vitamin B$_3$). Cleary concluded that alcoholism might be a manifestation of niacin deficiency in some people and recommended that alcoholics consider supplementation with 500 mg of niacin per day.[4] Without specifying the amount of niacin used, Cleary's preliminary research findings suggested that niacin supplementation helped wean some alcoholics away from alcohol.[5] Activated vitamin B$_3$ used intravenously has also helped alcoholics quit drinking.[6] Niacinamide—a safer form of the same vitamin—might have similar actions and has been reported to improve alcohol metabolism in animals.[7]

Deficiencies of other **B-complex** (page 603) vitamins are common with chronic alcohol use.[8] The situation is exacerbated by the fact that alcoholics have an increased need for B vitamins.[9] It is possible that successful treatment of B-complex vitamin deficiencies may actually reduce alcohol cravings, because animals crave alcohol when fed a B-complex-deficient diet.[10] Many doctors recommend 100 mg of B-complex vitamins per day.

Alcoholics may be deficient in a substance called prostaglandin E$_1$ (PGE$_1$) and in gamma-linolenic acid (GLA), a precursor to PGE$_1$.[11] In a double-blind study of alcoholics who were in a detoxification program, supplementation with 4 grams per day of **evening primrose oil** (page 511) (containing 360 mg of GLA) led to greater improvement than did placebo in some, but not all, parameters of liver function.[12]

The daily combination of 3 grams of **vitamin C** (page 604), 3 grams of **niacin** (page 598), 600 mg of **vitamin B$_6$** (page 600), and 600 IU of **vitamin E** (page 609) has been used by researchers from the University of Mississippi Medical Center in an attempt to reduce **anxiety** (page 30) and **depression** (page 145) in alcoholics.[13] Although the effect of vitamin supplementation was no better than placebo in treating alcohol-associated depression, the vitamins did result in a significant drop in anxiety within three weeks of use. Because of possible side effects, anyone taking such high amounts of niacin and vitamin B$_6$ must do so only under the care of a doctor.

Although the incidence of B-complex deficiencies is

known to be high in alcoholics, the incidence of other vitamin deficiencies remains less clear.[14] Nonetheless, deficiencies of **vitamin A** (page 594), **vitamin D** (page 607), **vitamin E** (page 609), and **vitamin C** (page 604) are seen in many alcoholics. While some reports have suggested it may be safer for alcoholics to supplement with **beta-carotene** (page 469) instead of vitamin A,[15] potential problems accompany the use of either vitamin A or beta-carotene in correcting the deficiency induced by alcoholism.[16] These problems result in part because the combinations of alcohol and vitamin A or alcohol and beta-carotene appear to increase potential damage to the liver. Thus, vitamin A-depleted alcoholics require a doctor's intervention, including supplementation with vitamin A and beta-carotene accompanied by assessment of liver function. Supplementing with vitamin C, on the other hand, appears to help the body rid itself of alcohol.[17] Some doctors recommend 1 to 3 grams per day of vitamin C.

Kenneth Blum and researchers at the University of Texas have examined neurotransmitter deficiencies in alcoholics. Neurotransmitters are the chemicals the body makes to allow nerve cells to pass messages (of **pain** [page 338], touch, thought, etc.) from cell to cell. **Amino acids** (page 465) are the precursors of these neurotransmitters. In double-blind research, a group of alcoholics were treated with 1.5 grams of **D,L-phenylalanine** (page 568) (DLPA), 900 mg of **L-tyrosine** (page 544), 300 mg of **L-glutamine** (page 530), and 400 mg of L-tryptophan (now available only by prescription) per day, plus a **multivitamin-mineral** (page 559) supplement.[18] This nutritional supplement regimen led to a significant reduction in withdrawal symptoms and decreased stress in alcoholics compared to the effects of placebo.

The amino acid, **L-glutamine** (page 530), has also been used as an isolated supplement. Animal research has shown that glutamine supplementation reduces alcohol intake, a finding that has been confirmed in double-blind human research.[19] In that trial, 1 gram of glutamine per day given in divided portions with meals decreased both the desire to drink and anxiety levels.

Alcoholics are sometimes deficient in **magnesium** (page 551), and some researchers believe that symptoms of withdrawal may result in part from this deficiency.[20] Nonetheless, a double-blind trial reported that magnesium injections did not reduce symptoms of alcohol withdrawal.[21]

Because of the multiple nutrient deficiencies associated with alcoholism, most alcoholics who quit drinking should supplement with a high-potency multivitamin-mineral for at least several months after the detoxification period. Whether or not the supplement should include iron should be discussed with a doctor.

Are there any side effects or interactions?
Refer to the individual supplement for information about any side effects or interactions.

Herbs that may be helpful
Milk thistle (page 710) extract is commonly recommended to counteract the harmful effects of alcohol on the liver.[22] Milk thistle extracts have been shown in one double-blind study to reduce death due to alcohol-induced **cirrhosis of the liver** (page 290),[23] though another double-blind study did not confirm this finding.[24] Milk thistle extract may protect the cells of the liver by both blocking the entrance of harmful toxins and helping remove these toxins from the liver cells.[25, 26] Milk thistle has also been reported to regenerate injured liver cells.[27]

Kudzu (page 700) is most famous as a quick-growing weed in the southern United States. Alcoholic hamsters (one of the few animals to become so besides humans) were found to have decreased interest in drinking when fed kudzu extract.[28] Traditional Chinese medicine practitioners generally recommend 3 to 5 grams of root three times per day; some herbal practitioners also suggest that 3 to 4 ml of tincture taken three times per day may also be helpful to reduce alcohol cravings. Nonetheless, a double-blind trial using 1.2 grams of powdered kudzu root twice per day failed to show any benefit in helping alcoholics remain abstinent from alcohol.[29]

Are there any side effects or interactions?
Refer to the individual herb for information about any side effects or interactions.

ALLERGIES AND SENSITIVITIES

What do I need to know?
Self-care for allergies and sensitivities can be approached in a number of ways—but it can be hard to know just where to start. To make it easier, our doctors recommend trying these simple steps first:

Watch what you eat
 Work with a professional who specializes in food sensitivities to see if certain foods are causing your allergies

Clean it up
 Control household allergens like dust, mold, and animal dander to reduce your overall allergic load
See an allergist
 Find a health professional to help you manage your allergies
Help children avoid allergies with beneficial bacteria
 Take a supplement containing high-potency beneficial bacteria (probiotics) during pregnancy and give them to newborns to help reduce the risk of children developing allergies

About allergies
Allergies are responses mounted by the immune system to a particular food, inhalant (airborne substance), or chemical. In popular terminology, the terms "allergies" and "sensitivities" are often used to mean the same thing, although many sensitivities are not true allergies. The term "sensitivity" is general and may include true allergies, reactions that do not affect the immune system (and therefore are not technically allergies), and reactions for which the cause has yet to be determined.

Some non-allergic types of sensitivity are called intolerances and may be caused by toxins, enzyme inadequacies, drug-like chemical reactions, psychological associations, and other mechanisms.[1] Examples of well-understood intolerances are **lactose intolerance** (page 288) and **phenylketonuria** (page 354). Environmental sensitivity or intolerance are terms sometimes used for reactions to chemicals found either indoors or outdoors in food, water, medications, cosmetics, perfumes, textiles, building materials, and plastics. Detecting allergies and other sensitivities and then eliminating or reducing exposure to the sources is often a time-consuming and challenging task that is difficult to undertake without the assistance of an expert.

CHECKLIST FOR ALLERGIES		
Rating	**Nutritional Supplements**	**Herbs**
★★☆	**Probiotics** (page 575) (food allergy) **Thymus extracts** (page 591)	
★☆☆	**Betaine hydrochloride** (page 473) (food allergy) **Enzymes** (page 506) (food allergy) **Flavonoids** (page 516) **Quercetin** (page 580)	

What are the symptoms of allergies?

Common symptoms may include itchy, watery eyes; sneezing; headache; fatigue; postnasal drip; runny, stuffy, or itchy nose; sore throat; dark circles under the eyes; an itchy feeling in the mouth or throat; abdominal pain; **diarrhea** (page 163); and the appearance of an itchy, red skin rash. Life-threatening allergic reactions—most commonly to peanuts, nuts, shellfish, and some drugs—are uncommon. When they do occur, initial symptoms may include trouble breathing and difficulty swallowing.

Medical treatments

Over the counter drugs include antihistamines such as diphenhydramine (Benadryl), loratadine (Claritin), and chlorpheniramine (Chlor-Trimeton), as well as the decongestant pseudoephedrine (Sudafed). Topical nasal decongestants such as Oxymetazoline (Afrin) and Phenylephrine (Neo-Synephrine) may be used for a few days without harmful side effects. Saline-based nasal sprays such as Ocean, Ayr, and Dristan Saline Spray may be used to soothe inflamed tissue due to allergies. The nasal solution cromolyn sodium (Nasalcrom) may be used to prevent future allergy attacks.

Prescription treatments include antihistamines, such as fexofenadine (Allegra), cetirizine (Zyrtec), anddesloratadine (Clarinex); bronchodilators, such as albuterol (Proventil, Ventolin); nasal corticosteroids, such as fluticasone (Flonase), triamcinolone (Nasacort AQ), mometasone (Nasonex), and flunisolide (Nasalide); and weekly allergy shots (desensitization immunotherapy). Individuals who have experienced severe allergic reactions should carry an auto-injector syringe of epinephrine (EpiPen) for use during an attack.

People with allergies and sensitivities are typically advised to avoid exposure to particular allergens, such as tree and grass pollens, dust mites, molds, specific foods, latex, or environmental and household irritants. Those who have experienced severe reactions should wear a medical alert tag listing their allergens.

What conditions are related to allergies?

According to J. C. Breneman, M.D., author of the book *Basics of Food Allergy,*[2] many health conditions are related to allergies and have been the subject of independent studies. Even so, any relationship between the condition and the allergy needs to be considered with the aid of a doctor. More information about the relationship between specific health conditions and allergies or other sensitivities can be found in the following articles:

- **Arthritis (rheumatoid)** (page 387)[3, 4, 5, 6, 7]
- **Asthma** (page 32)[8, 9, 10]
- **Attention deficit-hyperactivity disorder** (page 55)[11, 12, 13]
- Bladder infection (**Urinary tract infection** [page 436])[14, 15, 16]
- **Candidiasis (vaginal)** (page 109)[17, 18]
- **Canker sores** (page 90)[19, 20, 21, 22]
- **Celiac disease** (page 102)[23, 24, 25, 26, 27]
- **Colic** (page 121)[28, 29, 30, 31, 32]
- **Constipation** (page 137)[33, 34, 35]
- **Crohn's disease** (page 141)[36]
- **Depression** (page 145)[37, 38]
- **Diarrhea** (page 163)[39]
- **Ear infections** (page 383) (recurrent)[40, 41, 42]
- **Eczema** (page 177) (including atopic dermatitis)[43, 44, 45, 46, 47]
- **Gallbladder attacks** (page 193)[48]
- **Gastroesophageal reflux disease** (page 198) (GERD)[49, 50, 51, 52, 53, 54, 55, 56]
- **Glaucoma** (page 205)[57, 58]
- **Hay fever** (page 211)[59, 60, 61]
- **High blood pressure** (page 246)[62]
- **Hives** (page 245)[63, 64, 65, 66, 67, 68, 69]
- **Hypoglycemia** (page 251)[70]
- **Infection** (page 265)[71, 72, 73, 74, 75, 76]
- **Irritable bowel syndrome** (page 280) (IBS)[77, 78]
- **Migraine headaches** (page 316)[79, 80, 81, 82]
- **MSG sensitivity** (page 322)[83, 84, 85]
- **Obesity** (page 446)[86]
- **Psoriasis** (page 379)[87]
- **Sinusitis** (page 407)[88, 89, 90, 91, 92]
- **Sinus congestion** (page 405)[93, 94, 95, 96]
- **Ulcer** (page 433), duodenal[97, 98]

The following conditions may also be related to allergies and other sensitivities:

Bed-wetting (Nocturnal enuresis)

If there is no medical cause for bed-wetting, allergies should be investigated. Several researchers have reported that allergies appear to be an important cause of bed-wetting.[99, 100]

Cyclic vomiting syndrome

Allergies to foods, especially cows' milk, may play a role in cyclic vomiting syndrome, a disorder characterized by repeated unpredictable, explosive and unexplained bouts of vomiting.[101] This condition affects nearly 2% of school-aged children.[102]

Gastrointestinal symptoms

Vague gastrointestinal (GI) symptoms (such as abdominal pain, bloating, **gas** [page 195], and **diarrhea** [page

163]) that are not caused by serious disease can sometimes be triggered by food sensitivities. In one double-blind trial, people with vague GI problems believed to be caused by dairy were given dairy to see how their bodies would react.[103] These people were not lactose intolerant. Various indicators of immunity changed as a result of the dairy challenge, showing their bodies were reacting to the dairy in an abnormal way. However, the indicator of a true dairy allergy (milk-specific immunoglobulin E) was normal in most of these people. This study suggests that vague GI symptoms unrelated to serious disease can be caused by food sensitivities that reflect neither lactose intolerance nor true allergies.

IgA nephropathy (autoimmune kidney disease)
In a small, preliminary trial, people with IgA nephropathy consumed a hypoallergenic diet (rice, olive oil, turkey, rabbit, lamb, green vegetables, potatoes, pears, apples, salt, and water) for 14 to 23 weeks. Laboratory parameters for kidney function improved significantly, and all participants remained relapse-free while maintaining the diet.[104]

Multiple Food Protein Intolerance (MFPI) of infancy
Many infants who are intolerant to one food have been found to also be intolerant to several other food proteins, including soy formula and extensively hydrolyzed formula. This syndrome has recently been dubbed Multiple Food Protein Intolerance (MFPI) of infancy. As a group, these infants tend to have symptoms of severe **colic** (page 121), **gastroesophageal reflux** (page 198) and esophagitis (inflammation of the esophagus due to irritation by stomach acids from repeated episodes of reflux), or atopic dermatitis (**eczema** [page 177]). As many as 30% of infants may suffer from these symptoms, but it is not yet clear how many of them may be suffering from this syndrome.[105]

Multiple chemical sensitivity
Multiple chemical sensitivity, also known as idiopathic environmental intolerances, is a poorly understood and controversial chronic disorder in which a person may have a variety of recurring symptoms believed to be due to reactions to very small amounts of substances in the environment.[106, 107, 108] Avoidance of these substances, though often difficult, has been reported to bring at least partial relief,[109] and psychological counseling has also been reported to be helpful.[110]

*Musculoskeletal **pain** (page 338) (including **back pain** [page 293])*
Ingestion of allergenic foods has been reported to produce a variety of musculoskeletal syndromes in susceptible people.[111]

Nephrotic syndrome
Several studies have found a link between nephrotic syndrome (a kidney disease) and allergies. In one study nephrotic syndrome patients responded when the allergens were removed from their diet;[112] however, in another study patients did not respond.[113]

Leaky gut syndrome
Allergy to food has been associated with increased permeability, or "leakiness," of the intestine.[114, 115] Some alternative health practitioners believe that this increased permeability, sometimes referred to as the "leaky gut syndrome," is an important treatable cause of food allergy. However, the reverse may also be possible. Allergic reactions in the intestine tend to cause temporary increases in permeability,[116, 117] which would explain the apparent connection between the two. More research is needed to better understand the role of intestinal permeability in the development and treatment of food allergies.

Dietary changes that may be helpful
A low-allergen diet, also known as an elimination diet or a hypoallergenic diet is often recommended to people with suspected food allergies to find out if avoiding foods that commonly trigger allergies will provide relief from symptoms.[118] This diet eliminates foods and food additives considered to be common allergens, such as wheat, dairy, eggs, corn, soy, citrus fruits, nuts, peanuts, tomatoes, food coloring and preservatives, coffee, and chocolate. Some popular books offer guidance to people who want to attempt this type of diet.[119, 120] The low-allergen diet is not a treatment for people with food allergies, however. Rather, it is a diagnostic tool used to help discover which foods a person is sensitive to. It is maintained only until a reaction to a food or foods has been diagnosed or ruled out. Once food reactions have been identified, only those foods that are causing a reaction are subsequently avoided; all other foods that had previously been eaten are once again added to the diet. While individual recommendations regarding how long a low-allergen diet should be adhered to vary from five days to three weeks, many nutritionally oriented doctors believe that a two-week trial is

generally sufficient for the purpose of diagnosing food reactions.

Strict avoidance of allergenic foods for a period of time (usually months or years) sometimes results in the foods no longer causing allergic reactions.[121] Restrictive elimination diets and food reintroduction should be supervised by a qualified healthcare professional.

Lifestyle changes that may be helpful

People with inhalant allergies are often advised to reduce exposure to common household allergens like dust, mold, and animal dander, in the hope that this will reduce symptoms even if other, non-household allergens cannot be avoided.[122] Strategies include removing carpets, frequent cleaning and vacuuming, using special air filters in the home heating system, choosing allergen-reducing bed and pillow coverings, and limiting household pets' access to sleeping areas.

Nutritional supplements that may be helpful

Probiotics (page 575) may be important in the control of food allergies because of their ability to improve digestion, by helping the intestinal tract control the absorption of food allergens and/or by changing immune system responses to foods.[123, 124, 125] One group of researchers has reported using probiotics to successfully treat infants with food allergies in two trials: a double-blind trial using Lactobacillus GG bacteria in infant formula, and a preliminary trial giving the same bacteria to nursing mothers.[126] Probiotics may also be important in non-allergy types of food intolerance caused by imbalances in the normal intestinal flora.[127]

Thymomodulin (page 591) is a special preparation of the thymus gland of calves. In a double-blind study of allergic children who had successfully completed an elimination diet, 120 mg per day of thymomodulin prevented allergic skin reactions to food and lowered blood levels of antibodies associated with those foods.[128] These results confirmed similar findings in an earlier, controlled trial.[129]

According to one theory, allergies are triggered by partially undigested protein. Proteolytic **enzymes** (page 506) may reduce allergy symptoms by further breaking down undigested protein to sizes that are too small to cause allergic reactions.[130] Preliminary human evidence supports this theory.[131] **Hydrochloric acid** (page 260) secreted by the stomach also helps the digestion of protein, and preliminary research suggests that some people with allergies may not produce ade-

quate amounts of stomach acid.[132, 133, 134] However, no controlled trials have investigated the use of enzyme supplements to improve digestion as a treatment for food allergies.

Many of the effects of allergic reactions are caused by the release of histamine, which is the reason antihistamine medication is often used by allergy sufferers. Some natural substances, such as **vitamin C** (page 604)[135, 136] and **flavonoids** (page 516),[137] including **quercetin** (page 580),[138, 139] have demonstrated antihistamine effects in test tube, animal, and other preliminary studies. However, no research has investigated whether these substances can specifically reduce allergic reactions in humans.

Are there any side effects or interactions?
Refer to the individual supplement for information about any side effects or interactions.

Herbs that may be helpful

See the articles on specific health conditions listed above for information on the effectiveness of herbs for each condition.

Are there any side effects or interactions?
Refer to the individual herb for information about any side effects or interactions.

Holistic approaches that may be helpful

Acupuncture may be helpful in the treatment of some types of allergy. Studies of mice treated with acupuncture provide evidence of an anti-allergic effect with results similar to treatment with corticosteroids (cortisone-like drugs).[140, 141, 142] A preliminary trial found a significant decrease in allergy symptoms following acupuncture treatment. It was found that the decline in symptoms coincided with a decline in laboratory measures of allergy. Relief persisted for two months following the treatment.[143] Other preliminary trials have also demonstrated positive results.[144] One controlled trial reported a reduction in allergic complaints following acupuncture treatment, but the results were not statistically significant.[145] In the future, controlled trials with larger numbers of subjects may help to determine conclusively whether allergies can be successfully treated with acupuncture therapy.

Provocation-neutralization is a controversial method of both allergy testing and treatment. Treatment consists of injecting minute dilutions of foods, inhalants, or (in some cases) chemicals into the lower layers of the skin. This approach is not the same as traditional desensitization injections given by medical allergy specialists. Preliminary[146, 147] and double-blind[148, 149] research suggests treatment of allergies by provocation-neutralization may be effective, though negative double-blind research also exists.[150]

Allergy treatment using extracts of allergens taken orally is another controversial method advocated by some alternative healthcare practitioners.[151] Most[152, 153, 154, 155] but not all double-blind trials[156, 157] have found this approach effective for house dust allergy. Preliminary[158] and double-blind[159, 160, 161] trials have reported success using this method for other allergies as well.

Treatment of food allergy using very small but increasing daily doses of actual foods has been reported,[162] and in one controlled trial[163] 12 of 14 patients successfully completed the program and could tolerate previously allergenic foods.

All desensitization programs require the guidance of a healthcare professional. While none of these approaches has been unequivocally proven, several show promise that people with allergies may be treatable by means other than simple avoidance of the offending food or inhalant substance.

What tests can detect allergies? Several tests or procedures are used by physicians to detect allergies. Most of these tests remain controversial.[164] Some clinicians (cited below), however, believe some of these tests can be effective.

Scratch testing This form of testing is one of the most widely used. A patient's skin is scratched with a needle that contains a portion of the food, inhalant, or chemical that is being tested. After a period of time, the skin is examined for reactions. If there is a reaction, it is determined that an allergy exists. Although this test is accepted by most allergists, scratch testing is subject to a relatively high incidence of inaccurate results, some tests showing positive when the person is not truly allergic to the substance (false positive) and some tests showing negative when an allergy really exists (false negative).

RAST/MAST/PRIST/ELISA (and other tests that measure immunoglobulins) The radioallergosorbent test (RAST) indirectly measures antibodies in the blood that react to specific foods. It is used by many physicians and has been shown to be a somewhat reliable indicator of allergies.[165, 166] It does not, however, help diagnose non-allergic food sensitivities and is therefore associated with a high risk of false negative readings. In an attempt to avoid this problem, a variety of modifications have been made to tests related to RAST (such as MAST, PRIST, and ELISA). Some of these changes may have reduced the risk of false negative readings somewhat but are likely to have increased the risk of false positive readings. A number of conditions associated with food sensitivities, such as **migraine headaches** (page 316) and **irritable bowel syndrome** (page 280), have shown remarkably poor correlation between RAST results and the actual sensitivities of patients.

Cytotoxic testing The cytotoxic test views a patient's serum under a microscope to see whether it is reacting to certain substances. The test is subject to numerous errors and is not generally considered to be reliable.[167]

Clinical ecology (provocation-neutralization; endpoint titration) This branch of medicine is considered very controversial. Testing is done using intra-dermal (under the skin) injections of minute dilutions of foods, inhalants or (in some cases) chemicals. Based on reactions, additional dilutions are used. This test not only determines whether an allergy exists but also operates on the theory that one dilution can trigger a reaction while another can neutralize a reaction. Preliminary research suggests this approach may have beneficial effects,[168, 169] A similar method uses these dilutions under the tongue to test for allergies.[170] Double-blind research has not found this method effective.[171]

Elimination and reintroduction The most reliable way to determine a food allergy is to have the patient eliminate a suspected food from the diet for a period of time and then reintroduce it later. Once a food is eliminated, the symptoms it may be causing either improve or resolve, typically after several days to three weeks. The body then becomes more sensitive to the food, so when the food is reintroduced, the symptom is more likely to recur. This tool shows with a high degree of certainty which foods are problem foods. The testing requires a great deal of patience and, as with all other forms of allergy testing, is best undertaken with the help of a physician who can monitor the diet.[172] Reintroduction of an allergenic food has been reported to lead occasionally to dangerous reactions in some people with certain conditions, particularly asthma—another reason this approach should not be attempted without supervision.

Other tests

Bioelectric tests are controversial procedures that attempt to measure changes in electrical activity at acupuncture points when a potential allergen is brought into proximity. A preliminary study reported that the EAV (Electroacupuncture According to Voll) device, also called the Vega test, identified the same allergens as RAST testing in 70.5 percent of tests.[173] Another preliminary study found the Vega test identified the same neutralization doses as clinical ecology testing (see above) in 66% of tests.[174] More research is needed to better evaluate these testing techniques.

ALZHEIMER'S DISEASE

Alzheimer's disease is a brain disorder that occurs in the later years of life. People with Alzheimer's develop progressive loss of memory and gradually lose the ability to function and to take care of themselves.

The cause of this disorder is not known, although the problem appears to involve abnormal breakdown of acetylcholine (an important neurotransmitter in the brain). Some studies suggest it may be related to an accumulation of aluminum in the brain.[1] Despite this suggestion, aluminum toxicity has been studied in humans, and it is quite distinct from Alzheimer's disease.[2] Therefore, the importance of aluminum in causing Alzheimer's disease remains an unresolved issue.

What are the symptoms of Alzheimer's disease?

Symptoms of Alzheimer's include a pattern of forgetfulness, short attention span, difficulty in performing routine tasks, language problems, disorientation, poor judgment, problems with thinking, misplacing things, **depression** (page 145), irritability, paranoia, hostility, and lack of initiative.

Medical treatments

Over the counter aspirin (Bayer Children's Aspirin, Ecotrin Adult Low Strength, Halfprin 81), in low daily doses, might be beneficial in the treatment of Alzheimer's disease.

Though prescription medications neither stop nor slow the progression of Alzheimer's dementia, cholinesterase inhibitors such as tacrine (Cognex), donepezil (Aricept), and Rivastigmine (Exelon) might improve symptoms in people with mild to moderate cases.

CHECKLIST FOR ALZHEIMER'S DISEASE		
Rating	Nutritional Supplements	Herbs
★★★		*Ginkgo biloba* (page 681)
★★☆	**Acetyl-L-carnitine** (page 461) **Vitamin B₁** (page 597) **Vitamin E** (page 609)	**Huperzine A** (page 694) **Lemon Balm** (page 701) **Periwinkle** (page 727) **Sage** (page 740)
★☆☆	**Coenzyme Q₁₀** (page 496) (in combination with **iron** [page 540] and **vitamin B₆** [page 600]) **DHEA** (page 503) **DMAE (2-dimethylaminoethanol)** (page 508) **Folic acid** (page 520) **Lecithin** (page 546) **NADH** (page 564) **Phosphatidylserine** (page 569) (bovine brain PS only; soy-derived PS does not appear to be effective) **Vitamin B₁₂** (page 599)	**Bacopa** (page 632)

Dietary changes that may be helpful

Whether aluminum in the diet can cause Alzheimer's disease remains controversial.[3, 4] A preliminary study found Alzheimer's disease patients are more likely to have consumed foods high in aluminum additives (e.g., some grain product desserts, American cheese, chocolate pudding, chocolate beverages, salt, and some chewing gum), compared to people without the disease.[5] Until this issue is resolved, it seems prudent for healthy people to take steps to minimize exposure to this unnecessary and potentially toxic metal by reducing intake of foods cooked in aluminum pots, foods that come into direct contact with aluminum foil, beverages stored in aluminum cans, and foods containing aluminum additives. Aluminum is added to some municipal water supplies to prevent the accumulation of particulates. In such areas, bottled water may be preferable. It appears unlikely, however, that avoidance of aluminum exposure after the diagnosis of Alzheimer's disease could significantly affect the course of the disease.

In population studies, high dietary intake of fat and calories was associated with an increased risk for Alzheimer's disease, whereas high intake of fish was associated with a decreased risk.[6, 7, 8] Whether these associations represent cause and effect is unknown.

Lifestyle changes that may be helpful

Keeping active outside of one's work, either physically or mentally, during midlife may help prevent Alzheimer's disease. People with higher levels of non-occupational activities, such as playing a musical instrument, gardening, physical exercise, or even playing board games, were less likely to develop Alzheimer's later in life, according to one study.[9]

Nutritional supplements that may be helpful

Several clinical trials have found that **acetyl-L-carnitine** (page 461) supplementation delays the progression of Alzheimer's disease,[10] improves memory,[11, 12, 13] and enhances overall performance in some people with Alzheimer's disease.[14, 15] However, in one double-blind trial, people who received acetyl-L-carnitine (1 gram three times per day) deteriorated at the same rate as those given a placebo.[16] Overall, however, most short-term studies have shown clinical benefits, and most long-term studies (one year) have shown a reduction in the rate of deterioration.[17] A typical supplemental amount is 1 gram taken three times per day.

In a preliminary study, people who used **antioxidant** (page 467) supplements (**vitamin C** [page 604] or **vitamin E** [page 609]) had a lower risk of Alzheimer's disease compared with people who did not take antioxidants.[18] Other preliminary research shows that higher blood levels of vitamin E correlate with better brain functioning in middle-aged and older adults.[19] The possible protective effect of antioxidants may be explained by the observation that oxidative damage appears to play a role in the development of dementia.[20] Large amounts of supplemental vitamin E may slow the progression of Alzheimer's disease. A double-blind trial found that 2,000 IU of vitamin E per day for two years extended the length of time people with moderate Alzheimer's disease were able to continue caring for themselves (e.g., bathing, dressing, and other necessary daily functions), compared with people taking a placebo.[21]

Vitamin B₁ (page 597) is involved in nerve transmission in parts of the brain (called cholinergic neurons) that deteriorate in Alzheimer's disease.[22, 23] The activity of vitamin B₁-dependent enzymes has been found to be lower in the brains of people with Alzheimer's disease.[24] It has therefore been suggested that vitamin B₁ supplementation could slow the progression of Alzheimer's disease. Two double-blind trials have reported small but significant improvements of mental function in people with Alzheimer's disease who took 3 grams a day of vitamin B₁, compared to those who took a placebo.[25, 26] However, another double-blind trial using the same amount for a year found no effect on mental function.[27]

Phosphatidylserine (page 569) (PS), which is related to **lecithin** (page 546), is a naturally occurring compound present in the brain. Although it is not a cure, 100 mg of PS taken three times per day has been shown to improve mental function, such as the ability to remember names and to recall the location of frequently misplaced objects, in people with Alzheimer's disease.[28] However, subsequent studies have not validated these results. In one double-blind trial, only the most seriously impaired participants received benefits from taking PS; people with moderate Alzheimer's disease did not experience significant improvements in cognitive function.[29] In another double-blind trial, people with Alzheimer's disease who took 300 mg of PS per day for eight weeks had better improvement in overall well-being than those who took placebo, but there were no significant differences in mental function tests.[30] In another double-blind trial, 200 mg of PS taken twice daily produced short-term improvements in mental function (after six to eight weeks), but these effects faded toward the end of the six-month study period.[31]

A further concern is that the PS used in these studies was obtained from cow brain, which has been found in some instances to be infected with the agents that cause mad-cow disease. The human variant of mad cow disease, called Creutzfeldt-Jakob disease, is rare, but fatal and is thought to be transmitted to people who consume organs and meat from infected cows. A plant source of PS is also available. However, the chemical structure of the plant form of PS differs from the form found in cow brain. In a preliminary study, plant-derived PS was no more effective than a placebo at improving the memory of elderly people.[32] Soy-derived PS was also ineffective in a double-blind study of elderly people with **age-related cognitive decline** (page 8).[33]

A double-blind trial of 20 to 25 grams per day of **lecithin** (page 546) failed to produce improvements in mental function in people with Alzheimer's disease.[34] However, there were improvements in a subgroup of people who did not fully comply with the program, suggesting that lower amounts of lecithin may possibly be helpful. Lecithin supplementation has also been studied in combination with a cholinesterase inhibitor drug called tacrine, with predominantly negative results.[35, 36, 37, 38]

DMAE (2-dimethylaminoethanol) (page 508) may increase levels of the brain neurotransmitter acetylcholine. In one preliminary trial, people with senile dementia were given DMAE supplements of 600 mg three times per day for four weeks. The participants did not show any changes in memory, though some did show positive behavior changes.[39] However, a subsequent double-blind trial found no significant benefit from DMAE supplementation in people with Alzheimer's disease.[40]

In a preliminary report, two people with a hereditary form of Alzheimer's disease received daily: **coenzyme Q₁₀** (page 496) (60 mg), **iron** (page 540) (150 mg of sodium ferrous citrate), and **vitamin B₆** (page 600) (180 mg). Mental status improved in both patients, and one became almost normal after six months.[41]

Studies in the test tube have shown that **zinc** (page 614) can cause biochemical changes associated with Alzheimer's disease.[42] For that reason, some scientists have been concerned that zinc supplements might promote the development of this disease. However, in a study of four people with Alzheimer's disease, supplementation with zinc (30 mg per day) actually resulted in improved mental function.[43] In a recent review article, one of the leading zinc researchers concluded that zinc does not cause or worsen Alzheimer's disease.[44]

A small, preliminary trial showed that oral **NADH** (page 564) (10 mg per day) improved mental function in people with Alzheimer's disease.[45] Further studies are necessary to confirm these early results.

Some researchers have found an association between Alzheimer's disease and deficiencies of **vitamin B₁₂** (page 599) and **folic acid** (page 520);[46, 47] however, other researchers consider such deficiencies to be of only minor importance.[48] In a study of elderly Canadians, those with low blood levels of folate were more likely to have dementia of all types, including Alzheimer's disease, than those with higher levels of folate.[49] Little is known about whether supplementation with either vitamin would significantly help people with this disease. Nonetheless, it makes sense for people with Alzheimer's disease to be medically tested for vitamin B₁₂ and folate deficiencies and to be treated if they are deficient.

Most,[50, 51, 52, 53] but not all,[54, 55] studies have found that people with Alzheimer's disease have lower blood **DHEA** (page 503) levels than do people without the condition. Emerging evidence suggests a possible benefit of DHEA supplementation in people with Alzheimer's disease. In one double-blind trial, participants who took 50 mg twice daily for six months had significantly better mental performance at the three-month mark than those taking placebo. At six months, statistically significant differences between the two groups were not seen, but results still favored DHEA.[56] In another clinical trial, massive amounts of DHEA (1,600 mg per day for four weeks) failed to improve mental function or mood in elderly people with or without Alzheimer's disease.[57] It is likely that the amount of DHEA used in this trial was far in excess of an appropriate amount, illustrating that more is not always better.

Are there any side effects or interactions?
Refer to the individual supplement for information about any side effects or interactions.

Herbs that may be helpful
An extract made from the leaves of the *Ginkgo biloba* tree is an approved treatment for early-stage Alzheimer's disease in Europe. While not a cure, ***Ginkgo biloba*** (page 681) extract (GBE) may improve memory and quality of life and slow progression in the early stages of the disease. In addition, four double-blind trials have shown that GBE is helpful for people in early stages of Alzheimer's disease, as well as for those experiencing another form of dementia known as multi-infarct dementia.[58, 59, 60, 61] One trial reported no effect of GBE supplementation in the treatment of Alzheimer's disease, vascular dementia or age-associated memory impairment.[62] However, the results of this trial have been criticized, since analysis of the results does not separate those patients with Alzheimer's disease or vascular dementia from those with age-associated memory impairment. A comparison of placebo-controlled trials of ginkgo for Alzheimer's disease concluded that the herb compared favorably with two prescription drugs, donepezil and tacrine, commonly used to treat the condition.[63] Research studies have used 120 to 240 mg of

GBE, standardized to contain 6% terpene lactones and 24% flavone glycosides per day, generally divided into two or three portions. GBE may need to be taken for six to eight weeks before desired actions are noticed.

Huperzine A is a substance found in **huperzia** (page 694) *(Huperzia serrata),* a Chinese medicinal herb. In a placebo-controlled trial, 58% of people with Alzheimer's disease had significant improvement in memory and mental and behavioral function after taking 200 mcg of huperzine A twice per day for eight weeks—a statistically significant improvement compared to the 36% who responded to placebo.[64] Another double-blind trial using injected huperzine A confirmed a positive effect in people with dementia, including, but not limited to, Alzheimer's disease.[65] Yet another double-blind trial found that huperzine A, given at levels of 100 to 150 mcg two to three times per day for four to six weeks, was more effective at improving minor memory loss associated with **age-related cognitive decline** (page 8) than the drug piracetam.[66] This study found that huperzine A was *not* effective in relieving symptoms of Alzheimer's disease. Clearly, more research is needed before the usefulness of huperzine A for Alzheimer's disease is confirmed.

Lesser periwinkle (page 727) contains the alkaloid vincamine. Supplementation with a semi-synthetic derivative of vincamine, known as vinpocentine, showed no benefit for people with Alzheimer's disease in a preliminary study,[67] but vincamine itself was shown to be beneficial in a later double-blind trial.[68]

In a double-blind trial, supplementation with an extract of lemon balm *(Melissa officinalis)* for 16 weeks significantly improved cognitive function and significantly reduced agitation, compared with a placebo, in people with Alzheimer's disease.[69] The amount of lemon balm used was 60 drops per day of a 1:1 tincture, standardized to contain at least 500 mcg per ml of citral.

In a double-blind study of people with Alzheimer's disease, supplementing with **sage** (page 740) for four months resulted in a significant improvement in cognitive function, compared with a placebo.[70] The amount of sage used was 60 drops per day of a 1:1 tincture. Although it is not known for sure how sage improves cognitive function, it appears to have an effect on acetylcholine, one of the chemical messengers (neurotransmitters) in the brain.

Animal studies have found the Ayurvedic herb **bacopa** (page 632) has constituents that enhance several aspects of mental function and learning ability.[71, 72, 73] A controlled study found that a syrup containing an extract of dried bacopa herb given to children improved several measures of mental performance.[74] A double-blind trial in adults found that a standardized extract of bacopa (300 mg per day for people weighing under 200 lbs and 450 per day for people over 200 lbs) improved only one out of several measures of memory function after three months.[75] Another double-blind trial lasting twelve weeks found 300 mg per day of bacopa improved four out of fifteen measures of learning, memory, and other mental functions in adults.[76] A third double-blind study found no effects on mental function in a group of healthy adults given 300 mg of standardized bacopa and tested two hours later. Bacopa has not been tested on people with memory problems.[77]

Are there any side effects or interactions?
Refer to the individual herb for information about any side effects or interactions.

AMENORRHEA

Amenorrhea is the absence of menstrual cycles.

Amenorrhea is called primary when a woman has not started to menstruate by the age of 16 years, while secondary amenorrhea refers to the abnormal cessation of menstruation in a woman who previously has had menstrual cycles.[1] In amenorrheic women, the levels of female reproductive hormones are not sufficient to stimulate menstruation. This condition is sometimes associated with malnutrition, such as that which occurs in **anorexia nervosa** (page 174), or with extreme exercise, which puts excessive nutritional and other demands on the body.[2, 3] An association between stress and amenorrhea has also been demonstrated.[4] Amenorrhea may also result from potentially serious disorders of the ovaries, the hypothalamus, or the pituitary gland; therefore, a physician should always evaluate chronic absence of menstrual cycles. Prolonged amenorrhea can result in early bone loss and increased risk of **osteoporosis** (page 333).[5] Amenorrhea occurs naturally in women who are breast-feeding,[6] but in these circumstances it does not put the bones at risk.[7]

What are the symptoms of amenorrhea?
Women with amenorrhea may have symptoms of absent periods, increased facial hair, decreased pubic and

armpit hair, deeper voice, decreased breast size, and secretions from the breast.

CHECKLIST FOR AMENORRHEA

Rating	Nutritional Supplements	Herbs
★★☆	Progesterone (page 577)	
★☆☆	Acetyl-L-carnitine (page 461)	Blue cohosh (page 642)
	Calcium (page 483) and vitamin D (page 607) for preventing bone loss	Motherwort (page 712)
		Rue
		Partridge berry
	Vitamin B₆ (page 600)	Vitex agnus-castus (page 757)
	Vitamin C (page 604)	
	Zinc (page 614)	Yarrow (page 763)

Medical treatments

Prescription medications used to treat amenorrhea include birth control pills (Ortho Novum, Loestrin, Mircette, Triphasil), clomiphene (Clomid, Serophene), or gonadotropin-releasing hormone (GnRH) therapy using nafarelin (Synarel) and histrelin (Supprelin).

Dietary changes that may be helpful

It has long been known that extreme dietary restriction can cause amenorrhea.[8, 9] When such restriction is due to eating disorders (page 174), such as anorexia and bulimia,[10] professional treatment is necessary. Athletic amenorrheic women may have low intakes of calories and other nutrients, and there are reports of some athletes resuming menstruation after adding to their diet a daily nutritional beverage containing additional calories, protein, carbohydrate, fat, vitamins, and minerals.[11, 12] However, these women also decreased their exercise intensity, which likely contributed to normalization of their menstrual function.

When compared with women who menstruate regularly, women who menstruate infrequently or not at all often have lower dietary intakes of fat (especially saturated fat), protein, and total calories, as well as a greater proportion of carbohydrate and fiber in their diet.[13, 14, 15] In preliminary studies of normal-weight women with no obvious eating disorders, women who experienced amenorrhea had diets described as "close to normal" but significantly low in fat. These women had lower percentages of body fat as well.[16, 17] In one of these studies, regular menstruation returned in women who increased their fat intake and percentage of body fat to normal over four months.[18]

Specific diets may be associated with increased risk of amenorrhea. A strict raw foods diet was found in one preliminary study to be strongly associated with weight loss and amenorrhea.[19] Vegetarians have been studied for their susceptibility to amenorrhea, but the results so far have been inconsistent.[20] Vegetarian diets tend to be rich in the antioxidant nutrients known as **carotenes** (page 488). Women with excessive carotene levels in their blood appear to be at higher risk of amenorrhea than women with normal levels,[21, 22] and, while research has not shown high carotene levels to directly cause amenorrhea, they may constitute a contributing factor.[23] In one preliminary study, women with high levels of both carotenes and amenorrhea had predominantly vegetarian diets, and reducing dietary intake of carotenes led to lower carotene levels and improvement in their amenorrhea.[24] Women vegetarians often rely heavily on soy foods as sources of protein, and a number of studies have found that increasing dietary intake of soy reduces levels of estrogen and progesterone in premenopausal women,[25, 26, 27, 28, 29, 30] although some studies have not found these changes.[31, 32] Changes in menstrual cycles were not consistent in these studies, and none found an increase in missed menses with high-soy diets. The only well-controlled comparison study found that the number of cases of amenorrhea among healthy, stable-weight vegetarian women was not different from that of healthy, stable-weight non vegetarian women.[33] The authors of this study speculated that, after reviewing all of the evidence, a vegetarian diet is likely not to contribute to amenorrhea.

Lifestyle changes that may be helpful

Moderate exercise has many benefits to the overall health of premenopausal women, but intensive or excessive exercise can contribute to amenorrhea and increase the risk of early **bone loss** (page 333) due to detrimental effects on hormone balance.[34] Exercise typically increases bone density, but a study of dancers with amenorrhea found that bone density measurements remained below normal for the entire two-year duration of the study.[35] The demands placed upon women performers and athletes are believed to contribute to the high incidence of eating disorders among them. This, along with the increased physical and nutritional demands of intensive exercise, can lead to nutrient deficiencies and lowered body-fat percentages that may contribute to amenorrhea and bone loss in women athletes.[36, 37, 38] Running and ballet dancing are among the activities most closely associated with amenorrhea,[39] with as many as 66% of women long-distance runners and ballet dancers experiencing amenorrhea.[40] Among women bodybuilders in one study, 81% experienced amenorrhea, and many had nutritionally deficient diets.[41] While some amenorrheic athletes have been reported to resume menstruation after adding one day of rest per week and consuming a daily nutritional beverage containing additional calories, protein, carbohydrate, fat, vitamins, and minerals,[42, 43] no controlled trials have investigated this approach.

Hormonal changes associated with breast-feeding prevent menstruation in healthy women.[44] The duration of this interruption in menstruation, known as lactational or postpartum amenorrhea, depends on many factors, including the nutritional health of the mother. Poor maternal nutritional status has been associated with longer periods of lactational amenorrhea in developing countries[45, 46, 47, 48] as well as in Great Britain among poor nursing women.[49] Better maternal nutritional status was found to be associated with shorter lactational amenorrhea in well-nourished nursing mothers in the United States.[50] When malnourished nursing mothers are given food supplements, the length of lactational amenorrhea can be shortened, according to preliminary studies.[51] However, one controlled trial found dietary supplementation with skim milk did not shorten the duration of amenorrhea in well-nourished nursing mothers.[52] Although prolonged lactational amenorrhea prevents another pregnancy, it has not been shown to result in permanent bone loss.[53]

Excessive stress causes the body to produce increased amounts of the adrenal hormone cortisol, and several studies have linked high cortisol levels to low levels of reproductive hormones and to amenorrhea.[54, 55, 56] In one study, amenorrheic women showed a greater increase in cortisol in response to stress than did women with normal menstrual cycles.[57] No research has been done to evaluate stress reduction interventions for the treatment of amenorrhea.

Smoking may contribute to amenorrhea. A survey study found that young women smoking one pack or more per day were more likely to be amenorrheic than other women.[58] However, whether smoking cessation will normalize menstrual function in amenorrheic women is unknown.

Nutritional supplements that may be helpful

Oral, micronized **progesterone** (page 577) (200 to 300 mg per day) has been shown in at least one double-blind trial to successfully induce normal menstrual bleeding in women with secondary amenorrhea.[59] Use of this natural hormone should always be supervised by a doctor.

A preliminary trial showed that **bone loss** (page 333) occurred over a one-year period in amenorrheic exercising women despite daily supplementation with 1,200 mg of **calcium** (page 483) and 400 IU of **vitamin D** (page 607).[60] In a controlled study of amenorrheic nursing women, who ordinarily experience brief bone loss that reverses when menstruation returns, bone loss was not prevented by a multivitamin supplement providing 400 IU of vitamin D along with 500 mg twice daily of calcium or placebo.[61] Despite the lack of evidence that calcium and vitamin D supplements alone are helpful to amenorrheic women, they are still generally recommended to prevent the added burden of calcium and vitamin D deficiency from further contributing to bone loss.[62] Amounts typically recommended are 1,200 to 1,500 mg calcium and 400 to 800 IU vitamin D daily.

Acetyl-L-carnitine (page 461) is an amino acid that may have effects on brain chemicals and hormones that control female reproductive hormones. In a preliminary trial, 2 grams daily of acetyl-L-carnitine was given to amenorrheic women who had either low or normal blood levels of female hormones. Hormone levels improved in the women with low initial levels, and half of all the women resumed menstruating within three to six months after beginning supplementation.[63] Controlled trials are needed to confirm these promising results.

Vitamin C (page 604) alone, at 400 mg daily, had no effect on amenorrhea in one preliminary trial, although it was associated with the return of ovulation in some women who were menstruating regularly but not ovulating. In a second phase of the trial, the same amount of vitamin C was combined with a drug that affects female hormone levels, and this combination was associated with return of ovulation in almost half of amenorrheic women who had not benefited from the drug alone.[64] More studies of the effect of vitamin C on amenorrhea are needed.

Prolactin is a hormone that may be elevated in some cases of amenorrhea. A preliminary trial of 200 to 600 mg daily of **vitamin B$_6$** (page 600) restored menstruation and normalized prolactin levels in three amenorrheic women with high initial prolactin levels; however, 600 mg daily of vitamin B_6 had no effect on amenorrheic women who did not have high prolactin levels.[65] A number of other small, preliminary trials have not demonstrated an effect of either oral or injected vitamin B_6 on prolactin levels,[66, 67, 68, 69, 70] and they also have reported inconsistent effects on restoring menstruation.[71, 72, 73] Larger, controlled trials are needed to better determine the usefulness of vitamin B_6 in amenorrhea.

While **zinc** (page 614) is known to be important for many aspects of reproductive function, little research has investigated its role in amenorrhea.[74] In a controlled study of intense exercisers, zinc deficiency was equally common between amenorrheic and menstruating exercisers.[75] More research is needed.

Are there any side effects or interactions?
Refer to the individual supplement for information about any side effects or interactions.

Herbs that may be helpful
Blue cohosh (page 642) is a traditional remedy for lack of menstruation. It is considered an emmenagogue (agent that stimulates menstrual blood flow) and a uterine tonic. No clinical trials have validated this traditional use.

Other herbal emmenagogues traditionally regarded as stimulating absent or diminished menses are **motherwort** (page 712), rue, partridge berry, and **yarrow** (page 763). None of these herbs has undergone modern clinical trials to determine their efficacy. All emmenagogues should be avoided in pregnancy, as they may possibly cause a spontaneous abortion.

In herbal medicine, *Vitex agnus-castus* (page 757) (chaste tree) is sometimes used to treat **female infertility** (page 187) and amenorrhea.[76] Elevation of prolactin can be a cause of amenorrhea, and vitex has been shown in animals to reduce elevated prolactin levels.[77] In a controlled trial, prolactin production was normalized in women with high prolactin levels after three months of treatment with vitex.[78] Vitex has also been found to raise levels of luteinizing hormone and subsequent progesterone levels in women with luteal phase defect—a condition that can also lead to menstrual cycle abnormalities, including amenorrhea.[79] To date, only one small preliminary trial has studied the effects of vitex on amenorrhea. This study found that ten of fifteen women with amenorrhea began having a normal period after taking 40 drops of a liquid vitex preparation once daily for six months.[80] Further research is

needed to determine what role vitex may play in the management of amenorrhea.

Are there any side effects or interactions?
Refer to the individual herb for information about any side effects or interactions.

Holistic approaches that may be helpful
In a number of preliminary trials,[81, 82, 83] acupuncture has been shown to induce ovulation in women with disorders involving lack of ovulation. Preliminary studies show that levels of estrogen and progesterone, as well as levels of the related hormones LH (luteinizing hormone) and FSH (follicle-stimulating hormone), may all be affected by acupuncture.[84, 85] Few studies have looked at the use of acupuncture for treatment of amenorrhea, but one preliminary trial found it helpful for women who have widely separated menstrual cycles.[86] In one controlled trial, amenorrheic women showed a trend toward normalizing hormone levels following acupuncture.[87]

ANEMIA

Anemia is a general term for a category of blood conditions that affect the red blood cells or the oxygen-carrying hemoglobin they contain.

In anemia, there is either a reduction in the number of red blood cells in circulation or a decrease in the amount or quality of hemoglobin. There are many causes of anemia, including severe blood loss, genetic disorders, and serious diseases. (See **iron-deficiency anemia** [page 278], **pernicious anemia** [page 601] [vitamin B_{12}-related], and **sickle cell anemia** [page 403].) Anyone with unexplained anemia should have the cause determined by a qualified doctor.

Some athletes appear to have anemia when their blood is tested, but this may be a normal adaptation to the stress of exercise,[1] which does not need treatment. Further evaluation by a qualified doctor is necessary.

What are the symptoms of anemia?
Some common symptoms of anemia include fatigue, lethargy, weakness, poor concentration, and frequent colds. A peculiar symptom of iron-deficiency anemia, called pica, is the desire to eat unusual things, such as ice, clay, cardboard, paint, or starch. Advanced anemia may also result in lightheadedness, headaches, ringing in the ears (**tinnitus** [page 430]), irritability, pale skin,

Anemia

unpleasant sensations in the legs with an uncontrollable urge to move them, and getting out of breath easily.

	CHECKLIST FOR ANEMIA	
Rating	Nutritional Supplements	Herbs
★★★	**Copper** (page 499) (if deficient) **Iron** (page 540) (when iron deficiency is diagnosed) **Vitamin A** (page 595) (if deficient) **Vitamin B₁** (page 597) (for genetic thiamine-responsive anemia) **Vitamin B₂** (page 598) (if deficient) **Vitamin B₆** (page 600) (if deficient and for genetic vitamin B₆-responsive anemia) **Vitamin B₁₂** (page 601) (if deficient) **Vitamin C** (page 604) (if deficient) **Vitamin E** (page 609) (if deficient)	
★★☆	**Folic acid** (page 520) (for thalassemia if deficient) **L-carnitine** (page 543) (for thalassemia) **Magnesium** (page 551) (for thalassemia) **Taurine** (page 590) (if deficient in iron) **Vitamin B₁₂** (page 601) (for thalassemia if deficient) **Vitamin E** (page 609) (injections for thalassemia, orally for glucose-6-phosphate dehydrogenase deficiency [G6PD] anemia and anemia caused by kidney dialysis) **Zinc** (page 614) (for thalassemia if deficient)	
★☆☆	**Antioxidants** (page 467) (for thalassemia) **Vitamin C** (page 604) (for thalassemia if deficient)	

Medical treatments

Over the counter treatment of anemia includes **iron** (page 540) (Feosol, Fergon), **vitamin B₁₂** (page 601),

and **folic acid** (page 520), though a correct diagnosis is necessary to determine which nutrient is deficient.

Medications requiring a prescription include injectable forms of iron (InFeD, Ferrlecit), vitamin B₁₂, and folic acid, as well as a high dose oral form of folic acid. Individuals with non-nutrient-deficient anemia may be prescribed epoetin (Epogen, Procrit).

Blood transfusions may be required to treat severe anemia.

Dietary changes that may be helpful

Severe protein deficiency can cause anemia because protein is required for normal production of hemoglobin and red blood cells.[2] However, this deficiency is uncommon in healthy people living in developed countries.

Thalassemia is an inherited type of anemia that is most common in people of Mediterranean descent. Children with severe thalassemia often have reduced growth rates that may be partially due to inadequate diets. This problem is primarily found in developing countries.[3]

Nutritional supplements that may be helpful

Deficiencies of **iron** (page 540), **vitamin B₁₂** (page 601), and **folic acid** (page 520) are the most common nutritional causes of anemia.[4] Although rare, severe deficiencies of several other vitamins and minerals, including **vitamin A** (page 595),[5, 6] **vitamin B₂** (page 598),[7] **vitamin B₆** (page 600),[8, 9] **vitamin C** (page 604),[10] and **copper** (page 499),[11, 12] can also cause anemia by various mechanisms. Rare genetic disorders can cause anemias that may improve with large amounts of supplements such as **vitamin B₁** (page 597).[13, 14]

Taurine has been shown, in a double-blind study, to improve the response to iron therapy in young women with iron-deficiency anemia.[15] The amount of taurine used was 1,000 mg per day for 20 weeks, given in addition to iron therapy, but at a different time of the day. The mechanism by which taurine improves iron utilization is not known.

Hemolytic anemia refers to a category of anemia in which red blood cells become fragile and undergo premature death. **Vitamin E** (page 609) deficiency, though quite rare, can cause hemolytic anemia because vitamin E protects the red blood cell membrane from oxidative damage. Vitamin E deficiency anemia usually affects only premature infants and children with **cystic fibrosis** (page 143).[16, 17] Preliminary studies have reported

Angina

that large amounts (typically 800 IU per day) of vitamin E improve hemolytic anemia caused by a genetic deficiency of the enzyme glucose-6-phosphate dehydrogenase (G6PD)[18, 19, 20] and anemia caused by kidney dialysis.[21, 22]

People with severe thalassemia who receive regular blood transfusions become overloaded with **iron** (page 540), which increases damaging **free radical** (page 467) activity and lowers **antioxidant** (page 467) levels in their bodies.[23, 24, 25, 26] Some people with milder forms of thalassemia may also have iron overload.[27] Iron supplements should be avoided by people with thalassemia unless **iron deficiency** (page 278) is diagnosed. Preliminary studies have found that oral supplements of 200 to 600 IU per day of **vitamin E** (page 609) reduce free radical damage to red blood cells in thalassemia patients.[28, 29, 30] However, only injections of vitamin E have reduced the need for blood transfusions caused by thalassemia.[31, 32]

Test tube studies have shown that propionyl-L-carnitine (a form of **L-carnitine** [page 543]) protects red blood cells of people with thalassemia against free radical damage.[33] In a preliminary study, children with beta thalassemia major who took 100 mg of L-carnitine per 2.2 pounds of body weight per day for three months had a significantly decreased need for blood transfusions.[34] Some studies have found people with thalassemia to be frequently deficient in **folic acid** (page 520), **vitamin B$_{12}$** (page 601),[35] and **zinc** (page 614).[36, 37] Researchers have reported improved growth rates in zinc-deficient thalassemic children who were given zinc supplements of 22.5 to 90 mg per day, depending on age.[38, 39] **Magnesium** (page 551) has been reported to be low in thalassemia patients in some,[40, 41] but not all,[42] studies. A small, preliminary study reported that oral supplements of magnesium, 7.2 mg per 2.2 pounds of body weight per day, improved some red blood cell abnormalities in thalassemia patients.[43]

Sideroblastic anemia refers to a category of anemia featuring a buildup of iron-containing immature red blood cells (sideroblasts). One type of sideroblastic anemia is due to a genetic defect in an enzyme that uses **vitamin B$_6$** (page 600) as a cofactor.[44, 45] Vitamin B$_6$ supplements of 50 to 200 mg per day partially correct the anemia, but must be taken for life.[46]

Are there any side effects or interactions?
Refer to the individual supplement for information about any side effects or interactions.

ANGINA

Angina, or angina pectoris, is chest pain due either to reduced blood flow to the heart or to certain other abnormalities of heart function.

Hardening (atherosclerosis) of the coronary arteries that feed the heart is usually the underlying problem. Spasms of the coronary arteries may also cause angina.

There are three main types of angina. The first is called stable angina. This type of chest pain comes on during exercise and is both common and predictable. Stable angina is most often associated with atherosclerosis. A second type, called variant angina, can occur at rest or during exercise. This type is primarily due to sudden coronary artery spasm, though atherosclerosis may also be a component. The third, most severe type is called unstable angina. This angina occurs with no predictability and can quickly lead to a **heart attack** (page 212). Anyone with significant, new chest pain or a worsening of previously mild angina must seek medical care immediately.

It is important for treatment and prevention of angina (and for overall health) to learn more about **atherosclerosis** (page 38).

Rating	Nutritional Supplements	Herbs
★★★	**Coenzyme Q$_{10}$** (page 496) **L-carnitine** (page 543)	
★★☆	**Arginine** (page 467) **Magnesium** (page 551) **N-acetyl cysteine** (page 562) **Ribose** (page 582) **Vitamin E** (page 609)	**Hawthorn** (page 689)
★☆☆	**Bromelain** (page 481) **Fish oil** (page 514) (EPA/**DHA** [page 514])	Khella **Kudzu** (page 700)

CHECKLIST FOR ANGINA

What are the symptoms of angina?
Common symptoms of angina include a squeezing pressure, heaviness, ache, or burning pain (like indigestion) in the chest that occur for 5 to 30 minutes at a time. These sensations are usually felt behind the breastbone but may also be felt in the jaw, neck, arms, back, or upper abdomen. Some people may also have

Angina

difficulty in breathing or may become pale and sweaty. Symptoms of angina usually appear during physical exertion, after heavy meals, and with heightened emotional states, such as anger, frustration, shock, and excitement.

Medical treatments

Aspirin (Bayer Low Adult Strength, Ecotrin Adult Low Strength) reduces the risk of death or nonfatal heart attack in patients with a previous history of **heart attack** (page 212) or unstable angina.

Many classes of prescription drugs are use to treat angina. Calcium channel blocking agents, such as verapamil (Calan, Verelan), diltiazem (Cardizem, Tiazac), and amlodipine (Norvasc). Nitrates, such as nitroglycerin, are available as tablets to be placed under the tongue (Nitrostat), applied topically as an ointment (Nitro-Bid), or as a patch to be applied to the skin (Nitro-Dur, Transderm-Nitro). Other nitrates include isosorbide dinitrate (Isordil) and isosorbide mononitrate (ISMO, Imdur). The last major category used to treat angina is the beta-adrenergic blocking agents, such as atenolol (Tenormin), metoprolol (Lopressor, Toprol XL), and propranolol(Inderal).

Smoking is discouraged, since nicotine prevents proper blood flow. In advanced stages, surgical repair of the blood vessels in the heart may be recommended. Treatment may be directed toward underlying medical conditions, such as **high cholesterol** (page 223), **high blood pressure** (page 246), **anemia** (page 25), hyperthyroidism, **obesity** (page 446), or lung disease.

Dietary changes that may be helpful

Coffee should probably be avoided. Drinking five or more cups of coffee per day has been shown to increase the risk of angina, although effects of different forms of coffee on angina are unclear.[1]

Lifestyle changes that may be helpful

Cigarette smoking causes damage to the coronary arteries and, in this way, can contribute to angina. It is critical for anyone with angina who smokes to stop smoking. Smoking has also been shown to reduce the effectiveness of treatments for angina.[2] Secondhand smoke should be avoided as well.[3]

Increasing physical exercise has been clearly demonstrated to reduce symptoms of angina, as well as to relieve its underlying causes. One study found that intense exercise for ten minutes daily was as effective as beta-blocker drugs in a group of patients with angina.[4] Anyone with angina or any other heart condition, as well as anyone over the age of 40, should consult a doctor before beginning an exercise program.

Nutritional supplements that may be helpful

L-carnitine (page 543) is an **amino acid** (page 465) needed to transport fats into the mitochondria (the place in the cell where fats are turned into energy). Adequate energy production is essential for normal heart function. Several studies using 1 gram of L-carnitine two to three times per day showed an improvement in heart function and a reduction in symptoms of angina.[5, 6, 7] **Coenzyme Q$_{10}$** (page 496) also contributes to the energy-making mechanisms of the heart. Angina patients given 150 mg of coenzyme Q$_{10}$ each day have experienced greater ability to exercise without experiencing chest pain.[8] This has been confirmed in independent investigations.[9]

Low levels of **antioxidant** (page 467) vitamins in the blood, particularly **vitamin E** (page 609), are associated with greater rates of angina.[10] This is true even when smoking and other risk factors for angina are taken into account. Early short-term studies using 300 IU (International Units) per day of vitamin E could not find a beneficial action on angina.[11] A later study supplementing small amounts of vitamin E (50 IU per day) for longer periods of time showed a minor benefit in people suffering angina.[12] Those affected by variant angina have been found to have the greatest deficiency of vitamin E compared with other angina patients.[13]

Nitroglycerin and similar drugs cause dilation of arteries by interacting with nitric oxide, a potent stimulus for dilation. Nitric oxide is made from **arginine** (page 467), a common amino acid. Blood cells in people with angina are known to make insufficient nitric oxide,[14] which may in part be due to abnormalities of arginine metabolism. Taking 2 grams of arginine three times per day for as little as three days has improved the ability of angina sufferers to exercise.[15] Seven of ten people with severe angina improved dramatically after taking 9 grams of arginine per day for three months in an uncontrolled study.[16] Detailed studies have investigated the mechanism of arginine and have proven it operates by stimulating blood vessel dilation.[17]

N-acetyl cysteine (page 562) (NAC) may improve the effects of nitroglycerin in people with angina.[18] People with unstable angina who took 600 mg of NAC three times daily in combination with a nitroglycerin transdermal (skin) patch for four months had significantly lower rates of subsequent heart attacks than did people who used either therapy alone or placebo.[19]

Magnesium (page 551) deficiency may be a contributing factor for spasms that occur in coronary arteries, particularly in variant angina.[20, 21] While studies have used injected magnesium to stop such attacks effectively,[22, 23] it is unclear whether oral magnesium would be effective in preventing or treating blood vessel spasms. One double-blind study of patients with exercise-induced angina, however, showed that oral magnesium supplementation (365 mg twice a day) for 6 months significantly reduced the incidence of exercise-induced chest pain, compared with a placebo.[24]

In a controlled study, men with severe coronary heart disease were given an exercise test, after which they took either 15 grams of **ribose** (page 582) or a placebo four times daily for three days. Compared with the initial test, men taking ribose were able to exercise significantly longer before experiencing chest pain and before abnormalities appeared on their electrocardiogram (ECG), but only the ECG changes were significantly improved compared with those in the placebo group.[25] Sports supplement manufacturers recommend 1 to 10 grams per day of ribose, while heart disease patients and people with rare enzyme deficiencies have been given up to 60 grams per day.

Bromelain (page 481) has been reported in a preliminary study to relieve angina. In that study, 600 people with **cancer** (page 87) were receiving bromelain (400 to 1,000 mg per day). Fourteen of those individuals had been suffering from angina. In all 14 cases, the angina disappeared within 4 to 90 days after starting bromelain.[26] However, as there was no control group in the study, the possibility of a placebo effect cannot be ruled out. Bromelain is known to prevent excessive stickiness of blood platelets,[27] which is believed to be one of the triggering factors for angina.

Fish oil (page 514), which contains the fatty acids known as EPA and **DHA** (page 509), has been studied in the treatment of angina. In some studies, enough fish oil to provide a total of about 3 grams of EPA and 2 grams of DHA has reduced chest pain as well as the need for nitroglycerin;[28] other investigators could not confirm these findings.[29] People who take fish oil may also need to take **vitamin E** (page 609) to protect the oil from undergoing potentially damaging oxidation in the body.[30] It is not known how much vitamin E is needed to prevent such oxidation; the amount required would presumably depend on the amount of fish oil used. In one study, 300 IU of vitamin E per day prevented oxidation damage in individuals taking 6 grams of fish oil per day.[31]

Are there any side effects or interactions?
Refer to the individual supplement for information about any side effects or interactions.

Herbs that may be helpful

The fruit, leaves, and flowers of the **hawthorn** (page 689) tree contain **flavonoids** (page 516), including oligomeric procyanidins, which may protect blood vessels from damage. A 60 mg hawthorn extract containing 18.75% oligomeric procyanidins taken three times per day improved heart function and exercise tolerance in angina patients in a small clinical trial.[32]

Khella is an African plant that contains spasm-relieving compounds, including khellin. Purified khellin was shown to be helpful in relieving angina in preliminary studies in the 1940s and 1950s.[33, 34] It is unknown whether the whole herb would have the same effects. Due to the potential side effects of khella, people with angina should consult with a physician knowledgeable in botanical medicine before taking it.

Kudzu (page 700) is used in modern Chinese medicine as a treatment for angina. Standardized root tablets (10 mg tablet is equivalent to 1.5 grams of the crude root) are sometimes used for angina pectoris in the amount of 30 to 120 mg per day.

Are there any side effects or interactions?
Refer to the individual herb for information about any side effects or interactions.

Holistic approaches that may be helpful

People suffering from angina may find acupuncture to reduce symptoms, the need for medication, and even the need for invasive surgery. While some studies of acupuncture treatment for angina found no benefit,[35] others have demonstrated positive results. An uncontrolled trial of 49 angina patients found that acupuncture resulted in 58% less nitroglycerin use and a 38% decrease in the number of angina attacks.[36] In another study, 69 patients suffering with severe angina were treated with a combination of acupuncture, shiatsu (acupressure), and lifestyle changes. The results were compared to patients with severe angina treated with coronary artery bypass grafting (CABG). The incidence of heart attack and death was 21% among those treated with CABG and 7% among those treated with the combined therapy including acupuncture. In addition, 61% of those treated with the combination therapy, because of their improved health, postponed any further invasive treatment.[37] In a single-blind study of 26 pa-

Angina

tients, a reduction in angina attack rate and nitroglycerin use, as well as an improvement in exercise performance, occurred in the treatment group compared to a sham (fake) acupuncture group.[38] Findings from a controlled trial comparing acupuncture treatment (three treatments per week for four weeks) to placebo tablets support these results, demonstrating a reduction in the number of angina attacks, improved exercise performance, and corresponding improvements in ECG readings.[39]

Transcendental meditation (20 minutes twice daily of silently chanting a mantra with eyes closed) was found in a small controlled trial to reduce angina-like chest pain and to normalize electrocardiograms (ECGs) in patients with cardiac syndrome X, a form of angina in people with otherwise normal coronary arteries.[40] While these patients did not have angina in the classic sense, their chest pain was thought to result from anxiety, which may reduce blood flow to the heart, and their ECGs resembled those of classic angina patients. It is not yet known whether transcendental meditation would have the same effect on patients with angina pectoris.

Evidence from preliminary[41, 42, 43] and controlled[44] studies suggests that there may be a relationship between the presence of **heart disease** (page 98) and changes to the muscles and joints of the spine that are detectable by practitioners of spinal manipulation. In a double-blind study, patients with proven coronary disease were more likely to have specific changes in their spine detectable by palpating or "feeling" their backs than were subjects who were healthy.[45] Controlled studies have demonstrated that manipulation of the joints in the middle of the neck can increase heart rate, respiratory rate, and blood pressure,[46, 47] but manipulation of the lower neck does not appear to have the same effect.[48] Despite these intriguing findings, there is no research investigating whether manipulation reduces angina symptoms or otherwise benefits the heart and cardiovascular system.

ANXIETY

What do I need to know?

Self-care for anxiety can be approached in a number of ways—but it can be hard to know just where to start. To make it easier, our doctors recommend trying these simple steps first:

Address your stress
> Reduce stress with meditation, counseling, and other methods

Avoid caffeine
> If you are anxious, avoid stimulants such as caffeine

Try valerian and passion flower
> Calm the nervous system by taking a combination of valerian (100 to 200 mg) and passion flower (45 to 90 mg) three times a day

Aim for better nutrition with a multivitamin-mineral
> Taking one a day may help reduce anxiety and feelings of stress

About anxiety

Anxiety describes any feeling of worry or dread, usually about events that might potentially happen. Some anxiety about stressful events is normal. However, in some people, anxiety interferes with the ability to function.

Some people who think they are anxious may actually be **depressed** (page 145). Because of all these factors, it is important for people who are anxious to seek expert medical care. Natural therapies can be one part of the approach to helping relieve mild to moderate anxiety.

What are the symptoms of anxiety?

Physical symptoms of anxiety include fatigue, **insomnia** (page 270), stomach problems, sweating, racing heart, rapid breathing, shortness of breath, and irritability.

Medical treatments

Prescription drug treatment includes anti-anxiety agents such as lorazepam (Ativan), alprazolam (Xanax), and buspirone (Buspar). Antidepressants, such as fluoxetine (Prozac), paroxetine (Paxil), and venlafaxine (Effexor), are often prescribed to treat generalized anxiety and panic attacks.

Underlying medical conditions, such as excess hormone secretion from the thyroid or adrenal glands, should be treated when present. Psychological counseling often accompanies drug therapy.

Dietary changes that may be helpful

All sources of caffeine should be avoided, including coffee, tea, chocolate, caffeinated sodas, and caffeine-containing medications. People with high levels of anxiety appear to be more susceptible to the actions of caffeine.[1]

CHECKLIST FOR ANXIETY		
Rating	Nutritional Supplements	Herbs
★★☆	Inositol (page 537) Multivitamin-mineral (page 559)	Passion flower (page 722) (in combination with valerian) Valerian (page 756) (in combination with passion flower)
★☆☆	Magnesium (page 551) Vitamin B₃ (niacinamide) (page 598)	American scullcap (page 626) Bacopa (page 632) Chamomile (page 656) Hops (page 690) Linden (page 704) Motherwort (page 712) Oats (page 716) (oat straw) Pennyroyal (page 723) St. John's wort (page 747) Wood betony (page 761)

Nutritional supplements that may be helpful

Inositol (page 537) has been used to help people with anxiety who have panic attacks. Up to 4 grams three times per day was reported to control such attacks in a double-blind trial.[2] Inositol (18 grams per day) has also been shown in a double-blind trial to be effective at relieving the symptoms of obsessive-compulsive disorder.[3]

An isolated double-blind trial found that supplementation with a **multivitamin-mineral supplement** (page 559) for four weeks led to significant reductions in anxiety and perceived stress compared to placebo.[4]

Many years ago, **magnesium** (page 551) was reported to be relaxing for people with mild anxiety.[5] Typically, 200 to 300 mg of magnesium are taken two to three times per day. Some doctors recommend soaking in a hot tub containing 1–2 cups of magnesium sulfate crystals (Epsom salts) for 15 to 20 minutes, though support for this approach remains anecdotal.

Niacinamide (a form of **Vitamin B₃** [page 598]) has been shown in animals to work in the brain in ways

similar to drugs such as benzodiazepines (Valium-type drugs), which are used to treat anxiety.[6] One study found that niacinamide (not niacin) helped people get through withdrawal from benzodiazepines—a common problem.[7] A reasonable amount of niacinamide to take for anxiety, according to some doctors, is up to 500 mg four times per day.

Are there any side effects or interactions?
Refer to the individual supplement for information about any side effects or interactions.

Herbs that may be helpful

Several plants, known as "nervines" (nerve tonics), are used in traditional herbal medicine for people with anxiety, with few reports of toxicity. Most nervines have not been rigorously investigated by scientific means to confirm their efficacy. However, one study found that a combination of the nervines **valerian** (page 756) and **passion flower** (page 722) reduced symptoms in people suffering from anxiety.[8] In a double-blind study, 45 drops per day of an extract of passion flower taken for four weeks was as effective as 30 mg per day of oxazepam (Serax), a medication used for anxiety.[9]

Other nervines include **oats** (page 716) (oat straw), **hops** (page 690), **passion flower** (page 722), **American scullcap** (page 626), **wood betony** (page 761), **motherwort** (page 712), **pennyroyal** (page 723), and **linden** (page 704).

Bacopa (page 632), a traditional herb used in Ayurvedic medicine, has been shown to have anti-anxiety effects in animals.[10] A preliminary study reported that a syrup containing an extract of dried bacopa herb reduced anxiety in people with anxiety neurosis.[11] A double-blind trial in healthy adults found that 300 mg per day of a standardized bacopa extract reduced general feelings of anxiety, as assessed by a questionnaire.[12]

St. John's wort (page 747) has been reported in one double-blind study to reduce anxiety.[13]

An old folk remedy for anxiety, particularly when it causes **insomnia** (page 270), is **chamomile** (page 656) tea. There is evidence from test tube studies that chamomile contains compounds with a calming action.[14] There are also animal studies that suggest a benefit from chamomile for anxiety,[15] but no human studies support this belief. Often one cup of tea is taken three or more times per day.

Anxiety

Warning: Kava should only be taken with medical supervision. Kava is not for sale in certain parts of the world.

Until recently, the preeminent botanical remedy for anxiety was **kava** (page 698), an herb from the South Pacific. It has been extensively studied for this purpose.[16] One 100 mg capsule standardized to 70% kavalactones is given three times per day in many studies. Preliminary[17] and double-blind trials[18, 19] have validated the effectiveness of kava for people with anxiety, including **menopausal** (page 311) women.[20] A previous study found kava to be just as effective as benzodiazepines over the course of six weeks.[21] The latest research shows that use of kava for up to six months is safe and effective compared with placebo.[22] Although kava rarely causes side effects at the given amount, it may cause problems for some people if combined for more than a few days with benzodiazepines.[23]

Are there any side effects or interactions?
Refer to the individual herb for information about any side effects or interactions.

Holistic approaches that may be helpful

Reducing exposure to stressful situations can help decrease anxiety. In some cases, meditation, counseling, or group therapy can greatly facilitate this process.[24]

Acupuncture has been the subject of limited research as a therapy for anxiety. In an uncontrolled study, eight patients suffering from anxiety were treated with acupuncture three times per week for eight sessions. Six of the eight patients achieved good to moderate improvement.[25] However, a trial of acupuncture treatment for anxiety associated with quitting smoking did not provide any evidence of benefit.[26] A double-blind study of acupuncture for the treatment of anxiety associated with dental procedures reported that acupuncture and placebo were equally effective.[27] Acupuncture remains unproven in the treatment of people with anxiety.

A form of counseling known as Cognitive-Behavioral Therapy (CBT) has been shown to be superior to placebo for managing the symptoms of panic disorder.[28] In a controlled trial, six months of CBT produced a response rate of 39.5%, compared to only 13% in the placebo group. When combined with the tricyclic antidepressant drug imipramine (Tofranil), response rates were even higher (57.1%). For long-term management of panic disorder, imipramine produced a superior quality of response, but CBT had more durability and was better tolerated.

ASTHMA

What do I need to know?

Self-care for asthma can be approached in a number of ways—but it can be hard to know just where to start. To make it easier, our doctors recommend trying these simple steps first:

Clean it up
> To avoid triggering asthma attacks, control household and workplace irritants such as dust, mold, smoke, chemicals, and animal dander, and dietary triggers like certain food additives

See an allergy specialist
> Find a healthcare professional to help you build tolerance to allergens

Watch your sodium intake
> Avoid aggravating symptoms by limiting use of table salt and salty fast foods, and by reading labels to find low-sodium groceries

Keep a healthy body weight
> Shed extra pounds to improve breathing and decrease the need for medications

Check out carotenoids
> 30 mg a day of lycopene or 64 mg a day of natural beta-carotene can help prevent exercise-related asthma attacks

Aim for good nutrition
> Avoid deficiencies common in asthmatics and improve intake of important antioxidants by eating plenty of fruits, vegetables, and other plant foods and taking a daily multivitamin-mineral supplement

Try proven herbal remedies
> Supplements containing boswellia extract (900 mg a day), ivy leaf extract (50 drops a day), or tylophora leaf (200 to 400 mg a day) may improve breathing symptoms; children should be given one-half of these amounts or less, depending on body weight

About asthma

Asthma is a lung disorder in which spasms and inflammation of the bronchial passages restrict the flow of air in and out of the lungs.

The number of people with asthma and the death rate from this condition have been increasing since the late 1980s. Environmental pollution may be one of the causes of this growing epidemic. Work exposure to flour or cotton dust, animal fur, smoke, and a wide variety of chemicals has been linked to increased risk of asthma.[1]

Findings from animal and human studies confirm that DTP (diphtheria and tetanus toxoids and pertussis) and tetanus vaccinations can induce **allergic** (page 14) responses,[2, 3, 4, 5, 6] and can increase the risk of allergies, including allergic asthma. An analysis of data from nearly 14,000 infants and children revealed that having a history of asthma is twice as great among those who were vaccinated with DTP or tetanus vaccines than among those who were not.[7]

CHECKLIST FOR ASTHMA

Rating	Nutritional Supplements	Herbs
★★☆	**Fish oil (EPA)** (page 514)	Amrita Bindu
	Green-lipped mussel (page 533) (Lyprinol)	**Boswellia** (page 644)
		Coleus (page 660)
	Lycopene (page 548)	**Ivy leaf** (page 697)
	Magnesium (page 551)	Picrorhiza
	Selenium (page 584)	(page 728)
	Vitamin B₆ (page 600)	Tylophora
	Vitamin C (page 604)	(page 754)
★☆☆	**Beta-carotene** (page 469)	Elecampane (page 671)
	Betaine HCl (page 472)	*Ginkgo biloba* (page 681)
	Bromelain (page 481)	
	Molybdenum (page 559)	**Hyssop** (page 695)
	Quercetin (page 580)	Khella
	Thymus extracts (page 591)	**Licorice** (page 702)
		Lobelia (page 705)
	Vitamin B₁₂ (page 601)	**Marshmallow** (page 708)
		Mullein (page 713)
		Onion (page 718)
		Saiboku-to

What are the symptoms of asthma?

An asthma attack usually begins with sudden fits of wheezing, coughing, or shortness of breath. However, it may also begin insidiously with slowly increasing manifestations of respiratory distress. A sensation of tightness in the chest is also common.

Medical treatments

Over the counter treatment includes oral expectorant combinations containing ephedrine (Primatene Tablets) and inhalers containing epinephrine (Primatene Mist).

Several classes of prescription drugs are commonly used for short-term symptom relief and long-term control. Inhaled beta-adrenergic agonist drugs albuterol (Proventil, Ventolin), salmeterol (Serevent), and metaproterenol (Alupent) are used to treat acute asthma attacks. Oral theophylline (Slo-Bid, Theolair, Theo-Dur) and oral corticosteroids, such as prednisone (Deltasone) and prednisolone (Prelone, Pediapred), can either be used for acute symptom relief or prevention. Long-term control primarily involves the use of inhaled corticosteroids and oral leukotriene receptor antagonists. Commonly prescribed inhaled corticosteroids include fluticasone (Flovent), triamcinolone (Azmacort), budesonide (Pulmicort), and flunisolide (AeroBid). Oral leukotriene receptor antagonists include zafirlukast (Accolate) and montelukast (Singulair). Cromolyn sodium (Intal), a synthetic flavonoid, is also used for long-term care to prevent bronchial asthma. Although anticholinergic drugs, such as atropine, are less frequently used, a chemically related drug, ipratropium bromide (Atrovent), is currently useful for long-term treatment.

Medical management of asthma includes controlling environmental factors that can trigger an attack (animal dander, dust mites, airborne molds and pollens, and certain foods).

Dietary changes that may be helpful

A vegan (pure vegetarian) diet given for one year in conjunction with many specific dietary changes (such as avoidance of caffeine, sugar, salt, and chlorinated tap water) and combined with a variety of herbs and supplements led to significant improvement in one group of asthmatics.[8] Although 16 out of 24 people who continued the intervention for the full year were much better and one person was actually cured, it remains unclear how much of the action was purely a result of the dietary changes compared with the many other therapies employed.

Vitamin C (page 604), an **antioxidant** (page 467) present in fruits and vegetables, is a powerful antioxidant and anti-inflammatory. This anti-inflammatory activity may influence the development of asthma symptoms. A large preliminary study has shown that young children with asthma experience significantly less wheezing if they eat a diet high in fruits rich in vitamin C.[9]

Studies suggest that high salt intake may have an adverse effect on asthma, particularly in men. In a small, preliminary trial, doubling salt intake for one month led to a small increase in airway reactivity (indicating a worsening of asthma) in men with asthma, as well as in non-asthmatics.[10] Several double-blind trials have provided limited evidence of clinical improvement following a period of sodium restriction.[11, 12, 13, 14] It is difficult to compare the results of these studies because they used different amounts of sodium restriction. However, they consistently suggest that increased dietary sodium may aggravate asthma symptoms, especially in men.[15]

Although most people with asthma do not suffer from **food allergies** (page 14),[16] unrecognized food allergy can be an exacerbating factor.[17] A medically supervised "allergy elimination diet," followed by reintroduction of the eliminated foods, often helps identify problematic foods. A healthcare professional must supervise this allergy test because of the possibility of triggering a severe asthma attack during the reintroduction.[18]

Some asthmatics react to food additives, such as sulfites, tartrazine (yellow dye #5), and sodium benzoate, as well as natural salicylates (aspirin-like substances found in many foods).[19, 20] A doctor or an allergist can help determine whether chemical sensitivities are present.

Lifestyle changes that may be helpful

Being overweight increases the risk of asthma.[21] Obese people with asthma may improve their lung-function symptoms and overall health status by engaging in a **weight-loss** (page 446) program. A controlled study found that weight loss resulted in significant decreases in episodes of shortness of breath, increases in overall breathing capacity, and decreases in the need for medication to control symptoms.[22]

Nutritional supplements that may be helpful

Lycopene (page 548), an **antioxidant** (page 467) related to **beta-carotene** (page 469) and found in tomatoes, helps reduce the symptoms of asthma caused by exercising. In one double-blind trial,[23] over half of people with exercise-induced asthma had significantly fewer asthma symptoms after taking capsules containing 30 mg of lycopene per day for one week compared to when they took a placebo.

Vitamin B$_6$ (page 600) deficiency is common in asthmatics.[24] This deficiency may relate to the asthma itself or to certain asthma drugs (such as theophylline and aminophylline) that deplete vitamin B$_6$.[25] In a double-blind trial, 200 mg per day of vitamin B$_6$ for two months reduced the severity of asthma in children

and reduced the amount of asthma medication they needed.[26] In another trial, asthmatic adults experienced a dramatic decrease in the frequency and severity of asthma attacks while taking 50 mg of vitamin B$_6$ twice a day.[27] Nonetheless, the research remains somewhat inconsistent, and one double-blind trial found that high amounts of B$_6$ supplements did not help asthmatics who required the use of steroid drugs.[28]

Magnesium (page 551) levels are frequently low in asthmatics.[29] Current evidence suggests that high dietary magnesium intake may be associated with better lung function and reduced bronchial reactivity. Intravenous injection of magnesium has been reported in most,[30, 31, 32, 33] but not all,[34] double-blind trials to rapidly halt acute asthma attacks. Magnesium supplements might help prevent asthma attacks because magnesium can prevent spasms of the bronchial passages. In a preliminary trial, 18 adults with asthma took 300 mg of magnesium per day for 30 days and experienced decreased bronchial reactivity.[35] However, a double-blind trial investigated the effects of 400 mg per day for three weeks and found a significant improvement in symptoms, but not in objective measures of airflow or airway reactivity.[36] The amount of magnesium used in these trials was 300 to 400 mg per day (children take proportionately less based on their body weight).

Supplementation with 1 gram of **vitamin C** (page 604) per day reduces the tendency of the bronchial passages to go into spasm,[37] an action that has been confirmed in double-blind research.[38] Beneficial effects of short-term vitamin C supplementation (i.e., less than three days) have been observed. In one double-blind trial, 500 mg of vitamin C per day for two days prevented attacks of exercise-induced asthma.[39] Two other preliminary trials found that vitamin C supplementation reduced bronchial reactivity to metacholine, a drug that causes bronchial constriction.[40, 41] However, other studies,[42] including two double-blind trials,[43, 44] have failed to corroborate these findings. The only double-blind trial of a long duration found that vitamin C supplementation (1 gram per day for 14 weeks) reduced the severity and frequency of attacks among Nigerian adults with asthma.[45] A buffered form of vitamin C (such as sodium ascorbate or calcium ascorbate) may work better for some asthmatics than regular vitamin C (ascorbic acid).[46]

People with low levels of **selenium** (page 584) have a high risk of asthma.[47, 48, 49, 50, 51] Asthma involves **free-radical** (page 467) damage[52] that selenium might protect against. In a small double-blind trial, supplementation with 100 mcg of sodium selenite (a form of selenium) per day for 14 weeks resulted in clinical improvement in six of eleven patients, compared with only one of ten in the placebo group.[53] Most doctors recommend 200 mcg per day for adults (and proportionately less for children)—a much higher, though still safe, level.

Double-blind research shows that **fish oil** (page 514) partially reduces reactions to **allergens** (page 14) that can trigger attacks in some asthmatics.[54] Although a few researchers report small but significant improvements when asthmatics supplement with fish oil,[55, 56] reviews of the research show that most fish oil studies with asthmatics come up empty-handed.[57, 58] It is possible that some of these trials failed because they did not last long enough to demonstrate an effect. There is evidence that children who eat oily fish may have a much lower risk of getting asthma.[59] Moreover, in a double-blind trial, children who received 300 mg per day of fish oil (providing 84 mg of EPA and 36 mg of DHA) experienced significant improvement of asthma symptoms.[60] It should be noted that these benefits were obtained under circumstances in which exposure to food allergens and environmental allergens was strictly controlled. Though the evidence supporting the use of fish oil remains somewhat conflicting, eating more fish and supplementing with fish oil may still be worth considering, especially among children with asthma.

In a double-blind study of people with asthma, supplementation with a proprietary extract of New Zealand green-lipped mussel (Lyprinol) twice a day for 8 weeks significantly decreased daytime wheezing and improved airflow through the bronchi.[61] Each capsule of Lyprinol contains 50 mg of omega-3 fatty acids.

A study conducted many years ago showed that 80% of children with asthma had hypochlorhydria (**low stomach acid** [page 260]). Supplementation with hydrochloric acid (HCl) in combination with avoidance of known food allergens led to clinical improvement in this preliminary trial.[62] In more recent times, HCl has usually been supplemented in the form of **betaine HCl** (page 472). The amount needed depends on the severity of hypochlorhydria and on the size of a meal. Because it is a fairly strong acid, betaine HCl should be used only with medical supervision.

In some people with asthma, symptoms can be triggered by ingestion of food additives known as sulfites. Pretreatment with a large amount of **vitamin B$_{12}$** (page 601) (1,500 mcg orally) reduced the asthmatic reaction

to sulfites in children with sulfite sensitivity in one preliminary trial.[63] The trace mineral **molybdenum** (page 559) also helps the body detoxify sulfites.[64] While some doctors use molybdenum to treat selected patients with asthma, there is little published research on this treatment, and it is not known what an appropriate level of molybdenum supplementation would be. A typical American diet contains about 200 to 500 mcg per day,[65] and preliminary short-term trials have used supplemental amounts of 500 mcg per day.[66] People who suspect sulfite-sensitive asthma should consult with a physician before taking molybdenum.

Quercetin (page 580), a **flavonoid** (page 516) found in most plants, has an inhibiting action on lipoxygenase, an enzyme that contributes to problems with asthma.[67] No clinical trials in humans have confirmed whether quercetin decreases asthma symptoms. Some doctors are currently experimenting with 400 to 1,000 mg of quercetin three times per day.

Bromelain (page 481) reduces the thickness of mucus, which may be beneficial for those with asthma,[68] though clinical actions in asthmatics remain unproven.

Some researchers have suggested that asthma attacks triggered by exercise might be caused by free-radical damage caused by the exercise. **Beta-carotene** (page 469) is an **antioxidant** (page 467) that protects against free-radical damage. Israeli researchers reported that 64 mg per day of natural beta-carotene for one week in a double blind trial protected over half of a group of asthmatics who experienced attacks as a result of exercise.[69] More research is needed to confirm this promising finding.

The oral administration of a **thymus extract** (page 591) known as thymomodulin has been shown in preliminary and double-blind clinical trials to improve the symptoms and course of asthma.[70, 71, 72, 73] Presumably this clinical improvement is the result of restoration of proper control over **immune function** (page 255).

Are there any side effects or interactions?
Refer to the individual supplement for information about any side effects or interactions.

Herbs that may be helpful
There are two categories of herbs generally used for people with asthma. These are herbs that help dilate the airways and herbs that are anti-inflammatory. Herbs in each category are summarized in the table below.

Asthma

Category	Herbs with Support from Human Trials	Herbs Used Traditionally for Asthma (No Human Trials Available)
Anti-spasmodic, bronchodilating	**Coleus** (page 660)	Fennel (page 676), khella, **lobelia** (page 705)
Anti-inflammatory	Amrita Bindu (antioxidant), **Boswellia** (page 644), **ginkgo** (page 681), **onion** (page 718) (weak evidence), **picrorhiza** (page 728), saiboku-to formula, **tylophora** (page 754) (mechanism of action not clear)	**Elecampane** (page 671), **hyssop** (page 695), **licorice** (page 702), **marshmallow** (page 708), **mullein** (page 713)

Amrita Bindu is an Ayurvedic herbal preparation that contains a mixture of 13 salts and spices. It has been shown to have **antioxidant** (page 467) activity. In a preliminary study, children with severe asthma received 250 to 500 mg (depending on their age) of Amrita Bindu twice a day after meals.[74] After three months of treatment, most of the children were able to stop their prescription asthma medications and were no longer having asthma attacks. While these results are impressive, they should be followed up with a double-blind study, to rule out the possibility that the benefit was due to a placebo effect.

One double-blind trial has investigated the effects of the Ayurvedic herb **boswellia** (page 644) in people with acute bronchial asthma.[75] Participants took 300 mg of powdered boswellia resin extract or placebo three times daily for six weeks. By the end of the study, the number of asthma attacks was significantly lower in the group taking boswellia. Moreover, objective measurements of breathing capacity were also significantly improved by boswellia.

A small double-blind trial found that a constituent of **coleus** (page 660), called forskolin, when inhaled, could decrease lung spasms in asthmatics compared to placebo.[76] Coleus extracts standardized to 18% forskolin are available, and 50 to 100 mg can be taken two to three times per day. Fluid extract can be taken in the amount of 2 to 4 ml three times per day. Most trials

have used injected forskolin, so it is unclear whether oral ingestion of coleus extracts will provide similar benefits in the amounts recommended above.

A controlled trial on children with bronchial asthma suggested that 25 drops of **ivy leaf** (page 697) extract given twice daily was effective in increasing the amount of oxygen in the lungs after only three days of use. However, the frequency of cough and shortness of breath symptoms did not change during the short trial period.[77]

Two preliminary trials have shown **picrorhiza** (page 728) to be of benefit in asthma.[78, 79] However, a follow-up double-blind trial did not confirm these earlier results.[80] A range of 400 to 1,500 mg of powdered, encapsulated picrorhiza per day has been used in a variety of trials. It remains unclear how effective picrorhiza is for people with asthma.

Different preparations of **tylophora** (page 754), including crude leaf, tincture, and capsule, have been tested in human clinical trials. One double-blind trial had people with bronchial asthma chew and swallow one tylophora leaf (150 mg of the leaf by weight) per day for six days. Participants were also given a comparable placebo to be chewed and swallowed during a different six-day period. When consuming tylophora, over half of the people reported experiencing moderate to complete relief of their asthma symptoms, compared to only about 20% reporting relief when consuming the placebo.[81] In a follow-up double-blind trial, an alcoholic extract of crude tylophora leaves had comparable effects to that of chewing the crude leaf.[82] Another double-blind trial found 350 mg of tylophora leaf powder per day increased the lungs' capacity for oxygen and reduced nighttime shortness of breath, but was not as effective as an antiasthmatic drug combination.[83] A fourth double-blind trial found no significant changes in lung volume measurements or asthmatic symptoms after treatment with 400 mg per day tylophora.[84]

Traditionally, herbs that have a soothing action on bronchioles are also used for asthma. These include **marshmallow** (page 708), **mullein** (page 713), **hyssop** (page 695), and **licorice** (page 702). **Elecampane** (page 671) has been used traditionally to treat coughs associated with asthma.[85]

Ginkgo biloba (page 681) extracts (GBE) have been considered a potential therapy for asthma. This is because the extracts block the action of platelet-activating factor (PAF), a compound the body produces that in part causes asthma symptoms. A trial using isolated ginkgolides from ginkgo (not the whole extract) found they reduced asthma symptoms.[86] A controlled trial used a highly concentrated tincture of ginkgo leaf and found this preparation helped decrease asthma symptoms.[87] For asthma, 120 to 240 mg of standardized GBE or 3 to 4 ml of regular tincture three times daily can be used.

In three preliminary trials on people with asthma, a traditional Japanese herbal formula known as saiboku-to has been shown to reduce symptoms and enable some people to reduce their use of steroid medication.[88, 89, 90] Saiboku-to has been extensively studied in the laboratory and has been shown to have numerous anti-inflammatory actions.[91] Some of these studies used 2.5 grams three times per day of saiboku-to. A traditional Chinese or Japanese medicine practitioner should be consulted for more information. Saiboku-to contains **bupleurum** (page 647), hoelen, pinellia, magnolia, **Asian ginseng** (page 630), **Chinese scullcap** (page 658), **licorice** (page 702), perilla, **ginger** (page 680) and jujube.

Eclectic physicians—doctors in turn-of-the-century North America who used herbs as their main medicine—considered **lobelia** (page 705) to be one of the most important plant medicines.[92] Traditionally, it was used by Eclectics to treat **coughs** (page 139) and spasms in the lungs from all sorts of causes.[93] A plant that originates in Africa, khella, is also considered an antispasmodic like lobelia. Though it is not strong enough to stop acute asthma attacks, khella has been recommended by German physicians practicing herbal medicine as possibly helpful for chronic asthma symptoms.[94]

Onion (page 718) may act as an anti-inflammatory in people with asthma. Human studies have shown onion can be a strong anti-inflammatory.[95] However, some people with asthma may experience an exacerbation of symptoms if they are allergic to onion and are exposed to it.[96]

Are there any side effects or interactions?
Refer to the individual herb for information about any side effects or interactions.

Holistic approaches that may be helpful

A set of breathing exercises called Buteyko breathing techniques has been reported to significantly reduce the need for prescription drugs for people with asthma.[97] Although the people in this controlled trial experienced an improved quality of life while doing these exercises, objective measures of breathing capacity did not improve, despite the decreased need for drugs.

Antibiotic use during the first year or two of life has been associated with an increased risk of asthma in preliminary studies.[98, 99] Whether this association might result from **allergic** (page 14) versus non-allergic effects remains unknown. However, the association does suggest that, until more is known, gratuitous use of antibiotics in early childhood (e.g., to inappropriately treat viral diseases) should be reconsidered. Of course, the appropriate use of antibiotics in the treatment of **infections** (page 265) as necessary should not be avoided. Concerns should be discussed with the prescribing physician.

Acupuncture might be useful for some asthmatics. Case reports[100, 101] and preliminary trials[102, 103, 104] have suggested acupuncture may be helpful for people with asthma, either as a treatment for an acute attack or as a longer term therapy for reducing the number or severity of attacks, decreasing the need for medications, and so on. Placebo-controlled trials using sham ("fake") acupuncture, however, have been quite contradictory, many of them showing a strong placebo effect that is not significantly improved upon by real acupuncture.[105, 106, 107, 108] It is possible that needle insertion in non-acupuncture points has a stimulating effect that benefits asthma. The success of acupuncture may also depend on other factors, such as the type of asthma being treated and certain characteristics of the patient. Nonetheless, since some controlled research has demonstrated positive effects of real acupuncture, people with asthma may want to consider a trial of acupuncture treatment to see if it helps their individual cases.

Chiropractic physicians have reported that manipulation may be helpful for patients with asthma.[109, 110, 111] In a controlled study, chronic asthmatics received either real or sham chiropractic manipulations for four weeks, after which the treatments were switched for another four weeks. No improvement in measurements of lung function was found at the end of the study. In addition, while both the manipulation and the sham treatment groups reported significant decreases in asthma frequency and severity, there were no differences between the treatments.[112] A larger controlled study compared chiropractic manipulation to sham manual treatments in children whose asthma was still a problem despite usual medical management.[113] Both groups experienced a significant decrease in symptoms and need for medication, as well as small increases in ability to breathe. These benefits lasted for four months after the treatments were discontinued. Although there was no additional benefit of chiropractic compared to the sham treatments, it is possible that improvements in both groups were real, rather than placebo effects. The sham therapy, which consisted of "soft tissue massage and gentle palpation [touching]," may have had real effects. More research is needed to address this confusing issue.

ATHEROSCLEROSIS

Atherosclerosis is hardening of the arteries, a common disease of the major blood vessels characterized by fatty streaks along the vessel walls and by deposits of cholesterol and calcium.

Atherosclerosis of arteries supplying the heart is called coronary artery disease. It can restrict the flow of blood to the heart, which often triggers **heart attacks** (page 212)—the leading cause of death in Americans and Europeans. Atherosclerosis of arteries supplying the legs causes a condition called **intermittent claudication** (page 276), which is characterized by pain in the legs after walking short distances.

People with elevated **cholesterol** (page 223) levels are much more likely to have atherosclerosis than people with low cholesterol levels. Many important nutritional approaches to protecting against atherosclerosis are aimed at lowering serum cholesterol levels.

People with **diabetes** (page 152) are also at very high risk for atherosclerosis, as are people with elevated **triglycerides** (page 235) and **high homocysteine** (page 234).

What are the symptoms of atherosclerosis?
Atherosclerosis is typically a silent disease until one of the many late-stage vascular manifestations intervenes. Some people with atherosclerosis may experience **angina** (page 27) (chest pain) or **intermittent claudication** (page 276) (leg cramps and pain) on exertion. Symptoms such as these develop gradually as the disease progresses.

Medical treatments
Prevention is still the best treatment for atherosclerosis. Once established, treatment is directed toward the various complications, such as **angina** (page 27), heart attacks, **heart failure** (page 134), **stroke** (page 419), kidney failure, and **peripheral vascular disease** (page 352).

CHECKLIST FOR ATHEROSCLEROSIS

Rating	Nutritional Supplements	Herbs
★★★	**Tocotrienols** (page 593)	**Garlic** (page 679)
★★☆	**Fish oil** (page 514) **Folic acid** (page 520) **Selenium** (page 584) **Vitamin C** (page 604) **Vitamin E** (page 609)	**Fenugreek** (page 676) **Green tea** (page 686) **Guggul** (page 688) **Psyllium** (page 732)
★☆☆	**Betaine (trimethylglycine)** (page 472) **Chondroitin sulfate** (page 492) **Evening primrose oil** (page 511) **Lycopene** (page 548) (prevention only) **Quercetin** (page 580) **Resveratrol** (page 581) **Vitamin B₆** (page 600) **Vitamin B₁₂** (page 601)	**Bilberry** (page 634) **Butcher's broom** (page 649) **Ginger** (page 680) *Ginkgo biloba* (page 681) **Peony** (page 724) (red peony root) **Rosemary** (page 739) **Turmeric** (page 753)

Dietary changes that may be helpful
The most important dietary changes in protecting arteries from atherosclerosis include avoiding meat and dairy fat and avoiding foods that contain trans fatty acids (margarine, some vegetable oils, and many processed foods containing vegetable oils). Increasingly, the importance of avoiding trans fatty acids is being accepted by the scientific community.[1] Leading researchers have recently begun to view the evidence linking trans fatty acids to markers for **heart disease** (page 98) as "unequivocal."[2]

People who eat diets high in alpha-linolenic acid (ALA), which is found in canola and **flaxseed oils** (page 517), have higher blood levels of omega-3 fatty acids than those consuming lower amounts,[3, 4] which may confer some protection against atherosclerosis. In 1994, researchers conducted a study in people with a history of heart disease, using what they called the "Mediterranean" diet.[5] The diet differed significantly from what people from Mediterranean countries actually eat, in that it contained little olive oil. Instead, the diet included a special margarine high in ALA. Those people assigned to the Mediterranean diet had a remarkable 70% reduced risk of dying from heart disease compared with the control group during the first 27 months. Similar results were also confirmed after almost four years.[6] The diet was high in beans and peas, fish, fruit, vegetables, bread, and cereals, and low in meat, dairy fat, and eggs. Although the authors believe that the high ALA content of the diet was partly responsible for the surprising outcome, other aspects of the diet may have been partly or even totally responsible for decreased death rates. Therefore, the success of the Mediterranean diet does not prove that ALA protects against heart disease.[7]

A systematic review of 20 years of research evaluated the association between dietary **fiber** (page 512) and coronary heart disease.[8] The meta-analysis portion of this review showed that regular whole grain foods are associated with a coronary heart disease risk reduction of about 26%. In general, the fibers most linked to the reduction of cholesterol levels are found in **oats** (page 716), **psyllium** (page 732) seeds, fruit (pectin) and beans (guar gum).[9] An analysis of many soluble fiber trials proves that a **cholesterol** (page 223) lowering effect exists, but the amount the cholesterol falls is quite modest.[10] For unknown reasons, however, diets higher in *in*soluble fiber (found in whole grains and vegetables and mostly unrelated to cholesterol levels) have been reported to correlate better with protection against **heart disease** (page 98) in both men and women.[11, 12] Some trials have used 20 grams of additional fiber per day for several months to successfully lower cholesterol.[13]

Independent of their action on serum cholesterol, foods that contain high amounts of cholesterol—mostly egg yolks—can induce atherosclerosis.[14] It makes sense to reduce the intake of egg yolks. However, eating eggs does not increase serum cholesterol as much as eating saturated fat, and eggs may not increase serum cholesterol at all if the overall diet is low in fat. A decrease in atherosclerosis resulting from a pure vegetarian diet (no meat, poultry, dairy or eggs), combined with exercise and stress reduction, has been proven by controlled medical research.[15]

Preliminary evidence has suggested that excessive salt consumption is a risk factor for heart disease and death from heart disease in **overweight** (page 446) people.[16] Controlled trials are needed to confirm these observations.

Eating a diet high in refined carbohydrates (e.g., white flour, white rice, simple sugars) appears to increase the risk of coronary heart disease, and thus of **heart attacks** (page 212), especially in overweight women.[17] However, controlled trials of reducing refined carbohydrate intake to prevent heart disease have not been attempted to confirm these preliminary findings.

Lifestyle changes that may be helpful

Virtually all doctors acknowledge the abundant evidence that smoking is directly linked to atherosclerosis and **heart disease** (page 98).[18] Quitting smoking protects many people from atherosclerosis and heart disease, and is a critical step in the process of disease prevention.[19, 20]

Obesity (page 446),[21] type A behavior (time conscious, impatient, and aggressive), stress,[22] and sedentary lifestyle[23] are all associated with an increased risk of atherosclerosis; interventions designed to change these risk factors are linked to protection from this condition.[24]

Aggressive verbal or physical responses when angry have been consistently related to coronary atherosclerosis in numerous preliminary studies.[25, 26, 27] A low level of social support, especially when combined with a high level of outwardly expressed anger has also been associated with accelerated progression of coronary atherosclerosis.[28]

Nutritional supplements that may be helpful

Tocotrienols (page 593) may offer protection against atherosclerosis by preventing oxidative damage to LDL cholesterol.[29] In a double-blind trial in people with severe atherosclerosis of the carotid artery—the main artery supplying blood to the head—tocotrienol administration (200 mg per day) reduced the level of lipid peroxides in the blood. Moreover, people receiving tocotrienols for 12 months had significantly more protection against atherosclerosis progression, and in some cases reductions in the size of their atherosclerotic plaques, compared with those taking a placebo.[30]

Supplementation with **fish oil** (page 514), rich in omega-3 fatty acids, has been associated with favorable changes in various risk factors for atherosclerosis and heart disease in some,[31, 32, 33, 34, 35, 36] but not all, studies.[37, 38, 39] A double-blind trial showed that people with atherosclerosis who took fish oil (6 grams per day for 3 months and then 3 grams a day for 21 months) had significant regression of atherosclerotic plaques and a decrease in cardiovascular events (e.g., **heart attack** [page 212] and **stroke** [page 419]) compared with those who did not take fish oil.[40] These results contradict the findings of an earlier controlled trial in which fish oil supplementation for two years (6 grams per day) did not promote major favorable changes in the diameter of atherosclerotic coronary arteries.[41]

In some studies, people who consumed more **selenium** (page 584) in their diet had a lower risk of heart disease.[42, 43] In one double-blind report, people who

Atherosclerosis

had already had one **heart attack** (page 212) were given 100 mcg of selenium per day or placebo for six months.[44] At the end of the trial, there were four deaths from heart disease in the placebo group but none in the selenium group; however, the number of people was too small for this difference to be statistically significant. Some doctors recommend that people with atherosclerosis supplement with 100–200 mcg of selenium per day.

Experimentally increasing **homocysteine** (page 562) levels in humans has led to temporary dysfunction of the cells lining blood vessels. Researchers are concerned this dysfunction may be linked to atherosclerosis and heart disease. **Vitamin C** (page 604) has been reported in one controlled study to reverse the dysfunction caused by increases in homocysteine.[45] Vitamin C also protects LDL.[46]

Despite the protective mechanisms attributed to vitamin C, some research has been unable to link vitamin C intake to protection against **heart disease** (page 98). These negative trials have mostly been conducted using people who consume 90 mg of vitamin C per day or more—a level beyond which further protection of LDL may not occur. Studies of people who eat foods containing lower amounts of vitamin C *have* been able to show a link between dietary vitamin C and protection from heart disease. Therefore, leading vitamin C researchers have begun to suggest that vitamin C may be important in preventing heart disease, but only up to 100–200 mg of intake per day.[47] In a double-blind trial,[48] supplementation with 250 mg of timed-release vitamin C twice daily for three years resulted in a 15% reduction in the progression of atherosclerosis, compared with placebo. Many doctors suggest that people take vitamin C—often 1 gram per day—despite the fact that research does not yet support levels higher than 500 mg per day.

Vitamin E (page 609) is an **antioxidant** (page 467) that serves to protect LDL from oxidative damage[49] and has been linked to prevention of heart disease in double-blind research.[50] Many doctors recommend 400–800 IU of vitamin E per day to lower the risk of atherosclerosis and **heart attacks** (page 212). However, some leading researchers suggest taking only 100–200 IU per day, as studies that have explored the long-term effects of different supplemental levels suggest no further benefit beyond that amount, and research reporting positive effects with 400–800 IU per day have not investigated the effects of lower intakes.[51] In a double-

blind trial, people with high cholesterol who took 136 IU of natural vitamin E per day for three years had 10% less progression of atherosclerosis compared with those taking placebo.[52]

Blood levels of an **amino acid** (page 465) called **homocysteine** (page 562) have been linked to atherosclerosis and heart disease in most research,[53, 54] though uncertainty remains about whether elevated homocysteine actually causes heart disease.[55, 56] Although some reports have found associations between homocysteine levels and dietary factors, such as coffee and protein intakes,[57] evidence linking specific foods to homocysteine remains preliminary. Higher blood levels of **vitamin B$_6$** (page 600), **vitamin B$_{12}$** (page 601), and **folic acid** (page 520) are associated with low levels of homocysteine[58] and supplementing with these vitamins lowers homocysteine levels.[59, 60]

While several trials have consistently shown that B$_6$, B$_{12}$, and folic acid lower homocysteine, the amounts used vary from study to study. Many doctors recommend 50 mg of vitamin B$_6$, 100–300 mcg of vitamin B$_{12}$, and 500–800 mcg of folic acid. Even researchers finding only inconsistent links between homocysteine and heart disease have acknowledged that a B vitamin might offer protection against heart disease independent of the homocysteine-lowering effect.[61] In one trial, people with normal homocysteine levels had demonstrable reversal of atherosclerosis when supplementing B vitamins (2.5 mg folic acid, 25 mg vitamin B$_6$, and 250 mcg of vitamin B$_{12}$ per day).[62]

For the few cases in which vitamin B$_6$, vitamin B$_{12}$, and folic acid fail to normalize homocysteine, adding 6 grams per day of **betaine (trimethylglycine)** (page 472) may be effective.[63] Of these four supplements, folic acid appears to be the most important.[64] Attempts to lower homocysteine by simply changing the diet rather than by using vitamin supplements have not been successful.[65]

Quercetin (page 580), a **flavonoid** (page 516), protects LDL cholesterol from damage.[66] While several preliminary studies have found that eating foods high in quercetin lowers the risk of heart disease,[67, 68, 69] the research on this subject is not always consistent,[70] and some research finds no protective link.[71] Quercetin is found in apples, onions, black tea, and as a supplement. In some studies, dietary amounts linked to protection from heart disease are as low as 35 mg per day.

Though low levels (2 grams per day) of **evening primrose oil** (page 511) appear to be without action,[72]

3–4 grams per day have lowered **cholesterol** (page 223) in double-blind research.[73] Lowering cholesterol levels should in turn reduce the risk of atherosclerosis.

Preliminary research shows that **chondroitin sulfate** (page 492) may prevent atherosclerosis in animals and humans and may also prevent **heart attacks** (page 212) in people who already have atherosclerosis.[74, 75] However, further research is needed to determine the value of chondroitin sulfate supplements for preventing or treating atherosclerosis.

Preliminary studies have found that people who drink red wine, which contains **resveratrol** (page 581), are at lower risk of death from heart disease. Because of its **antioxidant** (page 467) activity and its effect on platelets, some researchers believe that resveratrol is the protective agent in red wine.[76, 77, 78] Resveratrol research remains very preliminary, however, and as yet there is no evidence that the amounts found in supplements help prevent atherosclerosis in humans.

In 1992, a Finnish study found a strong link between unnecessary exposure to **iron** (page 540) and increased risk for **heart disease** (page 98).[79] Since then many studies have not found that link,[80, 81, 82] though perhaps an equal number have been able to confirm the outcome of the original report.[83, 84] One 1999 analysis of 12 studies looking at iron status and heart disease found no overall relationship,[85] though another 1999 analysis of published studies came to a different conclusion.[86] While the effect of unnecessary exposure to iron, including iron supplements, on the risk of heart disease remains unclear, there is no benefit in supplementing iron in the absence of a diagnosed deficiency.

The carotenoid, **lycopene** (page 548), has been found to be low in the blood of people with atherosclerosis, particularly if they are smokers.[87] Although no association between atherosclerosis and blood level of any other **carotenoid** (page 488) (e.g., **beta-carotene** [page 469]) was found, the results of this study suggested a protective role for lycopene. Lycopene is present in high amounts in tomatoes.

Are there any side effects or interactions?
Refer to the individual supplement for information about any side effects or interactions.

Herbs that may be helpful
Many actions associated with herbal supplements may help prevent or potentially alleviate atherosclerosis. Herbs such as **garlic** (page 679) and **ginkgo** (page 680)

appear to directly affect the hardened arteries by multiple mechanisms. Herbs such as **psyllium** (page 732), **guggul** (page 688), and **fenugreek** (page 676) reduce cholesterol and other lipid levels in the blood—known risk factors for hardened arteries. A related group are herbs, including **green tea** (page 686), prevents the oxidation of cholesterol, an important step in protecting against atherosclerosis. Finally, there are herbs such as **ginger** (page 680) and **turmeric** (page 753) that reduce excessive stickiness of platelets, thereby reducing atherosclerosis.

Herbs	Action
Garlic (page 679)	Directly anti-atherosclerotic
Fenugreek (page 676), **garlic** (page 679), **guggul** (page 688), **psyllium** (page 732)	Cholesterol-lowering
Green tea (page 686)	Block oxidation of cholesterol
Garlic (page 679), **ginger** (page 680), **ginkgo** (page 681), **peony** (page 724), **turmeric** (page 753)	Decrease excessive platelet stickiness
Butcher's broom (page 649), **rosemary** (page 739)	Traditionally considered circulatory stimulant

Garlic has been shown to prevent atherosclerosis in a four-year double-blind trial.[88] The preparation used, standardized for 0.6% allicin content, provided 900 mg of standardized garlic powder per day. The people in this trial were 50 to 80 years old, and the benefits were most notable in women. This trial points to the long-term benefits of garlic to both prevent and possibly slow the progression of atherosclerosis in people at risk.

Garlic has also lowered **cholesterol** (page 223) levels in double-blind research,[89] though more recently, some double-blind trials have not found garlic to be effective.[90, 91, 92] Some of the negative trials have flaws in their design.[93] Nonetheless, the relationship between garlic and cholesterol-lowering is somewhat unclear.[94]

Garlic has also been shown to prevent excessive platelet adhesion in humans.[95] Allicin, often considered the main active component of garlic, is not alone in this action. The constituent known as ajoene has also shown beneficial effects on platelets.[96] Aged garlic extract, but not raw garlic, has been shown, to prevent oxidation of LDL cholesterol in humans,[97] an event believed to be a significant factor in the development of atherosclerosis.

Ginkgo (page 681) may reduce the risk of athero-sclerosis by interfering with a chemical the body sometimes makes in excess, called platelet activating factor (PAF).[98] PAF stimulates platelets to stick together too much; ginkgo stops this from happening. Ginkgo also increases blood circulation to the brain, arms, and legs.[99]

Garlic and ginkgo also decrease excessive blood co-agulation. Both have been shown in double-blind[100] and other controlled[101] trials to decrease the overactive coagulation of blood that may contribute to athero-sclerosis.

Guggul (page 688) has been less extensively studied, but double-blind evidence suggests it can significantly improve cholesterol and **triglyceride** (page 235) levels in people.[102] Numerous medicinal plants and plant compounds have demonstrated an ability to protect LDL cholesterol from being damaged by **free radicals** (page 467). Garlic,[103] ginkgo,[104] and guggul[105] are of particular note in this regard. Garlic and ginkgo have been most convincingly shown to protect LDL choles-terol in humans.

Several other herbs have been shown in research to lower lipid levels. Of these, **psyllium** (page 732) has the most consistent backing from multiple double-blind trials showing lower cholesterol and triglyceride lev-els.[106] The evidence supporting the ability of **fenugreek** (page 676) to lower lipid levels is not as convincing, coming from preliminary studies only.[107]

Since oxidation of LDL cholesterol is thought to be important in causing or accelerating atherosclerosis, and **green tea** (page 686) protects against oxidation, this herb may have a role in preventing atherosclerosis. However, while some studies show that green tea is an **antioxidant** (page 467) in humans,[108] others have not been able to confirm that it protects LDL cholesterol from damage.[109] Much of the research documenting the health benefits of green tea is based on the amount of green tea typically drunk in Asian countries—about three cups per day (providing 240–320 mg of polyphe-nols).

The research on **ginger** (page 680)'s ability to reduce platelet stickiness indicates that 10 grams (approximately 1 heaping teaspoon) per day is the minimum necessary amount to be effective.[110] Lower amounts of dry ginger,[111] as well as various levels of fresh ginger,[112] have not been shown to affect platelets.

Turmeric (page 753)'s active compound curcumin has shown potent anti-platelet activity in animal stud-ies.[113] It has also demonstrated this effect in preliminary

human studies.[114] In a similar vein, **bilberry** (page 634) has been shown to prevent platelet aggregation[115] as has **peony** (page 724).[116] However, none of these three herbs has been documented to help atherosclerosis in human trials.

Butcher's broom (page 649) and **rosemary** (page 724) are not well studied as being circulatory stimu-lants but are traditionally reputed to have such an ac-tion that might impact atherosclerosis. While butcher's broom is useful for various diseases of veins, it also ex-erts effects that are protective for arteries.[117]

Are there any side effects or interactions?
Refer to the individual herb for information about any side effects or interactions.

ATHLETE'S FOOT

What do I need to know?
Self-care for athlete's foot can be approached in a num-ber of ways—but it can be hard to know just where to start. To make it easier, our doctors recommend trying these simple steps first:

Try tea tree oil
  Apply a 10% concentration in a cream base as a natural alternative to antifungal medications
Keep it dry down there
  To discourage fungal growth, dry feet thor-oughly after showering or bathing, use foot powders, and change socks frequently
Let your feet see the light
  Wear sandals or other open footwear to expose skin to sunlight's antifungal effects

About athlete's foot
Athlete's foot is a fungal infection of the foot that can be caused by a number of different skin fungi.

Generally, athlete's foot does not cause serious prob-lems; however, the disruption of the skin barrier can be a source of significant infections in people with im-paired blood flow to the feet (such as people with **dia-betes** [page 152]) or in those with impaired **immune systems** (page 255). Infections of the nails are more dif-ficult to treat than those affecting only the skin.

What are the symptoms of athlete's foot?
Symptoms of athlete's foot include a persistent, burning itch that often starts between the toes. The skin on the

feet may be damp, soft, red, cracked, or peeling; the feet may also show patches of dead skin. The feet often have a strong or unusual smell, and sometimes small blisters occur on the feet.

Rating	Nutritional Supplements	Herbs
★★☆		Tea tree (page 751) oil
★☆☆		Garlic (page 679)

CHECKLIST FOR ATHLETE'S FOOT

Medical treatments

Over the counter agents used to treat athlete's foot are available as creams, powders, and sprays. Available drugs include clotrimazole (Lotrimin), miconazole (Micatin), terbinafine (Lamisil), undecylenic acid (Desenex) and tolnaftate (Tinactin, Aftate).

Topical prescription drugs used to treat athlete's foot include econazole (Spectazole), ketoconazole (Nizoral), and ciclopirox (Loprox).

Drying powders can be used inside the socks and shoes to help keep the feet dry during the day.

Lifestyle changes that may be helpful

Keeping the feet dry is very important for preventing and fighting athlete's foot. After showering or bathing, thorough drying or careful use of a hair dryer is recommended. Light is also an enemy of fungi. People with athlete's foot should change socks daily to decrease contact with the fungus and should wear sandals occasionally to get sunlight exposure.

Herbs that may be helpful

Tea tree (page 751) oil has been traditionally used to treat athlete's foot. One trial reported that application of a 10% tea tree oil cream reduced symptoms of athlete's foot just as effectively as drugs and better than placebo, although it did not eliminate the fungus.[1]

The compound known as ajoene, found in **garlic** (page 679), is an antifungal agent. In a group of 34 people using a 0.4% ajoene cream applied once per day, 79% of them saw complete clearing of athlete's foot after one week; the rest saw complete clearing within two weeks.[2] All participants remained cured three months later. One trial found a 1% ajoene cream to be more effective than the standard topical drug terbinafine for treating athlete's foot.[3] Ajoene cream is

not yet available commercially, but topical application of crushed, raw garlic may be a potential alternative application.

Are there any side effects or interactions?
Refer to the individual herb for information about any side effects or interactions.

ATHLETIC PERFORMANCE

What do I need to know?

Self-care for athletic performance can be approached in a number of ways—but it can be hard to know just where to start. To make it easier, our doctors recommend trying these simple steps first:

Eat more carbs
Supply the body with efficient energy fuel found in grains, starchy vegetables, fruits, low-fat dairy products, and carbohydrate-replacement drinks

Don't worry about protein
A normal diet provides enough protein for most athletes

Get enough water and electrolytes
Water is crucial for all sports activities—electrolytes are only important for extreme endurance exercise

Check out creatine monohydrate
Take 15 to 20 grams a day for five or six days to improve performance of high-intensity, short duration exercise (like sprinting) or sports with alternating low- and high-intensity efforts

Take a multivitamin-mineral supplement
When your diet isn't enough, extra vitamins and minerals will help your body get the nutrition it needs for exercise

Try vitamin C
Take 400 mg a day for several days before and after intense exercise to reduce pain and speed muscle strength recovery

About athletic performance

Aside from training, nutrition may be the most important influence on athletic performance.[1] However, in seeking a competitive edge, athletes are often susceptible to fad diets or supplements that have not been scientifically validated. Nevertheless, there is much useful research to guide the exerciser toward optimum health and performance.

Athletic Performance

CHECKLIST FOR ATHLETIC PERFORMANCE

Rating	Nutritional Supplements	Herbs
★★★	**Creatine monohydrate** (page 501) (for high-intensity, short duration exercise or sports with alternating low- and high-intensity efforts) **Multivitamin-mineral supplements** (page 559) (if deficient) **Vitamin C** (page 604) (to reduce pain and speed muscle strength recovery after intense exercise)	
★★☆	Citrate (for high-intensity, short- to intermediate-duration exercise) **Creatine monohydrate** (page 501) (for non-weight bearing endurance exercise) **DHEA** (page 503) (for improving strength in older men only) Electrolyte replacement (for ultra-endurance competition only) **Glutamine** (page 530) (for reducing risk of post-exercise **infection** [page 265] only) **HMB** (page 534) (for improving body composition with strength training in untrained people only) **Iron** (page 544) (for **iron deficiency** [page 278] only) **Pyruvate** (page 580) (for exercise performance) Sodium bicarbonate (for performance enhancement in events of specific durations only) **Soy** (page 587) (for exercise recovery only) **Vitamin C** (page 604) (for deficiency only) **Vitamin E** (page 609) (for exercise recovery and high-altitude exercise performance only) **Whey protein** (page 613)	**Asian ginseng** (page 630) (for endurance exercise and muscle strength only) **Eleuthero** (page 672) **Rhodiola** (page 738) (to improve endurance)
★☆☆	**Arginine** (page 467)/ **Ornithine** (page 565) (for body composition and strength) Aspartic acid **Beta-sitosterol** (page 471)/Beta-sitosterol glucoside (in combination for reducing the risk of post-exercise infection) **Branched-chain amino acids** (page 479) (for high altitude and extreme temperature, for reducing the risk of post-exercise infection, or for preventing decline of mental functioning during exercise) **Chromium** (page 493) **CLA** (page 499) **Coenzyme Q$_{10}$** (page 496) **Copper** (page 499) **Eucalyptus** (page 673) (topical) **Gamma oryzanol** (page 525) **L-carnitine** (page 543) **Magnesium** (page 551) **Medium chain triglycerides** (page 554) **Methoxyisoflavone** (page 558) **Octacosanol** (page 565) **Ornithine alpha-ketoglutarate** (page 566) (OKG) **Phosphorus** (page 570) **Pyruvate** (page 580) (for improving body composition with strength training in untrained people only) **Ribose** (page 582) **Vitamin B-complex** (page 603) **Zinc** (page 614)	**American ginseng** (page 625) **Cayenne** (page 654) (topical capsaicin) **Eucalyptus** (page 673) (topical) **Guaraná** (page 687) Kola Tribulus **Yohimbe** (page 764)

Medical treatments

Athletic performance may be improved by ensuring adequate and balanced nutrition, sufficient fluid intake, and proper rest. The avoidance of performance-reducing drugs such as alcohol and tobacco is also commonly recommended.

Dietary changes that may be helpful

Calories

Calorie requirements for athletes depend on the intensity of their training and performance. The athlete who trains to exhaustion on a daily basis needs more fuel than one who performs a milder regimen two or three times per week. Calorie requirements can be as much as 23 to 39 calories per pound of body weight per day for the training athlete who exercises vigorously for several hours per day.[2, 3] Many athletes compete in sports having weight categories (such as wrestling and boxing), sports that favor small body size (such as gymnastics and horse racing), or sports that may require a specific socially accepted body shape (such as figure skating). These athletes may feel pressured to restrict calories to extreme degrees to gain a competitive edge.[4] Excessive calorie restriction can result in chronic fatigue, sleep disturbances, reduced performance, impaired ability for intensive training, and increased vulnerability to injury.[5]

Carbohydrates

Carbohydrates are the most efficient fuel for energy production and can also be stored as glycogen in muscle and liver, functioning as a readily available energy source for prolonged, strenuous exercise. For these reasons, carbohydrates may be the most important nutrient for sports performance.[6] Depending on training intensity and duration, athletes require up to 4.5 grams of carbohydrates per day per pound of body weight or 60 to 70% of total dietary calories from carbohydrates, whichever is greater.[7, 8] Emphasizing grains, starchy vegetables, fruits, low-fat dairy products, and carbohydrate-replacement beverages, along with reducing intake of fatty foods, results in a relatively high-carbohydrate diet.

Carbohydrate beverages should be consumed during endurance training or competition (30 to 70 grams of carbohydrate per hour) to help prevent carbohydrate depletion that might otherwise occur near the end of the exercise period. Standard sport drinks containing 6 to 8% carbohydrates can be used during exercise to support both carbohydrate and fluid needs, but these should not contain large amounts of fructose, which can cause gastrointestinal distress.[9] At the end of endurance exercise, body carbohydrate stores must be replaced to prepare for the next session. This replacement can be achieved most rapidly if 40 to 60 grams of carbohydrate are consumed right after exercise, repeating this intake every hour for at least five hours after the event.[10] High-density carbohydrate beverages containing 20 to 25% carbohydrate are useful for immediate post-exercise repletion.

Adding protein to carbohydrate intake immediately after exercise may be helpful for improving recovery of glycogen (carbohydrate) stores after exercise according to some,[11, 12, 13] though not all,[14, 15, 16, 17, 18] controlled studies. It appears that adding protein during the post-exercise period is not necessary when carbohydrate intake is high enough (about 0.55 grams per pound of body weight).[19]

Carbohydrate loading, or "super-compensation," is a pre-event strategy that improves performance for some endurance athletes.[20, 21] Carbohydrate-loading can be achieved by consuming a 70% carbohydrate diet (or 4.5 grams per pound of body weight) for three to five days before competition, while gradually reducing training time, and ending with a day of no training while continuing the diet until the event date.

Glycemic index

The glycemic index (GI) is a measure of the ability of a food to raise blood sugar levels after it is eaten. Attention to the GI of carbohydrate sources may be helpful for increasing sports performance. Within one hour before exercise, consuming low GI carbohydrates (such as most fruits, pasta, legumes, or rice) provides carbohydrate without triggering a rapid rise in insulin that could result in hypoglycemia and prevent release of energy sources from fat cells.[22] Some controlled studies of cycling endurance have found that eating a pre-exercise meal of low-GI foods (lentils, rolled oats, or a combination of low GI foods) is more effective than consuming high-GI foods (potatoes, puffed rice, or a combination of high GI foods),[23, 24, 25] but most studies have found no significant advantage of low GI foods or fructose (a low-GI sugar) compared with other carbohydrate sources in a pre-exercise meal. [26, 27, 28, 29, 30, 31, 32, 33] After exercise, on the other hand, high-GI foods and beverages may be most helpful for quickly restoring depleted glycogen stores.[34]

Protein

Protein requirements are often higher for both strength and endurance athletes than for people who are not exercising vigorously; however, the increased food intake needed to supply necessary calories and carbohydrates also supplies extra protein. As long as the diet contains at least 12 to 15% of calories as protein, or up to 0.75 grams per day per pound of body weight, protein supplements are neither necessary, nor likely to be of benefit.[35, 36] Concerns have been raised that the very high-protein diets sometimes used by body builders could put stress on the kidneys, potentially increasing the risk of kidney disease later in life. A preliminary study of male athletes consuming at least 2.77 grams per pound of body weight per day showed no evidence of kidney impairment; however, the study was limited to one month, and evidence of long-term kidney problems associated with chronic protein loading were not examined.[37]

Preliminary studies have suggested that increased protein intake may have biological effects that could improve muscle growth resulting from strength training, especially if liquid supplements (typically containing at least 6 grams of protein or amino acids in addition to varying amounts of carbohydrate) are taken either immediately after exercise or just before exercise.[38, 39, 40, 41, 42, 43, 44] However, controlled studies have found no advantage of protein supplementation (up to about 100 grams per day or about 14 grams immediately following exercise) for improving strength or body composition as long as the diet already supplies typical amounts of protein and calories.[45, 46, 47]

Fat

Some athletes have speculated that consuming a high-fat diet for two or more weeks prior to endurance competition might cause the body to shift its fuel utilization toward more abundant fat stores ("fat adaptation").[48] However, neither short- nor long-term use of high-fat diets has been found to improve endurance performance compared with high-carbohydrate diets, and may even be detrimental due to depletion of glycogen stores.[49, 50]

Following a high-fat diet with at least 24 hours of high carbohydrate intake has been suggested as a way to achieve fat adaptation while restoring glycogen levels before endurance competition.[51, 52] While this concept is supported by physiological studies on athletes, no actual performance enhancement was shown when athletes were tested in competitive situations after a five- to six-day high-fat diet followed by 24 hours of high carbohydrate intake.[53, 54, 55] However, one controlled study found a small, significant benefit of ten days of high fat intake followed by three days of high carbohydrate intake.[56]

Water

Water is the most abundant substance in the human body and is essential for normal physiological function. Water loss due to sweating during exercise can result in decreased performance and other problems. Fluids should be consumed prior to, during, and after exercise, especially when extreme conditions of climate, exercise intensity, and exercise duration exist.[57] Approximately two glasses of fluid should be consumed two hours before exercise and at regular intervals during exercise; fluid should be cool, not cold (59 to 72° F, 15 to 22.2° C). Flavored sports drinks containing electrolytes are not necessary for fluid replacement during brief periods of exercise, but they may be more effective in encouraging the athlete to drink frequently and in larger amounts.[58, 59]

Lifestyle changes that may be helpful

Many athletes use exercise and weight-modifying diets as tools to change their body composition, assuming that a lower percentage of body fat and/or higher lean body mass is desirable in any sport. There is no single standard for body weight and body composition that applies to all types of athletic activities. Different sports, even different roles in the same sport (e.g., running vs. blocking in football), require different body types. These body types are largely determined by genetics. However, within each athlete's genetic predisposition, variations result from diet and exercise that may affect performance. In general, excess weight is a disadvantage in activities that require quickness and speed. However, brief, intense bursts of power depend partly on muscle size, so this type of activity may favor athletes with greater muscle mass. On the other hand, participants in endurance sports, which require larger energy reserves, should not attempt to lower their body fat so much as to compromise their performance.[60]

Nutritional supplements that may be helpful

Creatine

Creatine (page 501) (creatine monohydrate) is used in muscle tissue for the production of phosphocreatine, a factor in the formation of ATP, the source of energy for muscle contraction and many other functions in the body.[61, 62] Creatine supplementation increases phosphocreatine levels in muscle, especially when accompanied by exercise or carbohydrate intake.[63, 64] It may also increase exercise-related gains in lean body mass, though it is unclear how much of these gains represents added muscle tissue and how much is simply water retention.[65]

Over 40 double-blind or controlled studies have found creatine supplementation (typically 136 mg per pound of body weight per day or 15 to 25 grams per day for five or six days) improves performance of either single or repetitive bouts of short-duration, high-intensity exercise lasting under 30 seconds each.[66, 67, 68, 69, 70, 71, 72] Examples of this type of exercise include weightlifting; sprinting by runners, cyclists, or swimmers; and many types of athletic training regimens for speed and power. About 15 studies did not report enhancement by creatine of this type of performance. These have been criticized for their small size and other research design problems, but it is possible that some people, especially elite athletes, are less likely to benefit greatly from creatine supplementation.[73]

Fewer studies have investigated whether creatine supplementation benefits continuous high-intensity exercise lasting 30 seconds or longer. Five controlled studies have found creatine beneficial for this type of exercise,[74] but one study found no benefit on performance of a military obstacle course run.[75] Most studies of endurance performance have found no advantage of creatine supplementation, except perhaps for non-weight bearing exercise such as cycling. [76, 77, 78]

Long-term use of creatine supplementation is typically done using smaller daily amounts (2 to 5 grams per day) after an initial loading period of several days with 20 grams per day. Very little research has been done to investigate the exercise performance effects of long-term creatine supplementation. One study reported that long-term creatine supplementation improved sprint performance.[79] Four controlled long-term trials using untrained women,[80] trained men,[81] or untrained older adults found that creatine improved gains made in strength and lean body mass from weight-training programs.[82, 83] However, two controlled trials found no advantage of long-term creatine supplementation in weight-training football players.[84, 85]

Creatine supplementation appears to increase body weight and lean body mass or fat-free mass, but these measurements do not distinguish between muscle growth and increased water content of muscle.[86, 87] A few double-blind studies using more specific muscle measurements have been done and found that combining creatine supplementation with strength training over several weeks does produce greater increases in muscle size compared with strength training alone.[88, 89, 90]

Multivitamin-mineral supplements

Many athletes do not eat an optimal diet, especially when they are trying to control their weight while training strenuously.[91] These athletes may experience micronutrient deficiencies that, even if marginal, could affect performance or cause health problems.[92, 93, 94, 95] However, athletes who receive recommended daily allowances of vitamins and minerals from their diet do not appear to benefit from additional **multivitamin-mineral supplements** (page 559) with increased performance.[96, 97, 98]

Very little research has been done to evaluate the ergogenic effects of most vitamins or minerals other than those discussed in this article. Supplementation with **selenium** (page 584) (180 mcg per day for 10 weeks) had no effect on the results of endurance training in one double-blind trial.[99] Vanadyl sulfate, a form of **vanadium** (page 594) that may have an insulin-like action, was given to weight-training athletes in a double-blind trial, using 225 mcg per pound of body weight per day, but no effect on body composition was seen after 12 weeks, and effects on strength were inconsistent.[100] The importance of other individual vitamins and minerals is discussed elsewhere in this section.

Antioxidants

Most research has demonstrated that strenuous exercise increases production of harmful substances called **free radicals** (page 467), which can damage muscle tissue and result in inflammation and muscle soreness. Exercising in cities or smoggy areas also increases exposure to free radicals. **Antioxidants** (page 467), including **vitamin C** (page 604) and **vitamin E** (page 609), neutralize free radicals before they can damage the body, so antioxidants may aid in exercise recovery. Regular exercise increases the efficiency of the antioxidant defense system, potentially reducing the amount of supplemental antioxidants that might otherwise be needed for protection. However, at least theoretically, supplements of antioxidant vitamins may be beneficial for older or untrained people or athletes who are undertaking an especially vigorous training protocol or athletic event.[101, 102]

Placebo-controlled research, some of it double-blind, has shown that taking 400 to 3,000 mg of vitamin C per day for several days before and after intense exercise may reduce pain and speed up muscle strength recovery.[103, 104, 105] However, taking vitamin C only after such exercise was not effective in another double-blind study.[106] While some research has reported that vitamin E supplementation in the amount of 800 to 1,200 IU per day reduces biochemical measures of free radical activity and muscle damage caused by strenuous exercise,[107, 108, 109] several studies have not found such benefits,[110, 111, 112, 113] and no research has investigated the effect of vitamin E on performance-related measures of strenuous exercise recovery. A combination of 90 mg per day of **coenzyme Q₁₀** (page 496) and a very small amount of vitamin E did not produce any protective effects for marathon runners in one double-blind trial,[114] while in another double-blind trial a combination of 50 mg per day of **zinc** (page 614) and 3 mg per day of **copper** (page 499) significantly reduced evidence of post-exercise free radical activity.[115]

In most well-controlled studies, exercise performance has not been shown to improve following supplementation with vitamin C, unless a deficiency exists, as might occur in athletes with unhealthy or irrational eating patterns.[116, 117] Similarly, vitamin E has not benefited exercise performance, [118, 119] except possibly at high altitudes. [120, 121]

Alkalinizing agents

The use of alkalinizing agents, such as sodium bicarbonate, sodium citrate, and phosphate salts (potassium phosphate, sodium acid phosphate, and tribasic sodium phosphate) to enhance athletic performance is designed to neutralize the acids produced during exercise that may interfere with energy production or muscle contraction.[122] Some double-blind studies, though not all, have found that sodium bicarbonate or sodium citrate typically improves exercise performance for events lasting either 1 to 10 minutes or 30 to 60 minutes.[123, 124, 125, 126, 127, 128, 129, 130, 131] The amounts used are 115 to 180 mg of sodium bicarbonate or 135 to 225 mg of sodium citrate per pound of body weight. These amounts are dissolved in at least two cups of fluid and are taken either as a single ingestion at least one hour before exercise or divided into smaller amounts and taken over several hours before exercise. Performance during periods of less than one minute or between 10 and 30 minutes is not improved by taking alkalinizing agents.[132, 133, 134, 135, 136] Sodium citrate may be preferable to sodium bicarbonate because it causes less gastrointestinal upset.[137] Another alkalinizing agent, phosphate salts, has been investigated primarily as an endurance performance enhancer, with very inconsistent results.[138, 139]

DHEA

Dehydroepiandrosterone (DHEA) is a hormone produced by the adrenal glands that is used by the body to make the male sex hormone testosterone. In one double-blind trial, 100 mg per day of DHEA was effective

for improving strength in older men,[140] but 50 mg per day was ineffective in a similar study of elderly men and women.[141] DHEA has not been effective for women or younger men in other studies.[142, 143]

Electrolytes

Electrolyte replacement is not as important as water intake in most athletic endeavors. It usually takes several hours of exercise in warm climates before sodium depletion becomes significant and even longer for depletions of **potassium** (page 572), chloride, and **magnesium** (page 551) to occur.[144] However, the presence of sodium in fluids will often make it easier to drink as well as to retain more fluid.[145] Athletes participating in several hours of exercise, especially in hot, humid conditions, should use sodium-containing fluids to reduce the risk of performance-diminishing and possibly dangerous declines in blood sodium levels.[146, 147]

Glutamine

The **amino acid glutamine** (page 465) appears to play a role in several aspects of human physiology that might benefit athletes, including their muscle function and immune system.[148] Intense exercise lowers blood levels of glutamine, which can remain persistently low with overtraining.[149] Glutamine supplementation raises levels of growth hormone at an intake of 2 grams per day,[150] an effect of interest to some athletes because of the role of growth hormone in stimulating muscle growth,[151] and glutamine, given intravenously, was found to be more effective than other amino acids at helping replenish muscle glycogen after exercise.[152] However, glutamine supplementation (30 mg per 2.2 pounds body weight) has not improved performance of short-term, high-intensity exercise such as weightlifting or sprint cycling by trained athletes,[153, 154] and no studies on endurance performance or muscle growth have been conducted. Although the effects of glutamine supplementation on **immune function** (page 255) after exercise have been inconsistent,[155, 156] double-blind trials giving athletes glutamine (5 grams after intense, prolonged exercise, then again two hours later) reported 81% having no subsequent **infection** (page 265) compared with 49% in the placebo group.[157]

HMB

HMB (beta hydroxy-beta-methylbutyrate) is a metabolite (breakdown product) of leucine, one of the essential **branched-chain amino acids** (page 479). Biochemical and animal research show that HMB has a role in protein synthesis and might, therefore, improve muscle growth and overall body composition when given as a supplement. However, double-blind human research suggests that HMB may only be effective when combined with an exercise program in people who are not already highly trained athletes. Double-blind trials found no effect of 3 to 6 grams per day of HMB on body weight, body fat, or overall body composition in weight-training football players or other trained athletes.[158, 159, 160, 161, 162] However, one double-blind study found that 3 grams per day of HMB increased the amount of body fat lost by 70-year old adults who were participating in a strength-training program for the first time.[163] A double-blind study of young men with no strength-training experience reported greater improvements in muscle mass (but not in percentage body fat) when HMB was used in the amount of 17 mg per pound of body weight per day.[164] However, another group of men in the same study given twice as much HMB did not experience any changes in body composition.

Inosine

Inosine (page 537) is a nucleic acid derivative that appears in exercising muscle tissue. Its role in various cellular functions has led to suggestions that it may have ergogenic effects.[165] However, three controlled studies demonstrated no beneficial effects on performance and suggested that inosine may impair some aspects of exercise performance.[166, 167, 168] Therefore, use of inosine is discouraged.

Iron

Iron (page 539) is important for an athlete because it is a component of hemoglobin, which transports oxygen to muscle cells. Some athletes, especially women, do not get enough iron in their diet. In addition, for reasons that are unclear, endurance athletes, such as marathon runners, frequently have low body-iron levels.[169, 170, 171] However, **anemia** (page 25) in athletes is often not due to iron deficiency and may be a normal adaptation to the stress of exercise.[172] Supplementing with iron is usually unwise unless a deficiency has been diagnosed. People who experience undue fatigue (an early warning sign of iron deficiency) should have their iron status evaluated by a doctor. Athletes who are found to be iron deficient by a physician are typically given 100 mg per day until blood tests indicate they are no longer deficient. Supplementing iron-deficient athletes with 100 to 200 mg per day of iron increased aerobic exercise performance in some,[173, 174, 175] though not all,[176, 177] double-blind studies. A recent double-blind trial found that iron-deficient women who took 20 mg per day of iron for six weeks were able to perform knee strength exercises for a longer time without muscle fatigue compared with those taking a placebo.[178]

Protein

Certain **amino acids** (page 465), the building blocks for protein, might be ergogenic aids as discussed in this article. However, while athletes have an increased need for protein compared with non-exercising adults, the maximum amount of protein suggested by many researchers—0.75 grams per pound of body weight per day—is already in the diet of most athletes as long as they are not restricting calories. Preliminary studies have suggested that supplementing with combinations of amino acids, typically along with carbohydrate, immediately after exercise increases muscle protein synthesis.[179, 180, 181, 182, 183] However, long-term controlled trials in young adult men,[184] older men,[185] and women have found no benefits in strength gains from supplementing with amino acids after weight training exercise.[186]

In one preliminary study, elderly men participating in a 12-week strength training program took a liquid supplement containing 10 grams of protein (part of which was soy protein), 7 grams of carbohydrate, and 3 grams of fat either immediately following exercise or two hours later.[187] Men taking the supplement immediately following exercise experienced significantly greater gains in muscle growth and lean body mass than those supplementing two hours later, but strength gains were no different between the two groups. A controlled study of female gymnasts found that adding 0.45 grams of soy protein (0.45 grams per pound of body weight per day) to a diet that was adequate in protein during a four-month training program did not improve lean body mass compared with a placebo.[188] No research has compared different sources of protein to see whether one source, such as soy protein, has a better or more consistent effect on exercise recovery or the results of strength training.

Animal studies suggest that **whey protein** (page 613) can increase gains in lean body mass resulting from exercise.[189] A controlled trial found that six weeks of strength training while taking 1.2 grams of whey protein per 2.2 pounds of body weight per day resulted in greater gains in lean body mass, but improved only one out of four strength tests.[190] Another controlled study found that people taking 20 grams per day of whey protein for three months performed better on a test of short-term intense cycling exercise than people taking a similar amount of milk protein (casein).[191] However, a double-blind trial found that men taking 1.5 grams per 2.2 lbs of body weight per day of predigested whey protein for 12 weeks along with a strength training exercise program gained only half as much lean body mass and had significantly smaller increases in strength compared with men using a similar amount of predigested casein along with strength training.[192] A controlled study of HIV-infected women found that adding whey protein to strength training exercise was no more effective than exercise alone for increasing strength or improving body composition.[193]

Pyruvate

One group of researchers in two small, controlled trials has reported that 100 grams of a combination of dihydroxyacetone and **pyruvate** (page 580) enhanced the endurance of certain muscles in untrained men.[194, 195] Three controlled studies of untrained individuals using a combination of 6 to 10 grams per day of pyruvate and an exercise program reported greater effects on weight loss and body fat compared with those taking a placebo with the exercise program.[196, 197, 198] However, in a study of healthy untrained women undergoing an exercise program, supplementing with 5 grams of pyruvate twice a day had no effect on exercise performance.[199] Studies of pyruvate supplementation on exercise performance in trained athletes have also failed to demonstrate any beneficial effect. Seven grams per day did not improve aerobic exercise performance in cyclists,[200] and an average of 15 grams per day did not improve anaerobic performance or body composition in football players.[201] More recently, evidence has appeared casting doubt on the ability of high levels (an average exceeding 15 grams per day depending upon body weight) of pyruvate to improve exercise capacity in a weight-lifting study.[202]

Zinc

Exercise increases **zinc** (page 614) losses from the human body, and severe zinc deficiency can compromise muscle function.[203, 204] Athletes who do not eat an optimal diet, especially those who are trying to control their weight or use fad diets while exercising strenuously, may become deficient in zinc to the extent that performance or health is compromised.[205, 206] One double-blind trial in women found that 135 mg per day of zinc for two weeks improved one measure of muscle strength.[207] Whether these women were zinc deficient was not determined in this study. A double-blind study of male athletes with low blood levels of zinc found that 20 mg per day of zinc improved the flexibility of the red blood cells during exercise, which could benefit blood flow to the muscles.[208] No other studies of the effects of zinc supplementation in exercising people have been done. A safe amount of zinc for long-term use is 20 to 40 mg per day along with 1 to 2 mg of copper. Higher amounts should be taken only under the supervision of a doctor.

Arginine/Ornithine

At very high intakes (approximately 250 mg per 2.2 pounds of body weight), the **amino acid arginine** (page 467) has increased growth hormone levels,[209] an effect that has interested body builders due to the role of growth hormone in stimulating muscle growth.[210] However, at lower amounts recommended by some manufacturers (5 grams taken 30 minutes before exercise), arginine failed to increase growth hormone release and may even have impaired the release of growth hormone in younger adults.[211] Large quantities (170 mg per 2.2 pounds of body weight per day) of a related amino acid, **ornithine** (page 566), have also raised growth hormone levels in some athletes.[212] High amounts of arginine or ornithine do not appear to raise levels of insulin,[213, 214] another anabolic (bodybuilding) hormone. More modest amounts of a combination of these amino acids have not had measurable effects on any anabolic hormone levels during exercise.[215, 216]

Nonetheless, double-blind trials conducted by one group of researchers, combining weight training with either arginine and ornithine (500 mg of each, twice per day, five times per week) or placebo, found the amino-acid combination produced decreases in body fat,[217] resulted in higher total strength and lean body mass, and reduced evidence of tissue breakdown after only five weeks.[218]

Aspartic acid

Aspartic acid is a non-essential amino acid that participates in many biochemical reactions relating to energy and protein. Preliminary, though conflicting, animal and human research suggested a role for aspartic acid (in the form of potassium and magnesium aspartate) in reducing fatigue during exercise.[219] However, most studies have found aspartic acid useless in improving either athletic performance or the body's response to exercise.[220, 221, 222, 223, 224]

B-complex vitamins

The **B-complex vitamins** (page 603) are important for athletes, because they are needed to produce energy from carbohydrates. Exercisers may have slightly increased requirements for some of the B vitamins, including **vitamin B₂** (page 598), **vitamin B₆** (page 600), and vitamin B₅ (**pantothenic acid** [page 568]);[225] athletic performance can suffer if these slightly increased needs are not met.[226] However, most athletes obtain enough B vitamins from their diet without supplementation,[227] and supplementation studies have found no positive effect on performance measures for vitamin B₂,[228, 229] vitamin B₃ (**niacin** [page 598]),[230] or vitamin B₆.[231] On the contrary, large amounts of niacin have been shown to impair endurance performance.[232]

Beta-sitosterol

Beta-sitosterol (page 471), (BSS) a natural sterol found in many plants, has been shown in a double-blind trial to improve **immune function** (page 255) in marathon runners when combined with a related substance called B-sitosterol glucoside (BSSG).[233] This implies that beta-sitosterol might reduce **infections** (page 265) in athletes who engage in intensive exercise, though studies are still needed to prove this. The usual amount of this combination used in research is 20 mg of BSS and 200 mcg of BSSG three times per day.

Branched-chain amino acids

Some research has shown that supplemental **branched-chain amino acids** (page 479) (BCAA) (typically 10 to 20 grams per day) do not result in meaningful changes in body composition,[234] nor do they improve exercise performance or enhance the effects of physical training.[235, 236, 237, 238, 239, 240] However, BCAA supplementation may be useful in special situations, such as preventing muscle loss at high altitudes and prolonging endurance performance in the heat.[241, 242] One controlled study gave triathletes 6 grams per day of BCAA for one month before a competition, then 3 grams per day from the day of competition until a week following. Compared with a placebo, BCAA restored depleted glutamine stores and immune factors that occur in elite athletes, and led to a reported one-third fewer symptoms of infection during the period of supplementation.[243] Studies by one group of researchers suggest that BCAA supplementation may also improve exercise-induced declines in some aspects of mental functioning.[244, 245, 246]

Bromelain

Bromelain (page 481) is effective for shortening the healing time of such injuries as sprains and strains.[247] Typically, two to four tablets or capsules are taken sev-

eral times per day. Other uses of bromelain for sports and fitness have not been studied.

Caffeine

Caffeine is present in many popular beverages and appears to have an effect on fat utilization.[248] Caffeine does not benefit short-term, high-intensity exercise, according to most,[249, 250] but not all, studies.[251, 252] However, controlled research, much of it double-blind, has shown that endurance performance lasting at least 30 minutes does appear to be enhanced by caffeine in many athletes.[253, 254, 255, 256, 257] Inconsistency in reported effectiveness of caffeine in some trials can be explained by differences in caffeine sensitivity among athletes, variable effects of caffeine on different forms of exercise and under different environmental conditions, and effects of other dietary components on the response to caffeine.[258, 259] Effective amounts of caffeine appear to range from 1.4 to 2.7 mg per pound of body weight, taken one hour before exercise.[260] While this amount of caffeine could be obtained in 1 to 3 cups of brewed coffee, most research has used caffeine supplements in capsules, and a recent study found caffeine was not effective when taken as coffee.[261] Caffeine consumption is banned by the International Olympic Committee at levels that produce urinary concentrations of 12 mg per milliliter or more. These levels would require ingestion of considerably more than 2.5 mg per pound of body weight, or several cups of coffee, over a short period of time.[262]

Calcium

Calcium (page 483) is important for achieving and maintaining optimum bone density. Some athletes, especially women with low body weight and/or amenorrhea, are at risk for serious bone loss and fractures.[263, 264] Contributing to this risk are the diets of these athletes, which are frequently deficient in calcium.[265] All athletes should try to achieve the recommended intakes of calcium, which are 1,300 mg per day for teenagers and 1,000 mg per day for adults. Other uses of calcium for sports and fitness, including prevention or relief of sports-related muscle cramps, have not been studied.

Chromium

Chromium (page 493), primarily in a form called chromium picolinate, has been studied for its potential role in altering body composition. Preliminary research in animals and humans suggested that chromium picolinate might increase fat loss and lean muscle tissue gain when used with a weight-training program.[266, 267, 268] However, most studies have found little to no effect of chromium on body composition or strength.[269, 270, 271, 272, 273] One group of researchers has reported significant reductions in body fat in double-blind trials using 200 to 400 mcg per day of chromium for six to twelve weeks in middle-aged adults,[274, 275] but the methods used in these studies have been criticized.[276]

Chondroitin sulfate

Chondroitin sulfate (page 492), 800 to 1,200 mg per day, is effective for reducing joint pain caused by osteoarthritis.[277, 278] Other uses of chondroitin sulfate for sports and fitness, including prevention of joint pain or treatment of sports injuries, have not been studied.

CLA

Conjugated linoleic acid (page 499) (CLA) is a slightly altered form of the essential fatty acid linoleic acid. Animal research suggests an effect of CLA supplementation on reducing body fat.[279, 280] Controlled human research has reported that 5.6 to 7.2 grams per day of CLA produces only non-significant gains in muscle size and strength in experienced and inexperienced weight-training men.[281, 282, 283] A double-blind study of a group of trained men and women reported reduced body fat in the upper arm after 12 weeks of supplementation with 1.8 grams per day of CLA.[284] Further research using more accurate techniques for measuring body composition is needed to confirm these findings.

Coenzyme Q10

Strenuous physical activity lowers blood levels of **coenzyme Q10** (page 496) (CoQ10).[285] However, the effects of CoQ10 on how the healthy body responds to exercise have been inconsistent, with several studies finding no improvement.[286, 287, 288, 289] A few studies, using at least four weeks of CoQ10 supplementation at 60 to 100 mg per day, have reported improvements in measures of work capacity ranging from 3 to 29% in sedentary people and from 4 to 32% in trained athletes.[290] However, recent double-blind and/or placebo-controlled trials in trained athletes, using performance measures such as time to exhaustion and total performance, have found either no significant improvement or significantly poorer results in those taking CoQ10.[291, 292, 293]

Gamma oryzanol

Gamma oryzanol (page 525) is a mixture of sterols and ferulic acid esters. Despite claims that gamma oryzanol or its components increase testosterone levels, stimulate the release of endorphins, and promote the growth of lean muscle tissue, research has provided little support for these claims and has also shown gamma-oryzanol to be poorly absorbed.[294] A recent nine-week, double-blind trial of 500 mg per day of gamma-oryzanol in weight lifters found no benefit compared with placebo in strength performance gains or circulating anabolic hormones.[295] However, a small, double-blind trial using 30 mg per day of ferulic acid for eight weeks in trained weight lifters did find significantly more weight gain (though lean body mass was not measured) and increased strength in one of three measures compared with placebo.[296]

Glucosamine

Glucosamine sulfate, 1,500 mg per day, is effective for reducing joint pain caused by osteoarthritis according to most studies.[297, 298, 299] Whether other forms of glucosamine, such as glucosamine hydrochloride, are as effective for joint pain as glucosamine sulfate is unclear at this time, but studies have found some benefits from the use of the hydrochloride form.[300, 301] Other uses of glucosamine for sports and fitness, including prevention of joint pain or treatment of sports injuries, have not been studied.

L-carnitine

L-carnitine (page 543), which is normally manufactured by the human body, has been popular as a potential ergogenic aid (i.e., having the ability to increase work capacity), because of its role in the conversion of fat to energy.[302] However, while some studies have found that L-carnitine improves certain measures of muscle physiology, research on the effects of 2 to 4 grams of L-carnitine per day on performance have produced inconsistent results.[303] L-carnitine may be effective in certain intense exercise activities leading to exhaustion,[304] but recent studies have reported that L-carnitine supplementation does not benefit non-exhaustive or even marathon-level endurance exercise,[305, 306] anaerobic performance,[307] or lean body mass in weight lifters.[308]

Magnesium

Magnesium (page 551) deficiency can reduce exercise performance and contribute to muscle cramps, but suboptimal intake does not appear to be a problem among most groups of athletes.[309, 310] Controlled trials suggest that magnesium supplementation might improve some aspects of physiology important to sports performance in some athletes,[311, 312] but controlled and double-blind trials focusing on performance benefits of 212 to 500 mg per day of magnesium have been inconsistent.[313, 314, 315, 316, 317, 318] It is possible that magnesium supplementation benefits only those who are deficient or who are not highly trained athletes.[319, 320]

Medium chain triglycerides

Medium chain triglycerides (page 554) (MCT) contain a class of fatty acids found only in very small amounts in the diet; they are more rapidly absorbed and burned as energy than are other fats.[321] For this reason, athletes have been interested in their use, especially during prolonged endurance exercise. However, no effect on carbohydrate sparing or endurance exercise performance has been shown with moderate amounts of MCT (30 to 45 grams over two to three hours).[322, 323] Controlled trials using very large amounts of MCT (approximately 85 grams over two hours) have resulted in both increased and decreased performance,[324, 325] while a double-blind trial found that 60 grams per day of MCT for two weeks had no effect on endurance performance.[326] A controlled study found increased performance when MCTs were added to a 10% carbohydrate solution,[327] but another study found no advantage of adding MCT,[328] and a third trial actually reported decreased performance with this combination, probably due to gastrointestinal distress, in athletes using MCTs.[329]

Octacosanol

Wheat germ oil, which contains a waxy substance known as **octacosanol** (page 565), has been investigated as an ergogenic agent. Preliminary studies have suggested that octacosanol improves endurance, reaction time, and other measures of exercise capacity.[330] In another preliminary trial, supplementation with 1 mg per day of octacosanol for eight weeks improved grip strength and visual reaction time, but it had no effect on chest strength, auditory reaction time, or endurance.[331]

Ornithine alpha-ketoglutarate

Ornithine alpha-ketoglutarate (page 566) (OKG) is formed from the amino acids ornithine and glutamine and is believed to facilitate muscle growth by enhancing the body's release of anabolic hormones. While this effect has been found in studies on hospitalized patients and elderly people,[332, 333] no studies on muscle growth in athletes using OKG have been published.

Methoxyisoflavone

Methoxyisoflavone (page 558) is a member of the family **flavonoids** (page 516) (isoflavones). In a U.S.

Patent, the developers of this substance claim, based on preliminary animal research, that it possesses anabolic (muscle-building and bone-building) effects without the side effects seen with either androgenic (male) hormones or estrogenic (female) hormones.[334] A preliminary controlled trial found that strength-training athletes who took 800 mg per day of methoxyisoflavone for eight weeks experienced a significantly greater reduction in percentage body fat than those who took a placebo.[335] Double-blind research is needed to confirm these findings. The U.S. patent also claims methoxyisoflavone reduces appetite and lowers blood cholesterol levels. Whether this claim is true has not yet been demonstrated in published scientific research.

Ribose

Ribose (page 582) is a type of sugar used by the body to make the energy-containing substance adenosine triphosphate (ATP). Intense exercise depletes muscle cells of ATP as well as the ATP precursors made from ribose,[336, 337] though these deficits are typically replaced within minutes.[338] Unpublished reports suggested that ribose supplementation might increase power during short, intense bouts of exercise.[339, 340] However, in a double-blind study, exercisers took four grams of ribose four times per day during a six-day strength-training regimen, and no effects on muscle power or ATP recovery in exercised muscles were found.[341] In two other controlled studies, either 10 grams of ribose per day for five days or 8 grams every 12 hours for 36 hours resulted in only minor improvements in some measures of performance during repetitive sprint cycling.[342, 343]

Are there any side effects or interactions?

Refer to the individual supplement for information about any side effects or interactions.

Herbs that may be helpful

Ginseng

Extensive but often poorly designed studies have been conducted on the use of Asian ginseng (*Panax ginseng*) to improve athletic performance.[344, 345] While some early controlled studies suggested there might be benefits, several recent double-blind trials have found no significant effects of Asian ginseng on endurance exercise.[346, 347, 348] In many studies, it is possible that ginseng was used in insufficient amounts or for an inadequate length of time; a more effective regimen for enhancing endurance performance may be 2 grams of powdered root per day or 200 to 400 mg per day of an extract standardized for 4% ginsenosides, taken for eight to twelve weeks.[349] Short-term intense exercise has also not been helped by Asian ginseng according to double-blind trials,[350, 351] but one controlled study reported increased pectoral and quadricep muscle strength in non-exercising men and women after taking 1 gram per day of Asian ginseng for six weeks.[352] An extract of a related plant, **American ginseng** (page 625) (*Panax quinquefolius*), was found ineffective at improving endurance exercise performance in untrained people after one week's supplementation in a double-blind study.[353]

Eleuthero

Eleuthero (page 672) *(Eleutherococcus senticosus)* supplementation may improve athletic performance, according to preliminary Russian research.[354] Other studies have been inconclusive and two recent double-blind studies showed no beneficial effect on endurance performance in trained men.[355, 356, 357] Eleuthero strengthens the immune system and thus might reduce the risk of post-exercise infection. Although some doctors suggest taking 1 to 4 ml (0.2 to 0.8 tsp) of fluid extract of eleuthero three times per day, evidence supporting the use of this herb to enhance athletic performance remains weak.

Rhodiola

In a double-blind trial, healthy volunteers received 200 mg of an extract of **Rhodiola rosea** (page 738) (standardized to contain 3% rosavin plus 1% salidroside) or a placebo one hour prior to an endurance-exercise test. Compared with placebo, rhodiola significantly increased endurance, as measured by the time it took to become exhausted.[358] However, after daily use of rhodiola for four weeks, the herb no longer enhanced short-term endurance. Consequently, if rhodiola is being considered as an exercise aid, it should be used only occasionally.

Arnica

Arnica-containing ointments are recommended by many practitioners for the treatment of sprains and strains and other traumatic injuries.[359] Homeopathic arnica tablets are also used by some practitioners for similar conditions.[360] One uncontrolled trial showed that arnica gel applied twice daily reduced symptoms of osteoarthritis of the knee and a double-blind study reported that a combination of topical arnica ointment and oral homeopathic arnica tablets reduced pain in people recovering from hand surgery.[361, 362] No other

studies of topical arnica have been done, but several studies of homeopathic arnica have found it ineffective for treating muscle and joint pain.[363, 364, 365]

Cayenne (topical capsaicin)

Capsaicin ointment (page 654), applied four times per day over painful joints in the upper or lower limbs, reduces pain caused by osteoarthritis,[366] and a plaster containing capsaicin applied to the low back for several hours per day provided relief from chronic low back pain in one study.[367] Other uses of cayenne or capsaicin for sports and fitness have not been studied.

Eucalyptus

Eucalyptus (page 673)-based rubs have been found to warm muscles in athletes.[368] This suggests that eucalyptus may help relieve minor muscle soreness when applied topically, though studies are needed to confirm this possibility.

Guaraná and kola

Some athletes take **guaraná** (page 687) during their training; however, there is no scientific research to support this use. Guaraná contains caffeine. Another caffeine-containing herb sometimes used during training is kola nut.

Tribulus

Extracts of *Tribulus terrestris* (puncture vine) have been reported in preliminary studies to affect anabolic hormones in men.[369] However, a double-blind trial found no effect of 1.5 mg per day of tribulus per pound of body weight in improving body composition or strength performance results from an eight-week strength training program.[370]

Yohimbine

The ability of **yohimbine** (page 764), a chemical found in yohimbe bark, to stimulate the nervous system,[371, 372] promote the release of fat from fat cells,[373, 374] and affect the cardiovascular system [375] has led to claims that yohimbe might help athletic performance or improve body composition. However, a double-blind study of men who were not dieting reported no effect of up to 43 mg per day of yohimbine on weight or body composition after six months.[376] No research has tested yohimbe herb for effects on body composition, and no human research has investigated the ability of yohimbine or yohimbe to affect athletic performance. Other studies have determined that a safe daily amount of yohimbine is 15 to 30 mg.[377] However, people with kidney disorders should not take yohimbe, and side effects of nausea, dizziness, or nervousness may occur that necessitate reducing or stopping yohimbe supplementation.

Are there any side effects or interactions?
Refer to the individual herb for information about any side effects or interactions.

ATTENTION DEFICIT–HYPERACTIVITY DISORDER

What do I need to know?

Self-care for ADHD/ADD can be approached in a number of ways—but it can be hard to know just where to start. To make it easier, our doctors recommend trying these simple steps first:

Check out L-carnitine
   To improve behavior, take 100 mg for each 2.2 pounds of body weight a day, with a maximum of 4 grams a day

Supplement with essential fatty acids
   Getting approximately 186 mg of EPA (eicosapentaenoic acid), 480 mg of DHA (docosahexaenoic acid), 96 mg of GLA (gamma-linolenic acid), 864 mg of linoleic acid, and 42 mg of arachidonic acid supplies fatty acids important to brain function

Try the Feingold diet
   Work with the Feingold Association or a knowledgeable practitioner to reduce or eliminate additives and other food issues that may affect ADHD

Give magnesium a go
   200 mg a day can address possible magnesium deficiency that may influence ADHD

About ADHD

Attention deficit-hyperactivity disorder (ADD or ADHD) is defined as age-inappropriate impulsiveness, lack of concentration, and sometimes excessive physical activity.

ADHD has been associated with learning difficulties and lack of social skills. Obviously what constitutes "normal" in these areas covers a wide spectrum; thus it is unclear which child suffers true ADHD and which child is just more rambunctious or rebellious than another. No objective criteria exist to accurately confirm the presence of ADHD. ADHD often goes undiag-

nosed if not caught at an early age, and it affects many adults who may not be aware of their condition.

CHECKLIST FOR ATTENTION DEFICIT–HYPERACTIVITY DISORDER		
Rating	Nutritional Supplements	Herbs
★★☆	Essential fatty acids **L-carnitine** (page 543) **Magnesium** (page 551) **Zinc** (page 614)	
★☆☆	**B vitamins** (pages 597–604) **Evening primrose oil** (page 511) **Vitamin B$_6$** (page 600)	

What are the symptoms of ADHD?

ADHD is generally recognized by a pattern of inattention, distractibility, impulsivity, and hyperactivity estimated to affect 3 to 5% of school-aged children. Learning disabilities or emotional problems often accompany ADHD. Children with ADHD experience an inability to sit still and pay attention in class, and they often engage in disruptive behavior.

Medical treatments

The most commonly prescribed prescription drugs, methylphenidate (Ritalin, Metadate) and amphetamine mixtures (Adderall), are considered stimulant drugs, though they produce a paradoxical calming effect in people with ADHD. Another medication less frequently used is pemoline (Cylert).

Dietary changes that may be helpful

The two most studied dietary approaches to ADHD are the Feingold diet and a hypoallergenic diet. The Feingold diet was developed by Benjamin Feingold, M.D., on the premise that salicylates (chemicals similar to aspirin that are found in a wide variety of foods) are an underlying cause of hyperactivity. In some studies, this hypothesis does not appear to hold up.[1] However, in studies where markedly different levels of salicylates were investigated, a causative role for salicylates could be detected in some hyperactive children.[2] As many as 10 to 25% of children may be sensitive to salicylates.[3] Parents of ADHD children can contact local Feingold Associations for more information about which foods and medicines contain salicylates.

The Feingold diet also eliminates synthetic additives,

dyes, and chemicals, which are commonly added to processed foods. The yellow dye tartrazine has been specifically shown to provoke symptoms in controlled studies of ADHD-affected children.[4] Again, not every child reacts, but enough do so that a trial avoidance may be worthwhile. The Feingold diet is complex and requires guidance from either the Feingold Association or a healthcare professional familiar with the Feingold diet.

In one study, children diagnosed with ADHD were put on a hypoallergenic diet, and those children who improved (about one-third) were then challenged with food additives. All of them experienced an aggravation of symptoms when given these additives.[5] Other studies have shown that eliminating individual allergenic foods and additives from the diet can help children with attention problems.[6, 7]

Some parents believe that consuming sugar may aggravate ADHD. One study found that avoiding sugar reduced aggressiveness and restlessness in hyperactive children.[8] Girls who restrict sugar have been reported to improve more than boys.[9] However, a study using large amounts of sugar and aspartame (NutraSweet) found that negative reactions to these substances were limited to just a few children.[10] While most studies have not found sugar to stimulate hyperactivity, except in rare cases,[11] the experimental design of these studies may not have been ideal for demonstrating an adverse effect of sugar on ADHD, if one exists. Further studies are needed.

Lifestyle changes that may be helpful
Smoking during **pregnancy** (page 363) should be avoided, as it appears to increase the risk of giving birth to a child who develops ADHD.[12]

Lead[13] and other heavy-metal exposures[14] have been linked to ADHD. If other therapies do not seem to be helping a child with ADHD, the possibility of heavy-metal exposure can be explored with a health practitioner.

Nutritional supplements that may be helpful
Some children with ADHD have lowered levels of **magnesium** (page 551). In a preliminary, controlled trial, children with ADHD and low magnesium status were given 200 mg of magnesium per day for six months.[15] Compared with 25 other magnesium-deficient ADHD children, those given magnesium supplementation had a significant decrease in hyperactive behavior.

In a double-blind study, children with ADHD who received 15 mg of **zinc** (page 614) per day for six weeks showed significantly greater behavioral improvement, compared with children who received a placebo.[16] This study was conducted in Iran, and zinc deficiency has been found to be quite common in certain parts of that country. It is not clear, therefore, to what extent the results of this study apply to children living in other countries.

In a double-blind study, supplementation with **L-carnitine** (page 543) for eight weeks resulted in clinical improvement in 54% of a group of boys with ADHD, compared with a 13% response rate in the placebo group.[17] The amount of L-carnitine used in this study was 100 mg per 2.2 pounds of body weight per day, with a maximum of 4 grams per day. No adverse effects were seen, although one child developed an unpleasant body odor while taking L-carnitine. Researchers have found that this uncommon side effect of L-carnitine can be prevented by supplementing with riboflavin. Although no serious side effects were seen in this study, the safety of long-term L-carnitine supplementation in children has not been well studied. This treatment should, therefore, be monitored by a physician.

A deficiency of several essential fatty acids has been observed in some children with ADHD compared with unaffected children.[18, 19] One study gave children with ADHD **evening primrose oil** (page 511) supplements in an attempt to correct the problem.[20] Although a degree of benefit was seen, results were not pronounced. In a 12-week double-blind study, children with ADHD were given either a placebo or a fatty-acid supplement providing daily: 186 mg of eicosapentaenoic acid (EPA), 480 mg of docosahexaenoic acid (DHA), 96 mg of gamma-linolenic acid (GLA), 864 mg of linoleic acid, and 42 mg of arachidonic acid. Compared with the placebo, the fatty-acid supplement produced significant improvements in both cognitive function and behavioral problems.[21] No adverse effects were seen.

Iron (page 540) status, as measured by the serum ferritin concentration, was significantly lower in a group of children with ADHD than in healthy children. Ferritin levels were below normal in 84% of the children with ADHD, compared with 18% of the healthy children.[22] Since iron deficiency can adversely affect mood and cognitive function, iron status should be assessed in children with ADHD, and those who are deficient should receive an iron supplement.

B vitamins (pages 597–604), particularly **vitamin B$_6$** (page 600), have also been used for ADHD. Deficient levels of vitamin B$_6$ have been detected in some ADHD patients.[23] In a study of six children with low blood levels of the neurotransmitter (chemical messenger) serotonin, vitamin B_6 supplementation (15–30 mg per 2.2 pounds of body weight per day) was found to be more effective than methylphenidate (Ritalin). However, lower amounts of vitamin B_6 were not beneficial.[24] The effective amount of vitamin B_6 in this study was extremely large and could potentially cause nerve damage, although none occurred in this study. A practitioner knowledgeable in nutrition must be consulted when using high amounts of vitamin B_6. High amounts of other B vitamins have shown mixed results in relieving ADHD symptoms.[25, 26]

Are there any side effects or interactions?
Refer to the individual supplement for information about any side effects or interactions.

AUTISM

Autism is a developmental disorder of the brain that appears in early childhood. The condition causes impairment of social interaction and communication, as well as unusual behaviors.

Rating	Nutritional Supplements	Herbs
CHECKLIST FOR AUTISM		
★★★	**Vitamin B_6** (page 600)	
★★☆	**Vitamin C** (page 604)	
★☆☆	**Magnesium** (page 551)	

What are the symptoms of autism?

Symptoms vary but are characterized by a difficulty in relating to people, objects, and events. Communication problems may be present, such as a lack of eye contact or response when their name is called; fixation on specific subjects or toys; difficulty with changes to routine or surroundings; and repetitive body movements, such as head banging or hand flapping.

Medical treatments

There is no established treatment for autism. Medications, such as antidepressants, stimulants, and antipsychotics are used to manage the symptoms of associated disorders, which include **attention deficit** (page 55), hyperactivity, obsessions, compulsions, tics, irritability, seizures, and **depression** (page 145).

Dietary changes that may be helpful

Preliminary research suggests that some autistic children may be **allergic** (page 14) or sensitive to certain foods and that removal of these foods from the diet has appeared to improve some behaviors.[1] As a result, one prominent doctor has recommended a trial hypoallergenic diet.[2] Such a trial requires supervision by a doctor.

Nutritional supplements that may be helpful

Uncontrolled and double-blind research shows that **vitamin B_6** (page 600) can be helpful for autistic children.[3, 4, 5] In these trials, children typically took between 3.5 mg and almost 100 mg of B_6 for every 2.2 pounds of body weight, with some researchers recommending 30 mg per 2.2 pounds of body weight. Although toxicity was not reported, such amounts are widely considered to have potential toxicity that can damage the nervous system; these amounts should only be administered by a doctor. One prominent researcher has suggested that vitamin B_6 is better supported by research than is drug treatment in dealing with autism.[6]

Some researchers have added **magnesium** (page 551) to vitamin B_6, reporting that taking both nutrients may have better effects than taking B_6 alone.[7] The amount of magnesium—10 to 15 mg per 2.2 pounds of body weight—is high enough to cause **diarrhea** (page 163) in some people and should be administered by a doctor. Doctors will often try vitamin B_6 or the combination of B_6 and magnesium for at least three months to see whether these nutrients help autistic children.

In one double-blind trial lasting ten weeks, autistic children given 1 gram **vitamin C** (page 604) for each 20 pounds of body weight showed a reduction in symptom severity compared with placebo.[8] The authors speculate that vitamin C may play a positive role because of its known effects on a hormone pathway typically disturbed in children with autism.

Are there any side effects or interactions?
Refer to the individual supplement for information about any side effects or interactions.

BELL'S PALSY

Bell's palsy is a disorder of the nerve that controls certain muscles of the face.

People with Bell's palsy lose control of some or all of the muscles on one half of the face; consequently, the face looks asymmetrical. Rarely are both sides of the face affected. The cause is unknown, and the disorder usually resolves without treatment within six to twelve months.

People with **diabetes** (page 152) or **hypertension** (page 246) have greater-than-average risk for Bell's palsy.[1, 2, 3] While no research has investigated whether better control of these conditions may help prevent Bell's palsy, people with Bell's palsy should be checked for diabetes and hypertension, especially if the palsy occurs repeatedly or affects both sides of the face.

CHECKLIST FOR BELL'S PALSY		
Rating	Nutritional Supplements	Herbs
★★☆	Vitamin B$_{12}$ (page 601) (injections)	

What are the symptoms of Bell's palsy?

Some common symptoms of Bell's palsy include a rapid onset of weakness, numbness, heaviness, or paralysis of one side of the face. People with Bell's palsy may also have symptoms of pain behind the ear, inability to completely close one eye, drooling, and speech difficulties.

Medical treatments

Over the counter treatment with artificial tear solutions might help with symptoms involving the eye. Drugs used include polyvinyl alcohol (Hypotears, Murine, Liquifilm Tears), hydroxypropyl methylcellulose (LubriTears, Tears Naturale Free, Moisture Drops), and carboxymethylcellulose (Refresh Plus, Celluvisc).

Prescription drug therapy involves the use of steroids, such as prednisone (Deltasone), methylprednisolone (Medrol), and prednisolone (Prelone, Pediapred).

Skin tape or an eye patch may be used to help the eye stay closed and lubricated. Difficult cases may require a surgical procedure in which the eyelids are stitched together.

Nutritional supplements that may be helpful

Vitamin B$_{12}$ (page 601) deficiency can cause nerve degeneration,[4] and both oral[5] and injected[6, 7] vitamin B$_{12}$ have been used to treat many types of nerve disorders.[8] One older case report described successful treatment of chronic Bell's palsy with vitamin B$_{12}$ injections of 500 to 1,000 mcg given every one to two days.[9] A more re-

cent trial compared the effect of 500 mcg of injected vitamin B$_{12}$ (in the form of methylcobalamin) given three times weekly for at least eight weeks—steroid medication, or both. Researchers found significantly faster recovery in the groups given B$_{12}$ injections with or without steroids, compared to those given steroids alone.[10] These findings agree with earlier reports on the effectiveness of methylcobalamin injections for Bell's palsy.[11, 12] It is unlikely that oral vitamin B$_{12}$ would be similarly effective. People seeking B$_{12}$ injections should consult a physician.

Are there any side effects or interactions?
Refer to the individual supplement for information about any side effects or interactions.

Holistic approaches that may be helpful

Many reports claim that acupuncture speeds recovery from Bell's palsy,[13, 14, 15, 16] but no controlled trials have been done to confirm this is neither a placebo effect nor the natural course of healing.

Hyperbaric oxygen therapy (HBT) is a procedure in which the patient breaths 100% oxygen at pressures up to three times greater than normal atmospheric pressure. A well controlled study of Bell's palsy patients compared HBT plus a placebo tablet with fake oxygen therapy plus steroid medication.[17] HBT produced significantly faster recovery (22 vs. 34 days) compared to the use of steroids.

Biofeedback techniques (using simple electronic devices to measure and report information about a person's biological system) have been reported to help limit the deterioration of muscle function and speed recovery in Bell's palsy.[18, 19] However, a controlled trial of patients with chronic facial paralysis (including some with Bell's palsy) found that using a mirror as feedback was as effective as a mirror plus electrical biofeedback for improving facial symmetry and muscle function.[20]

BENIGN PROSTATIC HYPERPLASIA

Benign prostatic hyperplasia (BPH) is a non-malignant enlargement of the prostate gland.

The prostate is a small gland that surrounds the neck of the bladder and urethra in men. Its major function is to contribute to seminal fluid. If the prostate enlarges, pressure may be put on the urethra, acting like a partial clamp and causing a variety of urinary symptoms. Half of all 50-year-old men have BPH, and the prevalence of the condition increases with advancing age. The name "benign prostatic hyperplasia" has replaced the older term "benign prostatic hypertrophy"; both terms refer to the same condition.

Rating	Nutritional Supplements	Herbs
★★★	**Beta-sitosterol** (page 471) **Rye Pollen** (page 571) extract	**Saw palmetto** (page 743)
★★☆	**Amino acids** (page 465) (**alanine** [page 463], **glutamic acid** [page 529], **glycine** [page 532])	Garlic (Kastamonu Garlic) **Nettle** (page 714) **Pumpkin seeds** (page 733) **Pygeum** (page 734)
★☆☆	**Copper** (page 499) **Flaxseed oil** (page 517) **Zinc** (page 614)	

CHECKLIST FOR BENIGN PROSTATIC HYPERPLASIA

What are the symptoms of BPH?

A man with BPH has to urinate more often, especially at night, and experiences less force and caliber while urinating, often dribbling. If the prostate enlarges too much, urination is difficult or impossible, and the risk of **urinary tract infection** (page 436) and kidney damage increases. A doctor can usually detect an enlarged prostate during a rectal exam.

Medical treatments

Prescription medications used to treat BPH include finasteride (Proscar), terazosin (Hytrin), and tamsulosin (Flomax). Though these drugs can reduce urinary symptoms in men with BPH, it is not clear whether they slow the progression of the disease.

Doctors often recommend surgery when symptoms are severe or when there is a high risk of urinary obstruction. Though prostate surgery has a high success rate, it also has a higher rate of complications than drug therapy.

Lifestyle changes that may be helpful

More physically active men have a lower frequency of symptoms related to BPH. In a preliminary study, physical activity was associated with a decrease in occurrence of BPH, surgery for BPH, and symptoms of BPH.[1] Walking, the most prevalent activity among men in this study, was related to a decreased risk of BPH. Men who exercised by walking two to three hours per week had a 25% lower risk of BPH compared with men who didn't use walking for exercise.

Nutritional supplements that may be helpful

Beta-sitosterol (page 471), a compound found in many edible plants, has also been found to be helpful for men with BPH. In one double-blind trial, 200 men with BPH received 20 mg of beta-sitosterol three times a day or a placebo for six months. Men receiving beta-sitosterol had a significant improvement in urinary flow and an improvement in symptoms, whereas no change was reported in men receiving the placebo.[2] Another double-blind study reported similarly positive results using 130 mg per day of beta-sitosterol.[3]

Rye pollen (page 571) extract has improved the symptoms of BPH in preliminary trials.[4, 5, 6] Double-blind trials have also reported that rye pollen extract is effective for reducing symptoms of BPH[7, 8] This rye pollen extract was shown to be comparable in effect to an **amino acid** (page 465) mixture used for BPH in a double-blind study.[9] A double-blind comparison with **pygeum** (page 734) resulted in significant subjective improvement in 78% of those given the rye pollen extract compared with 55% using pygeum.[10] Research on this commercial rye pollen extract has used three to six tablets, or four capsules, per day; the effect of other pollens in men with prostate conditions has not yet been studied.

In a controlled trial, men with BPH received a supplement containing three **amino acids** (page 465) (**glycine** [page 532], **alanine** [page 463], and **glutamic acid** [page 529]) totaling about 760 mg three times per day for two weeks, then 380 mg three times per day for a total of three months. After three months, about half of these men reported reduced urgency, frequency, and/or less delay starting urine flow, compared to 15% or less of the men who received a placebo.[11] Another similar controlled trial of this combination also reported positive results[12] Although it is not known how the amino acid combination works, it is believed to reduce the amount of swelling in prostate tissue.

In a 1941 preliminary report, 19 men with BPH were given an essential fatty acid (EFA) supplement.[13] In every case, the amount of retained urine was reduced, and nighttime urination problems stopped in

69% of cases. Dribbling was eliminated in 18 of the 19 men. All men also reported improved libido and a reduction in the size of the enlarged prostate, as determined by physical examination. Because this study did not include a control group and the amount given was surprisingly small, the possibility of a placebo effect cannot be ruled out.

Despite the lack of good published research, many doctors have been impressed with the effectiveness of essential fatty acids (EFAs) in cases of BPH. A typical recommendation is one tablespoon of **flaxseed oil** (page 517) per day, perhaps reduced to one or two teaspoons per day after several months. Because taking EFAs increases the requirement for **vitamin E** (page 609), most doctors recommend taking a vitamin E supplement along with EFAs. However, controlled research is needed to establish whether EFAs are helpful for BPH.

Prostatic secretions are known to contain a high concentration of **zinc** (page 614); that observation suggests that zinc plays a role in normal prostate function. In one preliminary study, 19 men with benign prostatic hyperplasia took 150 mg of zinc daily for two months, and then 50 to 100 mg daily. In 74% of the men, the prostate became smaller.[14] Because this study did not include a control group, improvements may have been due to a placebo effect. Zinc also reduced prostatic size in an animal study but only when given by local injection.[15] Although the research supporting the use of zinc is weak, many doctors recommend its use. Because supplementing with large amounts of zinc (such as 30 mg per day or more) may potentially lead to **copper** (page 499) deficiency, most doctors recommend taking 2 to 3 mg of copper per day along with zinc.

Are there any side effects or interactions?
Refer to the individual supplement for information about any side effects or interactions.

Herbs that may be helpful

In many parts of Europe, herbal supplements are considered standard medical treatment for BPH. Although herbs for BPH are available without prescription, men wishing to take them should be monitored by a physician.

The fat-soluble (liposterolic) extract of the **saw palmetto** (page 743) berry has become the leading natural treatment for BPH. This extract, when used regularly, has been shown to help keep symptoms in check.[16] Saw palmetto appears to inhibit 5-alpha-reductase, the enzyme that converts testosterone to its more active form, dihydrotestosterone (DHT). Saw palmetto also blocks DHT from binding in the prostate.[17] Studies have used 320 mg per day of saw palmetto extract that is standardized to contain approximately 80 to 95% fatty acids.

A three-year preliminary study in Germany found that 160 mg of saw palmetto extract taken twice daily reduced nighttime urination in 73% of patients and improved urinary flow rates significantly.[18] In a double-blind trial at various sites in Europe, 160 mg of saw palmetto extract taken twice per day treated BPH as effectively as finasteride without side effects, such as loss of libido.[19] A one-year dose-comparison study found that 320 mg once per day was as effective as 160 mg twice per day in the treatment of BPH.[20] A review of all available double-blind trials has concluded that saw palmetto is effective for treatment of men with BPH and is just as effective as, with fewer side effects than, the drug finasteride.[21]

In a preliminary study, supplementation with a special aged garlic extract (Kastamonu Garlic) in the amount of 1 ml per 2.2 pounds of body weight per day for one month resulted in a 32% reduction in the size of the prostate gland and a significant improvement in urinary symptoms.[22] It is not known whether other forms of garlic would have the same effect.

Pygeum (page 734), an extract from the bark of the African tree, has been approved in Germany, France, and Italy as a remedy for BPH. Controlled studies published over the past 25 years have shown that pygeum is safe and effective for men with BPH of mild or moderate severity.[23] These studies have used 50 to 100 mg of pygeum extract (standardized to contain 13% total sterols) twice per day. This herb contains three compounds that may help the prostate: pentacyclic triterpenoids, which have a diuretic action; phytosterols, which have anti-inflammatory activity; and ferulic esters, which help rid the prostate of any cholesterol deposits that accompany BPH.

Another herb for BPH is a concentrated extract made from the roots of the **nettle** (page 714) plant. This extract may increase urinary volume and the maximum flow rate of urine in men with early-stage BPH.[24] It has been successfully combined with both **saw palmetto** (page 743) and pygeum to treat BPH in double-blind trials.[25] An appropriate amount appears to be 120 mg of nettle root extract (in capsules or tablets) twice per day or 2 to 4 ml of tincture three times per day.

Pumpkin (page 733) seed oil has been used in combination with saw palmetto in two double-blind human studies to effectively reduce symptoms of benign prostatic hyperplasia (BPH).[26, 27] Only one group of researchers has evaluated the effectiveness of pumpkin seed oil alone for BPH, but the results of their large preliminary trials have been favorable.[28, 29] Researchers have suggested the zinc, free fatty acid, or plant sterol content of pumpkin seeds may account for their benefit in men with BPH, but this has not been confirmed. Animal studies have shown that pumpkin seed extracts may improve the function of the bladder and urethra; this might partially account for BPH symptom relief.[30] Pumpkin seed oil extracts standardized for fatty acid content have been used in BPH studies in the amount of 160 mg three times per day with meals.

Are there any side effects or interactions?
Refer to the individual herb for information about any side effects or interactions.

BIPOLAR DISORDER

Bipolar disorder is a mood disorder characterized by alternating states of **depression** (page 145) and mania that follow each other in a repeating cycle.

People with bipolar disorder may cycle through these states quickly or may experience long periods of depression or mania. Often one mood state predominates, while the other occurs only infrequently or briefly. The cause of bipolar disorder is unknown.

CHECKLIST FOR BIPOLAR DISORDER		
Rating	**Nutritional Supplements**	**Herbs**
★★☆	Vitamin-mineral-amino acid formula (currently proprietary) **Fish oil** (page 514)	
★☆☆	**5-HTP** (page 459) **Choline** (page 546) **Folic acid** (page 520) **Inositol** (page 537) **SAMe** (page 583) **Vitamin B$_{12}$** (page 601) **Vitamin C** (page 604)	

What are the symptoms of bipolar disorder?
Symptoms of the elevated mood stage of bipolar disorder include an exaggerated sense of confidence and well-being, racing thoughts, excessive talking, distractibility, increased desire for pleasurable activity, decreased need for sleep, impulsivity, irritability, and impairment in judgment. The depressed phase includes symptoms of sadness, fatigue, pessimism, feelings of helplessness, low self-esteem, and loss of interest in life, possibly with thoughts of suicide.

Medical treatments
Prescription drug treatment of bipolar disorder includes lithium carbonate (Eskalith, Lithobid), valproic acid (Depakote, Depakene), carbamazepine (Tegretol), and lamotrigine (Lamictal). Antianxiety drugs, antidepressants, and antipsychotics are also common components of treatment.

Psychological counseling and sleep management is sometimes recommended. Severe cases requiring hospitalization due to rapid or pronounced mood swings might also require electroconvulsive therapy (electrical impulses applied to the brain).

Lifestyle changes that may be helpful
Exercise influences the production and use of neurotransmitters and hormones in the body, and its antidepressant effect is well known.[1] A preliminary study of the effects of vigorous exercise on the body chemistry of patients with bipolar disorder found that exercise increased a specific chemical associated with better mood.[2] However, exercise may adversely influence the effectiveness of some medications used for bipolar disorder. Many people with bipolar disorder take lithium, and because lithium is lost in sweat, exercise that involves significant sweating may change blood levels of lithium. Such a change has been reported in one person;[3] therefore, people taking lithium who intend to start a vigorous exercise program should be monitored by their doctor.

Nutritional supplements that may be helpful
People diagnosed with **depression** (page 145) may have lower blood levels of omega-3 fatty acids.[4, 5] A double-blind trial found that bipolar patients taking 9.6 grams of omega-3 fatty acids from **fish oil** (page 514) per day in addition to their conventional medications had significant improvements compared with those taking placebo.[6]

L-tryptophan is the **amino acid** (page 465) used by the body to produce serotonin, a chemical messenger important for proper brain function. Supplementation with L-tryptophan has led to improvement in depression in many studies,[7, 8] but information is limited about its effect on bipolar disorder. Case reports on two bipolar patients treated with lithium or an antidepressant drug described marked improvements when they were given 12 grams daily of L-tryptophan.[9, 10] Two trials using 6 grams of L-tryptophan daily for acute mania in patients with bipolar disorder found little or no improvement,[11, 12] but another double-blind, controlled study using 9.6 grams daily reported better results.[13]

L-tryptophan is converted to **5-hydroxytryptophan** (page 459) (5-HTP) before it becomes serotonin in the body. In a controlled trial, 200 mg daily of supplemental 5-HTP had antidepressant effects in bipolar patients, though it was not as effective as lithium.[14] In a double-blind trial, patients with bipolar disorder had greater improvement with a combination of 5-HTP at 300 mg daily plus an antidepressant drug than with 5-HTP alone.[15]

S-adenosylmethionine (page 583) (SAMe) is another amino acid that has an impact on serotonin levels, and it has demonstrated significant antidepressant effects in clinical trials.[16, 17, 18] In both controlled and preliminary studies, SAMe has been shown to be helpful for the depressive symptoms of bipolar disorder. However, some patients have switched from depression to mania while using SAMe at 500 to 1,600 mg daily.[19, 20] This is a known side effect of other antidepressant medications.[21] The mania induced by SAMe resolved when the supplement was discontinued, and in one case resolved spontaneously while the patient continued taking SAMe.[22] Therefore, people with bipolar disorder should supplement with SAMe only under the supervision of a qualified healthcare practitioner.

Both **folic acid** (page 520) and **vitamin B$_{12}$** (page 601) are used in the body to manufacture serotonin and other neurotransmitters. It is well known that deficiency of either nutrient is associated with depression.[23, 24] There is some evidence that patients diagnosed with mania are also more likely to have folate deficiencies than healthy controls.[25] Other studies, however, have found that folic acid deficiency was not more common in bipolar patients taking lithium than in healthy people.[26, 27, 28] Some studies have found that people who take lithium long term, and who also have high blood levels of folic acid, respond better to lithium.[29, 30] Not all studies have confirmed these findings, however.[31] A double-blind study of patients receiving lithium therapy showed that the addition of 200 mcg of folic acid per day resulted in clinical improvement, whereas placebo did not.[32]

There have been case reports of both mania and depression associated with vitamin B$_{12}$ deficiency, and these symptoms cleared after treatment with injections of B$_{12}$.[33, 34] However, B$_{12}$ deficiency has not been reported in bipolar disorder patients, and no studies have been published investigating the effects of vitamin B$_{12}$ supplementation in people with bipolar disorder.

Vitamin C (page 604) helps the body to reduce its load of vanadium and this has been studied for its possible role in treatment of bipolar disorder.[35] A double-blind trial found that both manic and depressed bipolar patients were significantly improved after one-time administration of 3 grams of vitamin C, compared with a placebo.[36] The same study found that both manic and depressed patients did better on a reduced-vanadium diet compared to a normal diet. Another double-blind study reported that 4 grams per day of vitamin C in combination with a drug known as EDTA (which also helps remove elements such as vanadium from the body) was helpful to depressed bipolar patients but not to those experiencing mania.[37] Until more is known, people with bipolar illness should avoid supplements containing vanadium and consider supplementing with vitamin C.

Inositol (page 537) is a nutrient found in large amounts in the brain, but its possible role in mood disorders is unclear. Inositol levels may be reduced in certain parts of the brains of depressed and bipolar patients.[38] However, lithium reduces normal brain levels of inositol, and this may be one of the ways lithium helps people with bipolar disorder.[39, 40, 41] Although inositol is known to have significant antidepressant properties when administered in large amounts of 12 grams per day,[42, 43] case reports involving bipolar patients have reported either no benefit,[44] some benefit,[45] or worsening of symptoms from inositol supplementation.[46] Until controlled research clarifies the effects of inositol in people with bipolar illness, it should only be used under the supervision of a qualified healthcare practitioner.

Acetylcholine levels in the brain may affect mood disorders, and supplemental **choline** (page 546) can increase acetylcholine levels. In a preliminary trial, six people with bipolar disorder were given 1 to 2 grams of choline twice per day (2 to 4 grams per day). Five of the six had a significant reduction in manic symptoms, and four of the six had a reduction in all mood symptoms.[47] No properly controlled trials have yet investigated the effects of choline in treating people with bipolar disorder.

Restriction of dietary **calcium** (page 483) was reported to alleviate manic episodes in one bipolar patient, and calcium supplementation (approximately 800 mg per day) increased mania symptoms slightly in six manic-depressive patients, according to another uncontrolled report.[48] Therefore, if calcium supplementation is desired by people with bipolar disorder, it should be taken with caution.

Lithium is a mineral contained in certain drugs used in the medical treatment of bipolar disorder. Lithium may be present in some trace mineral supplements, but amounts are too small to have any effect on bipolar disorder.

Vanadium (page 594) is a trace mineral nutrient that may adversely influence bipolar disorder. Elevated blood and hair levels of vanadium have been reported in people with mania and depression, and one effect of the bipolar medication lithium is to interrupt a biochemical action of vanadium in the body.[49] Vanadium is therefore one suspect in the search for a cause of bipolar disorder. People with bipolar disorder should avoid supplements containing vanadium until more is known.

In a preliminary trial, 11 patients with bipolar disorder were treated for six months with a moderate-potency vitamin-mineral formula (E.M. Power+ manufactured by Evince International, of Farmington, Utah) that also contained a proprietary blend of amino acids and other nutrients. The severity of depression decreased on average by 71% and the severity of mania decreased by 60% during the study.[50] A double-blind study is needed to confirm these promising results.

Are there any side effects or interactions?
Refer to the individual herb for information about any side effects or interactions.

BIRTH DEFECTS PREVENTION

See also: Pregnancy and Postpartum Support (page 363)

Birth defects affect about 120,000 babies born in the United States each year. Birth defects account for more than 20% of infant deaths and contribute substantially to life-long disabilities.

The causes of about 70% of all birth defects are unknown. Various occupational hazards, dietary factors, medications, personal habits, and environmental exposures may contribute to birth defects, but many questions remain about the exact nature of their influence.

Neural tube defects (NTDs) are one of the most common birth defects. NTDs result when the neural tube (which includes the spinal cord and brain) fails to close during the first month of embryonic development. NTDs include several disorders ranging from spina bifida (incomplete closure of the bones around the spinal cord that can lead to paralysis) to a lack of a cranium (the bones of the head) and its contents, called anencephaly. Approximately 4,000 pregnancies in the United States are affected by NTDs each year.

CHECKLIST FOR BIRTH DEFECTS PREVENTION		
Rating	Nutritional Supplements	Herbs
★★★	**Folic acid** (page 520)	
★★☆	**Choline** (page 546) **Multivitamin** (page 559) **Zinc** (page 614)	

Dietary changes that may be helpful
Drinking beverages containing caffeine may increase the risk of miscarriage among non-smoking women, according to one study.[1] Women who miscarried during the first 12 weeks of pregnancy were found to have significantly higher consumption of caffeine compared with women who carried their pregnancies to term. This association was limited to women who did not smoke cigarettes. Non-smoking women who consumed 500 mg of caffeine per day, or roughly five cups of coffee, were twice as likely to suffer a miscarriage compared with women who drank less than one cup of coffee per day. An increased risk of miscarriage was also found in women consuming as little of 100 mg of caffeine per day. This finding appears to indicate that there may be no "safe" amount of regular caffeine consumption during pregnancy.

One cup of coffee contains roughly 100 mg of caffeine, depending on how it is brewed (drip coffee contains the most caffeine and instant coffee the least). Black tea contains about 40–70 mg per cup, and a 12-oz. can of caffeinated soda may contain 30–55 mg of caffeine. Caffeine is also found in cocoa, chocolate, and certain over-the-counter medications.

Lifestyle changes that may be helpful
Pregnant women should avoid alcohol completely. Alcohol intake by pregnant women can lead to a spec-

trum of disorders, including fetal alcohol syndrome (FAS), alcohol-related neurodevelopmental disorder (ARND), and alcohol-related birth defects (ARBD). FAS is characterized by growth retardation, abnormal facial features, and mental retardation. In addition, about 80% of children with FAS have an abnormally small cranium, called microcephaly. Children with FAS also have serious lifelong disabilities, including learning disabilities and behavioral problems.[2, 3, 4] ARND and ARBD are milder versions of FAS.[5]

Drinking just one alcoholic beverage per day while pregnant has been associated with increased risk of having a child with impaired growth. The potential for harm increases as larger amounts of alcohol are consumed. Even minimal alcohol consumption during pregnancy can increase the risk of **hyperactivity** (page 55), **attention deficiency** (page 55), and emotional problems in the child.[6] No safe level of alcohol intake during pregnancy has been determined.[7, 8]

There are many medications that a woman should not use during pregnancy. A healthcare practitioner should review all over-the-counter and prescription medications, as well as any nutritional or herbal supplements. For example, the commonly prescribed acne medication, isotretinoin (Accutane), a synthetic form of vitamin A, can cause severe birth defects if used during pregnancy.

Excessive noise may have damaging effects on a developing fetus. Many pregnant women are exposed to noise in the workplace.[9, 10] In one study, the children of women exposed consistently to high levels of occupational noise during pregnancy were more likely to have high-frequency hearing loss (identified at four to ten years of age) than were children whose mothers were not exposed to such noise.[11] Noise exposure at these excessive levels (i.e., 85 to 90 decibels) occurs in many occupations, even among women wearing protective hearing devices. Other environmental sources of excessive noise include rock concerts, boom boxes, car stereos, and airport jet traffic.

Women who are **obese** (page 446) prior to pregnancy are at increased risk of having an NTD-affected pregnancy. One study showed a twofold or greater risk of NTD-affected pregnancy among women who were obese.[12]

Nutritional supplements that may be helpful
Several studies and clinical trials have shown that 50% or more of NTDs can be prevented if women consume a **folic acid** (page 520)-containing supplement before and during the early weeks of pregnancy.[13, 14] The United States Department of Public Health, the Centers for Disease Control and Prevention (CDC), and the March of Dimes recommend that all women who are capable of becoming pregnant supplement with 400 mcg folic acid daily. Daily supplementation prior to pregnancy is necessary because most pregnancies in the United States are unplanned[15] and the protective effect of folic acid occurs in the first four weeks of fetal development,[16] before most women know they are pregnant.

For women who have had a previous NTD-affected pregnancy, the CDC recommends daily supplementation with 4,000 mcg per day of folic acid. In a preliminary study, this amount of supplemental folic acid before and during early pregnancy resulted in a 71% reduction in the recurrence rate of NTDs.[17]

In a preliminary study of California mothers, those who had higher intakes of **choline** (page 546) during the three months prior to conception were significantly less likely to give birth to a child with an NTD, compared with women with lower choline intakes.[18] The possibility that choline may protect against NTDs is plausible, as choline has similar biochemical effects as folic acid, which is known to reduce NTD risk.

In a preliminary study, women with the highest total dietary **zinc** (page 614) intake before pregnancy (including zinc from both food and supplements) had a 35% decreased risk of having an NTD-affected pregnancy.[19] However, another preliminary study found no association between blood levels of zinc in pregnant women and the incidence of NTDs.[20] Zinc supplementation (15 mg per day) is considered safe for pregnant women. Given its safety and potential role in preventing NTDs, a zinc-containing multivitamin is recommended by many doctors to all women of childbearing age who may become pregnant.

Use of a **multivitamin** (page 559) supplement during the periconceptional period (defined as from the three months prior to pregnancy to the third month of pregnancy) can contribute significantly to a healthy pregnancy. Use of a multivitamin during these crucial months of fetal development has been associated with a reduced occurrence of many birth defects. In a preliminary study, periconceptional use of a multivitamin was associated with a lowered risk of heart defects in the offspring.[21] This association was not evident when use of the multivitamin began *after* the first month of pregnancy. The authors of this study concluded that approximately one in four major heart defects could be prevented by periconceptional multivitamin use. In another preliminary study, periconceptional use of a multivitamin was associated with a 43% reduction in the risk of having an infant with a severe heart defect.[22]

In a double-blind trial, women given a multivitamin containing folic acid starting at least one month before becoming pregnant to at least the second month of pregnancy were much less likely to have a child with a birth defect than were women given a trace mineral supplement.[23] The greatest reduction in risk was seen in the occurrence of urinary tract defects and heart defects. A preliminary study found that periconceptional use of a multivitamin reduced the risk for urinary tract defects and limb defects.[24] When multivitamin use was begun after the periconceptional period, there was a reduction in risk noted for cleft palate and again for urinary tract defects.

Childhood brain tumor rates may also be reduced by a mother's intake of a multivitamin while pregnant. In a preliminary study, use of a multivitamin by women for at least two-thirds of their pregnancy was associated with a decreased risk of brain tumor in the offspring compared to women who took a multivitamin for less than two-thirds of the pregnancy.[25] The greatest reduction of brain tumor risk (about 50%) was among children whose mothers took a multivitamin throughout the entire pregnancy.

A preliminary study, published in 1995 in the *New England Journal of Medicine (NEJM)*,[26] concluded that supplementation with more than 10,000 IU (3,000 mcg) per day of **vitamin A** (page 595) can increase the risk of certain birth defects. Since the publication of that report, women who are or could become pregnant have been told by doctors to consume no more than 10,000 IU per day of supplemental vitamin A. However, another study has challenged the findings of the *NEJM* report. In the new study, pregnancy outcome was determined in several hundred women who had consumed 10,000 to 300,000 IU (averaging about 50,000 IU) of supplemental vitamin A per day during early pregnancy.[27] No birth defects occurred in any of the infants exposed to maternal intakes of vitamin A greater than 50,000 IU per day. In fact, when compared with infants not exposed to vitamin A, a 50% *decreased* risk for birth defects was found in this high-exposure group.

A closer look at the recent study reveals a 32% higher-than-expected risk of birth defects in infants exposed to 10,000 to 40,000 IU of vitamin A per day but, paradoxically, a 37% decreased risk for those exposed to even higher levels. This suggests that both "higher" and "lower" risks may have been due to chance. At present, the level at which birth defects might be caused by vitamin A supplementation is not known, though it may well be higher than 10,000 IU per day. Nevertheless, women who are pregnant should talk with a doctor before supplementing with more than 10,000 IU per day.

Are there any side effects or interactions?
Refer to the individual supplement for information about any side effects or interactions.

BREAST CANCER

See also: Colon Cancer (page 123), **Lung Cancer** (page 298), **Prostate Cancer** (page 371), **Cancer Prevention and Diet** (page 87)

Breast cancer is a malignancy of the breast that is common in women and rare in men. It is characterized by unregulated replication of cells creating tumors, with the possibility of some of the cells spreading to other sites (metastasis).

This article includes a discussion of studies that have assessed whether certain vitamins, minerals, herbs, or other dietary ingredients offered in dietary or herbal supplements may be beneficial in connection with the reduction of risk of developing breast cancer, or of signs and symptoms in people who have this condition.

This information is provided solely to aid consumers in discussing supplements with their healthcare providers. It is not advised, nor is this information intended to advocate, promote, or encourage self prescription of these supplements for cancer risk reduction or treatment. Furthermore, none of this information should be misconstrued to suggest that dietary or herbal supplements can or should be used in place of conventional anticancer approaches or treatments.

It should be noted that certain studies referenced below, indicating the potential usefulness of a particular dietary ingredient or dietary or herbal supplement in connection with the reduction of risk of breast cancer, are preliminary evidence only. Some studies suggest an association between high blood or dietary levels of a particular dietary ingredient with a reduced risk of developing breast cancer. Even if such an association were established, this does not mean that dietary supplements containing large amounts of the dietary ingredient will necessarily have a cancer risk reduction effect.

Most breast cancer is not hereditary, although a small

percentage of women have a genetic weakness that dramatically increases their risk. Women with a strong family history of breast cancer may choose to explore the possibility of genetic testing with a geneticist, found on the staff of many major hospitals.

The incidence of postmenopausal breast cancer varies dramatically from one part of the world to the other, and those who move from one country to another will, on average, over time, begin to take on the risk of the new society to which they have moved. This evidence strongly suggests that most, though not all, breast cancer is preventable. However, great controversy exists about which factors are most responsible for the large differences in breast cancer incidence that separate high-risk populations from low-risk populations.

A few factors that affect the risk of having breast cancer are widely accepted:

- The later the age of the first menstrual cycle, the lower the risk.
- Full-term pregnancy at an early age (teens to early twenties) lowers the risk.
- Being overweight increases the risk of postmenopausal breast cancer.
- Use of hormone replacement therapy increases the risk, but this increase in risk has been reported to disappear shortly after hormone use is discontinued.
- Being older at the time of the last menstrual cycle (early fifties or older) confers a higher risk compared with women who have had their last menstrual cycle at a younger age (late forties or earlier).

Several other factors may affect a woman's risk of getting breast cancer. Many researchers and some doctors believe that long-term (greater than five years) use of oral contraceptives increases the risk of premenopausal breast cancer, but not the risk of postmenopausal breast cancer. Also, being overweight appears to slightly *reduce* the risk of premenopausal breast cancer, even though it increases the risk of postmenopausal breast cancer.

Almost all women with *noninvasive* breast cancer (ductal carcinoma in situ), along with a majority of women diagnosed with node-negative invasive breast cancer, are cured with appropriate conventional treatment. Even when breast cancer is diagnosed after it has spread to lymph nodes, many patients are curable. Once breast cancer has spread to a distant part of the body, conventional treatment sometimes extends life but cannot provide a cure.

CHECKLIST FOR BREAST CANCER

Rating	Nutritional Supplements	Herbs
★★☆	**Folic acid** (page 520) (reduces risk in women who consume alcohol)	
★☆☆	**Coenzyme Q$_{10}$** (page 494) **Conjugated linoleic acid** (page 499) **Melatonin** (page 555) **Vitamin D** (page 607) (reduces risk)	*Coriolus versicolor* **Eleuthero** (page 672) **European mistletoe** (page 711) **Green tea** (page 686) (reduces risk)

What are the symptoms of breast cancer?

The diagnosis of breast cancer is usually begun at the time a painless one-sided lump is discovered by the woman or her physician. In recent years, the diagnosis of breast cancer often begins with suspicious findings from a routine screening mammogram accompanied by no symptoms. In more advanced cases, changes to the contour of the affected breast may occur, and the lump may eventually become immovable.

If breast cancer spreads to a distant part of the body (distal metastasis), symptoms are determined by the location to which the cancer has spread. For example, if breast cancer spreads to bone, it frequently causes bone pain; if it spreads to the brain, it generally causes neurological symptoms, such as headaches that do not respond to aspirin. When it has spread to a distant part of the body, breast cancer also eventually causes severe weight loss, untreatable fatigue-inducing anemia, and finally death.

Medical treatments

Prescription drug treatment known as chemotherapy is commonly offered to most breast cancer patients, even many women with early-stage (node-negative) disease. Most chemotherapy is administered after surgery, although women with large tumors are sometimes treated before surgery. The chemotherapy drugs most commonly used to treat women with breast cancer include combinations of the following drugs: cyclophosphamide (Cytoxan, Neosar), methotrexate (Folex, Rheumatrex), fluorouracil (5-FU, Adrucil, Efudex, Fluoroplex), and doxorubicin (Adriamycin, Rubex, Doxil). Tamoxifen, an anti-estrogen (Nolvadex), is given to breast cancer patients whose disease is categorized as estrogen-receptor positive; other breast cancer patients generally do not receive tamoxifen. Some advanced breast cancer patients who have estrogen receptor-positive disease are also given aromatase-inhibitor drugs, which interfere with the body's ability to make estrogen. These drugs include letrozole (Femara), anastrozole (Arimidex), formestane (Lentaron), vorazole (Rizivor), and exemestane (Aromasin).

Increasingly, women with *non*invasive breast cancer (ductal carcinoma in situ) are treated with a variety of surgical and radiation options depending upon several factors (called Van Nuys criteria) that determine their risk of developing invasive (potentially life-threatening) breast cancer. Lobular carcinoma in situ is generally not considered to be breast cancer, only a risk factor for developing breast cancer. Most women with invasive breast cancer are initially offered one of two options: either removal of the lump (lumpectomy) combined with removal of axillary (arm pit) lymph nodes followed by radiation, or removal of the breast (mastectomy) combined with removal of axillary lymph nodes. In a minority of cases, patients receiving mastectomy are advised to receive radiation after the mastectomy.

Dietary changes that may be helpful
The following dietary changes have been studied in connection with breast cancer.

Avoidance of alcohol
An analysis of studies using the best available methodology found that women who drink alcohol have a higher risk of breast cancer compared with teetotalers.[1] Alcohol consumption during early adulthood may be more of a risk factor than alcohol consumption at a later age.[2]

Some,[3, 4] though not all,[5] studies have reported that alcohol increases estrogen levels. Increased estrogen levels might explain the increase in risk.

In a preliminary report, drinkers with low intake of **folic acid** (page 520) had a 32% increased risk of breast cancer compared with nondrinkers; however, the excess risk was only 5% in those drinkers who consumed adequate levels of folic acid.[6] In the same report, women taking **multivitamins** (page 559) containing folic acid and having at least 1.5 drinks per day had a 26% lower risk of being diagnosed with breast cancer compared with women drinking the same amount of alcohol but not taking folic acid-containing vitamins.[7]

Fiber (page 512)
Insoluble fiber from grains delays the onset of mammary (breast) cancer in animals.[8] In an analysis of the data from many studies, people who eat relatively high amounts of whole grains were reported to be at low risk for breast cancer.[9]

In some studies, the protective effect of fiber against the risk of breast cancer has been stronger in young women than in older women.[10] This finding might occur because fiber has been reported to lower estrogen levels in premenopausal women but not in postmenopausal women.[11, 12] Other researchers, however, report that fiber appears to equally reduce the risk of breast cancer in women of all ages.[13] One leading researcher has suggested the active components in fiber may be **phytate** (page 512) and isoflavones, substances that may provide protection even in the absence of a decrease in estrogen levels.[14] If these substances do protect against breast cancer, they might be as helpful in older women as in younger women.

Consuming a diet high in insoluble fiber is best achieved by switching from white rice to brown rice and from bakery goods made with white flour or mixed flours to 100% whole wheat bread, whole rye crackers, and whole grain pancake mixes. Refined white flour is generally listed on food packaging labels as "flour," "enriched flour," "unbleached flour," "durum wheat," "semolina," or "white flour." Breads containing only whole wheat are usually labeled "100% whole wheat."

Vegetarianism
Compared with meat eaters, most,[15] but not all,[16] studies have found that vegetarians are less likely to be diagnosed with cancer. Vegetarians have also been shown to have stronger **immune functioning** (page 255), possibly explaining why vegetarians may be partially protected against cancer.[17] Female vegetarians have been reported to have lower estrogen levels compared with meat-eating women, possibly explaining a lower incidence of breast cancer that has been reported in vegetarian women.[18]

Fruits and vegetables
An analysis of 17 studies on breast cancer risk and diet found that high consumption of vegetables was associated with a 25% decreased risk of breast cancer compared with low consumption.[19] The same report analyzed 12 studies that found high consumption of fruit was associated with a 6% reduction of breast cancer incidence compared with low consumption. However, when data from only the eight largest and best studies were combined, high intake of fruits and/or vegetables did not correlate with protection from breast cancer.[20] Therefore, the protective effect of fruit and

Breast Cancer

vegetable consumption against breast cancer remains unproven.[21]

Tomatoes

Tomatoes contain **lycopene** (page 548)—an **antioxidant** (page 467) similar in structure to **beta-carotene** (page 469). Most lycopene in our diet comes from tomatoes, though traces of lycopene exist in other foods. Lycopene has been reported to inhibit the proliferation of cancer cells in test tube research.[22]

A review of published research found that higher intake of tomatoes or higher blood levels of lycopene correlated with a reduced risk of a variety of cancers in 57 of 72 studies. Findings in 35 of these studies were statistically significant.[23] Evidence of a protective effect for tomato consumption was strongest for cancers other than breast cancer (**prostate** [page 371], **lung** [page 298], and stomach cancer), but some evidence of a protective effect also appeared for breast cancer.

Meat and how it is cooked

Most,[24, 25] but not all,[26] studies show that consumption of meat is associated with an increased risk of breast cancer. This association probably depends in part on how well the meat is cooked. Well-done meat contains more carcinogenic material than does lightly cooked meat.[27] Evidence from preliminary studies shows that women who eat well-done meat have a high risk of breast cancer.[28] Genetic factors may determine which women increase their risk of breast cancer by eating well-done meat.[29]

Fish

Fish eaters have been reported to have a low risk of breast cancer.[30] The **omega-3 fatty acids** (page 509) found in fish are thought by some researchers to be the components of fish responsible for protection against cancer.[31]

Coffee, unrelated to risk

Coffee drinking has been reported to increase breast pain associated with noncancerous lumps in the breast—a group of conditions commonly called **fibrocystic breast disease** (page 189). The presence of some forms of fibrocystic breast disease have been reported by some researchers to increase the risk of breast cancer.[32] As a result of these separate findings, some women may be concerned coffee drinking might increase the risk of breast cancer. However, most research has shown that coffee drinkers are at no higher risk of breast cancer than are women who do not drink coffee.[33, 34, 35]

Olive oil

Olive oil consumption has been associated with a reduced risk of breast cancer in several preliminary reports.[36, 37, 38] Oleic acid, the main fatty acid found in olive oil, does not appear to be the cause of this protective effect,[39] and scientists now guess that some as-yet undiscovered substance in olive oil might be responsible for the apparent protective effect of olive oil consumption.[40]

The dilemma over dietary fat

Olive oil and fish are two sources of dietary fat considered potentially helpful in protecting against breast cancer.[41, 42, 43, 44] Each has been discussed separately above. The information below discusses fat sources that some researchers are concerned might *increase* the risk of cancer.

High-fat diets increase the risk of mammary cancer in animals.[45] From country to country, breast cancer risk in women is proportionate to the level of total fat consumed in the diet.[46] Estrogen levels, body weight, and breast density have all been reported to decrease when women are put on low-fat diets—all changes that are thought to reduce the risk of breast cancer.[47, 48, 49, 50] Moreover, breast cancer patients have been reported to reduce their chances of survival by eating a diet high in saturated fat.[51] (Saturated fat is found mostly in meat and dairy fat.) Similarly, breast cancer patients have been reported to be at increased risk of suffering a recurrence if they eat higher levels of fatty foods, such as butter, margarine, red meat, and bacon.[52]

Analysis of human trials, using a research design dependent on the memories of subjects, also has shown women consuming high-fat diets to be at high risk of breast cancer.[53] In some cases, the correlation has been quite strong.[54] However, most,[55, 56, 57] but not all,[58] "prospective" studies—which avoid problems caused by faulty memories—have *not* found any association between fat intake and the risk of breast cancer.

Why do some research findings suggest that fat increases the risk of cancer and other studies find no association? Some studies finding dietary fat unrelated to cancer risks have not factored out the effects of olive oil or fish fat; both may *protect* against cancer.[59, 60, 61, 62] Adding them to the total dietary fat intake and then studying whether "more fat causes more cancer" is therefore misleading. Some studies finding no association between fat intake and breast cancer have made one or both of these errors.[63, 64]

Scientists know cancers caused by diet most likely occur many years after the causative foods are regularly consumed. When one group of researchers compared dietary intakes to cancer rates occurring ten years after the consumption of food, and also eliminated from consideration the effect of fat from fish consumption, they found a high degree of correlation between consumption of animal fat (other than from fish) and the risk of breast cancer death rates for women at least 50 years of age.[65]

In the debate over whether dietary fat increases breast cancer risks, only one fact is indisputable: women in countries that consume high amounts of meat and dairy fat have a high risk of breast cancer, while women in countries that mostly consume rice, soy, vegetables, and fish (instead of dairy fat and meat) have a low risk of breast cancer.[66]

The complex relationship between soy consumption and risk

Asian countries in which soy consumption is high generally have a low incidence of breast cancer. However, the dietary habits in these countries are so different from diets in high-risk countries that attributing protection from breast cancer specifically to soy foods on the basis of this evidence alone is premature.[67] Similarly, *within* a society, women who frequently consume tofu have been reported to be at low risk of breast cancer.[68] Consumption of tofu might only be a marker for other dietary or lifestyle factors that are responsible for protection against breast cancer.

Genistein, one of the isoflavones found in many soy foods, inhibits proliferation of breast cancer cells in test tube studies. Most animal studies report that soybeans and soy isoflavones protect against mammary cancer.[69] However, the protective effect in animals have occurred primarily when soy has been administered before puberty.[70] If the same holds true in humans, consuming soy products in adulthood might provide little, if any, protection against breast cancer.

The findings of several recent studies suggest that consuming soy might, under some circumstances, *increase* the risk of breast cancer.[71, 72, 73, 74, 75] When ovaries were removed from animals—a situation related to the condition of women who have had a total hysterectomy— dietary genistein was reported to *increase* the proliferation of breast cancer cells.[76] When pregnant rats were given genistein injections, their female offspring were reported to be at *greater* risk of breast cancer.[77] Although

premenopausal women have shown decreases in estrogen levels in response to soy consumption,[78, 79] *pro*estrogenic effects have also been reported.[80] When premenopausal women were given soy isoflavones, an increase in breast secretions resulted—an effect thought to *elevate* the risk of breast cancer.[81] In yet another trial, healthy breast cells from women previously given soy supplements containing isoflavones showed an *increase* in proliferation rates—an effect that might also increase the risk of breast cancer.[82]

The commonly held belief that consuming soybeans or isoflavones such as genistein will protect against breast cancer is, therefore, far from proven.[83, 84, 85, 86, 87] Possibly, consuming soybeans in childhood may ultimately be proven to have a protective effect.[88] Doing the same in adulthood, however, may have very different effects.[89, 90, 91, 92, 93]

Some scientists, at least under some circumstances, remain hopeful about the potential for soy to protect against breast cancer. These scientists recommend consumption of foods made from soy (such as tofu), as opposed to taking isoflavone supplements. Several substances in soybeans other than isoflavones have shown anticancer activity in preliminary research.[94]

Reduction in sugar

Preliminary studies have reported associations between an increased intake of sugar or sugar-containing foods and an increased risk of breast cancer,[95] though this link does not appear consistently in published research.[96] Whether these associations exist because sugar directly promotes cancer or because sugar consumption is only a marker for some other dietary or lifestyle factor remains unknown.

Lifestyle changes that may be helpful

The following lifestyle changes have been studied in connection with breast cancer.

Exercise and prevention

Girls who engage in a significant amount of exercise have been reported to be less likely to get breast cancer as adults.[97] Although some doctors speculate that exercise in preadolescent girls might reduce the risk of eventually getting breast cancer by reducing the number of menstrual cycles and therefore exposure to estrogen, these effects may occur only in girls engaging in very strenuous exercise.[98]

Most,[99, 100] but not all,[101] studies find that adult women who exercise are less likely to get breast cancer.

Women who exercise have also been reported to have a reduced risk of high-risk mammography patterns compared with inactive women.[102]

Exercise in adulthood might help protect against breast cancer by lowering blood levels of estrogen or by helping maintain ideal body weight. In addition to the preventive effects of exercise, aerobic exercise has been reported to reduce **depression** (page 145) and **anxiety** (page 30) in women already diagnosed with breast cancer.[103]

Smoking and risk

Some studies have found an association between smoking and an increased risk of breast cancer, including exposure to secondhand smoke.[104] However, several reports have either found no association[105] or have reported an association between smoking and an apparent *protection* against breast cancer.[106] Some of the studies reporting that smoking is detrimental have found that exposure to cigarette smoke during childhood appears to be most likely to increase the risk of breast cancer.[107]

The mind-body connection

In some studies, the risk of breast cancer has been reported to be higher in women who have experienced major (though not minor) **depression** (page 145) in the years preceding diagnosis.[108] Some,[109, 110] but not all,[111] studies have found that exposure to severely stressful events increases a woman's chance of developing breast cancer. In one study, breast cancer patients exposed to severely stressful events, such as death of a spouse or divorce, had more than five times the risk of suffering a recurrence compared with women not exposed to such stressors.[112] Although stress has long been considered as a possible risk factor, some studies have not found significant correlations between psychological stressors and breast cancer risk[113] or the risk of breast cancer recurrence.[114] Similarly, experiencing psychological distress (independent of external stressors) has, in some reports, not been associated with a reduction in survival or the risk of suffering a breast cancer recurrence.[115]

Exposure to psychological stress has been reported to weaken the **immune system** (page 255) of breast cancer patients.[116] Strong social support has been reported to increase immune function in breast cancer patients.[117] These findings suggest a possible way in which the mind might play a role in affecting the risk of a breast cancer recurrence.[118, 119]

In one study, breast cancer patients with strong social support in the months following surgery had only half the risk of dying from the disease during a seven-year period compared with patients who lacked anyone to confide in.[120] After 10[121] and 15 years,[122] breast cancer patients with a helpless and hopeless attitude or with an attitude of stoicism were much less likely to survive compared with women who had what the researchers called a "fighting spirit." In a five-year study, the same helpless/hopeless attitude correlated with an increased risk of recurrence or death in breast cancer patients, but a "fighting spirit" did not correlate with special protection against recurrence or death.[123] One trial reported that psychological therapy for hopeless/helpless breast cancer patients was capable of changing these attitudes and reducing psychological distress in only eight weeks.[124]

Several trials using a variety of psychological interventions have reported increased life expectancy in women receiving counseling or psychotherapy compared with women who did not receive psychological intervention[125]—even in women with late-stage disease.[126] In a now-famous trial, late-stage breast cancer patients in a year-long, 90-minute-per-week support group lived on average twice as long as a group of similar patients who did not receive such support.[127]

Finally, relaxation training has been reported to reduce psychological distress in breast cancer patients,[128] and group therapy and hypnosis have reduced pain in late-stage breast cancer patients.[129]

Even extensive psychological support (weekly peer support, family therapy, individual counseling, and use of positive mental imagery) has not led to a clear increase in breast cancer survival in every study.[130] Why some studies clearly find mind-body connections in regard to breast cancer risk, recurrence, or survival, while other studies find no such connection, remains unclear.

Overweight (page 446) and risk

Being overweight increases the risk of postmenopausal breast cancer, a fact widely accepted by the research community. Overweight does not increase the risk of *pre*menopausal breast cancer and even may be associated with a slightly reduced risk of breast cancer in young women.[131]

Nutritional supplements that may be helpful

The following nutritional supplements have been studied in connection with breast cancer.

Folic acid (page 520)

Among women who drink alcohol, those who consume relatively high amounts of folate from their diet have been reported to be at reduced risk of breast cancer, compared with women who drink alcohol but consumed less folate, according to a preliminary study.[132] In a similar report, consumption of folic acid-containing supplements was associated with a lower risk of breast cancer in women who drank alcohol, compared with women who drank alcohol but did not take such supplements.[133]

The damaging effect alcohol has on DNA—the material responsible for normal replication of cells—is partially reversed by folic acid. Therefore, a potential association between both dietary folate and folic acid supplements and protection against breast cancer in women who drink alcohol is consistent with our understanding of the biochemical effects of these substances. A combined intake from food and supplements of at least 600 mcg per day was associated with a 43% reduced risk of breast cancer in women who consumed 1.5 drinks per day or more, compared with women who drank the same amount but did not take folic acid-containing supplements.[134]

No research has yet explored the effect of folic acid supplementation in people who have already been diagnosed with cancer. Cancer patients taking the chemotherapy drug methotrexate must not take folic acid supplements without the direction of their oncologist.

Selenium (page 584)

The association between relatively higher blood levels of selenium and lower risks of cancer in men has been fairly consistent.[135, 136, 137] However, most,[138, 139, 140, 141] though not all,[142] studies have found selenium status to be unrelated to cancer risk in women, particularly in relation to cancers that strike only women. In fact, a few studies have reported that exposure to higher amounts of selenium[143]—including selenium from supplements[144]—is associated with a *higher* risk of several cancers in women, though these studies have been criticized.[145]

In a famous double-blind trial that reported dramatic reductions in the incidence of **lung** (page 298), **colon** (page 123), and **prostate** (page 371) cancers as a result of selenium supplementation, of the few women who got breast cancer during the trial, *more* were taking selenium than were taking placebo, though this difference may well have been due to chance.[146] Thus, the findings of this famous trial also do not support the idea that selenium supplementation protects against breast cancer.[147]

In contrast, animal studies generally find that selenium helps protect against mammary cancer,[148, 149]

and associations between higher selenium status and decreased risk of breast cancer in women have also occasionally been reported.[150, 151] Despite these hopeful findings, most studies suggest that higher selenium status confers no protection against breast cancer.[152, 153, 154, 155, 156, 157, 158]

Vitamin E (page 609)

Although some preliminary evidence suggests that vitamin E may protect against breast cancer,[159, 160] most research does not suggest a protective effect.[161, 162, 163] In a preliminary study, women taking vitamin E supplements had the same risk of breast cancer as did other women.[164] However, in one study, women with of low blood levels of *both* **selenium** (page 584) *and* vitamin E had a tenfold higher risk of breast cancer compared with women having higher levels of both nutrients.[165] Although vitamin E and selenium function together in the body, the meaning of this dramatic finding is not clear; most studies examining the effects of vitamin E or selenium separately have suggested that neither protects against breast cancer.

Although one form of vitamin E—alpha tocopheryl succinate—has been touted as a potential treatment for women with breast cancer, only test tube studies suggest that it may have anticancer activity,[166] and no trials have been conducted in breast cancer patients.

Vitamin D (page 607)

Breast cancer rates have been reported to be relatively high in areas of low exposure to sunlight.[167] Sunlight triggers the formation of vitamin D in the skin, which can be activated in the liver and kidneys into a hormone with great activity. This activated form of vitamin D causes "cellular differentiation"—essentially the opposite of cancer.

The following evidence indicates that vitamin D might have a protective role against breast cancer:

- Synthetic vitamin D-like molecules have prevented the equivalent of breast cancer in animals.[168]
- Activated vitamin D appears to have antiestrogenic activity.[169]
- Both sunlight and dietary exposure to vitamin D have correlated with a reduced risk of breast cancer.[170]

Activated vitamin D

Activated vitamin D comes in several forms. One of them—1,25 dihydroxycholecalciferol—is an exact duplicate of the hormone made in the human body.

The following preliminary, non-clinical evidence supports the idea that activated **vitamin D** (page 607) may be of help to some breast cancer patients:

- In combination with tamoxifen, a synthetic, activated-vitamin D-like molecule has inhibited the growth of breast cancer cells in test tube research.[171]
- Synthetic vitamin D-like molecules induce tumor cell death in breast cancer cells.[172]
- Activated vitamin D suppresses the growth of human cancer cells transplanted into animals.[173]
- In test tube research, activated vitamin D has increased the anticancer action of chemotherapy.[174]

In a preliminary trial, activated vitamin D was applied topically to the breast, once per day for six weeks, in 19 patients with breast cancer.[175] Of the 14 patients who completed the trial, three showed a large reduction in tumor size, and one showed a minor improvement. Those who responded had tumors that contained receptors for activated vitamin D. However, other preliminary reports have not found that high levels of these receptors consistently correlate with a better outcome.[176, 177, 178]

With a doctor's prescription, compounding pharmacists can put activated vitamin D, a hormone, into a topical ointment. Due to potential toxicity, use of this hormone, even topically, requires careful monitoring by a physician. Standard vitamin D supplements are unlikely to duplicate the effects of activated vitamin D in women with breast cancer. The patients in the breast cancer trial all had locally advanced disease.

Melatonin (page 555)

Melatonin has been reported to have anticancer activity against breast cancer cells in most[179, 180] though not all[181] test tube studies. In a preliminary trial, breast cancer patients were studied who previously had responded either not at all or only temporarily to treatment with the drug tamoxifen.[182] During the trial, these women were given tamoxifen again, this time with added melatonin. Blood levels of IGF-1, a marker for progression of breast cancer, declined significantly. Of fourteen patients, four showed evidence of tumor shrinkage that lasted an average of eight months.

Most cancer trials studying the effects of melatonin have used 20 mg of melatonin per 24 hours, all taken at bedtime.[183, 184, 185, 186, 187, 188, 189, 190, 191, 192, 193, 194] No one should take such a high amount of this hormone without the supervision of a healthcare professional.

Coenzyme Q10 (page 494) (CoQ10)

French researchers have reported that the lower the blood level of CoQ_{10} in breast cancer patients, the worse the chance of remaining free of disease.[195] For several years, researchers from Denmark and the United States have been studying the effects CoQ_{10} in a group of 32 breast cancer patients who were either at high risk of suffering a recurrence or had already been diagnosed with advanced disease.[196] After 18 months, only one patient had suffered a recurrence, all were still alive, those who did not have advanced disease at the beginning of the trial had not progressed to advanced disease, one patient with advanced disease had stabilized, and two patients with advanced disease had significantly improved.[197] Patients continued to do well after two years of supplementation,[198] and after three to five years, surprising improvements were reported in two patients who had had advanced disease at the beginning of the trial.[199]

At first, 90 mg of CoQ_{10} per day was used. In subsequent reports, the amount of CoQ_{10} was increased until some women were receiving 390 mg per day.[200] Initially, the CoQ_{10} was accompanied by the use of many other supplements.[201] The researchers of this trial have attributed the therapeutic effects observed primarily to CoQ_{10} and, in later reports, no further mention of other supplements was made.[202, 203, 204]

This preliminary investigation has been conducted with no control group, and published reports have provided only sketchy details about the conditions of most of the women being studied. Some of the patients were given conventional treatments along with CoQ_{10}. Therefore, CoQ_{10} remains unproven as a cancer treatment.

Fiber (page 512)

Although fiber is available in supplement form (such as Metamucil), most fiber consumption results from eating food. Preliminary evidence suggests that high fiber consumption may reduce the risk of breast cancer. See the discussion of fiber and possible prevention of breast cancer in Dietary changes, above.

Indole-3-carbinol (page 536)

Cruciferous vegetables—broccoli, Brussels sprouts, cauliflower, and cabbage—contain a substance called indole-3-carbinol (I3C). In preliminary research, I3C has been reported to affect the metabolism of estrogen in a way that might protect against breast cancer,[205] an idea supported by animal[206] and test tube research.[207] No research trials have yet investigated the effects of I3C supplementation in women with breast cancer.

Diindolylmethane
Diindolylmethane is a substance also found in cruciferous vegetables. Test tube[208] and animal studies[209] suggest that it may help protect against breast cancer. However, no clinical trials with cancer patients given diindolylmethane have yet been published.

Calcium D-glucarate *(page 486) (D-Glucaric acid)*
Calcium D-glucarate is available as a supplement, and it is also found in fruits and vegetables in a slightly altered form—D-glucaric acid.[210] Preliminary evidence suggests that calcium D-glucarate indirectly helps the body lower its burden of estrogen, an effect that may reduce the risk of breast cancer.[211] Although animal research supports such a possibility,[212] no human trials have been published to evaluate whether calcium D-glucarate has a therapeutic or preventive effect.

IP-6 *(page 539)*
IP-6 (also called inositol hexaphosphate, phytate, or phytic acid) is found in many foods, particularly oat bran, wheat bran, and unleavened (flat) bread. Until recently, most IP-6 research focused on interference with the absorption of minerals—a side effect of consuming IP-6. More recently, however, animal studies have found that IP-6 has anticancer activity.[213] No human trials using IP-6 supplements to prevent or treat breast cancer have yet been published.

Soy isoflavones *(page 587), including genistein*
No research has directly investigated whether soy isoflavone supplements prevent breast cancer or help people already diagnosed with this disease. Nonetheless, considerable preliminary information has been gathered about the relationship between soy isoflavones and breast cancer. For more information, see the discussion about soy in Dietary changes, above.

Conjugated linoleic acid *(page 499)*
Preliminary animal and test tube research suggests that CLA might reduce the risk of **cancers** (page 87) at several sites, including breast, **prostate** (page 371), **colorectal** (page 123), **lung** (page 298), skin, and stomach.[214, 215, 216, 217] Whether CLA will have a similar protective effect for people has yet to be demonstrated in human research.

Are there any side effects or interactions?
Refer to the individual supplement for information about any side effects or interactions.

Herbs that may be helpful
The following herbs have been studied in connection with breast cancer.

Garlic *(page 679) and* **onion** *(page 718)*
Preliminary studies hunting for associations between consumption of garlic *(Allium sativum)* and onion *(Allium cepa)* and a reduced risk of breast cancer have produced only mixed results;[218, 219] thus, there is no proof that consumption of either food helps prevent the risk of breast cancer.

Cloud mushroom (Coriolus versicolor)
Coriolus is a Chinese mushroom that has been reported to improve parameters of **immune function** (page 255).[220] A Japanese extract from this mushroom called Polysaccharide Krestin (PSK) has been studied in many trials with cancer patients, often in conjunction with conventional treatment.[221, 222, 223, 224, 225, 226, 227, 228, 229] PSK's effects in women with breast cancer have been somewhat inconsistent. One double-blind trial reported that some groups of women with breast cancer, given PSK along with chemotherapy, had better outcomes than those who took chemotherapy alone.[230] Another double-blind trial reported 81% survival in breast cancer patients given PSK plus chemotherapy, compared with 65% in those given chemotherapy alone, though this difference did not quite reach statistical significance.[231] A third double-blind trial did not find PSK to be beneficial for women with breast cancer.[232]

PSK is not readily available in the United States and is available in Japan only by prescription. Although hot water-extracted products made from Coriolus versicolor are available in the United States without prescription, the extent to which these herbal products produce the effects of Japanese PSK remains unknown.

Eleuthero *(page 672) (Eleutherococcus senticosus, Acanthopanax senticosus)*
Also known as Siberian ginseng, eleuthero has been shown to enhance **immune function** (page 255) in preliminary Russian trials studying people with cancer, particularly breast cancer.[233, 234] These trials typically used 1 to 2 ml of a fluid extract taken three times per

day for at least one month. Most of the people in these trials were also treated with chemotherapy, radiation therapy, and/or surgery.[235, 236] Several of the Russian trials showed fewer side effects from conventional therapies among those who also took eleuthero extracts. No information is available on the ability of eleuthero to prevent cancer, nor have clinical trials yet explored whether eleuthero extracts affect either recurrence of breast cancer or survival in women with breast cancer.

European mistletoe *(page 711) (Viscum album)*
Special extracts of European mistletoe injected under the skin has been studied in several positive and negative double-blind trials with cancer patients.[237, 238, 239, 240, 241] A double-blind trial of women with breast cancer (all treated with chemotherapy) found that those who received mistletoe injections had improved immunity and quality of life compared with those who took a placebo.[242] The use of oral mistletoe preparations has not been studied in breast cancer patients. Mistletoe injections (usually of a product called Iscador) are available only through physicians and are not readily available in the United States. It is unknown if American mistletoe *(Phoradendron leucarpum)* would provide the same effect as European mistletoe.

Green tea *(page 686)*
In one Japanese study, green tea consumption was associated with increased survival time and decreased spread of cancer to lymph nodes in women with early stages of breast cancer, but not in breast cancer patients with more advanced disease.[243] Recurrence rates were found to be lowest in those who drank at least five cups per day.[244] Despite these associations, however, no proof yet exists that green tea consumption helps breast cancer patients or helps healthy women prevent breast cancer.

Are there any side effects or interactions?
Refer to the individual herb for information about any side effects or interactions.

BREAST-FEEDING SUPPORT

Human breast milk is the best food for newborn babies. In December 1997, the American Academy of Pediatrics issued a policy statement advocating breast milk as the ideal, exclusive food for babies in the first six months of life. They also recommended that breast-feeding continue for at least 12 months or longer if mutually desired.[1]

In the United States, only about 50% of new mothers giving birth in a hospital breast-feed their babies. This number declines rapidly, with only about 20% of women still breast-feeding at six months.[2] There is a large body of evidence on the benefits of breast-feeding for both mother and infant. With adequate support and good information on preventing some of the common problems associated with breast-feeding, a woman's chances of successfully breast-feeding her new baby are greatly improved.

CHECKLIST FOR BREAST-FEEDING SUPPORT

Rating	Nutritional Supplements	Herbs
★★☆	**Calcium** (page 483) **Cod liver fish oil** (page 514) **Docosahexaenoic acid** (page 509) (DHA) **Iron** (page 540) (for deficiency only) **Multivitamin-mineral** (page 559)	**Garlic** (page 679) (to increase duration of feedings)
★☆☆		**Anise** (page 627) **Chickweed** (page 658) (topical application, for sore nipples) **Comfrey** (page 662) (topical application, for sore nipples) Goat's rue (to stimulate milk production) **Marigold** (page 650) (topical application, for sore nipples) **Stinging nettle** (page 714) (to stimulate milk production) **Vitex** (page 757) (to stimulate milk production)

Why breast-feed?
Breast-feeding provides significant benefits for baby and mother.

Benefits for baby
Human milk contains the ideal balance of nutrients, enzymes, and anti-infective and immune supportive agents for babies.[3, 4] There are two kinds of breast milk: colostrum and mature milk. Colostrum, which is produced in the first few days after birth, has higher concen-

trations of protein and immune-enhancing agents and less sugar and fat than mature milk.[5] Mature human milk differs greatly from both infant formula and either cow or goat milk. Human milk, made specifically for the nutritional needs of the newborn, is superior to all alternatives.

One significant advantage of human breast milk is its abundance of immune-protective and anti-infective agents, including immunoglobulins (primarily immunoglobulin A, or IgA), lactoferrin, *Bifidobacterium bifidum,* white blood cells, and other factors. These agents are known to help the newborn fight a wide variety of illnesses. Many scientific studies in the United States and other developed countries have demonstrated the health protective benefits of breast milk.

Breast-feeding has been found to help prevent: **diarrhea** (page 163),[6, 7, 8, 9, 10] lower respiratory tract infection,[11, 12, 13, 14] **ear infections** (page 383) (otitis media),[15, 16, 17, 18, 19, 20] meningitis,[21, 22] **urinary tract infection** (page 436),[23] and other serious infections (botulism, necrotizing enterocolitis, bacteremia).[24, 25, 26, 27, 28] In addition, breast-feeding may possibly help prevent: sudden infant death syndrome (SIDS),[29, 30, 31] insulin-dependent **diabetes mellitus** (page 152),[32, 33] **inflammatory bowel disease** (page 269) (**Crohn's disease** [page 141], **ulcerative colitis** [page 433]),[34, 35] **cancer** (page 87) (lymphoma),[36, 37] allergic diseases,[38, 39, 40] and other chronic digestive diseases.[41, 42, 43] Breast-feeding may also enhance cognitive development.[44, 45]

The protein composition of breast milk is perfect for growing babies and is easy for them to digest. Breast milk also provides absorbable nutrients; the iron and zinc found in human milk is extremely easily absorbed (bioavailable) compared with **iron** (page 540) and **zinc** (page 614) from other foods. When infants are exclusively breast-fed, 50% of the iron is absorbed. By comparison, absorption of iron from cow's milk and iron-fortified commercial formula is much lower, only 10% and 4%, respectively.[46]

Breast milk is also quick, easy, and cost-effective. It's always available and does not need to be prepared, and the cost of providing the necessary additional nutrition to a breast-feeding mother is about half the cost of commercial formula.[47, 48, 49] And breast-feeding promotes bonding, allowing a mother and her baby to be in close physical contact, enhancing the formation of a close mother-baby bond.[50]

Benefits for mother
Breast-feeding a new baby has many important health benefits for the mother as well. Breast-feeding immediately after childbirth causes the release of a hormone called oxytocin, which causes the uterus to contract. This results in less postpartum (after pregnancy) blood loss and a more rapid return of the uterus to its pre-pregnancy size.[51] While breast-feeding, most women will not immediately resume their ovulation and menstrual periods. Delaying the return of ovulation may extend the time between pregnancies.[52, 53] Women who breast-feed for at least six months lose weight more quickly than women who continue breast-feeding for less than three months.[54] And, while breast-feeding can cause a short-term loss of bone density, it also seems to improve the body's ability to rebuild bones postpartum.[55] In addition, women who have breast-fed their babies may have fewer osteoporosis-linked hip fractures after they've passed through menopause.[56] Breast-feeding has also been associated with a lower risk of ovarian cancer and a reduced risk of **breast cancer** (page 65) in premenopausal women.[57, 58]

What conditions are related to breast-feeding?
Several problems common to breast-feeding mothers can be prevented or eased through simple techniques or addressed with common, simple treatment options.

Sore nipples
Most women will experience some degree of nipple soreness in the first days of breast-feeding. Discomfort that occurs at the onset of breast-feeding and is relieved by feeding is normal. It is caused by the stimulation of the nipple by the hormone oxytocin, which stimulates milk let-down. True nipple soreness, in which the nipples appear red and are tender to the touch, is rare and is probably caused by the baby's improper grasp on the nipple and areola (pigmented area surrounding the nipple) while feeding.

Correcting the baby's position on the breast is the most important tactic for preventing and relieving sore nipples. A physician, nurse, or lactation consultant can assist in assessing and correcting an infant's grasp of the nipple. Sore nipples can progress to more painful, cracked, and fissured nipples. As the condition worsens, the nipples are more susceptible to infection. In addition to correcting the baby's position, there are a number of self-help measures frequently recommended for the relief of sore nipples. These are most effective when begun at the onset of symptoms.

Check the position of the baby on the breast; the infant's tongue should be under the nipple and the mouth should grasp both the nipple and part of the areola. Vary the position of the breast-feeding infant with each feeding to avoid soreness of a particular area of the nipple.

The infant should be fed on demand; an overly hungry infant may suck harder, causing nipple soreness. Mothers with sore nipples should begin each feeding on the side that is least sore, switching to the sore breast after the let-down reflex has occurred. The infant should not be allowed to suck on an empty breast, which can cause damage to the nipple. If the nipples are sore, a breast-feeding session of ten minutes on each side should be sufficient to nourish the baby.

Ice packs applied to the breasts prior to breast-feeding can have a pain-relieving effect. Allowing nipples to air-dry after nursing can help to reduce nipple soreness.

In the case of cracked nipples, the application of an ointment or cream can aid healing. Ointments or creams allow the skin's internal moisture to heal deep cracks and fissures while keeping the skin pliable.[59] A frequently recommended and safe ointment for cracked nipples is medical grade, purified anhydrous lanolin (derived from wool fat). The nipples should be patted dry prior to application of a small amount of lanolin.

Engorgement

Engorgement is a common condition that occurs as blood and lymphatic flow to the breasts greatly increases, leading to congestion and discomfort. The pain associated with engorgement can range from mild to severe. Engorgement typically occurs on the first full day of milk production and lasts only about 24 hours. The breasts may feel firm and hot to the touch and the skin may appear reddened. As with other conditions, the best remedy is prevention. Many health professionals believe frequent breast-feeding (at least every three hours) will successfully prevent engorgement. This is probably true for most women. However, the physical changes associated with initiation of breast-feeding may eventually lead to engorgement in some women. If engorgement occurs, the best remedy is to breast-feed frequently. This can relieve the engorgement and prevent the condition from worsening.

Doctors often recommend additional options for women with engorgement. A well-fitted bra can relieve some of the discomfort of engorgement. Applications of moist heat may encourage flow of milk from the breasts. Women may apply hot packs to the breasts just prior to breast-feeding. Other suggestions include frequent warm showers or alternating hot and cold showers. Cold packs applied to the breasts after breast-feeding can provide a slight pain-relieving effect.

Some infants will have a difficult time correctly latching on to an engorged breast. This can lead to inadequate nourishment and sore nipples. Expressing some excess milk, manually or with a pump, just prior to breast-feeding may relieve this difficulty. Women may also express milk after the infant has finished feeding to relieve any remaining sense of fullness. Massaging the breasts while breast-feeding may encourage milk flow from all the milk ducts and help to relieve engorgement.

Mastitis

Mastitis is inflammation of the breast that is frequently caused by an infection. The infected breast may feel hot and swollen. The breast may be tender to the touch, and fever, fatigue, chills, headache, and nausea may be present. Some women feel as though they have the flu. A breast infection requires prompt medical attention. Complete bed rest is important for a speedy recovery, and antibiotics are frequently prescribed. In addition, doctors often provide further guidelines for treating mastitis.

A woman should continue breast-feeding from both breasts; the milk from the infected breast is still good for the baby. Moist heat over the painful breast can be helpful, and cold applications after breast-feeding can help alleviate swelling and pain. Breast-feeding women should also avoid constricting or under-wire bras that may irritate the infected breast.

Who can breast-feed?

Breast-feeding is the best food for babies, and most mothers will be able to breast-feed their infants. However, there are some uncommon situations in which breast-feeding is not in the best interest of the infant.

Galactosemia is a rare metabolic condition that leads to an inability to break down galactose, one of the components of milk sugar (lactose). Infants with galactosemia should not breast-feed, but should be fed a special formula without lactose.[60]

Phenylketonuria (page 354) (PKU) is another rare metabolic disorder, in which a newborn is unable to break down the amino acid **phenylalanine** (page 568). The resulting build-up of phenylalanine in the system can be harmful. There is some disagreement regarding whether it is safe to breast-feed infants with PKU. Some sources recommend against breast-feeding the infant with PKU.[61] However, breast milk is low in phenylalanine and there is evidence that the exclusively breast-fed infant with PKU will not have damaging levels of phenylalanine accumulate in the bloodstream. A mother interested in breast-feeding her infant with PKU should work closely with a doctor. Close monitoring of the infant's blood phenylalanine levels will be necessary.[62]

For infants in the United States and other developed countries born to mothers infected with the human immunodeficiency virus (**HIV** [page 239]) it may be safer not to breast-feed.[63] However, there is controversy over this issue. Some researchers have found HIV in human milk, indicating that there is the potential for passing the virus to a healthy baby while breast-feeding. Other studies indicate a very low risk of actually passing the infection to the baby through the breast milk.[64]

Additionally, a mother with untreated active tuberculosis should not breast-feed her infant. And the infant whose mother abuses drugs should not be breast-fed.[65]

Dietary changes that may be helpful

Pregnant and breast-feeding women should choose a well-balanced and varied diet that includes fresh fruits and vegetables, whole grains, legumes, and fish. Many doctors recommend limiting intake of refined sugars, white flour, fried foods, processed foods, and chemical additives.

The caloric needs of a breast-feeding woman are even higher than during pregnancy. An extra 400 to 500 calories per day above pregnancy requirements are needed. Most women should consume approximately 2,800 calories per day to meet the energy needs of breast-feeding.[66] Therefore, under most circumstances, doctors discourage dieting (i.e., calorie restriction). Weight loss following pregnancy usually occurs naturally, particularly if a woman can engage in moderate exercise. Breast-feeding uses up fat stores, and is a natural way to lose weight.

A woman should continue to take prenatal vitamins in order to meet the nutrient requirements of breast-feeding. Especially important is continued intake of **calcium** (page 483) and calcium-rich foods.

Breast milk contains essential fatty acids. The fat composition of breast milk varies with a woman's diet. If a woman consumes foods that provide essential fatty acids (e.g., vegetable oils such as canola oil, corn oil, and safflower oil; nut and seed oils; and fish), the breast milk she produces will contain higher quantities of essential fatty acids.[67]

Drinking to quench thirst is enough to support a healthy milk supply.[68] Women are frequently instructed to drink extra fluids to increase milk supply. This is a common misunderstanding, however, and excessive fluid intake should be avoided.[69]

Lifestyle changes that may be helpful

It is best to avoid all unnecessary medications, herbs, and nutritional supplements when breast-feeding. Most prescribed and over-the-counter medications, when taken by a breast-feeding mother, are considered safe for the infant. However, a doctor should always be consulted before any medication is taken. There are a few medications that mothers may need to take that may make it necessary to interrupt breast-feeding temporarily.

Caffeine

Caffeine, which is considered a drug, is excreted into breast milk. It is estimated that an infant receives 1.5 to 3.1 mg of caffeine after the mother drinks a cup of coffee (a cup of coffee typically contains 60 to 50 mg of caffeine). Because this amount is fairly low, a morning cup of coffee is not likely to cause any problems. However, if the mother is a heavy caffeine user, caffeine can accumulate in the infant.[70] Infants have immature livers that are unable to adequately process caffeine. A baby who is irritable and sleeping poorly may be reacting to caffeine in the mother's diet. A woman can switch to decaffeinated coffees and teas to effectively reduce the amount of caffeine her baby receives through her milk.

Alcohol (page 12)

Alcohol reaches maternal milk in concentrations similar to those in the mother's blood.[71] It is therefore best for breast-feeding mothers to minimize or eliminate alcohol consumption. It is commonly believed that drinking beer can increase a woman's milk supply. In fact, drinking beer intake does increase secretion of prolactin (the hormone that stimulates production of breast milk) in both men and women.[72] However, research has shown that infants breast-fed after their mothers drank alcoholic beer consumed less milk than when their mothers drank non-alcoholic beer.[73]

Smoking

Breast-feeding mothers should not smoke. Nicotine passes to the baby through the breast milk and can cause feeding problems and illness, especially in newborns. Babies should also be protected from the dangers of second-hand smoke. Second-hand smoke has been shown to increase the risk of SIDS (sudden infant death syndrome)[74, 75, 76, 77, 78] and **colic** (page 121) in newborns.[79]

Initiating the breast-feeding relationship

There are many reasons why women decide not to breast-feed or discontinue breast-feeding earlier than the recommended six months. These include a lack of family, societal, or medical support;[80] misinformation or lack of education about breast-feeding;[81] marketing of commercial formulas to new mothers;[82] and the difficulties often encountered in returning to work or school.[83] In addition, there are some common difficulties that could interfere with a healthy breast-feeding relationship. These include fear of not having enough milk to nourish the baby, sore nipples, engorgement, and mastitis (inflammation of the breast, frequently caused by infection).

A new mother should try to breast-feed her baby as soon as possible after delivery, ideally within the first hour of life.[84] An infant should be fed on demand. A hungry infant will first get fussy, with increased activity and rooting (a reflex wherein the infant appears to be searching for the breast with his or her mouth) or mouthing behavior. Crying is a late sign of hunger. To get into the habit of feeding their babies, new mothers are often instructed to follow a schedule of breast-feeding every four hours around the clock. However, these imposed schedules, if followed beyond the first few weeks of life, often lead to frustration and confusion. The only infant who needs to be breast-fed on such a schedule is the infant who does not demand to be fed. Feeding on demand is the best way to increase milk supply. Most infants will empty the breast in 10 to 15 minutes. Some doctors advise gradually increasing the duration of breast-feeding over the first week of life. If this regimen is followed, it is important to breast-feed for at least five minutes on each side to get the benefit of the let-down reflex (which promotes the release of milk from the storage ducts in the breasts).[85]

Infants need no additional foods or liquids, if exclusively breast-feeding. Early introduction of these items may make successful breast-feeding difficult. Most breast-fed infants will not require any supplemental vitamins or minerals to meet daily requirements until at least six months of age.[86] **Vitamin D** (page 607) may be required for infants whose mothers are vitamin D-deficient or those infants not exposed to adequate sunlight. **Iron** (page 540) may be required for infants with low iron stores or **anemia** (page 25).[87]

Anxiety over milk supply

Breast milk is made on demand. The more often a baby feeds, the more milk will be produced. If breast-feeding sessions are frequent and long enough, the milk supply will rarely be inadequate. Parents can be reassured that their infants are receiving enough milk if they have six or more wet diapers a day while exclusively breast-feeding. If a parent still feels anxious about the adequacy of the nourishment provided by breast-feeding alone, weekly weighing may allay fears. A weight gain of 0.38 pound (190 grams) per week is evidence of sufficient nourishment and growth.

Some low-birth-weight infants will require intensive care and ventilation in the hospital. Mothers of these infants often have difficulty continuing to produce breast milk. These mothers must rely on expressing breast milk manually because their babies cannot effectively breast-feed. Pumping milk is much less efficient than breast-feeding. Due to the inadequacy of pumping milk, milk production can decline. In low-birth-weight infants in an intensive care setting, skin-to-skin holding over a four-week period postpartum has increased a mother's milk supply.[88] In contrast, women who did not participate in skin-to-skin holding of their low-birth-weight infants did not experience an increase in milk production. These findings may have implications for all mothers experiencing a diminishing milk supply. In addition, some doctors will prescribe a day of rest to busy mothers whose milk supply seems to be lessening.[89] Spending a day in close and relaxed contact with one's newborn, with its associated increase in frequency of feedings, can effectively increase milk supply.

Stress and fatigue can greatly inhibit the let-down reflex, lessening the production of milk. In a clinical trial involving mothers of premature infants, mothers who listened to an audiocassette tape based on relaxation and imagery techniques increased milk production by more than 60%, compared with mothers not listening to the tape.[90] Whether relaxation techniques would increase milk supply in the mothers of full-term infants is not known.

Nutritional supplements that may be helpful

Docosahexaenoic acid (page 509) (DHA), an omega-3 fatty acid present in **cod liver oil** (page 514) and other fish oils, is important for normal development of the brain and eyes. Studies have shown that higher concentrations of DHA in mothers' milk are associated with better visual acuity in the infants.[91] Other studies have suggested that DHA improves the development of infants, although not all research agrees.[92] Because DHA in the mother's diet passes into the breast milk,[93] some doctors advise nursing mothers to supplement their diet with cod liver oil or another fish-oil supplement. Women wishing to use this or any supplement while breast-feeding should consult their doctors and use only under the supervision of a qualified healthcare practitioner.

Are there any side effects or interactions?
Refer to the individual supplement for information about any side effects or interactions.

Herbs that may be helpful
Numerous herbs are used traditionally around the world to promote production of breast milk.[94] Herbs that promote milk production and flow are known as galactagogues. **Stinging nettle** (page 714) *(Urtica dioica)* enriches and increases the flow of breast milk and restores the mother's energy following childbirth.[95] **Vitex** (page 757) *(Vitex agnus castus)* is one of the best-recognized herbs in Europe for promoting lactation. An older German clinical trial found that 15 drops of a vitex tincture three times per day could increase the amount of milk produced by mothers with or without pregnancy complications compared with mothers given **vitamin B$_1$** (page 597) or nothing. Vitex should not be taken during **pregnancy** (page 363).[96] Goat's rue *(Galega officinalis)* also has a history of use in Europe for supporting breast-feeding. Taking 1 teaspoon of goat's rue tincture three times per day is considered by European practitioners to be helpful in increasing milk volume.[97] Studies are as yet lacking to support the use of goat's rue as a galactagogue. In two preliminary trials, infants have been shown to nurse longer when their mothers ate **garlic** (page 679) than when their mothers took placebos.[98, 99] However, some infants may develop **colic** (page 121) if they consume garlic in breast milk.

For sore nipples, some healthcare practitioners may recommend a warm, moist poultice of herbs with demulcent (soothing) properties. Demulcents are traditionally used to aid healing and soothe any irritated tissue. Examples of herbs traditionally used as demulcents to relieve sore nipples are **marigold** (page 650) *(Calendula officinalis)*, **comfrey** (page 662) *(Symphytum officinalis)*, and **chickweed** (page 658) *(Stellaria media)*. To prepare a poultice, the dried herbs are moistened with boiling water and wrapped within two layers of gauze. The poultice is then applied to the breasts. Application of a hot water bottle over the poultice will keep the poultice warm longer. Any residue should be washed from the breast before the baby breast-feeds. Individuals wishing to use herbs during breast-feeding should do so only under the supervision of a qualified healthcare practitioner.

The safety of using **anise** (page 627) during **pregnancy** (page 363) and breast-feeding is unknown, though it is very likely safe and has traditionally been used to support breast-feeding in some cultures.[100]

Are there any side effects or interactions?
Refer to the individual herb for information about any side effects or interactions.

BRITTLE NAILS

Brittle nails can be weak, thin, nails that peel or break easily, and/or grow slowly.

The common condition of brittle nails is often not definitively linked with any known cause. Nonetheless, natural medicine may be able to help strengthen brittle nails.

Most conditions that affect nails are unrelated to nutrition; they are caused by a lack of oxygen associated with lung conditions, hemorrhage due to infection, or inflammation around the nail due to infection. If there is any question about what the problem is, it is important to get a diagnosis from a healthcare practitioner.

Rating	Nutritional Supplements	Herbs
★★☆	**Biotin** (page 473) **Glucosamine** (page 528)	
★☆☆	Gelatin	**Horsetail** (page 693)

CHECKLIST FOR BRITTLE NAILS

What are the symptoms of brittle nails?
People with brittle nails may have frequent or easy breaking, cracking, splitting, or tearing of their nails.

Medical treatments
Therapy involves the intake of adequate nutrition; especially protein, **vitamin A** (page 595), **vitamin C** (page 604), **vitamin B$_6$** (page 600), **niacin** (page 598), **calcium** (page 483), and **iron** (page 539); the use of gloves when washing dishes, and the avoidance of drying chemicals, such as nail polish remover. Treatment of an underlying medical condition, such as thyroid deficiency or poor circulation, may be necessary.

Nutritional supplements that may be helpful

Nutrition can affect the health of nails in a variety of ways. **Iron deficiency** (page 278) may cause spoon-shaped nails.[1] For years, some doctors have believed **zinc** (page 614) deficiency causes white spots to appear on nails. In China, excessive **selenium** (page 584) has been linked to nails actually falling out.[2]

Biotin (page 473), a B vitamin, is known to strengthen hooves in animals. As a result, Swiss researchers investigated the use of biotin in strengthening brittle fingernails in humans, despite the fact that it remains unclear exactly how biotin affects nail structure. An uncontrolled trial of 2.5 mg biotin per day found improved firmness and hardness in almost all cases after an average treatment time of 5.5 months.[3] In a controlled trial using 2.5 mg of biotin per day, women with brittle nails, who had their nail thickness measured before and at six to fifteen months after, found their nail thickness increased by 25%. As a result, splitting of nails was reduced. In an uncontrolled study of people who had been taking biotin for brittle nails in America, 63% showed improvement from taking biotin.[4] Although the amount of research on the subject is quite limited and positive effects do not appear in all people, those people having brittle nails may want to consider a trial period of at least several months, using 2.5 mg per day of biotin.

Gelatin has been marketed as a remedy for brittle nails since the turn of the twentieth century and has been mentioned in medical journals at least since the 1950s.[5, 6, 7] Gelatin is a slaughterhouse byproduct, made from the hooves and other inedible connective tissue of cows. While some people claim success using gelatin to strengthen brittle nails, others claim that the remedy is ineffective,[8, 9] and that the real cause of brittle nails is lack of moisture, not protein deficiency.

One doctor has observed that supplementation with **glucosamine** (page 528) sulfate (amount not specified) can increase the growth rate and strength of fingernails and toenails;[10] however, no controlled trials have been done.

Are there any side effects or interactions?
Refer to the individual supplement for information about any side effects or interactions.

Herbs that may be helpful

Anecdotal reports suggest that **horsetail** (page 693) may be of some use in the treatment of brittle nails.[11]

This may be due to the high content of silicic acid and silicates in horsetail, which provide approximately 2 to 3% elemental **silicon** (page 586).

Are there any side effects or interactions?
Refer to the individual herb for information about any side effects or interactions.

BRONCHITIS

Bronchitis is an inflammation of the mucous membranes of the deep inner lung passages called the bronchial tree.

Bronchitis may be either acute or chronic. Acute bronchitis is frequently caused by a viral or bacterial **infection** (page 265). Acute bronchitis may also result from irritation of the mucous membranes by environmental fumes, acids, solvents, or tobacco smoke. Bronchitis usually begins with a dry, nonproductive cough. After a few hours or days, the cough may become more frequent and produce mucus. A secondary bacterial infection may occur, in which the sputum (bronchial secretions) may contain pus. People whose cough and/or fever continues for more than seven days should visit a medical practitioner.

Chronic bronchitis may result from prolonged exposure to bronchial irritants. Cigarette smoking, environmental toxins, and inhaled **allergens** (page 14) can all cause chronic irritation of the bronchi. The cells lining the bronchi produce excess mucus in response to the chronic irritation; this excess mucus production can lead to a chronic, productive cough.

Bronchitis can be particularly dangerous in the elderly and in people with compromised **immune systems** (page 255). These people should see a doctor if they develop a respiratory infection.

What are the symptoms of bronchitis?

Acute infectious bronchitis is often preceded by signs of an upper respiratory tract infection: stuffy or runny nose, malaise, chills, fever, muscle pain, and **sore throat** (page 129). The cough is initially dry and does not produce mucus. Later, small amounts of thick green or green-yellow sputum may be coughed up.

Chronic bronchitis is characterized by a productive cough that initially occurs only in the morning.

CHECKLIST FOR BRONCHITIS

Rating	Nutritional Supplements	Herbs
★★★	**N-acetyl cysteine** (page 562) **Thymus extracts** (page 591) **Vitamin C** (page 604)	
★★☆	**Vitamin A** (page 595) (for deficiency only) **Vitamin E** (page 609)	Geranium (*Pelargonium sidoides*) **Ivy leaf** (page 697) **Plantain** (page 729)
★☆☆		**Anise** (page 627) **Chinese scullcap** (page 658) **Echinacea** (page 669) **Elecampane** (page 671) **Eucalyptus** (page 673) **Horehound** (page 691) **Horseradish** (page 693) **Lobelia** (page 705) **Mullein** (page 713) **Pleurisy root** (page 730) **Thyme** (page 752)

Medical treatments

Over the counter drugs used to treat the symptoms of bronchitis include the expectorant guaifenesin (Robitussin) and the cough suppressant dextromethorphan (DM), which are usually found in combination (Robitussin DM, Vicks 44E Liquid, Benylin Expectorant Liquid).

Antibiotics, which require a prescription, are used when the sputum becomes dark green or yellow, indicating a bacterial infection. Agents used include the tetracycline doxycycline (Vibramycin), trimethoprim/sulfamethoxazole (Bactrim, Septra), amoxicillin/clavulanate (Augmentin), and azithromycin (Zithromax). Symptomatic treatment of cough may be given to aid sleep; however daytime use of antitussives (cough suppressants) should be limited in order to clear infected mucous from the lungs. Antitussives that require a prescription include codeine (Robitussin A-C Syrup) and hydrocodone (Vicodin Tuss Syrup, Tussionex).

Rest and increased fluid intake are recommended in the fever stage of acute bronchitis. Treatment of chronic bronchitis includes smoking cessation and a variety of drugs directed at relieving symptoms and treating superimposed bacterial infections.

Dietary changes that may be helpful

Dietary factors may influence both inflammatory activity and **antioxidant** (page 467) status in the body. Increased inflammation and decreased antioxidant activity may each lead to an increased incidence of chronic diseases, such as chronic bronchitis. People suffering from chronic bronchitis may experience an improvement in symptoms when consuming a diet high in anti-inflammatory fatty acids, such as those found in fish. In a double-blind study of children with recurrent respiratory tract infections, a daily essential-fatty-acid supplement (containing 855 mg of alpha-linolenic acid and 596 mg of linoleic acid) reduced both the number and the duration of recurrences.[1]

In people with bronchitis, lipids in the lung tissue may undergo oxidation damage (also called **free-radical** [page 467] damage), particularly when the bronchitis is a result of exposure to environmental toxins or cigarette smoke. A diet high in **antioxidants** (page 467) may protect against the free radical-damaging effect of these toxins. Studies comparing different populations have shown that increasing fruit and vegetable (and therefore, antioxidant) consumption may reduce the risk of developing chronic bronchitis.[2, 3]

Food and environmental **allergies** (page 14) may be triggering factors in some cases of chronic bronchitis.[4] Cows' milk allergy has been associated with bronchitis in children,[5, 6, 7] and some doctors believe that dairy products may increase mucus production and, therefore, that people suffering from either acute or chronic bronchitis should limit their intake of dairy products. Ingestion of simple sugars (such as sucrose or fructose) can lead to suppression of **immune function** (page 255);[8] therefore, some doctors believe simple sugars should be avoided during illness.

Lifestyle changes that may be helpful

Breast-feeding provides important nutrients to an infant and improves the functioning of the immune system. Studies have shown that breast-feeding prevents the development of lower respiratory tract infections during infancy.[9, 10] Whether that protective effect persists into adulthood is not known. Exposure to environmental

Bronchitis

chemicals, including passive smoke, can increase the incidence of respiratory illness among children.[11]

Chronic bronchitis is frequently associated with smoking and/or environmental exposure to chemicals or **allergens** (page 14). These exposures should be avoided to allow the cells of the bronchi to recover from chronic irritation and to decrease the burden on the **immune system** (page 255).

Nutritional supplements that may be helpful

In a double-blind study of elderly patients hospitalized with acute bronchitis, those who were given 200 mg per day of **vitamin C** (page 604) improved to a significantly greater extent than those who were given a placebo.[12] The **common cold** (page 129) may lead to bronchitis in susceptible people, and numerous controlled studies, some double-blind, have shown that vitamin C supplements can decrease the severity and duration of the common cold in otherwise healthy people.[13]

Vitamin C and **vitamin E** (page 609) may prevent oxidative damage to the lung lipids by environmental pollution and cigarette smoke exposure. It has been suggested that amounts in excess of the RDA (recommended dietary allowance) are necessary to protect against the air pollution levels currently present in North America,[14] although it is not known how much vitamin E is needed to produce that protective effect.

A review of 39 clinical trials of **N-acetyl cysteine** (page 542) (NAC) found that 400 to 600 mg per day was a safe and effective treatment for chronic bronchitis.[15] NAC supplementation was found to reduce the number of aggravations of the illness in almost 50% of people taking the supplement, compared with only 31% of those taking placebo. Smokers have also been found to benefit from taking NAC.[16] In addition to helping break up mucus, NAC may reduce the elevated bacterial counts that are often seen in the lungs of smokers with chronic bronchitis.[17] In another double-blind study, people with chronic bronchitis who took NAC showed an improved ability to expectorate and a reduction in cough severity.[18] These benefits may result from NAC's capacity to reduce the viscosity (thickness) of sputum.[19]

Vitamin A (page 595) levels are low in children with **measles** (page 307),[20] an **infection** (page 265) that can result in pneumonia or other respiratory complications. A number of studies have shown that supplementation with vitamin A decreased complications and deaths from measles in children living in developing countries where deficiencies of vitamin A are common.[21] However, little to no positive effect, and even slight *adverse* effects, have resulted from giving vitamin A supplements to prevent or treat infections in people living in countries where most people consume adequate amounts of vitamin A.[22, 23, 24, 25, 26, 27] Therefore, vitamin A supplements may only be useful for people with bronchial infections who are known to be deficient in vitamin A.

The thymus gland plays a number of important roles in the functioning of the **immune system** (page 255). **Thymus extract** (page 591) from calves, known as Thymomodulin, has been found, in a double-blind study, to decrease the frequency of respiratory infections in children who were prone to such infections.[28] The amount of Thymomodulin used in that study was 3 mg per kg of body weight per day.

Are there any side effects or interactions?
Refer to the individual supplement for information about any side effects or interactions.

Herbs that may be helpful

Several types of herbs may help people with bronchitis, either by treating underlying **infection** (page 265), by relieving inflammation, or by relieving symptoms such as cough. For clarity, the table below summarizes which herbs are in each category of action. Some herbs have more than one action. Herbs listed in the table have not necessarily been proven to be effective. The herbs are discussed in more detail following the table.

Action	Botanicals Supported by Clinical Trials	Botanicals Used Traditionally
Expectorant (helps remove mucus)		**Anise** (page 627), **horehound** (page 691), **horseradish** (page 693), **mullein** (page 713), **pleurisy root** (page 730)
Anti-inflammatory	**Chinese scullcap** (page 658), **ivy leaf** (page 697), **plantain** (page 729)	**Elecampane** (page 671), **marshmallow** (page 708), **mullein** (page 713), **slippery elm** (page 747)

Action	Botanicals Supported by Clinical Trials	Botanicals Used Traditionally
Fights infection	Echinacea (page 669) (by stimulating immune system), lavender (page 701), thyme (page 752)	Eucalyptus (page 673), horseradish (page 693)
Antitussive (relieves cough)		Lobelia (page 705), marshmallow (page 708)
Relieves broncho-spasms or spasmodic cough		Lobelia (page 705), thyme (page 752)

Expectorant herbs help loosen bronchial secretions and make elimination of mucus easier. Numerous herbs are traditionally considered expectorants, though most of these have not been proven to have this effect in clinical trials. **Anise** (page 627) contains a volatile oil that is high in the chemical constituent anethole and acts as an expectorant.[29]

Horehound (page 691) has expectorant properties, possibly due to the presence of a diterpene lactone in the plant, which is known as marrubiin.[30]

Mullein (page 713) has been used traditionally as a remedy for the respiratory tract, including bronchitis. The saponins in mullein may be responsible for its expectorant actions.[31]

Pleurisy root (page 730) is an expectorant and is thought to be helpful against all types of respiratory infections. It is traditionally employed as an expectorant for bronchitis. However, owing to the cardiac glycosides it contains, pleurisy root may not be safe to use if one is taking (heart medications.)[32] This herb should not be used by **pregnant** (page 363) women.

Anti-inflammatory herbs may help people with bronchitis. Often these herbs contain complex polysaccharides and have a soothing effect; they are also known as demulcents. **Plantain** (page 729) is a demulcent that has been documented in two preliminary trials conducted in Bulgaria to help people with chronic bronchitis.[33, 34] Other demulcents traditionally used for people with bronchitis include mullein, **marshmallow** (page 708), and **slippery elm** (page 747). Because demulcents can provoke production of more mucus in the lungs, they tend to be used more often in people with dry coughs.[35]

Elecampane (page 671) is a demulcent that has been used to treat coughs associated with bronchitis, **asthma** (page 32), and whooping cough. Although there have been no modern clinical studies with this herb, its use for these indications is based on its high content of soothing mucilage in the forms of inulin and alantalactone.[36] However, the German Commission E monograph for elecampane does not approve the herb for bronchitis.[37]

Geranium *(Pelargonium sidoides)* is an herbal remedy used in Germany, Mexico, Russia, and other countries for the treatment of **respiratory tract** (page 265) and **ear, nose, and throat infections** (page 383). In a double-blind study of adults with acute bronchitis, participants given an extract of geranium had a significantly shorter duration of illness, compared with those given a placebo.[38] No serious side effects were seen. The amount of the geranium extract used in this study was 30 drops three times per day, taken before or after meals for seven days.

Ivy leaf (page 697) is approved in the German Commission E monograph for use against chronic inflammatory bronchial conditions.[39] One double-blind human trial found ivy leaf to be as effective as the drug ambroxol for chronic bronchitis.[40] Ivy leaf is a nondemulcent anti-inflammatory.

Chinese scullcap (page 658) might be useful for bronchitis as an anti-inflammatory. However, the research on this herb is generally of low quality.[41]

Antimicrobial and immune stimulating herbs may also potentially benefit people with bronchitis. **Echinacea** (page 669) is widely used by herbalists for people with acute respiratory infections. This herb stimulates the **immune system** (page 255) in several different ways, including enhancing macrophage function and increasing T-cell response.[42] Therefore, echinacea may be useful for preventing a **cold** (page 129), **flu** (page 269), or viral bronchitis from progressing to a secondary bacterial infection.

Thyme (page 752) contains an essential oil (thymol) and certain **flavonoids** (page 516). This plant has antispasmodic, expectorant, and antibacterial actions, and it is considered helpful in cases of bronchitis.[43] One preliminary trial found that a mixture containing volatile oils of thyme, mint, clove, **cinnamon** (page 659), and **lavender** (page 701) diluted in alcohol, in the amount of 20 drops three times daily, reduced the number of recurrent **infections** (page 265) in people with chronic bronchitis.[44]

Horseradish (page 693) contains substances similar to mustard, such as glucosinolates and allyl isothiocynate.[45] In addition to providing possible antibacterial actions, these substances may also have expectorant properties that are supportive for persons with bronchitis.

Eucalyptus (page 673) leaf tea is used to treat bronchitis and inflammation of the throat,[46] and is considered antimicrobial. In traditional herbal medicine, eucalyptus tea or volatile oil is often used internally as well as externally over the chest; both uses are approved for people with bronchitis by the German Commission E.[47]

Lobelia (page 705) contains many active alkaloids, of which lobeline is considered the most active. Very small amounts of this herb are considered helpful as an antispasmodic and antitussive agent (a substance that helps suppress or ease coughs). Anti-inflammatory properties of the herb have been demonstrated, which may be useful, since bronchitis is associated with inflammation in the bronchi.[48] Lobelia should be used cautiously, as it may cause nausea and vomiting.

Are there any side effects or interactions?
Refer to the individual herb for information about any side effects or interactions.

BRUISING

Bruising occurs after traumatic injury and consists of swelling and discoloration under the skin but no disruption of the skin.

Bruising is a normal body response to trauma. It is only when bruising occurs often and from very minor (often unnoticed) trauma that a problem may exist. Refer to the **capillary fragility** (page 93) article for more information. While easy bruising is usually not a cause for concern, people who experience this problem should consult a physician to rule out more serious conditions that may cause bruising. Medical causes of easy bruising sometimes may be diagnosed from a few blood tests conducted by a doctor. More often, however, no clear cause for easy bruising is found.

What are the symptoms of bruising?
Bruises look like areas of blue to purple-colored skin that may turn yellow to dark brown over the course of a few days.

CHECKLIST FOR BRUISING

Rating	Nutritional Supplements	Herbs
★★★	**Vitamin C** (page 604) (only if deficient)	
★★☆	**Flavonoids** (page 516)	
★☆☆		Arnica (topical) **Comfrey** (page 662) (topical) Sweet clover

Medical treatments
The primary focus in the treatment of bruising is the diagnosis and management of any underlying medical condition. Conditions such as liver or kidney disease; blood disorders, such as hemophilia, platelet dysfunction, thrombocytopenia, leukemia, and multiple myeloma; connective tissue disorders including scurvy, Marfan's syndrome, and Ehlers-Danlos syndrome; or the use of blood-thinning medication, such as aspirin (Bayer, Ecotrin, Bufferin) and warfarin (Coumadin), should be considered.

Dietary changes that may be helpful
Even minor dietary deficiencies of **vitamin C** (page 604) can lead to increased bruising. People who experience easy bruising may benefit from eating more fruits and vegetables—common dietary sources of vitamin C and **flavonoids** (page 516).

Nutritional supplements that may be helpful
Doctors often suggest that people who experience easy bruising supplement with 100 mg to 3 grams of **vitamin C** (page 604) per day for several months. Controlled research is limited, but vitamin C supplements have been shown to reduce bruising in people with low vitamin C intake.[1] **Flavonoids** (page 516) are often recommended along with vitamin C. Flavonoids are vitamin-like substances that can help strengthen capillaries and therefore may also help with bruising.[2] Flavonoids may also increase the effectiveness of vitamin C; citrus flavonoids, in particular, improve the absorption of vitamin C. Older preliminary research suggested that vitamin C, 400–800 mg per day, in combination with 400–800 mg per day of the flavonoid, hesperidin, reduced bruising in **menopausal** (page 311) women.[3] A small, preliminary trial in Germany gave three people with

progressive pigmented purpura (a chronic bruising disorder) 1,000 mg per day of vitamin C and 100 mg per day of the flavonoid rutoside. After four weeks, noticeable bruising was no longer apparent and did not recur in the three month period after treatment was stopped.[4] Controlled research is needed to better establish whether vitamin C and flavonoids are effective for easy bruising.

Are there any side effects or interactions?
Refer to the individual supplement for information about any side effects or interactions.

Herbs that may be helpful

In traditional herbal medicine, a compress or ointment of sweet clover is applied to bruises.[5, 6] Enough should be applied to cover the bruise, and several applications per day may be necessary to improve healing.

Arnica is considered by some practitioners to be among the best vulnerary (wound-healing) herbs available.[7] As a homeopathic remedy, arnica is often recommended as both an internal and topical means to treat minor injuries. Some healthcare practitioners recommend mixing 1 tablespoon of arnica tincture in 500 ml water, then soaking thin cloth or gauze in the liquid and applying it to the injured area for at least 15 minutes four to five times per day.

Comfrey (page 662) is also widely used in traditional medicine as a topical application to help heal wounds.[8]

Are there any side effects or interactions?
Refer to the individual herb for information about any side effects or interactions.

BURNS

Burns are damage to tissue that can result from exposure to extreme heat, chemicals, electricity, or radioactive material.

For minor burns, natural medicine may be helpful after the burn is cleaned with soap and cold water and gently dried. Because of the risk of **infection** (page 265), topical applications should not be made to blistered or open burn wounds, unless under medical supervision. Extensive burns or burns causing more than minor discomfort should be treated by a healthcare professional.

CHECKLIST FOR MINOR BURNS		
Rating	Nutritional Supplements	Herbs
★★★	**Vitamin C** (page 604), in combination with **Vitamin E** (page 609) (for prevention of sunburn only)	
★★☆	**Vitamin D** (page 607) (for extensive burns)	**Aloe** (page 624)
★☆☆	**Colloidal silver** (page 498) **Vitamin E** (page 609) (topical, for minor burns)	**Calendula** (page 649) **Gotu kola** (page 684) **Plantain** (page 728) (topical)

What are the symptoms of burns?

Symptoms depend on the severity and cause of the burn but usually include **pain** (page 338) and sensitivity to touch. The skin may appear swollen, blistered, dried, charred, weeping, or red, gray, or black-colored.

Medical treatments

Over the counter lotions, creams, and sprays are used to provide temporary relief of pain due to minor burns. Some products contain a local anesthetic, such as lidocaine (Solarcaine Aloe Extra Burn Relief) and benzocaine (Solarcaine, Americaine Anesthetic, Lanacane, Dermoplast). Other products contain vitamins A, D, and E (A and D Ointment, Coppertone Cool Beads), as well as *Aloe vera* (page 624) (Pacquin Plus with Aloe, Coppertone Cool Beads).

The prescription medications silver sulfadiazine (Silvadene) and mafenide (Sulfamylon) are used topically to prevent and treat uncomplicated bacterial **infection** (page 265) in second and third degree burns, as are oral antibiotics such as levofloxacin (Levaquin) and cephalexin (Keflex).

Severe burns require hospitalization. They are typically treated by surgical removal of burned tissue followed by grafting of skin or synthetic substitutes.

Dietary changes that may be helpful

The body repairs and builds new tissues in a process called anabolism. Adequate amounts of calories and protein are required for anabolism, as the skin and underlying tissues are comprised of protein and energy is needed to fuel repair mechanisms. While major injuries requiring hospitalization raise protein and calorie requirements significantly, injuries such as minor burns should not require changes from a typical, healthful diet.[1]

Nutritional supplements that may be helpful

Antioxidants (page 467) may protect the skin from sunburn due to **free radical** (page 467)-producing ultraviolet rays.[2] Combinations of 1,000 to 2,000 IU per day of **vitamin E** (page 609) and 2,000 to 3,000 mg per day of **vitamin C** (page 604), but neither given alone, have a significant protective effect against ultraviolet rays, according to double-blind studies.[3, 4, 5] Oral synthetic **beta-carotene** (page 469) alone was not found to provide effective protection in a recent double-blind study,[6] it may be effective in combination with topical sunscreen.[7] However, other **carotenoids** (page 488) such as **lycopene** (page 548) may be more important for ultraviolet protection. One recent uncontrolled trial found 40 grams per day of tomato paste providing 16 mg per day lycopene for 10 weeks protected against burning by ultraviolet rays.[8] Another uncontrolled trial found 25 mg/day of natural mixed carotenoids also protected against ultraviolet radiation, especially when combined with 500 IU per day of vitamin E.[9]

Double-blind research has also shown that topical application of antioxidants protects against sunburn if used before,[10] but not after, exposure.[11, 12]

Despite a lack of research on the subject, using **vitamin E** (page 609) topically on minor burns is a popular remedy. This makes sense, because some of the damage done to the skin is oxidative, and vitamin E is an antioxidant. Some doctors suggest simply breaking open a capsule of vitamin E and applying it to the affected area two or three times per day. Vitamin E forms are listed as either "tocopherol" or "tocopheryl" followed by the name of what is attached to it, as in "tocopheryl acetate." While both forms are active when taken by mouth, the skin utilizes the tocopheryl forms very slowly.[13, 14] Therefore, those planning to apply vitamin E to the skin should buy the tocopherol form.

Burns affecting a large proportion of the body may result in **vitamin D** (page 607) deficiency[15], potentially increasing the risk of osteoporosis, which is a frequent long-term consequence of severe burns.[16]

Colloidal silver (page 498) has been used as a topical antiseptic for minor burns for over a century. Internal use of colloidal silver is not recommended for this condition.

Are there any side effects or interactions?
Refer to the individual supplement for information about any side effects or interactions.

Herbs that may be helpful

Aloe (page 624) is another popular remedy for minor burns and a small preliminary study found it more effective than Vaseline in treating burns.[17] The stabilized aloe gel is typically applied to the affected area of skin three to five times per day. Older case studies reported that aloe gel applied topically could help heal radiation burns,[18] but a large, double-blind trial did not find aloe effective in this regard.[19]

Calendula (page 649) cream may be applied to minor burns to soothe **pain** (page 338) and help promote tissue repair. It has been shown in animal studies to be anti-inflammatory[20] and to aid repair of damaged tissues.[21] The cream is applied three times per day. **Plantain** (page 728) is regarded as similar to calendula in traditional medicine, though usually the whole leaf is applied directly to the burn as a poultice.

Gotu kola (page 684) has been used in the medicinal systems of central Asia for centuries to treat numerous skin diseases. Saponins in gotu kola beneficially affect collagen (the material that makes up connective tissue) to inhibit its production in hyperactive scar tissue following burns or wounds.[22]

Are there any side effects or interactions?
Refer to the individual herb for information about any side effects or interactions.

Holistic approaches that may be helpful

Acupuncture may be useful in the treatment of serious burns. A report of patients suffering from extensive second-degree burns suggests acupuncture can reduce shock and **pain** (page 338) following the acute injury and may reduce **infection** (page 265) and pain when used as a part of post-injury wound care.[23] A preliminary report described ten patients with second-degree burns that did not respond to conventional medical treatment. A majority of these patients achieved greater than 90% recovery following electrical stimulation to the wound (similar to electroacupuncture).[24] Ear (auricular) acupuncture with electrical stimulation was studied in a small controlled trial, in which a significantly greater reduction in pain from burns was achieved with acupuncture. The relief lasted at least 60 minutes following acupuncture treatment.[25]

BURSITIS

Bursitis is an inflammation of one or more bursa (fluid-filled sacs that reduce friction around joints).

The most common bursa to become inflamed is in the shoulder. The cause of bursitis is mostly unknown, but trauma or arthritis may be involved.

Rating	Nutritional Supplements	Herbs
★☆☆	Vitamin B$_{12}$ (page 601)	Boswellia (page 644) Cayenne (page 654) Turmeric (page 753) Willow (page 760)

CHECKLIST FOR BURSITIS

What are the symptoms of bursitis?

Acute bursitis causes **pain** (page 338), tenderness over the inflamed bursa, and limited range of motion. Chronic bursitis attacks may follow acute bursitis, unusual exercise, or strain. Attacks may last a few days to several weeks and are characterized by pain, swelling, and tenderness.

Medical treatments

Over the counter nonsteroidal anti-inflammatory drugs (NSAIDs), including aspirin (Bayer, Ecotrin, Bufferin), ibuprofen (Advil, Motrin, Nuprin), and naproxen (Aleve), may be adequate to treat the pain associated with bursitis.

Prescription strength NSAIDs, such as celecoxib (Celebrex), valdecoxib (Bextra), ibuprofen (Motrin), naproxen (Anaprox, Naprosyn), etodolac (Lodine), and indomethacin (Indocin), are prescribed when over the counter products are ineffective. Narcotic pain-relievers including codeine (Tylenol with Codeine) and hydrocodone (Vicodin, Lortab) are also used. Oral corticosteroids such as prednisone (Deltasone) and methylprednisolone (Medrol) are often prescribed to reduce pain and inflammation. Corticosteroid injections such as methylprednisolone (Depo-Medrol) may be necessary to reduce inflammation in chronic, severe cases. For non-infected, acute bursitis, injections of the local anesthetic lidocaine (Xylocaine) may be used if other remedies don't adequately relieve pain.

Nutritional supplements that may be helpful

In a preliminary study, intramuscular injections of **vitamin B$_{12}$** (page 601)[1, 2] relieved the symptoms of acute subdeltoid (shoulder) bursitis and also decreased the amount of calcification in some cases. This mechanism is not understood. Oral B vitamins are unlikely to have the same effect, since the body's absorption of vitamin B$_{12}$ is quite limited. A doctor should be consulted regarding B$_{12}$ or B$_{12}$/**niacin** (page 598) injections.

Are there any side effects or interactions?
Refer to the individual supplement for information about any side effects or interactions.

Herbs that may be helpful

While there have been few studies on herbal therapy for bursitis, most practitioners would consider using anti-inflammatory herbs that have proven useful in conditions such as **rheumatoid arthritis** (page 387). These would include **boswellia** (page 644), **turmeric** (page 753), **willow** (page 760), and topical **cayenne** (page 654) ointment.

Are there any side effects or interactions?
Refer to the individual herb for information about any side effects or interactions.

CANCER PREVENTION AND DIET

See also: **Breast Cancer** (page 65), **Colon Cancer** (page 123), **Lung Cancer** (page 298), **Prostate Cancer** (page 371)

What do I need to know?

Self-care for cancer prevention can be approached in a number of ways—but it can be hard to know just where to start. To make it easier, our doctors recommend trying these simple steps first:

Get regular checkups
   Many cancers can be prevented or discovered in the early stages with screening tests available through your healthcare provider

Go vegetarian
   Eat more vegetables (especially tomatoes and cruciferous vegetables), fruits, whole grains, and legumes to help optimize body weight, immune function, hormone regulation, and to avoid

meat-related carcinogens, all of which may influence cancer risk

Focus on fiber

Eat foods rich in fiber, especially those made with whole grains, to help reduce the risk of several cancers

Find healthy fats

More meals containing olive oil or fish help protect against cancer, and avoiding fat from meat, dairy, and processed foods, may decrease cancer risk

Avoid alcohol

Use alcoholic beverages in moderation or not at all to reduce the risk of many cancers

About cancer prevention and diet

Cancer refers to a large number of diseases categorized by unregulated replication of cells.

The contents of this article are limited to information about diet and to a discussion of cancer prevention—not treatment. Prevention of cancer in a person who has never had cancer is called "primary" prevention. Primary prevention is the focus of this article.

This article includes a discussion of studies that have assessed whether certain dietary ingredients may be beneficial in connection with the reduction of risk of developing cancer.

This information is provided solely to aid consumers in discussing supplements with their healthcare providers. It is not advised nor is this information intended to advocate, promote, or encourage self-use of this information for cancer risk reduction. Some studies suggest an association between high blood or dietary levels of a particular dietary ingredient with a reduced risk of developing cancer. Even if such an association were established, this does not mean that dietary supplements containing large amounts of the dietary ingredient will necessarily have a cancer risk reduction effect.

Prevention of a recurrence in a cancer patient who is in remission is called "secondary" prevention. Whether the information in this article would be helpful to people interested in secondary prevention is, for the most part, unknown. However, of cancer patients who are in complete remission, the information presented here is unlikely to help people who were ever diagnosed with metastatic cancer (also known as stage IV, or advanced, cancer).

Cancer is the second leading cause of death in Americans. Information on the prevention of breast, colon, lung, and prostate cancers is not provided in this article. To find out more about these specific forms of cancer, read the **Breast Cancer** (page 65), **Colon Cancer** (page 123), **Lung Cancer** (page 298), and **Prostate Cancer** (page 371) articles.

Dietary changes that may be helpful

The following dietary changes have been studied in connection with cancer.

Alcohol and cancer

Alcohol consumption significantly increases the risk of cancers of the mouth (oral/oropharyngeal cancer), throat (esophageal cancer), and voice box (laryngeal cancer), particularly in conjunction with cigarette smoking.[1, 2, 3] Most studies documenting these associations also report that former drinkers have significantly lower risks for these cancers compared with current drinkers. Strong correlations between alcohol consumption and the risk of having liver cancer have also been reported.[4, 5]

Little is known about the effect of alcohol intake on the risk of female cancers other than breast cancer. Of the few published studies, findings have been inconsistent.[6, 7, 8, 9]

Fiber *(page 512)*

Whole grains (such as rye, brown rice, and whole wheat) contain high amounts of insoluble fiber—the type of fiber some scientists believe may help protect against a variety of cancers. In an analysis of the data from many studies, people who eat relatively high amounts of whole grains were reported to have low risks of lymphomas and cancers of the pancreas, stomach, colon, rectum, breast, uterus, mouth, throat, liver, and thyroid.[10] Most research focusing on the relationship between cancer and fiber has focused on breast and colon cancers.

Consuming a diet high in insoluble fiber is best achieved by switching from white rice to brown rice and from bakery goods made with white flour or mixed flours to 100% whole wheat bread, whole rye crackers, and whole grain pancake mixes. Refined white flour is generally listed on food packaging labels as "flour," "enriched flour," "unbleached flour," "durum wheat," "semolina," or "white flour." Breads containing only whole wheat are often labeled "100% whole wheat."

Vegetarianism

The following two possibilities are both strongly supported by research findings:

- Some foods consumed by vegetarians may protect against cancer.
- Eating meat may increase the risk of cancer.

Compared with meat eaters, most,[11] but not all,[12] studies have found that vegetarians are less likely to be diagnosed with cancer. Vegetarians have also been shown to have stronger **immune function** (page 255), possibly explaining why vegetarians may be partially protected against cancer.[13] Female vegetarians have been reported to have lower estrogen levels compared with meat-eating women, possibly explaining a lower incidence of uterine and breast cancers.[14] A reduced risk for various cancers is only partly,[15] not totally,[16] explained by differences in body weight, smoking habits, and other lifestyle issues.

Fruits and vegetables

Consumption of fruits and vegetables is widely accepted as lowering the risk of most common cancers.[17] Many doctors recommend that people wishing to reduce their risk of cancer eat several pieces of fruit and several portions of vegetables every day. Optimal intakes remain unknown.

Most doctors also recommend that people should not consider supplements as substitutes for the real thing. Some of the anticancer substances found in produce have probably not yet been discovered, while others are not yet available in supplement form. More important, some research, particularly regarding synthetic **beta-carotene** (page 469), does not support the idea that taking supplements has the same protective value against cancer as does consumption of fruits and vegetables.

Flavonoids *(page 516)*

Flavonoids are found in virtually all herbs and plant foods. Consumption of flavonoid-rich onions and apples contain large amounts of one flavonoid called **quercetin** (page 580). Consumption of flavonoids in general, or quercetin-containing foods in particular,[18] has been associated with protection against cancer in some,[19] but not all,[20] preliminary studies.

Tomatoes

Tomatoes contain **lycopene** (page 548)—an **antioxidant** (page 467) similar in structure to **beta-carotene** (page 469). Most lycopene in our diet comes from tomatoes, though traces of lycopene exist in other foods. Lycopene inhibits the proliferation of cancer cells in test tube research.[21]

A review of published research found that higher intake of tomatoes or higher blood levels of lycopene correlated with protection from cancer in 57 of 72 studies. Findings in 35 of these studies were statistically significant.[22] Evidence of a protective effect for tomato con-

sumption was strongest for cancers of the prostate, lung, and stomach, but some evidence of a protective effect also appeared for cancers of the pancreas, colon, rectum, esophagus (throat), mouth, breast, and cervix.

Cruciferous vegetables

Cabbage, Brussels sprouts, broccoli, and cauliflower belong to the Brassica family of vegetables, also known as "cruciferous" vegetables. In test tube and animal studies, these foods have been associated with anticancer activity,[23] possibly due to several substances found in these foods, such as **indole-3-carbinol** (page 536),[24] glucaric acid (**calcium D-glucarate** [page 486]),[25] and **sulforaphane** (page 589).[26] In a preliminary human study, people who ate cruciferous vegetables were reported to have a lower-than-average risk for bladder cancer.[27]

Meat (how it is cooked) and childhood cancers

In one report, high consumption of hot dogs was associated with an almost tenfold increase in the risk of childhood leukemia when compared with low consumption.[28] In another report, maternal consumption of hot dogs and childhood consumption of hamburgers or hot dogs at least once per week were associated with a doubling of the risk of cancers in children.[29] A review of nine studies found an association between consumption by pregnant women of cured meat and the risk of brain cancer in their offspring.[30] These associations do not yet constitute proof that eating hot dogs or hamburgers causes cancer in children, and evidence linking cured meat consumption to childhood cancers remains somewhat inconsistent.[31]

In the report studying the effects of eating hot dogs and hamburgers, the association between meat eating and leukemia was weakest among children who took **vitamin supplements** (page 559). Processed meats, such as hot dogs, contain nitrates and nitrites—precursors to carcinogens. **Antioxidants** (page 467) found in multivitamins keep nitrates and nitrites from converting into those carcinogens. Therefore, the association between vitamin consumption in children and protection against childhood cancers remains plausible, though unproven.

Fish

Fish eaters have been reported to have low risks of cancers of the mouth, throat, stomach, colon, rectum, pancreas,[32] lung,[33] breast,[34] and prostate.[35] The **omega-3 fatty acids** (page 509) found in fish are thought by some researchers to be the components of fish responsible for protection against cancer.[36]

Coffee

Years ago, researchers reported the greater the consumption of coffee in a country, the higher the risk of pancreatic cancer in that country.[37] An analysis of data from studies published between 1981 and 1993 did find some association between high consumption of coffee and an increased risk of pancreatic cancer.[38] Surprisingly, however, the same report found that people drinking only one or two cups of coffee per day had, on average, a *lower* risk of pancreatic cancer compared with people who never drink coffee.

Most,[39, 40, 41] but not all,[42] published reports have shown coffee drinkers are at increased risk of bladder cancer, though in one case the relationship was found only in men.[43] In another study, the association was found only with caffeinated coffee.[44] A review of 35 trials found a small (7%) increased risk of bladder cancer in coffee drinkers compared with people not drinking coffee—a difference not statistically significant.[45]

Calories

Scientists have known for many years that severe restriction of calories dramatically reduces the risk of cancer in laboratory animals.[46] Scientists speculate that caloric content of the human diet may also affect cancer rates,[47] though much less is known about the effect, if any, of moderate caloric restrictions in humans. In one report, adults with cancer were more likely to have consumed more calories during childhood compared with healthy adults.[48] In other reports, attempts to find associations between reduced intake of calories and cancer have produced mixed results.[49, 50, 51]

Only *severe* restriction in caloric intake provides significant protection in animal studies. As most people are unlikely to severely restrict calories, the association between caloric restriction and protection from cancer may ultimately prove to only be of academic interest.

Dietary fat

In studying data from country to country, incidence of ovarian cancer correlates with dietary fat intake.[52] According to preliminary research, consumption of saturated fat, dietary cholesterol (as found in eggs),[53] and animal fat in general[54] correlates with the risk of ovarian cancer.

Preliminary studies suggest dietary fat may correlate with the risk of uterine cancer.[55] Some of the excess risk appears to result from increased body weight that results from a high-fat diet.[56]

Many years ago, researchers reported that animals on a high-fat diet formed skin cancers more rapidly than did other animals.[57] Although some preliminary human research has found no relationship between dietary fat intake and the risk of skin cancer,[58] patients with basal cell and squamous cell skin cancers who were put on a low-fat diet for two years were reported to show a significant decrease in the number of new skin cancers compared with patients who maintained a high-fat diet.[59] Similarly, precancerous lesions of the skin have been prevented in people put on a low-fat diet.[60]

Polyunsaturated fats

A chain of carbon atoms in which several are not attached to the maximum possible amount of hydrogen is called "polyunsaturated"—in other words, unsaturated with hydrogen in several places. When nutrition researchers talk about polyunsaturated fatty acids, they are often referring primarily to linoleic acid—a fatty acid found in nuts and seeds and most vegetable oils.

In animal research, the consumption of polyunsaturated fatty acids increases the risk of some cancers.[61] However, in humans, most,[62, 63, 64] though not all,[65] reports do not find an association between polyunsaturates and cancer risks.

Sugar

A preliminary study has reported an association between an increasing intake of sugar or sugar-containing foods and an increased risk of gallbladder cancer.[66] Whether this association exists because sugar directly promotes cancer or because sugar consumption is only a marker for some other dietary or lifestyle factor remains unknown.

Salt

In preliminary research, increasing intake of salt correlates with increased risk of stomach cancer.[67, 68] Associations between foods preserved with salt and the risk of cancers of the head and neck have also been reported.[69]

Animal studies suggest that the antioxidant or immune-enhancing effect of **whey protein** (page 613) may produce anti-cancer effects.[70, 71, 72] Preliminary human case reports suggest that 30 grams per day of whey protein may improve responses to anti-cancer medications, but more research is needed.[73]

CANKER SORES

Canker sores are small ulcerations within the mouth.

Doctors call this common condition aphthous stomatitis.

CHECKLIST FOR CANKER SORES

Rating	Nutritional Supplements	Herbs
★★☆	**B-complex** (page 603) (**vitamin B$_1$** [page 597], **vitamin B$_2$** [page 598], **vitamin B$_6$** [page 600]) **Folic acid** (page 520) (for deficiency only) **Iron** (page 540) (for **iron deficiency** [page 278] only) *Lactobacillus acidophilus* (page 575) **Vitamin B$_{12}$** (page 601) (for deficiency only) **Zinc** (page 614) (for deficiency only)	**Aloe vera** (page 624) **Licorice** (page 702) (DGL)
★☆☆		Agrimony **Chamomile** (page 656) **Cranesbill** (page 665) **Echinacea** (page 669) **Goldenseal** (page 683) **Myrrh** (page 713) **Oak** (page 716) **Periwinkle** (page 727) Tormentil **Witch hazel** (page 760)

What are the symptoms of canker sores?

Canker sores appear alone or in clusters as shallow, **painful** (page 338) erosions in the mucous membrane inside the mouth. They typically have slightly raised, yellowish borders surrounded by a red zone, and are sometimes covered with a yellowish opaque material. Fatigue, fever, and swollen lymph nodes may be present in severe attacks.

Medical treatments

Over the counter treatment consists of local anesthetics, such as benzocaine (Anbesol, Num-Zit, Zilactin-B), which provide **pain relief** (page 338), and antiseptics containing carbamide peroxide (Gly-Oxide Liquid, Orajel Perioseptic).

Prescription drugs include antiseptic mouthwashes, such as chlorhexidine (Peridex, Periogard), and the oral anti-inflammatory products, amlexanox (Aphthasol), triamcinolone (Kenalog in Orabase), and hydrocortisone (Orabase-HCA). Occasionally, an antibiotic mouth rinse containing tetracycline is prescribed for individuals with multiple sores.

Dietary changes that may be helpful

Sensitivity to gluten, a protein found in wheat and other grains, has been associated with recurrent canker sores in some people. In preliminary trials, avoidance of gluten has reduced recurrent canker sores in people whether or not they had **celiac disease** (page 102),[1, 2, 3] but a double-blind trial did not find gluten avoidance helpful to people with recurrent canker sores who did not have celiac disease.[4] One preliminary trial suggested that people with recurrent canker sores, whose blood contains antibodies to gliadin (a component of gluten), may respond to a gluten-free diet even if they have no evidence of the tissue changes associated with celiac disease.[5]

Other **food sensitivities** (page 14) or **allergies** (page 14) may also make canker sores worse.[6, 7] One preliminary trial found evidence of food allergy in half of a group of people with recurrent canker sores; avoidance of the offending foods resulted in improvement in almost all cases.[8] While a double-blind study concluded that typical allergy mechanisms play only a minor role,[9] people with recurrent canker sores should discuss the diagnosis and treatment of food sensitivities with a doctor. For some people, treating allergies may be a key component to restoring health.

Lifestyle changes that may be helpful

Minor trauma from poor-fitting dentures, rough fillings, or braces can aggravate canker sores and should be remedied by a dentist.

Several reports have found sodium lauryl sulfate (SLS), a component of some toothpastes, to be a potential cause of canker sores.[10] In one trial, *most* recurrent canker sores were eliminated just by avoiding toothpaste containing SLS for three months.[11] Positive effects of eliminating SLS have been confirmed in double-blind research.[12] SLS is thought to increase the risk of canker sores by removing a protective coating (mucin) in the mouth. People with recurrent canker sores should use an SLS-free toothpaste for several months to see if such a change helps.

Measurements of stress were associated with recurrent canker sores in one preliminary study,[13] but not in another.[14] More research is needed to determine

Canker Sores

whether stress reduction techniques might reduce canker sore recurrences.

Nutritional supplements that may be helpful
Several preliminary studies,[15, 16, 17, 18] though not all,[19] have found a surprisingly high incidence of **iron** (page 540) and **B vitamin** (page 597) deficiency among people with recurrent canker sores. Treating these deficiencies has been reported in preliminary[20, 21] and controlled[22] studies to reduce or eliminate recurrences in most cases. Supplementing daily with B vitamins— 300 mg **vitamin B$_1$** (page 597), 20 mg **vitamin B$_2$** (page 598), and 150 mg **vitamin B$_6$** (page 600)—has been reported to provide some people with relief.[23] Thiamine (B$_1$) deficiency specifically has been linked to an increased risk of canker sores.[24] The right supplemental level of iron requires diagnosis of an **iron deficiency** (page 278) by a healthcare professional using lab tests.

Zinc (page 614) deficiency has also been linked with recurrent canker sores in preliminary studies[25] and in one case report.[26] A preliminary trial found that supplementation with up to 150 mg of zinc per day reduced recurrences of canker sores by 50 to 100%; participants who were zinc deficient experienced the most consistent benefit.[27] However, a double-blind trial (that did not test people for zinc deficiency) did not find zinc supplements helpful for recurrent canker sores.[28]

According to preliminary reports, some people with recurrent canker sores may respond to topical and/or oral use of *Lactobacillus acidophilus* (page 575)[29] and *Lactobacillus bulgaricus*.[30] However, a double-blind study found no effect of acidophilus bacteria on the healing time of canker sores.[31]

Are there any side effects or interactions?
Refer to the individual supplement for information about any side effects or interactions.

Herbs that may be helpful
Licorice (page 702) that has had the glycyrrhizic acid removed is called deglycyrrhizinated licorice (DGL). Glycyrrhizic acid is the portion of licorice root that can increase **blood pressure** (page 246) and cause **water retention** (page 180) in some people. The **wound-healing** (page 319) and soothing components of the root remain in DGL.

A mixture of DGL and warm water applied to the inside of the mouth may shorten the healing time for canker sores, according to a double-blind trial.[32] This DGL mixture is made by combining 200 mg of powdered DGL and 200 ml of warm water. It can then be swished in the mouth for two to three minutes, then spit out. This procedure may be repeated each morning and evening for one week. Chewable DGL tablets may be an acceptable substitute.

A gel containing the **aloe** (page 624) polysaccharide acemannon was found in one double-blind trial to speed the healing of canker sores better than the conventional treatment Orabase Plain.[33] The gel was applied four times daily. Because acemannon levels can vary widely in commercial aloe gel products, it is difficult to translate these results to the use of aloe gel for canker sores.

The antiviral, **immune-enhancing** (page 255), and wound-healing properties of **echinacea** (page 669) may make this herb a reasonable choice for canker sores. Liquid echinacea in the amount of 4 ml can be swished in the mouth for two to three minutes, then swallowed. This procedure may be repeated three times per day. However, no research has investigated the possible effects of this treatment.

Because of its soothing effect on mucous membranes (including the lining of the mouth) and its healing properties, **chamomile** (page 656) may be tried for canker sores and other mouth irritations.[34] A strong tea made from chamomile tincture can be swished in the mouth before swallowing, three to four times per day. **Goldenseal** (page 683) has also been used historically as a mouthwash to help heal canker sores.

Myrrh (page 713), another traditional remedy with wound-healing properties, has a long history of use for mouth and gum irritations. Some herbalists suggest mixing 200 to 300 mg of herbal extract or 4 ml of myrrh tincture with warm water and swishing it in the mouth before swallowing; this can be done two to three times per day.

Historically, herbs known as astringents have been used to soothe the **pain** (page 338) of canker sores. These herbs usually contain tannins that can bind up fluids and possibly relieve inflammation. They are used as a mouth rinse and then are spit out. None of these herbs has been studied in modern times. Examples of astringent herbs include agrimony, **cranesbill** (page 665), tormentil, **oak** (page 716), **periwinkle** (page 727), and **witch hazel** (page 760). Witch hazel is approved by the German Commission E for local inflammations of the mouth, presumably a condition that includes canker sores.

Are there any side effects or interactions?
Refer to the individual herb for information about any side effects or interactions.

CAPILLARY FRAGILITY

When the smallest blood vessels, capillaries, become weak, a person has capillary fragility.

There are no serious complications from having capillary fragility, but it may signify that a more serious, underlying problem exists. Therefore, people should consult a physician if there is bleeding in the skin.

CHECKLIST FOR CAPILLARY FRAGILITY		
Rating	Nutritional Supplements	Herbs
★★★	Vitamin C (page 604) (for deficiency only)	
★★☆	Proanthocyanidins (page 574)	
★☆☆	Flavonoids (page 516) (quercetin [page 580], rutin, hesperidin)	

What are the symptoms of capillary fragility?
Weak capillaries lead to small spots of bleeding in the skin and easy **bruising** (page 84). Bruises look like areas of blue to purple-colored skin that can turn yellow to dark brown over the course of a few days.

Medical treatments
The primary focus in the treatment of capillary fragility is the diagnosis and management of any underlying medical condition. Conditions such as liver or kidney disease; blood disorders, such as hemophilia, platelet dysfunction, thrombocytopenia, leukemia, and multiple myeloma; connective tissue disorders including scurvy, Marfan's syndrome, and Ehlers-Danlos syndrome; or the use of blood-thinning medication, such as aspirin (Bayer, Ecotrin, Bufferin) andwarfarin (Coumadin), should be considered.

Dietary changes that may be helpful
Eating plenty of fruits and vegetables will provide more of the nutrients mentioned in the Nutritional supplements information below that support the structure of capillaries.

Nutritional supplements that may be helpful
Severe **vitamin C** (page 604) deficiency (scurvy) is a well-recognized but uncommon cause of increased capillary fragility. Whether vitamin C supplementation can help capillary fragility in people who do not have scurvy is less clear. Patients undergoing dialysis may develop low levels of vitamin C,[1, 2] which can lead to capillary fragility, but giving dialysis patients 50 mg of vitamin C per day had no effect on capillary fragility in one study.[3] People with kidney failure and those undergoing dialysis should not supplement with more than 100 mg per day, unless supervised by a doctor.

According to preliminary studies, vitamin C may reduce capillary weakness in **diabetics** (page 152), who often have low blood levels of vitamin C compared to non-diabetics.[4, 5] In a double-blind trial, elderly people with low vitamin C levels and capillary fragility were helped with supplementation of one gram per day of vitamin C.[6]

Compounds called **flavonoids** (page 516) may help strengthen weakened capillaries. In test tube and animal studies, they have been shown to protect collagen, one of the most important components of capillary walls.[7, 8] A preliminary study found that **proanthocyanidins** (page 574) (flavonoids extracted from grape seeds), 150 mg per day, increased capillary strength in people with **hypertension** (page 246) and/or **diabetes** (page 152).[9] A double-blind trial found a combination of two flavonoids (900 mg per day of diosmin and 100 mg per day hesperidin) for six weeks reduced symptoms of capillary fragility.[10] Use of vitamin C with flavonoids, particularly **quercetin** (page 580), rutin, and hesperidin, is sometimes recommended for capillary fragility.[11] Doctors often recommend 400 mg of rutin or quercetin three times per day or 1 gram of citrus flavonoids three times per day.

Are there any side effects or interactions?
Refer to the individual supplement for information about any side effects or interactions.

CARDIAC ARRHYTHMIA

Cardiac arrhythmia is a term that denotes a disturbance of the heart rhythm.

Cardiac arrhythmias can range in severity from entirely benign to immediately life-threatening. If arrhythmia is suspected, a doctor should be consulted for

Cardiac Arrhythmia

confirmation. In addition, the use of natural substances for arrhythmia should always be supervised by a doctor.

CHECKLIST FOR CARDIAC ARRHYTHMIA

Rating	Nutritional Supplements	Herbs
★★★	**Magnesium** (page 551)	
★★☆	**Fish oil** (page 514) (do not take, or take only with a doctor's supervision, if there is a history of sustained ventricular tachycardia or ventricular fibrillation) **Potassium** (page 572)	
★☆☆	**Copper** (page 499) **Selenium** (page 584) **Vitamin D** (page 607)	**Corydalis** (page 663) **Hawthorn** (page 689)

What are the symptoms of cardiac arrhythmia?

Most arrhythmia does not result in symptoms, but people may experience **anxiety** (page 30), lightheadedness, dizziness, fainting, unusual awareness of the heartbeat, and sensations of fluttering or pounding in the chest.

Medical treatments

Prescription medications used to treat irregular heart rhythm, include quinidine (Quinidex, Quinaglute), procainamide (Pronestyl), disopyramide (Norpace), mexiletine (Mexitil), amiodarone (Cordarone, Pacerone), verapamil (Calan, Verelan), acebutolol (Sectral), and propranolol (Inderal).

Medical conditions that may cause arrhythmia, such as **anemia** (page 25), fever, **heart failure** (page 134), or electrolyte imbalance, are treated accordingly. In some cases, a synchronized electrical shock (defibrillation) is applied to the heart either externally or internally (from a previously implanted device that automatically activates when a life-threatening arrhythmia is detected). When a normal rhythm cannot be established by these methods, a pacemaker (an electronic device that controls the rhythm of the heart) may be implanted surgically. A newer procedure called radiofrequency ablation may be used to destroy small areas of the heart responsible for the arrhythmia.

Dietary changes that may be helpful

Excessive caffeine consumption has been associated with arrhythmia in human studies. Although most people do not experience arrhythmia as a result of caffeine consumption,[1] some healthy people appear to be susceptible to as little as one cup of coffee.[2]

Allergic reactions (page 14) to foods and environmental chemicals have been reported to trigger arrhythmias.[3] Consultation with a physician may help to pinpoint these sensitivities.

Nutritional supplements that may be helpful

A double-blind trial investigated the effect of oral **magnesium** (page 551) supplementation on arrhythmic episodes in people with **congestive heart failure** (page 134). Those people taking 3.2 grams per day of magnesium chloride (equivalent to 384 mg per day of elemental magnesium) had between 23% and 52% fewer occurrences of specific types of arrhythmia during the six-week study, compared with those taking placebo.[4] Lower serum concentrations of magnesium were found to be associated with a higher incidence of arrhythmia in a large population study.[5] The anti-arrhythmic properties of magnesium appear to be specific. For example, magnesium is clearly able to prevent a drug-induced arrhythmia called torsade de pointes,[6] but it does not appear to prevent atrial fibrillation.[7] A doctor should supervise any use of magnesium for cardiac arrhythmia.

In a double-blind trial, people with a type of arrhythmia known as ventricular premature complexes were supplemented for 16 weeks with either 15 ml (1 tbsp) per day of **fish oil** (page 514) or a similar amount of safflower oil as placebo. Patients taking the fish oil had a significantly reduced frequency of abnormal heartbeats compared with those receiving placebo, and 44% of those receiving fish oil experienced at least a 70% reduction in the frequency of abnormal beats.[8] In a separate study, however, men given 20 ml (4 tsp) of **cod liver oil** (page 514) per day for six weeks, beginning one week after a **heart attack** (page 212), had the same frequency of irregular heart beats as did men given no supplemental oil.[9] In a double-blind study, people who had a history of certain potentially life-threatening arrhythmias—sustained ventricular tachycardia or ventricular fibrillation—had an *increase* in the recurrence rate of these arrhythmias when they took fish oil.[10] Consequently, most people with a history of either of these arrhythmias should not take fish oil. The findings from that study may not apply to people who have had sustained ventricular tachycardia or ventricular fibrillation as a direct result of a heart attack or as a result of other reversible causes. Nevertheless, anyone who has had one of these arrhythmias should consult a doctor before taking fish oil supplements.

Patients taking hydrochlorothiazide for **high blood pressure** (page 246) had a significant reduction in arrhythmias when supplemented with 1 gram twice per day of potassium hydrochloride (supplying 1040 mg per day of elemental **potassium** [page 572]). Those results were not improved by adding 500 mg twice per day of magnesium hydroxide (supplying 500 mg per day of elemental magnesium) to the potassium.[11] Low serum concentrations of potassium were found to be associated with a higher incidence of arrhythmia in a large population study.[12]

Three cases have been reported in which ventricular premature beats disappeared after supplementation with **copper** (page 499) (4 mg per day in the two cases for which amounts were reported).[13] In one of these people, supplementing with **zinc** (page 614) made the arrhythmia worse, confirming previous observations that excessive zinc intake may lead to copper deficiency,[14] which in turn may lead to arrhythmia.

Gross deficiency of dietary **selenium** (page 524) may cause many heart problems, including arrhythmia. Based on this finding, one author has theorized that correction of low selenium status may improve many arrhythmias, even in the absence of overt deficiency symptoms.[15] Controlled research is needed to evaluate this possibility.

One case of long-standing sick-sinus syndrome (another type of arrhythmia) was reported to resolve upon supplementation with 800 IU per day of **vitamin D** (page 607) prescribed for an unrelated condition. However, it was not clear from that report whether the improvement was due to the vitamin D.[16] More research is needed.

Are there any side effects or interactions?
Refer to the individual supplement for information about any side effects or interactions.

Herbs that may be helpful
An animal study showed that an extract of **hawthorn** (page 689) significantly reduced the number of experimentally induced arrhythmias.[17] Although the use of hawthorn for arrhythmia in humans has not been stud-

ied scientifically, it traditionally has been used for this purpose.[18]

An active constituent in **corydalis** (page 663), dl-tetrahydropalmatine (dl-THP), may exert an antiarrhythmic action on the heart. This action was observed in a preliminary trial with 33 patients suffering from a specific type of arrhythmia called supraventricular premature beat or SVPB.[19] Each patient took 300 to 600 mg of dl-THP per day in tablet form, and the dl-THP was found to be significantly more effective than placebo in reducing arrhythmia.

Are there any side effects or interactions?
Refer to the individual herb for information about any side effects or interactions.

CARDIOMYOPATHY

Cardiomyopathy refers to abnormalities in the structure or function of the heart muscle. There are three major types of cardiomyopathy: dilated congestive, hypertrophic, and restrictive.

The most prevalent form is dilated congestive cardiomyopathy (DCM). In people with DCM, the heart muscle is damaged, most commonly by coronary artery disease (**atherosclerosis** [page 38]).[1] People with **diabetes** (page 152) have been reported to be at increased risk of DCM.[2] DCM can also be triggered by alcohol abuse, **infections** (page 265), exposure to certain drugs and toxins, nutritional deficiencies, connective tissue diseases, hereditary disorders, and **pregnancy** (page 363).

In DCM, the heart gradually loses its efficiency as a pump. Cardiomyopathy is a serious health condition and requires expert medical care rather than self-treatment. However, because of the associations between cardiomyopathy and diseases such as atherosclerosis, diabetes, **hypertension** (page 246), and **congestive heart failure** (page 134), lifestyle recommendations for the prevention of these conditions may also help prevent DCM.

Hypertrophic cardiomyopathy is usually a hereditary disorder, although the incidence of this form of cardiomyopathy may also be higher in people with hypertension.[3] Restrictive cardiomyopathy is usually due to a connective tissue disease, **cancer** (page 87), or an autoimmune condition. Both hypertrophic and restrictive cardiomyopathies are relatively uncommon.

Cardiomyopathy

CHECKLIST FOR CARDIOMYOPATHY

Rating	Nutritional Supplements	Herbs
★★☆	Coenzyme Q₁₀ (page 496)	Arjun Hawthorn (page 689) (if congestive heart failure [page 134] is also present)
★☆☆	L-carnitine (page 545) (only for children with inherited cardiomyopathy) Selenium (page 584) (only for Keshan's cardiomyopathy) Taurine (page 590) Vitamin B₁ (Thiamine) (page 597) (only for wet beri beri)	Coleus (page 660) Dan shen Hawthorn (page 689) (if congestive heart failure [page 134] is not present)

What are the symptoms of cardiomyopathy?
People with cardiomyopathy may have difficulty breathing during light exertion, and they may become fatigued easily. Other chronic symptoms are swelling around the ankles and an enlarged abdomen.

Medical treatments
Prescription drug therapy is directed toward treating any underlying cause. Medications used include ACE inhibitors, such as captopril (Capoten), enalapril (Vasotec), and lisinopril (Zestril, Prinivil); beta-blockers, such as atenolol (Tenormin) and metoprolol (Lopressor, Toprol XL); the combination of hydralazine (Apresoline) and isosorbide dinitrate (Isordil); digoxin (Lanoxin); and diuretics, such as hydrochlorothiazide (HydroDIURIL) and furosemide (Lasix).

Severe cases might require heart transplantation surgery.

Dietary changes that may be helpful
Protein-calorie malnutrition (PCM) may cause cardiomyopathy, though PCM is rare in U.S. society.

Lifestyle changes that may be helpful
Cardiomyopathy occurs with greater frequency in people who drink to excess.[4] Alcoholics are at significantly greater risk of developing a deficiency of thiamine (page 597) (vitamin B₁).[5, 6] They also may develop a form of thiamine deficiency called wet beri beri or

Shoshin beri beri, which frequently includes cardiomyopathy.[7, 8] See "Nutritional supplements that may be helpful," below, for more information.

Among alcoholics, the risk of developing DCM is greater for women than for men.[9] Many doctors suggest that people with cardiomyopathy abstain from alcohol consumption. People with alcohol-induced cardiomyopathy who avoid alcohol (page 12) may regain their health.

Moderate to heavy physical activity can be life-threatening for people with cardiomyopathy;[10] however, appropriate exercise often improves the condition.[11, 12, 13, 14] How much is "too much" varies from person to person. Any exercise program undertaken by someone with cardiomyopathy requires professional supervision.

The risk of being diagnosed with cardiomyopathy goes up with the number of cigarettes smoked per day.[15, 16] However, a few studies have reported a paradoxical *decrease* in the death rate among smokers with DCM compared with nonsmokers who have this disease.[17, 18] While the meaning of this association remains unclear, virtually all doctors recommend that smokers with DCM quit smoking for a wide variety of health-related reasons.

Nutritional supplements that may be helpful
People with DCM have been shown to be deficient in coenzyme Q₁₀ (page 496).[19] Most studies using coenzyme Q₁₀ in the treatment of cardiomyopathy have demonstrated positive results, including improved quality of life, heart function tests, and survival rates.[20, 21, 22] Coenzyme Q₁₀ also has been shown to improve cardiac function in people with hypertrophic cardiomyopathy—a less common form of cardiomyopathy.[23] A few studies, however, have found no benefit from CoQ₁₀ supplementation in treating people with cardiomyopathy.[24, 25] Despite a lack of consistency in the outcomes of published research, many doctors recommend that 100 to 150 mg be taken each day, with meals.

Deficiency of L-carnitine (page 545), an amino acid (page 465), is associated with the development of some forms of cardiomyopathy.[26] Inherited forms of cardiomyopathy seen in children may be the most responsive to therapy with L-carnitine.[27, 28] Whether carnitine supplementation helps the average person with cardiomyopathy remains unknown. Nonetheless, some doctors recommend 1 to 3 grams of carnitine per day for adults of average weight.

Several veterinary studies have demonstrated benefits from supplementation with **taurine** (page 590), another amino acid, in animals with cardiomyopathy. Most of these studies showed taurine deficiency to be a cause of cardiomyopathy. Taurine supplementation in animals with DCM has resulted in improvement of symptoms and survival rates.[29, 30] However, clinical studies in humans are lacking; thus, despite a good safety record, the benefits of taurine supplementation in people with any form of cardiomyopathy remain speculative. When taurine supplements are used by doctors to treat people with other conditions, 2 grams taken three times per day for a total of 6 grams per day is often recommended.

Selenium (page 584) deficiency has occasionally been reported as a cause of cardiomyopathy.[31, 32] Selenium deficiency is the probable cause of Keshan's disease, a form of cardiomyopathy found in China[33, 34] but only rarely reported in the United States.[35] Studies comparing populations in parts of the world other than mainland China have not supported a link between selenium deficiency and DCM,[36, 37] except in Taiwan.[38] Moreover, no clinical trials outside of China have explored the effects of supplementation with selenium for people with DCM, nor is there reason to believe that selenium supplementation would help most people outside of China and Taiwan suffering from cardiomyopathy.

The small proportion of people with cardiomyopathy whose disease is due to severe **vitamin B$_1$** (page 597) (thiamine) deficiency (known as wet beri beri) generally require intravenous vitamin B$_1$, followed by oral supplementation. Vitamin B$_1$ does not appear to be helpful for other types of cardiomyopathy. People requiring vitamin B$_1$ for cardiomyopathy must first be diagnosed as having wet beri beri, and treatment must be supervised by a healthcare professional.

Are there any side effects or interactions?
Refer to the individual supplement for information about any side effects or interactions.

Herbs that may be helpful
Many doctors expert in herbal medicine consider **hawthorn** (page 689) to be an effective and low-risk therapy for **congestive heart failure** (page 134), the main complication of cardiomyopathy. Rigorous clinical trials have now confirmed the effectiveness of hawthorn for the signs and symptoms of early-stage congestive heart failure,[39, 40, 41] though hawthorn stud-

ies with cardiomyopathy patients have yet to be conducted. The clinical trials with heart-failure patients have demonstrated efficacy using 80 to 300 mg of standardized extract of hawthorn leaves and flowers two to three times per day.

Two herbs used in the traditional medicine of India (Ayurveda) to treat people with cardiomyopathy and congestive heart failure have recently been supported by a small amount of clinical research. Arjun *(Terminalia arjuna)* has been shown to significantly improve the signs and symptoms of cardiomyopathy, as well as the objective measurements of heart function.[42] In a clinical trial, people with DCM and severe heart failure took 500 mg of arjun extract three times daily. After two weeks, significant improvement in heart function was observed, an effect that continued over the course of approximately two years.[43] The arjun used in this study was concentrated, but not standardized for any particular constituent. Commercial preparations are sometimes standardized to contain 1% arjunolic acid.

Another Ayurvedic herb, **coleus** (page 660), contains forskolin, a substance that may help dilate blood vessels and improve the forcefulness with which the heart pumps blood.[44] Recent clinical studies indicate that forskolin improves heart function in people with cardiomyopathy and congestive heart failure.[45, 46] A preliminary trial found that forskolin reduced blood pressure and improved heart function in people with cardiomyopathy. These trials used intravenous injections of isolated forskolin. It is unknown whether oral coleus extracts would have the same effect. While many doctors and practitioners of herbal medicine would recommend 200 to 600 mg per day of a coleus extract containing 10% forskolin, these amounts are extrapolations and have yet to be confirmed by direct clinical research.

Dan shen *(Salvia miltiorrhiza),* a Chinese herb, has been traditionally used to treat **angina** (page 27) and **coronary artery disease** (page 38). Some studies suggest that dan shen may improve the force of heart contractions and coronary circulation, and may prevent damage to the heart muscle that might lead to cardiomyopathy.[47, 48, 49] However, no clinical trials of dan shen for DCM have been reported. Doctors expert in Chinese herbal medicine typically recommend 1 to 6 grams per day of dried root.

Are there any side effects or interactions?
Refer to the individual herb for information about any side effects or interactions.

CARDIOVASCULAR DISEASE OVERVIEW

See also: Angina (page 27), **Atherosclerosis** (page 38), **Cardiac Arrhythmia** (page 93), **Cardiomyopathy** (page 95), **Chronic Venous Insufficiency** (page 116), **Diabetes** (page 152), **Heart Attack** (page 212), **High Cholesterol** (page 223), **High Homocysteine** (page 234), **High Triglycerides** (page 235), **Hypertension** (page 246), **Insulin Resistance Syndrome** (page 273), **Mitral Valve Prolapse** (page 319), **Stroke** (page 419)

What do I need to know?

Self-care for cardiovascular disease can be approached in a number of ways—but it can be hard to know just where to start. To make it easier, our doctors recommend trying these simple steps first:

Avoid cigarette smoke
> Quit smoking and stay clear of secondhand smoke to lower your risk of several types of cardiovascular disease (CVD)

Watch what you eat
> Eat lots of fruits, vegetables, legumes, whole grains, fish, and avoid fats from meat, dairy, and processed foods high in hydrogenated oils

Get moving
> Being a couch potato increases your CVD risk, so make sure you get regular exercise

Get tested
> See your doctor to find out if you have problems with high blood pressure or high blood levels of cholesterol, triglycerides, or glucose

About cardiovascular disease

Cardiovascular disease is a wide-encompassing category that includes all conditions that affect the heart and the blood vessels.

Cardiovascular disease is the number one cause of death in the United States. This introductory article briefly discusses several diseases that have a role in the development of cardiovascular disease. Many risk factors are associated with cardiovascular disease; most can be managed, but some cannot. The aging process and hereditary predisposition are risk factors that cannot be altered. Until age 50, men are at greater risk than women of developing heart disease, though once a woman enters **menopause** (page 311), her risk triples.[1]

Many people with cardiovascular disease have elevated or **high cholesterol** (page 223) levels.[2] Low HDL cholesterol (known as the "good" cholesterol) and high LDL cholesterol (known as the "bad" cholesterol) are more specifically linked to cardiovascular disease than is total cholesterol.[3] A blood test, administered by most healthcare professionals, is used to determine cholesterol levels.

Atherosclerosis (page 38) (hardening of the arteries) of the vessels that supply the heart with blood is the most common cause of **heart attacks** (page 212). Atherosclerosis and high cholesterol usually occur together, though cholesterol levels can change quickly and atherosclerosis generally takes decades to develop.

The link between **high triglyceride** (page 235) levels and heart disease is not as well established as the link between high cholesterol and heart disease. According to some studies, a high triglyceride level is an independent risk factor for heart disease in some people.[4]

High homocysteine (page 234) levels have been identified as an independent risk factor for heart disease.[5] Homocysteine can be measured by a blood test that must be ordered by a healthcare professional.

Hypertension (page 246) (high blood pressure) is a major risk factor for cardiovascular disease, and the risk increases as blood pressure rises.[6] Glucose intolerance and **diabetes** (page 152) constitute separate risk factors for heart disease. Smoking increases the risk of heart disease caused by hypertension.

Abdominal fat, or a "beer belly," versus fat that accumulates on the hips, is associated with increased risk of cardiovascular disease and heart attack.[7] **Overweight** (page 446) individuals are more likely to have additional risk factors related to heart disease, specifically hypertension, high blood sugar levels, high cholesterol, high triglycerides, and diabetes.

What are the symptoms of cardiovascular disease?

People with cardiovascular disease may not have any symptoms, or they may experience difficulty in breathing during exertion or when lying down, fatigue, lightheadedness, dizziness, fainting, **depression** (page 145), memory problems, confusion, frequent waking during sleep, chest pain, an awareness of the heartbeat, sensations of fluttering or pounding in the chest, swelling around the ankles, or a large abdomen.

Medical treatments

Over the counter aspirin (Bayer Children's Aspirin, Ecotrin Adult Low Strength, Halfprin 81) might be beneficial for reducing recurrent strokes and for reducing the risk of future heart attacks.

Use of prescription medications is directed toward any underlying causes. Drugs used may include ACE inhibitors, such as captopril (Capoten), enalapril (Vasotec), and lisinopril (Zestril, Prinivil); beta-blockers, such as atenolol (Tenormin), metoprolol (Lopressor, Toprol XL), and propranolol (Inderal); and the combination of hydralazine (Apresoline) and isosorbide dinitrate (Isordil). Other medications often prescribed include the blood thinner warfarin (Coumadin); digoxin (Lanoxin); nitroglycerin (Nitrostat, Nitro-Dur); and diuretics, such as hydrochlorothiazide (HydroDIURIL) and furosemide (Lasix).

Surgical treatments, such as angioplasty, bypass surgery, valve replacement, pacemaker installation, and heart transplantation, may be recommended for severe cases. Individuals with cardiovascular disease are strongly encouraged to stop smoking.

Dietary changes that may be helpful

Preliminary evidence has linked high salt consumption with increased cardiovascular disease incidence and death among overweight, but not normal weight, people. Among overweight people, an increase in salt consumption of 2.3 grams per day was associated with a 32% increase in **stroke** (page 419) incidence, an 89% increase in stroke mortality, a 44% increase in heart disease mortality, a 61% increase in cardiovascular disease mortality, and a 39% increase in death from all causes.[8] Intervention trials are required to confirm these preliminary observations.

Moderate alcohol consumption appears protective against heart disease.[9] However, regular, light alcohol consumption in men with established coronary heart disease is not associated with either benefit or deleterious effect.[10]

A high intake of **carotenoids** (page 488) from dietary sources has been shown to be protective against heart disease in several population-based studies.[11, 12] A diet high in fruits and vegetables,[13] **fiber** (page 512),[14] and possibly fish[15] appears protective against heart disease, while a high intake of saturated fat (found in meat and dairy fat) and trans fatty acids (in margarine and processed foods containing hydrogenated vegetable oils)[16] may contribute to heart disease. In a preliminary study, the total number of deaths from cardiovascular disease was significantly lower among men with high fruit consumption[17] than among those with low fruit consumption. A large study of male healthcare professionals found that those men eating mostly a "prudent" diet (high in fruits, vegetables, legumes, whole grains, fish, and poultry) had a 30% *lower* risk of **heart attacks** (page 212) compared with men who ate the fewest foods in the "prudent" category.[18] By contrast, men who ate the highest percentage of their foods from the "typical American diet" category (high in red meat, processed meat, refined grains, sweets, and desserts) had a 64% *increased* risk of heart attack, compared with men who ate the fewest foods in that category. The various risks in this study were derived after controlling for all other beneficial or harmful influencing factors.

A parallel study of female healthcare professionals showed a 15% reduction in cardiovascular risk for those women eating a diet high in fruits and vegetables—compared with those eating a diet low in fruits and vegetables.[19]

Lifestyle changes that may be helpful

Both smoking[20] and exposure to secondhand smoke[21] increase cardiovascular disease risk.

Moderate exercise protects both lean and **obese** (page 446) individuals from cardiovascular disease.[22]

CARPAL TUNNEL SYNDROME

Carpal tunnel syndrome (CTS) is a condition characterized by pain, tingling, and numbness into the areas of the fingers, hand, and sometimes radiating up into the elbow.

The painful sensations of CTS are caused by compression of the median nerve in the tunnel of bones in the wrist. In many cases, the condition results from long-term repetitive motions of the hands and wrists, such as from computer use. Although repetitive motion is often a culprit, it does not explain the frequent occurrence of CTS with non-motion-related conditions, such as **pregnancy** (page 363).

CHECKLIST FOR CARPAL TUNNEL SYNDROME		
Rating	Nutritional Supplements	Herbs
★★☆	**Vitamin B$_6$** (page 600)	

What are the symptoms of carpal tunnel syndrome?

Symptoms of CTS include recurrent numbness, tingling, weakness, or **pain** (page 338) in one or both hands in a characteristic location defined by the median nerve, which is compressed as it passes through the carpal tunnel in the wrist. Symptoms are usually worse at night and after prolonged use of the hands. Some people may experience clumsiness in handling objects, with a tendency to drop things, and may also have a decreased ability to feel hot and cold.

Medical treatments

Over the counter nonsteroidal anti-inflammatory drugs (NSAIDs), such as aspirin (Bayer, Ecotrin, Bufferin), naproxen sodium (Aleve), and ibuprofen (Motrin, Advil) are used to treat pain.

Prescription diuretic medications, such as hydrochlorothiazide (HydroDIURIL) and furosemide (Lasix), as well as injections of corticosteroids such as methylprednisolone (Depo-Medrol) into the wrist, might reduce swelling.

Splints are often recommended to immobilize the wrist, theoretically protecting it from repetitive motion injury. A physical therapy program of hand- and wrist-strengthening exercises, combined with the use of a wrist brace, is sometimes recommended. In more advanced cases, a surgical procedure called a "release" may be necessary. The procedure separates the ligaments covering the carpal tunnel in the wrist, which relieves painful pressure on the median nerve.

Nutritional supplements that may be helpful

Some, but not all, studies have found **vitamin B$_6$** (page 600) deficiency to be common in people with CTS.[1] Supplementation with vitamin B$_6$ has reportedly relieved the symptoms of CTS,[2] but some researchers have not found this treatment to be beneficial.[3, 4]

Several studies report that people with CTS are helped when given 100 mg of vitamin B$_6$ three times per day.[5, 6] Although some researchers have found benefits with lesser amounts,[7, 8, 9, 10] using *less* than 100 mg taken three times per day for several months has often failed.[11, 12, 13] Most doctors assume that people with CTS who respond to vitamin B$_6$ supplementation do so because of an underlying deficiency. However, at least one group of researchers has found vitamin B$_6$ to "dramatically" reduce pain in people with CTS who did not appear to be B$_6$-deficient.[14] Some doctors believe that

B$_6$ is therapeutic because it reduces swelling around the carpal tunnel in the wrist; this theory remains completely undocumented.

Very high levels of vitamin B$_6$ can damage sensory nerves, leading to numbness in the hands and feet as well as difficulty in walking; supplementation should be stopped if these symptoms develop after beginning vitamin B$_6$ supplementation. Vitamin B$_6$ is usually safe in amounts of 200 to 500 mg per day,[15] although occasional problems have been reported in this range.[16] Higher amounts are clearly toxic.[17] Any adult taking more than 200 mg of vitamin B$_6$ per day for more than a few months should consult a doctor.

In order to be effective, vitamin B$_6$ must be transformed in the body to pyridoxal-5'-phosphate (PLP). Some doctors have suggested that people who do not respond well to vitamin B$_6$ supplements should try 50 mg of PLP three times per day. There is no clear evidence that using PLP provides any advantage in reducing symptoms of CTS.

Are there any side effects or interactions?
Refer to the individual supplement for information about any side effects or interactions.

Holistic approaches that may be helpful

Acupuncture may be useful in the treatment of CTS. In a preliminary trial, people with CTS (some of whom had previously undergone surgery) received either acupuncture or electro-acupuncture (acupuncture with electrical stimulation). Eighty-three percent of the participants in this trial experienced complete relief that lasted through two to eight years of follow-up.[18] After reviewing all available scientific literature on the topic, a consensus conference convened in 1997 by the National Institutes of Health concluded that acupuncture for CTS "may be useful as an adjunct treatment or an acceptable alternative or be included in a comprehensive management program."[19]

Manipulative procedures may have a role in treating CTS by decreasing symptoms and improving function. A type of stretching treatment called myofascial release improved the symptoms of a patient with CTS in one published case report,[20] and similar treatments combined with specific wrist manipulations and self stretches were further tested in a small, preliminary trial.[21] Participants in this study experienced a decrease in **pain** (page 338), numbness, and weakness, and their nerve function improved as well.

A small, preliminary trial assessed a chiropractic treatment program consisting of exercises, soft tissue therapy, and manipulation of the wrist, the upper extremity, the spine, and the ribs.[22] The treatment resulted in improvement in grip and thumb strength, muscle function, flexibility, and overall function, as well as a decrease in pain among people with CTS. In a follow-up study six months later, most of the improvement had been maintained.[23] A controlled clinical trial compared traditional medical and chiropractic care for CTS.[24] People with CTS received either standard medical care (ibuprofen and nighttime wrist supports) or chiropractic care (manipulation of the wrist, elbow, shoulder, neck, and spine, as well as massage to the soft tissues). Ultrasound and nighttime splints were also used in the chiropractic treatments. People in both groups improved significantly and similarly in terms of pain reduction, increased function, and improved finger sensation and nerve function, but the chiropractic group reported fewer side effects.

CATARACTS

Cataract is a cloudiness in the lens of the eye caused by damage to the protein of the lens. This damage impairs vision.

Most people who live long enough will develop cataracts.[1] Cataracts are more likely to occur in those who smoke, have **diabetes** (page 152), or are exposed to excessive sunlight. All of these factors lead to oxidative damage. Oxidative damage to the lens of the eye appears to cause cataracts in animals[2] and people.[3]

It is unlikely that any nutritional supplements or herbs can reverse existing cataracts, although it is possible they might help prevent cataracts from becoming worse.

What are the symptoms of cataracts?

Cataracts usually develop slowly without any pain or redness of the eye. The most common symptoms of a cataract are fuzzy or blurred vision, increasing need for light when reading or doing other close work, visual disturbances caused by bright lights (e.g., sunlight, car headlights), faded color perception, poor night vision, and frequent need to change eyeglass or contact lens prescriptions. A cataract will not spread from one eye to the other, although many people develop cataracts in both eyes.

CHECKLIST FOR CATARACTS		
Rating	Nutritional Supplements	Herbs
★★☆	**Lutein** (page 548) **Vitamin B$_2$** (page 598) **Vitamin C** (page 604)	
★☆☆	**Beta-carotene** (page 469) **Carotenoids** (page 488) **Quercetin** (page 580) **Vitamin B$_3$** (page 598) **Vitamin E** (page 609)	Bilberry (page 633)

Medical treatments

In the beginning stages, magnifying lenses, stronger eyeglasses, and brighter lighting may compensate for the vision problems caused by cataracts. Once the vision problems affect daily activities, surgery may be necessary to replace the clouded lens with a clear artificial lens. For many people, the lens capsule remaining in the eye after surgery eventually turns cloudy, causing additional loss of vision.

Lifestyle changes that may be helpful

Obese men are significantly more likely to develop a cataract than are men of normal body weight.[4] To date, most,[5, 6, 7, 8] but not all,[9, 10] population studies have found an increased risk of cataracts as body mass increases.

Nutritional supplements that may be helpful

People with low blood levels of **antioxidants** (page 467) and those who eat few antioxidant-rich fruits and vegetables have been reported to be at high risk for cataracts.[11, 12]

Vitamin B$_2$ (page 598) and **vitamin B$_3$** (page 598) are needed to protect **glutathione** (page 531), an important antioxidant in the eye. Vitamin B$_2$ deficiency has been linked to cataracts.[13, 14] Older people taking 3 mg of vitamin B$_2$ and 40 mg of vitamin B$_3$ per day were partly protected against cataracts in one trial.[15] However, the intake of vitamin B$_2$ in China is relatively low, and it is not clear whether supplementation would help prevent cataracts in populations where vitamin B$_2$ intake is higher.

The major antioxidants in the lens of the eye are **vitamin C** (page 604)[16] and glutathione (a molecule composed of three **amino acids** [page 465]).[17] Vitamin C is needed to activate **vitamin E** (page 609),[18] which in turn activates glutathione. Both nutrients are important for healthy vision. People who take **multivitamins** (page 559) or any supplements containing vitamins C or E for more than 10 years have been reported to have a 60% lower risk of forming a cataract.[19]

Vitamin C levels in the eye decrease with age.[20] However, supplementing with vitamin C prevents this decrease[21] and has been linked to a lower risk of developing cataracts.[22, 23] Healthy people are more likely to take vitamin C and vitamin E supplements than those with cataracts according to some,[24] but not all,[25] studies. Dietary vitamin C intake has not been consistently associated with protection from cataracts.[26, 27] Nonetheless, because people who supplement with vitamin C have developed far fewer cataracts in some research,[28, 29] doctors often recommend 500 to 1,000 mg of vitamin C supplementation as part of a cataract prevention program. The difference between successful and unsuccessful trials may be tied to the length of time people actually supplement with vitamin C. In one preliminary study, people taking vitamin C for at least ten years showed a dramatic reduction in cataract risk, but those taking vitamin C for less than ten years showed no evidence of protection at all.[30]

Low blood levels of **vitamin E** (page 609) have been linked to increased risk of forming cataracts.[31, 32] Dietary vitamin E intake has not been consistently associated with protection from cataracts.[33, 34] Vitamin E supplements have been reported to protect against cataracts in animals[35] and people,[36] though the evidence remains inconsistent.[37] In one trial, people who took vitamin E supplements had less than half the risk of developing cataracts, compared with others in the five-year study.[38] Doctors typically recommend 400 IU of vitamin E per day as prevention. Smaller amounts (approximately 50 IU per day) have been proven in double-blind research to provide no protection.[39]

Some,[40] but not all,[41] studies have reported that people eating more foods rich in **beta-carotene** (page 469) had a lower the risk of developing cataracts. Supplementation with synthetic beta-carotene has not been found to reduce the risk of cataract formation.[42] It remains unclear whether natural beta-carotene from food or supplements would protect the eye or whether beta-carotene in food is merely a marker for other protective factors in fruits and vegetables high in beta-carotene.

People who eat a lot of spinach and kale, which are high in **lutein** (page 548) and zeaxanthin, carotenoids similar to beta-carotene, have been reported to be at low risk for cataracts.[43, 44] Lutein, zeaxanthin, and beta-carotene offer the promise of protection because they are antioxidants. It is quite possible, however, that lutein is more important than beta-carotene, because lutein is found in the lens of the eye, while beta-carotene is not.[45] In one preliminary study, lutein and zeaxanthin were the only carotenoids associated with protection from cataracts.[46] People with the highest intake of lutein and zeaxanthin were half as likely to develop cataracts as those with the lowest intake. In another study, supplementation with 15 mg of lutein three times a week for one year significantly improved visual function in a small group of people with age-related cataracts.[47]

The **flavonoid** (page 516) **quercetin** (page 580) may also help by blocking sorbitol accumulation in the eye.[48] This may be especially helpful for people with **diabetes** (page 152), though no clinical trials have yet explored whether quercetin actually prevents diabetic cataracts.

Are there any side effects or interactions?
Refer to the individual supplement for information about any side effects or interactions.

Herbs that may be helpful
Bilberry (page 633), a close relative of blueberry, is high in **flavonoids** (page 516) called anthocyanosides.[49] Anthocyanosides may protect both the lens and retina from oxidative damage. The potent **antioxidant** (page 467) activity of anthocyanosides may make bilberry useful for reducing the risk of cataracts.[50, 51] Doctors sometimes recommend 240 to 480 mg per day of bilberry extract, capsules or tablets standardized to contain 25% anthocyanosides.

Are there any side effects or interactions?
Refer to the individual herb for information about any side effects or interactions.

CELIAC DISEASE

Celiac disease (also called gluten enteropathy) is an intestinal disorder that results from an abnormal immunological reaction to gluten, a protein found in wheat, barley, rye, and, to a lesser extent, **oats** (page 716).

In addition to damaging the lining of the small intestine, celiac disease can sometimes affect other parts of the body, such as the pancreas (increasing the risk of diabetes), the thyroid gland (increasing the risk of thyroid disease), and the nervous system (increasing the risk of peripheral neuropathies and other neurological disorders). Occasionally, such damage occurs only in one or more of these parts of the body in the absence of damage to the intestines.

CHECKLIST FOR CELIAC DISEASE		
Rating	Nutritional Supplements	Herbs
★★☆	**Calcium** (page 483) (for deficiency only) **Enzymes** (page 506) **Folic acid** (page 520) (for deficiency only) **Iron** (page 540) (for deficiency only) **Magnesium** (page 551) (for deficiency only) **Multiple vitamin-mineral** (page 559) **Vitamin A** (page 595) (for deficiency only) **Vitamin D** (page 607) (for deficiency only) **Vitamin K** (page 612) (for deficiency only) **Zinc** (page 614) (for deficiency only)	
★☆☆	**Lipase** (page 550) **Vitamin B₆** (page 600) (for depression unresponsive to a gluten-free diet)	

What are the symptoms of celiac disease?

Celiac disease may not cause symptoms in some people. However, others may have a history of frequent **diarrhea** (page 163); pale, foul-smelling, bulky stools; abdominal pain, gas, and bloating; weight loss; fatigue; **canker sores** (page 90); muscle cramps; delayed growth or short stature; bone and joint pain; seizures; painful skin rash; or infertility. Microscopic examination of the small-intestinal lining reveals severe damage, especially in the jejunum (the central portion of the small intestines). People with untreated celiac disease may eventually experience malaise and weight loss and have an increased risk of developing **anemia** (page 25), **osteoporosis** (page 333), **osteomalacia** (page 392), and certain types of **cancer** (page 87). In addition to physical symptoms, some people may experience emotional disturbances, including feelings of **anxiety** (page 30) and **depression** (page 145).

Medical treatments

Prescription medications used to treat celiac disease include immunosuppressive and anti-inflammatory drugs. Agents prescribed include glucocorticoids, such as prednisone (Deltasone) and prednisolone (Prelone), and 6-mercaptopurine (Purinethol).

Strict adherence to a gluten-free diet is essential, although doctors are questioning the need for all celiac patients to avoid oats. People with severe damage to intestinal tissue may be prescribed intravenous nutritional supplements in order to replace unabsorbed nutrients.

Dietary changes that may be helpful

All doctors agree that consumption of the gluten-containing grains wheat, barley, and rye must be avoided in all celiac patients. Less consensus exists regarding the advisability of eating or restricting **oats** (page 716) and oat products. While oats contain a substance similar to gluten, modern research suggests that eating moderate amounts of oats does not cause problems for most people with celiac disease.[1] In one of these reports, approximately 95% of people with celiac disease tolerated 50 grams (almost two ounces) of oats per day for up to 12 months.[2]

Strict avoidance of wheat, barley, and rye, and of foods containing ingredients derived from these grains, usually results in an improvement in gastrointestinal symptoms within a few weeks, although in some cases the improvement may take many months. Tests of absorptive function usually improve after a few months on a gluten-free diet.[3]

Many people with celiac disease become symptom-free when following gluten-free diets. Others, however, continue to experience symptoms, often resulting from the presence of trace amounts of gluten either permitted in some gluten-free diets or consumed by mistake. Such mistakes are easy to make because many processed foods contain small amounts of gluten. For people with residual symptoms, a diet that truly eliminates all gluten, followed by open and double-blind challenges, resulted in symptomatic improvement in 77% of those studied.[4] A careful dietary analysis should ensure that all trace amounts of gluten are removed from the diet. If this fails to relieve symptoms after three months, then other food intolerances should be ruled out using an elimination diet.

Avoiding gluten may also reduce **cancer risk** (page 87). In one trial, 210 people with celiac disease were observed for 11 years. Those who followed a gluten-free diet had an incidence of cancer similar to that in the general population. However, those eating only a gluten-reduced diet or consuming a normal diet had an increased risk of developing cancer (mainly lymphomas and cancers of the mouth, pharynx, and esophagus).[5]

Children with untreated celiac disease have been reported to have abnormally low bone mineral density. However, after approximately one year on a gluten-free diet, bone mineral density increased rapidly and approximated the level seen in healthy children.[6] Long-term adherence to a gluten-free diet ensures normal bone density and is an important preventive measure in young people with celiac disease.[7]

Adults with celiac disease also have significantly lower bone mineral density than do healthy adults. After consumption of a gluten-free diet for one year, bone mineral density of the hip and lumbar spine has been reported to increase by an average of more than 15%.[8]

Infertility, which is common among people with celiac disease, has been reportedly reversed in both **men** (page 305) and **women** (page 187) after commencement of a gluten-free diet.[9]

Some people with celiac disease may be intolerant to other foods, in addition to gluten. Foods that have been reported to trigger symptoms include cows'milk[10] and soy.[11, 12, 13]

Lifestyle changes that may be helpful

In one study, children who were breast-fed for less than 30 days were four times more likely to develop celiac disease, compared with children who were breast-fed for more than 30 days.[14] Although this study does not prove that breast-feeding prevents the development of celiac disease, it is consistent with other research showing that breast-feeding promotes a healthier gastrointestinal tract than does formula-feeding.[15]

Nutritional supplements that may be helpful

The malabsorption that occurs in celiac disease can lead to multiple nutritional deficiencies. The most common nutritional problems in people with celiac disease include deficiencies of essential fatty acids, **iron** (page 540), **vitamin D** (page 607), **vitamin K** (page 612), **calcium** (page 483), **magnesium** (page 549), and **folic acid** (page 520).[16] **Zinc** (page 614) malabsorption also occurs frequently in celiac disease[17] and may result in zinc deficiency, even in people who are otherwise in remission.[18] People with newly diagnosed celiac disease should be as-

sessed for nutritional deficiencies by a doctor. Celiac patients who have not yet completely recovered should supplement with a high-potency **multivitamin-mineral** (page 559). Some patients may require even higher amounts of some of these vitamins and minerals—an issue that should be discussed with their healthcare practitioner. Evidence of a nutrient deficiency in a celiac patient is a clear indication for supplementation with that nutrient.

After commencement of a gluten-free diet, overall nutritional status gradually improves. However, deficiencies of some nutrients may persist, even in people who are strictly avoiding gluten. For example, magnesium deficiency was found in 8 of 23 adults with celiac disease who had been following a gluten-free diet and were symptom-free. When these adults were supplemented with magnesium for two years, their bone mineral density increased significantly.[19]

In another study, six people with diet-treated celiac disease had abnormal dark-adaptation tests (indicative of "night blindness"), even though some were taking a multivitamin that contained **vitamin A** (page 595). Some of these people showed an improvement in dark adaptation after receiving larger amounts of vitamin A, either orally or by injection.[20] People with celiac disease should discuss the possibility of vitamin A deficiency with a healthcare practitioner before taking vitamin A supplements.

Malabsorption-induced depletion of **vitamin D** (page 607) can lead to **osteomalacia** (page 392) (defective bone mineralization) in people with celiac disease.[21] Although supplementation with vitamin D appears to increase bone density, the excess risk of bone fracture may not be entirely eliminated.

It is possible that subtle deficiencies of other nutrients may exist in people with celiac disease who are on a gluten-free diet and are in remission. People who are not strictly avoiding gluten are likely to have more severe deficiencies. Because of the complexity of this condition and the multiple nutritional factors involved, people with celiac disease should be under the care of a doctor. Some doctors may recommend use of nutritional supplements, including a high-potency **multivitamin-mineral** (page 559) supplement, to reduce the risk of future deficiencies. No controlled trials have investigated the value of supplements in the minority of celiac disease patients who do not go into remission in response to a gluten-free diet.[22]

In one trial, 11 people with celiac disease suffered

from persistent **depression** (page 145) despite being on a gluten-free diet for more than two years. However, after supplementation with **vitamin B$_6$** (page 600) (80 mg per day) for six months, the depression disappeared.[23]

People with celiac disease often do not produce adequate digestive secretions from the pancreas, including **lipase enzymes** (page 547)[24] In a double-blind trial, children with celiac disease who received a **pancreatic enzyme** (page 506) supplement along with a gluten-free diet gained significantly more weight in the first month than those treated with only a gluten-free diet.[25] However, this benefit disappeared in the second month, suggesting enzyme supplements may only be useful at the beginning of dietary treatment.

Are there any side effects or interactions?
Refer to the individual supplement for information about any side effects or interactions.

CHILDHOOD DISEASES

Some of the most common illnesses of childhood cause skin eruptions and are known as exanthems. The childhood exanthems include rubeola (**measles** [page 307]), rubella (German measles), chicken pox, erythema infectiosum (fifth disease), and roseola infantum, all of which are viral infections, as well as scarlet fever, a bacterial infection. All of these infections affect the respiratory system and are highly contagious.

Children with these illnesses usually recover fully even without treatment; however, all of these conditions carry the possibility of severe complications, such as pneumonia, heart and kidney damage, and encephalitis (inflammation of the brain). Vaccinations and other changes in modern lifestyle have rendered several of these previously common illnesses virtually nonexistent in the developed world, though they are widespread and remain a major cause of childhood deaths in other parts of the world.

What are the symptoms of childhood diseases?
Children with a childhood disease may have symptoms including muscle aches, fatigue, fever, coughing, sneezing, sore throat, runny nose, nausea, and vomiting. There may also be an itchy skin rash with red bumps that may look like blisters.

CHECKLIST FOR CHILDHOOD DISEASES		
Rating	**Nutritional Supplements**	**Herbs**
★★★	**Vitamin A** (page 595)	
★☆☆	**Quercetin** (page 580) **Selenium** (page 584) **Vitamin C** (page 604) **Vitamin E** (page 609) **Zinc** (page 614)	

Medical treatments
Over the counter drugs focus on the treatment of symptoms, such as **pain** (page 338) and fever. The safest drug for this purpose is acetaminophen (Tylenol). Children with fever who are under the age of 19 are no longer given aspirin-containing products. Use in these circumstances has been linked to an increased risk of Reye's syndrome, a potentially serious illness that can affect the liver and brain.

Prescription antiviral medicines such as acyclovir (Zovirax) may be prescribed. Antibiotics may also be prescribed for some children in order to prevent a bacterial infection.

Children with an exanthem are commonly advised to rest and drink plenty of fluids. Doctors may also recommend limiting contact with other children to prevent transmission of the disease.

Dietary changes that may be helpful
Children who suffer from malnutrition have weakened immune systems and are more likely to acquire exanthemous infections and to experience more severe illness from them. Malnutrition contributes to half of all childhood deaths from infectious diseases worldwide.[1] **Measles** (page 307), a common childhood viral infection, is more likely to result in permanent blindness and is more likely to be fatal in children with poor nutritional status.[2, 3] Measles vaccinations are less effective in children who are malnourished.[4, 5]

Nutritional supplements that may be helpful
Preliminary research shows that supplemental **vitamin A** (page 595) improves the likelihood that the measles vaccine will provide protection.[6] Vitamin A has, since the 1920s, been the subject of much research into the prevention and treatment of childhood exanthems, particularly measles.[7] This nutrient has a critical role in

proper **immune function** (page 255), and there is evidence that supplementation with vitamin A reduces the incidence and severity of, and deaths from, childhood measles.[8, 9] The World Health Organization (WHO) has therefore recommended that children with signs of deficiency receive supplementation with vitamin A. The recommended amounts are 100,000 IU for children younger than one year and 200,000 IU for children older than one year, immediately upon diagnosis, and repeated once the next day and once in one to four weeks.[10] A controlled trial of African children given vitamin A supplementation according to the WHO's recommendations found that severity of measles and its long-term consequences were reduced by 82% on day eight, 61% in week six, and 85% six months after the onset.[11]

Another controlled trial found that giving approximately 200,000 IU of vitamin A once during measles illness was not adequate to provide any benefit in African children whose vitamin A status was unknown.[12] In a controlled prevention study, Indian children treated with 2,500 mcg (8,333 IU) of vitamin A weekly had fewer measles complications and less than half of the rate of death as compared with children receiving placebo;[13] but in another study, Indian children receiving 200,000 IU of vitamin A every six months did not have a different rate of total infectious illness nor rate of death as compared with children receiving placebo.[14]

An analysis of 20 controlled trials concluded that vitamin A supplementation reduced deaths from measles respiratory infection by 70%.[15] While vitamin A deficiency is widespread in developing countries, it has also been reported in the United States and has been linked with more severe cases of measles.[16] The American Academy of Pediatrics has recommended supplementation with vitamin A for children between the ages of six months and two years who are hospitalized with measles and its complications. The recommended amount is a single administration of 100,000 IU for children aged 6 to 12 months and 200,000 IU for children older than 1 year, followed by a second administration 24 hours later and a third after four weeks in children who are likely to have vitamin A deficiency.[17]

One trial showed that low levels of vitamin A are more prevalent in children with measles than in similar children without measles, with levels rising back to normal several days after the onset of the infection. This observation led the authors of the study to conclude that vitamin A deficiency is a consequence of infection with the measles virus and to recommend supplementa-

tion with vitamin A during measles infection even when prior deficiency is not suspected.[18] Vitamin A stores have also been shown to be depleted during chicken pox infection,[19] and some preliminary data supports its use in treatment of chicken pox. In a controlled trial, in which children without vitamin A deficiency were given either 200,000 IU of vitamin A or placebo one time during chicken pox, the children given vitamin A had shorter duration of illness and fewer severe complications. The researchers then treated the patients' siblings with vitamin A before chicken pox became evident, and they had an even shorter length of illness.[20]

Selenium (page 584) is a mineral known to have antioxidant properties and to be involved in healthy immune system activity. Recent animal and human research suggests that selenium deficiency increases the risk of viral infection and that supplementation prevents viral infection.[21, 22, 23, 24, 25] In a controlled trial, children with a specific viral infection (respiratory syncytial virus) who received a single supplement of 1 mg (1,000 mcg) of sodium selenite (a form of selenium) recovered more quickly than children who did not receive selenium.[26] While it is possible that childhood exanthemous viral infections might similarly be more severe in selenium-deficient children and helped through supplementation, none of the current research involves these specific viruses.

Zinc (page 614) is another mineral antioxidant nutrient that the immune system requires. Zinc deficiency results in lowered immune defenses, and zinc supplementation increases immune activity in people with certain illnesses.[27] As with vitamin A, zinc levels have been observed to fall during the early stages of measles infection and to return to normal several days later.[28] There is evidence that zinc supplements are helpful in specific viral infections,[29, 30, 31] but there are no data on the effect of zinc on childhood exanthemous infections.

Vitamin C (page 604) has been demonstrated in test tube, animal, and human studies to have immune-enhancing and direct antiviral properties.[32] Preliminary observations made on the effect of vitamin C on viral infections have involved both measles and chicken pox.[33] An active immune system uses vitamin C rapidly, and blood levels fall in children with bacterial or viral infections.[34] Reduced immune cell activity has been observed in people with measles, but in one preliminary study, supplementation with 250 mg daily of vitamin C in children 18 months to 3 years old had no impact on the course of the illness.[35] The authors of this study admit that this amount of vitamin C may have been too low to bring about an observable increase in immune cell activity and thus an increase in speed of recovery.

Healthy immune function also requires adequate amounts of **vitamin E** (page 609). Vitamin E deficiency is associated with increased severity of viral infections in mice.[36, 37, 38] Supplementation with vitamin E during viral infections has been shown to increase immune cell activity[39] and reduce virus activity[40] in mice. Research into the effects of vitamin E supplementation on childhood exanthems has not been done.

Flavonoids (page 516) are a group of compounds found in some plant foods and medicinal herbs. An antiviral action of some flavonoids has been observed in a number of test tube experiments.[41, 42, 43, 44, 45] **Quercetin** (page 580), one of the flavonoids, has shown particularly strong antiviral properties in the test tube;[46, 47, 48] however, one study did not find quercetin to be of benefit to mice with a viral infection.[49] It is not known whether flavonoids can be absorbed in amounts sufficient to exert an antiviral effect in humans, and therefore their possible role in the treatment of childhood exanthems remains unknown.

Are there any side effects or interactions?
Refer to the individual supplement for information about any side effects or interactions.

CHILDHOOD OBESITY

See also: Weight Loss and Obesity (page 446)

Excessive weight in children and adolescents is becoming an increasingly serious problem.[1, 2] In the United States, 13% of children aged 6 to 11 years and 14% of adolescents aged 12 to 19 years are overweight, and among adolescents the percentage is three times higher than it was 20 years ago.[3] Major contributors to childhood obesity include genetics, unhealthy diets, and sedentary lifestyles.[4, 5] Overweight children often become adults with weight problems that contribute to a wide variety of health problems,[6, 7] but even during childhood and adolescence, overweight can contribute to such disorders as **type 2 diabetes** (page 152), **high cholesterol** (page 223), **high blood pressure** (page 246), **insulin resistance** (page 273), and **liver disease** (page 290).[8, 9, 10] Being overweight also has social and psychological consequences for children in terms of social discrimination, poor self-esteem, and depression.[11, 12]

Parents, family members, and others who are important people in a child's life can either help or harm an obese child's situation. As with all children, those with weight problems need acceptance, support, and encouragement from their family, and the eating, exercising, and other health habits of family members play important roles in influencing the same behaviors in children.[13, 14]

CHECKLIST FOR CHILDHOOD OBESITY		
Rating	Nutritional Supplements	Herbs
★★☆	Glucomannan (page 526)	

What are the symptoms of childhood obesity?
The proper weight for a growing child or adolescent should be determined with the help of a doctor or other qualified health professional, who can also determine whether any unusual medical problems might be contributing to weight gain, whether any current health problems exist that are related to overweight, and appropriate weight control methods. Treating obesity should not include overly restrictive or fad diets that are missing essential nutrients. In fact, weight loss is not necessarily appropriate for a growing child. Often the best goal for an overweight child is to maintain their current weight as they grow taller.

Medical treatments
Treatment for childhood obesity involves screening for heart disease risk and other health risk factors, and providing information on improving diet and exercise habits. No medications are approved for treating childhood obesity.[15]

Dietary changes that may be helpful
Unhealthful eating patterns resulting in overconsumption of foods high in fat, calories, or added sugars are considered a major contributor to childhood obesity.[16] Since these patterns often include habits learned from the family, attention should be paid to providing healthful food to the entire family and encouraging good role modeling by other family members.[17]

Guiding healthful food choices when eating outside of the home is also a priority. To teach good lifetime eating habits, try the following:[18]

- Make healthful foods easy to see at home and keep unhealthful foods out of sight
- Plan meals and snacks ahead of time so that healthy choices will be available
- Avoid using food as a reward or withholding food as punishment
- Eat slowly and pay attention to when you are hungry and when you are satisfied
- Eat at a designated location such as a dining table, rather than in front of the TV
- Aim for several servings of fruits and vegetables every day
- Drink water when thirsty instead of beverages with added sugars
- Start the day with a healthful breakfast to prevent cravings later on

There is only limited research on the prevention of childhood obesity with diet. Preliminary studies have found that breast-feeding during infancy is usually associated with a reduced risk of developing obesity during early childhood, though the reasons for this effect are unclear.[19, 20, 21] In a controlled study of children between the ages of 7 and 12, a school-based education program designed to reduce carbonated-drink consumption resulted in a reduction in the number of overweight children after 12 months.[22]

Most authorities believe that the best diet for treating childhood obesity is a heart-healthy diet low in saturated fat and cholesterol, but high in vitamins, minerals, and other important nutrients.[23] However, few studies have actually compared different diets for their effectiveness in treating childhood obesity.

A recent 12-week controlled trial found that overweight adolescents lost more weight with a low-carbohydrate diet than with a low-fat diet.[24] Very-low-carbohydrate (ketogenic) diets have been shown to cause rapid weight loss in very obese children in short-term preliminary and controlled trials,[25, 26] but the long-term safety and benefits of this type of diet are unknown. More research is needed to evaluate low-carbohydrate diets for treating childhood obesity.

Glycemic index and glycemic load describe the tendency of foods to raise blood sugar. Eating meals containing foods that are low in glycemic index or glycemic load may influence appetite and other body mechanisms that affect excessive weight gain in children.[27, 28] A preliminary study reported that obese children using a low-glycemic-index diet lost more weight compared with a similar group using a low-fat diet.[29] A controlled trial found that obese adolescents eating freely on a low-glycemic-load diet lost more weight and body fat after six months than did a similar group following a typical low-calorie, low-fat diet.[30]

Very-low-calorie "modified fasting" diets, typically using high-protein meal replacement beverages, have been tried in preliminary and controlled studies of obese children with good short-term results.[31, 32] However, weight lost with these diets is often regained and there are health risks associated with their use.[33] Little is known about their effect on growth and other health issues in children.

Lifestyle changes that may be helpful
Lack of physical activity is considered a significant contributing factor in childhood obesity.[34] However, while the results of *treatment* of overweight children are usually enhanced by strategies to increase physical activity or decrease inactivity, attempts to improve physical activity levels have not been very successful in *preventing* childhood obesity according to most controlled research.[35] Nonetheless, watching television and playing computer or video games contributes to the sedentary lifestyle of many children, and controlled research has shown that weight control is more successful when these activities are controlled and healthier alternatives provided.[36, 37, 38] Children are recommended to get at least an hour of moderate physical activity most days of the week, and more may be necessary to offset genetic and other influences. Fun activities that involve other family members or other children will help make getting more exercise a positive experience.[39]

Weight-loss efforts that involve excessive restriction of calories or protein can inhibit a child's ability to gain lean body mass (such as muscle) during the normal growth process. Consequently, weight-loss diets for children should not be excessively restrictive. In addition, an appropriate exercise program can be a useful addition to a low-calorie diet for overweight children. A controlled trial found that strength training, when added to a low-calorie diet, resulted in a greater gain of lean body mass (while still promoting weight loss), compared with diet alone in obese children.[40] Another study of obese adolescents found that a physical exercise program combined with normal calorie intake resulted in reductions in body weight and body fat while allowing for normal growth and preservation of lean body mass.[41]

Nutritional supplements that may be helpful
Increased fiber intake is thought to have potential benefit in a weight-loss program since dietary fiber dilutes calories, slows down the eating process, and may make

people feel more full despite eating fewer calories.[42] However, research on using fiber in the treatment of childhood obesity has focused on using **fiber supplements** (page 512) rather than comparing low- and high-fiber diets. Supplementation for four months with 2 to 3 grams per day of a bulking agent called **glucomannan** (page 526), was effective in a group of obese adolescents in one controlled trial,[43] but another controlled trial found no significant effect of 2 grams per day for two months.[44]

Are there any side effects or interactions?
Refer to the individual supplement for information about any side effects or interactions.

Holistic approaches that may be helpful

Behavior-change techniques are considered useful for helping people break old habits and form more healthful habits. These techniques may be learned from counseling professionals, support groups, educational programs, or books. Many controlled studies have investigated various methods for using behavior-change techniques to prevent or treat childhood obesity, with several reporting success at reducing overweight compared with either no treatment or with conventional weight-loss approaches.[45, 46, 47]

Parental involvement in the treatment of childhood obesity is considered important for success, especially when parents are given adequate training in a wide range of behavior-change techniques that can be applied to the entire family.[48] Limited research suggests that training parents alone is superior to training either children alone or training both parents and children.[49, 50, 51] Some authorities suggest that training parents alone produces the best results because this avoids affecting the child's self-esteem and willingness to change, which might result from labeling him or her as "the patient."[52, 53]

Problem-solving techniques are used in some types of counseling to help people maintain changes in their behavior. In one controlled study, teaching problem-solving techniques to parents in addition to behavior-change techniques improved weight loss results in obese children compared with a group learning only behavior-change techniques.[54] However, another controlled study found no additional benefit when problem-solving training was given to either the child or to both child and parent.[55]

For support and information, parents can also try the following resources:

- The Surgeon General's Call to Action to Prevent and Decrease Overweight and Obesity: Over-

weight in Children and Adolescents (www. surgeongeneral.gov/topics/obesity/calltoaction/ fact_adolescents.htm)
- How Parents Can Fight the Obesity Epidemic (www.med.umich.edu/1libr/yourchild/ fightobesity.htm)
- Shapedown for Parents, Kids & Teens (www.shapedown.com/page2.htm)

CHRONIC CANDIDIASIS

See also: Yeast Infection (page 454)

What do I need to know?

Self-care for chronic candidiasis can be approached in a number of ways—but it can be hard to know just where to start. To make it easier, our doctors recommend trying these simple steps first:

Get a doctor's opinion
> Tests can help you make sure your symptoms are not the result of another health problem

Eat foods low in refined carbs and sugars
> White flour, refined sugars, and fruit juices may help yeast grow in the intestine, so cut them out of your diet

Avoid eating yeast and mold
> Eliminate foods produced with yeast and foods that may contain mold to reduce possible reactions due to sensitivities

Try some beneficial bacteria
> Take a supplement that contains 10 billion colony-forming units a day of acidophilus or bifidobacteria to control yeast in the intestine

Check out antifungal supplements
> To reduce yeast in the intestine, try caprylic acid (1,500 mg a day), garlic (5,000 mcg a day of allicin potential in an enteric-coated supplement), or oregano oil (0.2 to 0.4 ml a day of a coated supplement)

About chronic candidiasis

An overgrowth in the gastrointestinal tract of the usually benign yeast (or fungus) *Candida albicans* has been suggested as the origin of a complex medical syndrome called chronic candidiasis, or yeast syndrome.[1, 2]

Purported symptoms of chronic candidiasis are fatigue, **allergies** (page 14), **immune system malfunction** (page 255), **depression** (page 145), chemical sensitivities, and digestive disturbances.[3, 4] Conventional medical authorities do acknowledge the existence of a chronic Candida infection that affects the whole body and is sometimes called "chronic disseminated candidiasis."[5] However, this universally accepted disease is both uncommon, and decidedly more narrow in scope, than the so-called Yeast Syndrome—a condition believed by some to be quite common, particularly in people with a history of long-term antibiotic use. The term "chronic candidiasis" as used in this article refers to the as yet unproven Yeast Syndrome.

CHECKLIST FOR CHRONIC CANDIDIASIS

Rating	Nutritional Supplements	Herbs
★☆☆	**Betaine HCl** (page 473) Caprylic acid **Enzymes** (page 506) *Lactobacillus acidophilus* (page 575)	**Barberry** (page 632) *Echinacea purpurea* (page 669) **Garlic** (page 679) **Goldenseal** (page 683) Goldthread **Oregano** (page 719) oil **Oregon grape** (page 721) **Peppermint** (page 726) oil **Rosemary** (page 739) oil **Tea tree** (page 751) oil **Thyme** (page 752) oil

What are the symptoms of chronic candidiasis?

Symptoms attributed to chronic candidiasis include abdominal pain, **constipation** (page 137), **diarrhea** (page 163), **gas** (page 195), bloating, belching, **indigestion** (page 260), **heartburn** (page 260), recurrent vaginal **yeast infections** (page 454), **nasal congestion** (page 405), **sinus problems** (page 407), bad breath skin rashes, **allergies** (page 14), chemical sensitivies, rectal itching, muscle aches, cold hands and feet, fatigue, **depression** (page 145), irritability, difficulty concentrating, headaches, and dizziness.

Medical treatments

Chronic candidiasis is not a conventionally recognized medical condition, so no prescription drug treatment is standard. Treatment of chronic disseminated candidiasis usually consists of oral antifungal medications, such as nystatin (Mycostatin), ketoconazole (Nizoral), fluconazole (Diflucan), and itraconazole (Sporanox).

Dietary changes that may be helpful

Based on their clinical experience and on very preliminary research, several doctors have suggested that certain dietary factors may promote the overgrowth of *Candida albicans*. The most important of these factors are high intakes of sugar, milk, and other dairy products; foods with a high content of yeast or mold (e.g., alcoholic beverages, cheeses, dried fruits, and peanuts); and foods to which individual patients are **allergic** (page 14). However, few clinical trials have investigated whether these dietary factors affect people with conditions for which Candida is the causative agent.

One study compared levels of various sugars in urine of healthy women with levels found in women with chronic vaginal Candida infections.[6] Urine sugar levels correlated with dietary intakes of sugar, dairy, and artificial sweeteners. Among women who reduced their intake of sugar, 90% reported no vaginal yeast infections during the following year. These researchers reported a "dramatic reduction" in the incidence and severity of **vaginitis** (page 438) caused by Candida as a result of reducing intake of dairy, sugar, and artificial sweeteners.

Many apparently healthy people have some Candida in their gastrointestinal tract. In one trial, high-sugar diets given to healthy people had mixed effects on the concentration of Candida found in their stool, though some subjects did show an increase in Candida after eating more sugar.[7] These preliminary reports suggest, but do not prove, that diet might affect the ability of Candida to infect the body.

Yogurt that contains *Lactobacillus acidophilus* (page 575) has been reported to have a therapeutic effect in women with vaginal infections caused by Candida.

Nutritional supplements that may be helpful

Lactobacillus acidophilus (page 575) products are often used by people with candidiasis in an attempt to reestablish proper intestinal flora. Acidophilus produces natural factors that prevent the overgrowth of the yeast.[8, 9] Although there are no human trials, supplementation of acidophilus to immune-deficient mice infected with *C. albicans* produced positive effects on **immune function** (page 255) and reduced the number of Candida colonies.[10] The typical amount of acidophilus taken as a supplement is 1–10 billion live bacteria daily. Amounts exceeding this may induce mild gastrointestinal disturbances, while smaller amounts may not be able to sufficiently colonize the gastrointestinal tract.

Preliminary research from the 1940s and 1950s indicated that caprylic acid (a naturally occurring fatty acid) was an effective antifungal compound against Candida **infections** (page 265) of the intestines.[11, 12] Doctors sometimes recommend amounts of 500 to 1,000 mg three times a day.

It is unknown if taking **pancreatic enzymes** (page 506) or **betaine HCl** (page 473) (hydrochloric acid) tablets is beneficial for chronic candidiasis. Nonetheless, some doctors recommend improving digestive secretions with these agents. Hydrochloric-acid secretion from the stomach, pancreatic enzymes, and bile all inhibit the overgrowth of Candida and prevent its penetration into the absorptive surfaces of the small intestine.[13, 14, 15] Decreased secretion of any of these important digestive components can lead to overgrowth of Candida in the gastrointestinal tract. Consult a physician for more information.

In theory, the use of any effective anti-yeast therapy could result in what is referred to as the Herxheimer or "die-off" reaction.[16] The effective killing of the yeast organism can result in absorption of large quantities of yeast toxins, cell particles, and antigens. The Herxheimer reaction refers to a worsening of symptoms as a result of this die-off. Although this reaction has not been reported following use of any of the nutritional or herbal anti-Candida agents, the likelihood of experiencing this reaction can be minimized by starting any anti-yeast medications or nutritional supplements slowly, in lower amounts, and gradually increasing the amounts over one month to achieve full therapeutic intake.

Are there any side effects or interactions?
Refer to the individual supplement for information about any side effects or interactions.

Herbs that may be helpful
Garlic (page 679) has demonstrated significant antifungal activity against *C. albicans* in both animal and test tube studies.[17, 18, 19] Greater anti-Candida activity has resulted from exposing Candida to garlic, than to nystatin—the most common prescription drug used to fight Candida.[20] No clinical studies of garlic in the treatment of candidiasis have yet been conducted. However, some doctors suggest an intake equal to approximately one clove (4 grams) of fresh garlic per day; this would equal consumption of a garlic tablet that provides a total allicin potential of 4,000 to 5,000 mcg.

Volatile oils from **oregano** (page 719), **thyme** (page 752), **peppermint** (page 726), **tea tree** (page 751), and **rosemary** (page 739) have all demonstrated antifungal action in test tube studies.[21] A recent study compared the anti-Candida effect of oregano oil to that of caprylic acid.[22] The results indicated that oregano oil is over 100 times more potent than caprylic acid, against Candida. Since the volatile oils are quickly absorbed and associated with inducing **heartburn** (page 260), they must be taken in coated capsules, so they do not break down in the stomach but instead are delivered to the small and large intestine. This process is known as "enteric coating." Some doctors recommend using 0.2 to 0.4 ml of enteric-coated peppermint and/or oregano oil supplements three times per day 20 minutes before meals. However, none of these volatile oils has been studied for their anti-Candida effect in humans.

Berberine is an alkaloid found in various plants, including **goldenseal** (page 683), **barberry** (page 632), **Oregon grape** (page 721), and goldthread. Berberine exhibits a broad spectrum of antibiotic activity in test-tube, animal, and human studies.[23, 24] Berberine has shown effective antidiarrheal activity in a number of diarrheal diseases,[25, 26, 27] and it may offer the same type of relief for the **diarrhea** (page 163) seen in patients with chronic candidiasis. Doctors familiar with the use of berberine-containing herbs sometimes recommend taking 2 to 4 grams of the dried root (or bark) or 250 to 500 mg of an herbal extract three times a day. While isolated berberine has been studied, none of these herbs has been studied in humans with chronic candidiasis.

The fresh-pressed juice of *Echinacea purpurea* (page 669) has been shown to be helpful in preventing recurrence of vaginal **yeast infections** (page 454) in a double-blind trial; it may have similar benefit in Yeast Syndrome.[28] The typical recommendation for this effect is 2 to 4 ml of fluid extract daily.

Are there any side effects or interactions?
Refer to the individual herb for information about any side effects or interactions.

CHRONIC FATIGUE SYNDROME

What do I need to know?
Self-care for chronic fatigue syndrome can be approached in a number of ways—but it can be hard to

know just where to start. To make it easier, our doctors recommend trying these simple steps first:

Consult an expert

Find a healthcare professional experienced in treating CFS for help in managing this challenging disease

Gradually increase exercise

Even if you must begin with only a few minutes at a time, exercise can help you feel better

Get stress-reduction counseling

For help with coping strategies, find a qualified counselor experienced in helping people with CFS

Try NADH

10 mg per day of NADH (nicotinamide adenine dinucleotide, the active coenzyme form of vitamin B$_3$) may help your body produce more energy

Check out L-carnitine

Take 1 gram three times a day to provide a nutrient important for energy production

Consider vitamin B$_{12}$–injections

Consult a doctor for a trial of 2,500 to 5,000 mcg every two or three days for several weeks

About chronic fatigue syndrome

Chronic fatigue syndrome (CFS) is disabling fatigue lasting more than six months that reduces activity by more than half. CFS is a poorly understood disease involving many body systems. No single cause of CFS has been identified, therefore, it is diagnosed by symptoms and by ruling out other known causes of fatigue by a healthcare practitioner.

Suggested causes include chronic viral infections, **food allergy** (page 14), adrenal gland dysfunction, and many others. None of these have been convincingly documented in more than a minority of sufferers. In some people there is also difficulty sleeping, swollen lymph nodes, and/or mild fever. When there is muscle soreness, **fibromyalgia** (page 191) may be the actual problem. Although CFS is considered a modern diagnosis, it may have existed for centuries under other names, such as "the vapors," neurasthenia, "effort syndrome" (diagnosed in World War I veterans), **hypoglycemia** (page 251), and chronic mononucleosis.

What are the symptoms of chronic fatigue syndrome?

In addition to fatigue, there may also be muscle pain, joint pain not associated with redness or swelling,

short-term memory loss, and an inability to concentrate. Some people with chronic fatigue syndrome also experience **difficulty sleeping** (page 270), swollen lymph nodes, and/or mild fever.

CHECKLIST FOR CHRONIC FATIGUE SYNDROME		
Rating	**Nutritional Supplements**	**Herbs**
★★☆	**L-carnitine** (page 543) **NADH** (page 564) Potassium-magnesium aspartate **Vitamin B$_{12}$** (page 601)	
★☆☆	**DHEA** (page 503) **Fish oil (EPA/DHA)** (page 514) **Magnesium** (page 551)	Asian ginseng (page 630) Eleuthero (page 672) Licorice (page 702)

Medical treatments

Prescription medications such as anti-anxiety drugs (benzodiazepines), antidepressants, hydrocortisone (Cortef), and pain relievers might be beneficial.

Some healthcare providers recommend a combination of lifestyle changes (aerobic exercise, healthful diet, and stress reduction), light therapy, and psychological counseling.

Dietary changes that may be helpful

Some doctors believe that people with CFS who have low blood pressure should not restrict their salt intake. Among CFS sufferers who have a form of low blood pressure triggered by changes in position (orthostatic hypotension), some have been reported in a preliminary study to be helped by additional salt intake.[1] People with CFS considering increasing salt intake should consult a doctor before making such a change. (See the Herb information, below, for more information on blood pressure and CFS.)

Lifestyle changes that may be helpful

Exercise is important to prevent the worsening of fatigue. Many people report feeling better after undertaking a moderate exercise plan.[2, 3] However, most people with CFS are sensitive to overexertion, and excessive exercise may lead to consistently worsening fatigue and mental functioning.[4, 5, 6] Exercise should be attempted gradually, starting with very small efforts. One small study found that intermittent exercise, in which patients walked for three minutes followed by three minutes of rest for a total of 30 minutes, did not exacerbate their CFS symptoms.[7]

Nutritional supplements that may be helpful

The combination of potassium aspartate and magnesium aspartate has shown benefits for chronically fatigued people in double-blind trials.[8, 9, 10, 11] However, these trials were performed before the criteria for diagnosing CFS was established, so whether these people were suffering from CFS is unclear. Usually 1 gram of aspartates is taken twice per day, and results have been reported within one to two weeks.

Vitamin B$_{12}$ (page 601) deficiency may cause fatigue. However, some reports,[12] even double-blind ones,[13] have shown that people who are not deficient in B$_{12}$ have increased energy following a series of vitamin B$_{12}$ injections. Some sources in conventional medicine have discouraged such people from taking B$_{12}$ shots despite this evidence.[14] Nonetheless, some doctors have continued to take the limited scientific support for B$_{12}$ seriously.[15] In one preliminary trial, 2,500 to 5,000 mcg of vitamin B$_{12}$ given by injection every two to three days led to improvement in 50 to 80% of a group of people with CFS; most improvement appeared after several weeks of B$_{12}$ shots.[16] While the research in this area remains preliminary, people with CFS considering a trial of vitamin B$_{12}$ injections should consult a doctor. Oral or sublingual B$_{12}$ supplements are unlikely to obtain the same results as injectable B$_{12}$, because the body's ability to absorb large amounts is relatively poor.

A preliminary trial has shown that people with CFS have reduced functional B-vitamin status when compared to people without the condition.[17] The functional vitamin deficiency seen in this study was most pronounced for **vitamin B$_6$** (page 600). Double-blind trials are needed to establish whether **B-vitamin** (page 603) supplementation is effective in people with chronic fatigue syndrome.

L-carnitine (page 543) is required for energy production in the powerhouses of cells (the mitochondria). There may be a problem in the mitochondria in people with CFS. Deficiency of carnitine has been seen in some CFS sufferers.[18] One gram of carnitine taken three times daily for eight weeks led to improvement in CFS symptoms in one preliminary trial.[19]

NADH (page 564) (nicotinamide adenine dinucleotide) helps make ATP, the energy source the body runs on. In a double-blind trial, people with CFS received 10 mg of NADH or a placebo each day for four weeks.[20] Of those receiving NADH, 31% reported improvements in fatigue, decreases in other symptoms, and improved overall quality of life, compared with only 8% of those in the placebo group. Further double-blind research is needed to confirm these findings.

Magnesium (page 551) levels have been reported to be low in CFS sufferers. In a double-blind trial, injections with magnesium improved symptoms for most people.[21] Oral magnesium supplementation has improved symptoms in those people with CFS who previously had low magnesium levels, according to a preliminary report, although magnesium injections were sometimes necessary.[22] These researchers report that magnesium deficiency appears to be very common in people with CFS. Nonetheless, several other researchers report no evidence of magnesium deficiency in people with CFS.[23, 24, 25] The reason for this discrepancy remains unclear. If people with CFS do consider magnesium supplementation, they should have their magnesium status checked by a doctor before undertaking supplementation. It appears that only people with magnesium deficiency benefit from this therapy.

Dehydroepiandrosterone, more commonly known as **DHEA** (page 503), is a hormone now available as a supplement. In one report, DHEA levels were found to be low in people with CFS.[26] Another research group reported that, while DHEA levels were normal in a group of CFS patients, the ability of these people to increase their DHEA level in response to hormonal stimulation was impaired.[27] Whether supplementation with DHEA might help CFS patients remains unknown due to the lack of controlled research. DHEA should not be used without the supervision of a healthcare professional.

In a preliminary study, four patients with chronic fatigue syndrome reported an improvement in their symptoms after taking an **essential fatty acid** (page 514) supplement daily for at least 12 weeks.[28] The amount used was 10 to 18 capsules per day, and each capsule contained 93 mg of **eicosapentaenoic acid** (page 514) (EPA), 29 mg of **docosahexaenoic acid** (page 509) (DHA), and 10 mg of gamma-linolenic acid. Because there was no placebo group in this study and, because fatigue often improves after treatment with a placebo, additional research is needed to confirm this report.

Are there any side effects or interactions?
Refer to the individual supplement for information about any side effects or interactions.

Herbs that may be helpful

Some research suggests that CFS may be partially due to low adrenal function resulting from different stressors (e.g., mental stress, physical stress, and even viral illness) and impacting the normal communication between the hypothalamus, pituitary gland, and the adrenal glands.[29] **Licorice** (page 702) root is known to stimulate the adrenal glands and to block the breakdown of active cortisol in the body.[30] One case report described a man with CFS whose symptoms improved after taking 2.5 grams of licorice root daily.[31] While there have been no controlled trials to test licorice in patients with CFS, it may be worth a trial of six to eight weeks using 2 to 3 grams of licorice root daily.

Adaptogenic herbs such as **Asian ginseng** (page 630) and **eleuthero** (page 672) may also be useful for CFS patients—the herbs not only have an immunomodulating effect but also help support the normal function of the hypothalamic-pituitary-adrenal axis, the hormonal stress system of the body.[32] These herbs are useful follow-ups to the six to eight weeks of taking licorice root and may be used for long-term support of adrenal function in people with CFS. However, no controlled research has investigated the effect of adaptogenic herbs on CFS.

Are there any side effects or interactions?

Refer to the individual herb for information about any side effects or interactions.

Holistic approaches that may be helpful

Highly stressful situations should be avoided by people with CFS. Coping mechanisms for dealing with stress can sometimes be maximized by behavioral therapy, which has been shown helpful for people with CFS in several controlled studies.[33]

CHRONIC OBSTRUCTIVE PULMONARY DISEASE

Chronic obstructive pulmonary disease (COPD) refers to the combination of chronic **bronchitis** (page 80) and emphysema, resulting in obstruction of airways and poor oxygen transport in the lungs, respectively.

Although chronic bronchitis and emphysema are distinct conditions, smokers and former smokers often have aspects of both. In chronic bronchitis, the linings of the bronchial tubes are inflamed and thickened, leading to a chronic, mucus-producing **cough** (page 139) and shortness of breath. In emphysema, the alveoli (tiny air sacs in the lungs) are damaged, also leading to shortness of breath. COPD is generally irreversible and may even be fatal.

CHECKLIST FOR CHRONIC OBSTRUCTIVE PULMONARY DISEASE		
Rating	**Nutritional Supplements**	**Herbs**
★★★	**N-acetyl cysteine** (page 562) (for bronchitis)	
★★☆	**L-carnitine** (page 543)	**Ivy leaf** (page 697)
★☆☆	**Coenzyme Q$_{10}$** (page 496) **Fish oil** (page 514) (EPA/**DHA** [page 509]) **Magnesium** (page 551) **Vitamin C** (page 604)	**Anise** (page 627) **Elecampane** (page 671) **Eucalyptus** (page 673) Gumweed **Lobelia** (page 705) **Mullein** (page 713) **Wild cherry** (page 758) Yerba santa

What are the symptoms of COPD?

Symptoms of COPD develop gradually and may initially include shortness of breath during exertion, wheezing especially when exhaling, and frequent coughing that produces variable amounts of mucus. In more advanced stages, people may experience rapid changes in the ability to breathe, shortness of breath at rest, fatigue, **depression** (page 145), memory problems, confusion, and **frequent waking** (page 270) during sleep.

Medical treatments

Over the counter guiafenesin (Robitussin) may help to thin mucous.

Bronchodilators, such as albuterol (Proventil, Ventolin), salmeterol (Serevent), ipratropium (Atrovent), and metaproterenol (Alupent); oral corticosteroids, including prednisone (Deltasone); and inhaled corticosteroids, such as fluticasone (Flovent), triamcinolone (Azmacort), flunisolide (AeroBid), and budesonide (Pulmicort), are commonly used prescription drugs. Mucolytics such as Acetylcysteine (Mucomyst) are prescribed to help thin mucus secretions.

People with COPD should stop smoking and avoid secondhand smoke in order to slow the rate of lung function decline. Individuals with COPD should receive yearly pneumococcal (pneumonia) and flu vaccinations. Supplemental oxygen therapy and breathing rehabilitation programs are recommended in some situations. Severe cases might require lung volume reduction surgery or a lung transplant.

Dietary changes that may be helpful

Malnutrition is common in people with COPD and may further compromise lung function and the overall health of those with this disease.[1] However, evidence of malnutrition may occur despite adequate dietary intake of nutrients.[2] Researchers have found that increasing dietary carbohydrates increases carbon dioxide production, which leads to reduced exercise tolerance and increased breathlessness in people with COPD.[3] On the other hand, men with a higher intake of fruit (which is high in carbohydrates) over a 25-year period were at lower risk of developing lung diseases.[4] People with COPD should, therefore, consider eliminating most sources of refined sugars, but not fruits, from their diet.

Chronic **bronchitis** (page 80) has been linked to **allergies** (page 14) in many reports.[5, 6, 7] In a preliminary trial, long-term reduction of some COPD symptoms occurred when people with COPD avoided allergenic foods and, in some cases, were also desensitized to pollen.[8] People with COPD interested in testing the effects of a food allergy elimination program should talk with a doctor.

Lifestyle changes that may be helpful

Smoking is the underlying cause of the majority of cases of emphysema and chronic bronchitis. Anyone who smokes should stop, and, although quitting smoking will not reverse the symptoms of COPD, it may help preserve the remaining lung function. Exposure to other respiratory irritants, such as air pollution, dust, toxic gases, and fumes, may aggravate COPD and should be avoided when possible.

The **common cold** (page 129) and other respiratory infections may aggravate COPD. Avoiding exposure to **infections** (page 265) or bolstering resistance with **immune-enhancing** (page 260) nutrients and herbs may be valuable.

Nutritional supplements that may be helpful

N-acetyl cysteine (NAC) (page 562) helps break down mucus. For that reason, inhaled NAC is used in hospitals to treat bronchitis. NAC may also protect lung tissue through its **antioxidant** (page 467) activity.[9] Oral NAC, 200 mg taken three times per day, is also effective and improved symptoms in people with bronchitis in double-blind research.[10, 11] Results may take six months.

L-carnitine (page 543) has been given to people with chronic lung disease in trials investigating how the body responds to exercise.[12, 13] In these double-blind trials, 2 grams of L-carnitine, taken twice daily for two to four weeks, led to positive changes in breathing response to exercise.

A review of nutrition and lung health reported that people with a higher dietary intake of **vitamin C** (page 604) were less likely to be diagnosed with **bronchitis** (page 80).[14] As yet, the effects of supplementing with vitamin C in people with COPD have not been studied.

A greater intake of the omega-3 fatty acids found in **fish oils** (page 514) has been linked to reduced risk of COPD,[15] though research has yet to investigate whether fish oil supplements would help people with COPD.

Many prescription drugs commonly taken by people with COPD have been linked to **magnesium** (page 551) deficiency, a potential problem because magnesium is needed for normal lung function.[16] One group of researchers reported that 47% of people with COPD had a magnesium deficiency.[17] In this study, magnesium deficiency was also linked to increased hospital stays. Thus, it appears that many people with COPD may be magnesium deficient, a problem that might worsen their condition; moreover, the deficiency is not easily diagnosed.

Intravenous magnesium has improved breathing capacity in people experiencing an acute exacerbation of COPD.[18] In this double-blind study, the need for hospitalization also was reduced in the magnesium group (28% versus 42% with placebo), but this difference was not statistically significant. Intravenous magnesium is known to be a powerful bronchodilator.[19] The effect of oral magnesium supplementation in people with COPD has yet to be investigated.

Researchers have also given **coenzyme Q10** (page 496) (CoQ10) to people with COPD after discovering their blood levels of CoQ10 were lower than those found in healthy people.[20] In that trial, 90 mg of CoQ10 per day, given for eight weeks, led to no change in lung function, though oxygenation of blood improved, as did exercise performance and heart rate. Until more research is done, the importance of supplementing with CoQ10 for people with COPD remains unclear.

Antioxidants in general are hypothesized to be important for neutralizing the large amounts of free radicals associated with COPD. However, use of two antioxidant supplements (synthetic **beta-carotene** (page 469), 20 mg per day, and **vitamin E** (page 609), 50 IU per day) did not help smokers with COPD in a double-blind trial, despite the fact that people who ate higher amounts of these nutrients in their diets appeared to have lower risk.[21]

Are there any side effects or interactions?
Refer to the individual supplement for information about any side effects or interactions.

Herbs that may be helpful
One double-blind trial found an **ivy leaf** (page 697) extract to be as effective as the mucus-dissolving drug ambroxol for treating chronic **bronchitis** (page 80).[22]

Mullein (page 713) is classified in the herbal literature as both an expectorant, to promote the discharge of mucus, and a demulcent, to soothe and protect mucous membranes. Historically, mullein has been used as a remedy for the respiratory tract, particularly in cases of irritating **coughs** (page 139) with bronchial congestion.[23] Other herbs commonly used as expectorants in traditional medicine include **elecampane** (page 671), **lobelia** (page 705), yerba santa *(Eriodictyon californicum),* **wild cherry** (page 758) bark, gumweed *(Grindelia robusta),* **anise** (page 627) *(Pimpinella anisum),* and **eucalyptus** (page 673). Animal studies have suggested that some of these herbs increase discharge of mucus.[24] However, none have been studied for efficacy in humans.

Are there any side effects or interactions?
Refer to the individual herb for information about any side effects or interactions.

Holistic approaches that may be helpful
Negative ions may counteract the allergenic effects of positively charged ions on respiratory tissues and potentially ease symptoms of allergic **bronchitis** (page 80), according to preliminary research.[25, 26]

CHRONIC VENOUS INSUFFICIENCY

Chronic venous insufficiency (CVI) is poor return of blood from feet and legs back to the heart.

CVI may occur following excessive clotting and inflammation of the leg veins, a disease known as deep vein thrombosis. CVI also results from a simple failure of the valves in leg veins to hold blood against gravity, leading to sluggish movement of blood out of the veins, resulting in swollen legs.

CHECKLIST FOR CHRONIC VENOUS INSUFFICIENCY		
Rating	**Nutritional Supplements**	**Herbs**
★★★	**Flavonoids** (page 516) (rutin) **Proanthocyanidins** (page 574)	**Butcher's broom** (page 649) **Horse chestnut** (page 692)
★★☆		**Gotu kola** (page 684) Red vine leaf

What are the symptoms of chronic venous insufficiency?
CVI may cause feet and calves to become swollen, often accompanied by a dull ache made worse with prolonged standing. If CVI is allowed to progress, the skin tends to darken and ulcers may occur. CVI often causes **varicose veins** (page 440).

Medical treatments
Over the counter antibiotic products that contain bacitracin (Baciguent), neomycin (Myciguent), or a combination of the two with polymyxin B (Neosporin, Polysporin), might be useful if skin ulcers develop.

Topical prescription antibiotics such as mupirocin (Bactroban) and metronidazole (MetroGel) may be useful for the treatment of skin ulcers.

Health care practitioners typically advise patients to elevate the legs frequently, avoid prolonged standing or sitting, and wear graduated compression stockings with supportive shoes. Recurrent ulceration may be surgically treated with skin grafts. Surgical repair or bypass of the affected veins is sometimes necessary.

Lifestyle changes that may be helpful
People affected by chronic venous insufficiency should not sit or stand for long periods of time. When sitting, they should elevate their legs. Walking helps move blood out of the veins. Wearing tight-fitting compression stockings available from pharmacies further supports the veins.

Nutritional supplements that may be helpful

Flavonoids (page 516) promote venous strength and integrity. Most trials of flavonoids in patients with CVI have used a type of flavonoid called hydroxyethylrutoside (HR), which is derived from rutin. These double-blind and other controlled trials have consistently shown a beneficial effect of HR in clearing leg swelling and other signs of CVI.[1, 2, 3] Positive results from a double-blind trial have been obtained using 500 mg of HR taken twice per day for 12 weeks.[4] In this trial, the preparation was found to add further benefit to that provided by compression stockings commonly used to treat CVI. Similar results were obtained in another controlled trial.[5] It is unclear whether other flavonoids are as effective as HR for CVI. HR has also been used successfully as a topical preparation for the treatment of CVI.[6]

Proanthocyanidins (page 574) (OPCs), a group of flavonoids found in pine bark, grape seed, grape skin, **bilberry** (page 634), **cranberry** (page 664), black currant, **green tea** (page 686), black tea, and other plants, have also been shown to strengthen capillaries in double-blind research using as little as two 50 mg tablets per day.[7] In a double-blind trial using a total of 150 mg OPCs per day, French researchers reported reduced symptoms for women with CVI.[8] In another French double-blind trial, supplementation with 100 mg taken three times per day resulted in benefits within four weeks.[9]

Are there any side effects or interactions?
Refer to the individual supplement for information about any side effects or interactions.

Herbs that may be helpful

According to an extensive overview of clinical trials, standardized **horse chestnut** (page 692) seed extract, which contains the active compound aescin, has been shown to be effective in double-blind and other controlled research, supporting the traditional use of horse chestnut for venous problems.[10] In these trials, capsules of horse chestnut extract containing 50 mg of aescin were given two to three times daily for CVI. The positive effect results in part from horse chestnut's ability to strengthen capillaries, which leads to a reduction in swelling.[11]

Another traditional remedy for CVI is **butcher's broom** (page 649). One double-blind trial used a combination of butcher's broom, the **flavonoid** (page 516) hesperidin, and **vitamin C** (page 604). This was found

to be better than a placebo for treating CVI.[12] In a comparison study, a product combining butcher's broom extract, the flavonoid hesperidin, and vitamin C was more effective than a synthetic flavonoid product for treating CVI.[13] A double-blind study, in which Butcher's broom alone was used, has confirmed the beneficial effect of this herb.[14] Clinical trials have used one capsule, containing standardized extracts providing 15 to 30 mg of ruscogenins, three times each day. The amount of butcher's broom extract used in these trials is 150 mg two times per day. Other sources recommend standardized extracts providing 15 to 30 mg of ruscogenins, given three times each day.

Gotu kola (page 684) extracts, standardized to triterpenoid content, have been found successful in small preliminary trials to treat CVI.[15] The amount of extract used in these trials ranged from 60 to 120 mg per day.

A double-blind trial demonstrated that red vine leaf extract is effective at relieving the symptoms and swelling associated with CVI.[16] One group of participants took either 360 mg or 720 mg per day of a standardized extract for 12 weeks, and another group took a placebo. At the end of the treatment period, those who had taken the herb experienced significant improvement in symptoms of leg heaviness, tension sensation, tingling, and pain compared with those who had taken the placebo. Objective measurements of leg swelling were also significantly improved in the red vine group compared to the placebo group.

Are there any side effects or interactions?
Refer to the individual herb for information about any side effects or interactions.

CLUSTER HEADACHE

Cluster headaches are very painful one-sided headaches that tend to occur in clusters of several headaches in a short period of time, after which there may be no headaches for weeks or months. Cluster headaches that continue for more than one year without remission, or with remissions lasting less than 14 days, are considered to be chronic and are very difficult to treat.

What are the symptoms of cluster headaches?
Cluster headaches involve pain in the eye or upper face, tearing, runny nose with nasal congestion, and facial sweating.[1]

Cluster Headache

CHECKLIST FOR CLUSTER HEADACHE

Rating	Nutritional Supplements	Herbs
★★☆	**Melatonin** (page 555)	**Cayenne** (page 654)
★☆☆	**Magnesium** (page 551) (intravenous)	

Medical treatments

The prescription drugs used to treat cluster headaches include sumatriptan (Imitrex Injection), methysergide (Sansert), and dihydroergotamine (D.H.E. 45 Injection). Other agents that might be useful include a corticosteroid trial and indomethacin (Indocin).

Oxygen inhalation is especially beneficial when symptoms occur at night.

Dietary changes that may be helpful

Some doctors report that food sensitivities may trigger cluster headaches in some people.[2, 3] While the connection between diet and **migraine headache** (page 316) is well established, no controlled research has investigated the role of diet in cluster headache.

Many people with cluster headaches are heavy consumers of alcohol, and alcohol consumption has been reported to bring on cluster headache attacks.[4, 5] However, no research has investigated the effects of avoiding alcohol on cluster headache recurrences.

Lifestyle changes that may be helpful

Many people with cluster headaches are smokers.[6, 7, 8, 9, 10] While this does not necessarily mean quitting smoking will reduce cluster headache attacks, smoking should be avoided for many reasons.

Nutritional supplements that may be helpful

People who suffer from cluster headaches often have low blood levels of **magnesium** (page 551), and preliminary trials[11, 12] show that intravenous magnesium injections may relieve a cluster headache episode. However, no trials have investigated the effects of oral magnesium supplementation on cluster headaches.

Researchers have found low levels of the hormone **melatonin** (page 555) in cluster headache patients.[13, 14, 15, 16] In a small double-blind trial, a group of cluster headache sufferers took a 10 mg evening dose of melatonin for 14 days. About half of the group saw a significant decrease in the frequency of their headaches within three to five days, after which no further

headaches occurred until melatonin was discontinued.[17] Melatonin appears to be effective against both types of cluster headache (e.g., episodic and chronic).[18] More research is needed to establish the long-term effects of melatonin supplementation on cluster headache.

Are there any side effects or interactions?
Refer to the individual supplement for information about any side effects or interactions.

Herbs that may be helpful

Substance P is a nerve chemical involved in pain transmission that may cause some of the symptoms of cluster headache.[19, 20] Capsaicin, a constituent of **cayenne** (page 654) pepper can reduce the levels of substance P in nerves.[21] Preliminary clinical trials investigating the use of intranasal capsaicin for the prevention and treatment of cluster headaches report significant decreases in the number of cluster episodes in some of the participants.[22] The decreases usually lasted no more than 40 days after the end of treatment,[23] although a few patients have experienced relief for up to two years.[24] In a double-blind study, patients who received capsaicin intranasally twice daily for seven days during a cluster episode had a significant reduction in pain for the following 15 days.[25] As capsaicin can cause burning and irritation, this treatment should be utilized only under the supervision of a qualified doctor.

Are there any side effects or interactions?
Refer to the individual herb for information about any side effects or interactions.

Holistic approaches that may be helpful

Oxygen therapy has been found to be useful in treating cluster headaches. A double-blind trial compared breathing 100% oxygen with breathing air (nitrogen and oxygen) through a mask for 15 minutes or less during six headache episodes per person. The 100% oxygen significantly reduced the pain of acute cluster attacks in all subjects.[26] A controlled trial found that during acute episodes of cluster headaches, breathing 100% oxygen through a mask for 15 minutes significantly decreased pain in most of the people with episodic cluster headache and in over half of those with chronic cluster headache.[27] However, one-fourth of the study participants experienced cluster attacks soon after the treatment was stopped. While oxygen inhalation therapy is now considered a standard treatment,[28] treatments may need to be repeated, and they have not been shown to help prevent recurrences.

In controlled studies,[29, 30] a single treatment of hyperbaric oxygen therapy, in which the patient is placed in a chamber with highly concentrated oxygen, has been found to help decrease pain and prevent recurrence of cluster episodes in some patients for several days. Two studies have investigated the use of multiple treatments of hyperbaric oxygen in chronic cluster headache patients. In one small, preliminary trial,[31] ten 70-minute treatments over two weeks brought relief in most of the participants; headaches did not recur for 1 to 31 days after the end of treatment in those who responded. In another preliminary trial, chronic cluster headache patients received 15 hyperbaric oxygen treatment sessions (every other day for 30 minutes each); results showed a gradual decrease in episodes in some patients, which lasted for up to two weeks after treatment ended.[32]

COLD SORES

Cold sores are painful fluid-filled blisters that form on the borders of the lips caused by a herpes virus, most often the herpes simplex 1 virus.

Cold sores should not be confused with **canker sores** (page 90), which are small ulcerations in the mouth. The blisters, which are contagious, later break, ooze, and crust over before healing. Recurrences are common and can be triggered by stress, sun exposure, illness, and menstruation. **Genital herpes** (page 200) infection (usually caused by herpes simplex 2) is a related condition and potentially may be treated in much the same way as herpes simplex 1.

What are the symptoms of cold sores?

Cold sores may appear with colds, fevers, exposure to excessive sunlight, or menstrual periods, as well as during periods of stress or illness. The sores usually disappear within two weeks. Initially, there may be tingling or prickling at the site of the cold sores even before they are visible (called the prodrome); afterward, the blisters often weep a clear fluid and form a scab. If the **infection** (page 265) is transmitted to the eyes, it may lead to blindness.

Medical treatments

The over the counter topical agents docosanol (Abreva) and allantoin (Herpecin-L), as well as camphor and phenol combinations (Campho-Phenique), help relieve pain and might promote healing of cold sores. Analgesics, such as aspirin (Bayer, Ecotrin, Bufferin), ibuprofen (Motrin, Advil), and acetaminophen (Tylenol), might provide some pain relief.

Antiviral prescription medications such as topical acyclovir (Zovirax), topical penciclovir (Denavir), or oral acyclovir (Zovirax) might reduce the duration of the sores.

Rating	Nutritional Supplements	Herbs
★★★	Lysine (page 550) (recurrence prevention)	Lemon balm (page 701) (topical)
★★☆	Flavonoids (page 516) Vitamin C (page 604) Vitamin E (page 609) (topical) Zinc (page 614) (topical)	Witch hazel (page 760) (topical)
★☆☆	Boric acid (page 476) Propolis (page 579) (topical)	Chaparral (page 657) Echinacea (page 669) Elderberry (page 670), St. John's wort (page 747), Soapwort (in combination) Goldenseal (page 683) Licorice (page 702) (topical) Myrrh (page 713) St. John's wort (page 747) (topical)

CHECKLIST FOR HERPES SIMPLEX/COLD SORES

Dietary changes that may be helpful

The herpes simplex virus has a high requirement for the **amino acid** (page 465), **arginine** (page 467). On the other hand, the amino acid, **lysine** (page 550), inhibits viral replication.[1] Therefore, a diet that is low in arginine and high in lysine may help prevent or treat herpes outbreaks. Several studies have shown that increasing lysine intake can reduce the recurrence rate of cold sores.[2] Although people with herpes simplex reportedly consume about the same amount of arginine and lysine in their diet as do people without cold sores,[3] it is conceivable that adjusting the intake of these amino acids may be beneficial. For that reason, many doctors advise people with cold sores to avoid foods with high arginine-to-lysine ratios, such as nuts, peanuts, and chocolate. Nonfat yogurt and other nonfat dairy can be a healthful way to increase lysine intake.

Nutritional supplements that may be helpful

The **amino acid** (page 465), **lysine** (page 550), has been reported to reduce the recurrence rate of herpes simplex **infections** (page 265) in both preliminary[4, 5] and double-blind trials.[6, 7] The amount used in these studies was usually 1 to 3 grams per day, although some people received as little as 312 mg per day. In one double-blind trial, lysine supplementation (1,200 mg per day) failed to prevent recurrences better than placebo.[8] However, the results of that study may have been skewed by a large number of dropouts in the placebo group who fared poorly but were not included in the analysis.

When lysine has been used for acute outbreaks, the results have been mixed. In a preliminary study, 390 mg of lysine taken at the first sign of a herpes outbreak resulted in rapid resolution of the cold sores in all cases.[9] However, in a double-blind study, supplementing with 1 gram of lysine per day for five days did not increase the healing rate of the cold sores.[10]

Vitamin C (page 604) has been shown to inactivate herpes viruses in the test tube.[11] In one study, people with herpes infections received either a placebo or 200 mg of vitamin C plus 200 mg of **flavonoids** (page 516), each taken three to five times per day. Compared with the placebo, vitamin C and flavonoids reduced the duration of symptoms by 57%.[12]

Zinc (page 614) preparations have been shown to inhibit the replication of herpes simplex in the test tube.[13] In one study, people with recurrent herpes simplex infections applied a zinc sulfate solution daily to the sores. After healing occurred, the frequency of applications was reduced to once a week for a month, then to twice a month. During an observation period of 16 to 23 months, none of these people experienced a recurrence of their cold sores.[14]

Zinc oxide, the only commercially available form of zinc for topical application, is probably ineffective as a treatment for herpes simplex.[15] Other forms of topical zinc can be obtained by prescription, through a compounding pharmacist. However, because an excessive concentration of zinc may cause skin irritation, topical zinc should be used only with the supervision of a doctor knowledgeable in its use.

In a preliminary trial, a piece of cotton saturated with **vitamin E** (page 609) oil was applied to newly erupted cold sores and held in place for 15 minutes. The first application was performed in the dentist's office. Participants were instructed to repeat the procedure every three hours for the rest of that day, and then three times daily for two more days. In nearly all cases, pain disappeared in less than eight hours. Application of vitamin E oil appeared to accelerate healing of the cold sores.[16] Similar results were reported in another study.[17]

Application of an ointment containing **propolis** (page 579), the resin collected by bees from trees, has been shown to relieve genital herpes more effectively than topical acyclovir.[18] It is likely that this treatment might also benefit people with cold sores, although this has not been tested. Propolis ointment should be applied four times per day.

Boric acid (page 476) has antiviral activity. In a double-blind trial, topical application of an ointment containing boric acid (in the form of sodium borate) shortened the duration of cold sores by about one-third.[19] However, concerns about potential toxicity have led some doctors to avoid the use of boric acid for this purpose.

A preliminary study found that people with recurrent cold sores have lower **iron** (page 540) stores than healthy people.[20] This may mean that correcting an iron deficiency might help prevent herpes outbreaks, but more research is necessary. Most people should not take iron supplements unless they have an iron deficiency, confirmed by a blood test.

Are there any side effects or interactions?
Refer to the individual supplement for information about any side effects or interactions.

Herbs that may be helpful
Lemon balm (page 701) has antiviral properties. A cream containing an extract of lemon balm has been shown in double-blind trials to speed the healing of cold sores.[21] In one double-blind trial, topical application of a 1% 70:1 extract of lemon-balm leaf cream, four times daily for five days, led to significantly fewer symptoms and fewer blisters than experienced by those using a placebo cream.[22] In most studies, the lemon-balm cream was applied two to four times per day for five to ten days.

The **proanthocyanidins** (page 574) in **witch hazel** (page 760) have been shown to exert significant antiviral activity against herpes simplex 1 in the test tube.[23]

In a double-blind trial, people with acute cold sore outbreaks applied a topical cream containing 2% witch hazel bark extract or placebo six times a day for three to eight days.[24] By the end of the eighth day, those using the witch-hazel cream had a pronounced and statistically significant reduction in the size and spread of the inflammation when compared to the placebo group.

Licorice (page 702) in the form of a cream or gel may be applied directly to herpes sores three to four times per day. Licorice extracts containing glycyrrhizin or glycyrrhetinic acid should be used, as these are the constituents in licorice most likely to provide activity against the herpes simplex virus. There are no controlled trials demonstrating the effectiveness of this treatment, but a cream containing a synthetic version of glycyrrhetinic acid (carbenoxolone) was reported to speed healing time and reduce pain in people with herpes simplex.[25]

In traditional herbal medicine, tinctures of various herbs, including **chaparral** (page 657), **St. John's wort** (page 747), **goldenseal** (page 683), **myrrh** (page 713), and **echinacea** (page 669), have been applied topically to herpes outbreaks in order to promote healing.

An extract from **elderberry** (page 670) leaves, combined with St. John's wort and soapwort *(Saponaria officinalis)*, has been found to inhibit the herpes simplex virus in the test tube.[26] However, the effect of these herbs on cold sores has not been studied.

Are there any side effects or interactions?
Refer to the individual herb for information about any side effects or interactions.

COLIC

Colic is a common problem in infants in which the baby is healthy but has periods of inconsolable crying, apparently caused by abdominal pain. Colic usually develops within a few weeks of birth and disappears by the baby's fourth month.

What are the symptoms of colic?
Colic may cause infants, typically less than four months old, to cry inconsolably. The attacks usually occur in the late afternoon and evening, sometimes lasting for hours. During a colicky period, babies may bring their knees up, clench their fists, grimace, hold their breath, and generally be more active.

	CHECKLIST FOR COLIC	
Rating	Nutritional Supplements	Herbs
★★☆	**Probiotics** (page 575) (*Bifidobacterium lactis* and *Streptococcus thermophilus*)	**Chamomile** (page 656) **Chamomile** (page 656), **vervain** (page 756), **licorice** (page 702), **fennel** (page 676), **lemon balm** (page 701) (in combination) **Fennel** (page 676) (seed oil)
★☆☆		**Caraway** (page 651) **Cinnamon** (page 659) Fumitory Garden angelica **Hyssop** (page 695) **Peppermint** (page 726) **Yarrow** (page 763)

Medical treatments
Over the counter anti-gas medicine containing simethicone (Mylicon) may be used to reduce pain due to excess gas.

Treatment is directed toward providing comfort for the babies until they outgrow this difficult period. Feeding babies while they are sitting up, or burping them more frequently, may help prevent colic if too much air is being swallowed during feedings.

Dietary changes that may be helpful
Allergies (page 14) may be responsible for colic in some infants.[1, 2] If the child is fed with formula, the problem may be an intolerance to milk proteins from a cows' milk-based formula.[3] Switching to a soy formula may ease colic in such cases.[4] Infants who are sensitive to both milk and soy may be given a hypoallergenic formula containing extensively hydrolyzed proteins. However, some children are sensitive even to these formulas.

A true food protein intolerance in infants may result in persistent distress attributed to irritation of the esophagus caused by reflux (partial spitting up). These infants may respond to an **amino acid** (page 465)-based formula. In a clinical trial, infants who were intolerant of soy and extensively hydrolyzed formula, and who had failed to respond to various formula changes, were switched to an amino-acid formula (Neocate).[5] After two weeks, all the infants receiving the amino acid-based formula showed less distressed behavior and fewer symptoms of reflux.

If a baby is breast-fed, certain foods in the mother's diet may provoke an allergic reaction in the baby. Cows' milk consumed by a breast-feeding mother has been shown in some,[6] but not all,[7] studies to trigger colic. Cows' milk proteins, which may trigger allergic reactions, have been found at higher levels in milk from breast-feeding mothers with colicky infants than in milk from mothers with non-colicky infants.[8] Changing to a low-allergenic formula or restricting the mother's diet to exclude certain allergy-triggering foods significantly reduced colic symptoms in the infants in one double-blind trial. [9] A healthcare provider can help determine which foods eaten by breast-feeding mothers may be contributing to colic.

Lifestyle changes that may be helpful

All infants, particularly those with colic, need to be fed on demand and not by a specific clock schedule. Often a baby's cry is triggered by discomfort caused by **low blood sugar** (page 251). Unlike adults, infants do not have a carefully regulated ability to maintain healthy blood sugar levels in the absence of food. This physiological shortcoming of infants can be solved only by feeding on demand.

In one trial, parents were taught not to let babies cry unnecessarily but rather to attempt feeding right away in response to the infant's cry.[10] If that failed, parents were taught to try to respond to the cry in other ways, such as holding the infant or providing the opportunity to sleep. These parents were also given the solid medical advice that overfeeding is never caused by feeding on demand nor will the baby be "spoiled" by such an approach. As a result of this intervention, colic was dramatically (and statistically significantly) reduced, compared with a group of mothers given different instructions.

Nutritional supplements that may be helpful

In a double-blind study of infants, supplementation of a standard milk-based formula with **probiotic organisms** (page 575) (*Bifidobacterium lactis* and *Streptococcus thermophilus*) significantly reduced the frequency of colic, compared with the same formula without the probiotics.[11]

Are there any side effects or interactions?
Refer to the individual supplement for information about any side effects or interactions.

Herbs that may be helpful

Carminatives are a class of herbs commonly used for infants with colic. These herbs tend to relax intestinal spasms.

Chamomile (page 656) is a carminative with long history of use as a calming herb and may be used to ease intestinal cramping in colicky infants. A soothing tea made from chamomile, **vervain** (page 756), **licorice** (page 702), **fennel** (page 676), and **lemon balm** (page 701) has been shown to relieve colic more effectively than placebo.[12] In this study, approximately 1/2 cup (150 ml) of tea was given during each colic episode up to a maximum of three times per day.

In a double-blind study of infants with colic, supplementation with an emulsion of **fennel** (page 676) seed oil relieved colic in 65% of cases, compared with 24% of infants receiving a placebo, a statistically significant difference.[13] The amount used was 1 to 4 teaspoons, up to four times per day, of a water emulsion of 0.1% fennel seed oil.

Hyssop (page 695) has mild sedative properties and may also be helpful in relieving colic, but research is lacking. Though no definitive information on hyssop supplementation is available, 1 teaspoon of hyssop herb steeped in 1 cup of just-boiled water in a closed container for 15 to 20 minutes, then given in sips from a bottle over a period of 2 to 3 hours may help calm colic.

Caraway (page 651), like chamomile and fennel, relieves intestinal cramping and, in this way, may ease symptoms of colic. One tablespoon (15 grams) of caraway seed is mixed with 8 oz (240 ml) of just-boiled water and steeped in a closed container for at least 10 minutes. Three ounces of vegetable glycerin is added, and the resulting mixture is stored in a bottle in the refrigerator. Up to 1/2 teaspoon (2.5 ml) of the liquid may be given every 30 minutes to a colicky infant or given 15 minutes before feeding.[14]

Several other gas-relieving herbs used in traditional medicine for colic are approved in Germany for intestinal spasms.[15] These include **yarrow** (page 763), garden angelica (*Angelica archangelica*), **peppermint** (page 726), **cinnamon** (page 659), and fumitory (*Fumaria officinalis*). These herbs are generally given by healthcare professionals as teas or decoctions to the infant. Peppermint tea should be used with caution in infants and young children, as they may choke in reaction to the strong menthol.

Are there any side effects or interactions?
Refer to the individual herb for information about any side effects or interactions.

Holistic approaches that may be helpful

The symptoms of colic may be linked to mild biomechanical disturbances of the spinal joints and may respond to manipulation. A large, preliminary study of infants treated by chiropractic manipulation for colic reported marked improvement, often after one treatment.[16] This echoed an earlier study in which questionnaires sent to parents of 132 infants under chiropractic care revealed that 91% of the respondents observed improvement in their babies' symptoms after two to three manipulations.[17] In a controlled trial, infants were treated daily for two weeks either with a placebo medication or with a series of three to five treatments using gentle "fingertip" spinal manipulations.[18] Those treated with manipulation experienced a 67% reduction in daily hours of colic, compared with only a 38% reduction in infants on medication.

COLON CANCER

See also: Breast Cancer (page 65), **Lung Cancer** (page 298), **Prostate Cancer** (page 371), **Cancer Prevention and Diet** (page 87)

Colon cancer is a malignancy in the colon. It is characterized by unregulated replication of cells creating tumors, with the possibility of some of the cells spreading to other sites (metastasis).

This article includes a discussion of studies that have assessed whether certain vitamins, minerals, herbs, or other dietary ingredients offered in dietary or herbal supplements may be beneficial in connection with the reduction of risk of developing colon cancer, or of signs and symptoms in people who have this condition.

This information is provided solely to aid consumers in discussing supplements with their healthcare providers. It is not advised, nor is this information intended to advocate, promote, or encourage self prescription of these supplements for cancer risk reduction or treatment. Furthermore, none of this information should be misconstrued to suggest that dietary or herbal supplements can or should be used in place of conventional anticancer approaches or treatments.

It should be noted that certain studies referenced below, indicating the potential usefulness of a particular dietary ingredient or dietary or herbal supplement in connection with the reduction of risk of colon cancer, are preliminary evidence only. Some studies suggest an association between high blood or dietary levels of a

particular dietary ingredient with a reduced risk of developing colon cancer. Even if such an association were established, this does not mean that dietary supplements containing large amounts of the dietary ingredient will necessarily have a cancer risk reduction effect.

In Western countries, cancers of the colon and rectum account for more new cancer cases each year than any other site except the lung. Although the genetic susceptibility is low, some families have a predisposition for colon cancer that usually occurs before age 40. **Inflammatory bowel disease** (page 269), including both **ulcerative colitis** (page 433) and **Crohn's disease** (page 141) as well as familial polyposis, are disorders that, to varying degrees, increase the risk of colon cancer.

CHECKLIST FOR COLON CANCER		
Rating	**Nutritional Supplements**	**Herbs**
★★☆	**Folic acid** (page 520) (reduces risk) **Melatonin** (page 555) **Selenium** (page 584) (reduces risk)	**Garlic** (page 679) and **onion** (page 718) (reduces risk of stomach, esophageal, and colon cancers) **Green tea** (page 686) (reduces risk)
★☆☆	**Calcium** (page 483) (reduces risk) **Fish oil** (page 514) (reduces risk) **Glutathione** (page 531) **Vitamin C** (page 604) (reduces risk) **Vitamin D** (page 607) (reduces risk) **Vitamin E** (page 609) (reduces risk)	

What are the symptoms of colon cancer?

The initial symptoms of colon cancer depend on the location of the tumor. Cancer in the portion of the colon nearest the left side of the body and areas close to the rectum are the most common cause for a change in bowel habits and consistency of the stool. Cancer in this part of the colon may also cause a colicky pain that is made worse by eating. Blood mixed with the stool and bowel obstruction are other symptoms that characterize cancer at this site. Ineffectual and painful straining at stool may be a sign that the cancer is more advanced. Cancer localized to the part of the colon nearest the right side of the body may cause a generalized abdominal pain and brick red blood. It is commonly associated with **iron-deficiency anemia** (page 278), especially when no other cause can be identified. Cancers closer to the rectum often cause a steady gnawing pain and bright red blood coating the stool.

Medical treatments

Some forms of colon cancer have been successfully treated with the prescription medication fluorouracil or 5-FU (Adrucil) followed by levamisole (Ergamisol). Fluorouracil is also sometimes combined with folinic acid (Leucovorin).

The primary treatment for cancer of the colon is surgical removal of the cancer. The procedure will depend upon the location and invasiveness of the tumor. Radiation is sometimes used with surgery and chemotherapy, particularly for rectal cancer.

Dietary changes that may be helpful

The following dietary changes have been studied in connection with colon cancer.

Alcohol

Most,[1, 2, 3] but not all,[4] preliminary reports have found an association between beer drinking (though not consumption of other forms of alcohol) and rectal cancer. Beer drinking has also been associated with an increased risk of precancerous changes in the colon.[5] Nitrosamines—cancer-causing chemicals found in beer—may be partially responsible for these associations.[6] Several studies have found consumption of *any* form of alcohol to be associated with an increased risk of rectal and colon cancers, the link between rectal cancer and beer being only slightly stronger than the association between rectal cancer and consumption of other forms of alcohol.[7, 8]

Alcohol can indirectly damage DNA—the material that allows cells to replicate normally. Abnormal replication of cells can lead to cancer. **Folic acid** (page 520), a B vitamin, appears to protect against alcohol-induced DNA damage. Increasingly, researchers believe that folic acid may be able to protect against some of the colon cancer-causing effects of alcohol.[9, 10] Doctors recommend that people wishing to reduce their risks of colon and rectal cancers abstain from drinking alcohol.

Those who continue to drink should take folic acid supplements. In one report, women taking **multivitamins** (page 559) (often containing 400 mcg of folic acid per day) for at least 15 years had a 75% lower risk of colon cancer compared with women not taking such supplements.[11]

Fiber *(page 512)*

Until recently, most studies reported that people who ate a high-fiber diet were found to be at low risk for colon cancer.[12] Some researchers believed protection against colon cancer comes specifically from eating wheat bran[13, 14, 15] as opposed to other fibers. A clear understanding of how fiber might protect against colon cancer risk remains somewhat elusive.[16]

Recent research has begun to cast doubt on whether fiber provides significant protection against colon cancer,[17, 18] suggesting instead that consumption of meat and other animal products may be the primary culprit. Despite these recent reports, however, some doctors continue to believe that, until more definitive information is available, people wishing to reduce their risk of colon cancer should consume more fiber in their diets.

Consuming a diet high in insoluble fiber is best achieved by switching from white rice to brown rice and from bakery goods made with white flour or mixed flours to 100%-whole-wheat bread, whole-rye crackers, and whole-grain pancake mixes. Refined white flour is generally listed on food packaging labels as "flour," "enriched flour," "unbleached flour," "durum wheat," "semolina," or "white flour." Breads containing only whole wheat are often labeled "100% whole wheat."

Tomatoes

Tomatoes contain **lycopene** (page 548)—an **antioxidant** (page 467) similar in structure to **beta-carotene** (page 469). Most lycopene in our diet comes from tomatoes, though traces of lycopene exist in other foods. Lycopene inhibits the proliferation of cancer cells in test-tube research.[19]

A review of published research found that higher intake of tomatoes or higher blood levels of lycopene correlated with protection from cancer in 57 of 72 studies. Findings in 35 of these studies were statistically significant.[20] Evidence of a protective effect for tomato consumption was strongest for a variety of other **cancers** (page 87), but some evidence of a protective effect also appeared for colon cancer. Many doctors recommend that people who are not allergic to tomatoes increase their intake to reduce their risk of cancer.

Cruciferous vegetables

Cabbage, Brussels sprouts, broccoli, and cauliflower belong to the *Brassica* family of vegetables, also known as "cruciferous" vegetables. In test-tube and animal studies, these foods have been associated with anticancer activity,[21] possibly due to several substances found in these foods, such as **indole-3-carbinol** (page

536),[22] glucaric acid (**calcium D-glucarate** [page 486]),[23] and **sulforaphane** (page 589).[24] In a preliminary human study, people who eat cruciferous vegetables were reported to have lower-than-average risks for colon cancer.[25]

Meat and how it is cooked
Most, but not all, studies[26] show meat eaters have a high risk of colon cancer.[27, 28, 29] In some colon cancer studies, the association has been limited to consumption of sausage or other processed meats.[30, 31]

The association between cancer and consumption of meat depends in part on how well the meat is cooked. Well-done meat contains more carcinogenic material than does lightly cooked meat.[32] Recent evidence from preliminary studies shows that people who eat well-done,[33] fried or heavily-browned meat[34] have a high risk of colon cancer.

However, not every report has found that exposure to carcinogens found in well-done meat leads to an increased risk of colon cancer.[35] Some studies may have failed to find this link because they did not consider the effect of genetics. Susceptibility to the colon cancer-causing effects of well-cooked meat appears to be genetically determined.[36] Therefore, only some people appear to increase their risk of colon cancer by consuming well-cooked meat. However, people are rarely tested to see if they are "rapid acetylators"—meat-eaters considered to be at high risk of colon cancer[37]—except as subjects in a research experiment.

Most nutritionally oriented doctors tell people wishing to reduce their risk of colon cancers to stop eating meat, or at least significantly reduce consumption, and to limit intake to meat that is rare or medium-cooked. Removing all meat from the diet may be safest because consumption of even rare or medium-cooked meat has been associated with at least some increase in risk.[38]

Coffee
"Secondary bile acids" are substances in the gut that may increase the risk of colon and rectal cancers. Some researchers have hypothesized that coffee drinking might reduce the risks of colon and rectal cancers by decreasing the intestinal level of these substances.[39, 40] An analysis of preliminary studies suggests coffee drinkers have a significantly lower risk of these cancers compared to the risk in people who do not drink coffee.[41] However, only studies using the weakest methods of inquiry have found this protective effect. Due to the lack of support from studies using stronger methodology, the association between coffee drinking and pro-

tection against colon or rectal cancers remains unproven.[42]

Dietary fat
Dietary fat intake has long been regarded as an important nutritional influence on colon cancer development. Nevertheless, the association between colon cancer and total dietary fat remains inconsistent. Although there are known mechanisms by which a high dietary fat intake could promote tumor growth in the colon,[43] a review of the research shows the strongest dietary association with colon cancer to be the intake of meat, not necessarily the fat content of the meat.[44] See the discussion about Meat (how it is cooked), above.

Salt
Associations between salt intake and colon and rectal cancers are reported in some,[45] but not all, preliminary studies.[46] Doctors often do not mention salt restriction as part of a cancer-prevention diet because the only malignancy strongly associated with salt—stomach cancer—is no longer common in the United States despite our high intake of salt.

Sugar
Preliminary studies have reported associations between an increasing intake of sugar or sugar-containing foods and an increased risk colon cancer.[47, 48] Whether this association exists because sugar directly promotes cancer, or because sugar consumption is only a marker for some other dietary or lifestyle factor, remains unknown.

Lifestyle changes that may be helpful
The following lifestyle changes have been studied in connection with colon cancer.

Exercise and prevention
Most studies show that people who exercise are at lower risk of colon cancer or precancerous changes in the colon, compared with sedentary people.[49, 50, 51, 52] Regular exercise appears to be one factor that will predictably lower the risk of colon cancer.

***Obesity** (page 446) and risk*
Several studies suggest that obesity in men significantly increases the risk of colon cancer[53] or rectal cancer,[54] though some scientists believe that obesity may only be a surrogate for other risk factors such as a high-fat diet or lack of exercise.[55] Although the relationship between obesity and colon cancer risk in women is less clear, some researchers have found the increased risk of colon cancer in obese women as well as men.[56]

Smoking and risk

A history of smoking has been reported to significantly increase the risk of colon cancer in both men[57] and women.[58] Avoidance of tobacco is an important step in the prevention of colon cancer.

Nutritional supplements that may be helpful

The following nutritional supplements have been studied in connection with colon cancer.

Folic acid (page 520)

People with **ulcerative colitis** (page 433) (UC) are at increased risk for colon cancer. Many patients with this disease take the drug sulfasalazine, which depletes folic acid.[59] In a preliminary report, patients with long-standing UC who took folic acid supplements (at least 400 mcg per day) had a 62% lower incidence of colon cancer or precancerous changes in the colon, compared with those who did not supplement with folic acid.[60] Although this difference was not statistically significant, the researchers recommended that people who take sulfasalazine should supplement with folic acid to potentially reduce the risk of colon cancer.[61]

As dietary folate increases, the risks of precancerous polyps in the colon[62] and colon cancer itself decrease, according to some,[63] but not all, reports.[64] In one study, women who had taken folic acid supplements had a statistically significant 75% reduction in the risk of colon cancer, compared with women not taking folic acid supplements, but only when they had been supplementing with folic acid for more than 15 years.[65] In another report, the association between dietary folate and protection from precancerous polyps grew much stronger when use of folic acid supplements was considered (as opposed to studying only folate intake from food).[66]

The protection from colon cancer associated with high intake of folate has been reported to occur more in consumers of alcohol than in nondrinkers.[67] This finding fits well with evidence that folate reverses damage to DNA caused by alcohol consumption.[68] Damaged DNA can lead to abnormal cellular replication—a step toward cancer.

Some nutritionally oriented doctors recommend **folic acid** (page 520) supplementation for prevention of recurrences in patients who formerly had colon cancer but are now in complete remission. However, no research has yet explored the effect of folic acid supplementation in people who have already been diagnosed with cancer. Cancer patients taking the chemotherapy drug methotrexate must not take folic acid supplements without the direction of their oncologist.

Selenium (page 584)

Selenium has been reported to have diverse anticancer actions.[69, 70] Selenium inhibits cancer in animals.[71] Low soil levels of selenium, probably associated with low dietary intake, have been associated with increased cancer incidence in humans.[72] Blood levels of selenium have been reported to be low in patients with a variety of cancers,[73, 74, 75, 76, 77, 78, 79, 80] including colon cancer.[81] In preliminary reports, people with the lowest blood levels of selenium had between 3.8 and 5.8 times the risk of dying from cancer compared with those who had the highest selenium levels.[82, 83]

The strongest evidence supporting the anticancer effects of selenium supplementation comes from a double-blind trial of 1,312 Americans with a history of skin cancer who were treated with 200 mcg of yeast-based selenium per day or placebo for 4.5 years, then followed for an additional two years.[84] Although no decrease in *skin* cancers occurred, a dramatic 50% reduction in overall cancer deaths and a 37% reduction in total cancer incidence were observed. A statistically significant 58% decrease in cancers of the colon and rectum was reported.

Little is known about the effects of **selenium** (page 584) in the treatment of people with existing cancer. Selenium supplementation was reported to improve **immune function** (page 255) in colon cancer patients,[85] but no long-term follow-up was done to evaluate whether these patients ultimately lived longer or fared better.

In the double-blind study cited above,[86] the large reduction in cancer deaths found in such a short period of time (6.5 years) suggests that these researchers may have been successfully, though unknowingly, treating some people with undiagnosed cancer. However, this speculation has yet to be proven.

Melatonin (page 555)

The hormone melatonin is available as a supplement and is believed by some researchers to have anticancer activity because of its effects on the immune system.[87] In research trials, melatonin has been evaluated as a potential agent for use in connection with treatment for cancer patients—not to protect healthy people from getting cancer.

Patients with advanced colon cancer who had either not responded to chemotherapy, or who had relapsed after a response to chemotherapy, were given either no additional treatment (control group) or a combination of interleukin-2 and 40 mg of melatonin per day.[88] Nine of 25 patients given melatonin plus interleukin-2 survived for a year compared with only three of 25 patients in the control group, a difference that was statistically significant.

Many other controlled trials suggest that melatonin may extend survival, disease-free survival, and/or quality of life in cancer patients.[89, 90, 91, 92, 93, 94, 95, 96, 97, 98, 99, 100, 101] Most of these trials used 20 mg of melatonin taken at bedtime. Taking such a high amount of melatonin should be done only under the supervision of a doctor familiar with its use. Animal research suggests that the anticancer effects of this hormone may be reversed if melatonin is taken during the day. Therefore, melatonin should be taken only at night.

Calcium *(page 483)*

Through a variety of mechanisms, calcium may have anticancer actions within the colon. Most,[102, 103, 104] but not all,[105] preliminary studies have found associations between taking calcium supplements and a reduced risk of colon cancer or precancerous conditions in the colon. In double-blind trials, calcium supplementation has significantly protected against precancerous changes in the colon in some,[106, 107] but not all, reports.[108, 109] While most evidence examining the ability of calcium supplementation to help prevent colon cancer appears hopeful, no research findings yet support the use of calcium supplements in people already diagnosed with colon cancer.

Vitamin E *(page 609)*

In most,[110, 111] but not all, preliminary reports, people who take vitamin E supplements were found to have decreased risks of precancerous colon polyps and colon cancer, compared with those who do not take vitamin E.[112] Although a double-blind study of male smokers reported that those receiving low amounts of vitamin E (equivalent to approximately 50 IU per day) had a *higher* incidence of precancerous colon polyps than those assigned to placebo,[113] the same trial found a trend toward *lower* risk of colon cancer in the vitamin E group.[114] Insufficient information exists for making recommendations regarding the use of vitamin E in connection with the prevention of colon cancer.

Vitamin C *(page 604)*

Women, but not men, who took vitamin C supplements were reported to have a reduced risk of colon cancer, according to a preliminary report.[115]

Familial polyposis is a disease that usually leads to colon cancer. In a double-blind study, supplementation with 3 grams per day of vitamin C for nine months led to a reduction in the number of precancerous polyps in people with familial polyposis.[116] In another controlled trial, combining vitamin C with **vitamin A** (page 595) and **vitamin E** (page 609) led to a dramatic reduction in the recurrence of adenomatous polyps—another precancerous condition of the colon.[117] However, other trials attempting to prevent recurrence of adenomatous polyps using vitamin C alone or in combination with other vitamins have reported no therapeutic effect[118] or only weak trends favoring the group given supplements.[119, 120]

Therefore, the ability of vitamin C supplementation to reduce recurrences of precancerous polyps remains unproven. Whether long-term supplementation with vitamin C would directly help in the prevention of colon cancer has not yet been studied.

Cancer patients' white blood cells (WBCs) have been reported to contain low levels of vitamin C when compared with WBCs of healthy people.[121] In the 1970s, Linus Pauling and Ewan Cameron, a Scottish surgeon, gave 100 terminal cancer patients 10 grams of vitamin C per day (2.5 grams four times per day) and followed them until death.[122] These patients lived an average of 210 days, compared with an average of 50 days for similar cancer patients who did not receive vitamin C. A follow-up report on the same patients revealed an even greater gap in survival time between the two groups.[123]

Mayo Clinic researchers studied the effect of vitamin C in terminal cancer patients, but unlike Pauling and Cameron, they gave about half of the patients a placebo. The Mayo Clinic findings showed that vitamin C had no therapeutic effect.[124] Pauling claimed that his trial differed from the Mayo Clinic study because his patients had received much less chemotherapy. In theory, chemotherapy might inactivate vitamin C's anticancer effects.

The Mayo Clinic therefore conducted a second controlled study, this time in colon cancer patients who had not received chemotherapy.[125] Again, the Mayo Clinic reported that vitamin C was ineffective. In response, Pauling said that his patients had been given vitamin C supplements until they died. The Mayo Clinic's colon cancer patients, in contrast, were no longer given vitamin C once their cancers progressed. Thus Pauling's premise—that vitamin C would increase survival in terminal cancer patients if they continued to take vitamin C until they died—had not been adequately tested by the Mayo Clinic.

Pauling was also concerned that some of the colon cancer patients assigned to the placebo group may have been taking vitamin C supplements even though they had been instructed not to. The Mayo Clinic had made only limited attempts to monitor whether people in the control group were surreptitiously taking vitamin C.

In an attempt to duplicate Pauling's findings, Japanese researchers conducted a trial with terminal cancer patients.[126] As with the Pauling trial, a control group existed but was not given placebo. Patients assigned to vitamin C lived an average of 246 days compared with 43 days in those not receiving vitamin C. Thus, the Japanese research results independently confirmed the outcome of the Pauling and Cameron trial. Nonetheless, the negative reports from the controlled Mayo Clinic trials—despite criticisms of those trials—leave the issue unresolved. None of these studies investigated what effect, if any, vitamin C might have in patients with early stage colon cancer.

Vitamin D (page 607)

Ultraviolet light from sun exposure increases the risk of skin cancers and melanoma. Nonetheless, where sun exposure is *low*, rates of several cancers have been reported to be high.[127, 128, 129] An association between greater sun exposure and a reduced risk of colon cancer has appeared in some,[130] but not all, studies.[131]

In preliminary reports, people who take vitamin D supplements have been reported to be at low risk for colon cancer, though the differences between supplement takers and others might have been due to chance.[132, 133] More research is needed to determine whether vitamin D supplements may be useful in connection with the prevention of colon cancer.

Glutathione (page 531)

Glutathione is an **antioxidant** (page 467) made in the body, found in some foods, and available as a supplement. Preliminary research suggests that glutathione might have anticancer activity by binding with cancer causing agents or by acting as an antioxidant.

In a preliminary report, 11 patients with late-stage or terminal colon cancer were given 800 mg of glutathione twice per day for at least three months.[134] After an average of 21 weeks, three had died, four others did not improve, and four "recovered with normal diet [and] increased weight. . . . Three of the four were able to return home." In that report, glutathione was combined with the amino acid cysteine and with anthocyans—a type of flavonoid. More research is needed to evaluate whether glutathione is an effective agent for use in connection with treatment of people with late-stage colon cancer.

Fish oil (page 514)

Several human studies have found that supplementation with omega-3 fatty acids from fish oil leads to a reduction in markers for the risk of colon cancer.[135, 136, 137] In each case, enough fish oil was supplemented to supply several grams of omega-3 fatty acids per day, though the optimal amount remains unknown. Despite these promising reports, no trial has yet investigated whether supplementation with fish oil would actually help in the prevention of colon cancer, or be useful in connection with the treatment of people who already have been diagnosed with colon cancer.

IP-6 (page 539)

IP-6 (also called inositol hexaphosphate, phytate, or phytic acid) is found in many foods, particularly oat and wheat bran, and unleavened (flat) bread. Until recently most IP6 research focused on interference with the absorption of minerals—a side effect of consuming IP6. More recently, however, animal studies have found that IP6 has anticancer activity,[138] particularly in relation to colon cancer.[139] Although these animal studies look promising, no human trials using IP6 supplements to prevent or treat cancer have yet been published.

Fiber (page 512)

Although fiber is available in supplement form (such as Metamucil) most fiber consumption results from eating food. The commonly held belief that fiber might also reduce the risk of colon cancer has recently been challenged by several trials that do not support this hypothesis. A fuller discussion of fiber and possible prevention of cancer is found in the **Cancer Prevention and Diet** (page 87) article.

Beta-carotene (page 469)

In double-blind trials, synthetic beta-carotene supplements have had no effect on the incidence of precancerous polyps in the colon.[140, 141] Currently, no evidence shows that beta-carotene supplementation, either natural or synthetic, increases or reduces the risk of colon cancer.

Coenzyme Q$_{10}$ (page 496) (CoQ$_{10}$)

CoQ$_{10}$ has direct effects on the immune system.[142] Though high levels of CoQ$_{10}$ have been found in colon and rectal cancer tissue,[143] low blood levels of CoQ_{10} have been reported in patients with several other cancers.[144, 145, 146]

Are there any side effects or interactions?
Refer to the individual supplement for information about any side effects or interactions.

Herbs that may be helpful
The following herbs have been studied in connection with colon cancer.

Garlic *(page 679) (Allium sativum) and* **onion** *(page 718) (Allium cepa)*
These two herbs belong to the group of plants known as *Allium*. Many other edible plants are found in this group, including leeks and chives. Preliminary studies have investigated the association between eating *Allium* herbs and the incidence of cancer. The most consistent data come from research focusing on the protective effects of *Allium* consumption against cancers of the gastrointestinal tract.[147, 148, 149, 150, 151, 152] Several preliminary studies have found that people who consume more *Allium* vegetables appear to have a reduced risk of colon cancer[153, 154] and precancerous colon polyps.[155]

Constituents in garlic and onions prevent the conversion of nitrates (compounds found in vegetables and, to a lesser extent, in water) to cancer-causing nitrites and nitrosamines.[156]

Green tea *(page 686) and black tea (Camellia sinensis)*
Green and black tea have both been studied to determine whether they cause or prevent cancer. The evidence on the protective effect of either type of tea is inconsistent.[157, 158, 159, 160, 161, 162, 163, 164]

A number of preliminary studies have shown an association between drinking green tea and a reduced risk of several types of cancer,[165, 166, 167, 168] including colon cancer.[169] In contrast, preliminary studies found that consumers of *black* tea do not appear to have a reduced risk of any type of cancer.[170, 171, 172]

Other herbal therapies
No trials have investigated the effects of the Hoxsey herbal formula, *Coriolus versicolor* (PSK), the Essiac formula, or most other herbal therapies specifically for the treatment of people with colon cancer.

Are there any side effects or interactions?
Refer to the individual herb for information about any side effects or interactions.

COMMON COLD/ SORE THROAT

See also: Influenza (page 269) (Flu), **Sinus Congestion** (page 405), **Sinusitis** (page 407)

What do I need to know?
Self-care for common cold can be approached in a number of ways—but it can be hard to know just where to start. To make it easier, our doctors recommend trying these simple steps first:

Be sure to rest
> Give your body some down time to help it fight off the cold

Drink those fluids
> Get plenty of water and other clear fluids to help thin mucous

Take extra vitamin C
> Studies have shown 1 to 4 grams a day may make your cold shorter and less severe

Use zinc lozenges
> Use lozenges containing zinc gluconate, zinc gluconate-glycine, or zinc acetate, providing 13 to 25 mg every two hours, to help stop the virus and shorten the illness

Shorten sick time with echinacea
> At the first signs of a cold, take 3 to 5 ml of echinacea juice or tincture every two hours to make your cold less severe

Get some garlic
> Help prevent colds with 600 to 900 mg a day of a standardized garlic supplement

About the common cold
The common cold is an acute (short-term) viral infection of the upper respiratory tract that may be spread through the air (by sneezing, for example) or by contact with contaminated objects.

What are the symptoms of the common cold?
The common cold often causes runny nose, sore throat, and malaise (vague discomfort). Sore throat is sometimes a symptom of a more serious condition distinct from the common cold, such as strep throat, which may require medical diagnosis and treatment with appropriate antibiotics. Since it is a viral **infection** (page 265), antibiotics are not effective against the common cold.

	CHECKLIST FOR COMMON COLD/SORE THROAT	
Rating	Nutritional Supplements	Herbs
★★★	**Vitamin C** (page 604) **Zinc** (page 614) (as lozenges)	**Andrographis** (page 626) (for symptoms) **Echinacea** (page 669) (for symptoms; effective only for adults)
★★☆	**Propolis** (page 579) **Zinc** (page 614) (as nasal spray)	**Garlic** (page 679) Geranium (*Pelargonium sidoides*) Throat Coat (**marshmallow root** [page 708], **licorice root** [page 702], elm bark)
★☆☆		**Asian ginseng** (page 630) **Astragalus** (page 631) **Blackberry** (page 636) **Blueberry** (page 641) **Boneset** (page 644) Chinese artichoke **Coltsfoot** (page 661) **Elderberry** (page 670) **Eleuthero** (page 672) **Eucalyptus** (page 673) (oil) **Goldenseal** (page 683) Goldthread **Horseradish** (page 693) **Hyssop** (page 695) **Linden** (page 704) Malvia **Marshmallow** (page 708) **Meadowsweet** (page 709) **Mullein** (page 713) **Myrrh** (page 713) **Peppermint** (page 726) **Red raspberry** (page 735) **Sage** (page 740) **Schisandra** (page 744) **Slippery elm** (page 747) **Usnea** (page 754) **Wild indigo** (page 759) **Wood betony** (page 761) **Yarrow** (page 763)

Medical treatments

Over the counter products may help to reduce the symptoms associated with the common cold and sore throats, but they do not speed recovery. Analgesics, such as aspirin (Bayer, Ecotrin, Bufferin), ibuprofen (Motrin, Advil), and acetaminophen (Tylenol), reduce pain due to sore throats and headaches. Products containing local anesthetics such as benzocaine (Cepacol Maximum Strength, Spec-T) and phenol (Cepastat) provide temporary relief from sore throat pain. Topical nasal decongestants such as oxymetazoline (Afrin) and phenylephrine (NeoSynephrine) may provide relief from nasal congestion, but they should only be used for a few days. The oral decongestant pseudoephedrine (Sudafed) may help relieve nasal congestion, while antihistamines such as diphenhydramine (Benadryl), brompheniramine (Dimetapp), and chlorpheniramine (Chlor-Trimeton) might help dry excess mucous and reduce sneezing. Guaifenesin (Robitussin) is an expectorant used to remove mucous in the sinuses, lungs, and ears. The cough suppressant dextromethorphan (DM) may be recommended at bedtime to facilitate sleep; however, since expectoration of sputum is considered a valuable mechanism for expelling infectious organisms and congested secretions, a cough should not be suppressed during the day. Most products available over the counter to treat the common cold combine decongestants, antihistamines, analgesics, expectorants, and cough suppressants.

Though most symptoms of the common cold are controlled with over the counter products, some individuals might require prescription strength cough suppressants, such as codeine (Robitussin A-C) and hydrocodone (Vicodin Tuss, Tussionex, Hycodan). Individuals with sore throats that last for more than a few days should be checked by a healthcare practicioner as their condition might be caused by a bacterial infection, which requires oral antibiotics such as amoxicillin (Amoxil) and cephalexin (Keflex). Some health care practitioners may prescribe oral antibiotics to prevent a secondary bacterial infection in immune deficient patients.

A warm, humid environment created by a humidifier may provide comfort during the common cold. Rest is recommended, especially for people with severe symptoms. Increased fluid intake is necessary in order to maintain water balance and to thin secretions.

Dietary changes that may be helpful

Excessive sugar, dietary fat, and alcohol have been reported to impair **immune function** (page 255), although no specific information is available on how these foods may affect the course of the common cold.

Nutritional supplements that may be helpful

A review of 21 controlled trials using 1 to 8 grams of **vitamin C** (page 604) per day found that "in each of the twenty-one studies, vitamin C reduced the duration of episodes and the severity of the symptoms of the common cold by an average of 23%."[1] The optimum amount of vitamin C to take for cold treatment remains in debate but may be as high as 1 to 3 grams per day, considerably more than the 120 to 200 mg per day that has been suggested as optimal intake for healthy adults. A review of 23 controlled trials found that vitamin C supplementation produces a greater benefit for children than for adults.[2] The same review found that a daily amount of 2 grams or more was superior to a daily amount of 1 gram at reducing the duration of cold symptoms.

Zinc (page 614) interferes with viral replication in test tubes, may interfere with the ability of viruses to enter cells of the body, may help immune cells to fight a cold, and may relieve cold symptoms when taken as a supplement.[3] In double-blind trials, zinc lozenges have reduced the duration of colds in adults[4, 5] but have been ineffective in children.[6] Lozenges containing zinc gluconate, zinc gluconate-glycine, and, in most trials, zinc acetate[7, 8] have been effective; most other forms of zinc and lozenges flavored with citric acid,[9] tartaric acid, sorbitol, or mannitol have been ineffective.[10] Trials using these other forms of zinc have failed, as have trials that use insufficient amounts of zinc.[11] For the alleviation of cold symptoms, lozenges providing 13 to 25 mg of zinc (as zinc gluconate, zinc gluconate-glycine, or zinc acetate) are used every two hours while awake but only for several days. The best effect is obtained when lozenges are used at the first sign of a cold.

An analysis of the major zinc trials has claimed that evidence for efficacy is "still lacking."[12] However, despite a lack of *statistical* significance, this compilation of data from six double-blind trials found that people assigned to zinc had a 50% decreased risk of still having symptoms after one week compared with those given placebo. Some trials included in this analysis used formulations containing substances that may inactivate zinc salts. Other reasons for failure to show statistical significance, according to a recent analysis of these studies,[13] may have been small sample size (not enough people) or not enough zinc given. Thus, there are plausible reasons why the authors were unable to show sta-

tistical significance, even though positive effects are well supported in most trials using gluconate, gluconate-glycine, or acetate forms of zinc.

Zinc nasal sprays may be even more effective than zinc lozenges at speeding the resolution of cold symptoms. A double-blind trial showed a 74% reduction in symptom duration in people using a zinc nasal spray four times daily, compared with the 42 to 53% reduction reported in trials using zinc gluconate or zinc acetate lozenges.[14] The average duration of symptoms after the beginning of treatment was 2.3 days in the people receiving zinc, compared with 9.0 days in those receiving placebo. However, in another double-blind study, zinc nasal spray was no more effective than a placebo; in both groups the median duration of symptoms was seven days.[15] The beneficial effect of zinc nasal sprays should be weighed against a potentially serious side effect. At least ten cases have been reported of people with previously normal sense of smell who experienced severe or complete loss of smell function after using intranasal zinc gluconate. In some cases the loss of smell was long-lasting or permanent.[16]

Propolis (page 579) is the resinous substance collected by bees from the leaf buds and bark of trees, especially poplar and conifer trees. Propolis extracts may be helpful in preventing and shortening the duration of the common cold. A preliminary clinical trial reported propolis extract (daily dose not given) reduced upper respiratory infections in children.[17] In one small, double-blind trial of propolis for the common cold, the group taking propolis extract (amount unstated) became free of symptoms more quickly than the placebo group.[18] Most manufacturers recommend 500 mg of oral propolis products once or twice daily.

Are there any side effects or interactions?
Refer to the individual supplement for information about any side effects or interactions.

Herbs that may be helpful

Four different categories of herbs are used to help combat the common cold. First, herbs that stimulate the **immune system** (page 255) to fight the **infection** (page 265) are used during the onset of the common cold—echinacea (page 669) and **Asian ginseng** (page 630) are two examples. Second, herbs known as diaphoretics promote a mild fever and sweating both of which are useful for fighting infection. A fever is a sign that the immune system is working; thus, diaphoretics may also be immune stimulators—elder, **boneset** (page

644), and **yarrow** (page 763) are three examples. The third category includes herbs that, based on test tube studies, may directly kill the viruses that cause colds—**goldenseal** (page 683), **myrrh** (page 713), and **usnea** (page 754) are examples. Finally, a fourth category of herbs are used to alleviate cold symptoms, such as sore throats. These herbs tend to be high in mucilage and are soothing and anti-inflammatory, or have tannins that are astringent (i.e., that constrict boggy tissue, promoting healing)—**marshmallow** (page 708) and **red raspberry** (page 735) are two examples.

As the following chart shows, many herbs fit into more than one category; goldenseal is one example, as it has both immune-stimulating and antiviral properties.

Action Category	Herbs
Immune-stimulating	**Andrographis** (page 626), **Asian ginseng** (page 630), **astragalus** (page 631), **boneset** (page 644), **echinacea** (page 669), **eleuthero** (page 672), **garlic** (page 679), **goldenseal** (page 683), **hyssop** (page 695), **linden** (page 704), **schisandra** (page 744), **wild indigo** (page 759)
Diaphoretic	**Boneset** (page 644), elder flower, **hyssop** (page 695), **linden** (page 704), **yarrow** (page 763)
Antiviral (test tube studies only)	**Barberry** (page 632), **elderberry** (page 670), **goldenseal** (page 683), goldthread, **horseradish** (page 693), **myrrh** (page 713), **Oregon grape** (page 721), **usnea** (page 754), **wild indigo** (page 759)
Symptom-relieving	Soothe sore throat: **blackberry** (page 636), **blueberry** (page 641), **red raspberry** (page 735) (astringents), **coltsfoot** (page 661), mallow, **marshmallow** (page 708), **mullein** (page 713), **red raspberry** (page 735) (mucilage) Reduce nasal stuffiness: **eucalyptus** (page 673), **peppermint** (page 726) Relieve aches: **meadowsweet** (page 709) Miscellaneous sore throat relief: **sage** (page 740), **yarrow** (page 763)

Note: These actions have not necessarily been proven in clinical trials in humans and are intended only to clarify distinctions among herbs, not to give recommendations for use.

Double-blind trials have shown that various echinacea extracts shorten the duration of the common cold.[19, 20] Fresh pressed juice of **echinacea** (page 669) (*E. pur-*

purea) flowers preserved with alcohol, and tinctures of echinacea (*E. pallida*) root are the forms most commonly studied and proven effective. In addition, several double-blind trials have found that echinacea (*E. angustifolia*) root tinctures in combination with **wild indigo** (page 759), **boneset** (page 644), and homeopathic arnica reduce symptoms of the common cold.[21] In one double-blind trial, a proprietary formulation of echinacea, white cedar, and wild indigo, known as Esberitox, reduced the length and severity of cold symptoms significantly more than did placebo.[22] There is one, as yet unpublished, study that has found echinacea to be ineffective for the common cold,[23] and another double-blind study found that echinacea was not effective for the treatment of upper respiratory tract infections in children aged 2 to 11 years.[24]

Echinacea is believed to work primarily through **immune stimulation** (page 255). The minimum effective amount of echinacea tincture or juice appears to be 3 ml three times per day. Higher amounts, such as 3 to 5 ml every two hours, is generally better and is safe, even for children.[25] Encapsulated products may also be effective, according to a double-blind trial using the root of *E. pallida*.[26] Generally, capsules containing 300 to 600 mg are used three times per day. According to one double-blind trial, employees of a nursing home who consumed echinacea tea at the onset of a cold or **flu** (page 269) reduced the duration of their symptoms by about two days when compared with people consuming a placebo tea.[27] The participants drank five to six cups of tea on the first day of their symptoms and decreased this by one cup each day over the next five days.

Double-blind trials indicate that regular use of echinacea to *prevent* colds does not work.[28, 29, 30] Therefore, it is currently recommended to use echinacea at the onset of a cold, for a total of seven to ten days.

Andrographis (page 626) contains bitter constituents that are believed to have immune-stimulating and anti-inflammatory actions.[31] Several double-blind trials have found that andrographis may help reduce symptom severity in people with common colds.[32, 33, 34, 35] Though the earliest clinical trial among these showed modest benefits, later studies have tended to be more supportive. A combination of a standardized andrographis extract combined with **eleuthero** (page 672), known as Kan jang, has also been shown in a double-blind trial to reduce symptoms of the common cold.[36]

In a double-blind trial, participants took one capsule per day of a placebo or a **garlic** (page 679) supplement that contained stabilized allicin (the amount of garlic per capsule was not specified) for 12 weeks between November and February. During that time, the garlic group had 63% fewer colds and 70% fewer days ill than did the placebo group.[37]

Geranium (*Pelargonium sidoides*) is an herbal remedy used in Germany, Mexico, Russia, and other countries for the treatment of **respiratory** (page 405) tract and **ear, nose, and throat infections** (page 383). In a double-blind study of children with acute tonsillitis/pharyngitis that was not due to a Streptococcal infection, participants given an extract of geranium had significantly more rapid resolution of symptoms, compared with those given a placebo.[38] The amount of the geranium extract used in this study was 20 drops three times per day for six days.

In a double-blind study, a proprietary product containing **marshmallow root** (page 708), **licorice root** (page 702), and elm bark (Throat Coat) was effective in providing rapid, temporary relief of sore throat pain in people with acute pharyngitis.[39] Throat Coat was taken as a tea in the amount of 5 to 8 ounces, 4 to 6 times per day, for two to seven days.

Herbal supplements can help strengthen the immune system and fight infections. Adaptogens, which include eleuthero, **Asian ginseng** (page 630), **astragalus** (page 631), and **schisandra** (page 744), are thought to help keep various body systems—including the immune system—functioning optimally. They have not been systematically evaluated as cold remedies. However, one double-blind trial found that people who were given 100 mg of Asian ginseng extract in combination with a flu vaccine experienced a lower frequency of colds and flu compared with people who received only the flu vaccine.[40]

According to test tube experiments,[41] wild indigo stimulates **immune function** (page 255), which might account for its role in fighting the common cold and **flu** (page 269). In combination with echinacea, boneset, and homeopathic arnica, as mentioned above, wild indigo has prevented and reduced symptoms of the common cold in double-blind research. Wild indigo is traditionally considered a strong antimicrobial agent, though it has not yet been investigated as an agent against cold viruses.

Boneset is another immune stimulant and diaphoretic that helps fight off minor viral infections, such as the common cold. In addition, **linden** (page 704) and **hyssop** (page 695) may promote a healthy fever and the immune system's ability to fight **infections** (page 265). **Yarrow** (page 763) is another di-

aphoretic that has been used for relief of sore throats, though it has not yet been researched for this purpose.

Goldenseal (page 683) root contains two alkaloids, berberine and canadine, with antimicrobial and mild immune-stimulating effects.[42] However, due to the small amounts of alkaloids occurring in the root, it is unlikely these effects would occur outside the test tube. Goldenseal soothes irritated mucous membranes in the throat,[43] making it potentially useful for those experiencing a sore throat with their cold. Human research on the effectiveness of goldenseal or other berberine-containing herbs, such as **Oregon grape** (page 721), **barberry** (page 632), or goldthread *(Coptis chinensis),* for people with colds has not been conducted.

Goldenseal root should only be used for short periods of time. Goldenseal root extract, in capsule or tablet form, is typically taken in amounts of 4 to 6 grams three times per day. Using goldenseal powder as a tea or tincture may soothe a sore throat. Because goldenseal is threatened in the wild due to over-harvesting, substitutes such as **Oregon grape** (page 721) should be used whenever possible.

Elderberry (page 670) has shown antiviral activity and thus may be useful for some people with common colds. Elder flowers are a traditional diaphoretic remedy for helping to break fevers and promote sweating during a cold. **Horseradish** (page 693) has antibiotic properties, which may account for its usefulness in easing throat and upper respiratory tract infections. The resin of the herb **myrrh** (page 713) has been shown to kill various microbes and to stimulate macrophages (a type of white blood cell). **Usnea** (page 704) has a traditional reputation as an antiseptic and is sometimes used for people with common colds.

Herbs high in mucilage, such as **slippery elm** (page 747), mallow *(Malvia sylvestris),* and **marshmallow** (page 708), are often helpful for symptomatic relief of coughs and irritated throats. **Mullein** (page 713) has expectorant and demulcent properties, which accounts for this herb's historical use as a remedy for the respiratory tract, particularly in cases of irritating coughs with bronchial congestion. **Coltsfoot** (page 661) is another herb with high mucilage content that has been used historically to soothe sore throats. However, it is high in pyrrolizidine alkaloids—constituents that may damage the liver over time. It is best to either avoid coltsfoot or look for products that are free of pyrrolizidine alkaloids.

Red raspberry (page 735), **blackberry** (page 636), and **blueberry** (page 641) leaves contain astringent tannins that are helpful for soothing sore throats.[44] **Sage**

(page 740) tea may be gargled to soothe a sore throat. All of these remedies are used traditionally, but they are currently not supported by modern research.

Eucalyptus (page 673) oil is often used in a steam inhalation to help clear nasal and sinus congestion. It is said to work similarly to menthol, by acting on receptors in the nasal mucous membranes, leading to a reduction of nasal stuffiness.[45] **Peppermint** (page 726) may have a similar action and is a source of small amounts of menthol.

Meadowsweet (page 709) has been used historically for a wide variety of conditions. It is reputed to break fevers and to promote sweating during a cold or flu. Meadowsweet contains salicylates, which possibly give the herb an aspirin-like effect, particularly in relieving aches and pains during a common cold. While not as potent as **willow** (page 760), which has a higher salicin content, the salicylates in meadowsweet do give it a mild anti-inflammatory effect and the potential to reduce fevers during a cold or **flu** (page 269). However, this role is based on historical use and knowledge of the chemistry of meadowsweet's constituents; to date, no human studies have been completed with meadowsweet.

Traditional Chinese Medicine practitioners use Chinese artichoke *(Stachys sieboldii)*, a species similar to **wood betony** (page 761) *(Stachys betonica)*, for colds and flu.[46] It is unknown whether wood betony would be useful for people with the common cold.

Are there any side effects or interactions?
Refer to the individual herb for information about any side effects or interactions.

CONGESTIVE HEART FAILURE

Congestive heart failure (CHF) is a chronic condition that results when the heart muscle is unable to pump blood as efficiently as is needed.

High blood pressure (page 246) can cause congestive heart failure. Failure of the heart pump can also result from many other causes, such as severe **anemia** (page 25), hyperthyroidism, **heart attacks** (page 212), and **arrhythmias** (page 93) of the heart.

> **Caution:** Congestive heart failure is a serious medical condition that requires expert management rather than self-treatment.

CHECKLIST FOR CONGESTIVE HEART FAILURE

Rating	Nutritional Supplements	Herbs
★★★	**Magnesium** (page 551) **Propionyl-L-carnitine** (page 543) **Taurine** (page 590)	Berberine **Hawthorn** (page 689)
★★☆	**Arginine** (page 467) **Coenzyme Q₁₀** (page 496) **Potassium** (page 572)	Arjun (bark extract)
★☆☆	**Creatine monohydrate** (page 501)	**Coleus** (page 660)

What are the symptoms of congestive heart failure?
CHF leads to breathlessness, fatigue, and accumulation of fluid in the lungs or the veins (primarily in the legs) or both.

Medical treatments
Prescription medications used in the treatment of CHF are directed at improving the ability of the heart to pump blood. Drugs may also be used to regulate the heart's rhythm. Digitalis preparations, most commonly digoxin (Lanoxin), may be used to improve heart function and reduce the amount of diuretics needed. Loop diuretics such as furosemide (Lasix) and bumetanide (Bumex), and other diuretics including hydrochlorothiazide (HydroDIURIL) and metolazone (Zaroxolyn), are often used. ACE inhibitors are prescribed to improve heart and blood vessel function as well as exercise tolerance; they include captopril (Capoten), enalapril (Vasotec), lisinopril (Prinivil, Zestril), and quinapril (Accupril).

Lifestyle changes that may be helpful
Even with severe disease, appropriate exercise can benefit those with CHF.[1, 2] In a controlled trial, long-term (one year) exercise training led to improvements in quality of life and functional capacity in people with CHF.[3] Nonetheless, too much exercise can be life-threatening for those with CHF. How much is "too much" varies from person to person; therefore, any exercise program undertaken by someone with CHF requires professional supervision.

Non-steroidal anti-inflammatory drugs (NSAIDs) appear to significantly increase the risk of CHF. The use of NSAIDs in one preliminary study was found to double the likelihood of hospital admission with CHF the following week. This likelihood increased by more than 10 times for patients with a history of heart disease.[4] This study did not include people taking low-dose aspirin.

Nutritional supplements that may be helpful

People with CHF have insufficient oxygenation of the heart, which can damage the heart muscle. Such damage may be reduced by taking **L-carnitine** (page 543) supplements.[5] L-carnitine is a natural substance made from the **amino acids** (page 465), **lysine** (page 550) and **methionine** (page 557). Levels of L-carnitine are low in people with CHF;[6] therefore, many doctors recommend that those with CHF take 500 mg of L-carnitine two to three times per day.

Most L-carnitine/CHF research has used a modified form of the supplement called **propionyl-L-carnitine** (page 543) (PC). In one double-blind trial, people using 500 mg of PC per day had a 26% increase in exercise capacity after six months.[7] In double-blind research, other indices of heart function have also improved after taking 1 gram of PC twice per day.[8] It remains unclear whether propionyl-L-carnitine has unique advantages over L-carnitine, as limited research in animals and humans has also shown very promising effects of the more common L-carnitine.[9]

Magnesium (page 551) deficiency frequently occurs in people with CHF, and such a deficiency may lead to **heart arrhythmias** (page 93). Magnesium supplements have reduced the risk of these arrhythmias.[10] People with CHF are often given drugs that deplete both magnesium and **potassium** (page 572); a deficiency of either of these minerals may lead to an arrhythmia.[11] Many doctors suggest magnesium supplements of 300 mg per day.

Whole fruit and fruit and vegetable juice, which are high in potassium, are also recommended by some doctors; however, this dietary change should be discussed with a healthcare provider, because several drugs given to people with CHF may actually cause *retention* of potassium, making dietary potassium, even from fruit, dangerous.

Taurine (page 590), an amino acid, helps increase the force and effectiveness of heart-muscle contractions. Research (some double-blind) has shown that taurine helps people with CHF.[12, 13, 14, 15] Most doctors suggest taking 2 grams three times per day.

As is true for several other heart conditions, **coen-zyme Q$_{10}$** (page 496) (CoQ$_{10}$) has been reported to help people with CHF,[16] sometimes dramatically.[17] Positive effects have been confirmed in double-blind research[18] and in an overall analysis of eight controlled trials.[19] However, some double-blind trials have reported modest[20] or no improvement[21, 22, 23] in exercise capacity or overall quality of life. Most CoQ$_{10}$ research used 90–200 mg per day. The beneficial effects of CoQ$_{10}$ may not be seen until after several months of treatment. Discontinuation of CoQ$_{10}$ supplementation in people with CHF has resulted in severe relapses and should only be attempted under the supervision of a doctor.[24]

The body needs **arginine** (page 467), another amino acid, to make nitric oxide, which increases blood flow. This process is impaired in people with CHF. Arginine supplementation (5.6–12.6 grams per day) has been used successfully in double-blind trials to treat CHF.[25] A double-blind trial has also found that arginine supplementation (5 grams three times daily) improves kidney function in people with CHF.[26]

For people with congestive heart failure, intravenous injections of **creatine** (page 501) have been found to improve heart function; oral supplementation has not been effective, though it does improve skeletal muscle function.[27, 28]

In a preliminary study, blood levels of **DHEA** (page 503) (dehydroepiandrosterone) were found to be lower in people with CHF than in people without the disease. The lowered blood levels of DHEA among these people was proportional to the severity of their disease.[29] However, there is no evidence that DHEA supplementation can prevent or reverse CHF.

In a double-blind study of people with established **heart disease** (page 98) or **diabetes** (page 152), participants who took 400 IU of **vitamin E** (page 609) per day for an average of 4.5 years developed heart failure significantly more often than did those taking a placebo.[30] Hospitalizations for heart failure occurred in 5.8% of those in the vitamin E group, compared with 4.2% of those in the placebo group, a 38.1% increase. Considering that some other studies have shown a beneficial effect of vitamin E against heart disease, the results of this study are difficult to interpret. Nevertheless, individuals with heart disease or diabetes should consult their doctor before taking vitamin E.

Are there any side effects or interactions?
Refer to the individual supplement for information about any side effects or interactions.

Herbs that may be helpful

Berberine is used in Asia to treat congestive heart failure. In a double-blind trial, supplementation with berberine (300 to 500 mg, four times per day) for eight weeks significantly improved heart function and exercise capacity and reduced the frequency of arrhythmias in people with congestive heart failure.[31]

Clinical trials have shown that standardized extracts made from the leaves and flowers of **hawthorn** (page 689) are effective in helping people with early-stage CHF.[32, 33] Hawthorn extracts appear to increase blood flow to the heart, increase the strength of heart contractions, reduce resistance to blood flow in the extremities, and act as an **antioxidant** (page 467).[34, 35, 36] In a large preliminary trial, people with mild to moderate CHF were given 300 mg of hawthorn flower and leaf extract (standardized to contain 2.2% flavonoids) three times a day for two months.[37] Symptoms of CHF—including heart palpitations, chest pressure, and swelling in the extremities—decreased throughout the trial during the use of hawthorn. The efficacy of hawthorn for the treatment of CHF has been confirmed in a double-blind trial.[38]

Hawthorn extracts are available in capsules or tablets standardized to either total **flavonoid** (page 516) content (usually 2.2%) or **oligomeric procyanidins** (page 574) (usually 18.75%). Doctors who work with herbal medicine often suggest 80–300 mg two to three times per day. Hawthorn berry products that are not standardized may be weaker, and the recommended amount is typically 4 to 6 grams per day for the whole herb, or 4–5 ml of the tincture three times per day.

Coleus (page 660) contains forskolin, a substance that may help dilate blood vessels and improve the forcefulness with which the heart pumps blood.[39] Recent clinical trials indicate that forskolin improves heart function in people with congestive heart failure and **cardiomyopathy** (page 95).[40, 41] A preliminary trial found that forskolin reduced **blood pressure** (page 246) and improved heart function in people with cardiomyopathy. These trials have used intravenous infusions of isolated forskolin. It is unknown whether oral coleus extracts would have the same effect. While many doctors expert in herbal medicine would recommend 200–600 mg per day of a coleus extract containing 10% forskolin, these amounts are extrapolations and have yet to be confirmed by direct clinical research.

A small clinical trial found that supplementation with a bark extract of Arjun (*Terminalia arjuna*) improved heart function as well as lung congestion in patients with severe CHF.[42] Patients in the study took 500 mg of Arjun extract three times per day and began to exhibit significant improvement in heart function within two weeks; improvement continued over the course of approximately two years. The herb extract used in this study was concentrated but not standardized for any particular constituent. Commercial preparations are sometimes standardized to contain 1% arjunolic acid. Larger clinical trials are needed to confirm the results of this small study.

Are there any side effects or interactions?
Refer to the individual herb for information about any side effects or interactions.

CONJUNCTIVITIS AND BLEPHARITIS

Conjunctivitis is inflammation of the clear membrane that lines the eye.

Conjunctivitis is caused most commonly by **infection** (page 265) from viruses or bacteria, or by an **allergic reaction** (page 14), though other causes exist, such as overexposure to sun, wind, smog, chlorine, or contact lens solution. Pinkeye is the common name for conjunctivitis. Blepharitis is inflammation of the eyelid; most commonly, it is caused by a bacterial infection.

CHECKLIST FOR CONJUNCTIVITIS AND BLEPHARITIS		
Rating	**Nutritional Supplements**	**Herbs**
★☆☆	**Vitamin A** (page 595)	**Calendula** (page 650) **Chamomile** (page 656) **Comfrey** (page 662) **Eyebright** (page 674) **Goldenseal** (page 683) **Oregon grape** (page 721)

What are the symptoms of conjunctivitis?
Conjunctivitis and blepharitis may cause mild discomfort with tearing, itching, burning, light sensitivity, and

thickening of the eyelids. They may also produce a crust or discharge, occasionally causing the eyelids to stick together during sleep. The eyes and eyelids may become red, but usually there is no blurring or change in vision.

Medical treatments

Over the counter irrigating solutions containing boric acid (Eye Wash, Collyrium for Fresh Eyes Wash) might temporarily relieve irritation. Continued redness, irritation, or **pain** (page 338) requires medical treatment.

Prescription eye (ophthalmic) medications, available in ointment or drop form, often contain antibiotics such as erythromycin (Ilotycin), gentamicin (Garamycin), or sulfacetamide (Sodium Sulamyd, Bleph-10) to treat bacterial infection. Ophthalmic corticosteroids, in combination with antibiotics, include hydrocortisone (Cortisporin Ophthalmic Suspension), dexamethasone (TobraDex), and prednisolone (Poly-Pred Suspension) are often prescribed to treat inflammation and infection.

Individuals with diagnosed conjunctivitis should avoid irritants, such as contact lenses or allergy-causing agents.

Nutritional supplements that may be helpful

Vitamin A (page 595) deficiency has been reported in people with chronic conjunctivitis.[1] It is unknown whether vitamin A supplementation can prevent conjunctivitis or help people who already have the condition.

Are there any side effects or interactions?
Refer to the individual supplement for information about any side effects or interactions.

Herbs that may be helpful

Several herbs have been traditionally used to treat eye inflammation. Examples include **calendula** (page 650), **eyebright** (page 674), **chamomile** (page 656), and **comfrey** (page 662). None of these herbs has been studied for use in conjunctivitis or blepharitis. As any preparation placed on the eye must be kept sterile, topical use of these herbs in the eyes should only be done under the supervision of an experienced healthcare professional.

Goldenseal (page 683) and **Oregon grape** (page 721) contain the antibacterial constituent known as berberine. While topical use of berberine in eye drops has been clinically studied for eye infections,[2] the use of

the whole herbs has not been studied for conjunctivitis or blepharitis.

Are there any side effects or interactions?
Refer to the individual herb for information about any side effects or interactions.

CONSTIPATION

What do I need to know?

Self-care for constipation can be approached in a number of ways—but it can be hard to know just where to start. To make it easier, our doctors recommend trying these simple steps first:

Get a checkup
  Constipation that starts suddenly should be evaluated by a doctor to make sure no serious diseases are the cause

Get more fiber and water in your diet
  To increase stool bulk, include more vegetables, beans, bran, flaxseed, and whole grains in your diet; don't forget to drink more water when you increase fiber intake

Try a bulk laxative
  For results within 12 to 24 hours, take 5 to 10 grams per day of psyllium husk or 3 to 4 grams per day of glucomannan mixed in water, followed by a second glass of water

About constipation

Constipation is a condition in which a person experiences a change in normal bowel habits, characterized by a decrease in frequency and/or passage of hard, dry stools. Constipation can also refer to difficult defecation or to sluggish action of the bowels.

The most common cause of constipation is dietary, which is discussed below. However, constipation may be a component of **irritable bowel syndrome** (page 280) or other conditions ranging from drug side effects to physical immobility. Serious diseases, including **colon cancer** (page 123), may sometimes first appear as bowel blockage leading to acute constipation. However, constipation itself does not appear to increase the risk of colon cancer, contrary to popular opinion.[1]

Although dietary and other natural approaches discussed below are often effective, individuals with constipation should be evaluated by a doctor to rule out potentially serious causes.

Constipation

CHECKLIST FOR CONSTIPATION

Rating	Nutritional Supplements	Herbs
★★★	Fiber (page 512) Glucomannan (page 526)	Aloe (page 624) Cascara (page 652) Flaxseed (page 517) Psyllium (page 732) Senna (page 745)
★★☆		Alder buckthorn (page 622) Basil (page 633) Buckthorn (page 646) Rhubarb
★☆☆	Chlorophyll (page 492) Flaxseed oil (page 517)	Bladderwrack (page 639) Dandelion (page 666) Fenugreek (page 676) Fo-ti (page 678)

What are the symptoms of constipation?

Symptoms of constipation include infrequent stools, hard stools, and excessive straining to move the bowels. Frequency of bowel movements and severity of symptoms may vary from person to person.

Medical treatments

Over the counter products are best divided into fast- and slow-acting agents. Rapid relief of constipation is achieved with suppositories containing glycerin (Fleet) or bisacodyl (Dulcolax) enemas, and magnesium-containing products (Phillips' Milk of Magnesia, Magnesium Citrate Solution). Overnight relief is obtained with senna (Senokot, Fletcher's Castoria) and bisacodyl (Dulcolax) tablets. Bulk-forming laxatives containing psyllium (Metamucil, Konsyl-D), polycarbophil (Fibercon), and methylcellulose (Citrucel), as well as the stool softener docusate (Colace, Surfak), may require up to 72 hours for relief of symptoms.

Laxatives available with a prescription include lactulose (Chronulac), which acts within one to two days, and polyethylene glycol (Miralax), which may require two to four days of treatment before constipation is relieved. Large quantities of polyethylene glycol-electrolyte solution (CoLyte, GoLYTELY, NuLytely) might be prescribed for bowel cleansing the evening prior to intestinal examinations.

Healthcare practitioners often recommend increased dietary fiber (page 512) and fluid intake to shorten bowel transit time and increase stool weight. Use of laxatives beyond one week is discouraged, due to weakening of the colon and fluid retention. Laxative abuse is common in the elderly and among people with eating disorders (page 174).

Dietary changes that may be helpful

Fiber (page 512), particularly insoluble fiber, is linked with prevention of chronic constipation.[2] Insoluble fiber from food acts like a sponge, pulling water into the stool and making it easier to pass. Insoluble fiber comes mostly from vegetables, beans, brown rice, whole wheat, rye, and other whole grains. Switching from white bread and white rice to whole wheat bread and brown rice often helps relieve constipation. It is important to drink lots of fluid along with the fiber—at least 16 ounces of water per serving of fiber. Otherwise, the fiber may actually worsen the constipation.

In addition, wheat bran may be added to the diet. Doctors frequently suggest a quarter cup or more per day of wheat bran along with fluid. An easy way to add wheat bran to the diet is to put it in breakfast cereal or switch to high-bran cereals. Wheat bran often reduces constipation, although not all research shows it to be successful.[3] Higher amounts of wheat bran are sometimes more successful than lower amounts.[4]

A double-blind trial found that chronic constipation among infants and problems associated with it were triggered by intolerance to cows'milk in two-thirds of the infants studied.[5] Symptoms disappeared in most infants when cows' milk was removed from their diet. These results were confirmed in two subsequent, preliminary trials.[6, 7] Constipation triggered by other food allergies (page 14) might be responsible for chronic constipation in some adults. If other approaches do not help, these possibilities may be discussed with a physician.

Lifestyle changes that may be helpful

Exercise may increase the muscular contractions of the intestine, promoting elimination.[8] Nonetheless, the effect of exercise on constipation remains unclear.[9]

Nutritional supplements that may be helpful

Glucomannan (page 526) is a water-soluble dietary fiber that is derived from konjac root. Like other sources of fiber (page 512), such as psyllium (page 732) and fenugreek (page 676), glucomannan is considered a bulk-forming laxative. A preliminary trial[10] and several double-blind trials[11, 12, 13, 14] have found glucomannan to be an effective treatment for constipation. The amount of glucomannan shown to be effective as a laxative is 3 to 4 grams per day. In constipated people, glucomannan and other bulk-forming laxatives generally help produce a bowel movement within 12 to 24 hours.

Chlorophyll (page 492), the substance responsible for the green color in plants, may be useful for a number of gastrointestinal problems. In a preliminary trial, chlorophyll supplementation eased chronic constipation in elderly people.[15]

Are there any side effects or interactions?
Refer to the individual supplement for information about any side effects or interactions.

Herbs that may be helpful
The laxatives most frequently used world-wide come from plants. Herbal laxatives are either bulk-forming or stimulating.

Bulk-forming laxatives come from plants with a high **fiber** (page 512) and mucilage content that expand when they come in contact with water; examples include **psyllium** (page 732), **flaxseed** (page 517), and **fenugreek** (page 676). As the volume in the bowel increases, a reflex muscular contraction occurs, stimulating a bowel movement. These mild laxatives are best suited for long-term use in people with constipation.

Many doctors recommend taking 7.5 grams of psyllium seeds or 5 grams of psyllium husks, mixed with water or juice, one to two times per day. Some doctors use a combination of **senna** (page 745) (18%) and psyllium (82%) for the treatment of chronic constipation. This has been shown to work effectively for people in nursing homes with chronic constipation.[16]

Basil *(Ocimum basilicum)* seed has been found to relieve constipation by acting as a bulk-forming laxative in one preliminary study.[17] A similar study showed the seeds to be useful following major surgery for elderly people with constipation.[18] Alginic acid, one of the major constituents in **bladderwrack** (page 639) *(Fucus vesiculosus),* is a type of dietary fiber that may be used to relieve constipation. However, human studies have not been conducted on the effectiveness of bladderwrack for this condition.

Stimulant laxatives are high in anthraquinone glycosides, which stimulate bowel muscle contraction. The most frequently used stimulant laxatives are **senna** (page 745) leaves, **cascara** (page 652) bark, and **aloe** (page 624) latex. While senna is the most popular, cascara has a somewhat milder action. Aloe is very potent and should be used with caution. Other stimulant laxatives include **buckthorn** (page 646), **alder buckthorn** (page 622) *(Rhamnus frangula),* and rhubarb *(Rheum officinale, R. palmatum).*

The unprocessed roots of **fo-ti** (page 678) possess a mild laxative effect. The bitter compounds in **dandelion** (page 666) leaves and root are also mild laxatives.

Are there any side effects or interactions?
Refer to the individual herb for information about any side effects or interactions.

Holistic approaches that may be helpful
Anecdotal reports have claimed that acupuncture is beneficial in the treatment of constipation.[19, 20, 21, 22] However, a small, controlled study of eight people with constipation concluded that six acupuncture treatments over two weeks did not improve bowel function during the course of the study.[23] Placebo-controlled trials of longer duration are needed to determine whether acupuncture is a useful treatment for constipation.

Biofeedback techniques have been shown to significantly increase the frequency of bowel movements among women with chronic constipation.[24]

COUGH

A cough is a symptom of many diseases. Most coughs come from simple viral infections, such as the **common cold** (page 129). Sometimes, but not always, mucus is produced with the cough. If the color is green or yellow, it may be a hint of a bacterial **infection** (page 265), although this is not always a reliable indicator. If the color is red, there may be bleeding in the lungs. Any cough that produces blood or blood-stained mucus, as well as any cough that lasts more than two weeks, requires a visit to a medical professional for diagnosis.

Medical treatments
Over the counter drug treatment involves the use of the antitussive dextromethorphan (DM), which is best reserved for use at bedtime to facilitate sleep. Coughing forces the expectoration of infectious organisms and congested secretions; consequently, a cough should not be suppressed during the day.

Prescription drugs used to suppress cough include codeine (Robitussin AC) and hydrocodone (Vicodin Tuss, Tussionex, Hycodan).

Cough

Cough

A chronic, persistent cough requires medical attention in order to determine the underlying cause.

CHECKLIST FOR COUGH		
Rating	Nutritional Supplements	Herbs
★☆☆		**Anise** (page 627)
		Bloodroot (page 641)
		Catnip (page 653)
		Coltsfoot (page 661)
		Comfrey (page 662)
		Elecampane (page 671)
		Eucalyptus (page 673)
		Horehound (page 691)
		Hyssop (page 695)
		Ivy leaf (page 697)
		Licorice (page 702)
		Lobelia (page 705)
		Mallow (page 707)
		Marshmallow (page 708)
		Mullein (page 713)
		Onion (page 718)
		Pennyroyal (page 723)
		Plantain (page 729)
		Red clover (page 735)
		Slippery elm (page 747)
		Sundew (page 749)
		Thyme (page 752)
		Usnea (page 754)
		Wild cherry (page 758)

Herbs that may be helpful

A number of herbs have a rich history of use for treating coughs due to colds, **bronchitis** (page 80), or other mild conditions. Only a few studies have examined the effectiveness of these herbs. However, their effectiveness is well-known by practitioners of herbal medicine the world over. Among those herbs that have been shown to have some degree of cough-relieving activity are **marshmallow** (page 708),[1] **sundew** (page 749),[2] and **coltsfoot** (page 661).[3] Use of coltsfoot should be limited to preparations of the leaves and flowers only, as the root is high in pyrrolizidine alkaloids, constituents that may be toxic to the liver.

Thyme (page 752) has a long history of use in Europe for the treatment of dry, spasmodic coughs as well as for **bronchitis** (page 80).[4] Many constituents in thyme team up to provide its antitussive (preventing

and treating a cough), antispasmodic, and expectorant actions. The primary constituents are the volatile oils, which include the phenols thymol and carvacol.[5] These are complemented by the actions of **flavonoids** (page 516) along with saponins. Thyme, either alone or in combination with herbs such as **sundew** (page 749), continues to be one of the most commonly recommended herbs in Europe for the treatment of dry, spasmodic coughs as well as for whooping cough.[6] Because of its apparent safety, it has become a favorite for treating coughs in small children.

The active constituents in **anise** (page 627) *(Pimpinella anisum),* particularly the terpenoid anethole, give this plant a delightful flavor. As an antispasmodic, it helps in gently relieving spasmodic coughs.[7]

The mucilage of **slippery elm** (page 747) gives it a soothing effect for coughs. **Usnea** (page 754) also contains mucilage, which may be helpful in easing irritating coughs. There is a long tradition of using **wild cherry** (page 758) syrups to treat coughs. Other traditional remedies to relieve coughs include **bloodroot** (page 641), **catnip** (page 653), **comfrey** (page 662) (the above-ground parts, not the root), **horehound** (page 691), **elecampane** (page 671), **mullein** (page 713), **lobelia** (page 705), **hyssop** (page 695), **licorice** (page 702), **mallow** (page 707) *(Malvia sylvestris),* **red clover** (page 753), **ivy leaf** (page 697), **pennyroyal** (page 723) *(Hedeoma pulegioides, Mentha pulegium),* **onion** (page 718) *(Allium cepa),* and **plantain** (page 729) *(Plantago lanceolata, P. major).* None of these has been investigated in human trials, so their true efficacy for relieving coughs is unknown.

The early 19th-century Eclectic physicians in the United States (who used herbs as their main medicine) not only employed **eucalyptus** (page 673) oil to sterilize instruments and **wounds** (page 319) but also recommended a steam inhalation of the oil's vapor to help treat **asthma** (page 32), **bronchitis** (page 80), whooping cough, and emphysema.[8]

Are there any side effects or interactions?
Refer to the individual herb for information about any side effects or interactions.

Holistic approaches that may be helpful
Traditional Chinese Medicine (TCM) may be helpful in the treatment of a cough. Cupping (the use of a glass cup to create suction over a skin surface) is a traditional Chinese therapy, often used for patients to help relieve a cough. An uncontrolled study using cupping to relieve

coughs reported a curative response in 35 of 41 patients.[9] Other TCM therapies, including acupuncture and herbal medicine, may be helpful in cough-producing ailments such as **asthma** (page 32) and **bronchitis** (page 80).

CROHN'S DISEASE

Crohn's disease is a poorly understood inflammatory condition that usually affects the final part of the small intestine and the beginning section of the colon. It often causes bloody stools and **malabsorption** (page 304) problems.

CHECKLIST FOR CROHN'S DISEASE		
Rating	Nutritional Supplements	Herbs
★★★	**Fish oil** (page 514) (enteric-coated, free-fatty-acid form) **Vitamin D** (page 607)	
★★☆	**DHEA** (page 503) **Multivitamin-mineral** (page 559) (for prevention or treatment of deficiency only) *Saccharomyces boulardii* (page 575) **Vitamin K** (page 612) **Zinc** (page 614)	
★☆☆	**Enzymes** (page 506) **Folic acid** (page 520) **Lipase** (page 547) **Vitamin A** (page 595) **Vitamin B₁₂** (page 601)	Agrimony **Aloe** (page 624) **Chamomile** (page 656) **Cranesbill** (page 665) **Green tea** (page 686) **Licorice** (page 702) **Marshmallow** (page 708) **Oak** (page 716) **Slippery elm** (page 747) **Witch hazel** (page 760) **Yarrow** (page 763)

What are the symptoms of Crohn's disease?
Chronic **diarrhea** (page 163) with abdominal pain, fever, loss of appetite, weight loss, and a sense of full-

ness in the abdomen are the most common symptoms. About one-third of people with Crohn's have a history of anal fissures (linear ulcers on the margin of the anus) or fistulas (abnormal tube-like passages from the rectum to the surface of the anus).

Medical treatments
The over the counter antidiarrheal drug loperamide (Imodium A-D) may be used in Crohn's patients with **diarrhea** (page 163). Anal irritation and loose stools may sometimes be improved by giving bulk-forming laxative such as methylcellulose (Citrucel) or psyllium (Fiberall, Konsyl, Metamucil, Perdiem).

Diphenoxylate (Lomotil) is the prescription drug most often used to control diarrhea. Cramps may be treated with anticholinergic drugs, such as L-hyoscyamine (Levsin, Levbid) and belladonna (Belladonna Tincture). Sulfasalazine (Azulfidine) is used in patients with mild to moderate colitis. Oral corticosteroids, such as prednisone (Deltasone), may be used during acute flare-ups. However, long-term corticosteroid therapy does more harm than good. Certain immunosuppressive drugs may also be effective, including azathioprine (Imuran) and 6-mercaptopurine (Purinethol). Secondary bacterial **infections** (page 265) are managed with antibiotics such as tetracycline (Sumycin) and doxycycline (Vibramycin).

Dietary changes that may be helpful
A person with Crohn's disease might consume more sugar than the average healthy person.[1] A high-fiber, low-sugar diet led to a 79% reduction in hospitalizations compared with no dietary change in one group of people with Crohn's disease.[2] Another trial compared the effects of high- and low-sugar diets in people with Crohn's disease.[3] People with a more active disease were reported to fare better on the low-sugar diet than those eating more sugar. Several people on the high-sugar diet had to stop eating sugar because their disease grew worse. While details of how sugar injures the intestine are still being uncovered, doctors often suggest eliminating all sugar (including soft drinks and processed foods with added sugar) from the diets of those with Crohn's disease.

A diet high in animal protein and fat (from foods other than fish) has been linked to Crohn's disease in preliminary research.[4] As with many other health conditions, it may be beneficial to eat less meat and dairy fat and more fruits and vegetables.

Some people with Crohn's disease have **food aller-**

Crohn's Disease

gies (page 14) and have been reported to do better when they avoid foods to which they are allergic. One study found that people with Crohn's disease are most likely to react to cereals, dairy, and yeast.[5] Increasingly, baker's yeast (found in bread and other bakery goods) has been implicated as a possible trigger for Crohn's disease.[6] Yeast and some cheeses are high in histamine, which is involved in an allergenic response. People with Crohn's disease lack the ability to break down histamine at a normal rate,[7] so the link between yeast and dairy consumption and Crohn's disease occurrence may not be coincidental. However, the allergy theory cannot account for all, or even most, cases of Crohn's disease.

Elemental diets contain **amino acids** (page 465) (rather than whole proteins, which can stimulate allergic reactions) and are therefore considered hypoallergenic. They have been used extensively as primary therapy in people with Crohn's disease,[8, 9, 10] with remission rates comparable to those of steroid drugs. Nevertheless, diets containing intact proteins derived from dairy and wheat have proven equally effective at controlling the symptoms of Crohn's disease.[11, 12, 13] Until more is known, it is premature to conclude that food allergy plays a significant role in the development of Crohn's disease or that a hypoallergenic diet is any more likely to help than a diet whose protein is only partially broken down.

In one trial, people with Crohn's disease were asked which foods aggravated their symptoms.[14] Those without ileostomies found nuts, raw fruit, and tomatoes to be most problematic, though responses varied from person to person, and other reports have displayed different lists.[15] (Ileostomies are surgical passages through the wall of the abdomen into the intestine that allow the intestinal contents to bypass the rectum and drain into a bag worn on the abdomen.) People with Crohn's disease wishing to identify and avoid potential allergens should consult a doctor.

There is preliminary evidence that people who eat fast foods at least two times per week more than triple their risk of developing Crohn's disease.[16]

Lifestyle changes that may be helpful
People with Crohn's disease are more likely to smoke, and there is evidence that continuing to smoke increases the rate of disease relapse.[17]

Nutritional supplements that may be helpful
Vitamin D (page 607) malabsorption is common in Crohn's[18] and can lead to a deficiency of the vitamin.[19] Successful treatment with vitamin D for **osteomalacia**

(page 392) (bone brittleness caused by vitamin D deficiency) triggered by Crohn's disease has been reported.[20] Another study found 1,000 IU per day of vitamin D prevented bone loss in people with Crohn's, while an unsupplemented group experienced significant bone loss.[21] A doctor should evaluate vitamin D status and suggest the right level of vitamin D supplements.

Inflammation within the gut occurs in people suffering from Crohn's disease. EPA and **DHA** (page 509), the omega-3 fatty acids found in **fish oil** (page 514), have anti-inflammatory activity. A two-year trial compared the effects of having people with Crohn's disease eat 3.5 to 7 ounces of fish high in EPA and DHA per day or having them eat a diet low in fish.[22] In that trial, the fish-eating group had a 20% relapse rate compared with 58% among those not eating fish. Salmon, herring, mackerel, albacore tuna, and sardines are all high in EPA and DHA.

In a double-blind trial, people with Crohn's disease who took supplements providing 2.7 g of EPA/DHA per day had a recurrence rate of 26% after one year, compared to a 59% recurrence rate among those taking placebo. [23] Participants in this study used a special enteric-coated, "free-fatty-acid" form of EPA/DHA taken from fish oil. Other blinded trials using other fish oil supplements that were neither enteric-coated nor in the free-fatty-acid form have reported no clinical improvement.[24, 25] These disparate outcomes suggest that the enteric-coated, free-fatty-acid form may have important advantages, including the reported elimination of gastrointestinal symptoms that often result from taking regular fish oil supplements.[26] Unfortunately, enteric-coated "free-fatty-acid" fish oil is not commercially available at this time.

In a preliminary trial, six of seven people with Crohn's disease went into remission after taking 200 mg per day of **DHEA** (page 503) for eight weeks.[27] This large amount of DHEA has the potential to cause adverse side effects and should only be used under the supervision of a doctor.

In double-blind research, **diarrhea** (page 163) caused by Crohn's disease has partially responded to supplementation with the beneficial bacterium *Saccharomyces boulardii* (page 000).[28] Although the amount used in this trial, 250 mg taken three times per day, was helpful, as much as 500 mg taken four times per day has been administered in research successfully using *Saccharomyces boulardii* as a supplement with people suffering from other forms of diarrhea.[29]

In people with Crohn's disease, **vitamin K** (page 612) deficiency can result from malabsorption due to intestinal inflammation or bowel surgery, from chronic diarrhea, or from dietary changes necessitated by food intolerance. In addition, Crohn's disease is often treated with antibiotics that have the potential to kill beneficial vitamin K–producing bacteria in the intestines. Vitamin K levels were significantly lower in a group of people with Crohn's disease than in healthy people. Moreover, the rate of bone loss in the Crohn's disease patients increased with increasing degrees of vitamin K deficiency.[30] When combined with earlier evidence that vitamin K is required to maintain healthy bones, this study suggests that vitamin K deficiency is a contributing factor to the accelerated bone loss that often occurs in people with Crohn's disease.

Crohn's disease often leads to **malabsorption** (page 304). As a result, deficiencies of many nutrients are common. For this reason, it makes sense for people with Crohn's disease to take a high potency **multivitamin-mineral** (page 559) supplement. In particular, deficiencies in **zinc** (page 614), **folic acid** (page 520), **vitamin B$_{12}$** (page 601), **vitamin D** (page 607), and **iron** (page 540) have been reported.[31, 32, 33] Zinc, folic acid, and vitamin B$_{12}$ are all needed to repair intestinal cells damaged by Crohn's disease. Some doctors recommend 25 to 50 mg of zinc (balanced with 2 to 4 mg of copper), 800 mcg of folic acid, and 800 mcg of vitamin B$_{12}$. Iron status should be evaluated by a doctor before considering supplementation.

Vitamin A (page 595) is needed for the growth and repair of cells that line both the small and large intestine.[34] At least two case reports describe people with Crohn's disease who have responded to vitamin A supplementation.[35, 36] However, in one trial, vitamin A supplementation failed to maintain remission of the disease.[37] Therefore, although some doctors recommend 50,000 IU per day for adults with Crohn's disease, this approach remains unproven. An amount this high should never be taken without qualified guidance, nor should it be given to a woman who is or could become **pregnant** (page 363).

People with Crohn's disease may be deficient in **pancreatic enzymes** (page 506), including **lipase** (page 547).[38] In theory, supplementing with enzymes might improve the nutrient malabsorption that is often associated with Crohn's disease. However, people with Crohn's disease considering supplementation with enzymes should consult a doctor.

Are there any side effects or interactions?
Refer to the individual supplement for information about any side effects or interactions.

Herbs that may be helpful

Doctors sometimes use a combination of herbs to soothe inflammation throughout the digestive tract. One formula contains **marshmallow** (page 708), **slippery elm** (page 747), **cranesbill** (page 665), and several other herbs.[39] Marshmallow and slippery elm are mucilaginous plants that help soothe inflamed tissues. Cranesbill is an astringent. Clinical trials using this combination have not been conducted.

A variety of anti-inflammatory herbs historically have been recommended by doctors for people with Crohn's disease. These include **yarrow** (page 763), **chamomile** (page 656), **licorice** (page 702), and **aloe** (page 624) juice. Cathartic preparations of aloe should be avoided. No research has been conducted to validate the use of these herbs for Crohn's disease.

Tannin-containing herbs may be helpful to decrease **diarrhea** (page 163) during acute flare-ups and have been used for this purpose in traditional medicine. A preliminary trial using isolated tannins in the course of usual drug therapy for Crohn's disease found them to be more effective for reducing diarrhea than was no additional treatment.[40] Tannin-containing herbs of potential benefit include agrimony (*Agrimonia* spp.), **green tea** (page 686), **oak** (page 716), **witch hazel** (page 760), and **cranesbill** (page 665). Use of such herbs should be discontinued before the diarrhea is completely resolved; otherwise the disease may be aggravated.

Are there any side effects or interactions?
Refer to the individual herb for information about any side effects or interactions.

CYSTIC FIBROSIS

Cystic fibrosis (CF) is an inherited disease that results in impaired transport of chloride into and out of cells. The digestive and respiratory systems are most affected.

The most common manifestation of cystic fibrosis is frequent respiratory **infection** (page 265). Impaired digestion and **malabsorption** (page 304) due to **pancreatic insufficiency** (page 341) and blocked liver ducts is often seen as well. Management of this condition requires the help of a qualified doctor.

What are the symptoms of cystic fibrosis?

Symptoms include a persistent cough with thick and often greenish-colored mucus, failure to grow normally, recurrent **sinus** (page 407) and **bronchial infections** (page 80), and frequent, bulky, foul-smelling stools. Infants may experience a set of acute symptoms, including a distended abdomen, failure to pass stool, and vomiting. Although the course of the disease is highly variable, largely dependent upon the severity and frequency of respiratory infections, CF inevitably leads to debility and death. Average survival is to age 31.

CHECKLIST FOR CYSTIC FIBROSIS		
Rating	**Nutritional Supplements**	**Herbs**
★★★	Pancreatic enzymes (page 506) Vitamin A (page 595) Vitamin D (page 607)	
★★☆	Fish oil (page 514) (EPA) Taurine (page 590) Vitamin B₁₂ (page 601) Vitamin K (page 612)	
★☆☆	Vitamin E (page 609) Zinc (page 614)	

Medical treatments

Supplementation with over the counter fat-soluble **vitamin E** (page 609) and **vitamin K** (page 612) is recommended.

Prescription strength **pancreatic enzymes** (page 506) (Pancrease MT, Lipram, Viokase) to aid digestion are required. Healthcare practitioners might also prescribe antibiotics to prevent possible lung infections, enzymes (recombinant human DNAse) to thin the mucus in the airways, and oxygen therapy.

Treatment typically includes a daily regimen of physical therapy that consists of pounding on the chest to loosen mucus.

Dietary changes that may be helpful

People with CF are usually unable to digest food completely and therefore need to consume more calories than a healthy person of similar size and weight. Current guidelines recommend calorie intakes 20 to 50% above the recommended daily allowance.[1]

Children with CF lose a large amount of salt in their sweat and thus should be encouraged to salt their food liberally. In case of fever, an additional 2 to 4 grams (1/2 to 1 teaspoon) should be added to the daily diet.[2]

Lifestyle changes that may be helpful

Aerobic exercise appears to improve lung function in people with CF. In a three-year controlled trial, people with CF engaged in a home exercise program, during which they exercised for a minimum of 20 minutes, three times weekly, and attained a heart rate of approximately 150 beats per minute. A slower decline in lung function was observed in these people compared with non-exercisers.[3] Those who exercised also tended to feel better about themselves, had more energy, and/or experienced less chest congestion.

Nutritional supplements that may be helpful

People with CF tend to have **insufficient pancreas function** (page 341). Supplementation with **pancreatic enzymes** (page 506) will often lead to improved digestion, especially of fats. The current recommendation for people with cystic fibrosis is to supplement with pancreatic enzymes at meals. Amounts should not exceed 10,000 IU of **lipase** (page 547) per day per 2.2 pounds body weight[4] or 500 to 1,000 lipase units per gram of dietary fat consumed,[5] as larger amounts may damage the large intestine. A double-blind trial found enteric-coated microsphere enzyme preparations to be superior to enteric-coated capsules for reduction of abdominal pain and improvement of digestion.[6] Because pancreatin is rapidly emptied from the stomach during digestion, people taking these enzymes may obtain better results by spreading supplementation throughout the meal.[7]

Taurine (page 590) is an **amino acid** (page 465) and a component of bile acids, which are important for proper fat digestion. Some,[8, 9] but not all,[10] investigators have reported improvement in fat digestion among people with CF when they supplemented with 30 mg taurine per 2.2 pounds of body weight daily. Greater improvement was seen in people with the worst maldigestion.[11]

The impaired digestion of fats in people with CF often leads to a deficiency of essential fatty acids. This deficiency may in turn lead to lowered **immune function** (page 255), which makes people with CF more susceptible to respiratory infection.[12] This deficiency may be reversed by supplementation with corn oil (1 gram per 2.2 pounds body weight per day),[13] safflower oil (1 gram per 2.2 pounds body weight per day),[14] linoleic acid (7.7 grams per day),[15] and eicosapentaenoic acid (EPA from **fish oil** [page 514]) (2.7 grams per day).[16] EPA supplementation was particularly effective. In a double-blind trial, six weeks of supplementation with 2.7 grams of EPA per day led to a reduction in sputum and improvement in lung function in children with chronic respiratory infection due to CF.[17]

The fat malabsorption associated with CF often leads to a deficiency of fat-soluble vitamins. Oral supplementation of these nutrients is considered crucial to maintaining good nutritional status.[18] Current recommendations for supplementation are as follows: **vitamin A** (page 595), 5,000 to 10,000 IU/day; **vitamin D** (page 607), 1,000 to 2,000 IU/day; **vitamin E** (page 609), 100 to 300 IU/day; and **vitamin K** (page 612), 5 mg every three days. Of the water-soluble vitamins, only **vitamin B$_{12}$** (page 601) is poorly absorbed in cystic fibrosis,[19] and taking pancreatic enzymes helps prevent B$_{12}$ deficiencies.[20]

The malabsorption produced by CF may adversely affect mineral absorption as well. Blood concentrations of **zinc** (page 614) were low in a group of children with CF.[21] One child with CF was reported to have a severe generalized dermatitis that resolved upon correction of zinc and fatty acid deficiencies by using a formula containing zinc (about 3 mg per day) and **medium chain triglycerides** (page 554) (amount not reported).[22]

Children with slowed growth associated with CF were found, in a preliminary study, to have overgrowth of bacteria in the small intestine compared to healthy children.[23] There is as yet no evidence that elimination of this overgrowth will lead to improvement of CF symptoms.

Are there any side effects or interactions?
Refer to the individual supplement for information about any side effects or interactions.

DEPRESSION

What do I need to know?
Self-care for depression can be approached in a number of ways—but it can be hard to know just where to start. To make it easier, our doctors recommend trying these simple steps first:

Check out St. John's wort
Take 600 to 1,200 mg a day of a standardized extract (containing of 0.3% hypericin) to help with mild to moderate depression

Seek counseling
A mental health professional may help you make a full recovery

Move your body
Get exercise that increases your heart rate at least three hours a week (or 30 minutes a day) to boost your body's natural mood-enhancing compounds (endorphins)

Try B-vitamins
Take a B-vitamin supplement that contains folic acid and vitamins B$_{12}$ and B$_6$ to help correct deficiencies associated with depression

Get enough iron
A lack of iron can make depression worse; check with a doctor to find out if you are iron deficient

About depression
Depression is a condition characterized by unhappy, hopeless feelings. It can be a response to stressful events, hormonal imbalances, biochemical abnormalities, or other causes.

Mild depression that passes quickly may not require any diagnosis or treatment. However, when depression becomes recurrent, constant, or severe, it should be diagnosed by a licensed counselor, psychologist, social worker, or doctor. Diagnosis may be crucial for determining appropriate treatment. For example, depression caused by **low thyroid** (page 252) function can be successfully treated with prescription thyroid medication. Suicidal depression often requires prescription antidepressants. Persistent mild to moderate depression triggered by stressful events is often best treated with counseling and not necessarily with medications.

When depression is not a function of external events, it is called endogenous. Endogenous depression can be due to biochemical abnormalities. Lifestyle changes, nutritional supplements, and herbs may be used with people whose depression results from a variety of causes, but these natural interventions are usually best geared to endogenous depression.

What are the symptoms of depression?
A diagnosis of depression requires at least five of the following symptoms.
- Depressed mood.
- Diminished interest or pleasure in all or most activities, most of the day, nearly every day.
- Significant weight loss or gain when not dieting (e.g., more than 5% of body weight in a month).
- **Insomnia** (page 270) or excessive sleeping nearly every day.
- Agitation or depression in voluntary muscle movements nearly every day.
- Fatigue or loss of energy nearly every day.
- Feelings of worthlessness or excessive and inappropriate guilt nearly every day.
- Diminished ability to think or concentrate, or indecisiveness nearly every day.

Depression

- Recurrent thoughts of death (not just fear of death), recurrent suicidal ideation without a plan, or a suicide attempt or specific plan to commit suicide.

CHECKLIST FOR DEPRESSION

Rating	Nutritional Supplements	Herbs
★★★	Eicosapentaenoic acid (ethyl ester [E-EPA]) **Folic acid** (page 520) (for folate deficiency) **Iron** (page 540) (for iron deficiency) **Vitamin B$_{12}$** (page 601) (for B$_{12}$ deficiency) **Vitamin B$_6$** (page 600) (with oral contraceptives)	
★★☆	**5-HTP** (page 459) **Acetyl-L-carnitine** (page 461) (for elderly people) **DHEA** (page 503) (this supplement requires supervision by a healthcare professional) **Fish oil** (page 514) (EPA/DHA) **Inositol** (page 537) **L-phenylalanine/DLPA** (page 568) **L-tyrosine** (page 544) **Melatonin** (page 555) **SAMe** (page 583) **Selenium** (page 584) **Vitamin B$_6$** (page 600) (for **premenstrual syndrome** [page 368]) **Vitamin D** (page 607)	*Ginkgo biloba* (page 681) (for elderly people) **St. John's wort** (page 747)
★☆☆	**Calcium** (page 483) **Chromium** (page 493) **NADH** (page 564) **Phosphatidylserine** (page 569) (bovine brain PS only; soy-derived PS does not appear to be effective)	**Damiana** (page 666) **Pumpkin** (page 733) **Vervain** (page 756) **Yohimbe** (page 764)

Medical treatments

The most commonly prescribed antidepressants are the selective serotonin reuptake inhibitors (SSRIs), such as fluoxetine (Prozac), paroxetine (Paxil), sertraline (Zoloft), and citalopram (Celexa). The tricyclic antide-

pressants, such as amitriptyline (Elavil), imipramine (Tofranil), and doxepin (Sinequan), are still used on a regular basis, as are other agents, including trazodone (Desyrel), bupropion (Wellbutrin), and venlafaxine (Effexor). MAO inhibitors, such as phenelzine (Nardil) and tranylcypromine (Parnate), are rarely prescribed.

Psychological counseling is an essential component of therapy.

Dietary changes that may be helpful

Although some research has produced mixed results,[1] double-blind trials have shown that **food allergies** (page 14) can trigger mental symptoms, including depression.[2, 3] People with depression who do not respond to other natural or conventional approaches should consult a doctor to diagnose possible food sensitivities and avoid offending foods.

Restricting sugar and caffeine in people with depression has been reported to elevate mood in preliminary research.[4] How much of this effect resulted from sugar and how much from caffeine remains unknown. Researchers have reported that psychiatric patients who are heavy coffee drinkers are more likely to be depressed than other such patients.[5] However, it remains unclear whether caffeine can cause depression or whether depressed people were more likely to want the "lift" associated with drinking a cup of coffee. In fact, "improvement in mood" is considered an effect of long-term coffee consumption by some researchers, a concept supported by the fact that people who drink coffee have been reported to have a 58–66% decreased risk of committing suicide compared with non-coffee drinkers.[6] Nonetheless, a symptom of caffeine addiction can be depression.[7] Thus, consumption of caffeine (mostly from coffee) has paradoxically been linked with both improvement in mood and depression by different researchers. People with depression may want to avoid caffeine as well as sugar for one week to see how it affects their mood.

There is evidence that people with major depression may have insensitivity to insulin and impaired glucose tolerance.[8] Whether treatment of impaired glucose tolerance helps depression is unknown, but a doctor can order laboratory tests to detect such abnormalities, and initiate treatment as appropriate.

The amount and type of dietary fat consumed may influence the incidence of depression. Previous studies have found that diet regimens designed to lower **cholesterol** (page 223) levels may reduce death from **cardiovascular disease** (page 98), but may also heighten the incidence of depression.[9] Does low cholesterol cause depression? It appears not, since studies have shown no adverse effect on mood in people taking cholesterol-lowering drugs.[10, 11] The connection more likely has to do with the *balance* of fats in the diet. Diets to lower blood cholesterol usually focus on restricting total fat intake while increasing the intake of polyunsaturated fats (e.g., corn and soybean oils). These oils are very high in omega-6 fatty acids, but the recommended diets otherwise lack important omega-3 fatty acids (**EPA and DHA** [page 514]). A high intake of omega-6 fatty acids relative to omega-3 fatty acids and an inadequate intake of omega-3 fatty acids (e.g., from fish and **fish oils** [page 514]) have been associated with increased levels of depression.[12] People who eat diets high in omega-3 fatty acids from fish have a lower incidence of depression and suicide.[13, 14, 15, 16]

Lifestyle changes that may be helpful

Exercise increases the body's production of endorphins—chemical substances that can relieve depression. Scientific research shows that routine exercise can positively affect mood and help with depression.[17] As little as three hours per week of aerobic exercise can profoundly reduce the level of depression.[18] One trial compared the effects of an exercise training program with those of a prescription antidepressant drug in people over 50 years of age.[19] The researchers found the two approaches to be equally effective after 16 weeks of treatment.

Nutritional supplements that may be helpful

Iron deficiency (page 278) is known to affect mood and can exacerbate depression, but it can only be diagnosed and treated by a doctor. While iron deficiency is easy to fix with **iron** (page 540) supplements, people who have not been diagnosed with iron deficiency should not supplement iron.

Deficiency of **vitamin B$_{12}$** (page 601) can create disturbances in mood that respond to B$_{12}$ supplementation.[20] Significant vitamin B$_{12}$ deficiency is associated with a doubled risk of severe depression, according to a study of physically disabled older women.[21] Depression caused by vitamin B$_{12}$ deficiency can occur even if there is no B$_{12}$ deficiency-related anemia.[22]

Mood has been reported to sometimes improve with high amounts of vitamin B$_{12}$ (given by injection), even in the absence of a B$_{12}$ deficiency.[23] Supplying the body with high amounts of vitamin B$_{12}$ can only be done by injection. However, in the case of overcoming a diagnosed B$_{12}$ deficiency, one can follow an initial injection with oral maintenance supplementation (1 mg per day), even when the cause of the deficiency is a malabsorption problem such as **pernicious anemia** (page 601).

A deficiency of the B vitamin **folic acid** (page 520) can also disturb mood. A large percentage of depressed people have low folic acid levels.[24] Folic acid supplements appear to improve the effects of lithium in treating manic-depressives.[25] Depressed alcoholics report feeling better with large amounts of a modified form of folic acid.[26] Anyone suffering from chronic depression should be evaluated for possible folic acid deficiency by a doctor. Those with abnormally low levels of folic acid are sometimes given short-term, high amounts of folic acid (10 mg per day).

Preliminary evidence indicates that people with depression may have lower levels of **inositol** (page 537).[27] Supplementation with large amounts of inositol can increase the body's stores by as much as 70%.[28] In a double-blind trial, depressed people who received 12 grams of inositol per day for four weeks had a significant improvement in symptoms compared to those who took placebo.[29] In a double-blind follow-up to this trial, the antidepressant effects of inositol were replicated. Half of those who responded to inositol supplementation relapsed rapidly when inositol was discontinued.[30]

Oral contraceptives can deplete the body of **vitamin B$_6$** (page 600), a nutrient needed for maintenance of normal mental functioning. Double-blind research shows that women who are depressed and who have become depleted of vitamin B$_6$ while taking oral contraceptives typically respond to vitamin B$_6$ supplementation.[31] In one trial, 20 mg of vitamin B$_6$ were taken twice per day. Some evidence suggests that people who are depressed—even when not taking the oral contraceptive—are still more likely to be B$_6$ deficient than people who are not depressed.[32]

Several clinical trials also indicate that vitamin B$_6$ supplementation helps alleviate depression associated with **premenstrual syndrome** (page 368) (PMS),[33] although the research remains inconsistent.[34] Many doctors suggest that women who have depression associated with PMS take 100–300 mg of vitamin B$_6$ per day—a level of intake that requires supervision by a doctor.

Less than optimal intake of **selenium** (page 584) may have adverse effects on psychological function, even in the absence of signs of frank selenium deficiency. In a preliminary trial of healthy young men, consumption of a high-selenium diet (226.5 mcg selenium per day) was associated with improved mood (i.e., decreased confusion, depression, **anxiety** (page 30), and uncertainty), compared to consumption of a low-selenium diet (62.6 mcg selenium per day.)[35] In a double-blind trial, people who had a low selenium intake experienced greater improvement in depression symptoms after selenium supplementation (100 mcg per day) than did people with adequate selenium intake, suggesting that low-level selenium deficiency may contribute to depression.[36]

Vitamin D (page 607) supplementation may be associated with elevations in mood. In a double-blind trial, healthy people were given 400–800 IU per day of vitamin D3, or no vitamin D3, for five days during late winter. Results showed that vitamin D3 significantly enhanced positive mood and there was some evidence of a reduction in negative mood compared to a placebo.[37] In another double-blind trial, people without depression took 600 IU of vitamin D along with 1,000 mg of **calcium** (page 483), or a placebo, twice daily for four weeks.[38] Compared to the placebo, combined vitamin D and calcium supplementation produced significant elevations in mood that persisted at least one week after supplementation was discontinued.

Omega-3 fatty acids found in **fish oil** (page 514), particularly **DHA** (page 509), are needed for normal nervous system function. Depressed people have been reported to have lower omega-3 fatty acid levels (e.g., DHA) than people who are not depressed.[39, 40, 41, 42] Low levels of the other omega-3 fatty acid from fish, EPA, have correlated with increased severity of depression.[43] In a double-blind trial, people with manic depression were given a very high intake of supplemental omega-3 fatty acids (enough fish oil to contain 9.6 grams of omega-3 fatty acids per day) for four months.[44] Ten of 16 people in the placebo group eventually were forced to discontinue the trial due to worsening depression compared with only 3 of 14 taking omega-3 fatty acids. Some scores of depression levels fell as much as 48% in the omega-3 fatty acids group.

EPA alone has also been reported to be beneficial. There is one case report of a man with a long history of severe depression who showed clear improvement within one month of starting a purified EPA supplement (4 grams per day of the ethyl ester of eicosapentaenoic acid [E-EPA]).[45] In a double-blind study, supplementation with E-EPA for 12 weeks was significantly more effective than a placebo at relieving symptoms of depression.[46] E-EPA was beneficial, even though the participants in the study had failed to respond adequately to conventional antidepressant drugs. The conventional medications were continued during treatment with E-EPA or placebo. An effective level of intake was 1 gram per day, whereas larger amounts of E-EPA resulted in little or no benefit. The authors of the study suggested that taking too much E-EPA might cause an imbalance with other essential fatty acids, which could reduce the effectiveness of the treatment.

The amino acid **L-tyrosine** (page 544) can be converted into norepinephrine, a neurotransmitter that affects mood. Women taking oral contraceptives have lower levels of tyrosine, and some researchers think this might be related to depression caused by birth control pills.[47] L-tyrosine metabolism may also be abnormal in other depressed people[48] and preliminary research suggests supplementation might help.[49, 50] Several doctors recommend a 12-week trial of L-tyrosine supplementation for people who are depressed. Published research has used a very high amount—100 mg per 2.2 pounds of body weight (or about 7 grams per day for an average adult). It is not known whether such high amounts are necessary to produce an antidepressant effect.

L-phenylalanine (page 568) is another amino acid that converts to mood-affecting substances (including phenylethylamine and norepinephrine). Preliminary research reported that L-phenylalanine improved mood in most of the depressed people studied.[51] **DLPA** (page 568) is a mixture of the essential amino acid L-phenylalanine and its synthetic mirror image, D-phenylalanine. DLPA (or the D- or L- form alone) reduced depression in 31 of 40 people in a preliminary trial.[52] Some doctors suggest a one-month trial with 3–4 grams per day of phenylalanine for people with depression, although some researchers have found that even very low amounts—75 to 200 mg per day—were helpful in preliminary trials.[53] In one double-blind trial, depressed people given 150–200 mg of DLPA per day experienced results comparable to that produced by an antidepressant drug.[54]

Acetyl-L-carnitine (page 461) may be effective for depression experienced by the elderly. A preliminary trial found that acetyl-L-carnitine supplementation was effective at relieving depression in a group of elderly people, particularly those showing more serious clinical symptoms.[55] These results were confirmed in another similar clinical trial.[56] In that trial, participants received either 500 mg three times a day of acetyl-L-carnitine or a matching placebo. Those receiving acetyl-L-carnitine experienced significantly reduced symptoms of depression compared to those receiving placebo. At least two other clinical studies of acetyl-L-carnitine for depression in the elderly have reported similar results.[57, 58] The amount typically used is 500 mg three times daily, although one trial used twice that amount.

Some studies have reported lower **DHEA** (page 503) levels in groups of depressed patients.[59] However, this finding has not been consistent, and in one trial, severely depressed people were reported to show *increases* in blood levels of DHEA.[60]

Despite confusion regarding which depressed people might be DHEA-deficient, most double-blind trials lasting at least six weeks have reported some success in treating people with depression. After six months using 50 mg DHEA per day, "a remarkable increase in perceived physical and psychological well-being" was reported in both men and women in one double-blind trial.[61] After only six weeks, taking DHEA in levels up to 90 mg per day led to at least a 50% reduction in depression in five of 11 patients in another double-blind trial.[62]

Other researchers have reported dramatic reductions in depression at extremely high amounts of DHEA (90–450 mg per day) given for six weeks to adults who first became depressed after age 40 (in men) or at the time of **menopause** (page 311) (in women) in a double-blind trial.[63] Other double-blind research has shown that limiting supplementation to only two weeks is inadequate in treating people with depression.[64] Despite the somewhat dramatic results reported in clinical trials lasting at least six weeks, some experts claim that in clinical practice, DHEA appears to be effective for only a minority of depressed people.[65] Moreover, due to fears of potential side effects, most healthcare professionals remain concerned about the use of DHEA. Depressed people considering taking DHEA should consult a doctor well versed in the use of DHEA.

Melatonin (page 555) might help some people suffering from depression. Preliminary double-blind research suggests that supplementation with small amounts of melatonin (0.125 mg taken twice per day) may reduce **winter depression** (page 397).[66] People with major depressive disorders sometimes have sleep disturbances. A timed-release preparation of melatonin (5–10 mg per day for four weeks) was shown to be effective at improving the quality of sleep in people with major depression who were taking fluoxetine (Prozac), but melatonin did not enhance its antidepressant effect.[67] There is a possibility that melatonin could exac-

erbate depression, so it should only be used for this purpose under a doctor's supervision.

S-adenosyl methionine (**SAMe** [page 585]) is a substance synthesized in the body that has recently been made available as a supplement. SAMe appears to raise levels of dopamine, an important neurotransmitter in mood regulation. Higher SAMe levels in the brain are associated with successful drug treatment of depression, and oral SAMe has been demonstrated to be an effective treatment for depression in most,[68, 69, 70] but not all,[71] clinical trials. Most trials used 1,600 mg of SAMe per day. While it does not seem to be as powerful as full applications of antidepressant medications[72] or **St. John's wort** (page 747), SAMe's effects are felt more rapidly, often within one week.[73]

Disruptions in emotional well-being, including depression, have been linked to serotonin imbalances in the brain.[74] Supplementation with **5-hydroxytryptophan** (page 459) (5-HTP) may increase serotonin synthesis. Researchers are studying the possibility that 5-HTP might help people with depression. Some trials using 5-HTP with people suffering from depression have shown sign of efficacy.[75, 76, 77, 78, 79] However, much of the research was either uncontrolled or used 5-HTP in combination with antidepressant drugs. Depressed people interested in considering this hormone precursor should consult a doctor.

There have been five case reports of **chromium** (page 493) supplementation (200–400 mcg per day) significantly improving mood in people with a type of depression called dysthymic disorder who were also taking the antidepressant drug sertraline (Zoloft).[80] These case reports, while clearly limited and preliminary in scope, warrant further research to better understand the benefits, if any, of chromium supplementation in people with depression.

Phosphatidylserine (page 569) (PS), a natural substance derived from the amino acid serine, affects the levels of neurotransmitters in the brain related to mood. In a preliminary trial, elderly women suffering from depression who were given 300 mg of PS per day for 30 days experienced, on average, a 70% reduction in the severity of their depression.[81] Most research has been conducted with PS derived from bovine (cow) brain tissue. Due to concerns about the possibility of humans contracting infectious diseases (such as Creutzfeld-Jakob or "mad cow" disease), bovine PS is not available in the United States. The soy- and bovine-derived PS, are not structurally identical, and there is evidence that soy-derived PS may not have the same beneficial effects as bovine PS.[82]

An isolated preliminary trial suggests the supplement **NADH** (page 564) may help people with depression.[83] Controlled trials are needed, however, before any conclusions can be drawn.

A deficiency of other B vitamins not discussed above (including **vitamin B$_1$** [page 591], **vitamin B$_2$** [page 598], **vitamin B$_3$** [page 598], **pantothenic acid** [page 568] and **biotin** [page 473]) can also lead to depression. However, the level of deficiency of these nutrients needed to induce depression is rarely found in Western societies.

Are there any side effects or interactions?
Refer to the individual supplement for information about any side effects or interactions.

Herbs that may be helpful
St. John's wort (page 747) extracts are among the leading medicines used in Germany by medical doctors for the treatment of mild to moderate depression. Using St. John's wort extract can significantly relieve the symptoms of depression. People taking St. John's wort show an improvement in mood and ability to carry out their daily routine. Symptoms such as sadness, hopelessness, worthlessness, exhaustion, and poor sleep also decrease.[84, 85]

St. John's wort extract has been compared to the prescription tricyclic antidepressants imipramine (Tofranil),[86, 87, 88] amitriptyline (Elavil),[89] fluoxetine (Prozac),[90] and maprotiline (Ludiomil).[91] The improvement in symptoms of mild to moderate depression was similar, with notably fewer side effects, in people taking St. John's wort.

In a double-blind trial using standard amounts of fluoxetine (Prozac)—20 mg per day—St. John's wort extract in the amount of 400 mg twice daily was equally effective at relieving depression in people aged 60–80 years.[92] Another trial found that 250 mg of St. John's wort extract two times per day was also as effective as 20 mg of fluoxetine in treating adults with mild to moderate depression.[93] In both trials comparing St. John's wort to fluoxetine, there were far fewer side effects reported by people taking St. John's wort.

One clinical trial compared a higher amount of the St. John's wort extract LI 160 (1,800 mg per day) with a higher amount of imipramine (150 mg per day) in more severely depressed people.[94] Again, the improvement was virtually the same for both groups with far fewer side effects for the St. John's wort group. While this may point to St. John's wort as a possible treatment for more severe cases of depression, this treatment should only be pursued under the guidance of a healthcare professional.

Two well-publicized double-blind studies published in the *Journal of the American Medical Association* (*JAMA*) concluded that St. John's wort is not an effective treatment for depression. However, each of these studies had potential flaws. In the first study,[95] 900–1,200 mg of St. John's wort per day was slightly more effective than a placebo, as assessed by the Hamilton Rating Scale for Depression. However, the difference was not statistically significant. Although the remission rate was significantly greater with St. John's wort than with placebo, only 14.3% of the patients who received the herb went into remission, causing the authors of the report to question St. John's wort's efficacy. However, the 4.9% remission rate in the placebo group was far below the placebo response rate seen in other studies of depression. That finding suggests that many of the patients recruited for this study would have been unlikely to respond to any treatment.

In the second *JAMA* study, depressed patients were given one of three treatments: St. John's wort, placebo, or an antidepressant medication with proven efficacy (e.g., sertraline; Zoloft). Although St. John's wort was no more effective than the placebo, by many measures neither was sertraline.[96] The relatively poor outcome with sertraline makes one wonder whether the design of the study, or the criteria used to select participants, may have somehow skewed the results to make St. John's wort appear less effective than it really is.

Despite these two negative studies, the bulk of the scientific evidence indicates that St. John's wort is an effective treatment for mild to moderate depression.

Recent European trials have successfully treated mild to moderate depression using 500 to 1,050 mg of St. John's wort per day. As an antidepressant, St. John's wort should be taken for four to six weeks before judging its effectiveness.

Ginkgo biloba (page 681) (240 mg per day) may alleviate depression in depressed elderly people not responding to antidepressant drugs.[97] It is unknown if ginkgo could alleviate depression in other age groups. A small, preliminary trial has shown that ginkgo can reduce sexual problems caused by antidepressants like fluoxetine (Prozac), bupropion (Wellbutrin), venlafaxine (Effexor), and nefazodone (Serzone) in men and women.[98] Double-blind trials are now needed to determine whether ginkgo is truly effective for this purpose.

Damiana (page 666) has traditionally been used to treat people with depression. Yohimbine (the active component of the herb **yohimbe** [page 764]) inhibits monoamine oxidase (MAO) and therefore may be beneficial in depressive disorders. However, clinical research has not been conducted for its use in treating depression.

Pumpkin (page 733) seeds contain L-tryptophan, and for this reason have been suggested to help remedy depression.[99] However, research is needed before pumpkin seeds can be considered for this purpose. It is unlikely the level of L-tryptophan in pumpkin seeds would be sufficient to relieve depression.

Vervain (page 756) is a traditional herb for depression; however, there is no research to validate this use.

Are there any side effects or interactions?
Refer to the individual herb for information about any side effects or interactions.

Holistic approaches that may be helpful

Acupuncture may improve depression by affecting the synthesis of neurotransmitters that control mood.[100] Controlled trials[101, 102, 103] have found electro-acupuncture (acupuncture accompanied by electrical currents) equally effective as antidepressant drug therapy without causing side effects. However, a controlled trial found that both real and fake acupuncture improved depression equally well compared to no treatment.[104] It is well known that placebo effects are common in the treatment of depression,[105] so more controlled trials are needed before accepting the usefulness of acupuncture for depression.

Many people who are depressed seek counseling with a psychologist, social worker, psychiatrist, or other form of counselor. An analysis of four properly conducted trials of severely depressed patients comparing the effects of one form of counseling intervention, cognitive behavior therapy, with the effects of antidepressant drugs was published in 1999. In that report, cognitive behavior therapy was at least as effective as drug therapy.[106] While the outcome of counseling may be more variable than outcomes from drug or natural substance interventions, many healthcare professionals consider counseling an important part of recovery for depression not due to identifiable biochemical causes.

A rhythmic breathing technique called Sudarshan Kriya Yoga (SKY) may be an effective alternative to antidepressant drugs as an initial treatment for people with clinical depression. In a controlled trial, daily 45-minute SKY sessions six days per week produced a 67% remission rate among people with a diagnosis of depres-

sion.[107] This effect compared favorably with the effects of electro-shock therapy and the antidepressant drug imipramine; however, no placebo was used in this study. SKY technique is taught by the Art of Living Foundation.

In a controlled trial, magnetic stimulation to the front of the skull and underlying brain produced modest reductions of depressive symptoms in depressed people who had not responded adequately to standard treatment.[108] The procedure was performed by psychiatrists using sophisticated electromagnetic medical equipment, not a simple magnet.

DERMATITIS HERPETIFORMIS

Dermatitis herpetiformis (DH) is a chronic disease of the skin that may occur in people of any age, but is most common in the second to fourth decades of life.[1]

What are the symptoms of dermatitis herpetiformis?

DH is characterized by intensely itchy **hives** (page 245) or blister-like patches of skin located primarily on elbows, knees, and buttocks, although other sites may be involved. A burning or stinging sensation may accompany the itching.

	CHECKLIST FOR DERMATITIS HERPETIFORMIS	
Rating	Nutritional Supplements	Herbs
★★☆	**Selenium** (page 584) **Vitamin E** (page 609)	
★☆☆	**Betaine HCl** (page 473) **Folic acid** (page 520) (if deficient) **Iron** (page 540) (if deficient) **Multiple vitamin-mineral** (page 559) **PABA** (page 567) **Vitamin B$_{12}$** (page 601) (if deficient) **Vitamin B$_3$** (page 598) (nicotinamide, when combined with tetracycline) **Zinc** (page 614) (if deficient)	

Dermatitis Herpetiformis

Medical treatments

Prescription medications such as dapsone (Dapsone) and sulfapyridine are prescribed to treat the rash.

Strict adherence to a gluten-free diet is essential.

Dietary changes that may be helpful

The cause of DH is mainly an **allergic** (page 14) reaction (called hypersensitivity) to foods (wheat and other grains) containing a protein called gluten. People with DH are usually found to have abnormalities of the intestinal lining identical to that of **celiac disease** (page 102) (also called gluten-sensitive enteropathy or celiac sprue),[2] a serious intestinal disorder also due to gluten sensitivity. Unlike celiac disease however, gastrointestinal symptoms may be mild or absent in DH.[3, 4, 5, 6]

Strict adherence to a lifelong gluten-free diet (GFD) can eliminate symptoms of DH and the intestinal abnormalities, as well as reduce or eliminate the need for medication in most people. However, an average of 8 to 12 months of dietary restriction may be necessary before symptoms resolve.[7, 8, 9, 10, 11, 12, 13, 14, 15]

An increased incidence of lymphoma (**cancer** [page 87] of the lymph tissue),[16, 17, 18] and certain autoimmune and connective tissue disorders[19, 20] have also been reported in DH. Preliminary studies suggest a strict GFD of at least five years' duration may reduce the increased risk of developing lymphoma in DH.[21, 22, 23]

Not all people with DH improve on a GFD and/or medication. Preliminary studies indicate sensitivity to other dietary proteins may be involved.[24, 25, 26] Some practitioners would recommend an elimination diet and/or allergy testing to check for other food sensitivities.

A milk-free diet may improve symptoms of dermatitis herpetiformis, according to uncontrolled preliminary reports. In these reports, intake of milk products intensified symptoms of DH in two patients despite adherence to a gluten-free diet. The combination of a milk-free and gluten-free diet was effective, however.[27, 28]

Nutritional supplements that may be helpful

People with DH frequently have mild **malabsorption** (page 304) (difficulty absorbing certain nutrients) associated with **low stomach acid** (page 260) (hypochlorhydria) and inflammation of the stomach lining (atrophic gastritis).[29] Mild malabsorption may result in **anemia** (page 25)[30] and nutritional deficiencies of **iron** (page 540), **folic acid** (page 520),[31, 32] **vitamin B$_{12}$** (page 601),[33, 34] and **zinc** (page 614).[35, 36, 37] More se-

vere malabsorption may result in loss of bone mass.[38] Additional subtle deficiencies of vitamins and minerals are possible, but have not been investigated. Therefore, some doctors recommend people with DH have their nutritional status checked regularly with laboratory studies. These doctors may also recommend **multivitamin-mineral supplements** (page 559) and, to correct the low stomach acid, supplemental **betaine HCl** (page 473) (a source of hydrochloric acid).

Para-aminobenzoic acid (page 567) (PABA) in high amounts (9–24 grams per day) has been reported to reduce or eliminate the skin lesions of DH in one preliminary, clinical trial.[39] With continued administration, people with DH remained symptom-free for as long as 30 months. Since supplementation with such large amounts of PABA has the potential to cause side effects, these amounts should be used only with medical supervision.

A deficiency in the **selenium** (page 584)-containing **antioxidant** (page 467) enzyme known as glutathione peroxidase has been reported in DH.[40, 41] Preliminary[42] and double-blind[43] trials suggest that supplementation with 10 IU of **vitamin E** (page 609) and 200 mcg of selenium per day for six to eight weeks corrected this deficiency but did not lead to symptom improvement in the double-blind trial.

There is preliminary evidence that, when drug therapy with dapsone is not tolerated, people with DH may respond to a combination of the antibiotic, tetracycline, and **nicotinamide** (page 598) (a form of **vitamin B$_3$** [page 598]).[44, 45] However, this course of treatment should only be tried under the supervision of a physician.

Are there any side effects or interactions?
Refer to the individual supplement for information about any side effects or interactions.

DIABETES

What do I need to know?

Self-care for diabetes can be approached in a number of ways—but it can be hard to know just where to start. To make it easier, our doctors recommend trying these simple steps first:

Eat high-fiber foods
    Stabilize your blood sugar by eating fiber from whole grains, beans (legumes), vegetables, and

fruit, and consider using a fiber supplement such as glucomannan or psyllium

Slim down

If you are overweight, lose weight with a long-term program of exercise and healthier eating to improve your insulin sensitivity

Check out chromium

Taking 200 to 500 mcg a day may improve glucose tolerance

Improve and protect with alpha-lipoic acid

Take 600 to 1,200 mg a day to improve insulin sensitivity and help protect against diabetic complications such as nerve damage

Use capsaicin ointment

An ointment containing 0.025 to 0.075% capsaicin four times a day might help control nerve pain

Aim for total nutrition with a multivitamin-mineral supplement

Help ensure your body is getting the nutrition it needs to help prevent common infections

About diabetes

Diabetes mellitus is an inability to metabolize carbohydrates resulting from inadequate production or utilization of insulin. Other forms of diabetes (such as diabetes insipidus) are not included in this discussion.

People with diabetes cannot properly process glucose, a sugar the body uses for energy. As a result, glucose stays in the blood, causing blood glucose to rise. At the same time, however, the cells of the body can be starved for glucose. Diabetes can lead to poor **wound healing** (page 319), higher risk of **infections** (page 265), and many other problems involving the eyes, kidneys, nerves, and heart.

There are two types of diabetes mellitus. Childhood-onset diabetes is also called type 1, or insulin-dependent, diabetes. In type 1 diabetes, the pancreas cannot make the insulin needed to process glucose. Natural therapies cannot cure type 1 diabetes, but they may help by making the body more receptive to insulin supplied by injection. It is particularly critical for people with type 1 diabetes to work carefully with the doctor prescribing insulin before contemplating the use of any herbs, supplements, or dietary changes mentioned in this article. Any change that makes the body more receptive to insulin could require critical changes in insulin dosage that must be determined by the treating physician.

Adult-onset diabetes is also called type 2, or non-insulin-dependent, diabetes. With type 2 diabetes, the pancreas often makes enough insulin, but the body has trouble using the insulin. Type 2 diabetes frequently responds well to natural therapies.

People with diabetes have a high risk for **heart disease** (page 98) and **atherosclerosis** (page 38). In addition, those with diabetes have a higher mortality rate if they also have **high homocysteine** (page 234) levels.[1]

Medical treatments

Individuals diagnosed with type 1 diabetes, and occasionally some people with type 2 diabetes, are treated with insulin. Though most insulin is available over the counter, individuals should obtain an accurate diagnosis, as well as thorough guidance from their healthcare provider, before self-medicating. Insulin preparations are grouped according to onset and duration of action either as rapid-acting, such as regular (Humulin-R, Novolin-R); intermediate-acting, such as NPH (Humulin N, Novolin N) and lente (Humulin L, Novolin L); and long-acting, such as ultralente (Humulin U Ultralente). Oral glucose tablets (such as B-D Glucose) and gels (Glutose, Insta-Glucose, and Insulin Reaction) are available to treat low blood sugar resulting from insulin overdose.

Prescription-only insulin includes Insulin Analog Injection (Humalog). Common prescription medications used specifically to treat type 2 diabetes include sulfonylureas, such as glipizide (Glucotrol, Glucotrol XL), glimepiride (Amaryl), and glyburide (DiaBeta, Micronase, Glynase PresTab); the biguanide metformin (Glucophage); the meglitinide repaglinide (Prandin); and thiazolidinediones, such as rosiglitazone (Avandia) and pioglitazone (Actos). Injectable glucagon (Glucagon Emergency Kit) is used to treat severe hypoglycemia resulting from insulin overdose.

Dietary changes that may be helpful

The relationship between eating carbohydrates and type 2 diabetes is a complex issue. While eating carbohydrates increases the need for insulin to keep blood sugar normal, diets high in total carbohydrates do not necessarily increase the risk of type 2 diabetes.[2, 3] Researchers have found that diets very high in sugar may worsen glucose tolerance in nondiabetic animals[4] and humans.[5] However, the amount of sugar used in these studies in proportion to other foods is much larger than is typically found in human diets.

Diabetes

CHECKLIST FOR DIABETES

Rating	Nutritional Supplements	Herbs
★★★	**Alpha lipoic acid** (page 464) **Brewer's yeast** (page 480) (providing approximately 60 mcg of chromium per tablespoon) **Chromium** (page 493) **Evening primrose oil** (page 511) **Fiber** (page 512) **Glucomannan** (page 526) **Magnesium** (page 551)	**Cayenne** (page 654) (topical for neuropathy) **Fenugreek** (page 676) (seeds) **Psyllium** (page 732)
★★☆	**Biotin** (page 473) **Coenzyme Q₁₀** (page 496) **L-carnitine** (page 543) **Multiple vitamin– mineral supplement** (page 559) (for preventing infections) **Vitamin B₁ (Thiamine)** (page 597) **Vitamin B₆** (page 600) (gestational diabetes only) **Vitamin C** (page 604) **Vitamin E** (page 609) (for prevention of retrolental fibroplasia in premature infants, and for prevention of diabetic retinopathy) **Zinc** (page 614) (preferably for those with a documented deficiency)	**Aloe vera** (page 624) **American ginseng** (page 625) **Asian ginseng** (page 630) **Bilberry** (page 634) **Bitter melon** (page 635) **Cinnamon** (page 659) Crepe myrtle (*Lagerstroemia speciosa*) **Gymnema** (page 689) Hairy basil (seed) Holy basil (leaf) **Onion** (page 718)
★☆☆	**Fish oil** (page 514) (EPA/ DHA [page 509]) Following are associated with diabetic retinopathy: **Selenium** (page 584), **vitamin A** (page 595), **vitamin C** (page 604), and **vitamin E** (page 609) (combined) **Fructo-oligosaccharides** (page 522) (FOS) **Inositol** (page 537) **Manganese** (page 553) **Medium chain triglycerides** (page 554) **Quercetin** (page 580) **Starch blockers** (page 466) **Taurine** (page 590) **Vanadium** (page 594) (for type 2 diabetes) **Vitamin B₁₂** (page 601) **Vitamin B₃ (niacinamide)** (page 598) **Vitamin D** (page 607) **Vitamin E** (page 609) (associated with abetalipoproteinemia)	**Eleuthero** (page 672) *Ginkgo biloba* (page 681) **Mistletoe** (page 711) **Olive leaf** (page 717) **Reishi** (page 737)

Years ago, one researcher reported an increase in diabetes among Yemenite Jews who had migrated from a region where no sugar was eaten to one in which they ate a diet including sugar.[6] However, other factors, such as weight gain, may explain the increased risk of diabetes that occurred in this group.[7] Other studies have found no independent relationship between sugar intake and the development of glucose intolerance.[8]

Eating carbohydrate-containing foods, whether high in sugar or high in starch (such as bread, potatoes, processed breakfast cereals, and rice), temporarily raises blood sugar and insulin levels.[9] The blood sugar-raising effect of a food, called its "glycemic index," depends on how rapidly its carbohydrate is absorbed. Many starchy foods have a glycemic index similar to sucrose (table

sugar).[10] People eating large amounts of foods with high glycemic indices (such as those mentioned above), have been reported to be at increased risk of type 2 diabetes.[11, 12] On the other hand, eating a diet high in carbohydrate-rich foods with low glycemic indices is associated with a *low* risk of type 2 diabetes.[13, 14, 15] Beans, peas, fruit, and **oats** (page 716) have low glycemic indices, despite their high carbohydrate content, due mostly to the health-promoting effects of soluble **fiber** (page 512).

Diabetes disrupts the mechanisms by which the body controls blood sugar. Until recently, health professionals have recommended sugar restriction to people with diabetes, even though short-term high-sugar diets have been shown, in some studies, not to cause blood sugar problems in people with diabetes.[16, 17, 18] Currently, the American Diabetic Association (ADA) guidelines[19] do not prohibit the use of moderate amounts of sugar, as long as the goals of normalizing blood levels of glucose, **triglycerides** (page 235), and **cholesterol** (page 223) are being achieved.

Most doctors recommend that people with diabetes cut intake of sugar from snacks and processed foods, and replace these foods with high-**fiber** (page 512), whole foods. This tends to lower the glycemic index of the overall diet and has the additional benefit of increasing vitamin, mineral, and fiber intake. Other authorities also recommend lowering the glycemic index of the diet to improve the control of diabetes.[20]

A high-fiber diet has been shown to work better in controlling diabetes than the diet recommended by the ADA, and may control blood sugar levels as well as oral diabetes drugs.[21] In this study, the increase in dietary fiber was accomplished exclusively through the consumption of foods naturally high in fiber—such as leafy green vegetables, granola, and fruit—to a level beyond that recommended by the ADA. No fiber supplements were given. All participants received both the ADA diet (providing 24 grams of fiber per day) and the high-fiber diet (providing 50 grams of fiber per day) for a period of six weeks. After six weeks of following each diet, tests were performed to determine blood glucose, insulin, cholesterol, triglyceride, and other values. When glucose levels were monitored over a 24-hour period, participants eating the high-fiber diet had an average glucose level that was 10% lower than participants eating the ADA diet. Insulin levels were 12% lower in the group eating the high-fiber diet compared to the group eating the ADA diet, indicating a beneficial increase in the body's sensitivity to insulin. Moreover, people eating the high-fiber diet experienced significant reductions in total cholesterol, triglycerides, and LDL ("bad") cholesterol compared to those eating the ADA diet. They also had slight decreases in glycosylated hemoglobin, a measure of chronically high blood glucose levels.

High-fiber supplements, such as **psyllium** (page 732),[22, 23] guar gum (found in beans),[24] pectin (from fruit),[25] oat bran,[26] and **glucomannan** (page 526)[27, 28] have improved glucose tolerance in some studies. Positive results have also been reported with the consumption of 1–3 ounces of powdered **fenugreek seeds** (page 676) per day.[29, 30] A review of the research revealed that the extent to which moderate amounts of fiber help people with diabetes in the long term is still unknown, and the lack of many long-term studies has led some researchers to question the importance of fiber in improving diabetes.[31] Nonetheless, most doctors advise people with diabetes to eat a diet high in fiber. Focus should be placed on fruits, vegetables, seeds, **oats** (page 716), and whole-grain products.

Eating fish also may afford some protection from diabetes.[32] Incorporating a fish meal into a **weight-loss** (page 446) regimen was more effective than either measure alone at improving glucose and insulin metabolism and high cholesterol.[33]

Vegetarians have been reported to have a low risk of type 2 diabetes.[34] When people with diabetic nerve damage switch to a vegan diet (no meat, dairy, or eggs), improvements have been reported after several days.[35] In one trial, **pain** (page 338) completely disappeared in 17 of 21 people.[36] Fats from meat and dairy also contribute to **heart disease** (page 98), the leading killer of people with diabetes.

Vegetarians also eat less protein than do meat eaters. The reduction of protein intake has lowered kidney damage caused by diabetes[37, 38] and may also improve glucose tolerance.[39] However, in a group of 13 obese males with high blood-insulin levels (as is often seen in diabetes), a high-protein, low-carbohydrate diet resulted in greater weight loss and control of insulin levels, compared with that of a low-carbohydrate diet.[40] Switching to either a high- or low-protein diet should be discussed with a doctor.

Diets high in fat, especially *saturated fat*, worsen glucose tolerance and increase the risk of type 2 diabetes,[41, 42, 43, 44] an effect that is not simply the result of weight gain caused by eating high-fat foods. Saturated fat is found primarily in meat, dairy fat, and the dark meat and skins of poultry. In contrast, glucose intolerance has been improved by diets high in *monounsaturated* oils,[45, 46] which may be good for people with diabetes.[47] There is often difficulty in changing the overall percentage of calories from fat and carbohydrates in the diets of people with type 1 diabetes. However, modifying the *quality* of the dietary fat is achievable. In adolescents with type 1 diabetes, increasing monounsaturated fats relative to other fats in the diet is associated with better control over blood sugar and **cholesterol levels** (page 223).[48] The easiest way to incorporate monounsaturates into the diet is to use oils containing olive oil. However, those who are **overweight** (page 446) need to be aware—olive oil is high in calories.

Should children avoid milk to prevent type 1 diabetes? Worldwide, children whose dietary energy comes primarily from dairy (or meat) products have a significantly higher chance of developing type 1 diabetes than do children whose dietary energy comes primarily from vegetable sources.[49] Countries with high milk consumption have a high risk of type 1 diabetes.[50] Animal research also indicates that avoiding milk affords protection from type 1 diabetes.[51] Milk contains a protein related to a protein in the pancreas, the organ where in-

Diabetes

sulin is made. Some researchers believe that children who are **allergic** (page 14) to milk may develop antibodies that attack the pancreas, causing type 1 diabetes. Several studies have linked cows' milk consumption to the occurrence of type 1 diabetes in children.[52, 53, 54, 55] However, other studies have failed to find such a link.[56, 57] One study even reported a *protective* effect of higher intake of dairy products on diabetes risk in children.[58] One reason for the conflicting results of the research may be that different genetic strains of cows' milk protein (casein) are associated with different levels of risk.[59] Some children who drink cows' milk produce antibodies to the milk, and it has been hypothesized that these antibodies can cross-react with and damage the insulin-producing cells of the pancreas.[60]

Immune problems in people with type 1 diabetes have been tied to other **allergies** (page 14) as well,[61] and the importance of focusing only on the avoidance of dairy products remains unclear.[62] Preliminary studies have found that early introduction of cows' milk formula feeding increases the risk of developing type 1 diabetes, although contradictory results have also been published.[63, 64] A study of Finnish children (including full-term children with diabetes) showed that early introduction of cows' milk formula feeding before three months of age (vs. after three months of age) was associated with increased risk of type 1 diabetes.[65] This research supports abstaining from dairy products in infancy and early childhood, particularly for children with a family history of type 1 diabetes. Recent research also suggests a possible link between milk consumption in infancy and an increased risk of type 2 (non-insulin-dependent) diabetes.[66]

Lifestyle changes that may be helpful

Most people with type 2 diabetes are overweight.[67] Excess abdominal weight does not stop insulin formation,[68] but it does make the body less sensitive to insulin.[69] Excess weight can even make healthy people pre-diabetic.[70] **Weight loss** (page 446) reverses this problem.[71] In most studies, type 2 diabetes has improved with weight loss.[72, 73, 74]

Increased weight gain in infancy has been associated with a one-and-a-half-fold increase in the risk of developing type 1 diabetes in childhood.[75] Being overweight also increases the need for insulin. Therefore, people with type 1 diabetes should achieve and maintain appropriate body weight.

Exercise helps decrease body fat[76] and improve insulin sensitivity.[77] People who exercise are less likely to develop type 2 diabetes than those who do not.[78] People with type 1 diabetes who exercise require less insulin.[79] However, exercise can induce **low blood sugar** (page 251) or even occasionally *increased* blood sugar.[80] Moreover, a preliminary study has shown that long-term physical activity was not associated with control of blood glucose in people with type 1 diabetes.[81] Therefore, people with diabetes should never begin an intensive exercise program without consulting a healthcare professional.

Moderate drinking in *healthy* people improves glucose tolerance.[82, 83, 84, 85] However, alcohol has been reported to worsen glucose tolerance in the elderly[86] and in people with diabetes[87] in some studies. People with diabetes who drink have also been reported to have a high risk for eye[88] and nerve damage.[89]

Questions remain about where the line should be drawn regarding alcohol intake. For healthy people, light drinking will not increase the risk of diabetes, and may even reduce the risk of developing type 2 diabetes;[90] however, heavy drinking does increase the risk of developing diabetes and should be avoided.[91] People with diabetes should limit alcohol intake to two drinks per day. Total avoidance of alcohol in people with diabetes who are *not* suffering from **alcoholism** (page 12), liver disease (e.g., **cirrhosis** [page 290]), **gastritis** (page 195), **ulcers** (page 433), and other conditions made worse by alcohol might actually be counterproductive. In one report, older people with type 2 diabetes who drank daily, but moderately, had a dramatically lower incidence of deaths from **heart disease** (page 98) compared with nondrinkers.[92] This outcome is not surprising since moderate alcohol intake is associated with protection from heart disease in most other reports. This finding may be of particular importance because heart disease is the leading killer of people with diabetes. In another study, nondrinkers had a higher incidence of type 2 diabetes than did moderate drinkers.[93]

People with diabetes who smoke are at higher risk for kidney damage,[94] heart disease,[95] and other diabetes-linked problems. Smokers are also more likely to develop diabetes;[96] therefore, it is important to quit smoking.

Although most healthcare providers agree on the necessity of self-monitoring of blood glucose (SMBG) by people with type 1 diabetes, disagreement exists within the medical community regarding the efficacy and necessity of SMBG by people with type 2 diabetes. A controlled clinical trial found that home glucose monitoring strips did not affect the management of type 2 diabetes.[97] Moreover, a review of available literature concluded that the efficacy of SMBG in people with type 2 diabetes is questionable and should be tested in a rigorous high-quality trial.[98] Advocates of SMBG, such as the ADA, have observed that SMBG by people with diabetes has revolutionized management of the disease, enabling them to achieve and maintain specific goals.[99] These observations are well-supported in the medical literature.[100] Detractors point out that indiscriminate use of self-monitoring is of questionable value and adds enormously to healthcare costs.[101] The ADA acknowledges that accuracy of SMBG is instrument- and technique-dependent. Errors in technique and inadequate use of control procedures have been shown to lead to inaccurate test results.[102] Nevertheless, it is likely that self-monitoring of blood glucose, if used properly, can have a positive effect by increasing patient involvement in overall diabetes care.[103] Pharmacists and healthcare practitioners can teach people with diabetes certain skills that will enhance their ability to properly self-manage blood glucose.

Nutritional supplements that may be helpful
A variety of vitamins, minerals, amino acids, and other supplements may help with symptoms and deficiencies associated with diabetes.

Multiple vitamin–mineral supplement (page 559)
In a double-blind study, supplementation of middle-aged and elderly diabetics with a multiple vitamin and mineral preparation for one year reduced the risk of infection by more than 80%, compared with a placebo.[104]

Chromium (page 493)
Medical reports dating back to 1853, as well as modern research, indicate that chromium-rich **brewer's yeast** (page 480) (9 grams per day) can be useful in treating diabetes.[105, 106] In recent years, chromium has been shown to improve glucose and related variables in people with glucose intolerance and type 1, type 2, gestational, and steroid-induced diabetes.[107] Improved glucose tolerance with lower or similar levels of insulin have been reported in more than ten trials of chromium supplementation in people with varying degrees of glucose intolerance.[108] Chromium supplements improve glucose tolerance in people with both type 2[109] and type 1 diabetes, apparently by increasing sensitivity to insulin.[110] Chromium improves the processing of glucose in people with prediabetic glucose intolerance[111] and in women with diabetes associated with **pregnancy**

(page 363).[112] Chromium even helps healthy people,[113] although one such report found chromium useful only when accompanied by 100 mg of **niacin** (page 598).[114] Chromium may also lower total **cholesterol** (page 223), LDL cholesterol, and **triglycerides** (page 235) (risk factors in **heart disease** [page 98]).[115, 116]

A few trials have reported no beneficial effects from chromium supplementation.[117, 118, 119] All of these trials used 200 mcg or less of supplemental chromium, which is often not adequate for people with diabetes, especially if it is in a form that is poorly absorbed. The typical amount of chromium used in research trials is 200 mcg per day, although as much as 1,000 mcg per day has been used.[120] Many doctors recommend up to 1,000 mcg per day for people with diabetes.[121]

Supplementation with chromium or brewer's yeast could potentially enhance the effects of drugs for diabetes (e.g., insulin or other blood sugar-lowering agents) and possibly lead to **hypoglycemia** (page 251). Therefore, people with diabetes taking these medications should supplement chromium or brewer's yeast only under the supervision of a doctor.

Magnesium (page 551)
People with diabetes tend to have low magnesium levels.[122] Double-blind research indicates that supplementing with magnesium overcomes this problem.[123] Magnesium supplementation has improved insulin production in elderly people with type 2 diabetes.[124] However, one double-blind trial found no effect from 500 mg magnesium per day in people with type 2 diabetes, although twice that amount led to some improvement.[125] Elders without diabetes can also produce more insulin as a result of magnesium supplements, according to some,[126] but not all, trials.[127] In some trials, insulin requirements are lower in people with type 1 diabetes who supplement with magnesium.[128] However, in people with type 2 diabetes who nonetheless require insulin, Dutch researchers have reported no improvement in blood sugar levels.[129]

Diabetes-induced damage to the eyes is more likely to occur in magnesium-deficient people with type 1 diabetes.[130] In magnesium-deficient **pregnant** (page 363) women with type 1 diabetes, the lack of magnesium may even account for the high rate of spontaneous abortion and **birth defects** (page 63) associated with type 1 diabetes.[131] The American Diabetes Association admits "strong associations . . . between magnesium deficiency and insulin resistance" but will not say magnesium deficiency is a risk factor.[132] Many doctors, however, recommend that people with diabetes and normal kidney function supplement with 200–600 mg of magnesium per day.

Alpha lipoic acid (page 464)
Alpha lipoic acid is a powerful natural **antioxidant** (page 467). Preliminary[133, 134] and double-blind[135, 136, 137, 138, 139] trials have found that supplementing 600–1,200 mg of lipoic acid per day improves insulin sensitivity and the symptoms of diabetic neuropathy. In a preliminary study, supplementation with 600 mg of alpha-lipoic acid per day for 18 months slowed the progression of kidney damage in patients with type 1 and type 2 diabetes.[140]

Evening primrose oil (page 511)
Supplementing with 4 grams of evening primrose oil per day for six months has been found in double-blind research to improve nerve function and to relieve pain symptoms of diabetic neuropathy.[141]

Glucomannan (page 526)
Glucomannan is a water-soluble dietary fiber that is derived from konjac root *(Amorphophallus konjac)*. Glucomannan delays stomach emptying, leading to a more gradual absorption of dietary sugar. This effect can reduce the elevation of blood sugar levels that is typical after a meal.[142] After-meal blood sugar levels are lower in people with diabetes given glucomannan in their food,[143] and overall diabetic control is improved with glucomannan-enriched diets, according to preliminary[144] and controlled[145, 146] clinical trials. One preliminary report suggested that glucomannan may also be helpful in pregnancy-related diabetes.[147] For controlling blood sugar, 500–700 mg of glucomannan per 100 calories in the diet has been used successfully in controlled research.

Vitamin E (page 609)
People with low blood levels of vitamin E are more likely to develop type 1[148] and type 2 diabetes.[149] Vitamin E supplementation has improved glucose tolerance in people with type 2 diabetes in most,[150, 151, 152] but not all,[153] double-blind trials. Vitamin E has also improved glucose tolerance in elderly people without diabetes.[154, 155] Three months or more of supplementation may be required for benefits to become apparent. The amount used is at least 900 IU of vitamin E per day.

In one of the few trials to find vitamin E supplementation ineffective for glucose intolerance in people with type 2 diabetes, damage to nerves caused by the diabetes was nonetheless partially reversed by supplementing with vitamin E for six months.[156] Animal[157] and preliminary human[158] data indicate that vitamin E supplementation may protect against diabetic **retinopathy** (page 385) and nephropathy, serious complications of diabetes involving the eyes and kidneys, respectively, though no long-term trials in humans have confirmed this preliminary evidence.

Glycosylation is an important measurement of diabetes; it refers to how much sugar attaches abnormally to proteins. Vitamin E supplementation reduces this problem in many,[159, 160, 161, 162, 163] although not all,[164, 165, 166] studies.

In one report, vitamin E was found to *impair* glucose tolerance in **obese** (page 446) patients with diabetes.[167] The reason for the discrepancy between reports is not known.

Vitamin E appears to lower the risk of cerebral infarction, a type of **stroke** (page 419), in people with diabetes who smoke. A review of a large Finnish study of smokers concluded that smokers with diabetes (or **hypertension** [page 246]) represent a subset population that can benefit from small amounts of vitamin E (50 IU per day) *without* experiencing an increased risk of bleeding.[168]

Vitamin C (page 604)
People with type 1 diabetes appear to have low vitamin C levels.[169] As with vitamin E, vitamin C may reduce glycosylation.[170] Vitamin C also lowers sorbitol in people with diabetes.[171] Sorbitol is a sugar that can accumulate and damage the eyes, nerves, and kidneys of people with diabetes. Vitamin C may improve glucose tolerance in type 2 diabetes,[172, 173] although not every study confirms this benefit.[174] Vitamin C supplementation (500 mg twice daily for one year) has significantly reduced urinary protein loss in people with diabetes. Urinary protein loss (also called proteinuria) is associated with poor prognosis in diabetes.[175] Many doctors suggest that people with diabetes supplement with 1–3 grams per day of vitamin C. Higher amounts could be problematic, however. In one person, 4.5 grams per day was reported to *increase* blood sugar levels.[176]

One study examined antioxidant supplement intake, including both vitamins E and C, and the incidence of diabetic **retinopathy** (page 385) (damage to the eyes caused by diabetes).[177] Surprisingly, people with extensive retinopathy had a *greater* likelihood of having taken vitamin C and vitamin E supplements. The outcome of this trial, however, does not fit with most other published data and might simply reflect the fact that sicker people are more likely to take supplements in hopes of getting better. For the present, most doctors remain relatively unconcerned about the unexpected outcome of this isolated report.

B vitamins

Many people with diabetes have low blood levels of **vitamin B$_6$** (page 600).[178, 179] Levels are even lower in people with diabetes who also have nerve damage (neuropathy).[180] Vitamin B$_6$ supplementation has improved glucose tolerance in women with diabetes caused by pregnancy.[181, 182] Vitamin B$_6$ supplementation is also effective for glucose intolerance induced by birth control pills.[183] For other people with diabetes, 1,800 mg per day of a special form of vitamin B$_6$—pyridoxine alpha-ketoglutarate—has improved glucose tolerance dramatically in some research.[184] Standard vitamin B$_6$ has helped in some,[185] but not all, trials.[186]

Biotin (page 473) is a B vitamin needed to process glucose. When people with type 1 diabetes were given 16 mg of biotin per day for one week, their fasting glucose levels dropped by 50%.[187] Similar results have been reported using 9 mg per day for two months in people with type 2 diabetes.[188] Biotin may also reduce **pain** (page 338) from diabetic nerve damage.[189] Some doctors try 16 mg of biotin for a few weeks to see if blood sugar levels will fall.

Blood levels of **vitamin B$_1$** (page 597) (thiamine) have been found to be low in people with type 1 diabetes.[190] In the 1930s, a trial using 10 mg of vitamin B$_1$ per day for four weeks reported reduced blood sugar levels in six of eleven people with diabetes.[191] More recently, administration of both vitamin B$_1$ (25 mg per day) and **vitamin B$_6$** (page 600) (50 mg per day) led to significant improvement of symptoms of diabetic neuropathy after four weeks.[192] However, this was a trial conducted among people in a vitamin B$_1$-deficient developing country. Therefore, these improvements might not occur in other people with diabetes. Another trial found that combining vitamin B$_1$ (in a special fat-soluble form) and vitamin B$_6$ plus **vitamin B$_{12}$** (page 601) in high but variable amounts led to improvement in some aspects of diabetic neuropathy in 12 weeks.[193] As a result, some doctors recommend that people with diabetic neuropathy supplement with vitamin B$_1$, though the optimal level of intake remains unknown.

Coenzyme Q$_{10}$ (page 496)

Coenzyme Q$_{10}$ (CoQ$_{10}$) is needed for normal blood sugar metabolism. Animals with diabetes have been reported to be CoQ$_{10}$ deficient. People with type 2 diabetes have been found to have significantly lower blood levels of CoQ$_{10}$ compared with healthy people.[194] In one trial, blood sugar levels fell substantially in 31% of people with diabetes after they supplemented with 120 mg per day of CoQ7, a substance similar to CoQ$_{10}$.[195] In people with type 1 diabetes, however, supplementation with 100 mg of CoQ$_{10}$ per day for three months neither improved glucose control nor reduced the need for insulin.[196] The importance of CoQ$_{10}$ supplementation for people with diabetes remains an unresolved issue, though some doctors recommend approximately 50 mg per day as a way to protect against possible effects associated with diabetes-induced depletion.

L-carnitine (page 543)

L-carnitine is an **amino acid** (page 465) needed to properly utilize fat for energy. When people with diabetes were given L-carnitine (1 mg per 2.2 pounds of body weight), high blood levels of fats—both **cholesterol** (page 223) and **triglycerides** (page 235)—dropped 25–39% in just ten days in one trial.[197] In higher amounts (1 gram per day by injection), L-carnitine has been reported to reduce pain from diabetic nerve damage as well.[198]

Vitamin B$_{12}$ (page 601) is needed for normal functioning of nerve cells. Vitamin B$_{12}$ taken orally, intravenously, or by injection has reduced nerve damage caused by diabetes in most people studied.[199] In a preliminary trial, people with nerve damage due to kidney disease or to diabetes plus kidney disease received intravenous injections of 500 mcg of methylcobalamin (the main form of vitamin B$_{12}$ found in the blood) three times a day for six months in addition to kidney dialysis. Nerve pain was significantly reduced and nerve function significantly improved in those who received the injections.[200] Oral vitamin B$_{12}$ up to 500 mcg three times per day is recommended by some practitioners.

The intake of large amounts of **niacin** (page 598) (a form of vitamin B$_3$), such as 2–3 grams per day, may impair glucose tolerance and should be used by people with diabetes only with medical supervision.[201, 202] Smaller amounts (500–750 mg per day for one month followed by 250 mg per day) may help some people with type 2 diabetes,[203] though this research remains preliminary.

Preliminary trials have shown that **niacinamide** (page 598) (another form of vitamin B$_3$) supplementation might be useful in the very early stages of type 1 diabetes,[204] though not all trials support this claim.[205, 206, 207] Although an analysis of research shows that niacinamide does help preserve some function of

Diabetes

insulin-secreting cells in people recently diagnosed with type 1 diabetes, the amount of insulin required for those given niacinamide has remained essentially as high as for those given placebo.[208] A controlled trial found no beneficial effect of niacinamide supplementation (700 mg three times per day in addition to intensive insulin therapy) on pancreatic function and glucose tolerance in people newly diagnosed with type 1 diabetes.[209]

Some,[210] but not all,[211] reports suggest that *healthy* children at high risk for type 1 diabetes (such as the healthy siblings of children with type 1 diabetes) may be protected from the disease by supplementing with niacinamide. Parents of children with type 1 diabetes should consult their doctor regarding niacinamide supplementation as a way to prevent diabetes in their other children. Although the optimal amount of niacinamide is not known, recent evidence suggests that 25 mg per 2.2 pounds of body weight per day may be as effective as higher amounts.[212]

Zinc (page 614)

People with type 1 diabetes tend to be zinc-deficient,[213] which may impair **immune function** (page 255).[214] Zinc supplements have lowered blood sugar levels in people with type 1 diabetes,[215] though some evidence indicates that zinc supplementation in people with type 2 diabetes does not improve their ability to process sugar.[216] Nonetheless, people with type 2 diabetes also have low zinc levels, caused by excess loss of zinc in their urine.[217] Many doctors recommend that people with type 2 diabetes supplement with moderate amounts of zinc (15–25 mg per day) as a way to correct for the deficit.

Some doctors are concerned about having people with type 1 diabetes supplement with zinc because of a report that zinc supplementation increased glycosylation,[218] generally a sign of deterioration of the condition. This trial is hard to evaluate because zinc supplementation increases the life of blood cells and such an effect artificially increases the lab test results for glycosylation. Until this issue is resolved, those with type 1 diabetes should consult a doctor before considering supplementation with zinc.

Vitamin D (page 607)

Vitamin D is needed to maintain adequate blood levels of insulin.[219] Vitamin D receptors have been found in the pancreas where insulin is made and preliminary evidence suggests that supplementation can increase insulin levels in some people with type 2 diabetes;

prolonged supplementation might also help reduce blood sugar levels.[220] Not enough is known about optimal amounts of vitamin D for people with diabetes, and high amounts of vitamin D can be toxic. Therefore, people with diabetes considering vitamin D supplementation should talk with, and have vitamin D status assessed by, a doctor.

Inositol (page 537)

Inositol is needed for normal nerve function. Diabetes can cause a type of nerve damage known as diabetic neuropathy. This condition has been reported in some, but not all, trials to improve with inositol supplementation (500 mg taken twice per day).[221]

Taurine (page 590)

Taurine is an amino acid found in protein-rich food. People with type 1 diabetes have been reported to have low blood taurine levels, a condition that increases the risk of **heart disease** (page 98) by altering blood viscosity. Supplementing with taurine (1.5 grams per day) has restored blood taurine to normal levels and corrected the problem of blood viscosity within three months.[222] However, in a double-blind trial, taurine supplementation (2 grams per day for 12 months) failed to improve kidney complications associated with type 2 diabetes.[223]

Fish oil (page 514)

Glucose tolerance improves in *healthy* people taking omega-3 fatty acid supplements.[224] Some studies have found that fish oil supplementation improves glucose tolerance,[225] high **triglycerides** (page 235),[226] and **cholesterol** (page 223) levels in people with diabetes.[227] However, other studies have found that cholesterol increases[228] and diabetes worsens with fish oil supplementation.[229, 230, 231]

Until this issue is resolved, people with diabetes should feel free to increase their fish intake, but they should consult a doctor before taking fish oil supplements. Sometimes, such supplementation may be considered. In one trial, people with diabetic neuropathy and diabetic nephropathy experienced significant improvement when given 600 mg three times per day of purified EPA—one of the two major omega-3 fatty acids found in fish oil supplements—for 48 weeks.[232]

Doctors have suggested that **quercetin** (page 580) might help people with diabetes because of its ability to reduce levels of sorbitol—a sugar that accumulates in nerve cells, kidney cells, and cells within the eyes of people with diabetes—and has been linked to damage to those organs.[233] Clinical trials have yet to explore whether quercetin actually protects people with diabetes from neuropathy, nephropathy, or **retinopathy** (page 385).

Vanadium (page 594)

Vanadyl sulfate, a form of vanadium, may improve glucose control in people with type 2 diabetes,[234, 235, 236] though it may not help people with type 1 diabetes.[237] Over a six-week period, a small group of people with type 2 diabetes were given 75–300 mg of vanadyl sulfate per day.[238] Only in the groups receiving 150 mg or 300 mg was glucose metabolism improved, fasting blood sugar decreased, and another marker for chronic high blood sugar reduced. At the 300 mg level, total cholesterol decreased, although not without an accompanying reduction in the protective HDL cholesterol. None of the amounts improved insulin sensitivity. Although there was no evidence of toxicity after six weeks of vanadyl sulfate supplementation, gastrointestinal side effects were experienced by some of the participants taking 150 mg per day and by all of the participants taking 300 mg per day. The long-term safety of the large amounts of vanadium needed to help people with type 2 diabetes (typically 100 mg per day) remains unknown. Many doctors expect that amounts this high may prove to be unsafe in the long term.

Fructo-oligosaccharides (page 522)

In a preliminary trial, supplementation with fructo-oligosaccharides (FOS) (8 grams per day for two weeks) significantly lowered fasting blood-sugar levels and serum total-cholesterol levels in people with type 2 diabetes.[239] However, in another trial, supplementing with FOS (15 grams per day) for 20 days had no effect on blood-glucose or lipid levels in people with type 2 diabetes.[240] In addition, some double-blind trials showed that supplementing with FOS or galacto-oligosaccharides (GOS) for eight weeks had no effect on blood-sugar levels, insulin secretion, or blood lipids in healthy people.[241, 242] Because of these conflicting results, more research is needed to determine the effect of FOS and inulin on diabetes and lipid levels.

Manganese (page 553)

People with diabetes may have low blood levels of manganese.[243] Animal research suggests that manganese deficiency can contribute to glucose intolerance and may be reversed by supplementation.[244] A young adult with insulin-dependent diabetes who received oral manganese chloride (3–5 mg per day) reportedly experienced a significant fall in blood glucose, sometimes to dangerously low levels. In four other cases, manganese supplementation had no effect on blood glucose levels.[245] People with diabetes wishing to supplement with manganese should do so only with a doctor's close supervision.

Medium chain triglycerides (page 554)

Based on the results of a short-term clinical trial that found that medium chain triglycerides (MCT) lower blood glucose levels,[246] a group of researchers investigated the use of MCT to treat people with type 2 diabetes mellitus. Supplementation with MCT for an average of 17.5% of their total calorie intake for 30 days failed to improve most measures of diabetic control.[247]

Starch blockers (page 466)

Starch blockers are substances that inhibit amylase, the digestive enzyme required to break down dietary starches for normal absorption. Controlled research has demonstrated that concentrated starch blocker extracts, when given with a starchy meal, can reduce the usual rise in blood sugar levels of both healthy people and diabetics.[248, 249, 250, 251, 252] While this effect could be helpful in controlling diabetes, no research has investigated the long-term effects of taking starch blockers for this condition.

Are there any side effects or interactions?

Refer to the individual supplement for information about any side effects or interactions.

Herbs that may be helpful

Several herbs may help in managing symptoms associated with diabetes, including the control of blood sugar levels.

Cayenne (page 654)

Double-blind trials have shown that topical application of creams containing 0.025–0.075% capsaicin (from cayenne [Capsicum frutescens]) can relieve symptoms of diabetic neuropathy (numbness and tingling in the extremities caused by diabetes).[253, 254] Four or more applications per day may be required to relieve severe **pain** (page 338). This should be done only under a doctor's supervision.

Psyllium (page 732)

Supplementing with psyllium has been shown to be a safe and well-tolerated way to improve control of blood glucose and cholesterol. In a double-blind trial, men with type 2 diabetes who took 5.1 grams of psyllium per day for eight weeks lowered their blood glucose levels by 11% to 19.2%, their total cholesterol by 8.9%, and their LDL (bad) cholesterol by 13%, compared to a placebo.[255]

Asian ginseng *(page 630)*
Asian ginseng is commonly used in Traditional Chinese Medicine to treat diabetes. It has been shown in test tube and animal studies to enhance the release of insulin from the pancreas and to increase the number of insulin receptors.[256, 257] Animal research has also revealed a direct blood sugar-lowering effect of ginseng.[258] A double-blind trial found that 200 mg of ginseng extract per day improved blood sugar control, as well as energy levels in people with type 2 diabetes.[259]

American ginseng *(page 625)*
In a small preliminary trial, 3 grams of American ginseng was found to lower the rise in blood sugar following the consumption of a drink high in glucose by people with type 2 diabetes.[260] The study found no difference in blood sugar-lowering effect if the herb was taken either 40 minutes before the drink or at the same time. A follow-up to this study found that increasing the amount of American ginseng to either 6 or 9 grams did not increase the effect on blood sugar following the high-glucose drink in people with type 2 diabetes.[261] This study also found that American ginseng was equally effective in controlling the rise in blood sugar whether it was given together with the drink or up to two hours before.

Basil
Preliminary trials of holy basil *(Ocimim sanctum)* leaves and hairy basil *(Ocimum canum)* seeds have shown that these herbs may help people with type 2 diabetes control their blood sugar levels.[262, 263, 264] While the mechanism of action of holy basil leaf is not understood, hairy basil seed may work by replacing simple sugars in the diet (which rapidly and detrimentally elevate blood sugar levels) with dietary **fiber** (page 512) (which raises blood sugar levels more slowly for better control). It is unknown whether common culinary basil *(Ocimum basilicum)* would have similar effects.

Gymnema *(page 689)*
Gymnema may stimulate the pancreas to produce insulin in people with type 2 diabetes. Gymnema also improves the ability of insulin to lower blood sugar in people with both type 1 and type 2 diabetes. So far, no double-blind trials have confirmed the efficacy of gymnema for people with any type of diabetes. However, a preliminary study of type 2 diabetics reported that 400 mg per day of gymnema extract taken for periods of 18 months or more resulted in improvement, according to diabetes blood tests, and allowed reduction of diabetic medications.[265] In a controlled trial with type 1 (insulin-dependent) diabetics, a similar amount of gymnema extract reduced requirements for insulin.[266] Whether the extract used in these studies was standardized for active constituents is unclear. Recently, a preliminary trial found improved blood sugar levels after three months in a group of type 1 and type 2 diabetics who took 800 mg per day of an extract standardized for 25% gymnemic acids.[267] Gymnema is not a substitute for insulin, but insulin amounts may need to be lowered while taking gymnema to avoid hypoglycemia.

Bitter melon *(page 635)*
Whole, fried slices,[268] water extracts,[269] and juice[270] of bitter melon may improve blood-sugar control in people with type 2 diabetes, according to preliminary trials. However, double-blind trials are needed to confirm this potential benefit.

Cinnamon *(page 659)*
Test tube studies have suggested that cinnamon may improve the utilization of glucose. In a study of people with type 2 diabetes, supplementation with cinnamon in the amount of 1, 3, or 6 grams per day for 40 days was significantly more effective than a placebo at reducing blood glucose levels.[271] The reduction averaged 18 to 29% in the three treatments groups, and 1 gram per day was as effective as 3 and 6 grams per day.

Crepe myrtle
Lagerstroemia speciosa, commonly known as crepe myrtle, grows in various tropical countries and Australia. In folk medicine it has been used for the treatment of diabetes. In a preliminary study of people with type 2 diabetes, supplementation with an extract from the leaves of *Lagerstroemia speciosa* for two weeks resulted in a fall in blood-glucose levels averaging 20 to 30%.[272] The amount used was 32 or 48 mg of a product standardized to contain 1% corosolic acid (a putative active ingredient). The larger amount was somewhat more effect than the smaller amount. Although these results are promising, additional studies are needed to demonstrate the long-term safety and efficacy of this herbal preparation.

Onion (page 718)

Preliminary trials and at least one double-blind trial have shown that large amounts of onion can lower blood sugar levels in people with diabetes.[273, 274, 275] The mechanism of onion's blood sugar-lowering action is not precisely known, though there is evidence that constituents in onions block the breakdown of insulin in the liver. This would lead to higher levels of insulin in the body.[276]

Bilberry (page 634)

Bilberry may lower the risk of some diabetic complications, such as diabetic **cataracts** (page 101) and **retinopathy** (page 385). One preliminary trial found that supplementation with a standardized extract of bilberry improved signs of retinal damage in some people with diabetic retinopathy.[277]

Ginkgo biloba (page 681)

Ginkgo biloba extract may prove useful for prevention and treatment of early-stage diabetic neuropathy, though research is at best very preliminary in this area.[278] Other herbs that may help are **fenugreek** (page 676) seeds and **eleuthero** (page 672) (Siberian ginseng).

Mistletoe (page 711)

Mistletoe extract has been shown to stimulate insulin release from pancreas cells,[279] and animal research found that it reduces symptoms of diabetes.[280] No research in humans has yet been published; however, given mistletoe's worldwide reputation as a traditional remedy for diabetes, clinical trials are warranted to validate these promising preliminary findings. Traditionally, mistletoe is prepared by soaking 2–4 teaspoons of chopped mistletoe in two cups of water overnight. The mixture is drunk first thing in the morning and sweetened with honey if desired. Another batch may be left to steep during the day and drunk at bedtime.

Olive leaf (page 717)

Olive leaf extracts have been used experimentally to lower elevated blood-sugar levels in diabetic animals.[281] These results have not been reproduced in human clinical trials.

Reishi (page 737)

Animal studies[282] and some very preliminary trials in humans suggest reishi may have some beneficial action in people with diabetes.[283]

Are there any side effects or interactions?

Refer to the individual herb for information about any side effects or interactions.

Holistic approaches that may be helpful

Acupuncture may be helpful in the treatment of diabetes, or complications associated with diabetes. Preliminary trials have suggested that acupuncture can lower blood sugar[284, 285, 286] and improve insulin production[287] in people with type 2 diabetes, but trials on long-term effects have not been concluded. In a preliminary trial, 77% of people suffering from diabetic neuropathy experienced significant reduction in **pain** (page 338) following up to six acupuncture treatments over a ten-week period. Many were also able to reduce pain medications, but no long-term change in blood-sugar control was observed.[288] Bladder control problems, a complication of long-term diabetes, responded to acupuncture treatment with a significant reduction in symptoms in both controlled[289] and uncontrolled[290] trials.

DIARRHEA

Diarrhea is any attack of frequent, watery stools.

Diarrhea can be triggered by many different conditions. Acute diarrhea is often caused by an infection and may require medical management. The primary role of nutrition in acute diarrhea is to prevent depletion of fluid, sodium, **potassium** (page 572), and calories. Replenishment of all four has been achieved with "rehydration solutions" and with a variety of foods, from salted carrot soup to peeled scraped apple torice gruel. However, diarrhea severe enough to necessitate the use of rehydration solutions requires direct medical supervision. Therefore, nutritional approaches to overcoming depletion of fluid, sodium, potassium, and calories are not discussed here, but rather should be discussed with a doctor. Diarrhea-induced **low blood sugar** (page 251), dehydration, or electrolyte imbalance can be serious or even life-threatening, particularly if prolonged in children.

A healthcare provider should be consulted if diarrhea continues for more than a few days, as it may indicate a more serious health condition. Diarrhea alternating with constipation may be a sign of **irritable bowel syndrome** (page 280) (IBS).

Diarrhea

CHECKLIST FOR DIARRHEA

Rating	Nutritional Supplements	Herbs
★★★	**Lactase** (page 545) (for **lactose-intolerant** [page 288] people) **Multiple vitamin-mineral** (page 559) (to protect against deficiencies) **Probiotics** (page 575) (for infectious and antibiotic-associated diarrhea)	
★★☆	**Brewer's yeast** (page 480) (for infectious diarrhea) **Colostrum** (page 478) **Fiber** (page 520) **Glutamine** (page 530)	**Carob** (page 652) **Psyllium** (page 732) Sangre de drago Tormentil root extract (for rotavirus infection)
★☆☆	**Folic acid** (page 520) **Vitamin A** (page 595) **Zinc** (page 614)	**Barberry** (page 632) **Bilberry** (page 634) **Blackberry** (page 636) **Bladderwrack** (page 639) **Blueberry** (page 641) **Chamomile** (page 656) **Cranesbill** (page 665) **Goldenseal** (page 683) **Marshmallow** (page 708) **Oak** (page 716) **Oregon grape** (page 721) **Periwinkle** (page 727) **Red raspberry** (page 735) **Sweet Annie** (page 750) **Tylophora** (page 754)

What are the symptoms of diarrhea?

Normal bowel habits vary considerably from person to person depending on age, diet, cultural factors, and individual physiology. However, loose watery stools occurring three or more times in one day is generally considered abnormal. In some instances, diarrhea may be accompanied by cramping abdominal pain, nausea, vomiting, fever, loss of appetite, and bloody or foul-smelling stools.

Medical treatments

Over the counter antidiarrheal drugs include loperamide (Imodium A-D), bismuth subsalicylate (Pepto-Bismol), attapulgite (Kaopectate Advanced Formula), and charcoal (CharcoCaps).

Prescription medications used to stop diarrhea include diphenoxylate (Lomotil, Lonox, Motofen), and occasionally codeine.

Rest, along with fluid replacement using Pedialyte, Ceralyte, or Infalyte, is often recommended. Severe diarrhea, especially in children and the elderly, may require hospitalization for urgent fluid and electrolyte replacement in order to correct dehydration.

Dietary changes that may be helpful

Some foods contain sugars that are absorbed slowly, such as fructose in fruit juice or sorbitol in dietetic confectionery. Through a process called osmosis, these unabsorbed sugars hold onto water in the intestines, sometimes leading to diarrhea.[1] By reading labels, people with chronic non-infectious diarrhea can easily avoid fruit juice, fructose, and sorbitol to see if this eliminates the problem.

People who are **lactose intolerant** (page 288)—meaning they lack the enzyme needed to digest milk sugar—often develop diarrhea after consuming milk or ice cream. People whose lactose intolerance is the cause of diarrhea will rid themselves of the problem by avoiding milk and ice cream or in many cases by taking **lactase** (page 545), the enzyme needed to digest lactose. Lactase is available in a variety of forms in pharmacies (and in grocery stores in the form of lactase-treated milk).

Large amounts of **vitamin C** (page 604) or **magnesium** (page 551) found in supplements can also cause diarrhea, although the amount varies considerably from person to person. Unlike infectious diarrhea, diarrhea caused by high amounts of vitamin C or magnesium is not generally accompanied by other signs of illness. The same is true when the problem comes from sorbitol or fructose.[2] In these cases, avoiding the offending supplement or food brings rapid relief.

Drinking several cups of coffee per day causes diarrhea in some people.[3] People with chronic diarrhea who drink coffee should avoid all coffee for a few days to evaluate whether coffee is the culprit.

Allergies and food sensitivities (page 14) are common triggers for diarrhea.[4] For example, some infants suffer diarrhea when fed cow's milk-based formula but improve when switched to soy-based formula.[5] People with chronic diarrhea not attributable to other causes should discuss the possibility of food sensitivity with a doctor.

Some doctors recommend a diet called the BRAT diet for acute bouts of diarrhea. BRAT stands for bananas, rice, apples and toast. These foods are mild, well-tolerated and good sources of fiber, potassium and other nutrients that may be helpful in diarrhea. The efficacy of this diet has not been evaluated in clinical trials.

Nutritional supplements that may be helpful

An organism related to **brewer's yeast** (page 480), *Saccharomyces boulardii* (page 575) (Sb), is widely used in Europe to prevent antibiotic-induced diarrhea. It is also available as a supplement in the United States. Animal research with Sb shows interference with *Clostridium difficile,* a common bacterial cause of diarrhea.[6] In double-blind trials, Sb has prevented antibiotic-induced[7] and other forms of infectious diarrhea.[8] An intake of 500 mg four times per day has been used in some of this research. Sb has also helped tourists prevent traveler's diarrhea, according to double-blind research.[9] In one trial, positive results were obtained at amounts as low as 150–450 mg per day.[10] Even diarrhea caused by **Crohn's disease** (page 141) has partially responded to Sb supplementation in double-blind research.[11] While not every trial shows efficacy,[12] the preponderance of evidence clearly supports the use of Sb in people with diarrhea caused by antibiotics or **infection** (page 265). Seriously ill patients should consult with their doctor before supplementing with Sb, as rare but serious cases of infection caused by Sb in such patients has been reported.[13]

Beneficial bacteria, such as lactobacilli and bifidobacteria, normally live in a healthy colon, where they inhibit the over-growth of disease-causing bacteria.[14] Diarrhea flushes intestinal microorganisms out of the digestive tract, leaving the body vulnerable to opportunistic infections. Replenishing with acidophilus and other beneficial **probiotic** (page 575) bacteria can help resolve the diarrhea and prevent new infections.[15] The effective amount of probiotic bacteria depends on the strain used, as well as the concentration of viable organisms.

The combination of bifidobacteria and *Strep thermophilus* (found in certain yogurts) dramatically reduces the incidence of acute diarrhea in hospitalized children.[16] Active-culture yogurt, milk fermented with *Lactobacillus casei* and other sources of probiotic bacteria may prevent antibiotic-induced diarrhea.[17, 18, 19]

As mentioned in the dietary changes section above, if **lactose intolerance** (page 288) is the cause of diarrhea, supplemental use of **lactase** (page 545) prior to consuming milk or milk-containing products can be helpful.[20] Cheese rarely has enough lactose to cause symptoms in lactose-intolerant people. Lactase products are available that can be chewed while drinking milk or added to milk directly.

The malabsorption problems that develop during diarrhea can lead to deficiencies of many vitamins and minerals.[21] For this reason, it makes sense for people with diarrhea to take a **multivitamin-mineral supplement** (page 559). Two of the nutrients that may not be absorbed efficiently as a result of diarrhea are **zinc** (page 614) and **vitamin A** (page 595), both needed to fight infections. In third world countries, supplementation with zinc and vitamin A has led to a reduction in, or prevention of, infectious diarrhea in children.[22] Whether such supplementation would help people in better nourished populations remains unclear.

Brewer's yeast (page 480) supplementation has been shown to alter **immune function** (page 255) and the flora living in the intestine, and may relieve infectious diarrhea. Three capsules or tablets of brewer's yeast three times per day for two weeks was reported to improve three cases of infectious diarrhea caused by *Clostridium difficile.*[23] Animal research has confirmed that brewer's yeast helps fight this unfriendly bacterium.[24] (Note that real brewer's yeast is not identical to nutritional, or torula, yeast and that when asking for "brewer's yeast" in health food stores, people are often directed toward these other products. Real brewer's yeast is bitter, whereas other health food store yeasts have a more pleasant taste.)

Colostrum (page 478) might be useful for certain types of infectious diarrhea. In a double-blind trial, children with diarrhea caused by a rotavirus were treated with immunoglobulins extracted from colostrum derived from cows immunized with rotavirus. Compared with the placebo, colostrum extract significantly reduced the amount of diarrhea and the amount of oral rehydration solution required. The rotavirus was eliminated from the stool significantly more rapidly in the colostrum group than in the placebo group (1.5 days, vs. 2.9 days).[25]

In addition to a positive effect against acute rotavirus diarrhea,[26] there is also evidence that specific forms of colostrum (derived from specially immunized cows or those with confirmed presence of specific antibodies) are effective against diarrhea caused by *Cryp-*

tosporidium parvum, Helicobacter pylori, Escherichia coli, and *Clostridium difficile.*[27, 28, 29, 30, 31] However, it is not known whether commercially-available colostrum provides significant amounts of the specific immunoglobulins that are active against these organisms. Furthermore, unless the immunoglobulins are present in high enough concentrations, the preparation is not likely to be effective.[32]

In a double-blind study of children (ages six months to two years) with acute diarrhea, supplementing with **glutamine** (page 530) significantly reduced the duration of diarrhea by 26%.[33] Children were given 136 mg of glutamine per pound of body weight per day for seven days. Glutamine appeared to work by improving the health of the intestinal lining, rather than through any effect on the immune system.

While **fiber** (page 512) from dietary or herbal sources is often useful for constipation, it may also play a role in alleviating diarrhea.

Acute diarrhea can damage the lining of the intestine. **Folic acid** (page 520) can help repair this damage. In one preliminary trial, supplementing with very large amounts of folic acid (5 mg three times per day for several days) shortened the duration of acute infectious diarrhea by 42%.[34] However, a double-blind trial failed to show any positive effect with the same level of folic acid.[35] Therefore, evidence that high levels of folic acid supplementation will help people with infectious diarrhea remains weak.

It is known **vitamin A** (page 595) supplements support immune function and prevent infections. This is true, however, only under some circumstances. Vitamin A supplementation can also *increase* the risk of infections, according to the findings of a double-blind trial.[36] In a study of African children between six months and five years old, a 44% reduction in the risk of severe diarrhea was seen in those children given four 100,000–200,000 IU supplements of vitamin A (the lower amount for those less than a year old) during an eight-month period. On further investigation, the researchers discovered that the reduction in diarrhea occurred only in children who were very malnourished. For children who were not starving, vitamin A supplementation actually *increased* the risk of diarrhea compared with the placebo group. The vitamin A-supplemented children also had a 67% *increased* risk of coughing and rapid breathing, and signs of further lung infection, although this problem did not appear in children infected with the AIDS virus. These findings should be of concern to American parents, whose children are not

usually infected with HIV or severely malnourished. Such relatively healthy children fared poorly in the African trial in terms of both the risk of diarrhea and the risk of continued lung problems. Vitamin A provided no benefit to the well-nourished kids. Therefore, it makes sense *not* to give vitamin A supplements to children unless there is a special reason to do so, such as the presence of a condition causing **malabsorption** (page 303) (e.g., **celiac disease** [page 102]).

Are there any side effects or interactions?
Refer to the individual supplement for information about any side effects or interactions.

Herbs that may be helpful
The following recommendations are for milder forms of diarrhea. For more serious cases of diarrhea, proper medical evaluation and monitoring should occur before taking any herbal supplements.

Carob (page 652) is rich in tannins that have an astringent or binding effect on the mucous membranes of the intestinal tract. A double-blind trial has suggested it may be particularly useful for young children and infants with diarrhea.[37] Some healthcare professionals recommend 15 grams of carob powder is mixed with applesauce (for flavor) when given to children. Carob can also be used for treating adult diarrhea.

While **fiber** (page 512) from dietary or herbal sources is often useful for constipation, it may also play a role in alleviating diarrhea. For example, 9–30 grams per day of **psyllium seed** (page 732) (an excellent source of fiber) makes stool more solid and can help resolve symptoms of non-infectious diarrhea.[38] Alginic acid, one of the major constituents in **bladderwrack** (page 639) (*Fucus vesiculosus*), is a type of dietary fiber and as a result may potentially help relieve diarrhea. However, human studies have not been done on how effective bladderwrack is for this condition.

An extract from stem bark latex of Sangre de drago (*Croton lechleri*), an herb from the Amazon basin of Peru, has demonstrated significant anti-diarrheal activity in preliminary[39, 40] and double-blind trials. Double-blind research has demonstrated the extract's effectiveness for traveler's diarrhea,[41] non-specific diarrhea,[42] and diarrhea associated with **HIV** (page 239) infection and AIDS.[43, 44] For traveler's diarrhea and nonspecific diarrhea, amounts ranging from 125 mg to 500 mg taken four times daily for two days have proven effective. However, in one trial, only the 125 mg four times daily amount (but not higher amounts) was effective for acute nonspecific diarrhea.[45] The reasons for the failure of higher amounts in this study is not known. Very high amounts of these extracts (350–700 mg four times daily for seven or more days) were used in the trials involving people with HIV and AIDS. Such levels of supplementation should always be supervised by a doctor. Most of this research on Sangre de Drago is unpublished, and much of it is derived from manufacturers of the formula. Further double-blind trials, published in medical journals, are needed to confirm the efficacy reported in these studies.

Tormentil root *(Potentilla tormentilla)* is an herb that has been used for many years in different European folk medicines for the treatment of diarrhea. In a double-blind study of children with diarrhea caused by rotavirus infection, the duration of diarrhea averaged three days in children who received tormentil root extract, compared with five days in those who received a placebo.[46] No adverse effects were seen. The amount of tormentil root extract used was 3 drops for every year of life, taken three times a day until diarrhea stopped, or for a maximum of five days.

Other astringent herbs traditionally used for diarrhea include **blackberry** (page 636) leaves, blackberry root bark, **blueberry** (page 641) leaves, and **red raspberry** (page 735) leaves.[47] Raspberry leaves are high in tannins and, like blackberry, may relieve acute diarrhea. A close cousin of the blueberry, **bilberry** (page 634), has been used traditionally in Germany for adults and children with diarrhea.[48] Only dried berries or juice should be used—fresh berries may worsen diarrhea.

Cranesbill (page 665) has been used by several of the indigenous tribes of North America to treat diarrhea. The tannins in cranesbill likely account for the anti-diarrheal activity[49]—although there has been little scientific research to clarify cranesbill's constituents and actions.

In laboratory experiments, a tannin in **oak** (page 716), known as ellagitannin, inhibited intestinal secretion,[50] which may help resolve diarrhea. Oak is well regarded in Germany, where it is recommended (along with plenty of electrolyte-containing fluids) to treat mild, acute diarrhea in children.[51]

Due to of its supposed antimicrobial activity, **goldenseal** (page 683) has a long history of use for infectious diarrhea. Its major alkaloid, berberine (also found in **barberry** [page 632] and **Oregon grape** [page 721]), has been shown to improve infectious diarrhea in some double-blind trials.[52] Negative studies have generally focused on people with cholera, while positive studies

investigated viral diarrhea or diarrhea due to strains of *E. coli*. These studies generally used 400–500 mg berberine one to three times per day. Because of the low amount of berberine in most goldenseal products, it is unclear how effective the whole root or root extracts would be in treating diarrhea.

Chamomile (page 656) may reduce intestinal cramping and ease the irritation and inflammation associated with diarrhea, according to test tube studies.[53] Chamomile is typically taken as a tea. Many doctors recommend dissolving 2–3 grams of powdered chamomile or adding 3–5 ml of a chamomile liquid extract to hot water and drinking it three or more times per day, between meals. Two to three teaspoons (10–15 grams) of the dried flowers can be steeped in a cup of hot water, covered, for ten to fifteen minutes as well.

Tylophora (page 754) has been used traditionally in the Ayurvedic system for diarrhea probably due to its anti-inflammatory and antimicrobial actions, although human studies have not confirmed this use.

Herbs high in mucilage, such as **marshmallow** (page 708) or **slippery elm** (page 747), may help reduce the irritation to the walls of the intestinal tract that can occur with diarrhea. A usual amount taken is 1,000 mg of marshmallow extract, capsules, or tablets three times per day. Marshmallow may also be taken as a tincture in the amount of 5–15 ml three times daily.

Sweet Annie (page 750) has been used traditionally to treat infectious diarrhea and malaria. However, more modern studies have used the isolated constituent artemisinin and it is unclear how effective the herb is in managing diarrhea.

Are there any side effects or interactions?
Refer to the individual herb for information about any side effects or interactions.

Holistic approaches that may be helpful
Other integrative approaches that may be helpful: Acupuncture may be useful for the treatment of diarrhea, particularly in infants. A preliminary study of acupuncture treatment in 1,050 cases of infantile diarrhea found 95% were relieved with one to three treatments.[54] Similar results have been reported in other preliminary trials[55, 56] and case reports.[57, 58] A controlled trial of acupuncture for the treatment of infantile diarrhea compared scalp acupuncture or traditional body acupuncture with drug therapy, primarily antibiotics. The cure rate for scalp and body acupuncture was significantly higher (90% and 89%) than that of drug treatment (46%).[59]

Diverticular Disease

DIVERTICULAR DISEASE

Diverticular disease is a condition of abnormal pouches in portions of the colon.

High pressure inside the intestine may cause these outpouchings (called diverticula) to develop in areas of weakness within the wall of the colon.[1] The development of these pouches is called diverticulosis. Rarely, diverticula may also occur in the stomach or small intestine. When the pouches become inflamed (often as a result of bacterial **infection** [page 265]), symptoms such as cramping pains, fever, and nausea can result.[2] Such an infection (called diverticulitis) is potentially life-threatening and requires immediate medical intervention. Diverticular disease becomes increasingly common as people age and is a malady of 20th-century western society, primarily due to the consumption of a low-fiber diet.[3]

CHECKLIST FOR DIVERTICULAR DISEASE		
Rating	**Nutritional Supplements**	**Herbs**
★★★	**Fiber** (page 512)	**Psyllium** (page 732)
★☆☆	**Glucomannan** (page 526)	

What are the symptoms of diverticular disease?
People with diverticular disease may or may not have abdominal cramps, bloating, **constipation** (page 137), and tenderness or pain, especially along the lower left side of the abdomen. When there is an active infection, there may also be fever, chills, nausea, and vomiting.

Medical treatments
Over-the-counter fiber supplements such as methylcellulose (Citrucel), polycarbophil calcium (Fibercon), and psyllium (Metamucil) are often recommended.

Serious cases may be treated with prescription drugs, including intravenous antibiotics such as cefazolin (Ancef), cefamandole (Mandol), amikacin (Amikin); pain medication in combination with acetaminophen, such as codeine (Tylenol with Codeine), hydrocodone (Vicodin, Lortab), oxycodone (Percocet); and intestinal antispasmotics such as L-hyoscyamine (Levsin, Levbid). Injections of Vasopressin may be used to control bleeding diverticula.

For mild conditions, healthcare practitioners typically recommend adequate fluid intake and a high-fiber diet. Some severe cases might require a liquid diet or surgical removal of the affected portion of the colon. Giant diverticula always require surgery.

Dietary changes that may be helpful
Dietary factors influence the frequency and severity of diverticular disease recurrences. A diet high in **fiber** (page 512) has been shown to be protective against diverticular disease.[4] One study of food intake revealed a 50% increase in incidence of diverticular disease in people eating a diet high in meat and low in vegetables relative to those eating a high-vegetable and low-meat diet.[5] In addition to helping prevent the disease, a high-fiber diet may also be useful as a treatment for diverticular disease.[6]

Lifestyle changes that may be helpful
Obesity (page 446) may be associated with increased severity of diverticular disease.[7] Studies have yet to be conducted to determine if weight loss decreases signs and symptoms of diverticular disease in patients who are overweight.

Physical activity, specifically jogging or running, has been reported to protect against symptomatic diverticular disease.[8] While the reason for its positive effect is not known, exercise is associated with reduced symptoms of a variety of other diseases of the colon.

Nutritional supplements that may be helpful
In people with diverticular disease, a **fiber** (page 512) supplement may improve **constipation** (page 137). The results of double-blind of fiber supplementation for diverticular disease have been mixed. One study[9] demonstrated a beneficial effect of fiber supplementation in people who suffered from abdominal pain and pain with bowel movements; whereas a second study[10] indicated no improvement in these symptoms following fiber supplementation. Nevertheless, long-term fiber supplementation may protect against the complications of diverticular disease.[11]

Glucomannan (page 526) is a water-soluble dietary fiber that is derived from konjac root (*Amorphophallus konjac*). A preliminary clinical trial found that approximately one-third to one half of people with diverticular disease had reduced symptoms of diverticular disease after taking glucommanan.[12] The amount of glucomannan shown to be effective as a laxative is 3–4 grams per day.

Are there any side effects or interactions?
Refer to the individual supplement for information about any side effects or interactions.

Herbs that may be helpful

A preliminary trial of the herb **psyllium** (page 732) supports the use of this type of fiber in relieving the symptoms associated with diverticular disease and constipation.[13]

Are there any side effects or interactions?
Refer to the individual herb for information about any side effects or interactions.

DOWN'S SYNDROME

Down's syndrome is a genetic abnormality caused by a defect of chromosome 21. People with Down's syndrome are mentally retarded and suffer from a wide array of other symptoms, such as premature aging with development of **Alzheimer's disease** (page 19) before the age of 40, short stature and flaccid musculature, frequent infections, autoimmune disease, hypothyroidism, leukemia, and heart defects.[1]

Down's syndrome is the most common genetic disorder, occurring at a rate of about one in 700 to 800 births.[2]

What are the symptoms of Down's syndrome?

Newborns with Down's syndrome may be lethargic, rarely cry, and have extra skin around the neck. Children and adults with Down's syndrome may have slanted eyes, flattened nose, large tongue, small ears, short fingers, and broad hands, and may have difficulty performing routine activities of daily life.

CHECKLIST FOR DOWN'S SYNDROME		
Rating	Nutritional Supplements	Herbs
★★★	Zinc (page 614)	
★★☆	Acetyl-L-Carnitine (page 461) Vitamin E (page 609)	
★☆☆	Folic acid (page 520) Multivitamin (page 559) Selenium (page 584) Vitamin B₁₂ (page 601)	

Medical treatments

Treatment consists of management of medical conditions associated with this syndrome, such as thyroid deficiency, cardiac malformations, hearing loss, and difficulties with vision.

Lifestyle changes that may be helpful

A number of studies have examined the nutritional status of children with Down's syndrome. These children consume lower amounts of calories but are more likely to be obese and to have specific nutrient deficiencies in their diets.[3, 4] **Malabsorption** (page 304) is thought to contribute to the health consequences of Down's syndrome, such as **cardiovascular disease** (page 98) and **Alzheimer's disease** (page 19), and in a small preliminary study, stool analyses showed that all of four Down's syndrome patients examined had insufficient digestion.[5] Researchers have long suggested that gluten sensitivity may be a cause for malabsorption in many Down's syndrome patients.[6, 7] Many recent studies have established a link between Down's syndrome and **celiac disease** (page 102).[8, 9, 10, 11, 12, 13, 14, 15, 16, 17] The immune systems of individuals with celiac disease produce antibodies to gliadin, a protein from wheat gluten and some other grains, and these antibodies damage the intestines resulting in malabsorption and **diarrhea** (page 163). The treatment for celiac disease is complete avoidance of dietary gluten. The prevalence of celiac disease among people with Down's syndrome in these studies ranged between 3.9% and 16.9%, more than 100 times the prevalence in the general population. Antibodies to gliadin have been found to be elevated in many people with Down's syndrome who do not express the severe symptoms of celiac disease.[18, 19, 20, 21] One study found antibodies to proteins from egg and dairy to be elevated in a high percentage of Down's syndrome patients.[22] Patients with Down's syndrome should be evaluated by a doctor for these types of **food sensitivities** (page 14), as well as for celiac disease.

A comparison study found that children with Down's syndrome were likely to have less physical activity than other children, suggesting that the condition itself may not be responsible for the tendency toward **obesity** (page 446).[23] In another study, adults with Down's syndrome were more likely to be obese if they had poor social connections, even after the effects of physical activity and diet were taken into account.[24] People with Down's syndrome were found to have lower muscle strength and lower bone mineral density than both healthy individuals and people with mental retardation but without Down's syndrome. These findings have led researchers to emphasize the importance of physical training for individuals with Down's syndrome.[25] Although some studies have found that people with Down's syndrome do not benefit as much from exercise as people without Down's syndrome,[26, 27, 28] intervention trials have found that those who become physically active do improve in strength and endurance.[29, 30] Cardiac effects of Down's syndrome, such as **mitral valve prolapse** (page 319), may reduce the exercise capacity of these individuals.[31] Exercise has been suggested as a preventive measure to improve blood flow to the brain and to protect against Alzheimer's disease, because people with Down's syndrome have a high risk for developing this disease at a young age.[32] This potential benefit of exercise, however, has not yet been tested.

Nutritional supplements that may be helpful

In a double-blind trial, improvement was reported in the intellectual functioning of five children with Down's syndrome given a daily high-potency **multivitamin-mineral supplement** (page 559).[33] This sparked interest in further research, but in a larger double-blind trial that followed, no benefit was observed.[34] A later controlled trial found that multivitamin and mineral supplementation had no greater effect than did placebo in children with Down's syndrome.[35] A review of the research found no compelling reason to give multivitamin or **B vitamin** (pages 597–604) supplements to people with Down's syndrome.[36]

The red blood cells of people with Down's syndrome are unusual in ways that suggest either **vitamin B$_{12}$** (page 601) or **folic acid** (page 520) deficiency.[37, 38, 39] However, folic acid levels have been found to be normal in each of these studies, and only one study has found lower levels of vitamin B$_{12}$ in Down's syndrome as compared with healthy individuals.[40] Intervention trials using either vitamin B$_{12}$ or folic acid have not been done.

Alzheimer's disease (page 19), **cataracts** (page 101), autoimmune diseases, and a general increase in the pace of aging are all seen in people with Down's syndrome.[41] These associated conditions are similar in that they involve damage to body tissues by free radicals. It is believed that the genetic defect that produces Down's syndrome increases the need for **antioxidants** (page 467) (nutrients that prevent free-radical damage), and several studies of blood and urine biochemistry have shown this to be true.[42, 43] In a preliminary study, **vita-**

min E (page 609) protected cells of people with Down's syndrome from the oxidative damage to which they are most susceptible.[44] However, blood levels of **vitamin C** (page 604) and vitamin E, two antioxidant nutrients, have not been found to be different when compared with those of healthy individuals.[45, 46] The role of vitamin E and other antioxidants in treating Down's syndrome needs further exploration.

Blood levels of the antioxidant minerals **selenium** (page 584) and **zinc** (page 614) were normal in one study of people with Down's syndrome,[47] but others have found selenium[48, 49] and zinc[50, 51, 52] levels to be low. In some studies more than 60% of patients with Down's syndrome had low zinc levels.[53, 54] A preliminary study of selenium supplementation in children with Down's syndrome found that the antioxidant activity in the body improved; however, the implications of this finding on the long-term health of these people is unclear.[55] Zinc is critical for proper immune function, and in one preliminary study the majority of patients with Down's syndrome examined had low zinc levels and low immune cell activity. Supplementation with zinc resulted in improved immune cell activity.[56] In preliminary intervention trials, improved immune cell activity was associated with reduced rates of **infection** (page 265) in Down's syndrome patients given supplemental zinc in the amount of 1 mg per 2.2 pounds of body weight per day.[57, 58] A controlled trial, however, did not find zinc, at 25 mg daily for children under 10 years of age and 50 mg for older children, to have these benefits.[59] Zinc has other roles in the body; preliminary data have indicated that zinc supplementation, at 1 mg per 2.2 pounds of body weight per day, improved thyroid function in Down's syndrome patients,[60, 61, 62] and increased growth rate in children with Down's syndrome.[63]

Acetyl-L-carnitine (page 461) is a compound that occurs naturally in the brain and plays a role in the normal functioning of the nervous system. In a preliminary trial, patients with Down's syndrome were given 500 mg of L-acetyl-carnitine three times daily for 90 days and were observed to improve in visual memory and attention. Similar improvement was not seen in untreated patients, nor in patients with mental deficiency unrelated to Down's syndrome who were also given L-acetyl-carnitine.[64] More research into the effects of L-acetyl-carnitine in people with Down's syndrome is needed.

5-Hydroxytryptophan (page 459) (5-HTP) is an amino acid used in the body to make the neurotransmitter serotonin, which affects mood and sleep. 5-HTP is produced from the amino acid tryptophan, which occurs naturally in food proteins. Early data indicated that children with Down's syndrome have low levels of serotonin,[65] and several studies showed that infants given 5-HTP experienced improvement in muscle tone and reduction of tongue protrusion.[66, 67, 68] However, side effects from 5-HTP were common and included restlessness, diarrhea, vomiting, muscle spasms, and blood pressure elevation. One study reported seizures as a side effect of 5-HTP supplementation in infants.[69] Other studies have failed to find 5-HTP beneficial.[70, 71] Because of the high incidence side effects and the questionable benefits, supplementation with 5-HTP in infants and children with Down's syndrome is not recommended at this time.

Are there any side effects or interactions?
Refer to the individual supplement for information about any side effects or interactions.

DUPUYTREN'S CONTRACTURE

In Dupuytren's contracture, a fibrous tissue formation occurs in the palm of the hand that can cause the last two fingers to curl up.

The origin of this condition is not well understood.

What are the symptoms of Dupuytren's contracture?
Dupuytren's contracture is initially noticed as a tender, small, hardened nodule on the palm of the hand. As it progresses, a cordlike band develops along the palm and finger, which causes the affected finger to stay in a semiclosed position.

CHECKLIST FOR DUPUYTREN'S CONTRACTURE		
Rating	**Nutritional Supplements**	**Herbs**
★☆☆	**DMSO** (page 508) (topical) **Vitamin E** (page 609)	

Medical treatments
Corticosteroid injections such as methyprednisolone (Depo-Medrol) are commonly used.

Advanced contractures are treated with surgery; however, the recurrence rate is relatively high. Severe cases might require amputation of the affected finger.

Nutritional supplements that may be helpful
Many decades ago, researchers investigated the effects of taking **vitamin E** (page 609) to treat Dupuytren's contracture. Several studies reported that taking 200–2,000 IU of vitamin E per day for several months was helpful.[1] Other studies, however, did not find it useful.[2] Overall, there are more positive trials than negative ones,[3] although none of the published research is recent. Nonetheless, some doctors believe that a three-month trial using very high amounts of vitamin E (2,000 IU per day) is helpful in some cases.

DMSO (page 508) applied to the affected area may reduce pain by inhibiting transmission of pain messages, and may also soften the abnormal connective tissue associated with disorders such as Dupuytren's contracture, keloids, Peyronie's disease, and scleroderma. Research on the use of topical DMSO to treat Dupuytren's contracture remains preliminary and unproven.[4]

Are there any side effects or interactions?
Refer to the individual supplement for information about any side effects or interactions.

DYSMENORRHEA

Dysmenorrhea is painful menstruation. It is classified as either primary or secondary. Primary dysmenorrhea generally occurs within a couple of years of the first menstrual period. The pain tends to decrease with age and very often resolves after childbirth. Secondary dysmenorrhea is menstrual pain caused by another condition, commonly **endometriosis** (page 182). It starts later in life and tends to increase in intensity over time.

As many as half of menstruating women are affected by dysmenorrhea, and of these, about 10% have severe dysmenorrhea, which greatly limits activities for one to three days each month.[1]

What are the symptoms of dysmenorrhea?
Dysmenorrhea includes symptoms of abdominal bloating, frequent and intense cramps, **pain** (page 338) below the waistline, or a dull ache that may radiate to the lower back or legs. There may also be symptoms of headache, nausea, **diarrhea** (page 163) or **constipation**

Dysmenorrhea

(page 137), frequent urination, and, occasionally, vomiting. The symptoms usually occur just before or during the menstrual period.

Rating	Nutritional Supplements	Herbs
★★★	**Magnesium** (page 551)	
★★☆	**Vitamin B₃** (page 598) (niacin) **Vitamin B₃** (page 598) (niacin) (plus **vitamin C** [page 604] and **rutin** [page 580]) **Vitamin E** (page 609)	
★☆☆	**Calcium** (page 483) **Fish oil** (page 514) (EPA/ **DHA** [page 509]) **Progesterone** (page 577) (topical cream) **Vitamin B₁** (page 597)	**Black cohosh** (page 637) **Blue cohosh** (page 643) **Corydalis** (page 663) Cramp bark **Dong quai** (page 668) **False unicorn** (page 675) **Peony** (page 724) **Vervain** (page 756) **Vitex** (page 757)

CHECKLIST FOR DYSMENORRHEA

Medical treatments

Over the counter treatment includes pain medications, such as ibuprofen (Advil, Motrin, Midol PMS), naproxen (Aleve), and acetaminophen (Tylenol).

Prescription strength nonsteroidal anti-inflammatory drugs (NSAIDs) including celecoxib (Celebrex), valdecoxib (Bextra), ibuprofen (Motrin), diclofenac (Voltaren), ketoprofen (Orudis), and mefenamic acid (Ponstel) might be necessary for pain relief. Birth control pills (Ortho-Novum, Mircette, Loestrin, Triphasil) may be used to suppress ovulation. The anti-estrogen drug danazol (Danocrine) and progestins are also occasionally used. Severe cases involving nausea and vomiting might require the use of prochlorperazine (Compazine).

Dietary changes that may be helpful

Some physicians advise that alcohol should be avoided by women experiencing menstrual pain, because it depletes stores of certain nutrients and alters the metabolism of carbohydrates—which in turn might worsen muscle spasms. Alcohol can also interfere with the liver's ability to metabolize hormones. In theory, this might result in elevated estrogen levels, increased fluid and salt retention, and heavier menstrual flow.

Lifestyle changes that may be helpful

Many women feel the need to lie still while experiencing menstrual cramps, while others find that exercise helps relieve the pain of dysmenorrhea. This variation from woman to woman may explain why some researchers report that exercise makes symptoms worse,[2] though most studies report that exercise appears helpful.[3]

Nutritional supplements that may be helpful

The niacin form of **vitamin B₃** (page 598) has been reported to be effective in relieving menstrual cramps in 87% of a group of women taking 200 mg of niacin per day throughout the menstrual cycle. They then took 100 mg every two or three hours while experiencing menstrual cramps.[4] In a follow-up study, this protocol was combined with 300 mg of **vitamin C** (page 604) and 60 mg of the **flavonoid** (page 516) rutin per day, which resulted in a 90% effectiveness for relieving menstrual cramps.[5] Since these two preliminary studies were published many years ago, no further research has explored the relationship between niacin and dysmenorrhea. Niacin may not be effective unless taken for seven to ten days before the onset of menstrual flow.

In theory, **calcium** (page 483) may help prevent menstrual cramps by maintaining normal muscle tone. Muscles that are calcium-deficient tend to be hyperactive and therefore might be more likely to cramp. Calcium supplementation was reported to reduce pain during menses in one double-blind trial,[6] though another such study found that it relieved only *pre*menstrual cramping, not pain during menses.[7] Some doctors recommend calcium supplementation for dysmenorrhea, suggesting 1,000 mg per day throughout the month and 250–500 mg every four hours for pain relief, during acute cramping (up to a maximum of 2,000 mg per day).

Like calcium, **magnesium** (page 551) plays a role in controlling muscle tone and could be important in preventing menstrual cramps.[8, 9] Magnesium supplements have been reported in preliminary[10] and double-blind[11, 12] European research to reduce symptoms of dysmenorrhea. In one of these double-blind trials, women took 360 mg per day of magnesium for three days beginning on the day before menses began.[13]

Diets low in omega-3 fatty acids (EPA and **DHA** [page 509]) have been associated with menstrual pain.[14] In one double-blind trial, supplementation with **fish** oil (page 514), a good source of omega-3 fatty acids, led to a statistically significant 37% drop in menstrual symptoms. In that report, adolescent girls with dysmenorrhea took an unspecified amount of fish oil that provided 1,080 mg of EPA and 720 mg of DHA per day for two months to achieve this result.[15] A double-blind trial found that the same amount of EPA and DHA plus 7.5 mcg per day of vitamin B_{12} led to a greater than 50% decrease in menstrual symptoms, but a group taking only fish oil did not obtain as much relief.[16] Six grams of fish oil per day provides the approximate levels of EPA and DHA used in these trials.

In a double-blind trial, adolescents living in India who were suffering from dysmenorrhea took 100 mg of **vitamin B_1** (page 597) (thiamine) per day for three months. Eighty-seven percent of those treated experienced marked relief of dysmenorrhea symptoms.[17] However, vitamin B_1 deficiency is relatively common in India, whereas it is rare in the Western world, except among alcoholics. It is not known whether vitamin B_1 supplementation would relieve dysmenorrhea in women who are not B_1 deficient.

In a double-blind trial, supplementation with 500 IU of **vitamin E** (page 609) per day for two months, beginning two days before menstruation and continuing for three days after the onset of menstruation, was significantly more effective than a placebo at relieving menstrual pain.[18]

Some practitioners report success using topical **progesterone** (page 577) cream for dysmenorrhea.[19] To date, this approach lacks sufficient research.

Are there any side effects or interactions?
Refer to the individual supplement for information about any side effects or interactions.

Herbs that may be helpful
Corydalis (page 663) contains several alkaloids, and one called tetrahydropalmatine (THP) is considered to be the most potent. In laboratory research, THP has been shown to exhibit a wide number of pharmacological actions on the central nervous system, including pain-relieving and sedative effects.[20] According to a secondary reference, painful menstruation responded favorably to the administration of THP.[21] For a pain-relieving effect, the recommended amount for the crude dried rhizome is 5–10 grams per day. Alternatively, one can take 10–20 ml per day of a 1:2 extract.
Cramp bark *(Viburnum opulus)* has been a favorite traditional herb for menstrual cramps, thus its signature

name. Cramp bark may help ease severe cramps that are associated with nausea, vomiting, and sweaty chills. Research from animal studies shows that cramp bark blocks spasms of smooth muscle.[22] Cramp bark is traditionally prepared by placing two teaspoons of the dried bark into a cup of water and bringing it to a boil; it is then simmered gently for 10 to 15 minutes. The tea may be drunk three times per day.[23] Alternatively, 4–8 ml of tincture may be used three times per day.

Black cohosh (page 637) has a history as a folk medicine for relieving menstrual cramps. Black cohosh can be taken in several forms, including crude plant, dried root, or rhizome (300–2,000 mg per day), or as a solid, dry powdered extract (250 mg three times per day). Standardized extracts of the herb are available, though they have primarily been researched for use with **menopausal** (page 311) women suffering from hot flashes. The recommended amount is 20–40 mg twice per day.[24] The best researched form provides 1 mg of deoxyactein per 20 mg of extract. Tinctures can are also used (2–4 ml three times per day).[25] The Commission E Monograph recommends black cohosh be taken for up to six months, and then discontinued.[26]

Blue cohosh (page 643), although unrelated to black cohosh, has also been used traditionally for easing painful menstrual periods. Blue cohosh, which is generally taken as a tincture, should be limited to no more than 1–2 ml taken three times per day. The average single application of the whole herb is 300–1,000 mg. Blue cohosh is generally used in combination with other herbs. Women of childbearing age using this herb should cease using it as soon as they become **pregnant** (page 363)—the herb was shown to cause heart problems in an infant born following maternal use of blue cohosh.[27]

False unicorn (page 675) was used in the Native American tradition for a large number of women's health conditions, including painful menstruation. Generally, false unicorn root is taken as a tincture (2–5 ml three times per day). The dried root may also be used (1–2 grams three times daily). It is typically taken in combination with other herbs supportive of the female reproductive organs.

Dong quai (page 668) has been used either alone or in combination with other Traditional Chinese Medicine herbs to help relieve painful menstrual cramps. Many women take 3–4 grams per day. A Japanese herbal formulation known as toki-shakuyaku-san combines **peony** (page 724) root (*Paeonia* spp.) with dong quai and four other herbs and has been found to effectively reduce symptoms of cramping and pain associated with dysmenorrhea.[28]

Vervain (page 756) is a traditional herb for dysmenorrhea, however there is no research to validate this use. Tincture has been recommended at an amount of 5–10 ml three times per day.

Clinical reports from Germany have suggested that **vitex** (page 757) may help relieve different menstrual abnormalities associated with premenstrual syndrome, including dysmenorrhea.[29] These studies used 40 drops of a liquid preparation that delivers the equivalent of 40 mg of the dried berries of the plant.

Are there any side effects or interactions?
Refer to the individual herb for information about any side effects or interactions.

Holistic approaches that may be helpful

Relaxation techniques have been used with some success to alleviate dysmenorrhea in some young women. According to one preliminary study, the symptoms of menstrual cramps, nausea, irritability, and poor concentration greatly improved after 20-minute relaxation sessions twice per week.[30]

Acupuncture may be a useful therapy in the treatment of dysmenorrhea. A preliminary trial reported that 86% of women treated with acupuncture for dysmenorrhea had complete cessation of pain for three consecutive menstrual periods.[31] Other preliminary trials have demonstrated similar results.[32, 33, 34] A controlled clinical trial reported 91% efficacy with acupuncture compared to 36.4% efficacy with sham acupuncture (using fake acupuncture points) and 18% efficacy in an untreated control group.[35] A small trial compared a 30-minute TENS (transcutaneous electrical nerve stimulation) treatment to stimulate acupuncture points with a placebo pill for dysmenorrhea. There was a large placebo effect in this study, and pain relief over the next several hours was not significantly better in the treatment group compared to placebo.[36] More controlled trials are needed to determine whether acupuncture is a useful treatment for dysmenorrhea.

Spinal manipulation has been investigated as a treatment for dysmenorrhea. One small preliminary study reported improvement in symptoms measured by a questionnaire.[37] A controlled clinical trial compared a single treatment of spinal manipulation to the low back and pelvis to a sham manipulation that was designed to be ineffective. Women receiving real manipulation reported twice as much relief as those receiving sham treatment.[38] A recent, larger trial repeated the above study, testing a series of treatments over two months. Women reported less pain from both real and sham treatment, but there was no difference between the groups.[39] Whether there is a real benefit from spinal manipulation for women with dysmenorrhea remains unclear at this time.

EATING DISORDERS

Eating disorders are complex conditions involving psychological factors and nutritional deficiencies. The term eating disorders includes anorexia nervosa, bulimia, and binge-eating.

The psychological factors may include an inability to cope with stress, problems with family and other relationships, feelings of deprivation, and experiences of physical, sexual, or emotional abuse. Psychotherapy is an essential part of the treatment for eating disorders, along with nutrition counseling and medical care as needed.[1]

A person with anorexia does not eat enough to maintain a healthy weight; she views herself as overweight and is anxious about gaining weight. Anorexia typically begins in early adolescence, mainly among girls, though the numbers of boys developing this condition is increasing. People with anorexia weigh less than 85% of the normal weight for their age and height. Excessive exercise, vomiting, and abuse of laxatives and/or diuretics may also occur. Severe anorexia can be life threatening.

Bulimia, also known as bingeing and purging, is more common than anorexia, and usually affects teenage girls and women in their twenties. It involves a recurring, emotionally driven cycle of compulsive consumption of large quantities of high-calorie food in a short period of time, followed by induced vomiting. Some individuals also use laxatives, drugs that induce vomiting, diuretics, or excessive exercise in an attempt to purge. About 50% of anorexics also purge, and both bulimia and anorexia can coexist in the same person.[2] Unlike those with anorexia, some people affected by bulimia maintain normal or even excessive body weight.

Binge-eating disorder is similar to bulimia but no purging is done. It is more common than either bulimia or anorexia nervosa, and people with binge-eating disorder are usually overweight.[3]

CHECKLIST FOR EATING DISORDERS

Rating	Nutritional Supplements	Herbs
★★★	**Multivitamin-mineral** (page 559) (for prevention and treatment of deficiencies in restrictive eating disorders only)	
★★☆	**Vitamin K₂** (page 612) (for anorexia nervosa; with medical supervision only) **Zinc** (page 614) (for anorexia nervosa)	
★☆☆	**5-HTP** (page 459) L-tryptophan (for bulimia) **Vitamin B₆** (page 600) (for bulimia)	

What are the symptoms of eating disorders?

People with eating disorders may have a preoccupation with weight and food, anxiety about their body image, and/or a feeling that they lose control over how much they eat. They may also exercise compulsively and, in women, experience missed menstrual periods. They may also frequently use laxatives, diet pills, and medicines designed to induce vomiting or reduce fluid retention.

Medical treatments

Prescription medications commonly prescribed for bulimia include the selective serotonin reuptake inhibitors fluoxetine (Prozac), paroxetine (Paxil), sertraline (Zoloft), venlafaxine (Effexor), and fluvoxamine (Luvox), as well as the tricyclic antidepressants amitriptyline (Elavil), desipramine (Norpramin), and imipramine (Tofranil). Individuals with anorexia nervosa are sometimes prescribed the antihistamine cyproheptadine (Periactin) to stimulate appetite.

Treatment for eating disorders also includes psychological counseling, such as cognitive-behavioral, interpersonal, psychodynamic, and family therapy.

Dietary changes that may be helpful

The most important dietary change for people with eating disorders is to eat a sufficient amount of calories without purging. To accomplish this, most will need psychological as well as nutrition counseling.

Individuals with both bulimia and anorexia are likely to report a craving for sugar; people with bulimia eat more sweets and carbohydrates, particularly during binges, than do healthy individuals.[4, 5, 6, 7] In a double-blind study, bulimic subjects were reported to have significantly more mood changes after receiving glucose (corn sugar) injections compared to placebo injections.[8] Preliminary evidence suggests that purging results in low blood sugar, which might increase the incidence of repeated bingeing and purging by stimulating appetite or altering mood.[9]

In a preliminary trial, researchers fed ten bulimic women a diet free of all alcohol, caffeine, refined sugar, and foods containing white flour, added salt, monosodium glutamate, and flavor enhancers. They were also given 1 gram of **vitamin C** (page 604), 50 mg of a **vitamin B-complex** (page 603), and a **multiple vitamin and mineral** (page 559) supplement.[10] Cigarette smoking was not allowed during the trial. After three weeks, all women on this diet plan stopped bingeing whereas another ten bulimic women consuming a normal diet continued to binge. When the women who had been eating a normal diet were also placed on the more healthful diet plan, they too stopped bingeing. All 20 women remained binge-free for more than two and a half years.

Lifestyle changes that may be helpful

Although regular, moderate exercise offers important health benefits, for many people *excessive* exercise is a common component of eating disorders, especially anorexia nervosa.[11] In one controlled trial, a majority of the people with eating disorders reported that participation in competitive sports and exercise performed as part of a weight loss plan contributed to their condition.[12] For people with eating disorders, it is important to establish and maintain healthy exercise habits; these individuals should consult with a healthcare professional skilled in eating disorders.

Nutritional supplements that may be helpful

People with eating disorders who restrict their food intake are at risk for multiple nutrient deficiencies, including protein, **calcium** (page 483), **iron** (page 540), **riboflavin** (page 598), **niacin** (page 598),[13] **folic acid** (page 520),[14] **vitamin A** (page 595), **vitamin C** (page 604),[15] and **vitamin B₆** (page 600),[16] and essential fatty acids.[17] A general **multivitamin-mineral** (page 559) formula can reduce the detrimental health effects of these deficiencies.

In a preliminary study of women with anorexia nervosa, those who supplemented with 45 mg of **vitamin**

K₂ (page 612) per day for approximately one year experienced significantly less bone loss, compared with women who did not take the supplement.[18] This study suggests that supplementing with vitamin K₂ may help prevent **osteoporosis** (page 333), which is a common complication of anorexia nervosa. The amount of vitamin K₂ used in this study was much larger than the amount of vitamin K found in food and most supplements. Moreover, vitamin K₂ is not yet generally available as a supplement, although it can be obtained through some nutritionally oriented doctors. Individuals interested in using this treatment should be monitored by a doctor.

Zinc (page 614) deficiency has also been detected in people with anorexia or bulimia in most,[19, 20] though not all,[21] studies. In addition, some of the manifestations of zinc deficiency, such as reduced appetite, taste, and smell, are similar to symptoms observed in some cases of anorexia or bulimia.[22]

In an uncontrolled trial, supplementation with 45–90 mg per day of zinc resulted in weight gain in 17 out of 20 anorexics after 8–56 months.[23] In a double-blind study, 35 women hospitalized with anorexia, given 14 mg of zinc per day, achieved a 10% increase in weight twice as fast as the group that received a placebo.[24] In another report, a group of adolescent girls with anorexia, some of whom were hospitalized, was found to be consuming 7.7 mg of zinc per day in their diet—only half the recommended amount.[25] Providing these girls with 50 mg of zinc per day in a double-blind trial helped diminish their **depression** (page 145) and **anxiety** (page 30) levels, but had no significant effect on weight gain. Anyone taking zinc supplements for more than a few weeks should also supplement with 1 to 3 mg per day of **copper** (page 499) to prevent a zinc-induced copper deficiency.

Serotonin, a hormone that helps regulate food intake and appetite, is synthesized in the brain from the **amino acid** (page 465) L-tryptophan. Preliminary data suggest that some people with bulimia have low serotonin levels.[26] Researchers have reported that bulimic women with experimentally induced tryptophan deficiency tend to eat more and become more irritable compared to healthy women fed the same diet,[27, 28] though not all studies have demonstrated these effects.[29]

Weight-loss diets result in lower L-tryptophan and serotonin levels in women,[30] which could theoretically trigger bingeing and purging in susceptible people.

However, the benefits of L-tryptophan supplementation are unclear. One small, double-blind trial reported significant improvement in eating behavior, feelings about eating, and mood among women with bulimia who were given 1 gram of L-tryptophan and 45 mg of **vitamin B₆** (page 600) three times per day.[31] Other double-blind studies using only L-tryptophan have failed to confirm these findings.[32, 33] L-tryptophan is available by prescription only; most drug stores do not carry it, but "compounding" pharmacies do. Most cities have at least one compounding pharmacy, which prepares customized prescription medications to meet individual patient's needs.

Another serotonin precursor, **5-hydroxytryptophan** (page 459) (5-HTP), has been shown to reduce appetite in weight-control and **diabetes** (page 152) trials.[34, 35, 36] However, what effect 5-HTP has, if any, on people with binge eating disorder, bulimia, or anorexia is unknown. Unlike L-tryptophan, 5-HTP is available from health food stores and some pharmacies without prescription.

Are there any side effects or interactions?
Refer to the individual supplement for information about any side effects or interactions.

Holistic approaches that may be helpful
Psychological counseling, for both the individual and her family, and behavior modification training are also commonly used for people with eating disorders, often as part of a team approach that also includes nutrition counseling and medical care. Numerous preliminary and controlled studies have shown that the psychotherapy technique known as cognitive-behavioral therapy is effective in reducing the symptoms of bulimia.[37, 38] For example, one study found 69% of a group receiving cognitive-behavioral therapy were abstaining from binge-eating and purging six months later compared to only 15% of a group keeping a diary of their behavior.[39] Preliminary studies[40] and one controlled trial[41] suggest another technique, interpersonal psychotherapy, is equally effective for people with bulimia. Cognitive behavioral therapy and interpersonal psychotherapy have also been effective for people with binge-eating disorder in controlled trials,[42, 43] resulting in cessation of binge-eating in almost half of the subjects in one report.[44]

The effectiveness of psychotherapy for anorexia nervosa is less clear.[45, 46] One controlled trial found that psychotherapy (type unspecified) significantly improved weight gain compared to no treatment, and complete or nearly complete recovery occurred in 60% of the patients.[47] Two other studies comparing different types of psychotherapy for anorexia nervosa found comparable improvement from all types;[48, 49] one of these studies reported moderate improvement in 63% of cases.[50] Long-term effectiveness of psychotherapy for eating disorders has not been studied.

ECZEMA

What do I need to know?

Self-care for eczema can be approached in a number of ways—but it can be hard to know just where to start. To make it easier, our doctors recommend trying these simple steps first:

Avoid allergens and irritants
> Work with a qualified professional to identify airborne allergens, chemicals, foods, and irritants that make your condition worse

Take fatty acids
> Supply anti-inflammatory fatty acids missing in many people with eczema by taking 500 to 1,000 mg a day of GLA (gamma-linolenic acid) from evening primrose oil or borage oil, or 1,800 mg a day of EPA (eicosapentaenoic acid) from fish oils; children should take amounts proportionately less according to body weight

Help children avoid allergies with beneficial bacteria
> Pregnant women and newborns should get supplements that contain 10 billion colony-forming units a day of Lactobacillus-type bacteria to reduce risk of eczema in early life

About eczema

Eczema is a common inflammatory condition of the skin.

Many skin diseases cause symptoms similar to those of eczema, so it is important to have the disease properly diagnosed before it is treated.

What are the symptoms of eczema?

Eczema is characterized by scaling, thickened patches of skin that can become red and fissured. It may also appear as tiny blisters (called vesicles) that rupture, weep, and crust over. The most troublesome and prevalent symptom of eczema is itching, which may be constant.

CHECKLIST FOR ECZEMA		
Rating	Nutritional Supplements	Herbs
★★☆	**Borage oil** (page 475) **Evening primrose oil** (page 511) **Fish oil** (page 514) (EPA/ **DHA** [page 509]) **Probiotics** (page 575)	**Calendula** (page 650) (for radiation-induced dermatitis) **Chamomile** (page 656) **St. John's wort** (page 747) **Witch hazel** (page 760) Zemaphyte Chinese herbal formula
★☆☆	**Vitamin C** (page 604)	**Calendula** (page 650) **Chickweed** (page 658) **Licorice** (page 702) **Oak** (page 716) **Oats** (page 716) **Onion** (page 718) **Red clover** (page 735) **Sarsaparilla** (page 742) Shiunko (topical)

Medical treatments

Over the counter products for mild cases of eczema contain topical hydrocortisone (Cortaid, Cortizone). Emollients are often recommended to hydrate the excessively dry skin of eczema. Common emollients include white petrolatum and hydrogenated vegetable oil. Numerous emollient products are also available, such as Keri, Eucerin, Lubriderm, and Nivea.

Prescription strength topical corticosteroid creams or ointments are commonly prescribed. Drugs available include triamcinolone (Aristocort, Kenalog), fluocinonide (Lidex), betamethasone (Valisone, Diprosone, Diprolene), mometasone (Elocon), and clobetasol (Temovate). The nonsteroidal cream pimecrolimus (Elidel) may be used as well. Infected, weepy lesions might be treated with oral antibiotics, such as cephalexin (Keflex) and amoxicillin/clavulanate (Augmentin).

Avoidance of known **allergens** (page 14), as well as known irritants such as soap and hot water, is also recommended.

Eczema

Eczema

Dietary changes that may be helpful

Eczema can be triggered by **allergies** (page 14).[1, 2] Most children with eczema have food allergies, according to data from double-blind research.[3] A doctor should be consulted to determine whether allergies are a factor. Once the trigger for the allergy has been identified, avoidance of the allergen can lead to significant improvement.[4] However, "classical" food allergens (e.g., cows' milk, egg, wheat, soy, and nuts) are often not the cause of eczema in adults. A variety of substances have been shown, in a controlled trial, to trigger eczema reactions in susceptible individuals; avoidance of these substances has similarly been shown to improve the eczema. Triggers included food additives, histamine, salicylates, benzoates, and other compounds (such as aromatic compounds) found in fruits, vegetables, and spices.[5] These reactions do not represent true food allergies but are instead a type of food sensitivity reaction. The authors of this study did not identify which substances are the most common triggers.

It has been reported that when heavy coffee drinkers with eczema avoided coffee, eczema symptoms improved.[6] In this study, the reaction was to coffee, not caffeine, indicating that some people with eczema may be allergic to coffee. People with eczema who are using a hypoallergenic diet to investigate food allergies should avoid coffee as part of this trial.

Nutritional supplements that may be helpful

Researchers have reported that people with eczema do not have the normal ability to process fatty acids, which can result in a deficiency of gamma-linolenic acid (GLA).[7] GLA is found in **evening primrose oil** (page 511) (EPO), **borage oil** (page 475), and black currant seed oil. Some,[8, 9, 10] but not all,[11, 12, 13, 14] double-blind trials have shown that EPO is useful in the treatment of eczema. An analysis of nine trials reported that the effects for reduced itching were most striking.[15] Much of the research uses 12 pills per day; each pill contains 500 mg of EPO, of which 45 mg is GLA. Smaller amounts have been shown to lack efficacy.[16]

Supplementation with **borage** (page 475) oil, another source of GLA, has led to reductions in skin inflammation, dryness, scaliness, and itch in eczema patients in some,[17] but not all, preliminary[18] or double-blind trials.[19]

Many years ago, use of large amounts of vegetable oil (containing precursors to GLA) was reported to help treat people with eczema,[20, 21] but these studies were not controlled and do not meet modern standards of research.

Ten grams of **fish oil** (page 514) providing 1.8 grams of EPA (eicosapentaenoic acid) per day were given to a group of eczema sufferers in a double-blind trial. After 12 weeks, those using the fish oil experienced significant improvement.[22, 23] According to the researchers, fish oil may be effective because it reduces levels of leukotriene B4, a substance that has been linked to eczema.[24] The eczema-relieving effects of fish oil may require taking ten pills per day for at least 12 weeks. Smaller amounts of fish oil have been shown to lack efficacy.[25]

One trial using vegetable oil as the placebo reported that fish oil was barely more effective than the placebo (30% vs. 24% improvement).[26] As vegetable oil had previously been reported to have potential therapeutic activity, the apparent negative outcome of this trial should not dissuade people with eczema from considering fish oil.

Although supplementation with 400 IU of **vitamin E** (page 609) per day has been reported in anecdotal accounts to alleviate eczema,[27] research has not supported this effect.[28] Moreover, rare cases of topical vitamin E potentially *causing* eczema have appeared.[29] People with eczema should not expect vitamin E to be helpful with their condition.

A double-blind trial reported that use of a hypoallergenic infant formula plus **probiotics** (page 575) (500 million organisms of Lactobacillus GG bacteria per gram of formula, taken for one month) initially led to improvement in eczema symptoms in infants with suspected **allergy** (page 14) to cows'milk.[30] However, by the end of two months, both the group receiving Lactobacillus GG and the placebo group had improved approximately the same amount. In the same report, a preliminary trial giving 20 billion Lactobacilli twice per day to **breast-feeding** (page 74) mothers led to significant improvement of their allergic infants' eczema after one month. Probiotics may reduce allergic reactions by improving digestion, by helping the intestinal tract control the absorption of food allergens, and/or by changing immune system responses.

In 1989, *Medical World News* reported that researchers from the University of Texas found that **vitamin C** (page 604), at 50–75 mg per 2.2 pounds of body weight, reduced symptoms of eczema in a double-blind trial.[31] In theory, vitamin C might be beneficial in treating eczema by affecting the **immune system** (page 255), but further research has yet to investigate any role for this vitamin in people with eczema.

Are there any side effects or interactions?
Refer to the individual supplement for information about any side effects or interactions.

Herbs that may be helpful
The table below summarizes the three categories of herbs used for people with eczema: anti-inflammatories and herbs that affect the immune system (immunomodulators), astringents (herbs that bind fluids and exudates), and herbs that affect the liver (also called alteratives). Alterative herbs are poorly researched. Astringents are only helpful if applied topically when weeping eczema is present; they will not help people with dry eczema.

Mechanism of Action	Examples
Anti-inflammatory and/or immunomodulator	*Allium cepa*, **Calendula** (page 650), **chamomile** (page 656), **chickweed** (page 658), **licorice** (page 702), **onion** (page 718), Zemaphyte Chinese herbal formula
Astringent (helps dry up weeping lesions)	**Oak** (page 716), **witch hazel** (page 760) (also anti-inflammatory)
Alterative (liver-supportive)	**Burdock** (page 648), **red clover** (page 735), **sarsaparilla** (page 742), **wild oats** (page 716)

Zemaphyte, a traditional Chinese herbal preparation that includes **licorice** (page 702) as well as nine other herbs, has been successful in treating childhood and adult eczema in double-blind trials.[32, 33, 34] One or two packets of the combination is mixed in hot water and taken once per day. Because one study included the same amount of licorice in both the placebo and the active medicine, it is unlikely that licorice is the main active component of Zemaphyte.[35]

Several Chinese herbal creams for eczema have been found to be adulterated with steroids. The authors of one study found that 8 of 11 Chinese herbal creams purchased without prescription in England contained a powerful steroid drug used to treat inflammatory skin conditions.[36]

A cream prepared with **witch hazel** (page 760) and **phosphatidylcholine** (page 546) has been reported to be as effective as 1% hydrocortisone in the topical management of eczema, according to one double-blind trial.[37]

Topical applications of **chamomile** (page 656) have been shown to be moderately effective in the treatment of eczema.[38, 39] One trial found it to be about 60% as effective as 0.25% hydrocortisone cream.[40]

In a double-blind trial, people with eczema applied a cream containing an extract of **St. John's wort** (page 747) to the affected areas on one side of the body, and a placebo (the same cream without the St. John's wort) to the other side. The treatment was administered twice a day for four weeks. The severity of the eczema improved to a significantly greater extent on the side treated with St. John's wort than on the side treated with placebo.[41] Although the mechanism by which St. John's wort relieves eczema is not known, it might be due to the anti-inflammatory and antibacterial effects of hyperforin, one of its constituents. The cream used in this study contained 5% of an extract of St. John's wort (standardized to 1.5% hyperforin). As topical application of St. John's wort can cause sensitivity to the sun, care should be taken to avoid excessive sun exposure when using this treatment.

Onion (page 718) injections into the skin and topical onion applications have been shown to inhibit skin inflammation in people with eczema, according to one double-blind trial.[42] The quantity or form of onion that might be most effective is unknown.

A Japanese topical ointment called Shiunko has been reported to help improve symptoms of eczema, according to preliminary research.[43] The ointment contains sesame oil and four herbs (*Lithospermum* radix, *Angelica* radix, *Cera alba,* and *Adeps suillus*) and was applied twice daily along with petrolatum and 3.5% salt water for three weeks. Clinical improvement was seen in four of the seven people using Shiunko.

Topical preparations containing **calendula** (page 650), **chickweed** (page 658), or **oak** (page 716) bark[44] have been used traditionally to treat people with eczema but none of these has been studied in scientific research focusing on people with eczema.

Radiation therapy for breast cancer frequently causes painful dermatitis at the radiation site. In a study of women undergoing radiation therapy for breast cancer, those who topically applied ***Calendula officinalis*** (page 650) had significantly fewer cases of severe dermatitis, compared with those who used a standard medication.[45] Calendula treatment was begun after the first radiation session and was applied twice a day or more, depending on whether dermatitis or pain occurred.

Burdock (page 648), **sarsaparilla** (page 742), **red clover** (page 735), and **wild oats** (page 716) have been used historically to treat people with eczema, but without scientific investigation.

Are there any side effects or interactions?
Refer to the individual herb for information about any side effects or interactions.

Holistic approaches that may be helpful

Numerous trials have reported that hypnosis improves eczema in children and adults.[46] A preliminary trial emphasizing relaxation, stress management, and direct suggestion in hypnosis showed reduced itching, scratching, and sleep disturbance, as well as reduced requirements for topical corticosteroids. All of the patients studied had been resistant to conventional treatment.[47]

EDEMA

Abnormal accumulation of fluid beneath the skin is known as edema. This leads to a puffy appearance, often to a limb, most commonly a leg.

There are many causes of edema. In some cases, the underlying problem (for example, **congestive heart failure** [page 134] or **preeclampsia** [page 361] of pregnancy) must be medically treated in order for the edema to resolve. In other cases (such as **chronic venous insufficiency** [page 116], edema following **minor trauma** [page 319], or lymphedema resulting from damage to lymphatic vessels caused by surgery and other medical treatments), it is possible with both conventional and natural approaches to focus specifically on the edema. Unless edema is clearly due to minor trauma, it should never be treated until the underlying cause has been properly diagnosed by a healthcare professional. The discussion below deals only with situations in which it is safe to focus on the edema itself and not the underlying cause.

What are the symptoms of edema?

People with edema may notice that a ring on their finger feels tighter than in the past, or they might have difficulty in putting on shoes, especially toward the end of the day. They may also notice a puffiness of the face around the eyes, or in the feet, ankles, and legs. When edema is present, pressure on the skin, such as from the elastic band on socks, may leave an indentation that is slow to disappear. Edema of the abdomen, called ascites, may be a sign of serious underlying disease and must be immediately evaluated by a doctor.

Rating	Nutritional Supplements	Herbs
★★★	**Flavonoids** (page 516) (courmarin, hydroxyethyl-rutosides)	
★★☆	**Flavonoids** (page 516) (diosmin and hesperidin combination) **Selenium** (page 584) (for lymphedema)	
★☆☆	**Flavonoids** (page 516) (**quercetin** [page 580])	**Cleavers** (page 660) Corn silk **Dandelion** (page 666) (leaves) Goldenrod **Horse chestnut** (page 692) **Horsetail** (page 693) **Juniper** (page 698)

CHECKLIST FOR EDEMA (WATER RETENTION)

Medical treatments

Over the counter diuretics containing ammonium chloride and caffeine (Aqua-Ban) may be used to relieve symptoms related to edema or water retention when taken five to six days before menses. More severe edematous conditions require medical attention.

Treatment of edema with prescription medications is limited to the use of diuretics, commonly referred to as "water pills." Agents often used include the thiazide diuretics, such as hydrochlorothiazide (HydroDIURIL), indapamide (Lozol), and metolazone (Zaroxolyn); loop diuretics including furosemide (Lasix), bumetanide (Bumex), and torsemide (Demadex); and potassium-sparing diuretics, such as spironolactone (Aldactone), triamterene (Dyazide, Maxzide), and amiloride (Midamor).

Commonly, treatment consists of managing the underlying condition, which may include inadequate nutrition; liver, **heart** (page 98), and kidney disease; or obstruction of blood or lymph flow. In some cases, a salt-restricted diet may be recommended.

Dietary changes that may be helpful

High salt intake should be avoided, as it tends to lead to water retention and may worsen edema in some people. A controlled trial found that a low-salt diet (less than 2,100 mg sodium per day) resulted in reduced water retention after two months in a group of women with unexplained edema.[1]

Lifestyle changes that may be helpful

If the edema is affecting one limb, the limb should be kept elevated whenever possible. This allows fluid to drain more effectively from the congested area. To decrease fluid buildup in the legs, people should avoid sitting or standing for long periods of time without moving.

Nutritional supplements that may be helpful

Several double-blind trials[2, 3, 4, 5] have found that 400 mg per day of coumarin, a **flavonoid** (page 516) found in a variety of herbs, can improve many types of edema, including lymphedema after surgery. However, a large double-blind trial detected no benefit using 200 mg coumarin twice daily for six months in women who had arm edema after mastectomy (surgical breast removal).[6] (Coumarin should not be confused with the anticlotting drug Coumadin.)

A group of semi-synthetic **flavonoids** (page 516), known as hydroxyethylrutosides are also beneficial for some types of edema.[7] One double-blind trial found that 2 grams per day of hydroxyethylrutosides reduced ankle and foot edema in people with venous disorders after four weeks.[8] Another double-blind trial found that 3 grams per day of hydroxyethylrutosides significantly reduced lymphedema of the arm or leg and lessened the associated uncomfortable symptoms.[9]

A combination of the flavonoids diosmin (900 mg per day) and hesperidin (100 mg per day) has been investigated for the treatment of a variety of venous circulation disorders.[10] However, in a double-blind trial, this combination was not effective for lymphedema caused by **breast cancer** (page 65) treatments.[11]

In a preliminary study, individuals with lymphedema of the arm or head-and-neck region were treated with approximately 230 mcg of selenium per day, in the form of sodium selenite, for four to six weeks. A quality-of-life assessment showed an improvement of 59%, and the circumference of the edematous arm was reduced in 10 of 12 cases.[12]

Because coumarin, hydroxyethylrutosides, and diosmin are not widely available in the United States, other flavonoids, such as **quercetin** (page 580), rutin, or anthocyanosides (from **bilberry** [page 634]), have been substituted by doctors in an attempt to obtain similar benefits. The effect of these other flavonoids against edema has not been well studied. Also, optimal amounts are not known. However, in one study, quercetin in amounts of 30–50 mg per day corrected abnormal capillary permeability (leakiness),[13] an effect that might improve edema. A similar effect has been reported with rutin at 20 mg three times per day.[14] Doctors often recommend 80–160 mg of a standardized extract of bilberry, three times per day.

Whereas **vitamin B$_6$** (page 600) is sometimes recommended for reducing edema, no research has investigated its effectiveness.

Are there any side effects or interactions?
Refer to the individual supplement for information about any side effects or interactions.

Herbs that may be helpful

A double-blind trial found that a formula containing **butcher's broom** (page 649) extract, the **flavonoid** (page 516) hesperidin, and **vitamin C** (page 604), which is used in Europe to treat venous and lymphatic system disorders, was superior to placebo for reducing lymphedema.[15] The amount of butcher's broom extract typically used is 150 mg two or three times per day.

Herbs that stimulate the kidneys were traditionally used to reduce edema. Herbal diuretics do not work the same way that drugs do, thus it is unclear whether such herbs would be effective for this purpose. Goldenrod *(Solidago cnadensis)* is considered one of the strongest herbal diuretics.[16] Animal studies show, at very high amounts (2 grams per 2.2 pounds of body weight), that **dandelion** (page 666) leaves possess diuretic effects that may be comparable to the prescription diuretic furosemide (Lasix).[17] Human clinical trials have not been completed to confirm these results. Corn silk *(Zea mays)* has also long been used as a diuretic, though a human study did not find that it increased urine output.[18] Thus, diuretic herbs are not yet well supported for use in reducing edema.

Aescin, isolated from **horse chestnut** (page 692) seed, has been shown to effectively reduce post-surgical edema in preliminary trials.[19, 20] A form of aescin that is injected into the bloodstream is often used but only under the supervision of a qualified healthcare professional.

Horsetail (page 693) has a diuretic (urine flow increasing) action that accounts for its traditional use in reducing mild edema. Although there is no clinical research that yet supports its use for people with edema, the German government has approved horsetail for this use. The volatile oils in **juniper** (page 698) cause an increase in urine volume and in this way can theoretically lessen edema;[21] however, there is no clinical research that yet supports its use for people with edema.

Cleavers (page 666) is one of numerous plants considered in ancient times to act as a diuretic.[22] It was therefore used to relieve edema and to promote urine formation during bladder infections.

Are there any side effects or interactions?
Refer to the individual herb for information about any side effects or interactions.

ENDOMETRIOSIS

Endometriosis is a progressive and chronic condition in which endometrial tissue (the inner lining of the uterus that is shed each month during menses) is found outside of the uterus and implanted within the pelvic cavity.

Endometriosis is believed to affect as many as 10% of all women in the United States and is the third leading cause of gynecologic hospitalization and a leading cause of hysterectomy.[1] Although many theories exist, the cause of endometriosis is unclear. However, there does appear to be a genetic link—women who have a mother or sister with endometriosis are more likely to develop this condition.

What are the symptoms of endometriosis?
Women with endometriosis may have symptoms including pain before and during menstrual periods, pain with sexual intercourse, abdominal bloating, pain during urination or bowel movements, pelvic tenderness, premenstrual spotting, abnormally heavy or long menstrual periods, rectal bleeding during menstrual periods, and an inability to become pregnant.

Rating	Nutritional Supplements	Herbs
CHECKLIST FOR ENDOMETRIOSIS		
★★☆	**Vitamin C** (page 604) and **vitamin E** (page 609) (in combination)	
★☆☆	**Fish oil** (page 514)	**Vitex** (page 757)

Medical treatments
Over the counter drugs for inflamation, such as aspirin (Bayer, Ecotrin, Bufferin), ibuprofen (Motrin, Advil), and naproxen (Aleve), might be beneficial.

Prescription drug treatment focuses on controlling inflammation and reducing estrogen and progesterone blood levels. Prescription strength nonsteroidal anti-inflammatory drugs (NSAIDs), such as ibuprofen (Motrin), naproxen (Anaprox, Naprosyn), indomethacin (Indocin), ketoprofen (Orudis), and diclofenac (Voltaren), help control inflamation. Oral birth control pills (Ortho-Novum, Mircette, Loestrin, Triphasil), antiestrogens such as danocrine (Danazol), progestins including progesterone (Prometrium) and medroxyprogesterone (Provera), and gonadotropin-releasing hormones, such as leuprolide (Lupron) and goserelin (Zoladex), are prescribed to affect hormone levels.

Surgical treatments, such as removal of the endometrial areas, ovaries, or uterus may also be recommended.

Dietary changes that may be helpful
There has been no research investigating the effect of any specific diet in women with endometriosis. Preliminary research suggests that women who consume more than 5 grams of caffeine per month (about 1.5 cups of coffee a day) are more likely to have endometriosis.[2] No study has investigated whether avoiding caffeine improves the symptoms of endometriosis.

Lifestyle changes that may be helpful
Preliminary studies suggest that women who exercise two to four hours per week have less risk of developing endometriosis.[3, 4] However, the benefit seems to be limited to those women who participate in vigorous exercise, such as jogging or other activities that raise the heart rate. Whether exercise will reduce the symptoms of existing endometriosis is unknown.

Nutritional supplements that may be helpful
In a study of women with pelvic pain presumed to be due to endometriosis, supplementation with **vitamin E** (page 609) (1,200 IU per day) and **vitamin C** (page 604) (1,000 mg per day) for two months resulted in an improvement of pain in 43% of women, whereas none of the women receiving a placebo reported pain relief.[5]

Animal research suggests that **fish oils** (page 514) may reduce the severity of endometriosis,[6, 7] and fish oils have been shown to improve symptoms of **dysmenorrhea** (page 171) (painful menstruation),[8] which may be caused by endometriosis. Therefore, while no specific research has been done on the effects of fish oils in women with endometriosis, some health practitioners recommend several grams of fish oil per day for this condition.

Are there any side effects or interactions?
Refer to the individual supplement for information about any side effects or interactions.

Herbs that may be helpful

Vitex (page 757) is recommended either alone or in combination with other herbs, such as **dandelion root** (page 666), **prickly ash** (page 731), and **motherwort** (page 712), by some doctors to treat the symptoms of endometriosis.[9, 10] Although vitex affects hormones that in turn affect the severity of endometriosis,[11] and it may be effective for **premenstrual syndrome** (page 368),[12] no research has tested the effect of vitex supplementation on women with endometriosis. Similarly, no other botanical medicines have been scientifically researched for treating this disease.

Are there any side effects or interactions?
Refer to the individual herb for information about any side effects or interactions.

Holistic approaches that may be helpful

According to preliminary reports, regular meetings with other endometriosis sufferers may help women with endometriosis learn about the disease and cope better with the many psychological and emotional issues that often accompany this condition.[13] One preliminary study found that women who had the opportunity to speak with other women with endometriosis, as well as to meet with their physician, had a higher satisfaction with their overall care.[14]

Acupuncture has been reported anecdotally to help control the pain associated with some cases of endometriosis,[15] but no controlled studies have confirmed this claim. One small, preliminary study found that auricular acupuncture (acupuncture of the ear) was as effective as hormone therapy in treating infertility due to endometriosis.[16]

EPILEPSY

Epilepsy is a brain disorder in which abnormal bursts of electrical activity occur in cells of the brain, resulting in seizures.

There are many types of epilepsy, usually categorized by the symptoms that occur during seizures. The cause of many types of epilepsy is unknown, and frequently no cure is available. Rather, treatment focuses on reducing the frequency and severity of seizures.

CHECKLIST FOR EPILEPSY		
Rating	Nutritional Supplements	Herbs
★★★	**Vitamin E** (page 609) (for children)	
★★☆	**EPA and DHA** (page 514)	**Bupleurum** (page 647) in combination with **peony** (page 724) root, pinellia root, cassia bark, **ginger** (page 680) root jujube fruit, **Asian ginseng** (page 630) root, **Chinese scullcap** (page 658) root, and **licorice** (page 702) root
★☆☆	**Folic acid** (page 520) **Melatonin** (page 555) **Taurine** (page 590) **Vitamin B$_6$** (page 600) **Vitamin E** (page 609) (for adults)	**Bacopa** (page 632)

What are the symptoms of epilepsy?

There are many types of seizures in epilepsy. They are categorized as either partial or generalized, depending on how much of the brain is involved. Some types of epilepsy involve seizures characterized by convulsive muscle contractions of all or some parts of the body. Other types can involve momentary loss of consciousness, amnesia, unusual sensations or emotions, and other symptoms. Symptoms that indicate an imminent seizure (called auras) may occur. Similarly, non-convulsive symptoms, including deep sleep, headache, confusion, and muscle soreness (called a postictal state), may follow a generalized seizure.

Medical treatments

Prescription drug therapy focuses on reducing the frequency and severity of seizures. Agents prescribed depend on the type of seizures experienced by the patient. Multiple drug therapy might be necessary for some individuals. Commonly prescribed drugs include benzodiazepines, such as clonazepam (Klonipin), clorazepate (Tranxene), and diazepam (Valium), as well as phenytoin (Dilantin), lamotrigine (Lamictal), carbamazepine (Tegretol), oxcarbazepine (Trileptal), valproic acid (Depakene, Depakote), gabapentin (Neurontin), levetiracetam (Keppra), and phenobarbital.

Epilepsy

About 10 to 20% of epilepsy patients do not respond to drug therapy and may require surgery.

Dietary changes that may be helpful
The ketogenic diet was developed in the early twentieth century when few drug treatments for epilepsy were available; until recently, it had been used only when drug therapy was ineffective. The dietary approach was based on the observation that ketosis (increased blood levels of chemicals called ketones) is associated with reduction of seizures.[1] Ketosis can be produced by a diet high in fat and very low in carbohydrate and protein. The ketogenic diet has been evaluated in several preliminary and a few controlled trials. According to a 1996 review, the ketogenic diet appears to be very effective in one-third to one-half of epilepsy cases in children, and partially effective in another one-third of cases.[2]

Recent trials continue to support this success rate;[3, 4, 5] one preliminary trial demonstrated a 50% reduction in seizure activity in 71% of children in a group after 45 days on the diet. There is little research on the effects of the ketogenic diet in adults, but it may be effective in those who are able to comply with the strict dietary guidelines.[6, 7] The diet is usually initiated by fasting under close medical supervision, often in a hospital, followed by introduction of the diet and training of the family to ensure successful maintenance.

Possible side effects of the ketogenic diet include gastrointestinal upset, dehydration, **anemia** (page 25), low blood protein levels, high blood levels of fat and acidity, **kidney stones** (page 284), and signs of liver toxicity.[8, 9] Vitamin and mineral supplementation is necessary due to the many deficiencies of this unusual diet.[10] The ketogenic diet should not be attempted without the supervision of a qualified healthcare professional. Practical information about the ketogenic diet is available in recent texts [11] and articles,[12] as well as on the Internet.[13]

The Atkins diet is similar to the ketogenic diet, in that they are both high in fat and very low in carbohydrate. The Atkins diet, however, is easier to follow than the ketogenic diet, as it allows more liberal amounts of protein and has fewer calorie restrictions. Since the Atkins diet can produce ketosis, it has the potential to benefit people with epilepsy. In a preliminary study, three of six individuals with treatment-resistant epilepsy experienced marked improvement on the Atkins diet; two of these people became seizure-free.[14]

Allergic reactions (page 14) to food have been reported to trigger epileptic seizures in individual cases,[15, 16] some of which were proven with double-blind testing.[17] One report found people with epilepsy to have significantly more biochemical evidence of allergy than do non-epileptics.[18] A study of children who suffered from both epilepsy and **migraine headaches** (page 316) found that a diet low in potential food allergens reduced seizures in the majority of cases; however, children who had epilepsy alone without migraines did not respond to the diet.[19] Another report confirmed that children who have epilepsy without migraines do not improve on a low-allergen diet.[20] Some doctors recommend that people with epilepsy and other allergic symptoms, such as **asthma** (page 32) or **hay fever** (page 211), should be checked for food allergies that may be causing seizures.[21]

Nutritional supplements that may be helpful
Vitamin E (page 609) has been studied as a possible add-on to conventional drug treatment for epilepsy. A double-blind trial found that adding 400 IU per day of vitamin E reduced seizure frequency in children without side effects.[22] Other preliminary trials[23, 24] have reported similar results, and, while some preliminary research suggested this effect might also be achieved in adults,[25] a double-blind trial found no effect of vitamin E supplementation on adults with epilepsy.[26]

Folic acid (page 520) supplementation (5 mg per day) was reported to reduce epileptic seizure frequency, though the effect was not significantly better than with placebo.[27] Folic acid supplementation of as little as 800 mcg per day has also been reported to interfere with the action of anticonvulsant medications, resulting in an *increase* in the frequency and/or severity of seizures;[28, 29, 30, 31] this effect occurs only in a small number of cases.[32, 33] People taking anticonvulsant medications should consult with the prescribing physician before deciding whether to use folic acid.

Vitamin B$_6$ (page 600) has been used to treat infants and small children who have seizures related to a genetic enzyme defect.[34, 35, 36, 37] However, this condition is not considered true epilepsy, and whether people with epilepsy would benefit from taking vitamin B$_6$ supplements is unknown.

Taurine (page 590) is an **amino acid** (page 465) that is thought to play a role in the electrical activity of the brain; deficits of taurine in the brain have been associated with some types of epilepsy. However, while some short-term studies have suggested that taurine supplementation may reduce epileptic seizures in some people, the effect appears to be only temporary.[38]

Case reports have suggested that **evening primrose oil** (page 511) may worsen symptoms in people with temporal lobe epilepsy.[39] Until more is known, people with this type of epilepsy should avoid using evening primrose oil supplements, except perhaps under the supervision of a qualified physician.

In a preliminary study, supplementation with 3.25 grams per day of a mixture of **omega-3 fatty acids** (page 509) (primarily eicosapentaenoic acid [EPA] and docosahexaenoic acid [DHA]) for six months markedly reduced the frequency of seizures in five severely retarded epileptic patients.[40] Additional research is needed to confirm this report and to identify which people with epilepsy are most likely to benefit.

A small, preliminary trial found that 5 to 10 mg per day of **melatonin** (page 555) improved sleep and provided "clear improvement of the seizure situation" among children with one of two rare seizure disorders.[41] More research is needed to determine whether or not melatonin could benefit other people with epilepsy.

Two elderly individuals with well-controlled epilepsy reportedly developed recurrent seizures within two weeks of starting Ginkgo biloba extract.[42] Individuals with epilepsy should not, therefore, take Ginkgo biloba without medical supervision.

Are there any side effects or interactions?
Refer to the individual supplement for information about any side effects or interactions.

Herbs that may be helpful
The Chinese herb **bupleurum** (page 647) is included in two similar Chinese herbal formulae known as sho-saiko-to and saiko-keishi-to; these combinations contain the same herbs but in different proportions. The other ingredients are **peony** (page 724) root, pinellia root, cassia bark, **ginger** (page 680) root, jujube fruit, **Asian ginseng** (page 630) root, **Chinese scullcap** (page 658) root, and **licorice** (page 702) root. Both formulas have been shown in preliminary trials to be helpful for people with epilepsy.[43, 44, 45] No negative interactions with a variety of anticonvulsant drugs were noted in these trials. The usual amount taken of these formulas is 2.5 grams three times per day as capsules or tea. People with epilepsy should not use either formula without first consulting with a healthcare professional.

One older preliminary trial in India found an extract of **bacopa** (page 632), an Ayurvedic herb, reduced the frequency of epileptic seizures in a small group of peo-

ple.[46] However, another similar preliminary trial gave inconclusive results.[47] Controlled research is needed to properly evaluate whether bacopa is helpful for epilepsy.

Are there any side effects or interactions?
Refer to the individual herb for information about any side effects or interactions.

ERECTILE DYSFUNCTION

What do I need to know?
Self-care for erectile dysfunction can be approached in a number of ways—but it can be hard to know just where to start. To make it easier, our doctors recommend trying these simple steps first:

Get a checkup
    ED can be caused by some diseases and may be a side effect of certain medications
Consider counseling
    Psychological issues can be a cause, or an effect, of ED
Quit smoking
    Men who smoke have an increased ED risk
Check out Asian ginseng
    900 mg of a concentrated extract two or three times a day may improve libido and ability to maintain erection
Give ginkgo a go
    Take 240 mg a day of a standardized extract to increase blood flow to the penis

About erectile dysfunction
Erectile dysfunction (ED) is the inability of a male to attain or sustain an erection sufficient for sexual intercourse.

It can be a persistent condition; however, almost half of all men experience ED only occasionally. ED can have physical, psychological, or drug-induced causes.[1] Although some doctors used to believe differently, most researchers and doctors now believe that physical factors are responsible for the majority of ED cases.

Several conditions may contribute to ED by impairing blood flow to the penis. These include **atherosclerosis** (page 38), **diabetes** (page 152), **hypothyroidism** (page 252), **multiple sclerosis** (page 323), and chronic alcohol abuse.

CHECKLIST FOR ERECTILE DYSFUNCTION

Rating	Nutritional Supplements	Herbs
★★★		**Asian ginseng** (page 630) **Yohimbe** (page 764)
★★☆	**Arginine** (page 467) **DHEA** (page 503) Pycnogenol	*Butea superba* *Ginkgo biloba* (page 681) (for ED of vascular origin)
★☆☆		**Damiana** (page 666)

What are the symptoms of erectile dysfunction?

ED is defined by the symptoms listed above. Symptoms may also include loss of sexual desire (libido), premature ejaculation, or inability to achieve orgasm.

Medical treatments

Prescription drug treatments for ED include male hormone replacement therapy, such as testosterone (Delatestryl Injection, Depo-Testosterone Injection, Androderm Patch, Testoderm Patch), and dehydroepiandrosterone (**DHEA** [page 503]), as well as inhibitors of phosphodiesterase type 5, such as sildenafil (Viagra), tadalafil (Cialis), and vardenafil (Levitra). Other treatments include yohimbine (Yocon), and alprostadil (Caverject, Muse), which is inserted or injected into the penis.

Depending on the cause, therapy may include psychological and behavioral counseling, treatment of underlying **cardiovascular disease** (page 98), and avoidance of medications such as cimetidine, antihypertensives, and MAO inhibitors. Penile vacuum devices and surgical options, such as penile implants and vascular repair, are usually limited to those who have not responded to other treatments.

Lifestyle changes that may be helpful

Men who smoke have been shown to have an increased incidence of ED.[2]

In a study of obese men with erectile dysfunction, a two-year lifestyle program consisting of a low-calorie diet plus regular exercise resulted in a significant improvement in erectile function, which became normal in 31% of the participants.[3]

Nutritional supplements that may be helpful

Low blood levels of the hormone dehydroepiandrosterone (**DHEA** [page 503]) have been reported in some men with ED. In one double-blind trial, 40 men with low DHEA levels and ED were given 50 mg DHEA per day for six months.[4] Significant improvement in both erectile function and interest in sex occurred in the men assigned to take DHEA, but not in those assigned to take placebo. No significant change occurred in testosterone levels or in factors that could affect the prostate gland. Experts have concerns about the safe use of DHEA, particularly because long-term safety data do not exist.

Dilation of blood vessels necessary for a normal erection depends on a substance called nitric oxide, and nitric oxide formation depends on the amino acid **arginine** (page 467). In a preliminary trial, men with ED were given 2,800 mg of arginine per day for two weeks. Six of the 15 men in the trial were helped, though none improved while taking placebo.[5] In a larger double-blind trial, men with ED were given 1,670 mg of arginine per day or a matching placebo for six weeks.[6] Arginine supplementation was found to be particularly effective at improving ED in men with abnormal nitric oxide metabolism. Although little is known about how effective arginine will be for men with ED or which subset of these men would be helped, available research looks promising and suggests that at least some men are likely to benefit.

In a double-blind study of men with erectile dysfunction, supplementation with 120 mg per day of Pycnogenol, an extract of the bark of a certain tree *(Pinus pinaster)*, improved erectile function, whereas placebo treatment had no effect.[7]

Are there any side effects or interactions?

Refer to the individual supplement for information about any side effects or interactions.

Herbs that may be helpful

Yohimbine (the primary active constituent in **yohimbe** [page 764]) has been shown in several double-blind trials to help treat men with ED;[8, 9] negative results have also been reported, however.[10, 11] Yohimbe dilates blood vessels and may help, regardless of the cause of ED. A tincture of yohimbe bark is often used in the amount of 5 to 10 drops three times per day. Standardized yohimbe extracts are also available. A typical daily amount of yohimbine is 15 to 30 mg. It is best to use yohimbe and yohimbine under the supervision of a physician.

Asian ginseng (page 630) *(Panax ginseng)* has traditionally been used as a supportive herb for male potency. A double-blind trial found that 1,800 mg per day of Asian ginseng extract for three months helped improve libido and the ability to maintain an erection in men with ED.[12] The benefit of Asian ginseng confirmed in another double-blind study, in which 900 mg three times a day was given for eight weeks.[13]

Butea superba is a Thai plant that has been used traditionally to increase sexual vigor. In a preliminary trial, 82% of men with erectile dysfunction reported an improvement in erectile function while taking *Butea superba* for three months.[14] The amount used was 500 mg per day for the first four days, followed by 1,000 mg per day thereafter. The response rate in the placebo group could not be evaluated, because none of the men receiving the placebo returned for their follow-up visit.

Ginkgo biloba (page 681) may help some men with ED by increasing blood flow to the penis. One double-blind trial found improvement in men taking 240 mg per day of a standardized *Ginkgo biloba* extract (GBE) for nine months.[15] A preliminary trial, involving 30 men who were experiencing ED as a result of medication use (selective serotonin reuptake inhibitors and other medications), found that approximately 200 mg per day of GBE had a positive effect on sexual function in 76% of the men.[16]

Damiana (page 666) *(Turnera diffusa)* is a traditional herbal treatment for men with ED. However, no modern clinical trials have confirmed its effectiveness.

Are there any side effects or interactions?
Refer to the individual herb for information about any side effects or interactions.

Holistic approaches that may be helpful
ED that cannot be linked to physical causes has been successfully treated by hypnosis.[17] In one trial, three hypnosis sessions per week, later decreased to one per month, over a six-month period led to improvement in 75% of men in the trial.

Acupuncture might be of some benefit for men with ED. Electroacupuncture, which is acupuncture accompanied by electrical stimulation, was performed on various acupuncture points in men with ED in a preliminary trial of men with this condition.[18] Two treatments were administered every week for one month. An improvement in quality of erection was observed in 15% of the participants and an increase in sexual activity was reported by 31% of the men. Another preliminary trial[19] found good results in over half of the men treated, but the only controlled trial of electroacupuncture for ED[20] found that placebo also produced a large improvement in sexual function—an effect similar to that of acupuncture. Controlled trials with larger groups of men are necessary to better test the efficacy of acupuncture therapy for men suffering from ED.

FEMALE INFERTILITY

See also: Male Infertility (page 305)

Infertility is defined by doctors as the failure to become pregnant after a year of unprotected intercourse.

It can be caused by sex-hormone abnormalities, **low thyroid function** (page 252), **endometriosis** (page 182), scarring of the tubes connecting the ovaries with the uterus, or a host of other factors. Some of the causes of infertility readily respond to natural medicine, while others do not. The specific cause of infertility should always be diagnosed by a physician before considering possible solutions.

CHECKLIST FOR FEMALE INFERTILITY		
Rating	**Nutritional Supplements**	**Herbs**
★★☆	**Propolis** (page 579) (for infertility associated with endometriosis) **Vitamin C** (page 604) (for infertility associated with luteal phase defect)	**Vitex** (page 757)
★☆☆	**Arginine** (page 467) (for in vitro fertilization) **Iron** (page 540) (for deficiency) **Multivitamin-mineral** (page 559) **PABA** (page 567) **Vitamin E** (page 609)	

What are the symptoms of infertility?
For most infertile women, no symptoms accompany the infertility. Some women with symptoms of **obesity** (page 446), acne, and excessive facial hair; heavy, irregular, or absent menstrual periods; or fluid leaking from the breasts could have hormone imbalances that might interfere with fertility.

Medical treatments

Prescription fertility drugs such as clomiphene (Clomid, Serophene), gonadorelin (Factrel, Lutrepulse), human chorionic gonadotropin or "hCG" (A.P.L., Fullutein, Humegon, Pregnyl, Profasi), and human menopausal gonadotropins or "hMG" (Metrodin, Pergonal, Repronal) are commonly prescribed.

Artificial insemination can be used to place sperm directly in the cervix or uterus. Another more advanced procedure is called "in vitro fertilization," wherein the egg (collected from the ovary in a surgical procedure) and the sperm are combined under controlled conditions in a laboratory. The fertilized embryo is then implanted into the woman's uterus.

Dietary changes that may be helpful

Consumption of one to one and a half cups of coffee per day in one study[1] and about three[2] or four[3] cups per day in other studies has been associated with delayed conception in women trying to get **pregnant** (page 363). Caffeine consumption equivalent to more than two cups of coffee per day has been associated with an increased incidence of infertility due to tubal disease or endometriosis.[4] In another study, women who consumed more than one cup of coffee per day had a 50% reduction in fertility, compared with women who drank less coffee.[5]

Caffeine is found in regular coffee, black tea, **green tea** (page 686), some soft drinks, chocolate, cocoa, and many over-the-counter pharmaceuticals. While not every study finds that caffeine reduces female fertility,[6] many doctors recommend that women trying to get pregnant avoid caffeine.

In one study, consumption of three cups of decaffeinated coffee per day was associated with an increased risk of spontaneous abortion.[7] In another study, caffeine consumption compounded the negative effects of alcohol consumption on female fertility.[8] Some researchers suspect that the tannic acid found in any kind of coffee and black tea may contribute to infertility.[9]

Consumption of fish contaminated with polychlorinated biphenyls (PCBs) may reduce the ability of women to conceive. In one study, women who ate more than one fish meal per month of fish caught in Lake Ontario (known to be contaminated with PCBs) had reduced fecundity (meaning that it took longer for them to become pregnant) compared to women who ate less contaminated fish.[10]

Lifestyle changes that may be helpful

The more women smoke, the less likely they are to conceive.[11] In fact, women whose mothers smoked during *their* pregnancy are less likely to conceive compared with those whose mothers were nonsmokers.[12] Quitting smoking may enhance fertility.

Even moderate drinking of alcoholic beverages by women is linked to an increased risk of infertility in some,[13] although not all, research.[14] In a preliminary study, there was a greater than 50% reduction in the probability of conception in a menstrual cycle during which participants consumed alcohol. Caffeine appeared to enhance alcohol's negative effect in this study. Women who abstained from alcohol and consumed less than one cup of coffee per day were more than twice as likely to conceive (26.9 pregnancies per 100 menstrual cycles) compared with those who consumed any amount of alcohol and more than one cup of coffee per day (10.5 pregnancies per 100 menstrual cycles).[15] Based on this preliminary evidence, women who wish to improve their chances of conception should avoid alcohol and caffeine.

Being **excessively overweight** (page 446) or underweight may also contribute to infertility in females.[16] Infertile women who are overweight or underweight should consult a physician.

Some conventional medications can interfere with fertility. When in doubt, women taking prescription drugs should consult their physician or pharmacist.

Nutritional supplements that may be helpful

In a preliminary study of women with infertility and mild endometriosis, supplementation with **propolis** (page 579) (500 mg twice a day for six months) was associated with a pregnancy rate of 60%, compared with a rate of 20% in the placebo group (a statistically significant difference).[17] Whether propolis would be beneficial for infertile women who do not have endometriosis is not known.

In some women, infertility is due to a hormonal abnormality known as luteal phase defect. In this condition, the uterine lining does not develop and mature properly, presumably because of a deficiency of the hormone progesterone. In a study of infertile women with luteal phase defect, supplementation with 750 mg of **vitamin C** (page 604) per day for up to six months resulted in a pregnancy rate of 25%, compared with a rate of 11% in an untreated control group, a statistically significant difference.[18]

A double-blind trial found that taking a **multivita-**

min-mineral (page 559) supplement increased female fertility.[19]

Vitamin E (page 609) deficiency in animals leads to infertility.[20] In a preliminary human trial, infertile couples given vitamin E (200 IU per day for the female and 100 IU per day for the male) showed a significant increase in fertility.[21]

In preliminary research, even a subtle deficiency of **iron** (page 540) has been tentatively linked to infertility.[22] Women who are infertile should consult a doctor to rule out the possibility of iron deficiency.

Some previously infertile women have become pregnant after supplementing with **PABA** (page 567) (para-aminobenzoic acid), 100 mg four times per day.[23] PABA is believed to increase the ability of estrogen to facilitate fertility.

Supplementation with the **amino acid** (page 465), **L-arginine** (page 467) (16 grams per day), has been shown to improve fertilization rates in women with a previous history of failed attempts at *in vitro* (test tube) fertilization.[24]

Are there any side effects or interactions?
Refer to the individual supplement for information about any side effects or interactions.

Herbs that may be helpful

Vitex (page 757) is occasionally used as an herbal treatment for infertility—particularly in cases with established luteal phase defect (shortened second half of the menstrual cycle) and high levels of the hormone, prolactin. In one trial, 48 women (ages 23 to 39) who were diagnosed with infertility took vitex once daily for three months.[25] Seven women became pregnant during the trial, and 25 women experienced normalized **progesterone** (page 577) levels—which may increase the chances for pregnancy. In another double-blind trial, significantly more infertile women became **pregnant** (page 363) after taking a product whose main ingredient is vitex (the other ingredients were homeopathic preparations) than did those who took a placebo.[26] The amount used in this trial was 30 drops of fluid extract twice a day, for a total of 1.8 ml per day. This specific preparation is not available in the United States. Some doctors recommend taking 40 drops of a liquid extract of vitex each morning with water. Approximately 35–40 mg of encapsulated powdered vitex (one capsule taken in the morning) provides a similar amount. Vitex should be discontinued once a woman becomes pregnant.

Are there any side effects or interactions?
Refer to the individual herb for information about any side effects or interactions.

Holistic approaches that may be helpful

Acupuncture may be helpful in the treatment of some cases of female infertility due to problems with ovarian function. In a preliminary trial, women who did not ovulate were treated with acupuncture 30 times over three months. Effectiveness was determined by a combination of measures indicating ovulation was returning to normal. Acupuncture treatment resulted in a marked improvement in 35% and slight improvement in 48% of trial participants.[27] The beneficial results achieved with acupuncture may be due to alterations in the hormonal messages from the brain to the ovary.[28]

Auricular (ear) acupuncture has been studied in a preliminary trial and compared with standard hormone therapy for treatment of infertility. In both the acupuncture and hormone therapy groups, 15 out of 45 patients became pregnant. Although the **pregnancy** (page 363) rates were similar with either treatment, side effects occurred only in women taking hormones.[29] Still, double-blind trials are needed to conclusively determine whether acupuncture is a useful treatment for female infertility.

FIBROCYSTIC BREAST DISEASE

Fibrocystic breast disease (FBD) is a term given to a very common group of benign conditions affecting the breast in younger women.

What are the symptoms of fibrocystic breast disease?

Both breasts become tender or painful and lumpy, and these symptoms vary at different times in the menstrual cycle. Despite the fact that signs and symptoms of FBD appear to be quite distinct from textbook signs and symptoms of **breast cancer** (page 65), any lump in the breast should be diagnosed by a doctor to rule out the possibility of cancer.

Medical treatments

Over the counter pain relievers, such as aspirin (Bayer, Ecotrin, Bufferin), acetaminophen (Tylenol), and ibuprofen (Motrin, Advil), may be beneficial.

CHECKLIST FOR FIBROCYSTIC BREAST DISEASE

Rating	Nutritional Supplements	Herbs
★★☆	Evening primrose oil (page 511)	Vitex (page 757)
★☆☆	Iodine (page 538) Vitamin B₆ (page 600) Vitamin E (page 609)	

Some health care practitioners might prescribe oral contraceptives (Ortho-Novum, Mircette, Loestrin, and Triphasil) to reduce symptoms.

All women, including those with FBD, are encouraged to examine their breasts monthly and have regular medical evaluations, including mammograms after the age of 50.

Dietary changes that may be helpful

Some,[1, 2] but not all[3, 4] studies have found that women with FBD drink more coffee than women without the disease. Eliminating caffeine for less than six months does not appear to be effective at reducing symptoms of FBD.[5, 6] However, long-term and complete avoidance of caffeine does reduce symptoms of FBD.[7, 8] Some women are more sensitive to effects of caffeine than others, so benefits of restricting caffeine are likely to vary from woman to woman. Caffeine is found in coffee, black tea, green tea (page 686), cola drinks, chocolate, and many over-the-counter drugs. A decrease in breast tenderness can take six months or more to occur after caffeine is eliminated. Breast lumpiness may not go away, but the pain often decreases.

FBD has been linked to excess estrogen. When women with FBD were put on a low-fat diet, their estrogen levels decreased.[9, 10] After three to six months, the pain (page 338) and lumpiness also decreased.[11, 12] The link between dietary fat and symptoms appears to be most strongly related to saturated fat.[13] Foods high in saturated fat include meat and dairy products. Fish, nonfat dairy, and tofu are possible replacements.

Lifestyle changes that may be helpful

Exercise may decrease breast tenderness. In one study, women who ran 45 miles per menstrual cycle reported less breast tenderness as well as improvement in other symptoms, such as anxiety (page 30).[14]

Nutritional supplements that may be helpful

In double-blind research, evening primrose oil (page 511) (EPO) has reduced symptoms of FBD,[15, 16] though only slightly.[17] One group of researchers reported that EPO normalizes blood levels of fatty acids in women with FBD.[18] However, even these scientists had difficulty linking the improvement in lab tests with an actual reduction in symptoms. Nonetheless, most reports continue to show at least some reduction in symptoms resulting from EPO supplementation.[19, 20] Based on this research, many doctors recommend a trial of 3 grams per day of EPO for at least six months to alleviate symptoms of FBD.

While several studies report that 200–600 IU of vitamin E (page 609) per day, taken for several months, reduces symptoms of FBD,[21, 22] most double-blind trials have found that vitamin E does *not* relieve FBD symptoms.[23, 24] Nonetheless, many women take 400 IU of vitamin E for three months to see if it helps.

As with vitamin E, the effectiveness of vitamin B₆ (page 600) remains uncertain. Some,[25] but not all,[26] studies find that B₆ supplementation reduces symptoms. Since vitamin B₆ supplementation is effective for relieving the symptoms of premenstrual syndrome (page 361) (PMS), in addition to breast tenderness, women should discuss the use of vitamin B₆ with their healthcare provider.

Some doctors use iodine (page 538) to treat FBD symptoms. In animals, iodine deficiency can cause the equivalent of FBD.[27] What appears to be the most effective form—diatomic iodine[28]—is not readily available, however. Some people are sensitive to iodine and high amounts can interfere with thyroid function. Therefore, supplemental iodine should only be taken with the guidance of a healthcare practitioner.

Are there any side effects or interactions?
Refer to the individual supplement for information about any side effects or interactions.

Herbs that may be helpful

Since many women with FBD and cyclical breast tenderness also suffer from PMS (page 361), there is often an overlap in herbal recommendations for these two conditions despite a lack of research dealing directly with FBD.

In one double-blind trial, a liquid preparation containing 32.4 mg of vitex (page 757) and homeopathic ingredients was found to successfully reduce breast tenderness associated with the menstrual cycle (e.g. cyclic mastalgia).[29] Vitex is thought to reduce breast tenderness at menses because of its ability to reduce elevated levels of the hormone, prolactin.[30]

Doctors typically suggest 40 drops of a liquid, concentrated vitex extract or 35–40 mg of the equivalent dried, powdered extract to be taken once per day in the morning with some liquid. Vitex should be taken for at least three menstrual cycles to determine efficacy.

Are there any side effects or interactions?
Refer to the individual herb for information about any side effects or interactions.

FIBROMYALGIA

What do I need to know?
Self-care for fibromyalgia can be approached in a number of ways—but it can be hard to know just where to start. To make it easier, our doctors recommend trying these simple steps first:

Exercise
Low-intensity exercise (like walking or swimming) is the best known treatment

Address your stress
Reducing stress and unpleasant emotions may also reduce symptoms

Test a new therapy
Chiropractic treatment and acupuncture sometimes help

Try 5-HTP
100 mg of 5-HTP (hydroxytryptophane) three times a day may ease symptoms

About fibromyalgia
Fibromyalgia is a complex syndrome with no known cause or cure. Its predominant symptom is pain in the fibrous tissues, muscles, tendons, and ligaments, although other symptoms may be experienced.

Research has demonstrated that the axis connecting the three glands primarily responsible for the stress response (hypothalamus, pituitary, adrenals) may be dysfunctional in people with fibromyalgia.[1] Inflammation of the involved structures is generally absent in fibromyalgia.

Of the estimated three to six million people[2] affected by this disorder in the United States, the vast majority are women between 25 and 45 years of age.

CHECKLIST FOR FIBROMYALGIA		
Rating	Nutritional Supplements	Herbs
★★☆	**5-HTP** (page 459) **SAMe** (page 583)	chlorella
★☆☆	D-Ribose **Magnesium** (page 551) **Malic acid** (page 552) **Melatonin** (page 555) **Vitamin B₁** (page 597) **Vitamin E** (page 609)	

What are the symptoms of fibromyalgia?
Trigger-point pain at characteristic locations is the defining symptom of fibromyalgia. The most commonly affected locations are on the occiput (nape of the neck), the neck itself, shoulders, trunk, low back, and thighs. Other symptoms may also be experienced, including fatigue, chest pain, low-grade fever, swollen lymph nodes, **insomnia** (page 270), frequent abdominal pain, **irritable bowel syndrome** (page 280), and **depression** (page 145).[3]

Medical treatments
Over the counter pain relievers, such as aspirin (Bayer, Ecotrin, Bufferin), ibuprofen (Motrin, Advil), and acetaminophen (Tylenol), may be recommended. However, one double-blind trial found no difference between ibuprofen and placebo with respect to treating fibromyalgia symptoms.[4]

Treatment commonly involves a combination of medications, including one of several antidepressants, such as amitriptyline (Elavil), fluoxetine (Prozac), sertraline (Zoloft), paroxetine (Paxil), and fluvoxamine (Luvox), to help diminish pain and improve sleep. Some individuals might benefit from a muscle relaxant, such as cyclobenzaprine (Flexeril).

Low-impact exercise programs to improve aerobic fitness, stretching techniques to relax tense muscles, and cognitive therapy for coping with stress and emotional disorders are recommended treatments.

Dietary changes that may be helpful
A vegan diet (includes no animal products) that is also low in salt may help women with fibromyalgia. In a controlled clinical trial,[5] women with fibromyalgia were put on a special diet consisting only of raw foods—primarily fruits, vegetables, nuts, seeds, legumes, and cere-

Fibromyalgia

als (such as rolled oats). The diet also contained several fermented foods, including a fermented yogurt-food made from oats, a fermented beverage made from wheat berries (called Rejuvalac), and several types of fermented vegetables, particularly cabbage. During the three-month trial, women following the therapeutic diet experienced a significant reduction in body **weight** (page 446), **pain** (page 338), **morning sickness** (page 320), use of painkillers, **depression** (page 145), and the number of sore fibromyalgia points, compared with those who continued to eat their regular diet. Due to the liberal use of nuts and seeds, this diet was not low in fat; for example, 31% of all calories came from fat. Nonetheless, the total number of calories was relatively low (less than 1,900 calories per day), which was probably responsible for the decrease in body weight.

In a preliminary report, four women with fibromyalgia experienced marked improvement or complete resolution of their symptoms within months after eliminating monosodium glutamate (MSG) or MSG plus aspartame from their diet. In each case, symptoms recurred whenever MSG was ingested.[6]

Lifestyle changes that may be helpful

Low-intensity exercise may improve fibromyalgia symptoms. People with fibromyalgia who exercise regularly have been reported to suffer less severe symptoms than those who remain sedentary.[7, 8, 9] In a controlled trial, a program consisting of two 25-minute exercise classes plus two educational sessions per week for six weeks resulted in immediate and sustained improvement in walking distance, fatigue, and well-being in a group of people with fibromyalgia;[10] however, no reductions in **pain** (page 338), **anxiety** (page 30), or **depression** (page 145) were seen. In a more recent controlled trial, a 35-minute exercise program in a warm pool once a week for six months, coupled with counseling sessions, led to improvements in hand-grip strength and endurance, as well as to reductions in pain, distress, depression, and anxiety.[11] The results of this trial, and other similar trials, suggest that underwater exercise training, in combination with a counseling intervention, should be considered by people with fibromyalgia.

Nutritional supplements that may be helpful

People with fibromyalgia often have low serotonin levels in their blood.[12, 13, 14] Supplementation with **5-HTP** (page 459) may increase serotonin synthesis in these cases. Both preliminary[15, 16] and double-blind trials[17]

have reported that 5-HTP supplementation (100 mg three times per day) relieves some symptoms of fibromyalgia.

Some studies have found low **vitamin B$_1$** (page 597) (thiamine) levels and reduced activity of some thiamine-dependent enzymes among people with fibromyalgia.[18, 19] The clinical significance of these findings remains unknown.

One early preliminary study described the use of **vitamin E** (page 609) supplements in the treatment of "fibrositis"—the rough equivalent of what is today called fibromyalgia. Several dozen individuals were treated with vitamin E using amounts ranging from 100–300 IU per day. The results were positive and sometimes dramatic.[20] Double-blind trials are needed to confirm these preliminary observations.

Intravenous S-adenosylmethionine (**SAMe** [page 583]) given to people with fibromyalgia reduced pain and depression in two double-blind trials;[21, 22] but no benefit was seen in a short (ten-day) trial.[23] Oral SAMe (800 mg per day for six weeks) was tested in one double-blind trial and significant beneficial effects were seen, such as reduced **pain** (page 338), fatigue, and stiffness, and improved mood.[24]

A preliminary trial found that a combination of **magnesium** (page 551) and **malic acid** (page 552) might lessen muscle pain in people with fibromyalgia.[25] The amounts used in this trial were 300–600 mg of elemental magnesium and 1,200–2,400 mg of malic acid per day, taken for eight weeks. A double-blind trial by the same research group using 300 mg magnesium and 1,200 mg malic acid per day found no reduction in symptoms, however.[26] Though these researchers claimed that magnesium and malic acid appeared to have some effect at higher levels (up to 600 mg magnesium and 2,400 mg malic acid), the positive effects were not demonstrated under blinded study conditions. Therefore, the evidence supporting the use of these supplements for people with fibromyalgia remains weak and inconclusive.

Melatonin (page 555) supplementation may be useful in the treatment of fibromyalgia. In a preliminary trial, 3 mg of melatonin at bedtime was found to reduce tender points and to improve sleep and other measures of disease severity, though pain and fatigue improved only slightly.[27]

Are there any side effects or interactions?
Refer to the individual supplement for information about any side effects or interactions.

Holistic approaches that may be helpful

Stress is believed by some researchers to be capable of aggravating fibromyalgia symptoms. Stress-reduction techniques, such as meditation, have proven helpful in preliminary research.[28]

Acupuncture may be useful for short-term relief of fibromyalgia symptoms. In one preliminary trial, acupuncture produced a significant decrease in pain and point tenderness along with related biochemical changes measured in the fibromyalgia patients' blood.[29] Another uncontrolled trial used electroacupuncture (acupuncture with electrical stimulation) treatment in people with fibromyalgia who were unresponsive to conventional medical therapies. After an average of seven treatments per person, 46% claimed that electroacupuncture provided the best relief of symptoms when compared to all other therapies, and 64% reported using less medication for pain relief than prior to electroacupuncture.[30] A double-blind trial compared fake acupuncture to electroacupuncture and reported significant differences in improvement in five of eight outcome measurements among people with fibromyalgia.[31] Short-term pain reduction in people with fibromyalgia has been reported in other studies, some of which were at least partially controlled; however, long-term benefits have never been investigated in a controlled clinical trial.[32] Long-term controlled trials are necessary to conclusively determine whether acupuncture is a useful treatment for fibromyalgia.

Joint manipulation, chiropractic, and related treatments may be helpful for relieving some of the symptoms of fibromyalgia. A preliminary study[33] found that almost half of people with fibromyalgia who received chiropractic care had "moderate to good" improvement. A small preliminary trial[34] evaluated the effect of four weeks of chiropractic treatment (three to five times per week) consisting of soft tissue massage, stretching, spinal manipulation, and general advice and information. Treatment resulted in a significant decrease in pain and an increase in range of neck movement, but there was no improvement in tender points or in ability to function in daily life. Another preliminary trial[35] evaluated a longer treatment period (30 sessions) consisting of spinal manipulation and deep pressure massage to tender points in the muscles. More benefit was reported by this study, as 60% of the patients experienced significant pain reduction, reduced sensed of fatigue, and improved sleep. These benefits persisted one month after the treatment was completed. People who did not feel better after 15 treatments were not likely to benefit from this type of treatment. No controlled research has evaluated manipulation therapies for fibromyalgia.

GALLSTONES

Gallstones are hardened formations, composed primarily of cholesterol, that develop in the gallbladder.

Gallstones are commonly associated with bile that contains excessive cholesterol, a deficiency of other substances in bile (bile acids and **lecithin** [page 546]), or a combination of these factors.

CHECKLIST FOR GALLSTONES		
Rating	Nutritional Supplements	Herbs
★★☆	Wheat bran	
★☆☆	**Betaine HCl** (page 473) **Phosphatidylcholine** (page 546) **Vitamin C** (page 604)	**Milk thistle** (page 710) **Peppermint** (page 726) oil

What are the symptoms of gallstones?

Gallstone attacks cause extreme pain in the upper-right quarter of the abdomen, often extending to the back. This pain can be accompanied by nausea and vomiting.

Medical treatments

Prescription medications are used in certain specific situations to dissolve gallstones; they include ursodiol (Actigall) and monoctanoin (Moctanin).

The most common medical treatment for gallstones is surgical removal of the gallbladder (cholecystectomy). Mechanical shock waves (lithotripsy) may also be applied to break up the stones. Unfortunately, gallstones commonly recur following non-surgical forms of treatment.

Dietary changes that may be helpful

Cholesterol (page 223) is the primary ingredient in most gallstones. Some,[1] but not all,[2] research links dietary cholesterol to the risk of gallstones. Some doctors suggest avoiding eggs, either because of their high cholesterol content or because eggs may be allergenic. (See the discussion about gallstones and allergies below.) A recent study of residents of southern Italy found that a diet rich in sugars and animal fats and poor in vegetable fats and fibers was a significant risk factor for gallstone formation.[3]

Gallstones

Most studies report that vegetarians are at low risk for gallstones.[4] In some trials, vegetarians had only half the gallstone risk compared with meat eaters.[5, 6] Vegetarians often eat fewer calories and less cholesterol. They also tend to weigh less than meat eaters. All of these differences may reduce gallstone incidence. The specific factors in a vegetarian diet that account for a low risk of gallstone formation remain somewhat unclear and may only be present in certain vegetarian diets and not others. For example, some studies have found that vegetarians eating a high vegetable fat diet had elevated rather than reduced risks of gallstone formation.[7, 8]

Coffee increases bile flow and therefore might reduce the risk of gallstones. In a large study of men, those drinking two to three cups of regular coffee per day had a 40% lower risk of gallstones compared with men who did not drink coffee.[9] In the same report, men drinking at least four cups per day had a 45% reduced risk. Caffeine appears to be the protective ingredient, as decaffeinated coffee consumption was not linked with any protection. People at risk for gallstones who wish to consider increasing coffee drinking to reduce risks should talk with a doctor beforehand. Caffeinated beverages can aggravate symptoms of **insomnia** (page 270), **peptic ulcer** (page 349), **panic attacks** (page 30), and a variety of other conditions.

Constipation (page 137) has been linked to the risk of forming gallstones.[10] When constipation is successfully resolved, it has reduced the risk of gallstone formation.[11] Wheat bran, commonly used to relieve constipation when combined with fluid, has been reported to reduce the relative amount of cholesterol in bile of a small group of people whose bile contained excessive cholesterol (a risk factor for gallstone formation).[12] The same effect has been reported in people who already have gallstones.[13] Doctors sometimes recommend two tablespoons per day of unprocessed Miller's bran; an alternative is to consume commercial cereal products that contain wheat bran. Bran should always be accompanied by plenty of fluid. Adding more bran may cause gastrointestinal symptoms in some people. If this occurs, consult a doctor.

Gallbladder attacks (though not the stones themselves) have been reported to result from **food allergies** (page 14). The one study to examine this relationship found that all of the participants with gallbladder problems showed relief from gallbladder pain when allergy-provoking foods were identified and eliminated from the diet.[14] Eggs, pork, and onions were reported to be the most common triggers. Pain returned when the problem foods were reintroduced into the diet. Doctors can help diagnose food allergies.

Lifestyle changes that may be helpful

People with gallstones may consume too many calories[15] and are often overweight.[16, 17] Obese women have seven times the risk of forming gallstones compared with women who are not overweight.[18] Even slightly overweight women have significantly higher risks.[19] Losing weight is likely to help,[20] but *rapid* weight loss might increase the risk of stone formation.[21] Any weight-loss program to prevent or treat gallstones should be reviewed by a doctor. **Weight-loss** (page 446) plans generally entail reducing dietary fat, a change that itself correlates with protection against gallstone formation and attacks.[22, 23]

In women, recreational exercise significantly reduces the risk of requiring gallbladder surgery due to gallstones. In a study of over 60,000 women, an average of two to three hours per week of recreational exercise (such as cycling, jogging, and swimming) reduced the risk of gallbladder surgery by about 20%.[24]

Use of birth control pills significantly increases a woman's risk of developing gallstones.[25, 26]

Nutritional supplements that may be helpful

Vitamin C (page 000) is needed to convert cholesterol to bile acids. In theory, such a conversion should reduce gallstone risks. Women who have higher blood levels of vitamin C have a reduced risk of gallstones.[27] Although this does not prove that vitamin C supplements can prevent or treat gallstones, some researchers believe this is plausible.[28] One study reported that people who drink alcohol and take vitamin C supplements have only half the risk of gallstones compared with other drinkers, though the apparent protective effect of vitamin C did not appear in non-drinkers.[29] In another trial, supplementation with vitamin C (500 mg taken four times per day for two weeks before gallbladder surgery) led to improvement in one parameter of gallstone risk ("nucleation time"), though there was no change in the relative level of cholesterol found in bile.[30] While many doctors recommend vitamin C supplementation to people with a history of gallstones, supportive evidence remains preliminary.

According to one older report, people with gallstones were likely to have insufficient stomach acid.[31] Some doctors assess adequacy of stomach acid in people with gallstones and, if appropriate, recommend supplementation with **betaine HCl** (page 473). Nonetheless, no research has yet explored whether such supplementation reduces symptoms of gallstones.

Phosphatidylcholine (page 546) (PC)—a purified extract from **lecithin** (page 546)—is one of the components of bile that helps protect against gallstone formation. Some preliminary studies suggest that 300–2,000 mg per day of PC may help dissolve gallstones.[32, 33] Some doctors suggest PC supplements as part of gallstone treatment, though the supporting research is weak.[34]

Are there any side effects or interactions?
Refer to the individual supplement for information about any side effects or interactions.

Herbs that may be helpful

Milk thistle (page 710) extracts in capsules or tablets may be beneficial in preventing gallstones. In one study, silymarin (the active component of milk thistle) reduced cholesterol levels in bile,[35] which is one important way to reduce gallstone formation. People in the study took 420 mg of silymarin per day.

According to preliminary research, a mixture of essential oils dissolved some gallstones when taken for several months.[36] The greatest benefits occurred when the oils were combined with chenodeoxycholic acid, which is available by prescription.[37] However, only about 10% of people with gallstones have shown significant dissolution as a result of taking essential oils. **Peppermint** (page 726) oil is the closest available product to that used in the research described above. Use of peppermint or any other essential oil to dissolve gallstones should only be attempted with the close supervision of a doctor.

Are there any side effects or interactions?
Refer to the individual herb for information about any side effects or interactions.

GASTRITIS

Gastritis is a broad term for inflammation of the stomach lining, also called the gastric mucosa.

This condition can be caused by many factors and, in some cases, may lead to an **ulcer** (page 349). For that reason, many of the same nutrients, herbs, and lifestyle changes for a peptic ulcer might also help someone with gastritis.

Bacterial infection, most notably with *Helicobacter pylori*,[1] is a major cause of gastritis. *H. pylori* is the same bacterium responsible for most cases of peptic ulcer. When considering treatments for gastritis, many researchers now look for substances that eradicate *H. pylori,* including bismuth[2] and antibiotics.[3]

Other causes of gastritis include intake of caustic poisons, alcohol, and some medications (such as aspirin or adrenal corticosteroids), as well as physical stress from the **flu** (page 269), major surgery, severe burns, or **injuries** (page 319). For some people, a drug allergy or food poisoning can cause gastritis. Atrophic gastritis is a form of gastritis found particularly in the elderly, where stomach cells are destroyed, potentially leading to **pernicious anemia** (page 598).

CHECKLIST FOR GASTRITIS		
Rating	Nutritional Supplements	Herbs
★★☆	**Gamma oryzanol** (page 525) **N-acetyl cysteine** (page 562) **Vitamin C** (page 604)	
★☆☆	**Arginine** (page 467) **Beta-carotene** (page 469) **Glutamine** (page 530) **Vitamin A** (page 595) **Zinc** (page 614)	**Chamomile** (page 656) **Goldenseal** (page 683) **Licorice** (page 702) **Marshmallow** (page 708) **Slippery elm** (page 747) **Wood betony** (page 761)

What are the symptoms of gastritis?

Acute gastritis is typically characterized by nonspecific abdominal pain. Since gastritis often occurs in severely ill, hospitalized people, its symptoms may be eclipsed by other, more severe symptoms. Gastritis that is caused by *H. pylori* eventually leads to **peptic ulcers** (page 349), which are characterized by a dull ache in the upper abdomen that usually occurs two to three hours after a meal; the ache is typically relieved by eating.

Medical treatments

Over the counter antacids, such as magnesium hydroxide (Phillips' Milk of Magnesia), aluminum hydroxide (Amphojel), calcium carbonate (Tums), and the combi-

Gastritis

nation magnesium-aluminum hydroxide (Mylanta, Maalox), help relieve the symptoms of gastritis. The histamine H2 antagonists, such as cimetidine (Tagamet), ranitidine (Zantac), and famotidine (Pepcid), as well as the proton pump inhibitor omeprazole (Prilosec-OTC), are also beneficial.

Prescription drug therapy might involve antibiotics that eliminate *H. pylori* infection, such as amoxicillin (Amoxil), clarithromycin (Biaxin), metronidazole (Flagyl), and tetracycline (Sumycin), in combination with the proton pump inhibitors lansoprazole (Prevacid) and omeprazole (Prilosec). Bismuth subsalicylate (Pepto Bismol) may be added as well. Other medications may be prescribed to control stomach acidity, including prescription strength histamine H2 inhibitors, such as cimetidine (Tagamet), ranitidine (Zantac), and famotidine (Pepcid), as well as the prescription strength proton pump inhibitors omeprazole (Prilosec), lansoprazole (Prevacid), pantoprazole (Protonix), and rabeprazole (Aciphex).

Acute gastritis caused by trauma, stress, or severe illness usually heals rapidly when the underlying cause is resolved. Nonsteroidal anti-inflammatory drugs (NSAIDs) and ethanol are common stomach tissue irritants and their use should be limited in people with gastritis.

Dietary changes that may be helpful

Salt can irritate the stomach lining. Some research suggests that eating salty foods increases the risk of developing a *H. pylori* infection.[4] Researchers have speculated that increased salt intake may also increase the risk of other forms of gastritis.[5]

Doctors commonly suggest that people with gastritis avoid spicy foods. However, one study found that capsaicin, the pungent ingredient in **cayenne** (page 654) or chili pepper, protected against aspirin-induced gastritis in healthy persons. When people ate chili pepper followed by 600 mg of aspirin, stomach injury was considerably less than in people who took only aspirin.[6] The researchers of this study speculate that chili pepper helps by increasing blood flow to the stomach. Capsaicin has also been shown to protect against alcohol-induced gastritis in rats,[7] though this has yet to be tested in humans.

Some researchers have suggested that **food allergies** (page 14) or intolerance may cause gastritis.[8] In one double-blind trial, people with proven food sensitivities showed clear evidence of irritation of the stomach lining (including swelling, bleeding, and erosions) when

given foods to which they were known to react.[9] However, most of these people did not have abnormal results from standard blood tests for allergies. People suspecting food sensitivities or allergies should consider discussing an allergy elimination program with a healthcare professional.

Caffeine found in coffee, black tea, **green tea** (page 686), some soft drinks, chocolate, and many medications increases stomach acid,[10] as does decaffeinated coffee.[11] Avoiding these substances should therefore aid in the healing of gastritis.

Lifestyle changes that may be helpful

Gastritis is common among **alcoholics** (page 12).[12] Both heavy smoking and excessive alcohol consumption are known causes of acute gastritis.[13] While heavy alcohol intake is clearly damaging to the stomach lining, preliminary evidence suggests that moderate alcohol consumption (generally defined as two drinks per day in women or three drinks per day in men) may actually protect against the development of gastritis by facilitating the elimination of *H. pylori*.[14] When alcohol is consumed in greater than moderate amounts, it causes a wide variety of health problems.

Many medications, such as aspirin and non-steroidal anti-inflammatory drugs (NSAIDS, such as ibuprofen), can induce or aggravate stomach irritation.[15] People with a history of gastritis should never take aspirin or related drugs without first discussing the matter with their doctor.

Nutritional supplements that may be helpful

When *H. pylori* causes gastritis, free radical levels rise in the stomach lining.[16] These unstable molecules contribute to inflammation and damage to the stomach lining. **Vitamin C** (page 604), an antioxidant that helps quench free radical molecules, is low in the stomach juice of people with chronic gastritis. This deficiency may be the link between chronic gastritis and the increased risk of stomach cancer. When people with gastritis took 500 mg of vitamin C twice a day, vitamin C levels in their gastric juice rose, though not to normal levels.[17] In another trial, vitamin C supplementation (5 grams per day divided into several doses for four weeks) appeared to eliminate *H. pylori* infection.[18] While no direct evidence proves that taking vitamin C reduces gastritis symptoms, scientists widely believe that any agent capable of knocking out *H. pylori* should help people with this condition.

The results of several clinical trials suggest that

gamma oryzanol (page 525) supplementation can help people with gastritis and other gastrointestinal complaints. In one study, people with chronic gastritis were given 300 mg of gamma oryzanol per day.[19] After two weeks, 23% of people taking gamma oryzanol reported that it was "extremely effective" and 55% rated it as "moderately effective." Another study produced similar results: People with various types of gastritis received 300 mg of gamma oryzanol per day. After two weeks, more than 62% of those with superficial gastritis, more than 87% of those with atrophic gastritis, and all people with erosive gastritis experienced improvement. These results were confirmed in a large study involving approximately 2,000 people with various gastrointestinal complaints, including several forms of gastritis.[20] Some of these people required as much as 600 mg per day for symptoms to improve. People with gastritis wishing to take gamma oryzanol for more than six months, or in amounts exceeding 300 mg per day, should first consult with a physician.

Various amino acids (page 467) have shown promise for people with gastritis. In a double-blind trial, taking 200 mg of cysteine (page 502) four times daily provided significant benefit for people with bleeding gastritis caused by NSAIDs (such as aspirin).[21] Cysteine is a sulfur-containing amino acid that stimulates healing of gastritis. In a preliminary trial, 1–4 grams per day of N-acetyl cysteine (page 562) given to people with atrophic gastritis for four weeks appeared to increase healing.[22] Glutamine (page 530), another amino acid is a main energy source for cells in the stomach and supplementation may increase blood flow to this region.[23] Patients in surgical intensive care units often develop gastrointestinal problems related to a glutamine deficiency.[24] When burn victims were supplemented with glutamine, they did not develop stress ulcers, even after several operations.[25] Nevertheless, it remains unclear to what extent glutamine supplementation might prevent or help existing gastritis. Preliminary evidence suggests the amino acid arginine (page 467) may both protect the stomach and increase its blood flow,[26] but research has yet to investigate the effects of arginine supplementation in people with gastritis.

The antioxidant beta-carotene (page 469) may reduce free radical damage in the stomach,[27] and eating foods high in beta-carotene has been linked to a decreased risk of developing chronic atrophic gastritis.[28] Moreover, people with active gastritis have been reported to have low levels of beta-carotene in their stomachs.[29] In a preliminary trial, giving 30,000 IU of beta-carotene per day to people with ulcers (page 349) or gastritis led to the disappearance of gastric erosions.[30] In another study, combining vitamin C and beta-carotene also led to improvement in most people with chronic atrophic gastritis.[31]

Zinc (page 614) and vitamin A (page 595), nutrients that aid in healing, are commonly used to help people with peptic ulcers. For example, the ulcers of people taking 50 mg of zinc three times per day healed three times faster than those of people who took placebo.[32] Since some types of gastritis can progress to peptic ulcer, it is possible that taking it may be useful. Nevertheless, the research does not yet show that zinc specifically helps people with gastritis. The amount of zinc used in this study is very high compared with what most people take (15–40 mg per day). Even at these lower levels, it is necessary to take 1–3 mg of copper (page 499) per day to avoid a zinc-induced copper deficiency.

People with ulcers who took 50,000 IU of vitamin A three times a day experienced a significant decrease in both ulcer size and pain.[33] Because this amount of vitamin A is very high and can be quite toxic, usage requires the guidance of a doctor. A safe amount for women of childbearing age is 10,000 IU per day and probably 25,000 IU for other adults. In other preliminary research, using vitamin A together with drugs and proper nutrition eliminated erosive gastritis after three weeks in about 75% of affected people.[34] Research has not yet shown that vitamin A supplementation specifically helps people with gastritis.

People with pernicious anemia (page 601) due to atrophic gastritis require very high amounts of vitamin B$_{12}$ (page 601).

Are there any side effects or interactions?
Refer to the individual supplement for information about any side effects or interactions.

Herbs that may be helpful

Many of the same herbs that are helpful for peptic ulcers (page 349) may also aid people with gastritis. Licorice (page 702) root, for example, has been traditionally used to soothe inflammation and injury in the stomach. Its flavonoid constituents have been found to stall the growth of *H. pylori* in test tube studies.[35] However, there have been no clinical trials using licorice to treat gastritis. To avoid potential side effects, such as increasing blood pressure (page 246) and water weight gain, many physicians recommend deglycyrrhizinated licorice (DGL). This form of licorice retains its healing

Gastritis

qualities by removing the glycyrrhizin that causes problems in some people.

Goldenseal (page 683) is regarded as an herbal antibiotic and has been traditionally used for infections of the mucous membranes. While no specific research points to goldenseal as a treatment for gastritis, there is some evidence from test tube studies that berberine, an active ingredient in goldenseal, slows growth of *H. pylori*.[36] Modern herbal practitioners now prefer alternatives to goldenseal, since the plant is threatened with extinction due to overharvesting.

Chamomile (page 656), high in the **flavonoid** (page 516) apigenin, may soothe injured and inflamed mucous membranes. In addition, a test tube study has shown that apigenin inhibits *H. pylori*,[37] and chamazulene, another active ingredient in chamomile, reduces free radical activity,[38] both potential advantages for people with gastritis. Human clinical trials are needed to confirm chamomile's effectiveness for treating gastritis.

Demulcent herbs, such as **marshmallow** (page 708), **slippery elm** (page 747), and **bladderwrack** (page 639), are high in mucilage. Mucilage might be advantageous for people with gastritis because its slippery nature soothes irritated mucus membranes of the digestive tract. Marshmallow is used for mild inflammation of the gastric mucosa.[39]

Wood betony (page 761) *(Stachys betonica)* has been used in European traditional herbal medicine for the treatment of heartburn and gastritis.

Are there any side effects or interactions?
Refer to the individual herb for information about any side effects or interactions.

GASTROESOPHAGEAL REFLUX DISEASE

Gastroesophageal reflux disease (GERD) is a disorder of the esophagus that causes frequent symptoms of **heartburn** (page 260). The esophagus is the tube connecting the mouth to the stomach. GERD occurs when a muscular ring called the lower esophageal sphincter (LES) is weakened, which permits irritating stomach contents to pass up into the esophagus, resulting in heartburn.

Sometimes regurgitation of acid and food as high as the mouth can occur. Chronic irritation of the esophagus by stomach acid can eventually cause ulceration and scarring and might lead to **cancer** (page 87) of the esophagus, especially in people who smoke and/or consume large amounts of **alcohol** (page 12).[1]

CHECKLIST FOR GERD		
Rating	Nutritional Supplements	Herbs
★★☆		Licorice (page 702)
★☆☆	Digestive enzymes (page 506) Hydrochloric acid (page 260)	Aloe vera (page 624) Bladderwrack (page 639) Marshmallow (page 708) Slippery elm (page 747)

What are the symptoms of GERD?

People with GERD have heartburn, which usually feels like a burning pain that begins in the chest and may travel upward to the throat. Many people also feel a regurgitation of stomach contents into the mouth, leaving an acid or bitter taste. Some people with GERD may also have coughing while lying down, increased production of saliva, and difficulty sleeping after eating.

Medical treatments

Over the counter antacids, such as magnesium hydroxide (Phillips' Milk of Magnesia), aluminum hydroxide (Amphojel), calcium carbonate (Tums), and the combination magnesium-aluminum hydroxide (Mylanta, Maalox), help relieve the symptoms of GERD. The histamine H2 antagonists, such as cimetidine (Tagamet), ranitidine (Zantac), and famotidine (Pepcid), as well as the proton pump inhibitor omeprazole (Prilosec-OTC), are also beneficial.

Medications may be used to control stomach acidity, including prescription strength histamine H2 inhibitors, such as cimetidine (Tagamet), ranitidine (Zantac), and famotidine (Pepcid), as well as the prescription strength proton pump inhibitors omeprazole (Prilosec), lansoprazole (Prevacid), pantoprazole (Protonix), and rabeprazole (Aciphex).

Individuals with GERD should avoid stomach acid stimulants (e.g., coffee, alcohol), certain drugs (e.g., anticholinergics), specific foods (e.g., fats, chocolate), and smoking.

Dietary changes that may be helpful

Whether lowering dietary fat is important for people with GERD is somewhat unclear. Historically, low-fat diets have been recommended to patients with GERD because fatty foods appeared to be associated with increased heartburn and fatty foods had been shown to weaken the LES in both healthy people and people with GERD.[2, 3] A number of recent studies, however, have found no correlation between the fat content of a meal and subsequent symptoms of heartburn and reflux.[4, 5] Another study found that hospitalizations due to GERD were no more likely for people who ate high-fat diets than for those on low-fat diets.[6] One study compared different fast foods for their likelihood to cause reflux symptoms and found that chili and red wine caused more symptoms than higher-fat foods such as hamburgers and French fries.[7]

Eating foods or drinking beverages flavored with spearmint, **peppermint** (page 726), or other spices with strong aromatic oils causes relaxation of the LES and can contribute to symptoms in people with GERD.[8] Chocolate also relaxes the LES and can cause **heartburn** (page 260).[9, 10] Acidic beverages like juices, coffee, and tea have also been linked to increased heartburn pain, as have carbonated drinks, **alcohol** (page 12), and milk.[11]

Infants who suffer from GERD may have a true allergy to cows' milk.[12] Some small studies estimate that milk allergy is a cause in about 20% of infants with GERD,[13, 14, 15] but a larger study of 204 infants with GERD diagnosed cows' milk allergies in 41%.[16] For these infants, reflux symptoms improved with elimination of milk products from the diet. Some researchers advise a trial of cows' milk-elimination in all infants suffering from GERD.[17, 18] Infants with a condition known as multiple food protein intolerance in infancy (MFPI) have been shown to have a high incidence of GERD and may only improve when amino-acid based formula is used in place of other formulas.[19, 20]

Lifestyle changes that may be helpful

Smoking weakens the LES and is a strong risk factor for GERD.[21, 22, 23] A study of infants with GERD found that exposure to cigarette smoke in the environment is associated with reflux, leading the authors conclude that secondhand smoke contributes directly to GERD in infants.[24] No similar studies on environmental smoke have been done with adults. Psychological stress and alcohol have also been shown to be associated with the weakening of the LES and symptoms of GERD.[25, 26, 27, 28]

A number of studies have found that **obesity** (page 446) increases the risk of GERD,[29, 30] though one study found no association between severe obesity and GERD.[31] Obese people tend to have weaker sphincters,[32] and they more often develop a condition related to GERD called hiatal hernia, in which the upper part of the stomach protrudes above the diaphragm, resulting in a deformed LES.[33] It has been suggested that obesity may contribute to GERD by increasing abdominal pressure, but this mechanism has not been proven.[34] The benefit of weight loss for obese patients with GERD is controversial. Some researchers have found that symptoms of GERD are reduced with weight loss,[35] while others have seen no change with weight loss and even increased symptoms in patients with massive weight loss.[36]

Lying down prevents gravity from keeping the stomach contents well below the opening from the esophagus. For this reason, many authorities recommend that people with GERD avoid lying down sooner than three hours after a meal, and suggest elevating the head of the bed to prevent symptoms during sleep.[37, 38]

GERD occurs more frequently during exercise than at rest, and can be a cause of chest pain or abdominal pain during exertion.[39] One study found that increased intensity of exercise resulted in increased reflux in both trained athletes and untrained people.[40] In another study, running produced more reflux than less jarring activities, such as bicycling, while weight training produced few reflux symptoms.[41] Eating just before exercise has been found to further aggravate GERD.[42, 43] On the other hand, a recent survey found that people who participate in little recreational activity were more likely than active people to be hospitalized for GERD.[44] It makes sense for people with GERD to use exercise as part of a healthy lifestyle, perhaps choosing activities that are less likely to cause reflux symptoms.

Nutritional supplements that may be helpful

Hydrochloric acid (page 260) and **digestive enzymes** (page 506) are sometimes recommended by practitioners of natural medicine in the hope improved digestion will help prevent reflux.[45] However, these therapies have not been researched for their effectiveness.

Are there any side effects or interactions?
Refer to the individual supplement for information about any side effects or interactions.

Herbs that may be helpful

Licorice (page 702), particularly as chewable degly-cyrrhizinated licorice (DGL), has been shown to be an effective treatment for the healing of stomach and duodenal **ulcers** (page 349);[46, 47, 48] in an uncontrolled trial, licorice was effective as a treatment for aphthous ulcers (**canker sores** [page 90]).[49] A synthetic drug similar to an ingredient of licorice has been used as part of an effective therapy for GERD in both uncontrolled[50] and double-blind[51, 52] trials. In a comparison trial, this combination proved to be as effective as cimetidine (Tagamet), a common drug used to treat GERD.[53] However, licorice itself remains unexamined as a treatment for GERD.

Other herbs traditionally used to treat reflux and **heartburn** (page 260) include digestive demulcents (soothing agents) such as **aloe vera** (page 624), **slippery elm** (page 747), **bladderwrack** (page 639), and **marshmallow** (page 708).[54] None of these have been scientifically evaluated for effectiveness in GERD. However, a drug known as Gaviscon, containing magnesium carbonate (as an antacid) and alginic acid derived from bladderwrack, has been shown helpful for heartburn in a double-blind trial.[55] It is not clear whether whole bladderwrack would be as useful as its alginic acid component.

Are there any side effects or interactions?
Refer to the individual herb for information about any side effects or interactions.

GENITAL HERPES

Genital herpes is a common sexually transmitted viral infection characterized by fluid filled blisters or red bumps in the genital area.

Genital herpes is caused by either of two types of the herpes simplex virus (HSV). There is no known cure for herpes. Both conventional and alternative treatments only help in reducing the symptoms and frequency of outbreaks. Treatments effective for **cold sores** (page 119)—which are also caused by the herpes virus—may or may not also be effective for genital herpes, because of possible differences in the type of herpes virus causing infections in different body locations.

What are the symptoms of genital herpes?
People with genital herpes may have outbreaks of small, often painful, fluid-filled blisters (vesicles) in the genital

or anal region. Fever, general weakness, and painful urination often accompany the initial occurrence. Subsequent outbreaks may appear with colds, fevers, menstrual periods, or during periods of stress,[1] and usually disappear within two weeks. Initially there may be tingling or prickling at the site of the blisters even before they are visible, then the blisters often weep a clear fluid and form a scab.

CHECKLIST FOR GENITAL HERPES		
Rating	Nutritional Supplements	Herbs
★★☆	**Lysine** (page 550) **Propolis** (page 579) (topical) **Zinc** (page 614) (topical)	*Aloe vera* (page 624) (topical) **Lemon balm** (page 701) (topical)
★☆☆	Lithium (topical)	Cloves (topical) **Eucalyptus** (page 673) (topical) **Licorice root** (page 702) (topical) Seaweed (topical) **Turmeric** (page 753) (topical)

Medical treatments
Over the counter analgesics, such as aspirin (Bayer, Ecotrin, Bufferin), ibuprofen (Motrin, Advil), and acetaminophen (Tylenol), may provide symptomatic relief of pain.

Prescription antiviral medications, such as topical acyclovir (Zovirax Ointment) or oral acyclovir (Zovirax), famciclovir (Famvir), and valacyclovir (Valtrex), might accelerate healing and reduce the duration of pain.

Dietary changes that may be helpful
Many alternative healthcare practitioners recommend that people with herpes simplex infections eat a diet high in the amino acid **lysine** (page 550) and low in **arginine** (page 467). Foods high in lysine include red meat, poultry, fish, and dairy products, while foods such as chocolate, nuts, peas, and cereals are high in arginine. This recommendation is based on test tube research indicating that growth of the herpes virus is inhibited by lysine and promoted by arginine.[2] However, no research has investigated whether making these dietary changes helps prevent outbreaks of genital herpes. In fact, one preliminary study found that patients with and without genital herpes did not differ from each

other in how much dietary arginine and lysine they consumed.[3]

Lifestyle changes that may be helpful

Since genital herpes is highly contagious, people with active herpes infections should avoid direct sexual contact. Also, infected pregnant women should inform their obstetrician if their herpes becomes active around their delivery date, as HSV can be transmitted to the newborn during birth and cause a more serious infection in the child.

Nutritional supplements that may be helpful

Most research on **lysine** (page 550) has been done on people with **cold sores** (page 119) or on groups that include both cold sores and genital herpes sufferers. However, some evidence exists that supplemental lysine may be effective in the prevention and treatment of genital herpes. In one preliminary survey, 81% of people with HSV infections (including genital herpes) reported lysine was effective for reducing recurrences and shortening healing time in amounts averaging about 1,000 mg per day.[4] A small double-blind trial of people with oral and genital herpes examined the effects of 1,248 mg or 624 mg of lysine daily versus placebo.[5] The study found that 1,248 mg per day of lysine, but not the lower dose, was effective in reducing the recurrence rate of herpes outbreaks by 57% to 65%, while neither dose helped reduce the healing time. Another small double-blind trial found that using 3,000 mg per day of lysine in divided doses led to a decrease in severity of symptoms and a reduction in healing time of both oral and genital herpes.[6] One preliminary report found no benefit of lysine for a group of patients with either oral or genital herpes.[7]

In a test tube, **zinc** (page 614) is capable of inactivating the type of herpes virus responsible for the majority of genital herpes cases.[8] Topical zinc may therefore help prevent outbreaks of genital herpes. One preliminary study treated people (four of whom had genital herpes) with a 4% zinc sulfate solution applied to the site of the initial outbreak.[9] In all cases, the pain, burning, and tingling stopped within 24 hours of beginning the topical zinc therapy. The use of lower concentrations of zinc (0.025–0.05%) has also been shown effective against oral and genital herpes outbreaks.[10, 11] While topical zinc has been shown to be helpful, there is no convincing evidence that oral zinc offers the same benefits.[12]

Lithium is a mineral available in an ointment or in the prescription drug lithium carbonate. In small studies, pharmacological doses of lithium carbonate have helped prevent outbreaks of genital herpes.[13, 14] However, there is no evidence that smaller amounts of oral lithium in nonprescription supplements would be similarly effective. A controlled study using a topical ointment containing 8% lithium succinate with 0.05% zinc sulphate diminished the pain and discomfort of genital herpes and shortened the healing time.[15] In light of the known benefits of topical zinc, it is unclear whether lithium was an important component of this treatment

A test tube study found that **flavonoids** (page 516) present in **propolis** (page 579) are responsible for the supplement's antiviral action.[16] A controlled study found that an ointment containing propolis, used four times daily, was almost twice as effective as topical antiviral medication or a placebo ointment.[17]

Are there any side effects or interactions?
Refer to the individual supplement for information about any side effects or interactions.

Herbs that may be helpful

Licorice root (page 702) *(Glycyrrhiza glabra)* contains antiviral substances[18] and ointments containing related substances are effective in treating herpes infections.[19, 20] While the use of topical licorice preparations to prevent or treat genital herpes has not been studied, some alternative healthcare practitioners recommend applying creams or gels containing licorice three to four times a day.

A double-blind trial found that topical application of a cream containing a highly concentrated extract of **lemon balm** (page 701) *(Melissa officinalis)* four to five times a day helped heal oral and genital herpes sores faster than use of a placebo.[21]

Aloe vera (page 624) may also benefit those with genital herpes. A double-blind trial using a 0.5% *Aloe vera* cream found that applying the cream three times a day shortened the healing time of genital herpes outbreaks. All but 3 of 22 persons in the study who showed healing with the aloe cream had no recurrences 15 months after stopping treatment.[22]

Test tube and animal research suggests that substances found in **turmeric** (page 753), cloves, **eucalyptus** (page 673), and seaweed have potential benefit for topical prevention of genital herpes, but no human research using available herbal products has been performed.[23]

Are there any side effects or interactions?
Refer to the individual herb for information about any side effects or interactions.

Genital Herpes

Holistic approaches that may be helpful

Stress plays a major role in the recurrence of genital herpes outbreaks. One preliminary study found that persistent stress (stress lasting more than seven days) increased the recurrence rate by about 25%,[24] but another preliminary study found no connection between stress and genital herpes outbreaks.[25] In addition, short-term stress, mood changes, and menstrual cycles do not appear to affect herpes recurrences.[26] Treatments aimed in part at stress reduction may be helpful for treating genital herpes. One controlled trial showed that patients had fewer outbreaks, shorter episode duration, and less episode severity when they were treated with a series of sessions involving education about genital herpes, stress management, deep breathing exercises, and guided imagery.[27] A preliminary study suggested that applied relaxation (a technique that guides the participant through a series of muscle relaxation exercises) reduces recurrences of genital herpes outbreaks.[28] Two case reports indicate that self-hypnosis, practiced on a daily basis, helps ease the pain and severity of genital herpes lesions.[29]

GESTATIONAL HYPERTENSION

Gestational hypertension (GH) is high blood pressure that develops after the twentieth week of **pregnancy** (page 363) and returns to normal after delivery, in women with previously normal blood pressure.

GH may be an early sign of either **preeclampsia** (page 361) or chronic **hypertension** (page 246). If these complications do not develop, or if chronic hypertension develops but remains mild, the outcome of pregnancy is usually good for both the mother and newborn. GH has been shown to occur more frequently in women who are obese[1] or in those who are glucose-intolerant.[2, 3, 4]

CHECKLIST FOR GESTATIONAL HYPERTENSION		
Rating	**Nutritional Supplements**	**Herbs**
★★★	Calcium (page 483) Magnesium (page 551)	
★☆☆	Zinc (page 614)	

What are the symptoms of gestational hypertension?

Symptoms, which appear after the twentieth week of pregnancy, include swelling of the face and hands, visual disturbances, headache, high blood pressure, and a yellow discoloration of the skin and eyes.

Medical treatments

The category of prescription drugs known as diuretics are commonly used to treat hypertension. Agents often used include the thiazide diuretics, such as hydrochlorothiazide (HydroDIURIL), indapamide (Lozol), and metolazone (Zaroxolyn); loop diuretics including furosemide (Lasix), bumetanide (Bumex), and torsemide (Demadex); and potassium-sparing diuretics, such as spironolactone (Aldactone), triamterene (Dyazide, Maxzide), and amiloride (Midamor). Diuretics are usually combined with beta-blockers, such as propranolol (Inderal), metoprolol (Lopressor, Toprol XL), atenolol (Tenormin), and bisoprolol (Zebeta), or ACE inhibitors, including captopril (Capoten), benazepril (Lotensin), lisinopril (Zestril, Prinivil), enalapril (Vasotec), and quinapril (Accupril). In addition, calcium channel blockers such as amlodipine (Norvasc), verapamil (Calan SR, Verelan PM), and diltiazem (Cardizem CD) may be used either alone or in combination with diuretics to treat high blood pressure.

Treatment for GH includes bed rest, restriction of sodium intake, and, if necessary, hospitalization for observation. Intravenous **magnesium** (page 551) solutions are occasionally recommended. The definitive treatment is termination of the pregnancy by induced delivery or cesarean section.

Dietary changes that may be helpful

Unlike salt restriction in primary hypertension, a low-salt diet has not been shown to have a significant effect in reducing high blood pressure during pregnancy.[5, 6, 7] As a result, salt restriction is not recommended to women with GH.[8]

Increased consumption of fish was associated with reduced risk of GH in one preliminary study.[9] In this study, the incidence of hypertension during pregnancy was significantly higher in women from communities with lower consumption of fish and lower in women from communities with high fish consumption.

Lifestyle changes that may be helpful

In GH, regular checkups during pregnancy and after delivery are needed for the prevention and early detection of **preeclampsia** (page 361) and chronic **hypertension** (page 246).[10, 11, 12]

Job stress (lack of control over work pace and the timing and frequency of breaks) has been reported to be detrimental; therefore, reducing job stress may be beneficial in the prevention of GH.[13] In a preliminary study, women exposed to high job stress were found to be at greater risk of developing GH than were women with low job stress.[14]

The common practice of prescribing bed rest for women with GH has been questioned by some researchers.[15] In the few studies examining this issue, results have been inconsistent.[16, 17] While one controlled study found that bed rest reduced progression of GH to severe hypertension,[18] evidence is currently insufficient to determine whether bed rest reduces blood pressure in women with GH.

Nutritional supplements that may be helpful

Calcium (page 483) deficiency has been implicated as a possible cause of GH.[19, 20] In two preliminary studies, women who developed GH were found to have significantly lower dietary calcium intake than did pregnant women with normal blood pressure.[21, 22] Calcium supplementation has significantly reduced the incidence of GH in preliminary studies[23] and in many,[24, 25, 26, 27, 28, 29] though not all,[30] double-blind trials. Calcium supplements may be most effective in preventing GH in women who have low dietary intake of calcium. The National Institutes of Health (NIH) recommends an intake of 1,200 to 1,500 mg of calcium daily during normal pregnancy.[31] In women at risk of GH, studies showing reduced incidence have typically used 2,000 mg of supplemental calcium per day,[32, 33, 34, 35, 36, 37] without any reported maternal or fetal side effects.[38, 39] Nonetheless, many doctors continue to suggest amounts no higher than 1,500 mg per day.

Magnesium (page 551) deficiency has also been implicated as a possible cause of GH.[40, 41, 42] Dietary intake of magnesium is below recommended levels for many women during pregnancy.[43, 44] Magnesium supplementation has been reported to reduce the incidence of GH in preliminary[45] and many double-blind trials.[46, 47] In addition to preventing GH, magnesium supplementation has also been reported to reduce the severity of established GH in one study.[48] Amounts used in studies on GH range from 165 to 365 mg of supplemental magnesium per day.

Zinc (page 614) supplementation (20 mg per day) was reported to reduce the incidence of GH in one double-blind trial studying a group of low-income Hispanic pregnant women who were not zinc deficient.[49]

Antioxidant (page 467) levels in the blood of women with GH appear to be reduced in some,[50, 51, 52] but not all,[53] preliminary studies. No studies have yet been conducted evaluating the effects of antioxidant supplementation on the incidence or severity of GH.

Are there any side effects or interactions?
Refer to the individual supplement for information about any side effects or interactions.

GINGIVITIS

Gingivitis is an inflammation of the gums (gingivae), usually caused by bacteria.

Periodontitis is a deeper and more serious inflammation of both the gingivae and tissue that surrounds and supports the teeth.

Both common conditions are often progressive and can eventually result in loss of the underlying bone that supports the teeth. After age 30, periodontal disease is responsible for more tooth loss than are dental cavities. Severe periodontitis sometimes requires surgery to repair damaged gum tissue.

What are the symptoms of gingivitis?

Gingivitis is usually painless, although the gums may be red, swollen, and bleed easily with brushing. There can also be a bad taste in the mouth or persistent bad breath (**halitosis** [page 209]). In advanced stages of gingivitis, the gums recede, exposing the nerve roots, and the teeth may become loose. This may be an indication of periodontitis.

Medical treatments

Prescription antibacterial mouthwashes such as chlorhexidine (Peridex, PerioGard) are frequently used to treat gum inflammation.

Treatment usually involves a regimen of good oral hygiene, including correct tooth brushing, flossing, and professional cleanings. Severe cases might require gum surgery.

Nutritional supplements that may be helpful

A 0.1% solution of **folic acid** (page 520) used as a mouth rinse (5 ml taken twice a day for 30 to 60 days)

Gingivitis

CHECKLIST FOR GINGIVITIS (PERIODONTAL DISEASE)

Rating	Nutritional Supplements	Herbs
★★★	**Folic acid** (page 520) (rinse only) **Vitamin C** (page 604) (only if deficient)	
★★☆	**Coenzyme Q10** (page 496) **Vitamin C** (page 604) plus **flavonoids** (page 516)	**Bloodroot** (page 641) plus **zinc** (page 614) (toothpaste) Mouthwash containing **sage** (page 740) oil, **peppermint** (page 726) oil, menthol, **chamomile** (page 656) tincture, expressed juice from **echinacea** (page 669), **myrrh** (page 713) tincture, clove oil, and **caraway** (page 651) oil
★☆☆	**Calcium** (page 483) **Flavonoids** (page 516) **Folic acid** (page 520) (in pill form)	**Chamomile** (page 656) **Echinacea** (page 669)

has reduced gum inflammation and bleeding in people with gingivitis in double-blind trials.[1, 2] The folic acid solution is rinsed in the mouth for one to five minutes and then spit out. Folic acid was also found to be effective when taken in capsule or tablet form (4 mg per day),[3] though in another trial studying pregnant women with gingivitis, only the mouthwash—and not folic acid in pill form—was effective.[4] However, this may have been due to the body's increased requirement for folic acid during pregnancy.

Phenytoin (Dilantin) therapy causes gum disease (gingival hyperplasia) in some people. A regular program of dental care has been reported to limit or prevent gum disease in people taking phenytoin.[5, 6, 7] Double-blind research has shown that a daily oral rinse with a liquid folic acid preparation inhibited phenytoin-induced gum disease more than either folic acid in pill form or placebo.[8]

People who are deficient in **vitamin C** (page 604) may be at increased risk for periodontal disease.[9] When a group of people with periodontitis who normally consumed only 20–35 mg of vitamin C per day were given

an additional 70 mg per day, objective improvement of periodontal tissue occurred in only six weeks.[10] It makes sense for people who have a low vitamin C intake (e.g., people who eat few fruits and vegetables) to supplement with vitamin C in order to improve gingival health.

For people who consume adequate amounts of vitamin C in their diet, several studies have found that supplemental vitamin C has no additional therapeutic effect. Research,[11] including double-blind evidence,[12] shows that vitamin C fails to significantly reduce gingival inflammation in people who are not vitamin C deficient. In one study, administration of vitamin C plus **flavonoids** (page 516) (300 mg per day of each) did improve gingival health in a group of people with gingivitis;[13] there was less improvement, however, when vitamin C was given without flavonoids. Preliminary evidence has suggested that flavonoids by themselves may reduce inflammation of the gums.[14]

Preliminary evidence has linked gingivitis to a **coenzyme Q10** (page 496) (CoQ10) deficiency.[15] Some researchers believe this deficiency could interfere with the body's ability to repair damaged gum tissue. In a double-blind trial, 50 mg per day of CoQ10 given for three weeks was significantly more effective than a placebo at reducing symptoms of gingivitis.[16] Compared with conventional approaches alone, topical CoQ10 combined with conventional treatments resulted in better outcomes in a group of people with periodontal disease.[17]

Some,[18] but not all,[19] research has found that giving 500 mg of **calcium** (page 483) twice per day for six months to people with periodontal disease results in a reduction of symptoms (bleeding gums and loose teeth). Although some doctors recommend calcium supplementation to people with diseases of the gums, supportive scientific evidence remains weak.

Are there any side effects or interactions?
Refer to the individual supplement for information about any side effects or interactions.

Herbs that may be helpful

Bloodroot (page 641) contains alkaloids, principally sanguinarine, that are sometimes used in toothpaste and other oral hygiene products because they inhibit oral bacteria.[20, 21] Sanguinarine-containing toothpastes and mouth rinses should be used according to manufacturer's directions. A six-month, double-blind trial found that use of a bloodroot and **zinc** (page 614) toothpaste reduced gingivitis significantly better than placebo.[22] However, a similar study was unable to replicate these results.[23] Thus, at present, it is unknown who will respond to bloodroot toothpaste and who will not. Concerns also exist about the long-term safety of bloodroot.

In a double-blind trial, 1 gram of neem leaf extract in gel twice per day was more effective than chlorhexidine or placebo gel at reducing plaque and bacteria levels in the mouth in 36 Indian adults.[24] A similar trial found neem gel superior to placebo and equally effective as chlorhexidine at reducing plaque and bacteria levels in the mouth.[25] These promising early studies should be followed by studies regarding prevention of cavities and relief from gingivitis or periodontal disease.

A mouthwash combination that includes **sage** (page 740) oil, **peppermint** (page 726) oil, menthol, **chamomile** (page 656) tincture, expressed juice from **echinacea** (page 669), **myrrh** (page 713) tincture, clove oil, and **caraway** (page 651) oil has been successfully to treat gingivitis.[26] In cases of acute gum inflammation, 0.5 ml of the herbal mixture in half a glass of water three times daily is recommended by some herbalists. This herbal preparation should be swished slowly in the mouth before spitting out. To prevent recurrences, slightly less of the mixture can be used less frequently.

A toothpaste containing sage oil, peppermint oil, chamomile tincture, expressed juice from *Echinacea purpurea,* myrrh tincture, and rhatany tincture has been used to accompany this mouthwash in managing gingivitis.[27]

Of the many herbs listed above, chamomile, echinacea, and myrrh should be priorities. These three herbs can provide anti-inflammatory and antimicrobial actions critical to successfully treating gingivitis.

Are there any side effects or interactions?
Refer to the individual herb for information about any side effects or interactions.

GLAUCOMA

The term glaucoma describes a group of eye conditions that are usually associated with increased intraocular pressure (pressure within the eyeball).

In many cases, the cause of glaucoma is unknown. Conventional medications are frequently effective in reducing intraocular pressure. Therefore, it is important for people with glaucoma to be under the care of an ophthalmologist.

CHECKLIST FOR GLAUCOMA		
Rating	Nutritional Supplements	Herbs
★★★	Vitamin C (page 604)	*Ginkgo biloba* (page 681) (for normal tension glaucoma)
★★☆		Coleus (page 660)
★☆☆	Alpha lipoic acid (page 464) Fish oil and cod liver oil (page 514) (omega-3 fatty acids) Flavonoids (page 516) (rutin) Magnesium (page 551) Melatonin (page 555)	Dan shen Periwinkle (page 727)

What are the symptoms of glaucoma?
Because glaucoma may not cause any symptoms until it has reached an advanced and irreversible stage, regular eye exams are recommended, especially after age 40. In the later stages, symptoms include loss of peripheral (side) vision, blurred vision, blind spots, seeing halos around lights, and poor night vision. If left untreated, glaucoma may cause blindness.

Medical treatments
Several prescription medications are available to reduce pressure within the eye. Commonly used agents include dipivefrin (Propine), betaxolol (Betoptic), carteolol (Ocupress), timolol (Timoptic), pilocarpine (Isopto Carpine), and latanoprost (Xalatan).

Surgical procedures, such as laser trabeculoplasty and trabeculectomy, can increase fluid drainage from the eye to relieve pressure.

Dietary changes that may be helpful
At least two older reports claimed that **allergy** (page 14) can be a triggering factor for glaucoma.[1, 2] Although an association between allergy and glaucoma is not generally accepted in conventional medicine, people with glaucoma may wish to consult a physician to diagnose and treat possible allergies.

Nutritional supplements that may be helpful
Several studies have shown that supplementing with **vitamin C** (page 604) can significantly reduce elevated

intraocular pressure in individuals with glaucoma.[3] These studies used at least 2 grams per day of vitamin C; much larger amounts were sometimes given. Higher quantities of vitamin C appeared to be more effective than smaller amounts.

Doctors often suggest that people with glaucoma take vitamin C to "bowel tolerance."[4] The bowel-tolerance level is determined by progressively increasing vitamin C intake until loose stools or abdominal pain occurs, and then reducing the amount slightly, to a level that does not cause these symptoms. The bowel tolerance level varies considerably from person to person, usually ranging from about 5 to 20 or more grams per day. Vitamin C does not cure glaucoma and must be used continually to maintain a reduction in intraocular pressure.

Many years ago, the **flavonoid** (page 516) rutin was reported to increase the effectiveness of conventional medication in people with glaucoma.[5] The amount used—20 mg three times per day—was quite moderate. In that study, 17 of 26 eyes with glaucoma showed clear improvement. Modern research on the effects of rutin or other flavonoids in people with glaucoma is lacking.

Supplementing with 0.5 mg of **melatonin** (page 555) lowered intraocular pressure of healthy people,[6] but there have been no studies on the effects of melatonin in people with glaucoma.

Magnesium (page 551) can dilate blood vessels. One study looked at whether magnesium might improve vision in people with glaucoma by enhancing blood flow to the eyes. In that trial, participants were given 245 mg of magnesium per day. Improvement in vision was noted after four weeks, but the change did not reach statistical significance.[7]

Alpha lipoic acid (page 464) (150 mg per day for one month) improves visual function in people with some types of glaucoma.[8]

Surveys have shown that Inuit people, who consume large amounts of omega-3 fatty acids, have a much lower incidence of some types of glaucoma than do Caucasians. Although there have been no studies on the use of omega-3 fatty acids to treat glaucoma, one study found that **cod liver oil** (page 514) (a rich source of omega-3 fatty acids) reduced intraocular pressure in animals.[9]

Are there any side effects or interactions?
Refer to the individual supplement for information about any side effects or interactions.

Herbs that may be helpful
In a double-blind study, supplementation with a standardized extract of **Ginkgo biloba** (page 681) in the amount of 40 mg three times a day for four weeks partially reversed visual field damage in people with one type of glaucoma (normal tension glaucoma).[10]

Studies in healthy humans, including at least one double-blind trial, have repeatedly shown that intraocular pressure is lowered by direct application of forskolin, a constituent of the Ayurvedic herb **Coleus forskohlii** (page 660).[11, 12] Until ophthalmic preparations of coleus or forskolin are available, people with glaucoma should consult with a skilled healthcare practitioner to obtain a sterile fluid extract for use in the eyes. Direct application of the whole herb to the eyes has not been studied and is not advised.

Dan shen *(Salvia miltiorrhiza),* a traditional Chinese herb, used either alone or combined with other Chinese herbs for 30 days was reported to improve vision in people with glaucoma.[13] However, the herb was administered by muscular injection, a preparation that is not readily available in North America or Great Britain. It is not known whether oral use of the herb would have the same effect.

Are there any side effects or interactions?
Refer to the individual herb for information about any side effects or interactions.

GOITER

Goiter is an enlargement of the thyroid gland that often produces a noticeable swelling in the front of the neck.

This enlargement can be caused by iodine deficiency, inability of the body to use iodine correctly, or a variety of thyroid disorders, including **infection** (page 265), tumors, and autoimmune disease. Some environmental pollutants, heavy metal poisonings, and certain drugs can also contribute to goiter formation.[1, 2, 3] Both iodine deficiency and inability to use iodine properly make the thyroid gland unable to produce thyroid hormone, a hormone that helps to regulate the body's metabolic rate. This state is called **hypothyroidism** (page 252) and the symptoms include fatigue, weight gain, heavy menstrual bleeding in women, dry skin and hair, as well as goiter.

Iodine-deficiency goiter can be common in regions where the soils and foods have insufficient iodine.

Preschool children, adolescent girls, pregnant women, and the elderly are most vulnerable to goiter and other iodine-deficiency disorders.[4] Areas where iodine supplies are inadequate see high rates not only of goiter but also of birth defects and retardation of both mental and physical development.[5] While iodine deficiency is the leading cause of goiter worldwide, it is a rare cause of goiter in the developed world. For this reason, any goiter that occurs in the developed world must be evaluated by a healthcare provider and its cause determined before any treatment is given.

CHECKLIST FOR GOITER		
Rating	**Nutritional Supplements**	**Herbs**
★★★	**Iodine** (page 538)	
★☆☆	**Manganese** (page 553) (if deficient) **Vitamin A** (page 595) **Vitamin E** (page 609) **Zinc** (page 614) (if deficient)	

What are the symptoms of goiter?
People with goiter may notice a soft swelling in the front of the neck.

Medical treatments
Thyroid hormone replacement medications such as L-thyroxine (Synthroid, Levoxyl) and dessicated thyroid (Armour Thyroid) might be prescribed for individuals with goiter.

Other treatment includes the use of iodized table salt and the avoidance of goiter promoting (goitrogenic) foods, such as cabbage, Brussels sprouts, and soy. Surgical removal or radioactive iodine treatments may be necessary for cosmetic reasons or in individuals with large goiters that interfere with breathing or swallowing.

Dietary changes that may be helpful
The most important dietary concern in treating iodine-deficiency hypothyroidism and preventing goiter is ensuring adequate intake of **iodine** (page 538). Iodine is found naturally in foods from the ocean, such as fish and seafood, kelp, and sea vegetables, and in plant and animal products produced in areas where soil and water contain sufficient iodine.[6, 7] In developed countries, commercial table salt has been fortified with iodine

since the 1920s to prevent deficiency.[8] Iodized salt contains approximately 100 micrograms of iodine per gram of salt. This fortified salt is used directly and is incorporated into animal feeds and processed foods making it easy to achieve the Recommended Dietary Allowance (RDA) of 150 mcg for adolescents and adults and 200 mcg daily for pregnant and breast-feeding women.[9] Iodized salt has proven so effective it is recommended as the intervention of choice to eliminate iodine deficiency worldwide.[10, 11] Iodized oils, given as an annual injection or as food by mouth, have also been used effectively to treat iodine-deficiency goiter.[12, 13]

Although iodine deficiency and goiter are now quite uncommon in developed countries, recent studies have found that the average dietary iodine intake in the United States has fallen below RDA guidelines.[14] Long-term *excessive* dietary intake of iodine (1,000 to 2,000 micrograms daily), while less common than iodine deficiency, can occur in people who eat large amounts of kelp and other sea vegetables and can also cause goiter.[15, 16]

A number of commonly eaten foods have been shown to interfere with the use of iodine by the thyroid, thus reducing production of thyroid hormone and causing goiter. These foods, known as goitrogens, include vegetables in the *Brassica* family such as broccoli, cabbage, kale and mustard,[17] millet,[18] soybeans,[19] pine nuts[20] and some seed meals used in animal feeds.[21, 22] These foods can be safely eaten in moderate amounts by people who consume adequate iodine.[23] A combination of low iodine intake and high intake of goitrogenic foods increases the likelihood of goiter.[24, 25]

Nutrient deficiencies, including **zinc** (page 614),[26] **manganese** (page 553)[27] and **vitamin A** (page 595),[28, 29] and severe protein malnutrition[30] also contribute to an inability to use iodine well and to the development of goiter.[31, 32] In the presence of adequate iodine supplies, it is less common for such factors to cause goiter;[33, 34] however, when iodine intake becomes deficient, even mild malnutrition can have such a negative impact on thyroid function.[35, 36] High levels of minerals such as calcium and magnesium, and certain bacteria in drinking water, have also been shown to be goitrogenic.[37, 38] Therefore, proper nutrition and a healthy water supply are crucial in the prevention and treatment of goiter.

Nutritional supplements that may be helpful
Iodine (page 538) supplementation can be an effective treatment of iodine deficiency hypothyroidism and can

halt the growth of goiter if the cause is not complicated by malnutrition or environmental and dietary goitrogens.[39, 40] Iodine supplements will help to shrink goiters during early stages, but they have no effect in later stages.[41] Ingestion of 2,000 to 6,000 mcg of iodine daily over long periods of time can be toxic to the thyroid and can be a cause of goiter.[42, 43]

Blood levels of **vitamin A** (page 595) are lower in people with goiter than in similar people without goiter.[44, 45] The same relationship has been found for **vitamin E** (page 609) and goiter.[46] Animal research has found that, in iodine-deficient conditions, a supplement combination of **vitamin C** (page 604), vitamin E, and **beta-carotene** (page 469) prevented goiter formation (though hypothyroidism was not improved), and vitamin E alone had a similar effect.[47] No studies have been done to investigate this benefit in humans.

When iodine deficiency is present, other nutrient levels become important in the development of goiter. Deficiencies of **zinc** (page 614)[48] and **manganese** (page 553)[49] can both contribute to iodine-deficiency goiter; however, an animal study found that manganese excess can also be goitrogenic.[50] It has been suggested that selenium deficiency may contribute to goiter.[51] However, when selenium supplements were given to people deficient in both iodine and selenium, thyroid dysfunction was aggravated, and it has been suggested that selenium deficiency may provide some protection when there is iodine deficiency.[52, 53] A study of the effects of selenium supplementation at 100 mcg daily in women without selenium deficiency but with slightly low iodine intake found no effect on thyroid function.[54] The authors concluded that selenium supplementation seems to be safe in people with only iodine deficiency but not in people with combined selenium and iodine deficiencies. In those cases, iodine supplementation has been shown to be most useful.[55] No studies have been done to evaluate the usefulness of supplementation with zinc or manganese to prevent or treat goiter.

Are there any side effects or interactions?
Refer to the individual supplement for information about any side effects or interactions.

GOUT

Gout is a form of arthritis that occurs when crystals of uric acid accumulate in a joint, leading to the sudden development of **pain** (page 338) and inflammation.

People with gout either overproduce uric acid or are less efficient than other people at eliminating it. The joint of the big toe is the most common site to accumulate uric acid crystals, although other joints may be affected.

CHECKLIST FOR GOUT		
Rating	**Nutritional Supplements**	**Herbs**
★☆☆	**Folic acid** (page 520) **Quercetin** (page 580) **Vitamin C** (page 604)	Colchicine from autumn crocus

What are the symptoms of gout?
The **pain** (page 338) of gout can arise suddenly and is often very intense. The affected joint is usually red, swollen, and very tender to the touch. A low-grade fever may also be present.

Medical treatments
Over the counter analgesics, such as aspirin (Bayer, Ecotrin, Bufferin), ibuprofen (Motrin, Advil), and naproxen (Aleve), might provide temporary pain relief.

Acute gout attacks are typically treated with the prescription drug colchicine and prescription strength nonsteroidal anti-inflammatory drugs (NSAIDs) such as celecoxib (Celebrex), valdecoxib (Bextra), indomethacin (Indocin) and naproxen sodium (Anaprox). Occasionally corticosteroids, such as prednisone (Deltasone), are used to treat inflammation.

Individuals with gout are often prescribed allopurinol (Zyloprim) to prevent future acute attacks. Probenecid (Benemid) and sulfinpyrazone (Anturane) are available, yet less frequently used, to treat gout.

Healthcare practitioners recommend resting the affected joint during acute gout attacks.

Dietary changes that may be helpful
Foods that are high in compounds called purines raise uric acid levels in the body and increase the risk of gout. Restricting purine intake can reduce the risk of an attack in people susceptible to gout. Foods high in purines include anchovies, bouillon, brains, broth, consommé, dried legumes, goose, gravy, heart, herring, kidneys, liver, mackerel, meat extracts, mincemeat, mussels, partridge, fish roe, sardines, scallops, shrimp, sweetbreads, baker's yeast, **brewer's yeast** (page 480), and yeast extracts (e.g., Marmite, Vegemite).

Avoiding alcohol, particularly beer, or limiting alcohol intake to one drink per day or less may reduce the number of attacks of gout.[1, 2] Refined sugars, including sucrose (white table sugar) and fructose (the sugar found in fruit juice), should also be restricted, because they have been reported to raise uric acid levels.[3]

According to a 1950 study of 12 people with gout, eating one-half pound of cherries or drinking an equivalent amount of cherry juice prevented attacks of gout.[4] Black, sweet yellow, and red sour cherries were all effective. Since that study, there have been many anecdotal reports of cherry juice as an effective treatment for the **pain** (page 338) and inflammation of gout. The active ingredient in cherry juice remains unknown.

Lifestyle changes that may be helpful

People who are **overweight** (page 446) or have **high blood pressure** (page 246) are at greater risk of developing gout.[5] However, weight loss should not be rapid because restriction of calories can increase uric acid levels temporarily, which may aggravate the condition.

Nutritional supplements that may be helpful

Large amounts of supplemental **folic acid** (page 520) (up to 80 mg per day) have reduced uric acid levels in preliminary research.[6] However, other studies have failed to confirm the effectiveness of folic acid in treating people with gout.[7]

In one small study, people who took 4 grams of **vitamin C** (page 604) (but not lower amounts) had an increase in urinary excretion of uric acid within a few hours, and those who took 8 grams of vitamin C per day for several days had a reduction in serum uric acid levels.[8] Thus, supplemental vitamin C could, in theory, reduce the risk of gout attacks. However, the authors of this study warned that taking large amounts of vitamin C could also trigger an acute attack of gout by abruptly changing uric acid levels in the body. Despite this concern, some doctors recommend vitamin C supplementation (sometimes starting with one gram per day) as a method for reducing elevated uric acid levels.

In test tube studies, **quercetin** (page 580), a **flavonoid** (page 516), has inhibited an enzyme involved in the development of gout.[9, 10] However, it is not known whether taking quercetin by mouth can produce high enough quercetin concentrations in the body to achieve these effects. Although human research is lacking, some doctors recommend 150–250 mg of quercetin three times per day (taken between meals).

Are there any side effects or interactions?
Refer to the individual supplement for information about any side effects or interactions.

Herbs that may be helpful

Autumn crocus (*Colchicum autumnale*) is the herb from which the drug colchicine was originally isolated. Colchicine, a strong anti-inflammatory compound, is used as a conventional treatment for gout. Both the herb and the drug have significant toxicity and should only be used under the guidance of a physician.

Are there any side effects or interactions?
Refer to the individual herb for information about any side effects or interactions.

HALITOSIS

Halitosis is the technical term for bad breath, a condition estimated to affect 50 to 65% of the population.[1]

Up to 90% of cases are thought to originate from sources in the mouth, including poor oral hygiene, **periodontal disease** (page 203), coating on the tongue, impacted food, faulty dental restorations, and throat infections.[2, 3, 4] The remaining 10% are due to systemic disorders, such as **peptic ulcer** (page 349) (when associated with infection),[5, 6] lung infections (bad breath can be the first sign in some cases),[7] **liver** (page 290) or kidney disease,[8, 9] **diabetes mellitus** (page 152), **cancer** (page 87),[10] or even a person's imagination (healthy individuals sometimes complain of bad breath that cannot be smelled by anyone else and is not linked to any clinical disorder).[11]

In most cases, bad breath in the mouth can be traced to sulfur gases produced by bacteria in the mouth.[12, 13] Factors that support the growth of these bacteria will predispose a person to halitosis. Examples include accumulation of food within pockets around the teeth,[14] among the bumps at the back of the tongue,[15] or in small pockets in the tonsils; sloughed cells from the mouth; and diminished saliva flow. Mucus in the throat or sinuses can also serve as a breeding ground for bacteria. Conditions are most favorable for odor production during the night and between meals.[16]

Although bad breath primarily represents a source of embarrassment or annoyance, research has shown that the sulfur gases most responsible for halitosis (hydrogen sulfide and methyl mercaptan) are also potentially damaging to the tissues in the mouth, and can lead to **periodontitis** (page 203) (inflammation of the gums and ligaments supporting the teeth).[17, 18] As periodontal disease progresses, so may the halitosis, as bacteria accumulate in the pockets that form next to the teeth.

Halitosis

CHECKLIST FOR HALITOSIS

Rating	Nutritional Supplements	Herbs
★★☆	**Coenzyme Q₁₀** (page 496) (if gum disease) **Folic acid** (page 520) (if gum disease) **Zinc chloride** (page 614) (rinse or toothpaste)	
★☆☆	**Selenium** (page 584) (if gum disease) **Vitamin C** (page 604) (if gum disease and deficient) **Vitamin E** (page 609) (if gum disease and deficient)	**Bloodroot** (page 641) (rinse) **Caraway** (page 651) Clove oil (rinse or toothpaste) **Eucalyptus** (page 673) **Myrrh** (page 713) (rinse) **Peppermint** (page 726) **Sage** (page 740) **Tea tree oil** (page 751) (rinse or toothpaste) **Thyme** (page 752) oil (rinse)

Medical treatments

Improved oral hygiene and and treatment of underlying infections may be effective in some cases. Mouthwashes might help to control oral bacteria. Persistent halitosis requires professional dental care.

Lifestyle changes that may be helpful

Home oral hygiene is probably the most effective way to reduce accumulations of debris and bacteria that lead to halitosis. This includes regular tooth brushing and flossing, and/or the use of mechanical irrigators to remove accumulations of food after eating. Brushing the tongue or using a commercial tongue scraper, especially over the bumpiest region of the tongue, may help remove the odor-causing agents as well as lower the overall bacteria count in the mouth.

Because of the role of **gum disease** (page 203) in halitosis, regular dental care is recommended to prevent or treat gum disease. Treatment for a person with periodontal pockets might include scaling of the teeth to remove tartar.[19]

A reduced saliva flow increases the concentration of bacteria in the mouth and worsens bad breath.[20] One of the most common causes of dry mouth is medication, such as antihistamines, some antidepressants, and diuretics; however, chronic mouth breathing, radiation therapy, dehydration, and various diseases can also contribute.[21] Measures that help increase saliva production (e.g., chewing sugarless gum and drinking adequate water) may improve halitosis associated with poor saliva flow. Avoiding alcohol (ironically found in many commercial mouthwashes) may also help, because alcohol is drying to the mouth.

Access by oral bacteria to sulfur-containing amino acids will enhance the production of sulfur gases that are responsible for bad breath. This effect was demonstrated in a study in which concentrations of these sulfur gases in the mouth were increased after subjects used a mouth rinse containing the amino acid **cysteine** (page 502).[22] Cleaning the mouth after eating sulfur-rich foods, such as dairy, fish, and meat, may help remove the food sources for these bacteria.

Nutritional supplements that may be helpful

Because most halitosis stems from bacterial production of odiferous compounds, general measures to diminish bacteria as well as measures targeted at prevention or treatment of periodontitis and **gingivitis** (page 203) may be helpful. Mouthwashes or toothpastes containing a compound called stabilized chlorine dioxide appear to help eliminate bad breath by directly breaking down sulfur compounds in the mouth. One study showed reductions in mouth odor for at least four hours following the use of a mouthrinse containing this substance.[23]

Preliminary research has also demonstrated the ability of **zinc** (page 614) to reduce the concentration of volatile sulfur compounds in the mouth. One study found that the addition of zinc to a baking soda toothpaste lessened halitosis by lowering the levels of these compounds.[24] A mouthrinse containing zinc chloride was seen in another study to neutralize the damaging effect of methyl mercaptan on periodontal tissue in the mouth.[25, 26]

Nutritional supplements recommended by some doctors for prevention and treatment of periodontitis include **vitamin C** (page 604) (people with periodontitis are often found to be deficient),[27] **vitamin E** (page 609), **selenium** (page 584), zinc, **coenzyme Q₁₀** (page 496), and **folic acid** (page 520).[28] Folic acid has also been shown to reduce the severity of gingivitis when taken as a mouthwash.[29]

Are there any side effects or interactions?
Refer to the individual supplement for information about any side effects or interactions.

Herbs that may be helpful

The potent effects of some commercial mouthwashes may be due to the inclusion of thymol (from **thyme** [page 752]) and eukalyptol (from **eucalyptus** [page 673])—volatile oils that have proven activity against bacteria. One report showed bacterial counts plummet in as little as 30 seconds following a mouthrinse with the commercial mouthwash Listerine™, which contains thymol and eukalyptol.[30] Thymol alone has been shown in research to inhibit the growth of bacteria found in the mouth.[31, 32] Because of their antibacterial properties, other volatile oils made from **tea tree** (page 751),[33] clove, **caraway** (page 651), **peppermint** (page 726), and **sage** (page 740),[34] as well as the herbs **myrrh** (page 713)[35] and **bloodroot** (page 641),[36] might be considered in a mouthwash or toothpaste. Due to potential allergic reactions and potential side effects if some of these oils are swallowed, it is best to consult with a qualified healthcare professional before pursuing self-treatment with volatile oils that are not in approved over-the-counter products for halitosis.

Are there any side effects or interactions?
Refer to the individual herb for information about any side effects or interactions.

HAY FEVER

Hay fever is an **allergic condition** (page 14) triggered by the immune system's response to inhalant substances (frequently pollens).

Researchers have yet to clearly understand why some people's **immune systems** (page 255) overreact to exposure to pollens while other people do not suffer from this problem. Symptoms of hay fever are partly a result of inflammation that, in turn, is activated by the immune system.

What are the symptoms of hay fever?

Inhaled allergens trigger sneezing and inflammation of the nose and mucous membranes (conjunctiva) of the eyes. The nose, roof of the mouth, eyes, and throat begin to itch gradually or abruptly after the onset of the pollen season. Tearing, sneezing, and clear, watery nasal discharge soon follow the itching. Headaches and irritability may also occur.

CHECKLIST FOR HAY FEVER		
Rating	Nutritional Supplements	Herbs
★★☆	Thymus extracts (page 591) Vitamin E (page 609)	Butterbur *Tinospora cordifolia*
★☆☆	Quercetin (page 580) Vitamin C (page 604)	Nettle (page 714) Sho-seiryu-to (contains licorice [page 702], cassia bark, schisandra [page 744], ma huang, ginger [page 680], peony [page 724] root, pinellia, and asiasarum root) Tylophora (page 754)

Medical treatments

Over the counter topical nasal decongestants such as oxymetazoline (Afrin) and phenylephrine (NeoSynephrine) may provide relief from nasal congestion, but they should only be used for a few days. The oral decongestant pseudoephedrine (Sudafed) may help relieve nasal congestion, while antihistamines such as diphenhydramine (Benadryl), brompheniramine (Dimetapp), chlorpheniramine (Chlor-Trimeton), and loratadine (Claritin) might help dry excess mucous and reduce sneezing. Cromolyn sodium (Nasalcrom) is used as a nose spray to prevent hayfever symptoms.

Prescription antihistamines are often prescribed for relief of hay fever symptoms. These include cetirizine (Zyrtec), desloratadine (Clarinex), and fexofenadine (Allegra). Inhaled corticosteroids, such as flunisolide (Nasalide), triamcinolone (Nasacort), fluticasone (Flonase), and mometasone (Nasonex) may also be suggested to prevent and treat nasal symptoms.

Dietary changes that may be helpful

People with inhalant **allergies** (page 14) are likely to also have **food allergies** (page 14).[1, 2] A hypoallergenic diet has been reported to help some people with **asthma** (page 32) and allergic rhinitis,[3] but the effect of such a diet on hay fever symptoms has not been studied. Hay fever sufferers interested in exploring the possible effects of a food allergy avoidance program should talk with a doctor. Discovering and eliminating offending food allergens, should they exist, is likely to improve overall health even if such an approach has no effect on hay fever symptoms.

Nutritional supplements that may be helpful

Although **vitamin C** (page 604) has antihistamine activity, and supplementation, in preliminary research,[4, 5] has been reported to help people with hay fever, 2,000 mg of vitamin C per day did not reduce hay fever symptoms in a placebo controlled trial.[6] Thus, while some doctors recommend that hay fever sufferers take 1,000–3,000 mg of vitamin C per day, supportive evidence remains weak.

In a double-blind study of people with hay fever, adding 800 IU of **vitamin E** (page 609) per day to regular anti-allergy treatment during the pollen season significantly reduced the severity of hay fever symptoms by 23%, compared with placebo plus regular anti-allergy treatment.[7]

Quercetin (page 580) is an increasingly popular treatment for hay fever even though only limited preliminary clinical research has suggested that it is beneficial to hay fever sufferers.[8]

The oral administration of a **thymus extract** (page 591) known as Thymomodulin has been shown in preliminary studies and double-blind trials to improve the symptoms of hay fever and allergic rhinitis.[9, 10, 11] Presumably this clinical improvement is the result of restoration of proper control over **immune function** (page 255).

Are there any side effects or interactions?
Refer to the individual supplement for information about any side effects or interactions.

Herbs that may be helpful

In a double-blind study, an extract of the butterbur plant *(Petasites hybridus)* was significantly more effective than a placebo at improving symptoms in people suffering from seasonal allergic rhinitis.[12] The study used a preparation standardized to contain 8 mg of total petasin per tablet. One tablet was administered either two or three times a day for two weeks; the larger amount was found to be more effective than the smaller amount.

Tinospora cordifolia is an herb used in traditional Indian (Ayurvedic) medicine for increasing longevity, promoting intelligence, and improving memory and immune function. In a double-blind trial, an extract of

Tinospora cordifolia was significantly more effective than a placebo at relieving symptoms of allergic rhinitis, including sneezing, runny nose, nasal obstruction, and nasal itching. The study used 300 mg of a standardized extract three times a day for eight weeks.[13]

Tylophora (page 754) is an herb used by Ayurvedic doctors in India to treat people with **allergies** (page 14). It contains compounds that have been reported to interfere with the action of mast cells, which are key components in the process of inflammation responsible for most hay fever symptoms.[14] Mast cells are found in airways of the lungs (among other parts of the body). When mast cells are activated by pollen or other allergens, they release the chemical histamine, which in turn leads to a wide number of symptoms familiar to hay fever sufferers—itchy eyes, runny nose, and chest tightness. Ayurvedic doctors sometimes recommend 200–400 mg of the dried herb daily or 1–2 ml of the tincture per day for up to two weeks.

In an isolated double-blind trial, **nettle** (page 714) leaf led to a slight reduction in symptoms of hay fever—including sneezing and itchy eyes.[15] However, no other research has investigated this relationship. Despite the lack of adequate scientific support, some doctors suggest taking 450 mg of nettle leaf capsules or tablets two to three times per day, or a 2–4 ml tincture three times per day for people suffering from hay fever.

The Japanese herbal formula known as sho-seiryu-to has been shown to reduce symptom, such as sneezing, for people with hay fever.[16] Sho-seiryu-to contains **licorice** (page 702), cassia bark, **schisandra** (page 744), ma huang, **ginger** (page 680), **peony root** (page 724), pinellia, and asiasarum root.

Are there any side effects or interactions?
Refer to the individual herb for information about any side effects or interactions.

HEART ATTACK

Heart attacks occur when blood flow to a portion of the heart is severely reduced or cut off. The result is death of heart muscle cells (called an infarct).

Hardening and narrowing (**atherosclerosis** [page 38]) of the coronary arteries that feed the heart is usually the underlying problem. In some cases, a blood clot blocks blood flow; other times, the narrowing is caused by atherosclerosis alone. Spasm of the coronary arteries may also cause a heart attack.

Elevated **cholesterol** (page 223), **triglycerides** (page 235), or **homocysteine** (page 234); **angina pectoris** (page 27); and **diabetes** (page 152) are each associated with an increased risk of heart attack. **Congestive heart failure** (page 134) can occur in some people from severe damage to the heart resulting from a heart attack.

CHECKLIST FOR HEART ATTACK

Rating	Nutritional Supplements	Herbs
★★★	**Coenzyme Q₁₀** (page 496) **L-carnitine** (page 543) **Vitamin C** (page 604) (if deficient)	
★★☆	**Fish oil** (page 514) **Folic acid** (page 520) **Magnesium** (page 551) (IV immediately following an MI) **N-acetyl cysteine** (page 562) (IV immediately following an MI) **Selenium** (page 584) **Vitamin A** (page 595) **Vitamin E** (page 609)	
★☆☆	**Beta-carotene** (page 469) **Chondroitin sulfate** (page 492) **Magnesium** (page 551) (oral) **Vitamin B₁₂** (page 601) **Vitamin B₆** (page 600) **Vitamin C** (page 604) (for those not deficient)	**Astragalus** (page 631)

What are the symptoms of a heart attack?

The first symptom of a heart attack is usually deep aching or pressure-like chest pain that may radiate to the back, jaw, or left arm. Discomfort may be mild or severe. About 20% of heart attacks are silent (i.e., they cause no symptoms and may therefore be missed). Older people may experience shortness of breath. Nausea and vomiting may also occur. Restlessness, apprehension, pallor, and sweating are common.

Medical treatments

Aspirin (Bayer Low Adult Strength, Ecotrin Adult Low Strength) reduces the risk of death or nonfatal heart attack in patients with a previous history of heart attack or unstable **angina** (page 27)

Fifty percent of deaths from heart attack occur within three to four hours of the onset of symptoms. Therefore, treatment delay is potentially fatal. Optimal early management of heart attacks includes intravenous administration of thrombolytic (clot-dissolving) drugs, such as streptokinase (Kabikinase, Streptase), anistreplase (Eminase), or reteplase (Retavase). Other thrombolytic agents include heparin, hirudin (Hirulog), abciximab (ReoPro), and tirofiban (Aggrastat). Beta-blockers, such as atenolol (Tenormin), metoprolol (Lopressor), and isoproterenol (Isuprel) may reduce the potential for life-threatening **arrhythmias** (page 93). ACE inhibitors, including captopril (Capoten), lisinopril (Zestril, Prinivil), and enalapril (Vasotec), as well as vasodilators such as nitroglycerin (Nitrobid, Nitro-Dur) are also sometimes used.

Many hospitals perform a procedure called Primary Percutaneous Transluminal Cardiac Angioplasty (PTCA) in order to clear blocked arteries. Certain individuals might benefit more from this procedure than from thrombolytic agents.

Dietary changes that may be helpful

Dietary fat independently affects heart attack risk. The Nurses' Health Study found that eating foods high in saturated fats (meat and dairy fat) and trans fatty acids (margarine, hydrogenated vegetable oils, and many processed foods containing hydrogenated vegetable oils) was directly associated with many nonfatal heart attacks and deaths from **coronary heart disease** (page 98).[1] Consuming foods high in monounsaturated fat, such as olive oil, and polyunsaturated fat, as found in nuts and most vegetable oils, is linked to a decreased risk. This same study revealed that margarine increased the incidence of heart attack, particularly among women who had eaten margarine consistently for more than a decade.[2] Other studies report a direct association between frequent consumption of meat and butter and heart attack occurrence.[3]

Research consistently shows that people who frequently eat nuts have a dramatically reduced risk of heart disease;[4, 5] this could be because nut consumption lowers **cholesterol levels** (page 223).[6, 7] Of nuts commonly consumed, almonds and walnuts may be most effective at lowering cholesterol, and macadamia nuts may be least beneficial.[8] Hazelnuts[9] and pistachio nuts[10] may also help lower cholesterol.

Nuts contain many nutrients that could be responsible for protection against heart disease, including **fiber** (page 512), **vitamin E** (page 609), alpha-linolenic acid (found primarily in walnuts), oleic acid, **magnesium** (page 551), and **arginine** (page 467). Therefore, exactly how nuts lower cholesterol or lower the risk of heart disease remains somewhat unclear. Some doctors even believe that nuts may not be *directly* protective. Rather, people who eat nuts may not eat as much dairy, eggs, or trans fatty acids from margarine and processed food, the avoidance of which would reduce both cholesterol levels and the risk of **heart disease** (page 98).[11, 12] Nonetheless, the remarkable consistency of research outcomes strongly suggests that nuts directly protect against heart disease. Although nuts are loaded with calories, a recent preliminary study reported that adding hundreds of calories per day from nuts for six months did not increase body weight in humans[13]—an outcome supported by several other reports.[14] Even when increasing nut consumption has led to weight gain, the amount of added weight has been remarkably less than would be expected given the number of calories added to the diet.[15]

Several trials report that eating fish decreases heart attack deaths[16, 17] and reduces the size of the infarct,[18] though some researchers have not confirmed these findings.[19] The link between fish eating and heart attack prevention is supported by research showing that **fish oil** (page 514) supplements help reverse **atherosclerosis** (page 38).[20]

Eating eggs may increase heart attack risk. People who consume eggs have been reported to be more likely to die from all types of **heart disease** (page 98), including heart attack, in some,[21] although not all, research.[22] Increased oxidation, a state associated with heart attack risk, may be the key. Cooking or exposure to air oxidizes the cholesterol in eggs.[23] Eating eggs enhances LDL ("bad") cholesterol oxidation,[24] which may in turn contribute to heart attack risk.

Eating a diet high in refined carbohydrates (e.g., white flour, white rice, simple sugars) appears to increase the risk of coronary heart disease, and thus of heart attacks, especially in overweight women.[25]

A high-fiber diet, particularly water-soluble fiber (high in **oats** [page 716], **psyllium seeds** [page 732], fruit, vegetables, and legumes), is associated with decreased risk of both fatal and nonfatal heart attacks,[26] probably because these fibers are known to lower cholesterol.[27] However, large trials separately studying men and women who were followed for years, have linked the greatest protection to water-*insoluble* fiber (from cereals),[28, 29] though scientists have yet to understand why. Until the details are better understood, doctors

often recommend increasing intake of fruit, vegetables, beans, oats, and whole grains. In a preliminary study,[30] the total number of deaths from cardiovascular disease was found to be significantly lower among men with high fruit consumption.

Making positive dietary changes immediately following a heart attack is likely to decrease the chance of a second heart attack. In one study, individuals began eating more vegetables and fruits, and substituted fish, nuts, and legumes for meat and eggs 24–48 hours after a heart attack. Six weeks later, the diet group had significantly fewer fatal and nonfatal heart attacks than a similar group who did not make these dietary changes.[31] This trend continued for an additional six weeks.[32]

Many doctors tell people trying to reduce their risk of **heart disease** (page 98) to avoid all meat, margarine, and other processed foods containing hydrogenated oils and dairy fat. Fish are often suggested instead of meat; nuts instead of snack foods containing hydrogenated oils; olive oil instead of butter; nonfat yogurt, milk, and even cheese instead of full or reduced fat versions of the same foods; and oatmeal instead of eggs for breakfast.

People who eat diets high in alpha-linolenic acid (ALA), which is found in canola and **flaxseed oils** (page 517), have higher blood levels of omega-3 fatty acids than those consuming lower amounts,[33, 34] which may confer some protection against **atherosclerosis** (page 98). In 1994, researchers conducted a study in people with a history of heart disease, using what they called the "Mediterranean" diet.[35] The diet was significantly different from what people from Mediterranean countries actually eat, in that it contained little olive oil. Instead, the diet included a special margarine high in ALA. Those people assigned to the Mediterranean diet had a remarkable 70% reduced risk of dying from heart disease compared with the control group during the first 27 months. Similar results were also confirmed after almost four years.[36] The diet was high in beans and peas, fish, fruit, vegetables, bread, and cereals; and low in meat, dairy fat, and eggs. Although the authors believe that the high ALA content of the diet was partly responsible for the surprising outcome, other aspects of the diet may have been partially or even totally responsible for decreased death rates. Therefore, the success of the Mediterranean diet does not prove that ALA protects against heart disease.[37]

Most studies confirm that light to moderate alcohol consumption (one to three drinks per day) significantly reduces both fatal and nonfatal heart attack risk[38, 39, 40, 41] compared to heavy or no drinking,[42, 43] though a few reports find the link to protection both weak and statistically insignificant.[44] In France, abundant red wine drinking was assumed to be responsible for the country's remarkably low incidence of heart disease. However, a lower intake of animal fats in the French diet now appears to be the primary reason for what has been called the French paradox.[45] However, as animal fat intake continues to increase in France, a trend that began in the 1970s, researchers now speculate that heart disease and heart attacks will also increase.

Although red wine has been branded best for heart disease in a few reports, all types of alcoholic beverages appear to be beneficial.[46] Whether red wine has a clear advantage over other forms of alcohol remains unclear. Alcohol reduces the risk for heart attacks because it increases HDL ("good") cholesterol[47] and acts as a blood thinner.[48] High levels of another risk factor for heart attacks, lipoprotein(a), have also been reported to be lowered by drinking alcohol.[49]

Despite this healthful effect, alcohol consumption can cause liver disease (e.g., **cirrhosis** [page 290]), **cancer** (page 87), **high blood pressure** (page 246), **alcoholism** (page 12), and, at high intake, even an increased risk of heart attack. As a result, some doctors never recommend alcohol, even for people at risk for heart attack. Nevertheless, because limited intake of alcohol lowers heart attack risk, some people at high risk for heart attack who are not alcoholics, have healthy livers and normal blood pressure, and are not at an especially high risk for cancer, may benefit from light drinking. In fact, since **heart disease** (page 98) is the leading cause of death in the United States, and alcohol reduces that risk, most studies report that light drinkers live slightly longer on average than teetotalers. In an analysis of 16 trials, men who drank less than two drinks per day and women who averaged less than one drink per day were likely to slightly outlive those who did not drink at all.[50] In the same report, however, people who drank beyond these moderate levels in men and low levels in women were *more* likely to die sooner than were nondrinkers. In deciding whether light drinking might do more good than harm, people at high risk for heart attack should consult a doctor.

Drinking five cups of coffee or more per day has been shown to increase the risk of nonfatal heart attack in both men[51] and women.[52] Though many studies find such links,[53] many others do not.[54] Nevertheless, heavy coffee drinking should be avoided. This disparity may result in part from the fact that paper-filtered coffee does not raise **cholesterol** (page 223) but percolated, boiled, or French press coffees do. Several recent studies have linked coffee drinking to increased blood levels of **homocysteine** (page 234), another risk factor for **heart disease** (page 98).[55, 56] In this regard, research has yet to absolve paper-filtered coffee, because these studies have not examined separate effects for coffee prepared by different methods.

Recent preliminary evidence has implicated salt consumption as a risk factor for heart disease and death from heart disease in overweight people.[57] Among overweight persons, an increase in salt consumption of 2.3 grams per day was associated with a 44% increase in coronary heart disease mortality, a 61% increase in cardiovascular disease mortality, and a 39% increase in mortality from all causes. Blinded, intervention trials are still needed to confirm these preliminary observations.

Preliminary research conducted several decades ago suggested that high sugar consumption increased heart attack risk.[58] Some researchers at that time disagreed[59] and others have subsequently been unable to find a link. Nevertheless, sugar has been associated with reduced HDL ("good") cholesterol,[60] increased **triglycerides** (page 235),[61] as well as an increase in other risk factors linked to heart attacks.[62] As a result, many doctors recommend that people reduce their intake of sugar despite the fact that high sugar intake leads to only slightly higher risks of heart disease in most reports.[63]

Lifestyle changes that may be helpful

Two very large studies have confirmed that smoking increases the risk of a first heart attack by more than 100% in some people.[64, 65] Women were found to be at greater risk than men; "inhalers" were almost twice as susceptible as non-inhalers. Quitting smoking is critical for reversing this risk. According to one study, female ex-smokers who had not smoked for three or more years were "virtually indistinguishable" from women who had never smoked in terms of heart attack risk.[66] Exposure to secondhand smoke, which increases infarct size in animals[67] and impairs heart function and exercise tolerance in heart attack survivors,[68] should also be avoided. For people who have already had a heart attack, quitting smoking is associated with a significant decrease in mortality.[69]

Routine, moderate exercise is preferred over excessive exertion for people at risk for heart attacks. Research indicates that heart attack risk rises six-fold for one hour immediately following heavy physical activity (compared to moderate or no activity), particularly among people who are sedentary.[70] This risk is more than five times less in people who exercise four or more times per week.[71] Most studies show that regular, moderate exercise reduces overall heart attack risk. Therefore, researchers and doctors recommend that susceptible individuals engage in an exercise program.[72] Exercise recommendations for people who are at risk or who have a history of heart attack need to be custom tailored to the individual. Therefore, anyone with a heart condition or anyone over the age of 40 should consult a healthcare professional before beginning an exercise plan.

Although sexual activity can trigger a heart attack, the risk is very low and[73] is no greater for people with a history of **angina** (page 27) or **heart disease** (page 98). Doctors recommend regular, moderate exercise to further reduce this risk.

Obesity is associated with an increased risk for heart attack, particularly among younger people.[74] One study found this relationship increased in women who also had a history of **diabetes** (page 152) or **high cholesterol** (page 223).[75] Doctors encourage overweight people who are at risk for heart attack to **lose the extra weight** (page 446).

Type A behavior is typically defined by time-conscious, impatient, and aggressive feelings and the behavior that arises from those feelings. Type A behavior has been linked to increased heart attack risk in some,[76] but not all, studies.[77] The link between personality and heart attack remains unclear.[78] In the study with the most hopeful outcome, psychological intervention aimed at modifying type A behavior was reported to successfully change not only emotional state but also to significantly lower the risk of subsequent heart attacks.[79] Some healthcare professionals recommend that people at high risk for heart attacks who also have frequent feelings of impatience, lack of time, and hostility, seek counseling as a way to feel better and potentially reduce their risk of heart disease.

Researchers suggest that negative emotional states, such as hostility, distrust, anger,[80] worry,[81] and stress,[82] promote heart attacks. Results from the National Heart, Lung, and Blood Institute (NHLBI) Family Heart Study showed that hostility was significantly associated with an increased risk of having a heart attack (in women) and increased odds of having heart surgery (in men), when a family history of heart disease was also present.[83, 84] According to another study, women with a history of heart disease who report stressful relationships with their husbands or partners have almost triple the risk of suffering a heart attack, dying from heart disease,

or requiring bypass surgery or angioplasty, compared with women in positive relationships.[85]

Following a heart attack, bed rest is often recommended. However, a review of trials concluded that bed rest may actually worsen recovery from a heart attack.[86]

Nutritional supplements that may be helpful

L-carnitine (page 543) is an **amino acid** (page 465) important for transporting fats that can be turned into energy in the heart. Clinical trials have reported that taking L-carnitine (4–6 grams per day) increases the chance of surviving a heart attack.[87, 88, 89] In one double-blind trial, individuals with suspected heart attack were given 2 grams of L-carnitine per day for 28 days.[90] At the completion of this study, infarct size, as well as the number of nonfatal heart attacks, was lower in the group receiving L-carnitine versus the placebo group. Double-blind research using L-carnitine intravenously also shows promise.[91]

Vitamin C (page 604) has been reported to protect blood vessels from problems associated with heart attack risk in a variety of ways.[92, 93, 94] However, research attempting to link vitamin C directly to protection from heart attacks has been inconsistent.[95, 96] The reason for this discrepancy appears related to the amount of vitamin C intake investigated in these studies. True or marginal vitamin C deficiencies *do* appear to increase the risk of suffering heart attacks.[97, 98] However, in trials comparing acceptable (i.e., non-deficient) vitamin C levels to even higher levels, additional vitamin C has not been protective.[99] Therefore, though many doctors recommend that people at high risk for heart attack take vitamin C—often 1 gram per day—most evidence currently suggests that consuming as little as 100–200 mg of vitamin C per day from food or supplements may well be sufficient.

Coenzyme Q$_{10}$ (page 496) (CoQ$_{10}$) also contributes to the energy-making mechanisms of the heart and has been reported to lower lipoprotein(a), a risk factor for **heart disease** (page 98).[100] Animal studies confirm CoQ$_{10}$'s ability to protect heart muscle against reduced blood flow.[101, 102] In one double-blind trial, either 120 mg of CoQ$_{10}$ or placebo was given to people who had recently survived a heart attack. After 28 days, the CoQ$_{10}$ group had experienced significantly fewer repeat heart attacks, fewer deaths from heart disease, and less chest pain than the placebo group.[103] In another double-blind study of people suffering a heart attack, supplementation with 60 mg of coenzyme Q$_{10}$ twice a day for one year significantly reduced the incidence of recurrent cardiac events (fatal or non-fatal heart attack).[104] Treatment was begun within 72 hours of the onset of the heart attack. CoQ$_{10}$ used with **selenium** (page 584) (see below) has also been reported to increase the rate of heart attack survival.[105]

The relation between **selenium** (page 584) and protection from heart attacks remains uncertain. Low blood levels of selenium have been reported in people immediately following a heart attack,[106] suggesting that heart attacks may increase the need for selenium. However, other researchers claim that low selenium levels are present in people before they have a heart attack, suggesting that the lack of selenium might increase heart attack risk.[107] One report found that low blood levels of selenium increased the risk of heart attack only in smokers,[108] and another found the link only in *former* smokers.[109] Yet others have found no link between low blood levels of selenium and heart attack risk whatsoever.[110] In a double-blind trial, individuals who already had one heart attack were given 100 mcg of selenium per day or placebo for six months.[111] At the end of the trial, there were four deaths from **heart disease** (page 98) in the placebo group but none in the selenium group (although the numbers were too small for this difference to be statistically significant). In other controlled research, a similar group was given placebo or 500 mcg of selenium six hours or less after a heart attack followed by an ongoing regimen of 100 mcg of selenium plus 100 mg of **coenzyme Q$_{10}$** (page 496) per day.[112] One year later, six people had died from a repeat heart attack in the placebo group, compared with no heart attack deaths in the supplement group. Despite the lack of consistency in published research, some doctors recommend that people at risk for a heart attack supplement with selenium—most commonly 200 mcg per day.

Several studies[113, 114] including two double-blind trials[115, 116] have reported that 400 to 800 IU of natural **vitamin E** (page 609) reduces the risk of heart attacks. However, other recent double-blind trials have found either limited benefit,[117] or no benefit at all from supplementation with synthetic vitamin E.[118] One of the negative trials used 400 IU of natural vitamin E[119]—a similar amount and form to previous successful trials. In attempting to make sense of these inconsistent findings the following is clear: less than 400 IU of synthetic vitamin E, even when taken for years, does not protect against heart disease. Whether 400 to 800 IU of natural vitamin E is or is not protective remains unclear.

In one study, intravenous injections of **N-acetyl cys-teine** (page 562) (NAC) decreased the amount of tissue damage in people who had suffered a heart attack.[120] Whether oral NAC would have the same effect is unknown.

Fish oil (page 514) contains the beneficial omega-3 fatty acids EPA and **DHA** (page 509), which have led to partial reversal of **atherosclerosis** (page 38) in a double-blind trial.[121] In another double-blind trial, individuals were given either fish oil (containing about 1 gram of EPA and 2/3 gram of DHA) or mustard oil (containing about 3 grams alpha linolenic acid, another omega-3 fatty acid) 18 hours after a heart attack. Both groups experienced fewer nonfatal heart attacks compared to a placebo group, while the fish oil group also experienced fewer fatal heart attacks.[122] The largest published study on omega-3 fatty acids for heart attack prevention was the preliminary GISSI Prevenzione Trial,[123] which reported that 850 mg of omega-3 fatty acids from fish oil per day for 3.5 years resulted in a 20% reduction in total mortality and a 45% decrease in sudden death. Other investigators suggest that fish oil reduces the amount of heart muscle damage from a heart attack and enhances the effect of blood-thinning medication.[124] People wishing to supplement with fish oil should take fish oil supplements that include at least small amounts of **vitamin E** (page 609), which may protect this fragile oil against free radical damage.[125]

Blood levels of the **antioxidant** (page 467) nutrients vitamins A, C, and E, and beta-carotene are reported to be lower in people with a history of heart attack, compared with healthy individuals.[126] The number of free radical molecules is also higher, suggesting a need for antioxidants. Streptokinase, a drug therapy commonly used immediately following a heart attack, enhances the need for antioxidants.[127]

Taking antioxidant supplements may improve the outcome for people who have already had a heart attack. In one double-blind trial, people were given 50,000 IU of **vitamin A** (page 595) per day, 1,000 mg of **vitamin C** (page 604) per day, 600 IU of **vitamin E** (page 609) per day, and approximately 41,500 IU of **beta-carotene** (page 469) per day or placebo.[128] After 28 days, the infarct size of those receiving antioxidants was significantly smaller than the infarct size of the placebo group.

Blood levels of **magnesium** (page 551) are lower in people who have a history of heart attack.[129] Most trials have successfully used intravenous magnesium right after a heart attack occurs to decrease death and complications from heart attacks.[130] By far the largest trial did not find magnesium to be effective.[131] However, other researchers have argued that delaying the initial infusion of magnesium and administering the magnesium for too short a period may have caused this negative result.[132] People with a history of heart attack or who are at risk should consult with their cardiologist about the possible use of immediate intravenous magnesium should they ever suffer another heart attack.

Except for a link between high levels of magnesium in drinking water and a low risk of heart attacks,[133, 134] little evidence suggests that oral magnesium reduces heart attack risk. One trial found that magnesium pills taken for one year actually *increased* complications for people who had suffered a heart attack.[135] While another study reported that 400–800 mg of magnesium per day for two years decreased both deaths and complications due to heart attacks, results are difficult to interpret because those taking oral magnesium had previously received intravenous magnesium as well.[136] While increasing *dietary* magnesium has reduced the risk of heart attacks,[137] foods high in magnesium may contain other protective factors that might be responsible for this positive effect. Therefore, evidence supporting supplemental oral magnesium to reduce the risk of heart attacks remains weak.

High blood levels of the amino acid **homocysteine** (page 234) have been linked to an increased risk of heart attack in most,[138, 139, 140, 141] though not all,[142, 143] studies. A blood test screening for levels of homocysteine, followed by supplementation with 400 mcg of folic acid and 500 mcg of vitamin B_{12} per day could prevent a significant number of heart attacks, according to one analysis.[144] **Folic acid** (page 520)[145, 146] and vitamins **B_6** (page 600) and **B_{12}** (page 601) are known to lower homocysteine.[147]

There is a clear association between low blood levels of folate and increased risk of heart attacks in men.[148] Based on the available research, some doctors recommend 50 mg of vitamin B_6, 100–300 mcg of vitamin B_{12}, and 500–800 mcg of folic acid per day for people at high risk of heart attack.

Low levels of **beta-carotene** (page 469) in fatty tissue have been linked to an increased incidence of heart attacks, particularly among smokers.[149] One population study found that eating a diet high in beta-carotene is associated with a lower rate of nonfatal heart attacks.[150] However, beta-carotene supplementation may not offer the same protection provided by foods that contain beta-carotene. Most,[151, 152] but not all, trials[153] have found that supplemental beta-carotene is not associated with a reduced risk of heart attacks.

Years ago, researchers reported that taking **chondroitin sulfate** (page 492) for six years substantially reduced the risk of fatal and nonfatal heart attacks in people with **heart disease** (page 98).[154, 155, 156] Chondroitin may work by inhibiting **atherosclerosis** (page 38) and by acting as an anticoagulant. The few doctors aware of these older studies sometimes recommend that people with a history of heart disease or who are at risk for heart attack take approximately 500 mg of chondroitin sulfate three times per day.

The possibility that **vitamin D** (page 607) supplementation may increase the risk of heart disease remains an unproven and controversial issue. A preliminary trial suggested that a high intake of vitamin D from both dietary and supplemental sources increased heart attack risk.[157] However, other researchers have found that blood levels of vitamin D are no higher in people who had suffered a heart attack when compared to control groups.[158] Similarly, atherosclerosis does not appear to correlate with blood levels of vitamin D.[159] In fact, one trial found that higher levels of activated vitamin D correlated with *less* artery-clogging calcium deposits in humans.[160]

Relatively high blood levels of **calcium** (page 483)—sometimes a marker for high vitamin D intake—have been associated with high risk of heart attacks in Sweden.[161] However, high dietary vitamin D intake in Sweden often comes from high-fat dairy products, so the high calcium levels might simply reflect diets higher in dairy fat and have nothing to do with vitamin D.

Despite the lack of consistent evidence, some researchers continue to have concerns. **Vitamin D** (page 607) supplementation has reversed some of the beneficial effects of estrogen use in women with risk factors for **heart disease** (page 98),[162] an outcome confirmed by others using only 300 IU of vitamin D per day.[163] Further research is required to determine whether supplemental vitamin D increases heart attack risk.

Although several reports have linked **iron** (page 540) (both through diet and supplements) to an increased risk of heart disease, a recent analysis of 12 trials has found no link whatsoever between iron status and the risk of heart disease.[164] While it remains prudent for a variety of other reasons for people not to supplement iron unless a deficiency has been diagnosed, supplemental iron now appears unlikely to substantially increase the risk of suffering a heart attack.

Are there any side effects or interactions?
Refer to the individual supplement for information about any side effects or interactions.

Herbs that may be helpful

Preliminary clinical trials in China suggest that **astragalus** (page 631) may be of benefit in people after they have suffered a heart attack.[165, 166] These studies did not attempt to show any survival or symptom reduction benefit. Therefore, further research is needed to determine whether astragalus would be of benefit to people with heart attacks or **angina** (page 27).

Are there any side effects or interactions?
Refer to the individual herb for information about any side effects or interactions.

HEMORRHOIDS

Hemorrhoids are enlarged raised veins in the anus or rectum.

Common hemorrhoids are often linked to both **diarrhea** (page 163)[1] and **constipation** (page 137). Although the belief that hemorrhoids are caused by constipation has been questioned by researchers,[2] most doctors feel that many hemorrhoids are triggered by the straining that accompanies chronic constipation.[3] Therefore, natural approaches to hemorrhoids sometimes focus on overcoming constipation.

CHECKLIST FOR HEMORRHOIDS

Rating	Nutritional Supplements	Herbs
★★☆	**Fiber** (page 512) **Flavonoids** (page 516) (hydroxyethylrutosides derived from rutin)	**Horse chestnut** (page 692) **Psyllium** (page 732) **Witch hazel** (page 760)

What are the symptoms of hemorrhoids?

Symptoms of hemorrhoids may include painful swelling or a lump in the anus that can bleed and become inflamed, often causing discomfort and itching. There may also be bright red blood on the toilet paper, the stool, or in the toilet bowl.

Medical treatments

Over the counter products used to treat hemorrhoids include the use of rectal suppositories (Anusol), stool softeners (Colace, Surfak), topical preparations (Anusol, Preparation H), and medicated wipes (Tucks).

Prescription medications are available as creams, ointments, and suppositories. The hydrocortisone (Anusol-HC, Proctocort) contained in these products reduces inflammation, itching, and swelling.

Surgical treatment may be recommended for hemorrhoids that become very enlarged, protrude from the anus (prolapse), bleed frequently, or contain blood clots (thrombosis). Common procedures include freezing the affected tissue (cryotherapy), injecting chemicals into the hemorrhoid to shrink it (sclerosing solutions), surgically removing the hemorrhoid (hemorrhoidectomy), or placing rubber bands around the hemorrhoid for removal (ligation).

Dietary changes that may be helpful

Populations in which **fiber** (page 512) intake is high have a very low incidence of hemorrhoids. Insoluble fiber—the kind found primarily in whole grains and vegetables—increases the bulk of stool. Drinking water with a high-fiber meal or a fiber supplement results in softer, bulkier stools, which can move more easily. As a result, most doctors believe that fiber in combination with increased intake of liquids helps to treat people with hemorrhoids. Nonetheless, few clinical trials compare the effects of fiber supplementation against the effects of placebo in hemorrhoid sufferers.

Nutritional supplements that may be helpful

A number of **flavonoids** (page 516) have been shown to have anti-inflammatory effects and/or to strengthen blood vessels. These effects could, in theory, be beneficial for people with hemorrhoids. Most,[4, 5, 6, 7] but not all,[8] double-blind trials using a group of semisynthetic flavonoids (hydroxyethylrutosides derived from rutin) have demonstrated significant improvements in itching, bleeding, and other symptoms associated with hemorrhoids when people used supplements of 600–4,000 mg per day.

Other trials have evaluated Daflon, a product containing the food-derived flavonoids diosmin (90%) and hesperidin (10%). An uncontrolled trial reported that Daflon produced symptom relief in two-thirds of **pregnant** (page 363) women with hemorrhoids.[9] Double-blind trials have produced conflicting results about the effects of Daflon in people with hemorrhoids.[10, 11] Amounts of flavonoids used in Daflon trials ranged from 1,000 to 3,000 mg per day. Diosmin and hesperidin are available separately as dietary supplements.

Some doctors recommend flavonoid supplements for people with hemorrhoids. However, many different flavonoids occur in food and supplements, and additional research is needed to determine which flavonoids are most effective against hemorrhoids.

Are there any side effects or interactions?
Refer to the individual supplement for information about any side effects or interactions.

Herbs that may be helpful

Constipation (page 137) is believed to worsen hemorrhoid symptoms, and thus, bulk-forming fibers are often recommended for those with hemorrhoids. A double-blind trial reported that 7 grams of **psyllium** (page 732), an herb high in fiber, taken three times daily reduced the pain and bleeding associated with hemorrhoids.[12] Some healthcare professionals recommend taking two tablespoons of psyllium seeds or 1 teaspoon of psyllium husks two or three times per day mixed with water or juice. It is important to maintain adequate fluid intake while using psyllium.

Topically applied astringent herbs have been used traditionally as a treatment for hemorrhoids. A leading astringent herb for topical use is **witch hazel** (page 760),[13] which is typically applied to hemorrhoids three or four times per day in an ointment base.

Horse chestnut (page 692) extracts have been reported from a double-blind trial to reduce symptoms of hemorrhoids.[14] Some doctors recommend taking horse chestnut seed extracts standardized for aescin (also known as escin) content (16–21%), or an isolated aescin preparation, providing 90 to 150 mg of aescin per day.

Are there any side effects or interactions?
Refer to the individual herb for information about any side effects or interactions.

HEPATITIS

What do I need to know?

Self-care for hepatitis can be approached in a number of ways—but it can be hard to know just where to start. To make it easier, our doctors recommend trying these simple steps first:

See a doctor
> Get evaluated to determine the cause and best treatment for your condition

Reduce damage with milk thistle
> Take a standardized extract providing 420 mg a day of silymarin to help the liver

Try phyllanthus
> 900 to 2,700 mg a day may be beneficial for people with hepatitis B

About hepatitis

Hepatitis is a liver disease that can result from long-term **alcohol abuse** (page 12), **infection** (page 265), or exposure to various chemicals and drugs. Because hepatitis is potentially very dangerous, a healthcare professional should be involved in its treatment.

What are the symptoms of hepatitis?

Acute viral hepatitis varies from a minor flu-like illness to an overwhelming infection resulting in liver failure and death. The early phase is characterized by loss of appetite, malaise, nausea and vomiting, and fever. Signs include a darkening of the urine and jaundice (yellowing of the skin and whites of the eyes). Chronic hepatitis may be asymptomatic, or may manifest as malaise, fatigue, loss of appetite and a low-grade fever.

Rating	Nutritional Supplements	Herbs
★★★	**Flavonoids** (page 516) (catechin)	
★★☆	**Betaine** (page 472) (for nonalcoholic steatohepatitis) **Cordyceps** (page 663) **S-adenosylmethionine** (page 583) (SAMe) (for liver cholestasis) **Thiamine** (page 597) **Thymus extracts** (page 591) **Zinc** (page 614) (as zinc-L-**carnosine** [page 487], in combination with interferon, for hepatitis C)	**Bupleurum** (page 647) **Licorice** (page 702) (intravenous glycyrrhizin) **Milk thistle** (page 710) **Peony** (page 724) **Phyllanthus** (page 728)
★☆☆	**Alpha lipoic acid** (page 464) **Phosphatidylcholine** (page 546) **Selenium** (page 584) **Vitamin B$_{12}$** (page 601) **Vitamin C** (page 604) **Vitamin E** (page 609) **Whey protein** (page 613)	**Andrographis** (page 626) **Astragalus** (page 631) **Chinese scullcap** (page 658) **Licorice** (page 702) (oral glycyrrhizin) **Picrorhiza** (page 728) **Reishi** (page 737) **Schisandra** (page 744) **Shiitake** (page 746)

CHECKLIST FOR HEPATITIS

Medical treatments

Therapy for chronic hepatitis B and C is evolving and may include interferon (PEG-Intron, Roferon-A, Intron A, Infergen), antiviral (Rebetrol), and immune-modulating drugs. Autoimmune hepatitis is usually treated with corticosteroids, such as prednisone (Deltasone).

Acute hepatitis generally resolves without medications. Treatment of chronic hepatitis includes cessation of causative agents like alcohol. In the late stages of certain types of hepatitis (not hepatitis B, generally), liver transplantation may be required to preserve life.

Lifestyle changes that may be helpful

Avoiding alcohol (page 12) is the most obvious way to avoid the liver damage it causes.

A variety of prescription drugs can, on rare occasions, cause hepatitis, as can large amounts of **niacin** (page 598) or niacinamide (forms of vitamin B$_3$). Excessive intake of acetaminophen or other painkillers can damage the liver, so excessive intake of these drugs should be avoided. People with hepatitis C who failed to respond to interferon therapy have been found to have a higher amount of **iron** (page 540) within the liver.[1] People with hepatitis C should, therefore, avoid iron supplements. People with any type of hepatitis should ask their physician whether any medication they are taking poses a risk to the liver.

For infectious (viral) hepatitis, good hygiene is necessary to avoid spreading the infection. The hepatitis A virus can be spread very easily through food that is handled by infected individuals; therefore, people with hepatitis A should wash their hands very carefully after using the restroom and should not handle food at work. The hepatitis viruses B and C are both transmitted by blood and sexual contact.

Nutritional supplements that may be helpful

Catechin, a **flavonoid** (page 516), has helped people with acute viral hepatitis,[2] as well as individuals with chronic hepatitis,[3] though not all trials have found a benefit.[4] A typical amount used in successful trials is 500–750 mg three times per day. Although catechin is found in several plants, none contain sufficient amounts to reach the level used in the trials; thus, catechin supplements are needed. However, because of its potential to cause side effects on rare occasions,[5] catechin should be used only under medical supervision.

Proteins from the thymus gland, an important part of the **immune system** (page 255), may have a benefi-cial effect in people with chronic hepatitis B. Initial trials done in Poland used injected thymus proteins with good results.[6] Further trials using a variety of **thymus extracts** (page 591) by mouth have found that they can improve blood tests that measure liver damage as well as improve immune cell numbers.[7, 8] Preliminary evidence also suggests these extracts may help patients with hepatitis C.[9] The standard recommendation for supplementation is 200 mg three times per day of crude extracts or 40 mg three times per day of purified proteins.

S-adenosylmethionine (page 583) (SAMe) (1,600 mg/day orally or 800 mg/day intravenously) has been shown to aid in the resolution of blocked bile flow (cholestasis), a common complication of chronic hepatitis.[10, 11]

Taking 3 grams per day of **phosphatidylcholine** (page 546) (found in lecithin) was found to be beneficial in one investigation of people with chronic hepatitis B.[12] Signs of liver damage on biopsy were significantly reduced in this trial.

Vitamin E (page 609) levels have been shown to be low in people with hepatitis,[13] as well as in those who later develop liver cancer from long-standing hepatitis.[14] Vitamin E levels in the liver may also be decreased in some people with hepatitis.[15] In a controlled trial of individuals with hepatitis B, 600 IU of vitamin E per day for nine months resulted in all signs of hepatitis disappearing in five of twelve people.[16] In a preliminary trial of adults with hepatitis C, administering 1,200 IU per day of vitamin E for eight weeks appeared to reduce liver damage to some extent.[17] In a preliminary trial of people with hepatitis C, 544 IU of vitamin E per day for 24 weeks improved the response to interferon/**antioxidant** (page 467) therapy, although the results did not reach statistical significance.[18] However, in children with viral hepatitis, daily injections of vitamin E (300 IU) for seven days did not produce any benefit.[19]

Vitamin C (page 604) in the amount of 2 grams per day was reported in a preliminary trial to prevent hepatitis infection in individuals receiving blood transfusions.[20] This report was followed up by a double-blind trial, in which 3.2 grams per day of vitamin C was reported to have no protective effect against post-transfusion hepatitis.[21] (However, in the latter trial, vitamin C actually reduced the incidence of hepatitis by 29%, although this reduction was not statistically significant.) An older trial suggested that injections of vitamin C may be helpful in treating viral hepatitis.[22]

A potent antioxidant combination may protect the liver from damage in people with hepatitis C, possibly decreasing the necessity for a liver transplant. In a preliminary trial,[23] three people with **liver cirrhosis** (page 290) and esophageal varices (dilated veins in the esophagus that can rupture and cause fatal bleeding) caused by hepatitis C received a combination of **Alpha lipoic acid** (page 464) (300 mg twice daily), silymarin (from **milk thistle** (page 710); 300 mg three times daily), and **selenium** (page 584) (selenomethionine; 200 mcg twice daily). After five to eight months of therapy that included other "supportive supplements," such as vitamin C and **B vitamins** (page 603), all three people had significant improvements in their liver function and overall health. Larger clinical trials are needed to confirm these promising preliminary results.

Vitamin B$_{12}$ (page 601) (with or without **folic acid** [page 520]) has been reported in trials from the 1950s to help some people with hepatitis.[24, 25] Vitamin B$_{12}$ injections are likely to be more beneficial than oral administration, though 1,000 mcg (taken orally) each day can also be supplemented.

In a preliminary report, three patients with chronic hepatitis B had an improvement in the severity of their hepatitis after taking 100 mg of **thiamine** (page 591) (vitamin B$_1$) per day.[26]

In a preliminary trial, supplementation with **betaine** (page 472) (20 grams per day) for 12 months improved signs of liver inflammation in seven patients with non-alcoholic steatohepatitis, a type of liver inflammation. No significant side effects were seen.[27]

Supplementation with 17 mg of **zinc** (page 614) twice a day (in the form of a zinc complex of L-carnosine) enhanced the response to interferon therapy in patients with chronic hepatitis C, in a preliminary trial.[28] It is not known whether this benefit was due primarily to the zinc or the **carnosine** (page 487), or whether other forms of zinc would have the same effect.

A preliminary trial found 24 grams per day of **whey protein** (page 613) improved blood measures of liver dysfunction in people with hepatitis B, but not those with hepatitis C.[29]

Are there any side effects or interactions?
Refer to the individual supplement for information about any side effects or interactions.

Herbs that may be helpful

Preliminary trials have shown that the **bupleurum** (page 647)-containing formula sho-saiko-to can help reduce symptoms and blood liver enzyme levels in chil-

dren and adults with chronic active viral hepatitis.[30, 31, 32, 33] Most of theses trials were in people with hepatitis B infection, though one preliminary trial has also shown a benefit in people with hepatitis C.[34] Sho-saiko-to was also found, in a large preliminary trial to decrease the risk of people with chronic viral hepatitis developing liver cancer. However, people who had a sign of recent hepatitis B infection were not as strongly protected in this trial.[35] The usual amount of sho-saiko-to used is 2.5 grams three times daily. Sho-saiko-to should not be used together with interferon drug therapy as it may increase risk of pneumonitis—a potentially dangerous inflammation in the lungs.[36]

Cordyceps (page 663) has repeatedly been shown effective in clinical trials at reducing fibrosis and improving liver and immune function in people with chronic hepatitis B, including those with cirrhosis.[37, 38, 39] The usual amount taken is 3 to 4.5 grams twice daily as capsules or simmered for 10 to 15 minutes in water to make tea.

Silymarin, the flavonoid extracted from **milk thistle** (page 710), has been studied for treating all types of liver disease. The standard amount used in most trials has delivered 420 mg of silymarin per day. For acute hepatitis, double-blind trials have shown mixed results.[40, 41] A preparation of silymarin and **phosphatidylcholine** (page 546) was reported to help sufferers of chronic viral hepatitis. One small preliminary trial found that at least 420 mg of silymarin was necessary each day.[42] A controlled trial found that silymarin decreased liver damage.[43] One trial has suggested that silymarin may be more effective for hepatitis B as opposed to hepatitis C.[44]

Recent findings have shown that silymarin has the ability to block fibrosis, a process that contributes to the eventual development of **cirrhosis** (page 290) in persons with inflammatory liver conditions secondary to alcohol abuse or hepatitis.[45] While there are no published clinical trials in people with hepatitis C to date, this action makes milk thistle extract potentially attractive as a supportive treatment for the condition—particularly for those that have not responded to standard drug therapy. The effectiveness of silymarin (particularly its antifibrotic actions) needs to be studied in larger numbers of persons with hepatitis C to determine whether it is an effective treatment for this condition.

Phyllanthus (page 728) (*Phyllanthus amarus*), an Ayurvedic herb, has been studied primarily in carriers of the hepatitis B virus, as opposed to those with chronic active hepatitis. In one trial, administering this herb for 30 days appeared to eliminate the hepatitis B virus in 22 of 37 cases (59%).[46] However, other trials have failed to confirm a beneficial effect of *Phyllanthus amarus* against hepatitis B.[47, 48] A West Indian species, *Phyllanthus urinaria* (not widely available in the United States or Europe), has achieved much better results than Indian *Phyllanthus amarus*.[49] Thus, the specific plant species used may have a significant impact on the results. The amount of phyllanthus used in clinical trials has ranged from 900–2,700 mg per day.

A crude extract of red **peony** (page 724) root was shown in a small, preliminary trial to reduce cirrhosis in some people with chronic viral hepatitis.[50] Other preliminary trials published in Chinese demonstrated that red peony root was helpful (by reducing liver enzyme levels or symptoms or both) for people with viral hepatitis.[51]

One of the active constituents in **licorice** (page 702), glycyrrhizin, is sometimes used in Japan as an injected therapy for hepatitis B and C.[52, 53] Glycyrrhizin also blocks hepatitis A virus from replicating in test tubes.[54] One preliminary trial found that use of 2.5 grams licorice three times per day providing 750 mg glycyrrhizin was superior to the drug inosine polyIC in helping people with acute and chronic viral hepatitis.[55] Because glycyrrhizin can cause **high blood pressure** (page 246) and other problems, it should only be taken on the advice of a healthcare practitioner.

A series of cases of acute viral hepatitis were reported by one group in India, showing **picrorhiza** (page 728), combined with a variety of minerals, to be helpful in hastening recovery.[56] A variety of similar reports have appeared in the Indian literature over the years, although no double-blind clinical trials have yet been published. Between 400 and 1,500 mg of powdered, encapsulated picrorhiza per day has been used in a variety of trials. **Andrographis** (page 626), another traditional Indian herb, has shown preliminary benefit for people with chronic viral hepatitis.[57]

Preliminary human research demonstrates some efficacy for the mushroom **reishi** (page 737) in treating chronic hepatitis B; however, additional clinical trials are needed.[58]

An uncontrolled trial found that **shiitake** (page 746) formulations containing *Lentinus edodes* mycelium (LEM—the powdered mycelium of the mushroom before the cap and stem grow) may help decrease blood markers of liver inflammation.[59] One marker of hepatitis B infection in the blood (HBeAg) disappeared in 14% of the patients in this trial. Given the preliminary nature of the research, more information is needed to determine if LEM is effective for hepatitis.

Modern Chinese research suggests that compounds called lignans in **schisandra** (page 744) promote regeneration of liver tissue that has been damaged by harmful influences, such as hepatitis viruses or alcohol. In a controlled trial, Chinese patients with chronic viral hepatitis were given 500 mg schisandra extract three times daily or liver extract and B vitamins.[60] Among those given schisandra, serum glutamic pyruvic transaminase (SGPT) levels declined to normal levels in 68% compared to 44% of the control group. Lower SGPT levels suggest less liver inflammation. There was also a reduction in symptoms such as **insomnia** (page 270), fatigue, **loose stools** (page 163), and abdominal tension in the schisandra group. A preliminary trial in 5,000 people with various types of hepatitis found normalizations in SGPT or related liver enzymes in 75% of cases using an unspecified amount of schisandra.[61]

Early clinical trials in China suggest **astragalus** (page 631) root might benefit people with chronic viral hepatitis, though it may take one to two months to see results.[62] Textbooks on Chinese herbs recommend taking 9–15 grams of the crude herb per day in decoction form. A decoction is made by boiling the root in water for a few minutes and then brewing the tea.

Another Chinese herb, **Chinese scullcap** (page 658), might be useful for liver infections. However, the research on this is generally of low quality.[63]

Are there any side effects or interactions?
Refer to the individual herb for information about any side effects or interactions.

HIGH CHOLESTEROL

See also: Atherosclerosis (page 38)

What do I need to know?

Self-care for high cholesterol can be approached in a number of ways—but it can be hard to know just where to start. To make it easier, our doctors recommend trying these simple steps first:

Cut the bad fats
> Foods that contain saturated fat, hydrogenated fat, and cholesterol (such as animal products; fried foods; and sweet, baked snacks) can raise cholesterol

Reduce risk with fiber

Add whole grains, legumes, fruits, and vegetables to your meals to reduce heart disease risk

Raise "good" cholesterol with exercise

Start a regular exercise program to help raise HDL cholesterol

Add soy protein to your diet

30 grams (about one ounce) a day of powdered soy protein added to food or drinks can help lower cholesterol

Try plant sterols and stanols (natural vegetable fats)

Take 1.6 grams a day as a supplement or in specially fortified margarines to help reduce cholesterol

Check out policosanol

Take 10 to 20 mg a day of a product extracted from sugar cane to help lower cholesterol

Get some garlic

600 to 900 mg a day of a standardized garlic supplement may help lower cholesterol and prevent hardening of the arteries

About high cholesterol

Although it is by no means the only major risk factor, elevated serum (blood) cholesterol is clearly associated with a high risk of **heart disease** (page 98).

Most doctors suggest cholesterol levels should stay under 200 mg/dl. As levels fall below 200, the risk of heart disease continues to decline. Many doctors consider cholesterol levels of no more than 180 to be optimal. A low cholesterol level, however, is not a guarantee of good heart health, as some people with low levels do suffer **heart attacks** (page 212).

Medical laboratories now subdivide total cholesterol measurement into several components, including LDL ("bad") cholesterol, which is directly linked to heart disease, and HDL ("good") cholesterol, which is protective. The relative amount of HDL to LDL is more important than total cholesterol. For example, it is possible for someone with very high HDL to be at relatively low risk for heart disease even with total cholesterol above 200. Evaluation of changes in cholesterol requires consultation with a healthcare professional and should include measurement of total serum cholesterol, as well as HDL and LDL cholesterol.

The following discussion is limited to information about lowering serum cholesterol levels or increasing HDL cholesterol using natural approaches. Because high cholesterol is linked to atherosclerosis and heart

disease, people concerned about heart disease should also learn more about **atherosclerosis** (page 38).

CHECKLIST FOR HIGH CHOLESTEROL

Rating	Nutritional Supplements	Herbs
★★★	**Beta-glucan** (page 470) **Beta-hydroxy-beta-methylbutyrate (HMB)** (page 534) **Chromium** (page 493)/ **brewer's yeast** (page 480) **Fiber** (page 512) **Glucomannan** (page 526) **Policosanol** (page 571) Sitostanol **Soy** (page 587) **Vitamin B₃** (page 598) (niacin only) (see toxicity warnings) **Vitamin B₅** (page 603) (pantethine only) **Vitamin C** (page 604) (protection of LDL cholesterol)	**Fenugreek** (page 676) **Psyllium** (page 732) **Red yeast rice** (page 736)
★★☆	**Beta-sitosterol** (page 471) **Calcium** (page 483) **Copper** (page 499) **Flaxseed** (page 517) (raw) **Inositol hexaniacinate** (page 537) **Royal jelly** (page 582) **Tocotrienols** (page 593)	*Achillea wilhelmsii* **Artichoke** (page 628) **Garlic** (page 679) **Green tea** (page 686) **Green tea** (page 686) (enriched with theaflavins) **Guggul** (page 688)
★☆☆	**Chitosan** (page 491) **Chondroitin sulfate** (page 492) **Creatine monohydrate** (page 501) **L-carnitine** (page 543) **Lecithin** (page 546) **Magnesium** (page 551) **Vitamin E** (page 609)	**Alfalfa** (page 623) **Fo-ti** (page 678) **Maitake** (page 707) **Wild yam** (page 759)

What are the symptoms of high cholesterol?

This condition does not produce symptoms. Therefore, it is prudent to visit a health professional on a regular basis to have cholesterol levels measured.

Medical treatments

Cholesterol-lowering medications such as the HMG-CoA reductase inhibitors atorvastatin (Lipitor), fluvastatin (Lescol), lovastatin (Mevacor), pravastatin (Pravachol), and simvastatin (Zocor) are commonly prescribed. The bile acid sequestrants cholestyramine (Questran) and colestipol (Colestid) are occasionally used. Other available drugs include gemfibrozil (Lopid), fenofibrate (Tricor), and niacin (Niaspan). In women who have passed through **menopause** (page 311), high cholesterol might also be treated by hormone replacement therapy, such as conjugated estrogens (Premarin) and estradiol (Estrace).

People with high cholesterol are commonly advised to reduce their consumption of dietary cholesterol and saturated fats.

Dietary changes that may be helpful

Eating animal foods containing saturated fat is linked to high cholesterol levels[1] and **heart disease** (page 98).[2] Significant amounts of animal-based saturated fat are found in beef, pork, veal, poultry (particularly in poultry skins and dark meat), cheese, butter, ice cream, and all other forms of dairy products not labeled "fat free." Avoiding consumption of these foods reduces cholesterol and has been reported to reverse even existing heart disease.[3]

Unlike other dairy foods, skimmed milk, nonfat yogurt, and nonfat cheese are essentially fat-free. Dairy products labeled "low fat" are not particularly low in fat. A full 25% of calories in 2% milk come from fat. (The "2%" refers to the fraction of volume filled by fat, not the more important percentage of calories coming from fat.)

In addition to large amounts of saturated fat from animal-based foods, Americans eat small amounts of saturated fat from coconut and palm oils. Palm oil has been reported to elevate cholesterol.[4, 5] Research regarding **coconut oil** (page 494) is mixed, with some trials finding no link to **heart disease** (page 98),[6] while other research reports that coconut oil elevates cholesterol levels.[7, 8]

Despite the links between saturated fat intake and serum cholesterol levels, not every person responds to appropriate dietary changes with a drop in cholesterol. A subgroup of people with elevated cholesterol who have what researchers call "large LDL particles" has been reported to have no response even to dramatic reductions in dietary fat.[9] (LDL is the "bad" cholesterol most associated with an increased risk of heart disease.) This phenomenon is not understood. People who significantly reduce intake of animal fats for several months but do not see significant a reduction in cholesterol levels should discuss other approaches to lowering cholesterol with a doctor.

Yogurt, acidophilus milk, and kefir are fermented milk products that have been reported to lower cholesterol in most,[10, 11, 12, 13, 14, 15, 16] but not all, double-blind and other controlled research.[17, 18, 19] Until more is known, it makes sense for people with elevated cholesterol who consume these foods, to select nonfat varieties.

Eating fish has been reported to increase HDL cholesterol[20] and is linked to a reduced risk of heart disease in most,[21] but not all, studies.[22] Fish contains very little saturated fat, and **fish oil** (page 514) contains EPA and **DHA** (page 509), omega-3 fatty acids that appear to protect against heart disease.[23]

Vegetarians have lower cholesterol[24] and less heart disease[25] than meat eaters, in part because they avoid animal fat. Vegans (people who eat no meat, dairy, or eggs) have the lowest cholesterol levels,[26] and switching from a standard diet to a vegan diet, along with other lifestyle changes, has been reported to reverse heart disease in controlled research.[27, 28]

Dietary cholesterol

Most dietary cholesterol comes from egg yolks. Eating eggs has increased serum cholesterol in most studies.[29] However, eating eggs does not increase serum cholesterol as much as eating foods high in saturated fat, and eating eggs may not increase serum cholesterol at all if the overall diet is low in fat.[30]

Egg consumption does not appear to be totally safe, however, even for people consuming a low-fat diet. When cholesterol from eggs is cooked or exposed to air, it oxidizes. Oxidized cholesterol is linked to increased risk of **heart disease** (page 98).[31] Eating eggs also makes LDL cholesterol more susceptible to damage, a change linked to heart disease.[32]

Whether or not egg eaters are more likely to die from heart disease is a matter of controversy. In one preliminary study, egg eaters had a higher death rate from heart disease, even when serum cholesterol levels were not elevated.[33] However, another preliminary study found no evidence of an overall significant association between egg consumption, and risk of heart disease or **stroke** (page 419), except in people with **diabetes** (page 152).[34] Until more is known, limiting egg consumption may be a good idea, particularly for people with existing heart disease or diabetes.

While coconut oil is high in saturated fat, some evidence suggests it does not cause unhealthy changes in blood cholesterol levels compared with other saturated fats. In a controlled study of people with high cholesterol, coconut oil resulted in higher total and LDL cholesterol levels compared with safflower oil (a polyunsaturated oil), but lower levels compared with butter, while HDL levels were similar for all three diets.[35] Another controlled study compared coconut oil with canola oil,[36] and found that coconut oil raised total and LDL cholesterol in people with high cholesterol who were not taking cholesterol-lowering drugs, but did not affect these levels in people who were taking these drugs. HDL levels were not reported in this study.

Fiber (page 512)

Soluble fiber from beans,[37] **oats** (page 716),[38] **psyllium** (page 732) seed,[39] **glucomannan** (page 526), and fruit pectin[40] has lowered cholesterol levels in most trials.[41, 42] Doctors often recommend that people with elevated cholesterol eat more of these high-soluble fiber foods. However, even grain fiber (which contains *in*soluble fiber and does not lower cholesterol) has been linked to protection against heart disease, though the reason for the protection remains unclear.[43] It makes sense for people wishing to lower their cholesterol levels and reduce the risk of heart disease to consume more fiber of all types. Some trials have used 20 grams of additional fiber per day for several months to successfully lower cholesterol.[44]

Oat bran is rich in a soluble fiber called **beta-glucan** (page 470). In 1997, the U.S. Food and Drug Administration passed a unique ruling that allowed oat bran to be registered as the first cholesterol-reducing food at an amount providing 3 grams of beta-glucan per day, although some evidence suggests this level may not be high enough to make a significant difference.[45] Several double-blind and other controlled trials have shown that oat bran[46, 47, 48] and oat milk[49] supplementation may significantly lower cholesterol levels in people with elevated cholesterol, but only weakly lowers them in people with healthy cholesterol levels.[50]

Flaxseed (page 517), another good source of soluble fiber, has been reported to lower total and LDL cholesterol in preliminary studies.[51, 52] A double-blind trial found that while both flaxseed and sunflower seed lowered total cholesterol, only flaxseed significantly lowered LDL.[53] Amounts of flaxseed used in these trials

typically range from 30–50 grams per day. A controlled trial found that partially defatted flaxseed, containing 20 grams of fiber per day, significantly lowered LDL cholesterol, suggesting that at least one of the cholesterol-lowering components in flaxseed is likely to be the fiber in this product, as opposed to the oil removed from it.[54] Controlled trials of flaxseed oil alone have shown inconsistent effects on blood cholesterol.[55, 56, 57]

Alpha-linolenic acid

Doctors and researchers are interested in alpha-linolenic acid (ALA)—the special omega-3 fatty acid found in large amounts in flaxseeds and flaxseed oil. ALA is a precursor to EPA, a fatty acid from **fish oil** (page 514) that is believed to protect against heart disease. To a limited extent, ALA converts to EPA within the body.[58] However, unlike EPA, ALA does not lower **triglyceride** (page 235) levels (a risk factor for heart disease).[59] Preliminary research on the effects of ALA from flaxseed has produced conflicting results.

In 1994, researchers conducted a study in people with a history of heart disease, using what they called the "Mediterranean" diet.[60] The diet was significantly different from what people from Mediterranean countries actually eat, in that it contained little olive oil. Instead, the diet included a special margarine high in ALA. Those people assigned to the "Mediterranean" diet had a remarkable 70% reduced risk of dying from heart disease compared with the control group during the first 27 months. Similar results were also confirmed after almost four years.[61] Although cholesterol levels fell only modestly in the "Mediterranean" diet group, the positive results suggest that people with elevated cholesterol attempting to reduce the risk of heart disease should consider such a diet. The diet was high in beans and peas, fish, fruit, vegetables, bread, and cereals; and low in meat, dairy fat, and eggs. Although the authors believe that the high ALA content of the diet was partially responsible for the surprising outcome, other aspects of the diet may have been partly or even totally responsible for decreased death rates. Therefore, the success of the "Mediterranean" diet does not prove that ALA protects against heart disease.[62]

Soy

Tofu, tempeh, miso, and some protein powders in health food stores, are derived from soybeans. In 1995, an analysis of many trials proved that soy reduces both total and LDL cholesterol.[63] Since then, other double-blind and other controlled trials have confirmed these findings.[64, 65, 66, 67] Trials showing statistically significant reductions in cholesterol have generally used more than 30 grams per day of soy protein. However, if soy replaces animal protein in the diet, as little as 20 grams per day has been shown to significantly reduce both total and LDL cholesterol.[68] Isoflavones found in soy beans appear to be key cholesterol-lowering ingredients of the bean,[69, 70] but animal research suggests other components of soy are also important.[71, 72]

Sugar

Eating sugar has been reported to reduce protective HDL cholesterol[73] and increases other risk factors linked to heart disease.[74] However, higher sugar intake has been associated with only slightly higher risks of heart disease in most reports.[75] Although the exact relationship between sugar and heart disease remains somewhat unclear, many doctors recommend that people with high cholesterol reduce their sugar intake.

Coffee

Drinking boiled or French press coffee increases cholesterol levels.[76] Modern paper coffee filters trap the offending chemicals and keep them from entering the cup. Therefore, drinking paper-filtered coffee does not increase cholesterol levels.[77, 78] Espresso coffee has amounts of the offending chemicals midway between those of other unfiltered coffees and paper-filtered coffee,[79] but there is little research investigating the effect of espresso on cholesterol levels, and studies to date have produced conflicting results.[80, 81] The effects of decaffeinated coffee on cholesterol levels remain in debate.[82]

Alcohol

Moderate drinking (one to two drinks per day) increases protective HDL cholesterol.[83] This effect happens equally with different kinds of alcohol-containing beverages.[84, 85] Alcohol also acts as a blood thinner,[86] an effect that should lower heart disease. However, alcohol consumption may cause liver disease (e.g., **cirrhosis** [page 290]), **cancer** (page 87), **high blood pressure** (page 246), **alcoholism** (page 12), and, at high intake, an *increased* risk of **heart disease** (page 98). As a result, some doctors never recommend alcohol, even for people with high cholesterol. Nevertheless, those who have one to two drinks per day appear to live longer[87] and are clearly less likely to have heart disease.[88] Therefore, some people at very high risk of heart disease— those who are not alcoholics, who have healthy livers and normal blood pressure, and who are not at high risk for cancer, particularly **breast cancer** (page 65)—

are likely to receive more benefit than harm, from light drinking.

Olive oil

Olive oil lowers LDL cholesterol,[89, 90] especially when the olive oil replaces saturated fat in the diet.[91] People from countries that use significant amounts of olive oil appear to be at low risk for heart disease.[92] A double-blind trial showed that a diet high in monounsaturated fatty acids from olive oil, lowers cardiovascular disease risk by 25%, as compared with a 12% decrease from a low-fat (25% fat) diet.[93] The trial also found that low-fat diets decrease HDL cholesterol by 4%, which is undesirable, since HDL cholesterol is protective against heart disease. Diets high in monounsaturated fatty acids from olive oil do not adversely affect HDL levels. Although olive oil is clearly safe for people with elevated cholesterol, it is, like any fat or oil, high in calories, so people who are **overweight** (page 446) should limit its use.

Trans fatty acids and margarine

Trans fatty acids (TFAs) are found in many processed foods containing partially hydrogenated oils. The highest levels occur in margarine. Margarine consumption is linked to increased risk of unfavorable changes in cholesterol levels[94] and **heart disease** (page 98).[95] Margarine and other processed foods containing partially hydrogenated oils should be avoided.

However, special therapeutic margarines are now available that contain substances, called phytostanols, that block the absorption of cholesterol.[96] The FDA has approved some of these margarines as legitimate therapeutic agents for lowering blood cholesterol levels. The best-known of these products is Benecol. The cholesterol-lowering effect of these margarines has been demonstrated in numerous double-blind and other controlled trials.[97, 98, 99, 100, 101, 102, 103]

Garlic (page 679)

Garlic is available as a food, as a spice in powder form, and as a supplement. Eating garlic has helped to lower cholesterol in some research,[104] though several double-blind trials have not found garlic supplements to be thusly effective.[105, 106, 107] Although some of the negative reports have been criticized,[108] the relationship between garlic and cholesterol lowering remains unproven.[109] However, garlic is known to act as a blood thinner[110] and may reduce other risk factors for heart disease.[111] For these reasons, some doctors recommend eating garlic as food, taking 900 mg of garlic powder from capsules, or using a tincture of 2 to 4 ml, taken three times daily.

Nuts

Preliminary research consistently shows that people who eat nuts frequently have a dramatically reduced risk of **heart disease** (page 98).[112, 113] This apparent beneficial effect is at least partially explained by preliminary and controlled research demonstrating that nut consumption lowers cholesterol levels.[114, 115] Of nuts commonly consumed, almonds[116, 117] and walnuts[118, 119, 120] may be most effective at lowering cholesterol. Macadamia nuts have been less beneficial in most studies,[121, 122, 123] although one controlled trial found a cholesterol-lowering effect from macadamia nuts.[124] Hazelnuts[125] and pistachio nuts[126] have also been reported to help lower cholesterol.

Nuts contain many factors that could be responsible for protection against heart disease, including **fiber** (page 512), **vitamin E** (page 609), alpha-linolenic acid (found primarily in walnuts), oleic acid, **magnesium** (page 551), **potassium** (page 572), and **arginine** (page 467). Therefore, exactly how nuts lower cholesterol or lower the risk of heart disease remains somewhat unclear. Some doctors even believe that nuts may not be *directly* protective; rather, people busy eating nuts will not simultaneously be eating eggs, dairy, or trans fatty acids from margarine and processed food, the avoidance of which would reduce cholesterol levels and the risk of heart disease.[127, 128] Nonetheless, the remarkable consistency of research outcomes strongly suggests that nuts do help protect against heart disease. Although nuts are loaded with calories, a preliminary trial surprisingly reported that adding hundreds of calories per day from nuts for six months did not increase **body weight** (page 446) in humans[129]—an outcome supported by other reports.[130] Even when increasing nut consumption has led to weight gain, the amount of added weight has been remarkably less than would be expected, given the number of calories added to the diet.[131] Given the number of calories per ounce of nuts, scientists do not understand why moderate nut consumption apparently has so little effect on body weight.

Number and size of meals

When people eat a number of small meals, serum cholesterol levels fall compared with the effect of eating the same food in three big meals.[132, 133] People with elevated cholesterol levels should probably avoid very large meals and eat more frequent, smaller meals.

Lifestyle changes that may be helpful

Exercise increases protective HDL cholesterol,[134] an effect that occurs even from walking.[135] Total and LDL cholesterol are typically lowered by exercise, especially when weight-loss also occurs.[136] Exercisers have a relatively low risk of **heart disease** (page 98).[137] However, people over 40 years of age, or who have heart disease, should talk with their doctor before starting an exercise program; overdoing it may actually trigger **heart attacks** (page 212).[138]

Obesity (page 446) increases the risk of heart disease,[139] in part because weight gain lowers HDL cholesterol.[140] **Weight loss** (page 446) reduces the body's ability to make cholesterol, increases HDL levels, and reduces **triglycerides** (page 235) (another risk factor for heart disease).[141, 142] Weight loss also leads to a decrease in blood pressure.

Smoking is linked to a lowered level of HDL cholesterol[143] and is also known to cause heart disease.[144] Quitting smoking reduces the risk of having a heart attack.[145]

The combination of feelings of hostility, stress, and time urgency is called type A behavior. Men,[146, 147] but not women,[148] with these traits are at high risk for heart disease in most, but not all, studies.[149] Stress[150] or type A behavior[151] may elevate cholesterol in men. Reducing stress and feelings of hostility has reduced the risk of heart disease.[152]

Nutritional supplements that may be helpful

Glucomannan (page 526) is a water-soluble dietary **fiber** (page 512) that is derived from konjac root. Controlled[153, 154] and double-blind[155, 156] trials have shown that supplementation with glucomannan significantly reduced total blood cholesterol, LDL cholesterol, and **triglycerides** (page 235), and in some cases raised HDL cholesterol. Effective amounts of glucomannan for lowering blood cholesterol have been 4 to 13 grams per day.

Test tube and animal studies indicate that **policosanol** (page 571) is capable of inhibiting cholesterol production by the liver.[157, 158]

Extensive preliminary and double-blind research in Cuba and other countries in Latin America has demonstrated that taking 10 to 20 mg per day of policosanol extracted from sugar cane results in significant changes in blood cholesterol levels, including total cholesterol (17 to 21% lower on average), LDL cholesterol (21 to 29% lower), and HDL cholesterol (7 to 29% higher).[159, 160, 161, 162, 163, 164, 165, 166, 167, 168, 169]

The combined results of nine double-blind trials indicate that supplementation with **beta-hydroxy-beta-methylbutyrate (HMB)** (page 534) effectively lowers total and LDL cholesterol.[170] All trials used 3 grams per day, taken for three to eight weeks.

Vitamin C (page 604) appears to protect LDL cholesterol from damage.[171] In some clinical trials, cholesterol levels have fallen when people with elevated cholesterol supplement with vitamin C.[172] Some studies report that decreases in total cholesterol occur specifically in LDL cholesterol.[173] Doctors sometimes recommend 1 gram per day of vitamin C. A review of the disparate research concerning vitamin C and **heart disease** (page 98), however, has suggested that most protection against heart disease from vitamin C, is likely to occur with as little as 100 mg per day.[174]

Pantethine (page 568), a byproduct of **vitamin B5** (page 603) (pantothenic acid), may help reduce the amount of cholesterol made by the body. Several preliminary[175, 176, 177, 178, 179] and two controlled[180, 181] trials have found that pantethine (300 mg taken two to four times per day) significantly lowers serum cholesterol levels and may also increase HDL. However, one double-blind trial in people whose high blood cholesterol did not change with diet and drug therapy, found that pantethine was also not effective.[182] Common pantothenic acid has not been reported to have any effect on high blood cholesterol.

Chromium (page 493) supplementation has reduced total cholesterol,[183, 184] LDL cholesterol[185, 186] and increased HDL cholesterol[187, 188] in double-blind and other controlled trials, although other trials have not found these effects.[189, 190] One double-blind trial found that high amounts of chromium (500 mcg per day) in combination with daily exercise was highly effective, producing nearly a 20% decrease in total cholesterol levels in just 13 weeks.[191]

Brewer's yeast (page 480), which contains readily absorbable and biologically active **chromium** (page 493), has also lowered serum cholesterol.[192] People with higher blood levels of chromium appear to be at lower risk for heart disease.[193] A reasonable and safe intake of supplemental chromium is 200 mcg per day. People wishing to use brewer's yeast as a source of chromium should look for products specifically labeled "from the brewing process" or "brewer's yeast," since most yeast found in health food stores is not brewer's yeast, and does not contain chromium. Optimally, true brewer's yeast contains up to 60 mcg of chromium per

tablespoon, and a reasonable intake is 2 tablespoons per day.

High amounts (several grams per day) of niacin, a form of **vitamin B3** (page 598), lower cholesterol, an effect recognized in the approval of niacin as a prescription medication for high cholesterol.[194] The other common form of vitamin B3—niacinamide—does not affect cholesterol levels. Some niacin preparations have raised HDL cholesterol better than certain prescription drugs.[195] Some cardiologists prescribe 3 grams of niacin per day or even higher amounts for people with high cholesterol levels. At such intakes, acute symptoms (flushing, headache, stomachache) and chronic symptoms (liver damage, **diabetes** [page 152], **gastritis** [page 195], eye damage, possibly **gout** [page 208]) of toxicity may be severe. Many people are not able to continue taking these levels of niacin due to discomfort or danger to their health. Therefore, high intakes of niacin must only be taken under the supervision of a doctor.

Symptoms caused by niacin supplements, such as flushing, have been reduced with sustained-release (also called "time-release") niacin products. However, sustained-release forms of niacin have caused significant liver toxicity and, though rarely, liver failure.[196, 197, 198, 199, 200] One partial time-release (intermediate-release) niacin product has lowered LDL cholesterol and raised HDL cholesterol without flushing, and it also has acted without the liver function abnormalities typically associated with sustained-release niacin formulations.[201] However, this form of niacin is available by prescription only.

In an attempt to avoid the side effects of niacin, alternative health practitioners increasingly use **inositol hexaniacinate** (page 537), recommending 500 to 1,000 mg, taken three times per day, instead of niacin.[202, 203] This special form of niacin has been reported to lower serum cholesterol but so far has not been found to cause significant toxicity.[204] Unfortunately, compared with niacin, far fewer investigations have studied the possible positive or negative effects of inositol hexaniacinate. As a result, people using inositol hexaniacinate should not take it without the supervision of a doctor, who will evaluate whether it is helpful (by measuring cholesterol levels) and will make sure that toxicity is not occurring (by measuring liver **enzymes** [page 506], uric acid and glucose levels, and by taking medical history and doing physical examinations).

High Cholesterol

Soy (page 587) supplementation has been shown to lower cholesterol in humans.[205] Soy is available in foods such as tofu, miso, and tempeh and as a supplemental protein powder. Soy contains isoflavones, naturally occurring plant components that are believed to be soy's main cholesterol-lowering ingredients. A controlled trial showed that soy preparations containing high amounts of isoflavones effectively lowered total cholesterol and LDL ("bad") cholesterol, whereas low-isoflavone preparations (less than 27 mg per day) did not.[206] However, supplementation with either soy[207] or non-soy isoflavones (from red clover)[208] in pill form failed to reduce cholesterol levels in a group of healthy volunteers, suggesting that isoflavone may *not* be responsible for the cholesterol-lowering effects of soy. Further trials of isoflavone supplements in people with elevated cholesterol are needed to resolve these conflicting results. In a study of people with high cholesterol levels, a soy preparation that contained soy protein, soy fiber, and soy phospholipids lowered cholesterol levels more effectively than isolated soy protein.[209]

Soy contains phytosterols. One such molecule, **beta-sitosterol** (page 471), is available as a supplement. Beta-sitosterol alone, and in combination with similar plant sterols, has been shown to reduce blood levels of cholesterol in preliminary[210] and controlled[211] trials. This effect may occur because beta-sitosterol blocks absorption of cholesterol.[212] In studying the effects of 0.8, 1.6, and 3.2 grams of plant sterols per day, one double-blind trial found that higher intake of sterols tended to result in greater reduction in cholesterol, though the differences between the effects of these three amounts were not statistically significant.[213]

A synthetic molecule related to beta-sitosterol, sitostanol, is now available in a special margarine and has also been shown to lower cholesterol levels. In one controlled trial, supplementation with 1.7 grams per day of a plant-sterol product containing mostly sitostanol, combined with dietary changes, led to a dramatic 24% drop in LDL ("bad") cholesterol compared with only a 9% decrease in the diet-only part of the trial.[214] Other controlled and double-blind trials have confirmed these results.[215, 216, 217, 218, 219] A review of double-blind trials on sitostanol found that a reduction in the risk of **heart disease** (page 98) of about 25% may be expected from use of sitostanol-containing spreads, a larger clinical effect than that produced by people reducing their saturated fat intake.[220]

Tocotrienols (page 593), a group of food-derived compounds that resemble **vitamin E** (page 609), may lower blood levels of cholesterol, but evidence is conflicting. Although tocotrienols inhibited cholesterol synthesis in test-tube studies,[221, 222] human trials have produced contradictory results. Two double-blind trials found that 200 mg per day of either gamma-tocotrienol[223] or total tocotrienols[224] were more effective than placebo, reducing cholesterol levels by 13–15%. However, in another double-blind trial, 200 mg of tocotrienols per day failed to lower cholesterol levels,[225] and a fourth double-blind trial found 140 mg of tocotrienols and 80 mg of vitamin E (d-alpha-tocopherol) daily resulted in no changes in total cholesterol, LDL cholesterol, or HDL cholesterol levels.[226]

Deficiency of the trace mineral, copper, has been linked to high blood cholesterol.[227, 228] In a controlled trial, daily supplementation with 3 to 4 mg of **copper** (page 499) for eight weeks decreased blood levels of total cholesterol and LDL cholesterol, in a group of people over 50 years of age.[229]

Beta-glucan (page 470) is a type of soluble **fiber** (page 512) molecule derived from the cell wall of baker's yeast, **oats** (page 716) and barley, and many medicinal mushrooms, such as **maitake** (page 707). Beta-glucan is the key factor for the cholesterol-lowering effect of oat bran.[230, 231, 232, 233] As with other soluble-fiber components, the binding of cholesterol (and bile acids) by beta-glucan and the resulting elimination of these substances in the feces is very helpful for reducing blood cholesterol.[234, 235, 236] Results from a number of double-blind trials with either oat- or yeast-derived beta-glucan indicate typical reductions, after at least four weeks of use, of approximately 10% for total cholesterol and 8% for LDL ("bad") cholesterol, with elevations in HDL ("good") cholesterol ranging from zero to 16%.[237, 238, 239, 240, 241] For lowering cholesterol levels, the amount of beta-glucan used has ranged from 2,900 to 15,000 mg per day.

Some preliminary[242] and double-blind[243, 244] trials have shown that supplemental **calcium** (page 483) reduces cholesterol levels. Possibly the calcium is binding with and preventing the absorption of dietary fat.[245] However, other research has found no substantial or statistically significant effects of calcium supplementation on total cholesterol or HDL ("good") cholesterol.[246] Reasonable supplemental levels are 800 to 1,000 mg per day.

In one double-blind trial,[247] **vitamin E** (page 609) increased protective HDL cholesterol, but several other trials,[248, 249, 250] found no effect of vitamin E. However, vitamin E is known to protect LDL cholesterol from damage.[251] Most cardiologists believe that only damaged LDL increases the risk of heart disease. Studies of the ability of vitamin E supplements to prevent **heart disease** (page 98) have produced conflicting results,[252] but many doctors continue to recommend that everyone supplement 400 IU of vitamin E per day to lessen the risk of having a **heart attack** (page 212).

L-carnitine (page 543) is needed by heart muscle to utilize fat for energy. Some,[253, 254] but not all, preliminary trials report that carnitine reduces serum cholesterol.[255] HDL cholesterol has also increased in response to carnitine supplementation.[256, 257] People have been reported in controlled research to stand a greater chance of surviving a heart attack if they are given L-carnitine supplements.[258] Most trials have used 1 to 4 grams of carnitine per day.

Magnesium (page 557) is needed by the heart to function properly. Although the mechanism is unclear, magnesium supplements (430 mg per day) lowered cholesterol in a preliminary trial.[259] Another preliminary study reported that magnesium deficiency is associated with a low HDL cholesterol level.[260] Intravenous magnesium has reduced death following heart attacks in some, but not all, clinical trials.[261] Though these outcomes would suggest that people with high cholesterol levels should take magnesium supplements, an isolated double-blind trial reported that people with a history of heart disease assigned to magnesium supplementation experienced an *increased* number of heart attacks.[262] More information is necessary before the scientific community can clearly evaluate the role magnesium should play for people with elevated cholesterol.

Chondroitin sulfate (page 492) has lowered serum cholesterol levels in preliminary trials.[263, 264] Years ago, this supplement dramatically reduced the risk of heart attacks in a controlled, six-year follow-up of people with **heart disease** (page 98).[265] The few doctors aware of these older clinical trials sometimes tell people with a history of heart disease or elevated cholesterol levels, to take approximately 500 mg of chondroitin sulfate three times per day.

Although **lecithin** (page 546) has been reported to increase HDL cholesterol and lower LDL cholesterol,[266] a review of the research found that the positive effect of lecithin was likely due to the polyunsaturated fat content of the lecithin.[267] If this is so, it would make more sense to use inexpensive vegetable oil, rather than take lecithin supplements. However, an animal study found a cholesterol-lowering effect of lecithin independent of its polyunsaturate content.[268] A double-blind

trial found that 20 grams of soy lecithin per day for four weeks had no significant effect on total cholesterol, LDL cholesterol, HDL cholesterol, or **triglycerides** (page 235).[269] Whether taking lecithin supplements is a useful way to lower cholesterol in people with elevated cholesterol levels remains unclear.

The **fiber** (page 512)-like supplement **chitosan** (page 491) appears to reduce the absorption of bile acids or cholesterol; either of these effects may cause a lowering of blood cholesterol.[270] This effect has been repeatedly demonstrated in animals, and a preliminary human study showed that 3 to 6 grams per day of chitosan taken for two weeks resulted in a 6% drop in cholesterol and a 10% increase in HDL ("good") cholesterol.[271] Another preliminary trial showed a 43% lowering of total cholesterol in people being treated for kidney failure with dialysis who took 4 grams per day of chitosan for 12 weeks. These people also appeared to have improved kidney function and less severe anemia after chitosan treatment.[272] In a double-blind trial, however, administration of 2.4 grams of chitosan per day for three months to people with high cholesterol had no effect on their cholesterol levels.[273]

Chitosan in large amounts, given with **vitamin C** (page 604), has been shown to reduce dietary fat absorption in animals fed a high-fat diet.[274, 275, 276] However, the absorption of minerals and fat-soluble **vitamins** (page 603) was also reduced by feeding animals large amounts of chitosan.[277] In studies in humans, chitosan did not reduce the absorption of dietary fat.[278, 279]

Royal jelly (page 582) has prevented the cholesterol-elevating effect of nicotine[280] and has lowered serum cholesterol in animal studies.[281] Preliminary human trials have also found that royal jelly may lower cholesterol levels.[282, 283] An analysis of cholesterol-lowering trials shows that 50 to 100 mg per day is the typical amount used in such research.[284]

A double-blind trial found that 20 grams per day of **creatine** (page 501) taken for five days, followed by ten grams per day for 51 days, significantly lowered serum total cholesterol and triglycerides, but did not change either LDL or HDL cholesterol, in both men and women.[285] However, another double-blind trial found no change in any of these blood levels in trained athletes using creatine during a 12-week strength training program.[286] Creatine supplementation in this negative trial was lower—only 5 grams per day were taken for the last 11 weeks of the study.

Octacosanol (page 565), a substance found in wheat

germ oil, is sometimes available as a supplement. Small amounts (5 to 20 mg per day) of policosanol, an experimental supplement from Cuba consisting primarily of octacosanol, has led to large reductions in LDL cholesterol and/or increases in HDL.[287, 288, 289, 290] Octacosanol may lower cholesterol by inhibiting the liver's production of cholesterol.[291]

Homocysteine (page 234), a substance linked to **heart disease** (page 98) risk, may increase the rate at which LDL cholesterol is damaged.[292] While **vitamin B$_6$** (page 600), **vitamin B$_{12}$** (page 601), and **folic acid** (page 520) lower homocysteine,[293] a recent trial found no effect of supplements of these vitamins on protecting LDL cholesterol, even though homocysteine was lowered.[294]

Are there any side effects or interactions?
Refer to the individual supplement for information about any side effects or interactions.

Herbs that may be helpful
Researchers have determined that one of the ingredients in **red yeast rice** (page 736), called monacolin K, inhibits the production of cholesterol by stopping the action of the key **enzyme** (page 506) in the liver (i.e., HMG-CoA reductase) that is responsible for manufacturing cholesterol.[295] The drug lovastatin (Mevacor) acts in a fashion similar to this red-yeast-rice ingredient. However, the amount per volume of monacolin K in red yeast rice is small (0.2% per 5 mg) when compared to the 20 to 40 mg of lovastatin available as a prescription drug.[296]

The red yeast rice used in various studies was a proprietary product called Cholestin, which contains ten different monacolins. The sale of Cholestin has been banned in the United States, as a result of a lawsuit alleging patent infringement. Other red yeast rice products currently on the market differ from Cholestin in their chemical makeup. None contain the full complement of 10 monacolin compounds that are present in Cholestin, and some contain a potentially toxic fermentation product called citrinin.[297] Until further information is available, red yeast rice products other than Cholestin cannot be recommended.

Use of **psyllium** (page 732) has been extensively studied as a way to reduce cholesterol levels. An analysis of all double-blind trials in 1997 concluded that a daily amount of 10 grams psyllium lowered cholesterol levels by 5% and LDL cholesterol by 9%.[298] Since then, a large controlled trial found that use of 5.1 grams of psyllium two times per day significantly reduced serum cholesterol as well as LDL-cholesterol.[299] Generally, 5 to 10 grams of psyllium are added to the diet per day to lower cholesterol levels. The combination of psyllium and **oat** (page 716) bran may also be effective at lowering LDL cholesterol.[300]

Guggul (page 688), a mixture of substances taken from a plant, is an approved treatment for elevated cholesterol in India and has been a mainstay of the Ayurvedic approach to preventing **atherosclerosis** (page 38). One double-blind trial studying the effects of guggul reported that serum cholesterol dropped by 17.5%.[301] In another double-blind trial comparing guggul to the drug clofibrate, the average fall in serum cholesterol was slightly greater in the guggul group; moreover, HDL cholesterol rose in 60% of people responding to guggul, while clofibrate did not elevate HDL.[302] A third double-blind trial found significant changes in total and LDL cholesterol levels, but not in HDL.[303] However, in another double-blind trial, supplementation with guggul for eight weeks had no effect on total serum cholesterol, but significantly *increased* LDL-cholesterol levels, compared with a placebo.[304] Daily intakes of guggul are based on the amount of guggulsterones in the extract. The recommended amount of guggulsterones is 25 mg taken three times per day. Most extracts contain 5 to 10% guggulsterones, and doctors familiar with their use usually recommend taking guggul for at least 12 weeks before evaluating its effect.

In a double-blind trial, people with moderately high cholesterol took a tincture of *Achillea wilhelmsii,* an herb used in traditional Persian medicine.[305] Participants in the trial used 15 to 20 drops of the tincture twice daily for six months. At the end of the trial, participants experienced significant reductions in total cholesterol, LDL cholesterol and **triglycerides** (page 235), as well as an increase in HDL cholesterol compared to those who took placebo. No adverse effects were reported.

Reports on many double-blind **garlic** (page 679) trials performed through 1998 suggested that cholesterol was lowered by an average of 9 to 12% and triglycerides by 8 to 27% over a one-to-four month period.[306, 307, 308] Most of these trials used 600 to 900 mg per day of garlic supplements. More recently, however, several double-blind trials have found garlic to have minimal success in lowering cholesterol and triglycerides.[309, 310, 311, 312] One negative trial has been criticized for using a steam-distilled garlic "oil" that has no track record for this purpose,[313] while the others used the same standardized garlic products as the previous positive trials. Based on these findings, the use of garlic should not be considered a primary approach to lowering high cholesterol and triglycerides.[314]

Part of the confusion may result from differing effects from dissimilar garlic products. In most but not all trials, aged garlic extracts and garlic oil (both containing no allicin) have not lowered cholesterol levels in humans.[315, 316] Therefore, neither of these supplements can be recommended at this time for cholesterol lowering. Odor-controlled, enteric-coated tablets standardized for allicin content are available and, in some trials, appear more promising.[317] Doctors typically recommend 900 mg per day (providing 5,000 to 6,000 mcg of allicin), divided into two or three admininstrations.

Green tea (page 686) has been shown to lower total cholesterol levels and improve people's cholesterol profile, decreasing LDL cholesterol and increasing HDL cholesterol according to preliminary studies.[318, 319, 320, 321] However, not all trials have found that green tea intake lowers lipid levels.[322] Much of the research documenting the health benefits of green tea is based on the amount of green tea typically drunk in Asian countries—about three cups per day, providing 240 to 320 mg of polyphenols.

An extract of green tea, enriched with a compound present in black tea (theaflavins), has been found to lower serum cholesterol in a double-blind study of people with moderately high cholesterol levels.[323] The average reduction in total serum cholesterol during the 12-week study was 11.3%, and the average reduction in LDL cholesterol was 16.4%. The extract used in this study provided daily 75 mg of theaflavins, 150 mg of green tea catechins, and 150 mg of other tea polyphenols.

Artichoke (page 628) has moderately lowered cholesterol and triglycerides in some,[324] but not all,[325] human trials. One double-blind trial found that 900 mg of artichoke extract per day significantly lowered serum cholesterol and LDL cholesterol but did not decrease triglycerides or raise HDL cholesterol.[326] Cholesterol-lowering effects occurred when using 320 mg of standardized leaf extract taken two to three times per day for at least six weeks.

Berberine, a compound found in certain herbs such as goldenseal, barberry, and Oregon grape, has been found to lower serum cholesterol levels. In a study of people with high cholesterol levels, 500 mg of berberine taken twice a day for three months lowered the average cholesterol level by 29%. No significant side effects were reported, except for mild constipation.[327]

Fenugreek (page 676) seeds contain compounds known as steroidal saponins that inhibit both cholesterol absorption in the intestines and cholesterol production by the liver.[328] Dietary fiber may also contribute to fenugreek's activity. Multiple human trials (some double-blind) have found that fenugreek may help lower total cholesterol in people with moderate **atherosclerosis** (page 38) or those having insulin-dependent or non-insulin-dependent **diabetes** (page 152).[329, 330, 331] One human double-blind trial has also shown that defatted fenugreek seeds may raise levels of beneficial HDL cholesterol.[332] One small preliminary trial found that either 25 or 50 grams per day of defatted fenugreek seed powder significantly lowered serum cholesterol after 20 days.[333] Germination of the fenugreek seeds may improve the soluble fiber content of the seeds, thus improving their effect on cholesterol.[334] Fenugreek powder is generally taken in amounts of 10 to 30 grams three times per day with meals.

Preliminary Chinese research has found that high doses (12 grams per day) of the herb **fo-ti** (page 678) may lower cholesterol levels. Double-blind or other controlled trials are needed to determine fo-ti's use in lowering cholesterol. A tea may be made from processed roots by boiling 3 to 5 grams in a cup of water for 10 to 15 minutes. Three or more cups should be drunk each day. Fo-ti tablets containing 500 mg each are also available. Doctors may suggest taking five of these tablets three times per day.

Wild yam (page 759) has been reported to raise HDL cholesterol in preliminary research. Doctors sometimes recommend 2 to 3 ml of tincture taken three to four times per day, or 1 to 2 capsules or tablets of dried root taken three times per day. [335]

Animal studies suggest that the mushroom **maitake** (page 707) may lower fat levels in the blood.[336] This research is still preliminary and requires confirmation with controlled human trials.

Animal studies indicate that saponins in **alfalfa** (page 623) seeds may block absorption of cholesterol and prevent the formation of atherosclerotic plaques.[337] However, consuming the large amounts of alfalfa seeds (80 to 120 grams per day) needed to supply high doses of these saponins may potentially cause damage to red blood cells in the body.[338]

Are there any side effects or interactions?
Refer to the individual herb for information about any side effects or interactions.

HIGH HOMOCYSTEINE

Homocysteine, a normal breakdown product of the essential **amino acid methionine** (page 557), is believed to exert several toxic effects.

A growing body of evidence suggests that an elevated homocysteine level is a risk factor for **heart disease** (page 98), independent of other known risk factors, such as elevated serum **cholesterol** (page 223) and **hypertension** (page 246).[1, 2] The evidence is not all one-sided, however. In some research the link has appeared only in women,[3] and a few scientists still have doubts about the importance of elevations in homocysteine for anyone.[4] The clear association between elevated homocysteine levels and heart disease reported in most studies[5] does not conclusively prove that homocysteine *causes* heart disease. It might only be a marker for something else that is the real culprit.[6] Nonetheless, many cardiologists take seriously the association between elevations in homocysteine and increased risk of heart disease.

Anger and hostility correlate with the risk of **heart disease** (page 98).[7, 8] A preliminary study found a link between high homocysteine levels and hostility and repressed anger.[9] While anger, hostility, high homocysteine, and heart disease all appear to be tied together, which of these is cause and which is effect remains somewhat unclear.

Increased homocysteine levels may also be a risk factor for the development of many other conditions, including **stroke** (page 419),[10] thromboembolism[11] (blood clots that can dislodge and cause stroke, **heart attack** (page 212), and other complications), **osteoporosis** (page 333),[12] **inflammatory bowel disease** (page 269) (**Crohn's disease** [page 141] and **ulcerative colitis** [page 433]),[13] **Alzheimer's disease** (page 19),[14] death from **diabetes** (page 152),[15] miscarriage,[16, 17, 18, 19, 20] other complications of **pregnancy** (page 363),[21, 22, 23, 24, 25] and **hypothyroidism** (page 252).[26]

Scientists have yet to prove that elevated homocysteine levels cause any of these diseases. However, most doctors believe that high homocysteine increases the risk of at least heart disease. Fortunately, homocysteine levels can easily be reduced with safe and inexpensive B vitamin supplementation.

CHECKLIST FOR HIGH HOMOCYSTEINE		
Rating	**Nutritional Supplements**	**Herbs**
★★★	**Folic acid** (page 520), **vitamin B$_6$** (page 600), and **vitamin B$_{12}$** (page 601) (in combination)	
★★☆	**Betaine (trimethylglycine)** (page 472) **Choline** (page 546)	

What are the symptoms of high homocysteine?

Extremely high homocysteine can cause blood clots, rapid bone loss, and, in children, mental retardation. But in general, high homocysteine does not cause symptoms until and unless one of the diseases with which it is associated, appears.

Medical treatments

Over the counter supplementation with **vitamin B$_6$** (page 600), **vitamin B$_{12}$** (page 601), and **folic acid** (page 520) is recommended.

People with high homocysteine are typically advised to reduce their consumption of processed foods, meat, and saturated fats, because these dietary changes lower the risk of **heart disease** (page 98).

Dietary changes that may be helpful

Since homocysteine is produced from **methionine** (page 557), intake of large amounts of methionine would presumably increase homocysteine levels. Indeed, ingestion of supplemental methionine is used experimentally as a way to increase homocysteine levels.[27] Foods high in methionine that have also been linked with an increased risk of **heart disease** (page 98) include meat and eggs. The extent to which consumption of these foods affects the risk of heart disease as a result of their methionine content remains unknown.

A controlled trial showed that eating a diet high in fruits and vegetables containing **folic acid** (page 520), **beta-carotene** (page 469), and **vitamin C** (page 604) effectively lowered homocysteine levels.[28] Healthy people were assigned to either a diet containing a pound of fruits and vegetables per day, or to a diet containing three and a half ounces of fruits and vegetables per day. After four weeks, those eating the higher amount of fruits and vegetables had an 11% lower homocysteine level compared with those eating the lower amount of fruits and vegetables.

Another study of men with heart disease demonstrated that consumption of whole-grain and legume powder at breakfast, instead of their usual breakfast of refined rice, resulted in a significant reduction in homocysteine levels.[29]

Lifestyle changes that may be helpful

According to a recent study, both cigarette smoking and coffee consumption were associated with increased homocysteine levels.[30] These findings are consistent with studies that have found both smoking and caffeine consumption to be associated with an increased risk of both **cardiovascular disease** (page 98) and **osteoporosis** (page 333). The link between coffee and increased homocysteine has been confirmed by some researchers,[31] but not others.[32]

In one study, a diverse group of people participated in a week-long program that included a strict vegan diet, stress management and spirituality enhancement sessions, group support, and exclusion of tobacco, **alcohol** (page 12), and caffeine.[33] **B vitamin supplements** (page 603) known to reduce blood homocysteine levels were not provided. After only one week in the program, the average homocysteine level fell 13%.

Nutritional supplements that may be helpful

Vitamin B$_6$ (page 600), **folic acid** (page 520), and **vitamin B$_{12}$** (page 601) all play a role in converting homocysteine to other substances within the body. By so doing, they consistently lower homocysteine levels in research trials,[34, 35, 36] a finding that is now well accepted. Several studies have used (and some doctors recommend) 400–1,000 mcg of folic acid per day, 10–50 mg of vitamin B$_6$ per day, and 50–300 mcg of vitamin B$_{12}$ per day.

Of these three vitamins, **folic acid** (page 520) supplementation lowers homocysteine levels the most for the average person.[37, 38] It also effectively lowers homocysteine in people on kidney dialysis.[39] In 1996, the FDA required that all enriched flour, rice, pasta, cornmeal, and other grain products contain 140 mcg of folic acid per 3½ ounces.[40] This level of fortification has led to a measurable decrease in homocysteine levels.[41] However, even higher levels of food fortification with folic acid have been reported to be more effective in lowering homocysteine,[42] suggesting that the FDA-mandated supplementation is inadequate to optimally protect people against high homocysteine levels. Therefore, people wishing to lower their homocysteine levels should continue to take folic acid supplements despite the FDA-mandated fortification program.

Betaine (trimethylglycine) (page 472) (6 grams per day) and **choline** (page 546) (2 grams per day) have each been shown to lower homocysteine levels.[43, 44] More recently, 1.5 grams of betaine per day, an amount similar to that in a typical diet, also has been found to lower homocysteine levels.[45] Doctors usually consider supplementation with these nutrients only when supplementation with folic acid, vitamin B$_6$, and vitamin B$_{12}$ do not reduce homocysteine levels sufficiently. The results of this study, however, point to the potential benefit of increasing one's intake of foods rich in betaine (such as whole wheat, spinach, beets, and other plant foods).

Niacin (page 598), a form of vitamin B$_3$, is sometimes given in large amounts to people with elevated **cholesterol** (page 223) levels. A controlled study found that 1,000 mg or more per day of niacin raised homocysteine levels.[46] Since other actions of niacin lower **heart disease** (page 98) risk,[47, 48] the importance of this finding is unclear. Nonetheless, large amounts of niacin should never be taken without consulting a doctor.

Are there any side effects or interactions?
Refer to the individual supplement for information about any side effects or interactions.

HIGH TRIGLYCERIDES

Triglycerides (TGs) are a group of fatty compounds that circulate in the bloodstream and are stored in the fat tissue. Individuals who have elevated blood levels of TGs (known as hypertriglyceridemia) appear to be at increased risk of developing **heart disease** (page 98).

People with **diabetes** (page 152) often have elevated TG levels. Successfully controlling diabetes will, in some cases, lead to normalization of TG levels.

What are the symptoms of high triglycerides?

Very high triglycerides can cause pancreatitis, an enlarged liver and spleen, and fatty deposits in the skin called xanthomas. Otherwise, high triglycerides may not cause symptoms until and unless heart disease or other diseases of blood vessels develop.

Medical treatments

Prescription drug therapy includes niacin (Niaspan) and gemfibrozil (Lopid).

People with high triglycerides are typically advised to reduce their **weight** (page 446) and limit the consumption of processed foods, simple sugars, alcohol, and saturated fats. The latter is found predominantly in animal products, such as meat, eggs, and dairy products, and in tropical oils such as palm and coconut.

CHECKLIST FOR HIGH TRIGLYCERIDES		
Rating	**Nutritional Supplements**	**Herbs**
★★★	**Fish oil** (page 514) (EPA/**DHA** [page 509]) **Niacin** (page 598) (vitamin B$_3$) **Pantethine** (page 568)	**Guggul** (page 688) **Oats** (page 716)
★★☆	**Calcium** (page 483) **Chromium** (page 493) **Fructo-oligosaccharides** (page 522) (FOS) **Inositol hexaniacinate** (page 537) (vitamin B$_3$) **L-carnitine** (page 543) **Policosanol** (page 571)	*Achillea wilhelmsii* **Fenugreek** (page 676) **Garlic** (page 679) **Psyllium** (page 732) **Red yeast rice** (page 736)
★☆☆	**Creatine monohydrate** (page 501) **Fiber** (page 512)	**Green tea** (page 686) **Maitake** (page 707)

Dietary changes that may be helpful

While consuming moderate amounts of alcohol does not appear to affect TG levels, heavy drinking is believed to be an important cause of hypertriglyceridemia.[1] Alcoholics with elevated TG levels should deal with the disease of **alcoholism** (page 12) first.

Ingesting refined sugar increases TG levels, as well.[2, 3] People with elevated TGs should therefore reduce their intake of sugar, sweets, and other sugar-containing foods. There is also evidence that ingesting fructose in amounts that are found in a typical Western diet can raise TG levels, although not all studies agree on that point.[4] It should be noted that most studies of fructose investigated the refined form, not the fructose that occurs naturally in some fruits.

In a study of heavy caffeine users (individuals who were consuming an average of 560 mg of caffeine per day from coffee and tea), changing to decaffeinated coffee and eliminating all other caffeinated products for two weeks resulted in a statistically significant 25% reduction in TG levels.[5]

Diets high in **fiber** (page 512) have reduced TG levels in several clinical trials,[6] but have had no effect in other clinical trials.[7] Water-soluble fibers, such as pectin found in fruit, guar gum and other gums found in beans, and **beta-glucan** (page 470) found in **oats** (page 716), may be particularly helpful in lowering triglycerides.

Consumption of a low-fat, high-carbohydrate diet reduced TGs in one study.[8] However, in another study, populations that consumed a low-fat, high-carbohydrate diet had higher TG levels, compared with populations that consumed lower amounts of carbohydrates.[9] Suddenly switching to a high-carbohydrate, low-fat diet will generally increase TGs temporarily, but making the switch gradually protects against this short-term problem.[10]

The blood level of TGs *following* a meal may be a more important indicator of coronary heart disease risk than the fasting level.[11, 12] However, a low-fat diet (55% carbohydrates, 23% fats, 22% proteins) that succeeded in normalizing other blood lipids, including fasting TG levels, failed to normalize post-meal TG levels in a group of people with hypertriglyceridemia.[13] These results suggest that dietary reduction of fasting TGs, even if the diet controls other blood lipids, may not be enough to provide optimal protection against coronary heart disease. Many doctors recommend a diet low in saturated fat (meaning avoidance of red meat and all dairy except nonfat dairy) to reduce TGs and the risk of **heart disease** (page 98).[14]

Some,[15, 16] but not all,[17] studies have found that increasing consumption of fish is associated with a lower risk of **heart disease** (page 98). Significant amounts of TG-lowering omega-3 fatty acids (EPA and **DHA** [page 509]) can be found in the **fish oil** (page 514) of salmon, herring, mackerel, sardines, anchovies, albacore tuna, and black cod. Many doctors recommend that people with elevated TGs increase their intake of these fatty fish.

Lifestyle changes that may be helpful

Exercise lowers TG levels.[18] People who have **diabetes** (page 152), **heart disease** (page 98), or are over the age of 40, should talk with a doctor before beginning an exercise program.

Smoking has been linked to elevated TG levels.[19] As always, it makes sense for smokers to quit.

Obesity (page 446) increases TG levels.[20] Maintaining ideal body weight helps protect against elevated TG levels. Many doctors encourage people who have elevated TGs and who are overweight to lose the extra weight.

Nutritional supplements that may be helpful

Many double-blind trials have demonstrated that **fish oils** (page 514) (also called fish-oil concentrates) containing EPA and **DHA** (page 509) (mentioned above) lower TG levels.[21] The amount of fish oil used in much of the research was an amount that provided 3,000 mg per day of omega-3 fatty acids. To calculate how much omega-3 fatty acid is contained in a fish-oil supplement, add together the amounts of EPA and DHA. For example, a typical 1,000-mg capsule of fish oil provides 180 mg of EPA and 120 mg of DHA (total omega-3 fatty acids equals 300 mg). Ten of these capsules would contain 3,000 mg of omega-3 fatty acids. Other sources of omega-3 fatty acids, such as **flaxseed oil** (page 517), do not lower TGs. While flaxseed oil has other benefits, it should not be used for the purpose of reducing TGs.

Cod liver oil (page 514), another source of omega-3 fatty acids, has also been found to lower TGs.[22] Cod-liver oil is less expensive than the fish-oil concentrates discussed previously. However, cod-liver oil also contains relatively large amounts of **vitamin A** (page 595) and **vitamin D** (page 607); too much of either can cause side effects. In contrast, fish-oil concentrates have little or none of these vitamins. Individuals wishing to use cod liver oil as a substitute for a fish-oil concentrate should consult a doctor.

Omega-3 fatty acids from **fish oil** (page 514) and cod liver oil have been reported to affect blood in many other ways that might lower the risk of **heart disease** (page 98).[23] However, these supplements sometimes increase LDL **cholesterol** (page 223)—the bad form of cholesterol. A doctor can check to see if fish oil has this effect on an individual. Research shows that when 900 mg of **garlic** (page 679) extract is added to fish oil, the combination still dramatically lowers TG levels but no longer increases LDL cholesterol.[24] Therefore, it appears that taking garlic supplements may be a way to avoid the increase in LDL cholesterol sometimes associated with taking fish oil. People who take fish oil may also need to take **vitamin E** (page 609) to prevent the oil from undergoing potentially damaging oxidation in the body.[25] It is not known how much vitamin E is needed to prevent such oxidation. The amount required would presumably depend on the amount of fish oil used. In one clinical trial, 300 IU of vitamin E per day prevented oxidation damage in individuals taking 6 grams of fish oil per day.[26]

Pantethine (page 568) is a byproduct of pantothenic acid (vitamin B$_5$). Several clinical trials have shown that 300 mg of pantethine taken three times per day will lower TG levels.[27, 28, 29] Pantothenic acid, which is found in most B vitamins, does not have this effect.

The **niacin** (page 598) form of vitamin B$_3$ is used by doctors to lower **cholesterol** (page 223) levels, but niacin also lowers TG levels.[30] The amount of niacin needed to achieve worthwhile reductions in cholesterol and TG levels is several grams per day. Such quantities can cause side effects, including potential damage to the liver, and should not be taken without the supervision of a doctor. Some doctors recommend **inositol hexaniacinate** (page 537) (a special form of vitamin B$_3$) as an alternative to niacin. A typical amount recommended is 500 mg three times per day.[31, 32] This form of vitamin B$_3$ does not typically cause a skin flush and is said to be safer for the liver than niacin. However, the alleged safety advantage of inositol hexaniacinate needs to be confirmed by additional clinical trials. Moreover, it is not clear whether inositol hexaniacinate is as effective as niacin at lowering cholesterol and TG levels.

In a preliminary trial, supplementation with 800 mg of **calcium** (page 483) per day for one year resulted in a statistically significant 35% reduction in the average TG level among people with elevated cholesterol and triglycerides.[33] However, in another trial, calcium supplementation had no effect on TG levels.[34] One of the differences between these two trials was that more people in the former trial had initially elevated TG levels.

In a double-blind trial, 30 people with type 2 (non-insulin-dependent) **diabetes** (page 152) received 200 mcg of **chromium** (page 493) per day (as chromium picolinate) for two months and a placebo for an additional two months. The average TG level was significantly lower (by an average of 17.4%) during chromium supplementation than during the placebo period.[35] Some,[36, 37] but not all, trials[38, 39] support these findings. It is not clear whether chromium supplementation affects TG levels in non-diabetics, but some evidence suggests that it does not.[40, 41, 42, 43, 44]

L-carnitine (page 543) is another supplement that has lowered TGs in several clinical trials.[45, 46] However, the effect of carnitine is unpredictable, and some individuals have experienced an increase in triglyceride levels after receiving this supplement.[47] Some doctors recommend 1–3 grams of carnitine per day, in the form known as L-carnitine.

Several double-blind trials have evaluated the efficacy of **fructo-oligosaccharides** (page 522) (FOS) or inulin (a related compound) for lowering blood **cholesterol** (page 223) and triglyceride levels. These trials have shown that in individuals with elevated total cholesterol or triglyceride levels, including people with type 2 diabetes, FOS or inulin (in amounts ranging from 8 to 20 grams daily) produced significant reductions in triglyceride levels; however, the effect on cholesterol levels was inconsistent.[48, 49, 50, 51] In people with normal or low cholesterol or triglyceride levels, FOS or inulin produced little effect.[52, 53, 54]

The effect of **policosanol** (page 571) on serum triglycerides has been inconsistent, ranging from no effect up to as much as a 19% reduction.[55, 56, 57, 58, 59, 60, 61, 62, 63, 64] Several controlled studies have compared policosanol with cholesterol-lowering medications, such as statins, and have found policosanol similarly effective.[65, 66, 67, 68, 69, 70, 71] Policosanol extracted from beeswax or other sources differs from the sugar-cane-derived preparation in the proportions of long-chain alcohols, and whether these types of policosanol are as effective as sugar-cane-derived policosanol is unknown.

A double-blind trial found that a supplement of 5 grams of **creatine** (page 501) plus 1 gram of glucose taken four times per day for five days followed by twice a day for 51 days significantly lowered serum total triglycerides in both men and women.[72] However, another double-blind trial found no change in any of these blood levels in trained athletes using creatine during a 12-week strength training program.[73] Creatine supplementation in this negative trial was lower—only five grams per day was taken for the last 11 weeks of the study.

Are there any side effects or interactions?
Refer to the individual supplement for information about any side effects or interactions.

Herbs that may be helpful
Guggul (page 688), a mixture of ketonic steroids from the gum oleoresin of *Commiphora mukul*, is an approved treatment of hyperlipidemia in India and has been a mainstay of Ayurvedic herbal approaches to preventing **atherosclerosis** (page 38). Clinical trials indicate that guggul is effective in the treatment of high TGs; in one trial, serum TGs fell by 30.3%.[74]

However, these results have not been confirmed by large, controlled trials. The recommended daily intake of guggul is typically based on the amount of guggulsterones in the extract. The recommended amount of guggulsterones is 25 mg three times per day. Most extracts contain 5–10% guggulsterones. Guggul's effect on TGs should be monitored for three to four months,

and guggul may be taken long term if successful in lowering TGs.

Reports on many clinical trials of **garlic** (page 679) performed until 1998 suggested that triglycerides were lowered by an average of 8–27% and **cholesterol** (page 223) by 9–12% over a one- to four-month period.[75, 76, 77] Most of these trials used 600–900 mg per day of a garlic supplement standardized to alliin content and allicin potential. More recently, however, three double-blind clinical trials have found garlic to have minimal success in lowering triglycerides and cholesterol.[78, 79, 80] One negative trial has been criticized for using a steam distilled garlic "oil" that has no track record for this purpose,[81] while the others used the same standardized garlic products as the previous positive clinical trials. Based on these findings, the use of garlic should not be considered a primary approach to lowering high triglycerides and cholesterol.[82]

Odor-controlled, enteric-coated garlic tablets standardized for allicin content can be taken in the amount of 900 mg daily (providing 5,000–6,000 mcg of allicin), divided into two or three daily portions.

In a double-blind trial, people with moderately high triglycerides took a tincture of *Achillea wilhelmsii*, an herb used in traditional Persian medicine.[83] Participants in the trial used 15–20 drops of the tincture twice daily for six months. At the end of the trial, participants experienced significant reductions in triglycerides compared to those who took placebo. No adverse effects were reported.

Fenugreek (page 676) has been shown to lower total and LDL **cholesterol** (page 223) and triglyceride levels in people with high lipid levels in preliminary trials.[84] Bread made with 50 grams defatted fenugreek powder was used twice daily in the trial. Similar results have been seen at half that amount in people with **diabetes** (page 152) and elevated blood levels of various lipids.[85] A small randomized trial found similar results using 100 grams fenugreek seeds daily.[86] One small clinical trial found that either 25 grams or 50 grams per day of defatted fenugreek seed powder were effective in reducing triglycerides over a 20-day period.[87] Mild **diarrhea** (page 163) and gas can accompany the first few days of fenugreek use, though it almost always fades as the person taking it adapts.

Psyllium (page 732) seeds and husks have shown a modest ability to lower blood triglyceride levels in some,[88, 89] but not all,[90] clinical trials. Further research is needed to assess the effect of psyllium on triglyceride levels more closely, as much of the study so far has focused on lowering cholesterol levels.

Intake of three cups or less of **green tea** (page 686) daily has been shown not to affect blood triglyceride levels.[91] Intake of four or more cups per day has been correlated with lower triglyceride levels.[92] Overall, the evidence is unclear on how much of an effect high levels of intake of green tea has on triglyceride levels.

Although primarily used to lower high serum cholesterol, **red yeast rice** (page 736) extract, high in monacolins, has been found to significantly lower serum triglyceride levels.[93] People in the trial took 1.2 grams (approximately 13.5 mg total monacolins) of a concentrated red yeast rice extract per day for two months. The sale of Cholestin has been banned in the United States, as a result of a lawsuit alleging patent infringement. Other red yeast rice products currently on the market differ from Cholestin in their chemical makeup. None contain the full complement of 10 monacolin compounds that are present in Cholestin, and some contain a potentially toxic fermentation product called citrinin.[94] Until further information is available, red yeast rice products other than Cholestin cannot be recommended.

Animal studies suggest the mushroom **maitake** (page 707) may lower fat levels in the blood.[95] However, this research is still preliminary and requires confirmation by controlled human trials.

Are there any side effects or interactions?
Refer to the individual herb for information about any side effects or interactions.

HIV AND AIDS SUPPORT

Acquired immunodeficiency syndrome (AIDS) is a condition in which the **immune system** (page 255) becomes severely weakened and loses its ability to fight **infections** (page 265).

Although some scientists have questioned whether or not the human immunodeficiency virus (HIV) has actually been proven to cause AIDS,[1, 2, 3] most researchers do believe that HIV causes AIDS.

AIDS is an extremely complex disorder, and no cure is currently available. Certain drugs appear to be capable of slowing the progression of the disease. In addition, various nutritional factors may be helpful. However, because of the complicated nature of this disorder, medical supervision is strongly recommended with regard to dietary changes and nutritional supplements. People who have been infected with HIV are hereafter referred to as "HIV-positive."

CHECKLIST FOR HIV AND AIDS SUPPORT		
Rating	**Nutritional Supplements**	**Herbs**
★★☆	**Arginine** (page 467) (in combination with **HMB** [page 534] and **glutamine** [page 530]) for preservation of lean body mass **DHEA** (page 503) (for fatigue and **depression** [page 145]) **Glutamine** (page 530) (in combination with **HMB** [page 534] and **arginine** [page 467]) for preservation of lean body mass **Hydroxymethyl-butyrate** (page 534) (HMB) (in combination with **glutamine** [page 530] and **arginine** [page 467]) for preservation of lean body mass **Multiple vitamin-mineral** (page 559) **N-acetyl cysteine** (page 562) *Saccharomyces boulardii* (page 575) **Selenium** (page 584) **Zinc** (page 614)	Boxwood **Licorice** (page 702) Sangre de Drago (for HIV-associated **diarrhea** [page 163])
★☆☆	**Beta-carotene** (page 469) **Coenzyme Q$_{10}$** (page 496) **Folic acid** (page 520) **Glutamine** (page 530) **Iron** (page 540) **Methionine** (page 557) **Thymus extracts** (page 591) **Vitamin A** (page 595) **Vitamin B$_1$** (page 597) **Vitamin B$_{12}$** (page 601) **Vitamin B$_3$** (page 598) **Vitamin B$_6$** (page 600) **Vitamin C** (page 604) (oral and topical) **Vitamin E** (page 609) **Whey protein** (page 613)	**Andrographis** (page 626) **Asian ginseng** (page 630) **Bupleurum** (page 647) (in combination with **peony** [page 724] root, pinellia root, cassia bark, **ginger** [page 680] root, jujube fruit, Asian ginseng [page 630] root, **Chinese scullcap** [page 658] root, and **licorice** [page 702] root.) **Cat's claw** (page 653) **Echinacea** (page 669) **Eleuthero** (page 672) **Garlic** (page 679)

HIV and AIDS Support

Maitake (page 707)
Mistletoe (page 711)
Reishi (page 737)
Shiitake (page 746)
St. John's wort
(page 747)
Tea tree oil (page 751)
Turmeric (page 753)

What are the symptoms of HIV and AIDS?

HIV causes a broad spectrum of clinical problems, which often mimic other diseases. Within a few weeks of **infection** (page 265), some people may experience **flu** (page 269)-like signs and symptoms, including fever, malaise, rash, joint **pain** (page 338), and generalized swelling of the lymph nodes. These acute manifestations usually disappear, and many people remain asymptomatic for long periods. AIDS, the clinical syndrome associated with HIV infection, produces symptoms throughout the body related to opportunistic infections, tumors, and other immune-deficiency complications.

Medical treatments

Three main classes of prescription antiviral drugs are used to treat HIV infection. The first group, nucleoside analog reverse transcriptase inhibitors, includes zidovudine (ZDV, AZT, Retrovir), didanosine (ddI, Videx), zalcitabine (ddC, Hivid), stavudine (d4T, Zerit), and lamivudine (3TC, Epivir). The second class, non-nucleoside reverse transcriptase inhibitors, includes nevirapine (Viramune) and delavirdine (Rescriptor). The third group, protease inhibitors, includes saquinavir (Fortovase, Invirase), ritonavir (Norvir), indinavir (Crixivan), and nelfinavir (Viracept). Several other investigational drugs are also used. Treatment with two to four of these drugs is standard. Treatment of the complications of AIDS is specific to the **infection** (page 265) or complication present, and frequently includes antibiotics, antifungal medications, corticosteroids, and heart drugs.

Dietary changes that may be helpful

People with AIDS often lose significant amounts of weight or suffer from recurrent **diarrhea** (page 163). A diet high in protein and total calories may help a person maintain his or her body weight. In addition, whole foods are preferable to refined and processed foods. Whole foods contain larger amounts of many **vitamins and minerals** (page 559), and people with HIV infection tend to suffer from multiple nutritional deficiencies.

Nonetheless, no evidence currently suggests that dietary changes are curative for people with AIDS, or even that they significantly influence the course of the disease. In fact, a controlled trial comparing the efficacy of three nutritional regimens in the prevention of weight loss in HIV-positive people found no benefit from increasing caloric intake.[4] A 500-calorie per day caloric supplement with fatty acids plus a multivitamin and minerals did not promote increases in body weight beyond that offered by a **multivitamin-mineral** (page 559) supplement alone.

AIDS-related weight loss and chronic diarrhea are sometimes the result of abnormal intestinal function in the absence of an **infectious** (page 265) organism. This condition, called "HIV enteropathy" (pronounced "en-ter-OP-a-thee"), may respond to a gluten-free diet. In a preliminary trial,[5] men with HIV enteropathy were given a gluten-free diet for one week. During that week, the number of episodes of diarrhea decreased by nearly 40%. When gluten-containing foods were re-introduced for a week, the diarrhea returned. When they were eliminated a second time, again for one week, the episodes of diarrhea were again reduced. Participants in the study also experienced significant weight gain during the gluten-free periods.

Lifestyle changes that may be helpful

Loss of strength and lean body mass are frequent complications in people with AIDS. Drug therapy with anabolic steroids is sometimes used to counteract these losses. Preliminary trials suggest that progressive resistance training (i.e., weight training) may be used as an alternative or adjunct to steroids in this disease. In a preliminary trial, people with HIV who did progressive resistance training three times per week for eight weeks had significant increases in their lean body mass.[6] Exercise of any type three to four times per week or more has been associated with slower progression to AIDS at one year and with a slower progression to death from AIDS at one year in men.[7]

Nutritional supplements that may be helpful

Because people with HIV infection or AIDS often have multiple nutritional deficiencies, a broad-spectrum nutritional supplement may be beneficial. In one trial, HIV-positive men who took a **multivitamin-mineral supplement** (page 559) had slower onset of AIDS, compared with men who did not take a supplement.[8]

Use of a multivitamin by **pregnant** (page 363) and breast-feeding Tanzanian women with HIV did *not* affect the risk of transmission of HIV from mother to child, either in utero, during birth, or from breast-feeding.[9]

Selenium (page 584) deficiency is an independent factor associated with high mortality among HIV-positive people.[10] HIV-positive people who took selenium supplements experienced fewer **infections** (page 265), better intestinal function, improved appetite, and improved heart function (which had been impaired by the disease) than those who did not take the supplements.[11] The usual amount of selenium taken was 400 mcg per day.

Selenium deficiency has been found more often in people with HIV-related **cardiomyopathy** (page 95) (heart abnormalities) than in those with HIV and normal heart function.[12] People with HIV-related cardiomyopathy may benefit from selenium supplementation. In a small preliminary trial, people with AIDS and cardiomyopathy, 80% of whom were found to be deficient in selenium, were given 800 mcg of selenium per day for 15 days, followed by 400 mcg per day for eight days. Improvements in heart function were noted after selenium supplementation.[13] People wishing to supplement with more than 200 mcg of selenium per day should be monitored by a doctor.

The **amino acid** (page 465), **N-acetyl cysteine** (page 562) (NAC), has been shown to inhibit the replication of HIV in test tube studies.[14] In a double-blind trial, supplementing with 800 mg per day of NAC slowed the rate of decline in **immune function** (page 255) in people with HIV infection. NAC also promotes the synthesis of **glutathione** (page 531), a naturally-occurring **antioxidant** (page 467) that is believed to be protective in people with HIV infection and AIDS.[15]

The combination of **glutamine** (page 530), **arginine** (page 467), and the amino acid derivative, **hydroxymethylbutyrate** (page 534) (HMB), may prevent loss of lean body mass in people with AIDS-associated wasting. In a double-blind trial, AIDS patients who had lost 5% of their body weight in the previous three months received either placebo or a nutrient mixture containing 1.5 grams of HMB, 7 grams of L-glutamine, and 7 grams of L-arginine twice daily for eight weeks.[16] Those supplemented with placebo gained an average of 0.37 pounds, mostly fat, but lost lean body mass. Those taking the nutrient mixture gained an average of 3 pounds, 85% of which was lean body weight.

In a double-blind trial, the non-disease-causing yeast *Saccharomyces boulardii* (page 575) (1 gram three times per day) helped stop **diarrhea** (page 163) in HIV-positive people.[17] However, people with severely compromised immune function have been reported to develop **yeast infections** (page 454) in the bloodstream after consuming some yeast organisms that are benign for healthy people.[18, 19] For that reason, people with HIV infection who wish to take *Saccharomyces boulardii*, **brewer's yeast** (page 480) *(Saccharomyces cerevisiae),* or other live organisms should first consult a doctor.

A deficient level of dehydroepiandrosterone sulfate (DHEAS) in the blood is associated with poor outcomes in people with HIV.[20] Large amounts of supplemental **dehydroepiandrosterone** (page 503) (DHEA) may alleviate fatigue and depression in HIV-positive men and women. In a preliminary trial, men and women with HIV infection took 200–500 mg of DHEA per day for eight weeks.[21] All participants initially had both low mood and low energy. After eight weeks of DHEA supplementation, 72% of the participants reported their mood to be "much improved" or "very much improved," and 81% reported having significant improvements in energy level. DHEA supplementation had no effect on CD4 cell (helper T-cell) counts or testosterone levels.

Vitamin A (page 595) deficiency appears to be very common in people with HIV infection. Low blood levels of vitamin A are associated with greater disease severity[22] and increased transmission of the virus from a pregnant mother to her infant.[23] However, in preliminary[24] and double-blind[25, 26] trials, supplementation with vitamin A failed to reduce the overall mother-to-child transmission of HIV. HIV-positive women who took 5,000 IU per day of vitamin A (as retinyl palmitate) and 50,000 IU per day of **beta-carotene** (page 469) during the third trimester (13 weeks) of pregnancy, plus an additional single amount of 200,000 IU of vitamin A at delivery, had the same rate of transmission of HIV to their infants as those who did not take the supplement. However, lower rates of illness have been observed in the children of HIV-positive mothers when the children were supplemented with 50,000–200,000 IU of vitamin A every two to three months.[27]

Little research has explored whether vitamin A supplements are helpful at halting disease progression. HIV-positive children given two consecutive oral supplements of vitamin A (200,000 IU in a gelcap) in the two days following influenza vaccinations had a modest but significant decrease in viral load.[28] In one trial, giving people an extremely high (300,000 IU) amount of vitamin A one time only did not improve short-term measures of immunity in women with HIV.[29]

Beta-carotene levels have been found to be low in HIV-positive people, even in those without symptoms.[30] However, trials on the effect of beta-carotene supplements have produced conflicting results. In one double-blind trial, supplementing with 300,000 IU per day of beta-carotene significantly increased the number of CD4+ cells in people with HIV infection.[31] In another trial, the same amount of beta-carotene had no effect on CD4+ cell counts or various other measures of immune function in HIV-infected people.[32]

In HIV-positive people with B-vitamin deficiency, the use of **B-complex vitamin** (page 603) supplements appears to delay progression to and death from AIDS.[33] Thiamine (**vitamin B$_1$** [page 597]) deficiency has been identified in nearly one-quarter of people with AIDS.[34] It has been suggested that a thiamine deficiency may contribute to some of the neurological abnormalities that are associated with AIDS. **Vitamin B$_6$** (page 600) deficiency was found in more than one-third of HIV-positive men; vitamin B$_6$ deficiency was associated with decreased **immune function** (page 255) in this group.[35] In a population study of HIV-positive people, intake of vitamin B$_6$ at more than twice the recommended dietary allowance (RDA is 2 mg per day for men and 1.6 mg per day for women) was associated with improved survival.[36] Low blood levels of **folic acid** (page 520) and **vitamin B$_{12}$** (page 601) are also common in HIV-positive people.[37]

Preliminary observations suggest a possible role for **vitamin B$_3$** (page 598) in HIV prevention and treatment.[38] A form of vitamin B$_3$ (niacinamide) has been shown to inhibit HIV in test tube studies.[39] However, no published data have shown vitamin B$_3$ to inhibit HIV in animals or in people. One study did show that HIV-positive people who consume more than 64 mg of vitamin B$_3$ per day have a decreased risk of progression to AIDS or AIDS-related death.[40, 41] Clinical trials in humans are required to validate these preliminary observations.

Vitamin C (page 595) has been shown to inhibit HIV replication in test tubes.[42] Intake of vitamin C by HIV-positive persons may be associated with a reduced risk of progression to AIDS.[43] Some doctors recommend large amounts of vitamin C for people with AIDS. Reported benefits in preliminary research include greater resistance against infection and an improvement in overall well-being.[44] The amount of vitamin C used in that study ranged from 40 to 185 grams per day. Supplementation with such large amounts of vitamin C must be monitored by a doctor. This same researcher also reports some success in using a topical vitamin C paste to treat herpes simplex outbreaks and Kaposi's sarcoma in people with AIDS.

In test-tube studies, **vitamin E** (page 609) improved the effectiveness of the anti-HIV drug zidovudine (AZT) while reducing its toxicity.[45] Similarly, animal research suggests that **zinc** (page 614) and **NAC** (page 562) supplementation may protect against AZT toxicity.[46] It is not known whether oral supplementation with these nutrients would have similar effects in people taking AZT.

Blood levels of **coenzyme Q$_{10}$** (page 496) (CoQ$_{10}$) were also found to be low in people with HIV infection or AIDS. In a small preliminary trial, people with HIV infection took 200 mg per day of CoQ$_{10}$. Eighty-three percent of these people experienced no further infections for up to seven months, and the counts of **infection** (page 265)-fighting white blood cells improved in three cases.[47]

Blood levels of both zinc[48] and **selenium** (page 584)[49] are frequently low in people with HIV infection. Zinc supplements (45 mg per day) have been shown to reduce the number of infections in people with AIDS.[50]

Iron (page 540) deficiency is often present in HIV-positive children.[51] While iron is necessary for normal **immune function** (page 255), iron deficiency also appears to *protect* against certain bacterial **infections** (page 265).[52] Iron supplementation could therefore increase the severity of bacterial infections in people with AIDS. For that reason, people with HIV infection or AIDS should consult a doctor before supplementing with iron.

The **amino acid** (page 465), **glutamine** (page 530), is needed for the synthesis of **glutathione** (page 531), an important **antioxidant** (page 467) within cells that is frequently depleted in people with HIV and AIDS.[53] In well-nourished people, the body usually manufactures enough glutamine to prevent a deficiency. However, people with HIV or AIDS are often malnourished and may be deficient in glutamine.[54] In such people, glutamine supplementation may be needed, along with **NAC** (page 562), to maintain adequate levels of glutathione. It is not known how much glutamine is needed for that purpose; however, in other trials, 4–8 grams of glutamine per day was used.[55] In a double-blind trial, massive amounts of glutamine (40 grams per day) in combination with several antioxidants (27,000 IU per day of beta-carotene; 800 mg per day of vitamin C; 280 mcg per day of selenium; 500 IU per day of vitamin E) were given for 12 weeks to AIDS patients experiencing problems maintaining normal weight.[56] Those who took the glutamine-antioxidant combination experienced significant gains in body weight compared with those taking placebo. Larger trials are needed to determine the possible benefits of this nutrient combination on reducing opportunistic infections and long-term mortality.

People with AIDS have low levels of **methionine** (page 557). Some researchers suggest that these low methionine levels may explain some aspects of the disease process,[57, 58, 59] especially the deterioration that occurs in the nervous system and is responsible for symptoms such as dementia.[60, 61] A preliminary trial found that methionine (6 grams per day) may improve memory recall in people with AIDS-related nervous system degeneration.[62]

In a preliminary trial, a **thymus extract** (page 591) known as Thymomodulin improved several immune parameters among people with early HIV infection, including an increase in the number of T-helper cells.[63]

Whey protein (page 613) is rich in the amino acid cysteine, which the body uses to make glutathione, an important antioxidant. A double-blind trial showed that 45 grams per day of whey protein increased blood glutathione levels in a group of HIV-infected people.[64] Test tube[65] and animal[66] studies suggest that whey protein may improve some aspects of immune function.

Are there any side effects or interactions?
Refer to the individual supplement for information about any side effects or interactions.

Herbs that may be helpful
Many different herbs have been shown in test tube studies to inhibit the function or replication of HIV. Few of these studies have been followed up with any kind of investigation in HIV-positive humans. Some notable exceptions to this rule are discussed below.

There are three categories of herbs used in people with HIV infection. The first are herbs that are believed to directly kill HIV (antiretroviral herbs). The second are herbs that strengthen the **immune system** (page 255) to better withstand HIV's onslaught (immunomodulating herbs). The third are herbs that combat opportunistic **infections** (page 265) (antimicrobial herbs). The following table summarizes each category and herbs that belong in each. Note that some herbs fall into more than one category.

One double-blind trial has found that 990 mg per day of an extract of the leaves and stems of boxwood (*Buxus sempervirens*) could delay the progression of HIV infection (as measured by a decline in CD4 cell counts).[67] No adverse effects directly attributable to the extract were reported. Taking twice the amount of boxwood extract did not lead to further benefits and may have actually decreased its usefulness.

Category of Herb	Supporting Evidence from Human Trials	Supporting Evidence from Test Tube Studies
Antiretroviral	**Androgaphis** (page 626), boxwood, **licorice** (page 702), **St. John's wort** (page 747)	**Garlic** (page 679)
Immuno-modulators	**Androgaphis** (page 626) (possible antiretroviral), **Asian ginseng** (page 630), **bupleurum** (page 647), **echinacea** (page 669), **licorice** (page 702), **mistletoe** (page 711), Sangre de Drago, **turmeric** (page 753)	Herbs: **ashwagandha** (page 629), **eleuthero** (page 672), **schisandra** (page 744) Mushrooms: coriolus, **maitake** (page 707), **reishi** (page 737), **shiitake** (page 746)
Antimicrobial	**Garlic** (page 679), **tea tree oil** (page 751)	

Licorice (page 702) has shown the ability to inhibit reproduction of HIV in test tubes.[68] Clinical trials have shown that injections of glycyrrhizin (isolated from licorice) may have a beneficial effect on AIDS.[69] There is preliminary evidence that orally administered licorice also may be safe and effective for long-term treatment of HIV infection.[70] Amounts of licorice or glycyrrhizin used for treating HIV-positive people warrant monitoring by a physician, because long-term use of these substances can cause **high blood pressure** (page 246), **potassium** (page 572) depletion, or other problems. Approximately 2 grams of licorice root should be taken per day in capsules or as tea. Deglycyrrhizinated licorice (DGL) will not inhibit HIV.

An extract from stem bark latex of Sangre de Drago (*Croton lechleri*), an herb from the Amazon basin of Peru, has demonstrated significant anti-diarrheal activity in preliminary[71] and double-blind trials. Additional double-blind research has demonstrated the extract's effectiveness for **diarrhea** (page 163) associated with

HIV infection and AIDS.[72, 73] Very high amounts of this extract (350–700 mg four times daily for seven or more days) were used in the studies. Such levels of supplementation should always be supervised by a doctor. Most of this research on Sangre de Drago is unpublished, and much of it is derived from manufacturers of the formula. Further double-blind trials, published in peer-reviewed medical journals, are needed to confirm the efficacy reported in these studies.

A constituent from **St. John's wort** (page 747) known as hypericin has been extensively studied as a potential way to kill HIV. A preliminary trial found that people infected with HIV who took 1 mg of hypericin per day by mouth had some improvements in CD4+ cell counts, particularly if they had not previously used AZT.[74] A small number of people developed signs of mild liver damage in this study. Another much longer preliminary trial used injectable extracts of St. John's wort twice a week combined with three tablets of a standardized extract of St. John's wort taken three times per day by mouth. This study found not only improvements in CD4+ counts but only 2 of 16 participants developed opportunistic infections.[75] No liver damage or any other side effects were noted in this trial. In a later study, much higher amounts of injectable or oral hypericin (0.25 mg/kg body weight or higher) led to serious side effects, primarily extreme **sensitivity to sunlight** (page 356).[76] At this point, it is unlikely that isolated hypericin or supplements of St. John's wort extract supplying very high levels of hypericin can safely be used by people with HIV infection, particularly given St. John's wort's many drug interactions.

Garlic (page 679) may assist in combating opportunistic infections. In one trial, administration of an aged garlic extract reduced the number of infections and relieved **diarrhea** (page 163) in a group of patients with AIDS.[77] Garlic's active constituents have also been shown to kill HIV in the test tube, though these results have not been confirmed in human trials.[78]

A preliminary trial of isolated andrographolides, found in **andrographis** (page 626), determined that while they decreased viral load and increased CD4 lymphocyte levels in people with HIV infection, they also caused potentially serious liver problems and changes in taste in many of the participants.[79] It is unknown whether andrographis directly killed HIV or was having an immune-strengthening effect in this trial.

Other immune-modulating plants that could theoretically be beneficial for people with HIV infection include **Asian ginseng** (page 630), **eleuthero** (page 672),

and the medicinal mushrooms **shiitake** (page 746) and **reishi** (page 737). One preliminary study found that steamed then dried Asian ginseng (also known as red ginseng) had beneficial effects in people infected with HIV, and increased the effectiveness of the anti-HIV drug, AZT.[80] This supports the idea that immuno-modulating herbs could benefit people with HIV infection, though more research is needed.

The Chinese herb **bupleurum** (page 647), as part of the herbal formula sho-saiko-to, has been shown to have beneficial immune effects on white blood cells taken from people infected with HIV.[81] Sho-saiko-to has also been shown to improve the efficacy of the anti-HIV drug lamivudine in the test tube.[82] One preliminary study found that 7 of 13 people with HIV given sho-saiko-to had improvements in immune function.[83] Double-blind trials are needed to determine whether bupleurum or sho-saiko-to might benefit people with HIV infection or AIDS. Other herbs in sho-saiko-to have also been shown to have anti-HIV activity in the test tube, most notably **Chinese scullcap** (page 658).[84] Therefore studies on sho-saiko-to cannot be taken to mean that bupleurum is the only active herb involved. The other ingredients are **peony** (page 724) root, pinellia root, cassia bark, **ginger** (page 680) root, jujube fruit, **Asian ginseng** (page 630) root, Chinese scullcap root, and **licorice** (page 702) root.

Maitake (page 707) mushrooms, which are currently being studied, contain immuno-modulating polysaccharides (including **beta-D-glucan** [page 470]) that may be supportive for HIV infection.[85, 86]

A controversy has surrounded the use of **echinacea** (page 669) in people infected with HIV. Test tube studies initially showed that echinacea's polysaccharides could increase levels of a substance that might stimulate HIV to spread.[87] However, these results have not been shown to occur when echinacea is taken orally by humans.[88] In fact, one double-blind trial found that *Echinacea angustifolia* root (1 gram three times per day by mouth) greatly increased immune activity against HIV, while placebo had no effect.[89] Further studies are needed to determine the safety of using echinacea in HIV-positive people.

The story of European **mistletoe** (page 711) is similar to that of echinacea. Though originally believed to be a problem based on test tube studies, preliminary human clinical trials of mistletoe injections into the skin have shown only beneficial effects.[90, 91] Oral mistletoe is very unlikely to have the same effects as injected mistletoe. Injectable mistletoe should only be used under the supervision of a qualified healthcare professional.

Turmeric (page 753) may be another useful herb with immune effects in people infected with HIV. One preliminary trial found that curcumin, the main active compound in turmeric, helped improve CD4+ cell counts.[92] The amount used in this study was 1 gram three times per day by mouth. These results differed from those found in a second preliminary trial using 4.8 or 2.7 grams of curcumin daily. In that study, there was no apparent effect of curcumin on HIV replication rates.[93]

Cat's claw (page 653) is another immuno-modulating herb. Standardized extracts of cat's claw have been tested in small, preliminary trials in people infected with HIV, showing some benefits in preventing CD4 cell counts from dropping and in preventing opportunistic infections.[94, 95] Further study is needed to determine whether cat's claw is truly beneficial for people with HIV infection or AIDS.

A 5% solution of **tea tree oil** (page 751) has been shown to eliminate oral thrush in people with AIDS, according to one preliminary trial.[96] The volunteers in the study swished 15 ml of the solution in their mouths four times per day and then spit it out. This may cause mild burning for a short period of time after use.

A trial of a combination naturopathic protocol (consisting of multiple nutrients, **licorice** [page 702], **lomatium** [page 706], a combination Chinese herbal product, **lecithin** [page 546], calf **thymus extract** [page 591], lauric acid monoglycerol ester, and **St. John's wort** [page 747]) showed a possible slowing of the progression of mild HIV infection and a reduction of some symptoms.[97] Because there was no placebo group in this trial, the findings must be considered preliminary; controlled trials are needed to determine whether this protocol is effective.

Are there any side effects or interactions?
Refer to the individual herb for information about any side effects or interactions.

HIVES

Hives (urticaria) is an **allergic** (page 14) reaction in the skin characterized by white or pink welts or large bumps surrounded by redness.

These welts are known as *wheal* and *flare lesions* and are caused primarily by the release of histamine (an al-

lergy mediator) in the skin. About 50% of people with chronic hives develop angioedema—a deeper, more serious form of hives involving the tissue below the surface of the skin.

While the basic cause of hives involves the release of histamine from white blood cells, what actually triggers this release can be a variety of factors, such as physical contact or pressure, heat (prickly heat rash), cold, water, autoimmune reactions, **infectious** (page 265) organisms (e.g., **hepatitis B virus** [page 220], **Candida albicans** [page 109], and *streptococcal bacteria),* and **allergies or sensitivities** (page 14) to drugs (especially antibiotics and aspirin), foods, and food additives.

CHECKLIST FOR HIVES		
Rating	Nutritional Supplements	Herbs
★☆☆	Betaine HCl (page 473) Vitamin B-complex (page 603) Vitamin B$_{12}$ (page 601) Vitamin C (page 604)	Green tea (page 686)

What are the symptoms of hives?
Symptoms include an itchy skin rash with red bumps that can appear on the face, trunk of the body, and, sometimes, on the scalp, hands, or feet. Individual lesions usually last less than 24 hours and can change shape, fade, and then rapidly reappear. People with hives may also have wheezing, or swelling of the eyelids, lips, tongue, or throat.

Medical treatments
Over the counter antihistamines such as diphenhydramine (Benadryl) and loratadine (Claritin) are often recommended to treat hives.

Prescription medications used to relieve the rash and itching include antihistamines such as hydroxyzine (Atarax), cyproheptadine (Periactin), and cetirizine (Zyrtec). Severe cases might require oral corticosteroids such as prednisone (Deltasone, Orasone).

Dietary changes that may be helpful
Allergy (page 14) to foods and food additives is a common cause of hives, especially in chronic cases.[1] The foods most often reported to trigger hives are dairy products, eggs, chicken, cured meat, alcoholic beverages, chocolate, citrus fruits, shellfish, and nuts.[2, 3, 4] Food additives that have been shown to trigger hives in-

Hives

clude colorants (azo dyes), flavorings (salicylates), artificial sweeteners (aspartame), preservatives (benzoates, nitrites, sorbic acid), **antioxidants** (page 467) (hydroxytoluene, sulfite, gallate), and emulsifiers/stabilizers (polysorbates, vegetable gums).[5, 6, 7] Numerous clinical studies demonstrate that diets that are free of foods or food additives that commonly trigger allergic reactions typically produce significant reductions in symptoms in 50–75% of people with chronic hives.[8, 9, 10, 11] People with hives not clearly linked to a known cause should discuss the possibility of food allergies with a doctor.

Nutritional supplements that may be helpful

In theory, high amounts of **vitamin C** (page 604) might help people with hives by lowering histamine levels.[12] Amounts of at least 2,000 mg daily appear necessary to produce these effects.[13] No research trials have yet explored the clinical effects of vitamin C supplementation in people with hives.

Vitamin B$_{12}$ (page 601) has been reported to reduce the severity of acute hives as well as to reduce the frequency and severity of outbreaks in chronic cases.[14, 15] The amount used in these reported case studies was 1,000 mcg by injection per week. Whether taking B$_{12}$ supplements orally would have these effects remains unknown. On rare occasions, vitamin B$_{12}$ injections *cause* hives in susceptible people.[16] Whether such reactions are actually triggered by exposure to large amounts of vitamin B$_{12}$ or to preservatives and other substances found in most vitamin B$_{12}$ injections remains unclear.

According to preliminary studies from many years ago, lack of hydrochloric acid (HCl) secretion by the stomach was associated with chronic hives, presumably as a result of increasing the likelihood of developing **food allergies** (page 14). In one such study, 31% were diagnosed as having achlorhydria (no gastric acid output), and 53% were shown to be hypochlorhydric (having low gastric acid output).[17] In a related study, treatment with an HCl supplement and a **vitamin B-complex** (page 603) supplement helped to treat people with hives.[18] **Betaine HCl** (page 473) is the most common hydrochloric acid-containing supplement; it comes in tablets or capsules measured in grains or milligrams. One or more tablets or capsules, each containing 5–10 grains (325–650 mg) are typically taken with a meal that contains protein. Diagnosis of a deficiency of HCl and supplementation with HCl should be supervised by a doctor.

Are there any side effects or interactions?
Refer to the individual supplement for information about any side effects or interactions.

Herbs that may be helpful

Two components of **green tea** (page 686), the polyphenols epigallocatechin (EGC) and epicatechin gallate (ECG),[19] are reported to have an antihistamine effect. Some doctors recommend approximately 3 cups of green tea per day or about 3 grams of soluble components providing roughly 240 to 320 mg of polyphenols, although no human trials have studied the effects of green tea in people with hives.

Are there any side effects or interactions?
Refer to the individual herb for information about any side effects or interactions.

Holistic approaches that may be helpful

Psychological stress is often reported as a triggering factor in people with chronic hives.[20] Stress may play an important role by decreasing the effectiveness of **immune system** (page 255) mechanisms that would otherwise block allergic reactions. In a small preliminary trial of people with chronic hives, relaxation therapy and hypnosis were shown to provide significant benefit.[21] People were given an audio tape and asked to use the relaxation techniques described on the tape at home. At a follow-up examination 5 to 14 months after the initial session, six people were free of hives and an additional seven reported improvement.

HYPERTENSION

What do I need to know?

Self-care for hypertension can be approached in a number of ways—but it can be hard to know just where to start. To make it easier, our doctors recommend trying these simple steps first:

Maintain a healthy weight
Lose excess weight and keep it off with a long-term program of exercise and healthier eating

Side-step salt
Avoid using too much table salt, limit salty fast foods, and read labels to find low-sodium foods in your grocery store

Watch what you eat
Choose a diet low in cholesterol and animal fat; high in fruits, vegetables, whole grains,

legumes, and low-fat milk products; with some nuts and seeds

Try coenzyme Q₁₀

Taking 100 mg a day may have a significant impact on your blood pressure

Take minerals

Supplements of calcium (800 to 1,500 mg a day) and magnesium (350 to 500 mg a day) may be helpful

Boost heart health with garlic

A 600 to 900 mg a day standardized garlic supplement can improve heart and blood vessel health, and also has a mild blood pressure–lowering effect

CHECKLIST FOR HYPERTENSION

Rating	Nutritional Supplements	Herbs
★★★	**Coenzyme Q₁₀** (page 496) **Fish oil** (page 514) (EPA/ **DHA** [page 509]) **Potassium** (page 572) (for people *not* taking potassium-sparing diuretics)	
★★☆	**Calcium** (page 483) **Fiber** (page 512) **Magnesium** (page 551) (for people taking depleting diuretics) **Vitamin D** (page 607) (for deficiency only) **Vitamin E** (page 609)	*Achillea wilhelmsii* **Garlic** (page 679) Hibiscus Hibiscus tea
★☆☆	**Arginine** (page 467) **Taurine** (page 590) **Vitamin C** (page 604)	*Coleus forskohlii* (page 660) European **Mistletoe** (page 711) **Hawthorn** (page 689) Indian snakeroot **Olive leaf** (page 717) **Onion** (page 718) **Reishi** (page 737)

About hypertension

Approximately 90% of people with high blood pressure have "essential" or "idiopathic" hypertension, for which the cause is poorly understood. The terms "hypertension" and "high blood pressure" as used here refer *only* to this most common form and not to **pregnancy-induced hypertension** (page 202) or hypertension clearly linked to a known cause, such as Cushing's syndrome, pheochromocytoma, or kidney disease. Hypertension must always be evaluated by a healthcare professional. Extremely high blood pressure (malignant hypertension) or rapidly worsening hypertension (accelerated hypertension) almost always requires treatment with conventional medicine. People with mild to moderate high blood pressure should work with a doctor before attempting to use the information contained here, as blood pressure requires monitoring and in some cases the use of blood pressure-lowering drugs.

As with conventional drugs, the use of natural substances sometimes controls blood pressure if taken consistently but does not lead to a cure for high blood pressure. Thus, someone whose blood pressure is successfully reduced by **weight loss** (page 446), avoidance of salt, and increased intake of fruits and vegetables would need to maintain these changes permanently in order to retain control of blood pressure. Left untreated, hypertension significantly increases the risk of **stroke** (page 419) and **heart disease** (page 98).

What are the symptoms of hypertension?
Essential hypertension is usually without symptoms until complications develop. The symptoms of complications depend on the organs involved.

Medical treatments
The category of prescription drugs known as diuretics are commonly used to treat hypertension. Agents often used include the thiazide diuretics, such as hydrochlorothiazide (HydroDIURIL), indapamide (Lozol), and metolazone (Zaroxolyn); loop diuretics including furosemide (Lasix), bumetanide (Bumex), and torsemide (Demadex); and **potassium** (page 572)-sparing diuretics, such as spironolactone (Aldactone), triamterene (Dyazide, Maxzide), and amiloride (Midamor). Diuretics are usually combined with beta-blockers, such as propranolol (Inderal), metoprolol (Lopressor, Toprol XL), atenolol (Tenormin), and bisoprolol (Zebeta), or ACE inhibitors, including captopril (Capoten), benazepril (Lotensin), lisinopril (Zestril, Prinivil), enalapril (Vasotec), and quinapril (Accupril). The Angiotensin II receptor antagonists, such as losartan (Cozaar), valsartan (Diovan), irbesartan (Avapro), candesartan (Atacand), and telmisartan (Micardis), are commonly used either alone or in combination with other agents. Calcium-channel blockers, such as amlodipine (Norvasc), verapamil (Calan SR, Verelan PM), and diltiazem (Cardizem CD), may also be used either alone or in combination

with other drugs to treat high blood pressure. Another group of commonly used drugs, sympatholytic agents, includes prazosin (Minipress), doxazosin (Cardura), terazosin (Hytrin), and methyldopa (Aldomet).

Healthcare practitioners may also recommend lifestyle modifications, such as moderate **weight reduction** (page 446) and a decrease in salt intake. Though essential hypertension has no cure, treatment can modify its course and reduce the risk of complications.

Dietary changes that may be helpful

Primitive societies exposed to very little salt suffer from little or no hypertension.[1] Salt (sodium chloride) intake has also been definitively linked to hypertension in western societies.[2] Reducing salt intake in the diet lowers blood pressure in most people.[3] The more salt is restricted, the greater the blood pressure-lowering effect.[4] Individual studies sometimes come to differing conclusions about the relationship between salt intake and blood pressure, in part because blood pressure-lowering effects of salt restriction vary from person to person, and small to moderate reductions in salt intake often have minimal effects on blood pressure—particularly in young people and in those who do not have hypertension. Nonetheless, dramatic reductions in salt intake are generally effective for many people with hypertension.

With the prevalence of salted processed and restaurant food, simply avoiding the salt shaker no longer leads to large decreases in salt intake for most people. Totally eliminating salt is more effective, but is quite difficult to achieve. Moreover, while an overview of the research found "There is no evidence that sodium reduction presents any safety hazards,"[5] reports of short-term paradoxical *increases* in blood pressure in response to salt restriction have occasionally appeared.[6] Therefore, people wishing to use salt reduction to lower their blood pressure should consult with a doctor.

Vegetarians have lower blood pressure than do people who eat meat.[7] This occurs partly because fruits and vegetables contain **potassium** (page 572)—a known blood pressure-lowering mineral.[8] The best way to supplement potassium is with fruit, which contains more of the mineral than do potassium supplements. However, fruit contains so much potassium that people taking "potassium-sparing" diuretics can consume too much potassium simply by eating several pieces of fruit per day. Therefore, people taking potassium-sparing diuretics should consult the prescribing doctor before increasing fruit intake. In the Dietary Approaches to Stop Hypertension (DASH) trial, increasing intake of fruits

and vegetables (and therefore **fiber** [page 512]) and reducing cholesterol and dairy fat led to large reductions in blood pressure (in medical terms, 11.4 systolic and 5.5 diastolic) in just eight weeks.[9] Even though it did not employ a vegetarian diet itself, the outcome of the DASH trial supports the usefulness of vegetarian diets because diets employed by DASH researchers were related to what many vegetarians eat. The DASH trial also showed that blood pressure can be significantly reduced in hypertensive people (most dramatically in African Americans) with diet alone, without weight loss or even restriction of salt.[10] Nonetheless, restricting salt while consuming the DASH diet has lowered blood pressure even more effectively than the use of the DASH diet alone.[11]

Sugar has been reported to increase blood pressure in animals[12] and humans in short-term trials.[13] Though the real importance of this experimental effect remains unclear,[14] some doctors recommend that people with high blood pressure cut back on their intake of sugar.

Right after consuming caffeine from coffee or tea, blood pressure increases briefly.[15, 16] In trials lasting almost two months on average, coffee drinking has led to small increases in blood pressure.[17] The effects of long-term avoidance of caffeine (from coffee, tea, chocolate, cola drinks, and some medications) on blood pressure remain unclear. A few reports have even claimed that long-term coffee drinkers tend to have *lower* blood pressure than those who avoid coffee.[18] Despite the lack of clarity in published research, many doctors tell people with high blood pressure to avoid consumption of caffeine.

Several double-blind trials have shown that adding 6.5–7 grams of **fiber** (page 512) per day to the diet for several months leads to reductions in blood pressure.[19, 20, 21] However, other trials have not found fiber helpful in reducing blood pressure.[22, 23] The reasons for these discrepant findings is not clear.

Food allergy (page 14) was reported to contribute to high blood pressure in a study of people who had **migraine** (page 316) headaches.[24] In that report, all 15 people who also had high blood pressure experienced a significant drop in blood pressure when put on a hypoallergenic diet. People who suffer migraine headaches and have hypertension should discuss the issue of allergy diagnosis and elimination with a doctor.

Reusing vegetable oils for frying, especially oils with high concentrations of unsaturated fatty acids (such as sunflower or safflower oil) has been associated with an increased risk of high blood pressure.[25] Presumably, this increased risk is due to some of the degradation products (such as lipid peroxides or polymers) that result from the excessive heating of these oils. Frying with more stable oils, such as olive oil, is not associated with an increased risk of high blood pressure.

Exposure to lead and other heavy metals has been linked to high blood pressure in some,[26] but not all, research.[27] If other approaches to high blood pressure prove unsuccessful, it makes sense for people with hypertension to have their body's burden of lead evaluated by a healthcare professional.

Lifestyle changes that may be helpful

Smoking is particularly injurious for people with hypertension.[28] The combination of hypertension and smoking greatly increases the risk of **heart disease** (page 98)-related sickness and death. All people with high blood pressure need to quit smoking.

Consumption of more than about three alcoholic beverages per day appears to increase blood pressure.[29] Whether one or two drinks per day meaningfully increases blood pressure remains unclear.

Daily exercise can lower blood pressure significantly.[30] A 12-week program of Chinese T'ai Chi was reported to be almost as effective as aerobic exercise in lowering blood pressure.[31] Progressive resistance exercise (e.g., weight lifting) also appears to help reduce blood pressure.[32] At the same time, blood pressure has been known to increase significantly during the act of lifting heavy weights; for this reason, people with sharply elevated blood pressure, especially those with cardiovascular disease, should approach heavy strenuous resistance exercise with caution. In general, people over 40 years of age should consult with their doctors before starting any exercise regimen.

Most people with high blood pressure are overweight. **Weight loss** (page 446) lowers blood pressure significantly in those who are both overweight and hypertensive.[33] In fact, reducing body weight by as little as ten pounds can lead to a significant reduction in blood pressure.[34] Weight loss appears to have a stronger blood pressure-lowering effect than dietary salt restriction.[35]

Nutritional supplements that may be helpful

Both preliminary[36, 37, 38] and double-blind[39, 40] trials have reported that supplementation with **Coenzyme Q10** (page 496) (CoQ10) leads to a significant decrease in blood pressure in people with hypertension. Much of this research has used 100 mg of CoQ10 per day for at least ten weeks.

EPA and **DHA** (page 509), the omega-3 fatty acids found in **fish oil** (page 514), lower blood pressure, according to an analysis of 31 trials.[41] The effect was dependent on the amount of omega-3 oil used, with the best results occurring in trials using unsustainably high levels: 15 grams per day—the amount often found in 50 grams of fish oil. Although results with lower intakes were not as impressive, trials using over 3 grams per day of omega-3 (as typically found in ten 1,000 mg pills of fish oil) also reported significant reductions in blood pressure. One double-blind trial reported that DHA had greater effects on blood pressure than EPA or mixed fish oil supplements.[42] DHA is now available as a supplement separate from EPA.

Potassium (page 572) supplements in the amount of at least 2,400 mg per day lower blood pressure, according to an analysis of 33 trials.[43] However, potassium supplements greater than 100 mg per tablet require a prescription, and the low-dose potassium supplements available without a prescription can irritate the stomach if taken in large amounts. Moreover, some people, such as those taking potassium-sparing diuretics, should not take potassium supplements. Therefore, the use of potassium supplements for lowering blood pressure should only be done under the care of a doctor.

Some,[44] but not all,[45] trials show that **magnesium** (page 551) supplements—typically 350–500 mg per day—lower blood pressure. Magnesium appears to be particularly effective in people who are taking potassium-depleting diuretics.[46] Potassium-depleting diuretics also deplete magnesium. Therefore, the drop in blood pressure resulting from magnesium supplementation in people taking these drugs may result from overcoming a mild magnesium deficiency.

Calcium (page 483) supplementation—typically 800–1,500 mg per day—may lower blood pressure. However, while an analysis of 42 trials reported that calcium supplementation led to an average drop in blood pressure that was *statistically* significant, the actual decrease was small (in medical terms, a drop of 1.4 systolic over 0.8 diastolic pressure).[47] Results might have been improved had the analysis been limited to studies of people with hypertension, since calcium has almost no effect on the blood pressure of healthy people. In the analysis of 42 trials, effects were seen both with dietary calcium and with use of calcium supplements. A 12-week trial of 1,000 mg per day of calcium accompanied by blood pressure monitoring is a reasonable way to assess efficacy in a given person.

In a double-blind trial, women with low blood levels

Hypertension

of **vitamin D** (page 607) (measured as 25-hydroxyvitamin D$_3$) were given a calcium supplement, plus either 800 IU of vitamin D per day or a placebo for eight weeks. Compared with the placebo, vitamin D significantly reduced systolic blood pressure by an average of 9.3%, but did not affect diastolic blood pressure.[48]

Five double-blind trials have found that **vitamin C** (page 604) supplementation reduces blood pressure, but the reduction was statistically significant in only three of the five, and in most cases reductions were modest.[49, 50] Some doctors recommend that people with elevated blood pressure supplement with 1,000 mg vitamin C per day.

In a double-blind study of people with high blood pressure, 200 IU of **vitamin E** (page 609) per day taken for 27 weeks was significantly more effective than a placebo at reducing both systolic and diastolic blood pressure.[51] This study was done in Iran, and it is not clear whether the results would apply to individuals consuming a Western diet.

A deficiency of the amino acid **taurine** (page 590), is thought by some researchers to play an important role in elevating blood pressure in people with hypertension.[52] Limited research has found that supplementation with taurine lowers blood pressure in animals[53] and in people (at 6 grams per day),[54] possibly by reducing levels of the hormone epinephrine (adrenaline).

The amino acid **arginine** (page 467) is needed by the body to make nitric oxide, a substance that allows blood vessels to dilate, thus leading to reduced blood pressure. Intravenous administration of arginine has reduced blood pressure in humans in some reports.[55] In one controlled trial, people not responding to conventional medication for their hypertension were found to respond to a combination of conventional medication and oral arginine (2 grams taken three times per day.)[56]

Are there any side effects or interactions?
Refer to the individual supplement for information about any side effects or interactions.

Herbs that may be helpful
In a double-blind trial, people with mild hypertension took a tincture of *Achillea wilhelmsii,* an herb used in traditional Persian medicine.[57] Participants in the trial used 15–20 drops of the tincture twice daily for six months. At the end of the trial, participants experienced significant reductions in both systolic and diastolic blood pressure compared to those who took placebo. No adverse effects were reported.

Garlic (page 679) has a mild blood pressure-lowering effect, according to an analysis of ten double-blind trials.[58] All of these trials administered garlic for at least four weeks, typically using 600–900 mg of garlic extract per day. **Onion** (page 718)—closely related to garlic—may also have a mild blood pressure-lowering effect, according to preliminary research.[59]

Two controlled clinical trials have shown that hibiscus can lower blood pressure. In one, people with high blood pressure who went off their medications were given either 2 teaspoons (5 to 6 grams) *Hibiscus sabdariffa* infused in 1 cup (250 ml) water or black tea three times per day.[60] After 12 days the hibiscus group had significantly lower blood pressure than the black tea group. In another trial 10 grams of *Hibiscus sabdariffa* tea was compared to the drug captopril for four weeks in people with high blood pressure.[61] Blood pressures fell an equal amount in both groups, suggesting this herbal tea may be as potent as some blood pressure medications.

European mistletoe (page 711) *(Viscum album)* has reduced headaches and dizziness associated with high blood pressure, according to preliminary research.[62] Mistletoe may be taken as 0.5 ml tincture three times per day.[63] The blood pressure-lowering effect of mistletoe is small and may take weeks to become evident. Due to possible serious side effects, European mistletoe should only be taken under the careful supervision of a physician trained in its use.

Indian snakeroot *(Rauwolfia serpentina)* contains powerful alkaloids, including reserpine, that affect blood pressure and heart function. Indian snakeroot has been used traditionally to treat hypertension, especially when associated with stress and **anxiety** (page 30).[64] Due to possible serious side effects, Indian snakeroot should only be taken under the careful supervision of a physician trained in its use.

In animal studies oleuropein, one of the constituents of **olive leaf** (page 717), has decreased blood pressure and dilated arteries surrounding the heart, when given by injection or intravenously.[65] Olive leaf has been used traditionally to treat people with hypertension,[66] but controlled human trials are needed before a blood pressure-lowering effect can be established.

A double-blind trial reported that **reishi** (page 737) mushrooms significantly lowered blood pressure in humans.[67] The trial used a concentrated extract of reishi (25:1) in the amount of 55 mg three times per day for four weeks. It is unclear from the clinical report how long it takes for the blood pressure-lowering effects of reishi to be measured.

Hawthorn (page 689) leaf and flower extracts have been reported to have a mild blood pressure-lowering effect in people with early stage **congestive heart failure** (page 134).[68] This effect has not been studied in hypertensive people with normal heart functioning.

Human trials investigating the use of *Coleus forskohlii* (page 660) in blood pressure reduction have yet to be conducted. However, forskolin, the active ingredient in *Coleus forskohlii,* has lowered blood pressure in a small, preliminary trial with people suffering from **cardiomyopathy** (page 95).[69] Extracts of coleus standardized to contain 15–20% forskolin are available, but further trials are needed to determine effective levels for treating people with hypertension.

Most herbal reference books suggest that ginseng should not be used by people with hypertension. However, the results of a preliminary trial suggest that red ginseng root *(Panax ginseng radix rubra)* has either no effect on, or may actually slightly lower, blood pressure in hypertensive people.[70] However, many herbalists continue to believe that people with hypertension should avoid **Asian ginseng** (page 630) and **American ginseng** (page 625), and, while not a true ginseng, Siberian ginseng (**eleuthero** [page 672]) as well.

Are there any side effects or interactions?
Refer to the individual herb for information about any side effects or interactions.

Holistic approaches that may be helpful
Anxiety (page 30) in men (but not women) has been linked to development of hypertension.[71] Several research groups have also shown a relationship between job strain and high blood pressure in men.[72, 73, 74] Some researchers have tied blood pressure specifically to suppressed aggression.[75]

Although some kind of relationship between stress and high blood pressure appears to exist, the effects of *treatment* for stress remain controversial. An analysis of 26 trials reported that reductions in blood pressure caused by biofeedback or meditation were no greater than those seen with placebo.[76] Though some stress management interventions have not been helpful in reducing blood pressure,[77, 78] those trials that have reported promising effects have used combinations of yoga, biofeedback, and/or meditation.[79, 80, 81] Some doctors continue to recommend a variety of stress-reducing measures, sometimes tailoring them to the needs and preferences of the person seeking help.

Preliminary laboratory studies in animals[82] and humans[83, 84, 85] suggest that acupuncture may help regulate blood pressure. Most,[86, 87, 88, 89, 90, 91] but not all,[92] preliminary trials also suggest that acupuncture may be an effective way to lower blood pressure. Whether blood pressure goes back up after acupuncture is discontinued remains an unsettled question.

Auricular (ear) acupressure has been reported to be an effective treatment for hypertension,[93, 94, 95] though in one case the improvement was not significantly better than use of traditional herbal medicines.[96]

Spinal manipulation may lower blood pressure (at least temporarily) in healthy people, according to most preliminary[97, 98, 99] and controlled[100] trials. However, some research suggests the effect is no better than the blood pressure-lowering effect of sham ("fake") manipulation.[101] In hypertensive people, temporary decreases in blood pressure have also been reported after spinal manipulation.[102, 103, 104] However, most,[105, 106, 107] but not all,[108] trials suggest that manipulation produces only short-term decreases in blood pressure in hypertensive people.

HYPOGLYCEMIA

"Hypoglycemia" is the medical term for low blood sugar (glucose).

Occasionally, hypoglycemia can be dangerous (for example, from injecting too much insulin). It may also indicate a serious underlying medical condition, such as a tumor of the pancreas or liver disease. More often, however, when people say they have hypoglycemia, they are describing a group of symptoms that occur when the body overreacts to the rise in blood sugar that occurs after eating, resulting in a rapid or excessive fall in the blood sugar level. This is sometimes called "reactive hypoglycemia."

Many people who believe they have reactive hypoglycemia do not, in fact, have low blood sugar levels,[1] and many people who do have low blood sugar levels do not have any symptoms of reactive hypoglycemia.[2] Some evidence suggests that reactive hypoglycemia may be partly a psychological condition.[3] Consequently, some doctors believe that reactive hypoglycemia does not exist.[4] Most doctors, on the other hand, have found reactive hypoglycemia to be a common cause of the symptoms listed below.

What are the symptoms of hypoglycemia?
Common symptoms of hypoglycemia are fatigue, **anxiety** (page 30), headaches, difficulty concentrating,

sweaty palms, shakiness, excessive hunger, drowsiness, abdominal pain, and **depression** (page 145).

CHECKLIST FOR HYPOGLYCEMIA		
Rating	**Nutritional Supplements**	**Herbs**
★★★	**Chromium** (page 493)	
★☆☆	**Copper** (page 499) **Glucomannan** (page 526) **Magnesium** (page 551) **Manganese** (page 553) **Vitamin B₃** (page 598) (niacinamide) **Vitamin B₆** (page 600) **Vitamin C** (page 604) **Vitamin E** (page 609) **Zinc** (page 614)	

Medical treatments

A diet of frequent, small, high-protein, low-carbohydrate meals is often recommended. If illness prevents eating, hospitalization for intravenous glucose injections is typically required. In cases of pituitary or adrenal insufficiency, hormone replacement may be prescribed. For hypoglycemia due to an insulin-producing tumor, surgical removal of the tumor is usually recommended.

Dietary changes that may be helpful

Doctors find that people with hypoglycemia usually improve when they eliminate refined sugars and alcohol from their diet, eat foods high in **fiber** (page 512) (such as whole grains, fruits, vegetables, legumes, and nuts), and eat small, frequent meals. Few studies have investigated the effects of these changes, but the research that is available generally supports the observations of doctors.[5, 6, 7, 8] Some symptoms of low blood sugar may be related to, or made worse by, **food allergies** (page 14).[9]

Even modest amounts of caffeine may increase symptoms of hypoglycemia.[10] For this reason, caffeinated beverages (such as coffee, tea, and some soda pop) should be avoided.

Some people report an improvement in hypoglycemia episodes when eating a high-protein, low-carbohydrate diet. That observation appears to conflict with research showing that increasing protein intake can impair the body's ability to process sugar,[11] possibly because protein increases insulin levels[12] (insulin re-

duces blood sugar levels). However, some doctors have seen good results with high-protein, low-carbohydrate diets, particularly among people who do not improve with a high-fiber, high-complex-carbohydrate diet.

Nutritional supplements that may be helpful

Research has shown that supplementing with **chromium** (page 493) (200 mcg per day)[13] or **magnesium** (page 551) (340 mg per day)[14] can prevent blood sugar levels from falling excessively in people with hypoglycemia. **Niacinamide** (page 598) (vitamin B₃) has also been found to be helpful for hypoglycemic people.[15] Other nutrients, including **vitamin C** (page 604), **vitamin E** (page 609), **zinc** (page 614), **copper** (page 499), **manganese** (page 553), and **vitamin B₆** (page 600), may help control blood sugar levels in **diabetics** (page 152).[16] Since there are similarities in the way the body regulates high and low blood sugar levels, these nutrients might be helpful for hypoglycemia as well, although the amounts needed for that purpose are not known.

Glucomannan (page 526) is a water-soluble dietary fiber that is derived from konjac root (*Amorphophallus konjac*). In a preliminary trial,[17] addition of either 2.6 or 5.2 grams of glucomannan to a meal prevented hypoglycemia in adults with previous stomach surgery. A trial of glucomannan in children with hypoglycemia due to a condition known as "dumping syndrome" produced inconsistent results.[18]

Are there any side effects or interactions?
Refer to the individual supplement for information about any side effects or interactions.

HYPOTHYROIDISM

What do I need to know?

Self-care for hypothyroidism can be approached in a number of ways—but it can be hard to know just where to start. To make it easier, our doctors recommend trying these simple steps first:

Check your iodine intake
　　Consult with a nutritionist to learn whether you are getting too little or too much iodine from food, medications, and supplements
Limit foods high in goitrogens (like broccoli)
　　Consider limiting your intake of foods high in goitrogens (primarily foods from the Brassica

plant family, such as broccoli and kale); these foods are very nutritious, however, so don't avoid them unless it is necessary

About hypothyroidism

Hypothyroidism is a condition in which the thyroid gland fails to function adequately, resulting in reduced levels of thyroid hormone in the body. Cretinism is a type of hypothyroidism that occurs at birth and results in stunted physical growth and mental development. Severe hypothyroidism is called myxedema.

There are many causes of hypothyroidism. One common cause is Hashimoto's thyroiditis, an autoimmune disease of the thyroid gland. Another common cause of hypothyroidism is medical treatment, such as surgery or radiation to the thyroid gland, to treat hyperthyroidism (over-activity of the thyroid gland). Some drugs, such as lithium and phenylbutazone, may also induce hypothyroidism. Extreme **iodine** (page 538) deficiency, which is rare in the United States, is another possible cause. Failure of the pituitary gland or hypothalamus to stimulate the thyroid gland properly can cause a condition known as secondary hypothyroidism.

Some people with **goiter** (page 206) (an enlargement of the thyroid gland) also have hypothyroidism. Goiter can be caused by an iodine deficiency, by eating foods that contain goitrogens (goiter-causing substances), or by other disorders that interfere with thyroid hormone production. In many cases the cause of goiter cannot be determined. While natural therapies may help to some extent, thyroid hormone replacement is necessary for most people with hypothyroidism.

CHECKLIST FOR HYPOTHYROIDISM		
Rating	**Nutritional Supplements**	**Herbs**
★★☆	**Iodine** (page 538)	
★☆☆	**Selenium** (page 584) (if deficient) **Thyroid extract** (page 592) **Vitamin A** (page 595) **Vitamin B₃** (page 598) (niacin) **Zinc** (page 614)	**Bladderwrack** (page 639)

What are the symptoms of hypothyroidism?

The symptoms of hypothyroidism vary from person to person, but commonly include several of the following: fatigue, lethargy, intolerance to cold, **constipation** (page 137), weight gain, **depression** (page 145), **excessive menstruation** (page 314), dry skin, hair loss, and hoarseness. The onset of these symptoms may be so gradual as to evade detection by patient or physician.

Medical treatments

The preferred treatment for hypothyroidism is the synthetic thyroid hormone levothyroxine (Synthroid, Levothroid, Levoxyl). However, some healthcare practitioners prescribe dessicated thyroid (Armour Thyroid).

Dietary changes that may be helpful

Some foods, such as rapeseed (used to make canola oil) and Brassica vegetables (cabbage, Brussels sprouts, broccoli, and cauliflower), contain natural goitrogens, chemicals that cause the thyroid gland to enlarge by interfering with thyroid hormone synthesis.[1] Cooking has been reported to inactivate this effect in Brussels sprouts.[2] Cassava, a starchy root that is the source of tapioca, has also been identified as a goitrogenic food.[3] Other goitrogens include maize, sweet potatoes, lima beans, soy, and pearl millet.[4] While some practitioners recommend that people with hypothyroidism avoid these foods, none has been proven to cause hypothyroidism in humans.

Lifestyle changes that may be helpful

Preliminary studies have found an association between **multiple chemical sensitivities** (page 14) and hypothyroidism.[5] One study found a correlation between high blood levels of lead, a toxic heavy metal, and low thyroid hormone levels in people working in a brass foundry.[6] Many of these people also complained of **depression** (page 145), fatigue, **constipation** (page 137), and poor memory (symptoms of hypothyroidism).

Occupational exposure to polybrominated biphenyls and carbon disulfide has also been associated with decreased thyroid function.

Nutritional supplements that may be helpful

The relationship between **iodine** (page 538) and thyroid function is complex. Iodine is required by the body to form thyroid hormone, and iodine deficiency can lead to **goiter** (page 206) and hypothyroidism.[7] Severe and prolonged iodine deficiency can potentially lead to serious types of hypothyroidism, such as myxedema or cretinism. It is estimated that one and a half billion people living in 118 countries around the world are at risk for developing iodine deficiency.[8]

Today, most cases of iodine deficiency occur in developing nations. In industrialized countries where iodized salt is used, iodine deficiency has become extremely rare. On the other hand, iodine toxicity has become a concern in some of these countries.[9] Excessive iodine intake can result in either hypothyroidism[10] or hyperthyroidism (overactive thyroid).[11] Sources of iodine include foods (iodized salt, milk, water, seaweed, ground beef), dietary supplements (**multiple vitamin-mineral** [page 559] formulas, seaweed extracts), drugs (potassium iodide, amiodarone, topical antiseptics), and iodine-containing solutions used in certain laboratory tests. Many nutritional supplements contain 150 mcg of iodine. While that amount of iodine should prevent a deficiency, it is not clear whether supplementing with iodine is necessary or desirable for most people. Those wishing to take a nutritional supplement containing iodine should consult a doctor.

Laboratory animals with severe, experimentally induced **zinc** (page 614) deficiency developed hypothyroidism, whereas moderate zinc deficiency did not affect thyroid function.[12] In a small study of healthy people, thyroid hormone (thyroxine) levels tended to be lower in those with lower blood levels of zinc. In people with low zinc, supplementing with zinc increased thyroxine levels.[13] One case has been reported of a woman with severe zinc deficiency (caused by the combination of **alcoholism** [page 12] and **malabsorption** [page 304]) who developed hypothyroidism that was corrected by supplementing with zinc.[14] Although the typical Western diet is marginally low in zinc,[15] additional research is needed to determine whether zinc supplementation would be effective for preventing or correcting hypothyroidism.

Selenium (page 584) plays a role in thyroid hormone metabolism. Severe selenium deficiency has been implicated as a possible cause of goiter.[16] Two months of selenium supplementation in people who were deficient in both selenium and **iodine** (page 538) was shown to induce a dramatic fall of the already impaired thyroid function in clinically hypothyroid subjects.[17] Researchers have suggested that people who are deficient in both selenium and iodine should not take selenium supplements without first receiving iodine or thyroid hormone supplementation.[18] There is no research demonstrating that selenium supplementation helps people with hypothyroidism who are not selenium-deficient.

Preliminary data indicate that **vitamin B$_3$** (page 598) (niacin) supplementation may decrease thyroid hormone levels. In one small study, 2.6 grams of niacin per day helped lower blood fat levels.[19] After a year or more,

thyroid hormone levels had fallen significantly in each person, although none experienced symptoms of hypothyroidism. In another case report, thyroid hormone levels decreased in two people who were taking niacin for **high cholesterol** (page 223) and **triglycerides** (page 235); one of these two was diagnosed with hypothyroidism.[20] When the niacin was discontinued for one month, thyroid hormone levels returned to normal.

Desiccated thyroid, also called **thyroid extract** (page 592) (e.g., Armour Thyroid), is used by some doctors as an alternative to synthetic thyroid hormones (such as thyroxine [Synthroid or other brand names]) for people with hypothyroidism. Thyroid extract contains two biologically active hormones (thyroxine and triiodothyronine), whereas the most commonly prescribed thyroid-hormone preparations contain only thyroxine. One study has shown that the combination of the two hormones contained in desiccated thyroid is more effective than thyroxine alone for those with hypothyroidism.[21] One doctor reported that thyroid extract worked better than standard thyroid preparations for many of his patients with hypothyroidism.[22] Glandular thyroid products, which are available from health food stores, have had most of the thyroid hormone removed and would therefore not be expected to be effective for people with hypothyroidism. Intact desiccated thyroid is available only by prescription. Hypothyroidism sufferers who want to use desiccated thyroid must first consult with a physician.

People with hypothyroidism have been shown to have an impaired ability to convert **beta-carotene** (page 469) to **vitamin A** (page 595).[23, 24] For this reason, some doctors suggest taking supplemental vitamin A (approximately 5,000–10,000 IU per day) if they are not consuming adequate amounts in their diet.

Are there any side effects or interactions?
Refer to the individual supplement for information about any side effects or interactions.

Herbs that may be helpful
Bladderwrack (page 639) (*Fucus vesiculosus*) is a type of brown seaweed that contains variable amounts of **iodine** (page 538).[25] Hypothyroidism due to insufficient intake of iodine may possibly improve with bladderwrack supplementation, though human studies have not confirmed this.

Some Chinese herb formulations show promise for people with hypothyroidism. In one study, people with hypothyroidism were given a combination of Chinese herbs.[26] After one year, symptoms of hypothyroidism were markedly improved and blood levels of thyroid hormones had significantly increased. In an animal study, administration of certain Chinese herbs raised thyroid hormone levels in the blood.[27] Neither study listed the specific herbs used. People with hypothyroidism who wish to use Chinese herbs should consult with a physician skilled in their use.

Are there any side effects or interactions?
Refer to the individual herb for information about any side effects or interactions.

IMMUNE FUNCTION

What do I need to know?
Self-care for immune function can be approached in a number of ways—but it can be hard to know just where to start. To make it easier, our doctors recommend trying these simple steps first:

Update your vaccinations
> Consult your medical provider to see if you need vaccines for influenza, pneumonia, hepatitis, tetanus, and other infections

Avoid alcohol binges
> Keep your alcohol intake low or moderate to avoid damaging effects to your immune system

Aim for total nutrition with a multivitamin-mineral supplement
> Take daily to help prevent deficiencies that increase susceptibility to infections

Use exercise wisely
> Take advantage of the benefits of moderate exercise on immune function—but be careful about prolonged or intense exercise, which can temporarily increase your risk of infection

Get the good bacteria
> Stimulate the intestine's immune system and slow growth of infectious organisms in the intestine by regularly eating yogurt and other foods containing live cultures, or take a supplement containing 10 billion colony-forming units a day of acidophilus or bifidobacteria

About immune function
The immune system is an intricate network of specialized tissues, organs, cells, and chemicals. The lymph nodes, spleen, bone marrow, thymus gland, and tonsils all play a role, as do lymphocytes (specialized white blood cells), antibodies, and interferon.

Two types of immunity protect the body: innate and adaptive. Innate immunity is present at birth and provides the first barrier against microorganisms. The skin, mucus secretions, and the acidity of the stomach are examples of innate immunity that act as barriers to keep unwanted germs away from more vulnerable tissues.

Adaptive immunity is the second barrier to infection. It is acquired later in life, such as after an immunization or successfully fighting off an **infection** (page 265). The adaptive immune system retains a memory of all the invaders it has faced. This is why people usually get the measles only once, although they may be repeatedly exposed to the disease. Unfortunately some bugs—such as the viruses that cause the **common cold** (page 129)—"disguise" themselves and must be fought off time and again by the immune system.

	CHECKLIST FOR IMMUNE FUNCTION	
Rating	**Nutritional Supplements**	**Herbs**
★★★	**Multiple vitamin-mineral** (page 559) (for elderly people) **Vitamin E** (page 609) (for elderly people)	**Andrographis** (page 626)
★★☆	**Acidophilus** (page 575) **Beta-carotene** (page 469) **Fish oil** (page 514) (omega-3 fatty acids for critically ill and post surgery patients only) **Glutamine** (page 530) (for prevention of post-exercise infection in performance athletes) **Selenium** (page 584) (for elderly people) **Thymus extracts** (page 591) **Vitamin A** (page 595) **Vitamin C** (page 604) **Zinc** (page 614) (for elderly people)	**Ashwagandha** (page 629) **Asian ginseng** (page 630) **Echinacea** (page 669) **Eleuthero** (page 672)
★☆☆	**Beta-glucan** (page 470) **Cordyceps** (page 663) **DHEA** (page 503) **Lycopene** (page 548) **Vitamin B$_{12}$** (page 601) **Whey protein** (page 613) **Zinc** (page 614) (for non-elderly people)	**Astragalus** (page 631) **Cat's claw** (page 653) **Fo-ti** (page 678) **Green tea** (page 686) **Ligustrum** (page 704) **Maitake** (page 707) **Noni** (page 715)

What are the symptoms of low immune function?
Symptoms of decreased immune function include frequent **colds** (page 129) and **flus** (page 269), recurring **parasitic infections** (page 343), initially mild infections that become serious, opportunistic infections (infections by organisms that are usually well controlled by a healthy immune system, such as toxoplasmosis, cryptococcosis, and cytomegalovirus), and **cancer** (page 87).

Medical treatments
Prescription drug therapy includes preventative antibiotics, as well as immune-boosting medicines such as interferon (Roferon-A, Intron A, Infergen) and interleukin (Proleukin).

Treatment for decreased immune functioning also includes vaccination for the flu, pneumococcus (a cause of pneumonia), **hepatitis** (page 220), tetanus, and other infections combined with precautions to reduce exposure to infectious agents.

Dietary changes that may be helpful
All forms of sugar (including honey) interfere with the ability of white blood cells to destroy bacteria.[1, 2] Animal studies suggest diets high in sucrose (table sugar) impair some aspects of immune function.[3, 4] The importance of these effects in the prevention of infections in humans remains unclear.

Alcohol intake, including single episodes of moderate consumption, interferes with a wide variety of immune defenses.[5, 6] Alcohol's immune-suppressive effect may be one mechanism for the association between alcohol intake and certain **cancers** (page 87)[7] and **infections** (page 265).[8, 9] However, moderate alcohol consumption (up to three to four drinks per day) has been associated in preliminary studies with either no risk[10] or a *decreased* risk for upper respiratory infections in young nonsmokers.[11]

The effect of fats on the immune system is complex and only partially understood. Excessive intake of total dietary fat impairs immune response, but some types of fat may be neutral or even beneficial.[12] For example, monounsaturated fats, as found in olive oil, appear to have no detrimental effect on the immune system in humans at reasonable dietary levels.[13]

Research on the effect of the omega-3 fatty acids that are abundant in some fish, **fish oils** (page 514), and **flaxseed oil** (page 517) is conflicting. Liquid diets containing omega-3 fatty acids used in hospitals for critically ill people have been shown to improve immune

function and reduce **infections** (page 265).[14, 15] However, in one controlled study in healthy people, a low-fat diet improved or maintained immune function, but when fish was added to increase omega-3 fatty acid intake, immune function was significantly *inhibited*.[16]

Supplementation with **DHA** (page 509) (an omega-3 fatty acid found in fish oil) in healthy young men has been shown to decrease the activity of immune cells, such as natural killer (NK) cells, and to inhibit certain measures of inflammation in the test tube.[17] The anti-inflammatory effects of DHA may be useful in the management of autoimmune disorders; however, such benefits need to be balanced with the potential for increased risk of infections. Other studies suggest that increased oxidative damage might be the reason for the negative effects on the immune system sometimes caused by fish oil, and that increased intake of **antioxidants** (page 467), such as **vitamin E** (page 609), could correct the problem.[18]

As with omega-3 fatty acids, omega-6 fatty acids (as found in vegetable oils) have also produced conflicting effects on the immune system. Enriching a low-fat diet with omega-6 fatty acids did not impair immunity.[19] However, diets high in omega-6 fatty acids have suppressed immunity in other reports.[20, 21]

In summary, low-fat diets with moderate levels of monounsaturated fat from olive oil appear least likely to compromise immune function and may provide small benefits. Conclusions about the desirability of diets high in either omega-3 or omega-6 fatty acid supplementation await further research.

Many studies, in both animals and humans, have demonstrated immune-stimulating effects from yogurt which contains live cultures, such as *Lactobacillus acidophilus* (page 575) and other **probiotics** (page 575) (friendly bacteria). The effects of probiotics observed in humans include increasing the activity of several types of white blood cells. In preliminary human studies, consumption of live culture-containing yogurt has been associated with a reduced incidence of several immune-related diseases, including **cancer** (page 87), infections of the stomach and intestines, and some **allergic** (page 14) reactions.[22]

Lifestyle changes that may be helpful
Both excessive thinness and severe **obesity** (page 446) are associated with impaired immune responses.[23] Obesity increases the risk of **infection** (page 265), at least in hospitalized patients, according to preliminary research.[24] However, these effects may not occur with

mild to moderate obesity in otherwise healthy people, and attempts to lose weight through dietary restriction may actually be harmful to the immune system.[25] The detrimental effects of both excess weight and weight-loss diets appear to be offset when people regularly perform aerobic exercise.[26, 27]

The effects of exercise on immune function depend on many factors, including frequency and intensity of exercise.[28] Regular moderate physical activity has positive effects, at least on some measures of immunity, and has been shown to reduce risk of upper respiratory infection. However, very intense and prolonged exercise, such as running a marathon or overtraining, can, in the short term, actually increase the risk of developing infections.[29] The positive effects of moderate exercise on immunity may also partly explain the apparent reduced susceptibility to **cancer** (page 87) of physically active people.[30]

Nutritional supplements that may be helpful

Most,[31, 32] but not all,[33] double-blind studies have shown that elderly people have better immune function and reduced infection rates when taking a **multiple vitamin-mineral** (page 559) formula. In one double-blind trial, supplements of 100 mcg per day of **selenium** (page 584) and 20 mg per day of **zinc** (page 614), with or without additional **vitamin C** (page 604), **vitamin E** (page 609), and **beta-carotene** (page 469), reduced infections in elderly people, though vitamins without minerals had no effect.[34] Burn victims have also experienced fewer infections after receiving trace mineral supplements in double-blind research.[35] These studies suggest that trace minerals may be the most important micronutrients for enhancing immunity and preventing infections in the elderly.

Vitamin E enhances some measures of immune-cell activity in the elderly.[36] This effect is more pronounced with 200 IU per day compared to either lower (60 IU per day) or higher (800 IU per day) amounts, according to double-blind research.[37] Intakes under 200 IU per day have not boosted immune function in some reports.[38]

Beta-carotene and other **carotenoids** (page 488) have increased immune cell numbers and activity in animal and human research, an effect that appears to be separate from their role as precursors to vitamin A.[39, 40] Placebo-controlled research has shown positive benefits of beta-carotene supplements in increasing numbers of some white blood cells and enhancing cancer-fighting immune functions in healthy people at 25,000–100,000 IU per day.[41, 42]

In double-blind trials in the elderly, supplementation with 40,000–150,000 IU per day of **beta-carotene** (page 469) has increased natural killer (NK) cell activity,[43] but not several other measures of immunity.[44]

Controlled research has found that 50,000 IU per day of beta-carotene boosted immunity in people with **colon cancer** (page 123) but in not those with precancerous conditions in the colon.[45] Beta-carotene has also prevented immune suppression from ultraviolet light exposure.[46] Effects on immunodefiency in **HIV** (page 239)-positive people have been inconsistent using beta-carotene.[47, 48]

Vitamin C (page 604) stimulates the immune system by both elevating interferon levels[49] and enhancing the activity of certain immune cells.[50, 51] Two studies came to opposite conclusions about the ability of vitamin C to improve immune function in the elderly,[52, 53] and two other studies did not agree on whether vitamin C could protect people from **hepatitis** (page 220).[54, 55] However, a review of 20 double-blind studies concluded that while several grams of vitamin C per day has only a small effect in *preventing* **colds** (page 129), when taken at the onset of a cold, it does significantly reduce the duration of a cold.[56] In controlled reports studying people doing heavy exercise, cold frequency was reduced an average of 50% with vitamin C supplements ranging from 600 to 1,000 mg per day.[57] Thus, the overall effect of vitamin C on immune function is unclear, and its usefulness may vary according to the situation.

Vitamin A (page 595) plays an important role in immune system function and helps mucous membranes, including those in the lungs, resist invasion by microorganisms.[58] However, most research shows that while vitamin A supplementation helps people prevent or treat infections in developing countries where deficiencies are common,[59] little to no positive effect, and even slight *adverse* effects, have resulted from giving vitamin A supplements to people in countries where most people consume adequate amounts of vitamin A.[60, 61, 62, 63, 64, 65, 66] Moreover, vitamin A supplementation during infections appears beneficial only in certain diseases. An analysis of trials revealed that vitamin A reduces mortality from measles and **diarrhea** (page 163), but not from pneumonia, in children living in developing countries.[67] A double-blind trial of vitamin A supplementation in Tanzanian children with pneumonia confirmed its lack of effectiveness for this condition.[68] In general, parents in the developed world should *not* give vitamin A supplements to children unless there is a reason to believe vitamin A deficiency is likely, such as the presence of a condition causing **malabsorption** (page 304) (e.g., **celiac disease** [page 102]). However, the American Academy of Pediatrics recommends that all children with measles be given short-term supplementation with high-dose vitamin A in cases of hospitalization, malnutrition, and other special circumstances determined by a doctor.[69]

A combination of antioxidants **vitamin A** (page 595), **vitamin C** (page 604), and **vitamin E** (page 609) significantly improved immune cell number and activity compared with placebo in a group of hospitalized elderly people.[70] Daily intake of a 1,000 mg vitamin C plus 200 IU vitamin E for four months improved several measures of immune function in a preliminary study.[71] To what extent immune-boosting combinations of antioxidants actually reduce the risk of **infection** (page 265) remains unknown.

The amino acid **glutamine** (page 530) is important for immune system function. Liquid diets high in glutamine have been reported in controlled studies to be more helpful to critically ill people than other diets.[72, 73] Endurance athletes are susceptible to upper respiratory tract infections after heavy exercise, which depletes glutamine levels in blood.[74] Although the effects of glutamine supplementation on immune function after exercise have been inconsistent,[75, 76] a double-blind study giving athletes glutamine (2.5 grams after exercise and again two hours later) reported significantly fewer infections with glutamine.[77]

Supplements of **probiotics** (page 575) (friendly bacteria) such as *Lactobacillus acidophilus,* or the growth factors that encourage their development in the gastrointestinal tract may help protect the body from harmful organisms in the intestine that cause local or systemic **infection** (page 265) according to published research,[78, 79] including controlled[80] trials. The effective amount of probiotics depends on the strain used, as well as the concentration of viable organisms. Infectious **diarrhea** (page 163) in children has been successfully reduced with supplements of friendly bacteria in several trials, some of which were double-blind.[81, 82]

The thymus gland is responsible for many immune system functions. Preliminary studies suggest that a **thymus extract** (page 591) known as Thymomodulin may improve immune function, and double-blind trials in children and adults with a history of recurrent respiratory-tract infections have found reduced numbers of recurrent infections with Thymomodulin supplementation.[83, 84, 85, 86, 87] Thymomodulin has also been shown in a double-blind study to improve immune function in cases of exercise-induced immune suppression, and in preliminary studies to improve immune function in people with **diabetes** (page 152) and in elderly people.[88, 89, 90, 91]

Zinc (page 614) supplements have been reported to increase immune function.[92, 93] This effect may be especially important in the elderly according to double-blind studies.[94, 95] Some doctors recommend zinc supplements for people with recurrent **infections** (page 265), suggesting 25 mg per day for adults and lower amounts for children (depending on body weight). However, too much zinc (300 mg per day) has been reported to impair immune function.[96]

While zinc lozenges have been shown to be effective for reducing the symptoms and duration of the **common cold** (page 129) in some controlled studies, it is not clear whether this effect is due to an enhancement of immune function or to the direct effect of zinc on the viruses themselves.[97]

Large amounts of the carotenoid **lycopene** (page 548) have been shown to increase the activity of NK cells in the elderly. In a controlled trial, 15 mg of lycopene significantly increased NK cell concentration, but no other immune functions.[98]

A deficiency of **vitamin B$_{12}$** (page 601) has been associated with decreased immune function. In a controlled trial, people with **vitamin B$_{12}$ deficiency anemia** (page 601) were also found to have markedly decreased levels of white blood cells associated with immune function.[99] Restoration of vitamin B$_{12}$ stores by means of injections improved levels of these immune cells, suggesting an important role for vitamin B$_{12}$ in immune function.

Beta-glucan (page 470) is a fiber-type polysaccharide (complex sugar) derived from the cell wall of baker's yeast, oat and barley **fiber** (page 512), and many medicinal mushrooms, such as **maitake** (page 707). Numerous experimental studies in test tubes and animals have shown beta-glucan to activate white blood cells.[100, 101, 102, 103, 104] In fact, there have been hundreds of research papers on beta-glucan since the 1960s.[105] The research indicates that beta-1,3-glucan, in particular, is very effective at activating white blood cells known as macrophages and neutrophils. A beta-glucan–activated macrophage or neutrophil can recognize and kill tumor cells, remove cellular debris resulting from oxidative damage, speed up recovery of damaged tissue, and further activate other components of the immune system.[106, 107] Although the research in test tube and animal studies is promising, many questions remain about the effectiveness of beta-glucan as an oral supplement to enhance immune function in humans. Controlled trials are necessary to determine whether humans can benefit from beta-glucan, and in what amounts oral beta-glucan must be taken from meaningful effects.

The hormone **DHEA** (page 503) effects immunity. In a controlled trial, a group of elderly men with low DHEA levels who were given a high level of DHEA (50 mg per day) for 20 weeks, experienced a significant activation of immune function.[108] Postmenopausal women have also shown increased immune functioning in just three weeks when given DHEA in double-blind research.[109]

The effects of eating fish and other dietary sources of **omega-3 fatty acids** (page 509) is discussed above in the nutritional section. In terms of **fish oil** (page 514) supplements, except for effects in hospitalized patients, most studies have reported that additional omega-3 intake decreases immune function.[110, 111, 112, 113] **Antioxidants** (page 467) may correct this problem, according to preliminary research.[114]

Liquid diets containing supplemental **arginine** (page 467), omega-3 fatty acids, and nucleotides such as ribonucleic acid (RNA) have been more effective than other liquid diets in both maintaining immune function and reducing infections in critically ill and post-surgical hospital patients in most,[115, 116, 117, 118, 119] but not all,[120, 121] double-blind trials. Typical daily intakes in these trials are 3.3 grams of omega 3 fatty acids, 12.5 grams of arginine, and 1.2 grams of RNA. No research has studied the effects of these supplements in people with less severe health problems.

A double-blind trial showed that 45 grams per day of **whey protein** (page 613) increased blood glutathione levels in a group of HIV-infected people.[122] Test tube[123, 124] and animal[125] studies suggest that whey protein may improve some aspects of immune function.

Are there any side effects or interactions?
Refer to the individual supplement for information about any side effects or interactions.

Herbs that may be helpful
In general, human studies have found that **echinacea** (page 669) taken orally stimulates the function of a variety of immune cells, particularly natural killer cells.[126] The balance of evidence currently available from studies suggests that echinacea speeds recovery from the

common cold (page 129), via immune stimulation (as opposed to killing the cold virus directly).[127] Evidence on preventing the common cold with echinacea is largely negative, suggesting its immune-stimulating activity may be mild in generally healthy people. Other studies on oral echinacea have not found that it stimulates activity of the white blood cells known as neutrophils.[128] Many doctors recommend 3–5 ml of tincture three times per day to improve immune function. Echinacea in capsule form is also commonly available.

Andrographis (page 626) has been shown in a double-blind trial to successfully reduce the severity of the common cold.[129] A preliminary study also suggests it may prevent the onset of a cold in healthy people.[130] These actions are thought to be due to the immune system enhancing actions of the active constituents known as andrographolides.[131]

Asian ginseng (page 630) has a long history of use in traditional herbal medicine for preventing and treating conditions related to the immune system. A double-blind study of healthy people found that taking 100 mg of a standardized extract of Asian ginseng twice per day improved immune function.[132]

Eleuthero (page 672) (Siberian ginseng) has also historically been used to support the immune system. Preliminary Russian research has supported this traditional use.[133] A double-blind study has shown that healthy people who take 10 ml of eleuthero tincture three times per day had an increase in certain T lymphocytes important to normal immune function. These effects have not been studied in people with lowered immune function. The amount of eleuthero used in this trial is exceptionally high, though no side effects were seen.

Ashwagandha (page 629) is considered a general stimulant of the immune system,[134] and has been called a tonic or adaptogen[135]—an herb with multiple, non-specific actions that counteract the effects of stress and generally promote wellness. More research is needed to better evaluate these claims.

Complex polysaccharides present in **astragalus** (page 631) and in **maitake** (page 707) and coriolus mushrooms appear to act as "immunomodulators" and, as such, are being researched for their potential role in **AIDS** (page 239) and **cancer** (page 87). Presently, the only human studies on astragalus indicate that it can prevent white blood cell numbers from falling in people given chemotherapy and radiotherapy and can elevate antibody levels in healthy people.[136] Maitake has only been studied in animals as a way to increase immune function.[137] The primary immuno-activating polysaccharide found in these mushrooms, **beta-D-glucan** (page 470), is well absorbed when taken orally[138] and is currently under investigation as a supportive tool for HIV infection. Results from future research will improve the understanding of the possible benefits of these mushrooms and their constituents.

Substances found in **cat's claw** (page 653), called oxyindole alkaloids have been shown to stimulate the immune system.[139] However, little is known about whether this effect is sufficient to prevent or treat disease.

Cordyceps (page 663) has immune strengthening actions in human and animal studies.[140, 141] Further research is needed but it may be helpful in a wide range of conditions in which the immune system is weakened. The usual amount taken is 3 to 4.5 grams twice daily as capsules or simmered for 10 to 15 minutes in water for tea.

Green tea (page 686) has stimulated production of immune cells and has shown anti-bacterial properties in animal studies.[142, 143, 144] More research is needed to evaluate the effectiveness of green tea in protecting against infection and other immune system-related diseases.

Preliminary research suggests that **fo-ti** (page 678) plays a role in a strong immune system and has antibacterial action.[145] More research is needed to further understand the potential importance of these effects.

The main active compound in **ligustrum** (page 704) is ligustrin (oleanolic acid). Studies, mostly conducted in China, suggest that ligustrum stimulates the immune system.[146] Ligustrum is often combined with astragalus in traditional Chinese medicine. Although used for long-term support of the immune system in people with depressed immune function or cancer, more research is needed to demonstrate the optimal length of time to use ligustrum.

Animal and test tube studies show **noni** (page 715) to have some immune-enhancing activity. Specifically, the polysaccharide component has been shown to increase the release of immune-enhancing compounds that activate white blood cells to destroy tumor cells.[147] The usual recommendation is 4 ounces of noni juice 30 minutes before breakfast (effectiveness is thought to be best on an empty stomach). Human studies are needed to confirm the usefulness of noni.

Are there any side effects or interactions?
Refer to the individual herb for information about any side effects or interactions.

Holistic approaches that may be helpful
The immune system is suppressed during times of stress. Chronic mental and emotional stress can reduce immune function, but whether this effect is sufficient to increase the risk of **infection** (page 265) or **cancer** (page 87) is less clear.[148, 149] Nevertheless, immune function has been increased by stress-reducing techniques such as relaxation exercises, biofeedback, and other approaches,[150, 151] although not all studies have shown a significant effect.[152]

INDIGESTION, HEARTBURN, AND LOW STOMACH ACIDITY

What do I need to know?
Self-care for indigestion can be approached in a number of ways—but it can be hard to know just where to start. To make it easier, our doctors recommend trying these simple steps first:

Get a checkup
    See your healthcare provider to make sure your symptoms are not related to a medical problem
Try lactase enzymes
    If your symptoms seem to be brought on by milk products, try taking lactase digestive enzymes before eating those foods
Slow down at the table
    Take time to eat slowly and chew your food thoroughly
Check for food sensitivities
    Work with a knowledgeable health professional to see if certain foods make your symptoms worse
Help digestion with pancreatic enzymes
    Taking enzymes at each meal that provide 30,000 USP units (IU) of lipase and also include protease and amylase enzymes can improve digestion

About indigestion
"Indigestion" refers to any number of gastrointestinal complaints, which can include gas (belching, flatulence, or bloating) and upset stomach. "Heartburn" refers to a burning feeling that can be caused by stomach acid regurgitating into the esophagus from the stomach, by **gastritis** (page 195) (inflammation of the

lining of the stomach), or by an ulcer of the stomach or duodenum (also called **peptic ulcer** [page 349]). "Low stomach acidity" refers to the inability to produce adequate quantities of stomach acid that will affect digestion and absorption of nutrients.

In some cases, such as **lactose intolerance** (page 288), symptoms of indigestion are due to a specific cause that requires specific treatment. Sometimes symptoms associated with indigestion are caused by diseases unrelated to the gastrointestinal tract. For example, ovarian **cancer** (page 87) may cause a sensation of bloating. Anyone with symptoms of indigestion should be properly diagnosed by a healthcare professional before assuming that the information below is applicable to their situation.

The most common cause of heartburn is gastroesophageal reflux disease (**GERD** [page 198]), in which the sphincter between the esophagus and the stomach is not functioning properly. Another, related cause of heartburn is hiatal hernia, in which a small portion of the stomach protrudes through the aforementioned sphincter.

According to Jonathan Wright, MD, another cause of heartburn can be too *little* stomach acid.[1] This may seem to be a paradox, but based on the clinical experience of a few doctors such as Dr. Wright, supplementing with **betaine HCl** (page 473) (a compound that contains hydrochloric acid) often relieves the symptoms of heartburn and improves digestion, at least in people who have hypochlorhydria (low stomach acid). The amount of betaine HCl used varies with the size of the meal and with the amount of protein ingested. Typical amounts recommended by doctors range from 600 to 2,400 mg per meal. Use of betaine HCl should be monitored by a healthcare practitioner and should be considered only for indigestion sufferers who have been diagnosed with hypochlorhydria.

Medical researchers since the 1930s have been concerned about the consequences of hypochlorhydria. While all the health consequences are still not entirely clear, some have been well documented.

Many minerals and vitamins appear to require adequate concentrations of stomach acid to be absorbed optimally—examples are **iron** (page 540),[2] **zinc** (page 614),[3] and **B-complex vitamins** (page 603),[4] including **folic acid** (page 520).[5] People with achlorhydria (no stomach acid) or hypochlorhydria may therefore be at risk of developing various nutritional deficiencies, which could presumably contribute to the development of a wide range of health problems.

One of the major functions of stomach acid is to initiate the digestion of large protein molecules. If this digestive function is not performed efficiently, incompletely digested protein fragments may be absorbed into the bloodstream. The absorption of these large molecules may contribute to the development of **food allergies** (page 14) and immunological disorders.[6, 7]

In addition, stomach acid normally provides a barrier against bacteria, fungi, and other organisms that are present in food and water. People with inadequate stomach acidity may therefore be at risk of having "unfriendly" microorganisms colonize their intestinal tract.[8, 9] Some of these organisms produce toxic substances that can be absorbed by the body.

Some researchers have found that people with certain diseases are more likely to have an inability to produce normal quantities of stomach acid. However, this does not mean these diseases are caused by too little stomach acid. Jonathan Wright, MD, usually tests patients' stomach acid if they suffer from food **allergies** (page 14), arthritis (both **rheumatoid arthritis** [page 387] and **osteoarthritis** [page 328]), **pernicious anemia** (page 601) (too little **vitamin B_{12}** [page 601]), **asthma** (page 32), **diabetes** (page 152), **vitiligo** (page 443), **eczema** (page 177), tic douloureux, Addison's disease, **celiac disease** (page 102), **lupus erythematosus** (page 421), or thyroid disease.[10]

What are the symptoms of indigestion?

The symptoms of indigestion or upset stomach may include painful or burning sensations in the upper abdomen, bloating, belching, diffuse abdominal pain, heartburn, passing gas, nausea, and occasionally vomiting. The appearance of these symptoms is often associated with eating.

Medical treatments

Over the counter antacids, such as magnesium hydroxide (Phillips' Milk of Magnesia), aluminum hydroxide (Amphojel), calcium carbonate (Tums), and the combination magnesium-aluminum hydroxide (Mylanta, Maalox), help relieve the symptoms of heartburn due to excess acid. The histamine H2 antagonists, such as cimetidine (Tagamet), ranitidine (Zantac), and famotidine (Pepcid), as well as the proton pump inhibitor omeprazole (Prilosec-OTC), are also beneficial. Activated charcoal (CharcoCaps) or simethicone (Gas-X, Mylicon, Phazyme) may provide for relief of gas and bloating. Bismuth subsalicylate (Pepto-Bismol) might help treat indigestion and nausea.

CHECKLIST FOR INDIGESTION, HEARTBURN, AND LOW STOMACH ACIDITY

Rating	Nutritional Supplements	Herbs
★★★	Lactase (page 545) (for lactose intolerance only)	Artichoke (page 628) Greater celandine (page 684)
★★☆	Enzymes (page 506) (Lipase [page 547]) Vitamin B$_{12}$ (page 601) (for people with the combination of low vitamin B$_{12}$ levels, delayed gastric emptying, and *Helicobacter pylori* infection)	Bitter orange (page 635) Caraway (page 651) Fennel (page 676) Ginger (page 680) Linden (page 704) Peppermint (page 726) Sage (page 740) Turmeric (page 753)
★☆☆	Betaine HCl (page 473) (in cases of hypochlorhydria)	Andrographis (page 626) Anise (page 627) Barberry (page 632) Basil (page 633) Bitter melon (page 635) Bladderwrack (page 639) Blessed thistle (page 640) Boldo (page 643) Cardamom Centaury (page 655) Chamomile (page 656) Chaparral (page 657) Cinnamon (page 659) Cloves Coriander Dandelion (page 666) (leaves and root) Devil's claw (page 668) Dill Elecampane (page 671) European angelica Gentian (page 680) Goldenseal (page 683) Horehound (page 691) Juniper (page 698) Lavender (page 701) Lemon balm (page 701) Licorice (DGL) (page 702) Marshmallow (page 708) Oregano (page 719)

Oregon grape (page 721)
Picrorhiza (page 728)
Prickly ash (page 731)
Rooibos (page 739)
Rosemary (page 739)
Slippery elm (page 747) (symptom relief)
Thyme (page 752)
Vervain (page 756)
Wormwood (page 762)
Yarrow (page 763)
Yellow dock (page 763)

Medications may be used to control stomach acidity, including prescription strength histamine H2 inhibitors, such as cimetidine (Tagamet), ranitidine (Zantac) and famotidine (Pepcid), as well as the prescription strength proton pump inhibitors omeprazole (Prilosec), lansoprazole (Prevacid), pantoprazole (Protonix), and rabeprazole (Aciphex).

Treatment includes the avoidance of problem foods, such as citrus fruits, spicy foods, fatty foods, milk, and beans.

Dietary changes that may be helpful

Doctors have observed that heartburn and indigestion may be relieved in some people by avoiding or reducing the intake of caffeine and alcohol. In addition, some people with symptoms of indigestion appear to have food **allergies** (page 14) or intolerances. Avoiding such foods may improve digestive complaints in those people. While most doctors believe there is an important connection between diet and intestinal symptoms, there are few published data documenting such associations. Dietary modifications should be undertaken with the help of a healthcare practitioner.

People who eat too fast or fail to chew their food adequately may also experience symptoms of indigestion or heartburn.

Nutritional supplements that may be helpful

Lipase (page 547), a **pancreatic enzyme** (page 506), aids in the digestion of fats and may improve digestion in some people. In a double-blind trial, a timed-release form of pancreatic enzymes was shown to significantly reduce gas, bloating, and fullness after a high-fat meal.[11] Participants in this study took one capsule immediately before the meal and two capsules immediately after the meal. The three capsules together provided 30,000 USP units of **lipase** (page 547),

112,500 USP units of protease, and 99,600 USP units of amylase. However, the amount of pancreatic enzymes needed may vary from person to person, and should be determined with the help of a doctor.

Vitamin B$_{12}$ (page 601) supplementation may be beneficial for a subset of people suffering from indigestion: those with delayed emptying of the stomach contents in association with *Helicobacter pylori* infection and low blood levels of vitamin B$_{12}$. In a double-blind study of people who satisfied those criteria, treatment with vitamin B$_{12}$ significantly reduced symptoms of dyspepsia and improved stomach-emptying times.[12]

Are there any side effects or interactions?
Refer to the individual supplement for information about any side effects or interactions.

Herbs that may be helpful

Three major categories of herbs are used to treat indigestion when no cause for the condition is known: bitters (digestive stimulants), carminatives (gas-relieving herbs), and demulcents (soothing herbs). The effects of these different categories on heartburn and low stomach acid will be discussed individually. Although there is overlap in the conditions, the categories are helpful.

Action	Herbs
Bitter digestive stimulants	**Andrographis** (page 626), **Artichoke** (page 628), **Barberry** (page 632), **Bitter melon** (page 635), **Bitter orange** (page 635), **Blessed thistle** (page 640), **Boldo** (page 643), **Centaury** (page 655), **Dandelion** (page 666), **Devil's claw** (page 668), **Elecampane** (page 671), **Gentian** (page 680), **Goldenseal** (page 683), **Greater celandine** (page 684), **Horehound** (page 691), **Juniper** (page 698), **Oregon grape** (page 721), **Picrorhiza** (page 728), **Prickly ash** (page 731), **Vervain** (page 756), **Wormwood** (page 762), **Yarrow** (page 763), **Yellow dock** (page 763)
Carminatives	**Anise** (page 627), **Basil** (page 633), **Caraway** (page 651), Cardamom, **Chamomile** (page 656), **Cinnamon** (page 659), Cloves, Coriander, Dill, European angelica, **Fennel** (page 676), **Ginger** (page 680), **Lavender** (page 701), **Lemon balm** (page 701), **Linden** (page 704), **Oregano** (page 719), **Peppermint** (page 726), **Rosemary** (page 739), **Sage** (page 740), **Thyme** (page 752), **Turmeric** (page 753)

Action	Herbs
Demulcents	**Bladderwrack** (page 639), **Licorice** (page 702), **Marshmallow** (page 708), **Slippery elm** (page 747)
Multiple, unclear actions	**Chaparral** (page 657)

Bitter herbs are thought to stimulate digestive function by increasing saliva production and promoting both stomach acid and **digestive enzyme** (page 506) production.[13] As a result, they are particularly used when there is low stomach acid but not in heartburn (where too much stomach acid could initially exacerbate the situation). These herbs literally taste bitter. Some examples of bitter herbs include **greater celandine** (page 684), **wormwood** (page 762), and **gentian** (page 680). Bitters are generally taken either by mixing 1–3 ml tincture into water and sipping slowly 10–30 minutes before eating, or by making tea, which is also sipped slowly before eating.

A double-blind study found that a standardized extract of greater celandine could relieve symptoms of indigestion (such as abdominal cramping, sensation of fullness, and nausea) significantly better than placebo.[14] The study employed an extract standardized to 4 mg of chelidonine per capsule and gave 1–2 tablets three times daily for six weeks. However, recent reports of **hepatitis** (page 220) following intake of greater celandine have raised concerns about its safety for treating indigestion.[15]

Very little published research is available on the traditional uses of **bitter orange** (page 635) as a digestive aid and sedative. The German Commission E has approved the use of bitter orange for loss of appetite and dyspeptic ailments.[16] One test tube study showed bitter orange to potently inhibit rotavirus (a cause of diarrhea in infants and young children).[17] Bitter orange, in an herbal combination formula, reportedly normalized stool function and completely eased intestinal pain in 24 people with non-specific colitis and, again in an herbal combination formula, normalized stool function in another 32 people with constipation.[18, 19]

Artichoke (page 628), in addition to being an edible plant, is a mild bitter. Extracts of artichoke have been repeatedly shown in double-blind research to be beneficial for people with indigestion.[20] Artichoke is particularly useful when the problem is lack of bile production by the liver.[21] Extracts providing 500–1,000 mg per day of cynarin, the main active constituent of artichoke, are recommended by doctors.

Wormwood (page 762) is sometimes used in combination with carminative herbs for people with indigestion. One double-blind trial found that a combination with **peppermint** (page 726), caraway, and **fennel** (page 676) was useful in reducing gas and cramping in people with indigestion.[22] Other bitters are **gentian** (page 680), **dandelion** (page 666), **blessed thistle** (page 640), **yarrow** (page 763), **devil's claw** (page 668), bitter orange, **bitter melon** (page 635), **juniper** (page 698), **andrographis** (page 626), **prickly ash** (page 731), and **centaury** (page 655).[23] The amounts used are the same as the general recommendations for bitters when they are employed for the treatment of indigestion.

Some bitters widely used in traditional medicine in North America include **yarrow** (page 763), **yellow dock** (page 763), **goldenseal** (page 683), **Oregon grape** (page 721), and **vervain** (page 756). Oregon grape's European cousin **barberry** (page 632) has also traditionally been used as a bitter. Animal studies indicate that yarrow, barberry, and Oregon grape, in addition to stimulating digestion like other bitters, may relieve spasms in the intestinal tract.[24]

Boldo (page 643) has been used in South America for a variety of digestive conditions, although this may have stemmed from its impact on intestinal infections or liver function. Studies specifically showing a benefit from taking boldo in people with indigestion and heartburn have not been performed. **Picrorhiza** (page 728), from India, has a similar story to that of boldo. While it is clearly a bitter digestive stimulant, human studies to confirm this have not yet been completed.

Horehound (page 691) contains a number of constituents, including alkaloids, **flavonoids** (page 516), diterpenes (e.g., marrubiin), and trace amounts of volatile oils.[25] The major active constituent marrubiin and possibly its precursor, premarrubiin, are herbal bitters that increase the flow of saliva and gastric juice, thereby stimulating the appetite.[26] Similar to horehound, **elecampane** (page 671) has been used by herbalists to treat people with indigestion.

Carminatives (also called aromatic digestive tonics or aromatic bitters) may be used to relieve symptoms of indigestion, particularly when there is excessive gas. It is believed that carminative agents work, at least in part, by relieving spasms in the intestinal tract.[27]

Among the most notable and well-studied carminatives are **peppermint** (page 726), **fennel** (page 676), and **caraway** (page 651). Double-blind trials have shown that combinations of peppermint and caraway oil and a combination of peppermint, fennel, caraway, and **wormwood** (page 762) have been found to reduce gas and cramping in people with indigestion.[28, 29, 30] Generally, 3–5 drops of natural essential oils or 3–5 ml of tincture of any of these herbs, taken in water two to three times per day before meals, can be helpful. Alternately, a tea can be made by grinding 2–3 teaspoons of the seeds of fennel or caraway or the leaves of peppermint, and then simmering them in a cup of water (covered) for ten minutes. Drink three or more cups per day just after meals.

Linden (page 704) also has a long tradition of use for indigestion. Older clinical trials have shown that linden flower tea can help people who suffer from upset stomach or from excessive gas that causes the stomach to push up and put pressure on the heart (also known as the gastrocardiac syndrome.)[31, 32] The reputed antispasmodic action of linden, particularly in the intestines, has been confirmed in at least one human trial.[33] Linden tea is prepared by steeping 2–3 tsp of flowers in a cup of hot water for 15 minutes. Several cups per day are recommended.

In a double-blind trial, the spice **turmeric** (page 753) was found to relieve indigestion.[34] Two capsules containing 250 mg turmeric powder per capsule were given four times per day.

Chamomile (page 656) (German chamomile or *Matricaria recutita*) is effective in relieving inflamed or irritated mucous membranes of the digestive tract. Since heartburn sometimes involves reflux of stomach acid into the esophagus, the anti-inflammatory properties of chamomile may also be useful. In addition, chamomile promotes normal digestion.[35] However, modern studies to prove chamomile beneficial for people with heartburn or indigestion are lacking. Roman chamomile (*Anthemis nobilis*) has not been studied for indigestion though it has traditionally been used similarly to German chamomile.

Typically taken in tea form, chamomile is recommended three to four times per day between meals. Chamomile tea is prepared by pouring boiling water over dried flowers, and steeping for several minutes. Alternatively, 3–5 ml of chamomile tincture may be added to hot water or 2–3 grams of chamomile in capsule or tablet form may be taken three to four times per day between meals.

Lemon balm (page 701) is another carminative herb used traditionally for indigestion.[36] Lemon balm, usually taken as tea, is prepared by steeping 2–3 teaspoons of leaves in hot water for 10 to 15 minutes in a covered container. Three or more cups per day are consumed immediately after meals. Three to five milliliters of tincture can also be used three times per day.

There are numerous other carminative herbs, including European angelica root *(Angelica archangelica)*, **anise** (page 627), **basil** (page 633), cardamom, **cinnamon** (page 659), cloves, coriander, dill, **ginger** (page 680), **oregano** (page 719), **rosemary** (page 739), **sage** (page 740), **lavender** (page 701), and **thyme** (page 752).[37] Many of these are common kitchen herbs and thus are readily available for making tea to calm an upset stomach. Rosemary is sometimes used to treat indigestion in the elderly by European herbal practitioners.[38] The German Commission E monograph suggests a daily intake of 4–6 grams of sage leaf.[39] Pennyroyal is no longer recommended for use in people with indigestion, however, due to potential side effects.

Demulcents are the third category of herbs used to treat indigestion and heartburn. These herbs seem to work by decreasing inflammation and forming a physical barrier against stomach acid or other abdominal irritants. Examples of demulcent herbs include **ginger** (page 680), **licorice** (page 702), and **slippery elm** (page 747).

Ginger is a spice well known for its traditional use as a treatment for a variety of gastrointestinal complaints, ranging from flatulence to ulcers. Ginger has anti-inflammatory and anti-nausea properties. Ginger has been shown to enhance normal, spontaneous movements of the intestines that aid digestion.[40]

Licorice protects the mucous membranes lining the digestive tract by increasing the production of mucin, a compound that protects against the adverse effects of stomach acid and various harmful substances.[41] The extract of licorice root that is most often used by people with indigestion is known as deglycyrrhizinated licorice (DGL). Glycyrrhizin, which occurs naturally in licorice root, has cortisone-like effects and can cause **high blood pressure** (page 246), **water retention** (page 180), and other problems in some people. When the glycyrrhizin is removed to form DGL, the licorice root retains its beneficial effects against indigestion, while the risk of side effects is greatly reduced. The usual suggested amount of DGL is one or two chewable tablets (250–500 mg per tablet), chewed and swallowed 15 minutes before meals and one to two hours before bedtime.[42] Although many research trials show that DGL is helpful for people with **peptic ulcers** (page 349), the use of DGL for heartburn and indigestion is based primarily on anecdotal information.

The mucilage content in **slippery elm** (page 747) appears to act as a barrier against the damaging effects of acid on the esophagus in people with heartburn. It may also have an anti-inflammatory effect locally in the stomach and intestines. Two or more tablets or capsules (typically 400–500 mg each) may be taken three to four times per day. Alternatively, a tea is made by boiling 1/2–2 grams of the bark in 200 ml of water for 10 to 15 minutes, which is then cooled before drinking; three to four cups a day can be used. Tincture (5 ml three times per day) may also be taken but is believed to be less helpful. **Marshmallow** (page 708) and bladderwrack may be used the same way as slippery elm.

Rooibos (page 739) is traditionally used as a tea as a digestive aid. Unfortunately, no clinical trials have yet been published on this herb, so its efficacy is still unknown. Typically 1 to 4 teaspoons (5 to 20 mg) of rooibos is simmered in one cup of water (236 ml) for up to 10 minutes. Three cups of this tea can be drunk per day.

People in the southwestern United States and northern Mexico have long used **chaparral** (page 657) tea to help calm upset stomachs. It is unclear into which of the above categories—if any—chaparral fits. This strong tasting tea was used only in small amounts. Modern research has not confirmed the usefulness of chaparral for indigestion, and there are serious concerns about the safety of improper internal use of this herb. Before taking chaparral, consult with a knowledgeable healthcare professional.

Are there any side effects or interactions?
Refer to the individual herb for information about any side effects or interactions.

INFECTION

See also: Athlete's Foot (page 42), **Cold Sores** (page 119), **Common Cold/Sore Throat** (page 129), **Cough** (page 139), **Herpes Zoster (Shingles)** (page 401), **HIV and AIDS Support** (page 239), **Influenza** (page 269), **Parasites** (page 343), **Recurrent Ear Infections** (page 383), **Urinary Tract Infection** (page 436), **Yeast Infection** (page 454)

What do I need to know?

Self-care for infection can be approached in a number of ways—but it can be hard to know just where to start. To make it easier, our doctors recommend trying these simple steps first:

See a doctor
> Except for common infections such as a cold, see your doctor for help determining the cause and best treatment for your infection

Infection

Take a multivitamin-mineral supplement
  A daily multivitamin may help prevent deficiencies that increase your chances of getting an infection
Reduce stress
  Work with a counselor or with tapes and other self-help tools to reduce stress, which can impair your immune system

About infection

Infection is the result of invasion of the body by microorganisms, including bacteria, viruses, or fungi.

Not all microorganisms cause infections in the body, and exposure to a disease-causing microorganism does not always result in symptoms. The immune system plays a large role in determining the body's ability to fight off infection.

Some examples of infection are **common cold/sore throat** (page 129), **influenza** (page 269), **cough** (page 139), **recurrent ear infections** (page 383), **urinary tract infection** (page 436), **yeast infection** (page 454), **athlete's foot** (page 42), **cold sores** (page 119), **HIV** (page 239), **shingles** (page 401), and **parasites** (page 343).

CHECKLIST FOR INFECTION

Rating	Nutritional Supplements	Herbs
★★★	**Vitamin A** (page 595) **Vitamin C** (page 604)	**Andrographis** (page 626) **Licorice** (page 702)
★★☆	**Glutamine** (page 530) (for prevention of post exercise infection in **performance athletes** [page 43]) **Multiple vitamin-mineral** (page 559) (for elderly people) **Multiple vitamin–mineral supplement** (page 559) (for diabetics) **Probiotics** (page 575) **Selenium** (page 584) (for elderly people and to prevent hospital-acquired infections in very low birth weight infants) **Zinc** (page 614)	**Echinacea** (page 669) **Licorice** (page 702) (for viral infections)

| ★☆☆ | **American ginseng** (page 625) **Asian ginseng** (page 630) **Astragalus** (page 631) **Barberry** (page 632) **Chaparral** (page 657) Coriolus **Elderberry** (page 670) **Eleuthero** (page 672) **Eucalyptus** (page 673) **Garlic** (page 679) **Goldenseal** (page 683) **Green tea** (page 686) **Lemon Balm** (page 701) (antiviral) **Ligustrum** (page 704) **Lomatium** (page 706) **Maitake** (page 707) **Myrrh** (page 713) **Olive leaf** (page 717) **Onion** (page 718) **Oregano** (page 719) **Oregon grape** (page 721) Osha **Pau d'arco** (page 722) (for fungal infection only) **Picrorhiza** (page 728) **Reishi** (page 737) **Rosemary** (page 739) **Sage** (page 740) **Sandalwood** (page 741) **Schisandra** (page 744) **Shiitake** (page 746) **St. John's Wort** (page 747) **Tea tree oil** (page 751) (topical) **Thyme** (page 752) **Usnea** (page 754) **Wild Indigo** (page 759) |

What are the symptoms of infection?

Symptoms of infection include localized warmth, redness, swelling, discharge, foul-smelling odor, and **pain** (page 338) to the touch. In more serious cases, symptoms may also include fever, chills, nausea, vomiting, **diarrhea** (page 163), and fatigue.

Medical treatments

Over the counter agents available to treat minor bacterial skin infections include benzalkonium chloride (Zephiran), neosporin (Myciguent), bacitracin (Baciguent), and combination antibiotic formulas (Neosporin, Polysporin). Fungal skin infections may be treated with clotrimazole (Lotrimin AF), miconazole (Micatin), and terbinafine (Lamisil). Drugs used to treat vaginal yeast infections include clotrimazole (Gyne-Lotrimin, Mycelex), miconazole (Monistat), and butoconazole (Femstat 3). Individuals with infections that do not respond to over the counter medications should seek medical advice.

Prescription strength topical, oral, and intravenous antibiotic medicines are reserved for more serious bacterial infections; these include cephalosporins, such as cephalexin (Keflex), cefaclor (Ceclor), and cefazolin (Ancef); lincosamides, such as lincomycin (Lincocin) and clindamycin (Cleocin); macrolides, such as erythromycin (Ery-Tab), clarithromycin (Biaxin), and azithromycin (Zithromax); penicillins, such as penicillin VK (Veetids), amoxicillin (Amoxil), and dicloxacillin (Dynapen); and sulfonamides, such as sulfasoxazole (Gantrisin Pediatric) and sulfamethoxazole (Gantanol, Septra, Bactrim). Antiviral drugs are available to treat infections caused by herpes simplex and human immunodeficiency virus (HIV). Numerous drugs are available to treat topical and systemic infections caused by fungus and yeast.

Surgical treatment is recommended in some cases to remove diseased tissue, prevent the spread of infection, or drain pus from an infected area.

Dietary changes that may be helpful

Nutrition is a major contributor to the functioning of the immune system, which in turn influences whether or not the body is resistant to infection. Specifically, it makes sense to restrict sugar, because sugar interferes with the ability of white blood cells to destroy bacteria.[1] Alcohol also interferes with a wide variety of immune defenses,[2] and excessive dietary fat reduces natural killer cell activity.[3] However, there is no research investigating whether reducing sugar, alcohol, or fat intake decreases the risk of infection or improves healing.

Allergy (page 14), including food allergy, has been suggested to predispose people to recurrent infection,[4] and many doctors consider allergy treatment for people with recurrent infections. The links between allergy and **ear infections** (page 383),[5, 6] **urinary tract infections** (page 436) in children,[7] and **yeast vaginitis** (page 454) in women[8, 9] have been documented.

Lifestyle changes that may be helpful

Stress can depress the **immune system** (page 255), thus increasing the body's susceptibility to infection. Coping effectively with stress is important.[10] Exercise increases natural killer cell activity, which may also help prevent infections.[11]

Nutritional supplements that may be helpful

Nutrients useful for maintaining healthy immune function are also applicable for preventing infections. **Vitamin A** (page 595) plays an important role in immune system function and helps mucous membranes, including those in the lungs, resist invasion by microorganisms.[12] However, most research shows that while vitamin A supplementation helps people prevent or treat infections in developing countries where deficiencies are common,[13] little to no positive effect, and even slight *adverse* effects, have resulted from giving vitamin A supplements to people in countries where most people consume adequate amounts of vitamin A.[14, 15, 16, 17, 18, 19, 20] Moreover, vitamin A supplementation during infections appears beneficial only in certain diseases. An analysis of trials revealed that vitamin A reduces mortality from **measles** (page 307) and **diarrhea** (page 163), but not from pneumonia, in children living in developing countries.[21] A double-blind trial for vitamin A supplementation in Tanzanian children with pneumonia confirmed its lack of effectiveness for this condition.[22] In general, parents in the developed world should *not* give vitamin A supplements to children unless there is a reason to believe vitamin A deficiency is likely, such as the presence of a condition causing **malabsorption** (page 304) (e.g., **celiac disease** [page 102]). However, the American Academy of Pediatrics recommends that all children with measles should be given high-dose vitamin A for several days.

Vitamin C (page 604) has antiviral activity, and may help prevent viral infections[23] or, in the case of the **common cold** (page 129), reduce the severity and duration of an infection.[24] Most studies on the common cold used 1 to 4 grams of vitamin C per day.

Lactobacillus acidophilus (page 575) (the friendly bacteria found in yogurt) produces acids that kill invading bacteria.[25] The effective amount of acidophilus depends on the strain used, as well as the concentration of viable organisms. These and other friendly bacteria known as **probiotics** (page 575) inhibit the growth of potentially infectious organisms (pathogens) by producing acids, hydrogen peroxide, and natural antibiotics called bacteriocins and microcins, by utilizing nutrients needed by pathogens, by occupying attachment sites on the gut wall that would otherwise be available to pathogens, and by stimulating immune at-

Infection

tacks on pathogens. Infections that have been successfully prevented or treated with friendly bacteria include infectious **diarrhea** (page 163), **vaginitis** (page 438), and **urinary tract infections** (page 436).[26]

Marginal deficiencies of **zinc** (page 614) result in impairments of **immune function** (page 255).[27] Supplementation with 50 mg of zinc three times per day for 30 days has been shown to increase immune function in healthy people.[28] However, such large amounts of zinc can potentially cause adverse effects. Some doctors recommend lower amounts of supplemental zinc for people experiencing recurrent infections, such as 25 mg per day for adults and even lower amounts for children (depending on body weight). Zinc lozenges have been found helpful in some studies for the **common cold** (page 129). Zinc has not been studied as prevention or treatment for other types of infection.

A **multiple vitamin-mineral formula** (page 559) helped elderly people avoid infections in one double-blind trial, but not in another.[29, 30] In a double-blind study of middle-aged and elderly diabetics, supplementation with a multiple vitamin and mineral preparation for one year reduced the risk of infection by more than 80%, compared with a placebo.[31] In another double-blind trial, supplements of 100 mcg per day of **selenium** (page 584) and 20 mg per day of **zinc** (page 614), with or without additional **vitamin C** (page 604), **vitamin E** (page 609), and **beta-carotene** (page 469), reduced infections in elderly people, though vitamins without minerals had no effect.[32] That study suggests that trace minerals may be the most important components of a multiple vitamin and mineral formula for preventing infections.

Premature infants with very low birth weight have an increased susceptibility to infections. In a double-blind trial, premature infants were given either **selenium** (page 584) supplements (5–7 mcg per 2.2 pounds of body weight) or placebo. Those receiving the selenium supplements had fewer hospital-acquired infections.[33]

Athletes (page 43) who undergo intensive training or participate in endurance races (such as a marathon) are at increased risk of developing infections. In a double-blind study, marathon runners received either **glutamine** (page 530) (5 grams immediately after the race and 5 grams again two hours later) or a placebo. Compared with the placebo, supplementation with L-glutamine reduced the incidence of infections over the next seven days by 62%.[34]

Are there any side effects or interactions?
Refer to the individual supplement for information about any side effects or interactions.

Herbs that may be helpful
The main herbs for infection can be broken down into three basic categories: those that support a person's **immune system** (page 255) in the fight against microbes, those that directly attack microbes, and those that do both. These categories are summarized in the table below. Note that this table does not include herbs that are largely used for **parasitic** (page 341) infections of the intestines.

Mechanism of Action	Examples
Immune supportive	**American ginseng** (page 625), **andrographis** (page 626), **Asian ginseng** (page 630), **astragalus** (page 631), coriolus, **eleuthero** (page 672), **ligustrum** (page 704), **maitake** (page 707), **picrorhiza** (page 728), **reishi** (page 737), **schisandra** (page 744), **shiitake** (page 746)
Antimicrobial	**Chaparral** (page 657), **eucalyptus** (page 673), **garlic** (page 679), **green tea** (page 686), **lemon balm** (page 701) (antiviral), **lomatium** (page 706), **myrrh** (page 713), **olive leaf** (page 717), **onion** (page 718), **oregano** (page 719), **pau d'arco** (page 722) (antifungal), **rosemary** (page 739), **sage** (page 740), **sandalwood** (page 741), **St. John's wort** (page 747), **tea tree oil** (page 751), **thyme** (page 752), **usnea** (page 754)
Both immune supportive and antimicrobial	**Barberry** (page 632), **echinacea** (page 669), **elderberry** (page 670), **goldenseal** (page 683), **licorice** (page 702), **Oregon grape** (page 721), osha, **wild indigo** (page 759)

Are there any side effects or interactions?
Refer to the individual herb for information about any side effects or interactions.

INFLAMMATORY BOWEL DISEASE

Inflammatory bowel disease (IBD) refers to chronic disorders of the small and/or large intestine characterized by inflammatory changes in the intestinal tissue. The two major types of inflammatory bowel disease are Crohn's disease and ulcerative colitis.

Crohn's disease usually affects the small intestine but may extend into the large intestine as well. Ulcerative colitis occurs only in the large intestine. The function of the small intestine differs from that of the large intestine; therefore, while the health consequences and treatment of Crohn's disease and ulcerative colitis may be similar, there are important differences as well.

Irritable bowel syndrome (page 280) (IBS) is often confused with IBD, but IBS is a distinctly separate, non-inflammatory disease. For more information about specific types of inflammatory bowel disease, please refer to the following articles:

- **Crohn's disease** (page 141)
- **Ulcerative colitis** (page 433)

INFLUENZA

See also: Common Cold/Sore Throat (page 129), **Sinus Congestion** (page 405), **Sinusitis** (page 407)

Influenza is the name of a virus and the **infection** (page 265) it causes.

Although for most people the infection is mild, it can be severe and even deadly in those with compromised immune systems, including infants, the elderly, and people with diseases such as cancer and **AIDS** (page 239). In the past, huge epidemics of influenza have caused millions of deaths. Some nutritional and herbal recommendations for maintaining healthy **immune function** (page 255) are also applicable for treating influenza.

What are the symptoms of influenza?

Symptoms of influenza include fever, muscle aches, fatigue, nausea, and vomiting. Other symptoms include headache, chills, dry cough, sore throat, **pain** (page 338) when moving the eyes, sneezing, and runny nose. The onset of symptoms is often rapid and intense.

CHECKLIST FOR INFLUENZA

Rating	Nutritional Supplements	Herbs
★★☆	**Vitamin C** (page 604)	**Echinacea** (page 669) **Elderberry** (page 670)
★☆☆		**Asian ginseng** (page 630) **Boneset** (page 644) **Eleuthero** (page 672) **Goldenseal** (page 683) **Meadowsweet** (page 709) Thuja **Wild indigo** (page 759)

Medical treatments

Over the counter analgesics containing acetaminophen (Tylenol) are safe for individuals of all ages to treat fever, body aches, and headache associated with the flu. Aspirin-containing products are not given to people under 18 years old who have flu symptoms, since this practice has been linked to an increased risk of Reye's syndrome (brain and liver abnormalities that can lead to coma and death). People over 18 years old can take aspirin (Bayer, Ecotrin, Bufferin) and ibuprofen (Motrin, Advil) to reduce pain and fever associated with the flu.

Prescription antiviral medicines available include those taken orally, such as amantadine (Symmetrel), rimantadine (Flumadine), and oseltamivir (Tamiflu), or with an inhaler such as zanamivir (Relenza) and ribavirin (Virazole). Antibiotics are sometimes recommended to prevent secondary bacterial infections [1, 2] such as pneumonia.[3] Otherwise, antibiotics are not effective against viruses. Although early intervention with antibiotics may effectively prevent pneumonia [4] and reduce costs associated with influenza outbreaks,[5] some doctors believe the use of antibiotics to *prevent* (rather than to treat) bacterial infections is ill-advised[6] and should be limited to people who are most at risk of developing a secondary **infection** (page 265), such as the elderly and those with compromised **immune function** (page 255) (as in **AIDS** [page 239]). This is because overuse of antibiotics may lead to the development of antibiotic-resistant strains of bacteria that are more difficult to treat.[7]

People with flu symptoms are commonly advised to rest and drink plenty of fluids.

Nutritional supplements that may be helpful

Dockworkers given 100 mg of **vitamin C** (page 604) each day for ten months caught influenza 28% less often than did their coworkers not taking vitamin C. Of those who did develop the flu, the average duration of illness was 10% less in those taking vitamin C than in those not taking the vitamin.[8] Other trials have reported that taking vitamin C in high amounts (2 grams every hour for 12 hours) can lead to rapid improvement of influenza **infections** (page 265).[9, 10] Such high amounts, however, should only be used under the supervision of a healthcare professional.

Are there any side effects or interactions?
Refer to the individual supplement for information about any side effects or interactions.

Herbs that may be helpful

Echinacea (page 669) has long been used for colds and flu. Double-blind trials in Germany have shown that **infections** (page 265) associated with flu-like symptoms clear more rapidly when people take echinacea.[11] Echinacea appears to work by stimulating the **immune system** (page 255). The usual recommended amount of echinacea is 3–5 ml of the expressed juice of the herb or tincture of the herb or root, or 300 mg of dried root powder three times per day.

The effect of a syrup made from the berries of the black **elderberry** (page 670) on influenza has been studied in a small double-blind trial.[12] People receiving an elderberry extract (four tablespoons per day for adults, two tablespoons per day for children) appeared to recover faster than did those receiving a placebo.

Asian ginseng (page 630) and **eleuthero** (page 672) (Siberian ginseng) have immune-enhancing properties, which may play a role in preventing infection with the influenza virus. However, they have not yet been specifically studied for this purpose. One double-blind trial found that co-administration of 100 mg of Asian ginseng extract with a flu vaccine led to a lower frequency of colds and flu compared to people who just received the flu vaccine alone.[13]

Boneset (page 644) has been shown in test tube and other studies to stimulate immune-cell function,[14] which may explain it's traditional use to help fight off minor viral infections, such as the flu.

Wild indigo (page 759) contains polysaccharides and proteins that have been reported in test tube studies to stimulate the immune system. The immune-enhancing effect of wild indigo is consistent with its use in traditional herbal medicine to fight the flu.[15] However, wild indigo is generally used in combination with other herbs such as **echinacea** (page 669), **goldenseal** (page 683), or thuja.

While not as potent as **willow** (page 760), which has a higher salicin content, the salicylates in **meadowsweet** (page 709) do give it a mild anti-inflammatory effect and the potential to reduce fevers during a **cold** (page 129) or flu. However, this role is based on historical use and knowledge of the chemistry of meadowsweet's constituents; to date, no human studies have been completed with meadowsweet.

Are there any side effects or interactions?
Refer to the individual herb for information about any side effects or interactions.

Holistic approaches that may be helpful

Because family stress has been shown to increase the risk of influenza **infection** (page 265),[16] measures to relieve stressful situations may be beneficial.

INSOMNIA

What do I need to know?

Self-care for insomnia can be approached in a number of ways—but it can be hard to know just where to start. To make it easier, our doctors recommend trying these simple steps first:

Create a restful place to sleep
Remove or block noise, light, and other distractions and make sure your mattress is comfortable for you

Cut coffee and other stimulants
Eliminate or cut down on drinks and foods that have caffeine, ephedra, or pseudoephedrine; work with your doctor to find alternatives if you take medication with any of these ingredients

Learn to relax
A counselor experienced in treating insomnia or relaxation tapes and other self-help tools can help you let go of tension

Check out valerian
To fall asleep quicker and enjoy deeper sleep quality, take 300 to 600 mg of a concentrated root extract 30 minutes before bedtime, with or without other relaxing herbs such as lemon balm and passion flower

About insomnia

Insomnia refers to a prolonged inability to get adequate sleep. Not getting a good night's sleep can result from waking up in the middle of the night and having trouble getting back to sleep. It also occurs when people have a hard time falling asleep in the first place. Insomnia can be a temporary, occasional, or chronic problem.

CHECKLIST FOR INSOMNIA		
Rating	Nutritional Supplements	Herbs
★★★		**Valerian** (page 756)
★★☆	**5-HTP** (page 459) **Melatonin** (page 555)	**Corydalis** (page 663)
★☆☆	**Magnesium** (page 551) **Vitamin B$_{12}$** (page 601)	**American scullcap** (page 626) **Bitter orange** (page 635) **Catnip** (page 653) **Chamomile** (page 656) **Hops** (page 690) **Lavender** (page 701) **Lemon balm** (page 701) **Passion flower** (page 722)

What are the symptoms of insomnia?

Sleep-onset insomnia refers to the inability to fall asleep initially. Sleep-maintenance insomnia refers to the inability to stay asleep, with one or more awakenings during the night.

Medical treatments

Over the counter drugs include diphenhydramine (Sominex, Nytol, Excedrin PM) and doxylamine (Unisom).

The prescription medications most commonly used to treat insomnia include zolpidem (Ambien), zaleplon (Sonata), estazolam (ProSom), flurazepam (Dalmane), temazepam (Restoril), and triazolam (Halcion). Though these agents are beneficial, they often become less effective over time.

Behavioral or psychological counseling may be recommended for people with poor sleep habits or emotional disorders. People with insomnia are typically advised to avoid stimulants such as caffeine (found in coffee, tea, and soda), diet pills containing ephedra, and over the counter cold and allergy products containing pseudoephedrine.

Dietary changes that may be helpful

Caffeine is a stimulant.[1] The effects of caffeine can last up to 20 hours,[2] so some people will have disturbed sleep patterns even when their last cup of coffee was in the morning. Besides regular coffee, black tea, **green tea** (page 686), cocoa, chocolate, some soft drinks, and many over-the-counter pharmaceuticals also contain caffeine.

Doctors will sometimes recommend eating a high-carbohydrate food before bedtime, such as a slice of bread or some crackers. Eating carbohydrates can significantly increase levels of a neurotransmitter (chemical messenger) called serotonin,[3] which is known to reduce **anxiety** (page 30) and promote sleep.

Food **allergy** (page 14) may also contribute to insomnia. In a trial involving eight infants, chronic insomnia was traced to an allergy to cow's milk. Avoidance of milk resulted in a normalization of sleep patterns.[4]

Lifestyle changes that may be helpful

A steady sleeping and eating schedule combined with caffeine avoidance and counseling sessions using behavioral therapy has reduced insomnia for some people, as has listening to relaxation tapes.[5]

The effect of exercise on sleep has not been well studied. However, some healthcare practitioners recommend daily exercise as a way to reduce stress, which in turn can help with insomnia.

A naturopathic therapy for insomnia is take a 15- to 20-minute hot Epsom-salts bath before bedtime. One or two cups of Epsom salts (magnesium sulfate) in a hot bath are thought to act as a muscle relaxant.

Smokers are more likely to have insomnia than nonsmokers.[6] As with many other health conditions, it is important for people with insomnia to quit smoking.

Nutritional supplements that may be helpful

Melatonin (page 555) is a natural hormone that regulates the human biological clock. The body produces less melatonin with advancing age, which may explain why elderly people often have difficulty sleeping[7] and why melatonin supplements improve sleep in the elderly.[8]

Warning: Melatonin is a potent hormone and its long-term safety is not established. Melatonin should only be taken with medical supervision.

Insomnia

Middle-aged adults (average age, 54 years) with insomnia also have lower melatonin levels, compared with people of the same age without insomnia.[9] However, there is not much research on the use of melatonin for sleep problems in middle-aged people.

Double-blind trials have shown that melatonin facilitates sleep in young adults without insomnia,[10] but not in young people who suffer from insomnia.[11] However, one trial found that children with sleep disturbances stemming from school phobia had improved sleep after taking 1 mg of melatonin per night for one week, then 5 mg per night for one week, then 10 mg per night for a third week.[12]

The results of one double-blind trial also indicate that a controlled release melatonin supplement providing 2 mg per day improves sleep quality in people with schizophrenia.[13]

Normally, the body makes melatonin for several hours per night—an effect best duplicated with controlled-release supplements. Trials using timed-release melatonin for insomnia have reported good results.[14] Many doctors suggest taking 0.5 to 3 mg of melatonin one and a half to two hours before bedtime. However, because melatonin is a potent hormone, the long-term effects of which are unknown, it should be taken only with the supervision of a doctor.

The **amino acid** (page 465), L-tryptophan, has been used successfully for people with insomnia,[15] presumably because it is converted to the chemical messenger, serotonin. According to one preliminary trial, L-tryptophan supplementation was 100% effective at promoting sleep in people who awaken between three to six times per night, but not effective at all for people who only awaken once or twice, nor in people who doze on and off throughout the night in a state blurred between sleep and wakefulness.[16] However, L-tryptophan is no longer available over the counter in the United States. A related compound that occurs naturally in the body, 5-hydroxytryptophan (**5-HTP** [page 459]), is also converted into serotonin and might, therefore, be helpful for insomnia. In a double-blind trial of people without insomnia, supplementation with 5-HTP (200 mg at 9:15 p.m. and 400 mg at 11:15 p.m.) increased rapid-eye-movement (REM) sleep, presumably indicating improved sleep quality.[17] In a preliminary trial of people with **fibromyalgia** (page 191), supplementing with 100 mg of 5-HTP three times a day improved sleep quality.[18] However, additional research is needed to determine whether 5-HTP is safe and effective for people with insomnia.

In a preliminary study, 5-HTP was also found to be an effective treatment for "sleep terrors,"[19] a common problem in children that causes sudden awakening with persistent fear or terror, screaming, sweating, confusion, and increased heart rate.

Some people have difficulty sleeping because of a problem known as period limb movements during sleep (PLMS) or another condition called **restless legs syndrome** (page 384) (RLS). In a preliminary trial, people with PLMS or RLS who suffered from insomnia had a significant improvement in sleep efficiency after supplementing with **magnesium** (page 551) (about 300 mg each evening for four to six weeks).[20]

In two small preliminary trials, people with insomnia resulting from disorders of the sleep-wake rhythm improved after supplementing with **vitamin B$_{12}$** (page 601) (1,500 to 3,000 mcg per day).[21, 22]

Are there any side effects or interactions?
Refer to the individual supplement for information about any side effects or interactions.

Herbs that may be helpful
Herbal remedies have been used safely for centuries for insomnia. In modern herbal medicine, the leading herb for insomnia is **valerian** (page 756). Valerian root makes getting to sleep easier and increases deep sleep and dreaming. Valerian does not cause a morning "hangover," a side effect common to prescription sleep drugs in some people.[23, 24] A double-blind trial found that valerian extract (600 mg 30 minutes before bedtime for 28 days) is comparable in efficacy to oxazepam (Serax), a commonly prescribed drug for insomnia.[25] In a separate double-blind trial, the same amount of valerian extract was found to improve subjective assessments of sleep quality and certain aspects of brain function during sleep as well.[26] A concentrated (4–5:1) valerian root supplement in the amount of 300–600 mg can be taken 30 minutes before bedtime. Alternately, 2 to 3 grams of the dried root in a capsule or 5 ml tincture can be taken 30 minutes before bedtime.

A combination of valerian and **lemon balm** (page 701) has been tested for improving sleep. A small preliminary trial compared the effect of valerian root extract (320 mg at bedtime) and an extract of lemon balm (*Melissa officinalis*) with that of the sleeping drug triazolam (Halcion).[27] The effectiveness of the herbal combination was similar to that of Halcion, but only the Halcion group felt hung over and had trouble concentrating the next day. A double-blind trial found that a combination of valerian and lemon balm, taken over a two-week period, was effective in improving quality of sleep.[28]

Another double-blind trial found a combination of 360 mg valerian and 240 mg lemon balm taken before bed improved reported sleep quality in one-third of the participants.[29]

Combining valerian root with other mildly sedating herbs is common both in Europe and the United States. **Chamomile** (page 656), **hops** (page 690), **passion flower** (page 722), **lemon balm** (page 701), **American scullcap** (page 626), and **catnip** (page 653) are commonly recommended by doctors.[30] These herbs can also be used alone as mild sedatives for those suffering from insomnia or nervous exhaustion. Chamomile is a particularly good choice for younger children whose insomnia may be related to gastrointestinal upset. Hops and lemon balm are approved by the German government for relieving sleep disturbances.[31]

Bitter orange (page 635) has a history of use as a calming agent and to counteract insomnia. There is no clinical trial data to support its efficacy in this regard. The usual amount of tincture used is 2 to 3 ml at bedtime.

Corydalis (page 663) contains several ingredients, one of which has been shown to influence the nervous system, providing **pain** (page 338) relief and promoting relaxation. People with insomnia were able to fall sleep more easily after taking 100–200 mg per day of a corydalis extract (called dl-tetrahydropalmatine, or DHP), according to a preliminary report.[32] People taking the extract reported no drug hangover symptoms, such as dizziness or **vertigo** (page 441).

The volatile oil of **lavender** (page 701) contains many medicinal components, including perillyl alcohol, linalool, and geraniol. The aroma of the oil is known to be calming[33] and thus may be helpful in some cases of insomnia. One trial of elderly people with sleeping troubles found that inhaling lavender oil was as effective as tranquilizers.[34] Teas made from lavender flowers or from the oil (1–4 drops) are approved for internal use by the German Commission E for people with insomnia.[35] Internal use of essential oils can be dangerous and should be done only with the supervision of a trained herbalist or healthcare professional.

Are there any side effects or interactions?
Refer to the individual herb for information about any side effects or interactions.

Holistic approaches that may be helpful
Insomnia can be triggered by psychological stress. Dealing with stress, through counseling or other techniques, may be the key to a better night's rest. Many trials have shown that psychological intervention can be helpful for insomnia.[36] A combined program of counseling, sleep restriction methods (i.e., the only time spent in bed is when sleeping), and control of stimuli that might interfere with sleep, significantly increased sleep time in a group of people with insomnia.[37]

Acupuncture may be helpful for insomnia, possibly by increasing production of calming neurotransmitters such as serotonin and other substances.[38] A preliminary trial found one acupuncture treatment daily for seven to ten days resulted in complete recovery of normal sleep in 59% of patients and partial recovery in 21%.[39] A controlled trial treated patients with either acupuncture or fake acupuncture (insertion of needles at non-acupuncture points). The patients receiving true acupuncture had significant improvements in a laboratory measure of sleep quality compared to the placebo group.[40] The treatment of insomnia with auricular (ear) acupuncture may provide similar benefits to people with insomnia, according to a preliminary trial.[41] However, double-blind trials are necessary to conclusively determine the value of acupuncture in treating insomnia.

INSULIN RESISTANCE SYNDROME

The insulin resistance syndrome (IRS) is a group of health risk factors that increase the likelihood of **heart disease** (page 98),[1, 2, 3, 4] and perhaps other disorders, such as **diabetes** (page 152) and some **cancers** (page 87).[5, 6] The risk factors that make up IRS include insulin resistance, which refers to the reduced ability of the hormone insulin to control the processing of glucose by the body. Other major risk factors often associated with IRS include high blood sugar and high blood **triglycerides** (page 235), low HDL ("good") **cholesterol** (page 223), **high blood pressure** (page 246), and excessive body fat in the abdominal region. People with IRS do not always have every one of these risk factors, but they usually have many of them. A qualified doctor should make the diagnosis of IRS after a thorough examination and blood tests.

Most people with type 2 diabetes have insulin resistance, but many more people who are not diabetic also have insulin resistance.[7, 8, 9] Since insulin resistance itself often does not cause symptoms, these people may not be aware of their problem. Some authorities believe insulin resistance is partially inherited and partially due to lifestyle factors.

In addition to the recommendations discussed below, people with IRS may benefit from some of the recommendations given for type 2 **diabetes** (page 152). People with IRS should also benefit from health strategies that reduce the severity of the risk factors they possess, including **obesity** (page 446), high triglycerides, and high blood pressure.

CHECKLIST FOR INSULIN RESISTANCE SYNDROME

Rating	Nutritional Supplements	Herbs
★★★	Glucomannan (page 526)	
★★☆	Chromium (page 493) Guar gum	
★☆☆	Calcium (page 483) Coenzyme Q$_{10}$ (page 496) Magnesium (page 551) Vitamin E (page 609) Zinc (page 614)	

What are the symptoms of insulin resistance syndrome?

People with IRS may be **overweight** (page 446) (especially in the trunk area), feel sluggish after eating, and may have been told that they have **high blood pressure** (page 246) and **high cholesterol** (page 223).

Medical treatments

Though there are no specific prescription drugs available, medications commonly prescribed for **weight loss** (page 446) are beneficial. The most common agents used include orlistat (Xenical), sibutramine (Meridia), and phentermine (Fastin), though dextroamphetamine (Dexedrine) is occasionally prescribed. In addition, cholesterol lowering drugs, such as the bile acid sequestrants cholestyramine (Questran) and colestipol (Colestid), and the HMG-CoA Reductase Inhibitors atorvastatin (Lipitor), fluvastatin (Lescol), lovastatin (Mevacor), pravastatin (Pravachol), and simvastatin (Zocor), are often prescribed. Medications may also be prescribed to control high blood pressure.

Treatment typically includes dietary changes to limit fat and calories, increased exercise, and changes in habits or patterns of eating.

Dietary changes that may be helpful

Some authorities recommend people with IRS avoid high-carbohydrate diets, and some recommend a diet lower in carbohydrate than current public health guidelines suggest. The rationale is that high carbohydrate intake stimulates increased insulin levels, which can lead to **high triglycerides** (page 235), **low HDL** (page 223), and other adverse changes in the levels of blood fats that contribute to heart disease risk.[10] Other authorities disagree, however, because they believe a lower carbohydrate diet will result in higher calorie intake from fat, leading to more difficulties with overweight, insulin resistance, and heart disease risk.[11] A recent preliminary study suggested that a healthy, balanced diet low in fried foods and sausages, and high in vegetables, fruits, fish, and complex carbohydrates, such as whole grain rice and pasta, was associated with protection from many aspects of IRS.[12]

The effect of dietary fat on insulin resistance seems to depend on the type of fat eaten. Preliminary studies in animals and humans suggest that insulin resistance is worsened with increased use of saturated fat and improved with increased unsaturated **omega-3 fatty acids** (page 509) from fish, while the role of other unsaturated fats is less clear.[13] However, recent research has reported that diets high in monounsaturated fat improve insulin sensitivity in both healthy people and people with diabetes.[14] A diet low in saturated fat, but which allows both fish and monounsaturated fat makes sense for people with IRS, because such a diet is associated with protection from **heart disease** (page 98). Recently, a low-fat diet allowing fish was shown to decrease insulin resistance in people with IRS.[15]

High-carbohydrate diets have also been shown to improve insulin sensitivity; the reason for this may partly be that weight loss often occurs on this type of diet,[16] or that these diets are low in fats, such as saturated fat, that worsen insulin sensitivity.[17, 18] The type of carbohydrate consumed may influence the effect of a high-carbohydrate diet on insulin sensitivity. Animal research suggests that very high intake of fructose or sucrose worsens insulin sensitivity, but human studies have been inconsistent.[19, 20] "Glycemic index" refers to the blood sugar-raising effect of a food, and there is preliminary evidence from some,[21, 22, 23] though not all,[24] human research, that consumption of low glycemic index foods improves insulin sensitivity. Effects on glycemic index may be one reason dietary fiber is associated with better insulin sensitivity.[25] As with dietary fat intake, it makes sense for people with IRS to choose carbohydrates according to their effects on **heart disease** (page 98) risk. Therefore a diet low in refined carbohydrates and high in fiber appears most prudent.[26]

Very little research has investigated the effect of increasing dietary protein intake on insulin resistance in people with or without IRS. One controlled study found that people with some features of IRS lost more weight on a high protein diet than on a high-carbohydrate diet, although both diets produced similar improvements in a measurement of insulin sensitivity.[27] Preliminary and controlled trials in people without IRS have also shown that substituting protein for carbohydrate in a low-fat diet can improve blood lipids (**cholesterol** [page 223], **triglycerides** [page 235], and HDL) towards reduced heart disease risk.[28, 29] More research is needed on the effects of high protein diets in people with IRS.

In two controlled studies,[30, 31] a combined program of a weight-loss diet lower in fat and higher in fish, along with exercise three times per week, improved several measures of insulin resistance, blood triglycerides and cholesterol, and blood pressure in a group of people with IRS.

High salt intake decreases insulin sensitivity in young, healthy people,[32] but not in older people with **hypertension** (page 246),[33] according to preliminary studies. Moderate restriction of salt, however, also decreased insulin sensitivity in one preliminary study of healthy people,[34] but had no effect in other studies of people either with[35, 36, 37] or without[38, 39] hypertension. No studies have investigated the effect of salt intake or restriction in people with IRS.

Lifestyle changes that may be helpful

Obesity (page 446), especially when fat accumulates in the abdominal region, increases the severity of insulin resistance,[40, 41] and has been associated with IRS.[42, 43] Loss of excess weight tends to improve insulin sensitivity (i.e., reduce insulin resistance),[44, 45] and this has been recently shown to be true for people with IRS as well.[46] Weight loss also reduces many of the other health risk factors associated with IRS.[47]

Cigarette smoking, in most,[48, 49] though not all,[50] studies, as well as exposure to secondhand smoke[51] and use of nicotine replacement products,[52, 53] have been associated with insulin resistance. While smoking cessation has been shown to increase insulin sensitivity in healthy people,[54] no research has investigated the effect of quitting smoking on people with IRS.

Alcohol consumption in the light to moderate range is associated with better insulin sensitivity in healthy, nondiabetic people.[55, 56, 57, 58] Since alcohol consumption also reduces other risk factors for **heart disease** (page 98),[59, 60] it does not appear that people with IRS would benefit from avoiding alcohol if they are currently light to moderate drinkers. However, alcohol is potentially addicting and can increase the risk of other diseases, so people with IRS who are not users of alcohol should consult a doctor before starting regular consumption of alcoholic beverages.

Either aerobic exercise or strength training improves insulin sensitivity in both healthy and insulin-resistant people in most studies,[61, 62] though a recent controlled trial found that aerobic exercise alone did not affect insulin resistance in people with IRS.[63] Studies comparing strength training to aerobic exercise in insulin-resistant people have reported greater benefits from strength training,[64, 65] but a combination of the two will probably be more effective than either one alone.[66, 67] In addition, exercise has many benefits in reducing many of the risk factors associated with IRS.[68]

Some popular diet books claim that insulin resistance causes weight gain and prevents successful **weight loss** (page 446). However, one controlled study found no difference in the number of women experiencing successful short-term weight loss between women with or without insulin resistance.[69]

Insulin sensitivity decreases after certain stressful experiences, such as surgery,[70] and decreased insulin sensitivity is associated with work-related mental and emotional stress,[71] and other aspects of a stressful lifestyle.[72] However, these associations have not been explored in people with IRS, nor has stress reduction been investigated as a treatment for IRS.

Nutritional supplements that may be helpful

Glucomannan (page 526), a type of water-soluble dietary **fiber** (page 512), may reduce many risk factors in people with IRS. A double-blind trial found that 8–13 grams per day of glucomannan significantly improved several measures of blood cholesterol control and one measure of blood glucose control in people with IRS.[73] Another double-blind study of healthy people found that 30 grams per day of guar gum, a fiber similar to glucomannan, improved insulin sensitivity and many other components of IRS, including **blood pressure** (page 446) and blood glucose, **cholesterol** (page 223), and **triglycerides** (page 235), leading the authors to recommend guar gum for people with IRS.[74] However, in another study, **obese** (page 446) people taking 8–16 grams per day of guar gum for 6–12 weeks did not experience any change in insulin sensitivity.[75]

Vitamin E (page 609), 800–1,350 IU per day, has been shown to increase insulin sensitivity in both healthy[76] and hypertensive[77] people in double-blind studies. Research is needed to investigate this effect in people with IRS.

One double blind trial found that 1,500 mg per day of **calcium** (page 483) improved insulin sensitivity in people with hypertension.[78] No research on the effects of calcium in people with IRS has been done.

Magnesium (page 551) deficiency can reduce insulin sensitivity,[79] and low dietary intake[80] and low blood levels[81] of magnesium have been associated with greater insulin resistance in nondiabetic people. However, no studies of magnesium supplementation in people with IRS have been done.

Chromium (page 493) has long been known to be helpful to people with insulin-related disorders.[82, 83] While no chromium research has been done specifically on people with IRS, known mechanisms of chromium's effects indicate that chromium plays a role in promoting insulin sensitivity.[84, 85] Preliminary evidence also suggests that insulin resistance may cause loss of chromium from the body, increasing the likelihood of chromium deficiency.[86]

Preliminary studies have reported that low **zinc** (page 614) intake is associated with several of the risk factors common in IRS,[87] and a low blood level of zinc is associated with insulin resistance in overweight people.[88] However, people with IRS have not specifically been studied to determine whether they are zinc deficient or whether zinc supplements are helpful for them.

A double-blind trial showed that **coenzyme Q_{10}** (page 496), 120 mg per day, reduced glucose and insulin blood levels in people with **high blood pressure** (page 246) and **heart disease** (page 98).[89] These results suggest that coenzyme Q_{10} may improve insulin sensitivity in people with components of IRS, but more research is needed.

Are there any side effects or interactions?
Refer to the individual supplement for information about any side effects or interactions.

INTERMITTENT CLAUDICATION

See also: Atherosclerosis (page 38)

Intermittent claudication is pain in the legs caused by atherosclerosis (hardening of the arteries) of the lower extremities.

Because atherosclerosis decreases the supply of blood and oxygen to the legs, people with intermittent claudication experience leg pain after walking a certain distance. People with this condition should be monitored by a doctor. The natural treatments for intermittent claudication include many of those used for atherosclerosis; these include controlling **high cholesterol** (page 223), modifying dietary and lifestyle factors that might influence atherosclerosis, and taking various nutritional supplements and herbs.

You should also learn more about **atherosclerosis** (page 38) for more information about dietary changes that might favorably influence hardening of the arteries or the risk of **heart disease** (page 98) associated with it. What follows is a discussion limited to those aspects of lifestyle and natural medicine that have been studied specifically in relation to intermittent claudication.

CHECKLIST FOR INTERMITTENT CLAUDICATION

Rating	Nutritional Supplements	Herbs
★★★	**Inositol hexaniacinate** (page 537) (vitamin B_3) **Policosanol** (page 571) **Propionyl-L-carnitine** (page 543) **Vitamin E** (page 609)	*Ginkgo biloba* (page 681)
★★☆	**Arginine** (page 467) (intravenous only) **L-carnitine** (page 543)	**Garlic** (page 679) Padma 28
★☆☆	**Evening primrose oil** (page 511) **Magnesium** (page 551)	

What are the symptoms of intermittent claudication?

Initial symptoms of intermittent claudication are pain, aching, cramping, or fatigue of the muscles in the lower limbs that develop during walking and are quickly relieved by rest. Symptoms typically occur in the calf but may also be located in the foot, thigh, hip, or buttocks. In more advanced stages, the painful symptoms are present even at rest and are worsened by elevating the legs.

Medical treatments

Prescription medications used to treat intermittent claudication include pentoxifylline (Trental) and the antiplatelet drug Cilostazol (Pletal). In addition, cholesterol lowering drugs, such as the bile acid sequestrants cholestyramine (Questran) and colestipol (Colestid), and the HMG-CoA reductase inhibitors atorvastatin (Lipitor), fluvastatin (Lescol), lovastatin (Mevacor), pravastatin (Pravachol), and simvastatin (Zocor), are often prescribed in combination with anticlaudication medications.

Exercise rehabilitation therapy, weight loss, and smoking cessation are often recommended. Surgical options to restore blood supply, called "revascularization" procedures, are usually reserved for those with progressive or disabling symptoms.

Dietary changes that may be helpful

Important dietary changes for preventing atherosclerosis (and, consequently, intermittent claudication) include avoiding meat and dairy fat, increasing **fiber** (page 512), and possibly avoiding foods containing trans fatty acids.

Lifestyle changes that may be helpful

Smoking is directly linked to intermittent claudication.[1, 2] People who have intermittent claudication or wish to prevent it should not smoke.

Although exercise may be helpful in the treatment of intermittent claudication, it is important for all people with this condition to consult a healthcare practitioner before beginning an exercise program.[3, 4]

Nutritional supplements that may be helpful

Inositol hexaniacinate (page 537) (IHN), a special form of vitamin B_3, has been used successfully to treat intermittent claudication. The alleged advantage of IHN over niacin (another form of vitamin B_3) is a lower risk of toxicity. A double-blind trial explored the effect of 2 grams of IHN taken twice per day for three months.[5] In nonsmokers and in people with unchanged smoking habits, the increase in walking distance was significantly greater in the IHN group than in the placebo group. Other double-blind research has confirmed IHN's ability to improve symptoms of intermittent claudication compared with placebo.[6] This treatment should be monitored by a doctor.

In double-blind trials, supplementation with either **L-carnitine** (page 543) and propionyl-L-carnitine (a form of L-carnitine) has increased walking distance in people with intermittent claudication. Walking distance was 75% greater after three weeks of L-carnitine supplementation (2 grams taken twice per day), than after supplementation with a placebo, a statistically significant difference.[7] In the study using propionyl-L-carnitine, improvement occurred only in those who could not walk 250 meters to begin with. In that group, maximum walking distance increased by 78% with propionyl-L-carnitine supplementation compared with a 44% increase in the placebo group, also a statistically significant difference.[8] The amount of propionyl-L-carnitine used was 1 gram per day, increasing to 2 grams per day after two months, and 3 grams per day after an additional two months, if needed. The results of this trial have been confirmed in a large European trial.[9]

Policosanol (page 571), taken in the amount of 10 mg twice a day for at least six months, increases pain-free walking capacity by over 50% in people with intermittent claudication according to two double-blind trials.[10, 11] When policosanol was taken continuously for two years, walking capacity more than doubled.[12] This effect may be related to the ability of policosanol to reduce the stickiness of platelets,[13, 14, 15] which could result in improved circulation.

Vitamin E (page 609) supplementation has been shown in controlled trials to increase both walking distance and blood flow through arteries of the lower legs in people with intermittent claudication.[16, 17] Increasing dietary intake of vitamin E was also associated with better blood flow to the legs.[18] Some early studies did not find vitamin E useful. Possibly this failure was due to the short duration of the studies,[19] as one review article suggested that a minimum of four to six months of vitamin E supplementation may be necessary before significant improvement is seen.[20] Most clinical trials of vitamin E and intermittent claudication used 400 to 600 IU per day, although one study used 2,400 IU per day.

Intravenous injections of the amino acid **arginine** (page 467) have been shown to be remarkably effective at improving intermittent claudication. In a double-blind trial, 8 grams of arginine, injected twice daily for three weeks, improved pain-free walking distance by 230% and absolute walking distance by 155%, compared to no improvement with placebo.[21] To date, no trials have examined the effects of oral arginine supplementation on intermittent claudication.

Magnesium (page 551) may increase blood flow by helping to dilate blood vessels. A preliminary trial found that magnesium supplementation may increase walking distance in people with intermittent claudication.[22] Many doctors suggest that people with **atherosclerosis** (page 38), including those with intermittent claudication, take approximately 250 to 400 mg of magnesium per day.

In a preliminary trial, supplementing with **evening primrose oil** (page 511) (approximately 1,600 mg per day) led to a 10% increase in exercise tolerance in people with intermittent claudication.[23]

Caution: One study showed a slightly increased risk of vascular surgery among people with intermittent claudication who took **beta-carotene** (page 469) supplements.[24] Until more is known, people with intermittent claudication wishing to use beta-carotene supplements should first consult with their doctor.

Are there any side effects or interactions?
Refer to the individual supplement for information about any side effects or interactions.

Herbs that may be helpful

Extensive studies have been done with *Ginkgo biloba* (page 681) extracts (GBE) for treatment of intermittent claudication.[25, 26] Two double-blind trials found that 120 mg of GBE per day increased pain-free and total walking distance among people with intermittent claudication.[27, 28] Similar results were seen in another double-blind trial using 160 mg of GBE per day.[29] In yet another double-blind trial, two doses of ginkgo extract were compared for six months.[30] The researchers studied 60 vs. 120 mg twice daily and found that, while both amounts resulted in significant improvements in pain-free walking distance, the improvements were more pronounced at the higher dose.

A standardized extract of **garlic** (page 679) has been tested as a treatment for intermittent claudication. In a double-blind trial, the increase in walking distance was significantly greater in people receiving garlic powder extract (400 mg twice per day for 12 weeks) than in those given a placebo.[31]

In a double-blind trial, people with intermittent claudication received 760 mg twice daily of the Tibetan herbal formula Padma 28 or a placebo for 16 weeks. The average walking distance increased by 115% among people receiving Padma 28, compared with a 17% increase in the placebo group (a statistically significant difference). No side effects were reported.[32] Padma 28 was also found to increase walking distance in a second study.[33]

Are there any side effects or interactions?
Refer to the individual herb for information about any side effects or interactions.

IRON-DEFICIENCY ANEMIA

What do I need to know?

Self-care for iron-deficiency anemia can be approached in a number of ways—but it can be hard to know just where to start. To make it easier, our doctors recommend trying these simple steps first:

Find the cause
> Iron deficiency can have many non-nutritional causes, including some serious diseases, so work with your healthcare provider to investigate why you are low in iron

Take iron as directed
> Follow your doctor's instructions for using iron supplements

Know your iron level
> To avoid possible problems related to iron overload, have your blood tested regularly for both high and low iron while you are taking iron supplements

Don't mix iron with beverage breaks
> Drinking coffee or tea with iron supplements inhibits iron absorption

Get your vitamin C
> Eating vitamin C–rich foods with meals and taking 100 to 500 mg of vitamin C with iron supplements will improve your iron absorption

About iron-deficiency anemia

Anemia is a reduction in the number of red blood cells (RBCs); in the amount of hemoglobin in the blood (hemoglobin is the iron-containing pigment of the red blood cells that carry oxygen from the lungs to the tissues); and in another related index called hematocrit (the volume of RBCs after they have been spun in a centrifuge). All three values are measured on a complete blood count, also referred to as a CBC. Iron-deficiency anemia can be distinguished from most other forms of anemia by the fact that it causes RBCs to be abnormally small and pale, an observation easily appreciated by viewing a blood sample through a microscope.

Iron deficiency also can occur, even if someone is not anemic. Symptoms of iron deficiency without anemia may include fatigue, mood changes, and decreased cognitive function. Blood tests (such as serum ferritin, which measures the body's iron stores) are available to detect iron deficiency, with or without anemia.

Iron deficiency, whether it is severe enough to lead to anemia or not, can have many non-nutritional causes (such as **excessive menstrual bleeding** [page 314], bleeding **ulcers** [page 349], **hemorrhoids** [page 219], gastrointestinal bleeding caused by aspirin or related drugs, frequent blood donations, or **colon cancer** [page 123]) or can be caused by a lack of dietary **iron** (page 540). Menstrual bleeding is probably the leading cause of iron deficiency. However, despite common beliefs to the contrary, only about one premenopausal woman in ten is iron deficient.[1] Deficiency of **vitamin B12** (page 601), **folic acid** (page 520), **vitamin B6** (page 600), or **copper** (page 499) can cause other forms of anemia, and there are many other causes of anemia that are unrelated to nutrition. This article will only cover iron-deficiency anemia.

CHECKLIST FOR IRON-DEFICIENCY ANEMIA		
Rating	Nutritional Supplements	Herbs
★★★	**Iron** (page 540) **Liver extracts** (page 547)	
★★☆	**Taurine** (page 590) **Vitamin A** (page 595) (as an adjunct to supplemental iron) **Vitamin C** (page 604) (as an adjunct to supplemental iron)	
★☆☆	**Betaine HCl** (page 473) (as an adjunct to supplemental iron)	

What are the symptoms of iron-deficiency anemia?

Some common symptoms of anemia include fatigue, lethargy, weakness, poor concentration, and impaired **immune function** (page 255). In iron-deficiency, fatigue also occurs because **iron** (page 540) is needed to make optimal amounts of ATP—the energy source the body runs on. This fatigue usually begins long *before* a person is anemic. Said another way, a lack of anemia does not rule out iron deficiency in tired people. Another symptom of anemia, called pica, is the desire to eat unusual things, such as ice, clay, cardboard, paint, or starch. Advanced anemia may also result in lightheadedness, headaches, ringing in the ears (**tinnitus** [page 430]), irritability, pale skin, unpleasant sensations in the legs with an uncontrollable urge to move them (**restless legs syndrome** [page 384]), and getting winded easily.

Medical treatments

Over the counter products focus on replacing iron. Common forms of iron include ferrous sulfate (Feosol, Fer-In-Sol, Slow Fe), ferrous fumarate (Femiron, Feostat), ferrous gluconate (Fergon), and polysaccharide-iron complex (Niferex, Nu-Iron).

Injectable iron (InFeD, DexFerrum) is available with a prescription, and may be administered to those who cannot tolerate the oral forms.

Dietary changes that may be helpful

Iron deficiency is not usually caused by a lack of dietary iron alone. Nonetheless, a lack of iron in the diet is often part of the problem, so ensuring an adequate supply of iron is important for people with a documented deficiency. The most absorbable form of iron, called "heme" iron, is found in meat, poultry, and fish. Non-heme iron is also found in these foods, as well as in dried fruit, molasses, leafy green vegetables, wine, and most iron supplements. Acidic foods (such as tomato sauce) cooked in an iron pan can leech iron into the food and thus also be a source of dietary iron.

Vegetarians eat less iron than non-vegetarians, and the iron they eat is somewhat less absorbable. As a result, vegetarians are more likely to have reduced iron stores.[2] Vegetarians can increase their iron intake by emphasizing iron-containing foods within their diet (see above), or in some cases by supplementing iron, if needed.

Coffee interferes with the absorption of **iron** (page 540).[3] However, moderate intake of coffee (4 cups per day) may not adversely affect risk of iron-deficiency anemia when the diet contains adequate amounts of iron and **vitamin C** (page 604).[4] Black tea contains tannins that strongly inhibit the absorption of non-heme iron. In fact, this iron-blocking effect is so effective that drinking black tea can help treat hemochromatosis, a disease of iron overload.[5] Consequently, people who are iron deficient should avoid drinking tea.

Fiber (page 512) is another dietary component that can reduce the absorption of iron from foods. Foods high in bran fiber can reduce the absorption of iron from foods consumed at the same meal by half.[6] Therefore, it makes sense for people needing to take iron supplements to avoid doing so at mealtime if the meal contains significant amounts of fiber.

Nutritional supplements that may be helpful

Before iron deficiency can be treated, it must be diagnosed and the cause must be found by a doctor. In addition to addressing the cause (e.g., avoiding aspirin, treating a bleeding **ulcer** (page 349), etc.), supplementation with iron is the primary way to resolve iron-deficiency anemia.

If a doctor diagnoses iron deficiency, **iron** (page 540) supplementation is essential. Though some doctors use higher amounts, a common daily dose for adults is 100 mg per day. Even though symptoms of deficiency should disappear much sooner, iron deficient people usually need to keep supplementing with iron for six months to one year until the ferritin test is completely normal. Even after taking enough iron to overcome the deficiency, some people with recurrent iron deficiency—particularly some premenopausal women—need to continue to supplement with smaller levels of iron, such as the 18 mg present in most **multivitamin-mineral supplements** (page 559). This need for continual iron supplementation even after deficiency has been overcome should be determined by a doctor.

Liver extracts (page 547) from beef are a rich natural source of many vitamins and minerals, including iron. Bovine liver extracts provide the most absorbable form of iron—heme iron—as well as other nutrients critical in building blood, including **vitamin B$_{12}$** (page 601) and **folic acid** (page 520). Liver extracts can contain as much as 3–4 mg of heme iron per gram.

Taking **vitamin A** (page 595) and iron together has been reported to help overcome iron deficiency more effectively than iron supplements alone.[7] Although the optimal amount of vitamin A needed to help people with iron deficiency has yet to be established, some doctors recommend 10,000 IU per day.

Vitamin C (page 604) increases the absorption of non-heme iron.[8] Some doctors advise iron-deficient people to take vitamin C (typically 100–500 mg) at the same time as their iron supplement.[9]

Hydrochloric acid produced by the stomach improves the absorption of non-heme iron from food and supplements.[10, 11] Some practitioners recommend a hydrochloric acid supplement (e.g., **betaine hydrochloride** [page 473] [betaine HCl]), to enhance iron absorption in people with iron-deficiency anemia.

A high degree of association between iron-deficiency anemia and **vitamin D** (page 607) deficiency in Asian children has been previously reported.[12] In three different ethnic groups living in England, iron-deficiency anemia was found to be a significant risk factor for low vitamin D levels in children.[13] These findings suggest that children with iron-deficiency anemia should be screened for vitamin D deficiency and be given vitamin D supplements if necessary.

Taurine has been shown, in a double-blind study, to improve the response to iron therapy in young women with iron-deficiency anemia.[14] The amount of taurine used was 1,000 mg per day for 20 weeks, given in addition to iron therapy, but at a different time of the day. The mechanism by which taurine improves iron utilization is not known.

Caution: People who are not diagnosed with iron deficiency should not supplement with iron, because taking iron when it isn't needed has no benefit and may do some harm. Adult iron supplements are the most common cause of fatal poisonings in children. Keep all iron supplements out of the reach of children.

Are there any side effects or interactions?
Refer to the individual supplement for information about any side effects or interactions.

IRRITABLE BOWEL SYNDROME

What do I need to know?

Self-care for irritable bowel syndrome can be approached in a number of ways—but it can be hard to know just where to start. To make it easier, our doctors recommend trying these simple steps first:

Avoid problem foods
> Experiment with limiting dairy products and beans, as well as foods containing caffeine, fructose, or sorbitol, to see which restrictions may help reduce your symptoms

Explore food sensitivities
> Work with a qualified professional to identify other foods that aggravate your condition

Find the right fiber

Try different fiber sources, including high-fiber foods such as flaxseed, rye, brown rice, oatmeal, barley, and vegetables, as well as bulk-forming laxatives like psyllium husk and methylcellulose, to find the right balance of regularity without episodes of diarrhea

Try peppermint and caraway oils

Taking a coated product providing 0.2 to 0.4 ml of peppermint oil, preferably combined with 50 mg of caraway oil, three times a day may reduce gas production, ease intestinal cramping, and soothe the intestinal tract

Reduce stress

Managing stress and trying relaxation techniques can help improve IBS symptoms

About IBS

Irritable bowel syndrome (IBS) is a common gastrointestinal disorder that sometimes causes significant discomfort even though it is not a serious health threat.

The cause of IBS remains unknown. IBS is not related to inflammatory bowel diseases, such as **Crohn's disease** (page 141) or **ulcerative colitis** (page 433).

Rating	Nutritional Supplements	Herbs
CHECKLIST FOR IRRITABLE BOWEL SYNDROME		
★★★	**Lactase** (page 545) (for **lactose intolerant** [page 288] people)	**Caraway** (page 651) oil (combined with **peppermint** [page 726] oil) **Psyllium** (page 732)
★★☆		Chinese herbal combination formula containing **wormwood** (page 762), **ginger** (page 680), **bupleurum** (page 647), **schisandra** (page 744), dan shen, and other extracts **Peppermint** (page 726) oil
★☆☆	**Evening primrose oil** (page 511) (for premenstrual IBS) **Fiber** (page 512) (other than wheat) **Grapefruit seed extract** (page 532)	**Artichoke** (page 628) **Chamomile** (page 656) **Fennel** (page 676)

What are the symptoms of IBS?

Typical symptoms include abdominal bloating and soreness, gas, and alternating **diarrhea** (page 163) and **constipation** (page 137). People with IBS are more likely than others to have **backaches** (page 293), fatigue, and several other seemingly unrelated problems.

Medical treatments

Over the counter **fiber** (page 512) supplements or laxatives may be used to treat **constipation** (page 137). These products are best divided into fast- and slow-acting agents. Rapid relief of constipation is achieved with suppositories containing bisacodyl (Dulcolax) or glycerin (Fleet), enemas, and magnesium-containing products (Phillips' Milk of Magnesia, Magnesium Citrate Solution). Overnight relief is obtained with senna (Senokot, Fletcher's Castoria) and bisacodyl (Dulcolax) tablets. Bulk-forming laxatives containing **psyllium** (page 732) (Metamucil, Konsyl-D), polycarbophil (Fibercon), and methylcellulose (Citrucel), as well as the stool softener docusate (Colace, Surfak), may require up to 72 hours before relief is observed. The antidiarrheal product loperamide (Imodium A-D) may be used to treat episodes of **diarrhea** (page 163).

Though no prescription medications specifically treat irritable bowel syndrome (IBS), antidepressant and anti-anxiety drugs may be used for people with mental **depression** (page 145) or chronic **pain** (page 338), or for people who have symptoms that worsen during periods of stress. The anticholinergic drug L-hyoscyamine (Levsin, Levbid) may be used to treat colon muscle spasms and abdominal soreness.

A common treatment for IBS includes limiting the intake of dairy products and beans, as well as foods containing caffeine, fructose, or sorbitol. Concentrated amounts of fructose are found in dried fruit and fruit juice. Sorbitol is found primarily in dietetic foods, where it is used instead of sugar (sucrose). No conventional treatments of IBS have been proven to be effective in controlled trials.

Dietary changes that may be helpful

Several trials report that **food sensitivities** (page 14) occur in only a small percentage of people with IBS.[1, 2, 3] However, a leading researcher in the field claims at least 3.5 ounces of the offending food need to be consumed at frequent intervals to provoke IBS symptoms,[4] and the amount of test foods used in these studies was generally less than this amount. Therefore, inadequate quantities of food may have affected the outcomes of these trials. Other trials have reported that *most* IBS sufferers have food sensitivities, and that gas production and IBS symptoms diminish when the offending foods are discovered and avoided.[5, 6, 7, 8] Some researchers report that problem foods need to be eaten at every meal for at least two days to evaluate the potential of food sensitivity.[9]

Researchers have found that standard blood tests used to evaluate **allergies** (page 14) may not uncover food sensitivities associated with IBS, because IBS food sensitivities may not be true allergies.[10, 11] The only practical way to evaluate which foods might trigger IBS symptoms is to avoid the foods and then reintroduce them. Such a procedure requires the guidance of a healthcare practitioner. Attempts to find and avoid problem foods without professional help may fail and may aggravate symptoms.

Preliminary evidence suggests that some people with IBS have greater trouble absorbing the sugars lactose (as found in milk), fructose (as found in high concentration in fruit juice and dried fruit), and sorbitol (as found in some dietetic candy) than do healthy people.[12] In this report, restricting intake of these sugars led to reduction in symptoms in 40% of people with IBS.

Limited research has suggested that **fiber** (page 512) might help people with IBS.[13, 14] However, most studies find that IBS sufferers do not benefit by adding wheat bran to their diets,[15, 16, 17, 18] and some people feel worse as a result of wheat bran supplementation.[19] The lack of positive response to wheat bran may result from a wheat sensitivity,[20] which is one of the most common triggers for food sensitivity in people with IBS.[21] Rye, brown rice, oatmeal, barley, vegetables, and **psyllium** (page 732) husk are good sources of fiber and are less likely to trigger food sensitivities than is wheat bran. Except for psyllium, little is known about the effects of these other fibers in people with IBS.

Nutritional supplements that may be helpful

Double-blind research has shown that avoidance of lactose (present in milk and some other dairy products) by people with IBS who are also **lactose intolerant** (page 288) will relieve IBS symptoms.[22] Alternatively, **lactase** (page 545) enzyme may be used prior to consuming milk. Several different lactase products are commercially available and the amount needed depends on the specific preparation being used.

In one trial, women with IBS who experienced worsening symptoms before and during their menstrual period were helped by taking enough **evening primrose oil** (page 511) (EPO) to provide 360–400 mg of gamma linolenic acid (GLA) per day.[23] In that trial more than half reported improvement with EPO, but none was helped in the placebo group. The effects of EPO in other groups of IBS sufferers have not been explored.

A preliminary trial investigated the effectiveness of **grapefruit seed extract** (page 532) in people with **eczema** (page 177) and symptoms of IBS.[24] Participants received either 2 drops of a 0.5% oral solution of grapefruit seed extract twice daily or 150 mg of encapsulated grapefruit seed extract three times daily. After a month, IBS symptoms had improved in 20% of those taking the liquid, while all of the patients taking capsules noted definite improvement of constipation, flatulence, abdominal discomfort, and night rest. These results need confirmation in double-blind trials.

Are there any side effects or interactions?
Refer to the individual supplement for information about any side effects or interactions.

Herbs that may be helpful

Some people with IBS may benefit from bulk-forming laxatives. **Psyllium** (page 732) seeds (3.25 grams taken three times per day) have helped regulate normal bowel activity in some people with IBS.[25] Psyllium has improved IBS symptoms in double-blind trials.[26, 27]

In the intestinal tract, **peppermint** (page 726) oil reduces gas production, eases intestinal cramping, and soothes irritation.[28] Peppermint oil has been reported to help relieve symptoms of IBS in two analyses of controlled trials.[29, 30] Evidence supporting the use of peppermint oil has come from double-blind trials that typically have used enteric-coated capsules that supply 0.2–0.4 ml of peppermint oil taken three times per day.[31, 32, 33] Some trials have found peppermint oil ineffective.[34, 35] The reason for these conflicting findings remains unclear.

The combination of 90 mg of peppermint oil plus 50 mg of **caraway** (page 651) oil in enteric-coated capsules taken three times per day led to significant reduction in IBS symptoms in a double-blind trial.[36] In a similar trial, capsules that were not enteric-coated were as effective as enteric-coated capsules.[37] The same combination has compared favorably to the drug cisapride (Propulsid) in reducing symptoms of IBS.[38] The purpose of enteric coating is to protect peppermint oil while it is passing through the acid environment of the stomach.

Whole peppermint leaf is often used either alone or in combination with other herbs to treat abdominal discomfort and mild cramping that accompany IBS. The combination of peppermint, caraway seeds, **fennel** (page 676) seeds, and **wormwood** (page 762) was reported to be an effective treatment for upper abdominal complaints in a double-blind trial.[39]

In a preliminary study of people with irritable bowel syndrome who took an **artichoke** (page 628) leaf extract daily for two months, 26% reported an improvement in symptoms.[40] Because no placebo group was used in this study and because irritable bowel syndrome has a high rate of response to placebo, additional research is needed to confirm this report. The amount of artichoke leaf used in the study was 320 or 640 mg per day of a 1:5 standardized extract.

Chamomile's (page 656) essential oils have eased intestinal cramping and irritation in animals.[41] Chamomile is sometimes used by herbalists to relieve alternating bouts of **diarrhea** (page 163) and **constipation** (page 137), though research has yet to investigate these effects. This herb is typically taken three times per day, between meals, in a tea form by dissolving 2–3 grams of powdered chamomile or by adding 3–5 ml of herbal extract tincture to hot water.

A standardized Chinese herbal combination containing extracts from 20 plants (including wormwood *(Artemisia absinthium)*, **ginger** (page 680), **bupleurum** (page 647), **schisandra** (page 744), and dan shen *(Salvia miltiorrhiza)* reduced IBS symptoms.[42] In that double-blind trial, people were given five capsules of the herbal combination three times per day.

Are there any side effects or interactions?
Refer to the individual herb for information about any side effects or interactions.

Holistic approaches that may be helpful

IBS sufferers have increased sensitivity to rectal pain that has been linked to psychological factors.[43] Stress is known to increase symptoms of IBS.[44] Reducing stress or practicing stress management skills have been reported to be beneficial. In one trial, psychotherapy and relaxation combined with conventional treatment were more effective than conventional treatment alone in two-thirds of people with IBS.[45] Hypnosis for relaxation has dramatically and consistently relieved symptoms of IBS in some people.[46, 47, 48]

Traditional Chinese Medicine (TCM), which uses acupuncture and Chinese herbal therapies, has been reported to be helpful in the treatment of IBS,[49] although no formal research has evaluated this claim.

JET LAG

Jet lag is a disturbance of the sleep-wake cycle triggered by travel across time zones.

CHECKLIST FOR JET LAG		
Rating	Nutritional Supplements	Herbs
★★☆	Melatonin (page 555)	

What are the symptoms of jet lag?

Jet lag causes a combination of symptoms, including daytime sleepiness, disorientation, poor concentration, fatigue, gastrointestinal discomfort, headaches, **difficulty falling asleep** (page 270), and frequent waking from sleep. The symptoms can last from a day to a week or longer, depending on the person and the number of time zones crossed.

Medical treatments

Doctors usually recommend one to two days of rest or light activity upon arrival to allow for adjustment to the new time zone. Eating and sleeping patterns should be gradually shifted to fit the local time schedule during this period. In addition, medication schedules used for treating health conditions may need to be based on elapsed time rather than a specific time of day dosing.

Nutritional supplements that may be helpful

Melatonin (page 555) is a natural hormone that regulates the human biological clock and may be helpful in relieving symptoms of jet lag, according to some,[1, 2] though not all,[3, 4] double-blind studies. One double-blind trial, involving international flight crew members, found that melatonin supplementation was helpful when started after arriving at the destination but not when started three days before leaving.[5] Another double-blind study compared various amounts and forms of melatonin taken at bedtime for four days after the flight by people who traveled through six to eight time zones.[6] Fast-release melatonin supplements were found to be more effective than the controlled-release supplements. A 5 mg and 0.5 mg fast-release melatonin were almost equally effective for improving sleep quality, time it took to fall asleep, and daytime sleepiness.

Are there any side effects or interactions?
Refer to the individual supplement for information about any side effects or interactions.

KIDNEY STONES

What do I need to know?

Self-care for kidney stones can be approached in a number of ways—but it can be hard to know just where to start. To make it easier, our doctors recommend trying these simple steps first:

Drink plenty of fluids
Water, lemonade, and most fruit juices can help dilute the substances in the urine that form kidney stones; avoid grapefruit juice and soft drinks

Don't eat too much animal protein
Diets high in animal protein are linked to increased calcium in the urine

Avoid oxalate (organic acid in some foods that can help stones form)
Limit your intake of spinach, rhubarb, beet greens, nuts, chocolate, tea, bran, almonds, peanuts, and strawberries, which appear to significantly increase urinary oxalate levels

Try potassium
Potassium is linked with reduced risk of kidney stones, so eat plenty of fruits and vegetables

Protect yourself with vitamin B_6 and magnesium
Taking 50 mg a day of vitamin B_6 with 200 to 400 mg a day of magnesium (in the form of magnesium citrate) can inhibit stone formation

Check out calcium
If your healthcare provider has determined that you do not over-absorb calcium, take 800 mg a day of calcium (in the form of calcium citrate or calcium citrate-malate) with meals

About kidney stones

Kidney stones are hard masses that can grow from crystals forming within the kidneys. Doctors call kidney stones "renal calculi," and the condition of having such stones "nephrolithiasis."

Most kidney stones are made of calcium oxalate. People with a history of kidney stone formation should talk with their doctor to learn what type of stones they have—approximately one stone in three is made of something other than calcium oxalate and one in five

contains little if any **calcium** (page 483) in any form. Calcium oxalate stone formation is rare in primitive societies, suggesting that this condition is preventable.[1] People who have formed a calcium oxalate stone are at high risk of forming another kidney stone.

Caution: The information included in this article pertains to prevention of calcium oxalate kidney stone recurrence only—not to other kidney stones or to the treatment of acute disease. The term "kidney stone" will refer only to calcium oxalate stones. However, information regarding how natural substances affect urinary levels of calcium may also be important for people with a history of calcium phosphate stones.

Rating	Nutritional Supplements	Herbs
★★★	**Magnesium citrate** (page 551) and **Potassium citrate** (page 572) (in combination)	
★★☆	**IP-6** (page 539)	
★☆☆	**Calcium** (page 483) (for people who are not hyperabsorbers of calcium) **Chondroitin sulfate** (page 492) **Fiber** (page 512) Lemonade **Vitamin B_6** (page 600) **Vitamin E** (page 609)	**Pumpkin seeds** (page 733)

CHECKLIST FOR CALCIUM OXALATE KIDNEY STONES

What are the symptoms of kidney stones?

Kidney stones often cause severe back or flank **pain** (page 338), which may radiate down to the groin region. Sometimes kidney stones are accompanied by gastrointestinal symptoms, chills, fever, and blood in urine.

Medical treatments

Over the counter nonsteroidal anti-inflammatory drugs (NSAIDs), such as aspirin (Bayer, Ecotrin, Bufferin), ibuprofen (Motrin, Advil), and naproxen (Aleve), may help provide pain relief.

Prescription strength NSAIDs, such as ibuprofen

(Motrin), naproxen (Naprosyn, Anaprox), indomethacin (Indocin), diclofenac (Voltaren), and etodolac (Lodine), might be necessary. Moderate to severe pain might require the use of narcotics combined with acetaminophen, such as codeine (Tylenol with Codeine), hydrocodone (Vicodin, Lortab), oxycodone (Percocet). The diuretic trichlormethiazide (Diurese, Niazide, Trichlorex) is sometimes prescribed to prevent calcium oxalate stone formation.

Lithotripsy, an ultrasound treatment that breaks the stones into pieces small enough to pass in the urine, has largely replaced surgery as the preferred method for stone removal.

Dietary changes that may be helpful

Increasing dietary oxalate can lead to an increase in urinary oxalate excretion. Increased urinary oxalate increases the risk of stone formation. As a result, most doctors agree that kidney stone formers should reduce their intake of oxalate from food as a way to reduce urinary oxalate.[2] Many foods contain oxalate; however, only a few—spinach, rhubarb, beet greens, nuts, chocolate, tea, bran, almonds, peanuts, and strawberries—appear to significantly increase urinary oxalate levels.[3, 4]

Increased levels of urinary calcium also increases the risk of stone formation. Consumption of animal protein from meat, dairy, poultry, or fish increases urinary calcium. Perhaps for this reason, consumption of animal protein has been linked to an increased risk of forming stones[5, 6, 7, 8] and vegetarians have been reported to be at lower risk for stone formation in some reports.[9] As a result, many researchers and some doctors believe that people with a history of kidney stone formation should restrict intake of animal foods high in protein.

In one controlled trial, contrary to expectations, after 4.5 years of follow-up, those who restricted their dietary protein actually had an *increased* risk of forming a kidney stone, compared with the control group.[10] The findings of this trial conflict with the outcomes of most preliminary studies,[11, 12] and need to be confirmed by further clinical trials.[13] Other researchers have found that a low-protein diet *reduces* the risk of forming stones.[14, 15] Although *high*-protein diets should probably be avoided by people with kidney stones, the effect of restricting dietary protein to low levels (below the RDA level of 0.8 grams per 2.2 pounds of body weight per day) remains unclear. Until more is known, it makes sense to consume a diet with a moderate amount of protein, perhaps partially limiting animal protein, but not limiting protein from vegetarian sources, such as nuts and beans.

Salt increases urinary calcium excretion in stone formers.[16, 17, 18] In theory, this should increase the risk of forming a stone. As a result, some researchers have suggested that reducing dietary salt may be a useful way to decrease the chance of forming additional stones.[19, 20] Increasing dietary salt has also affected a variety of other risk factors in ways that suggest an increased chance of kidney stone formation.[21] Some doctors recommend that people with a history of kidney stones reduce salt intake. To what extent such a dietary change would reduce the risk of stone recurrence remains unclear.

Potassium (page 572) reduces urinary calcium excretion,[22] and people who eat high amounts of dietary potassium appear to be at low risk of forming kidney stones.[23] Most kidney stone research involving potassium supplementation uses the form potassium citrate. When a group of stone formers was given 5 grams of potassium citrate three times daily in addition to their regular drug treatment for 28 months, they had a significantly lower rate of stone recurrence compared to those taking potassium for only eight months and to those taking no potassium at all.[24] Although citrate itself may lower the risk of stone recurrence (see below), in some potassium research, a significant decrease in urinary calcium occurs even in the absence of added citrate.[25] This finding suggests that increasing potassium itself may reduce the risk of kidney stone recurrence. The best way to increase potassium is to eat fruits and vegetables. The level of potassium in food is much higher than the small amounts found in supplements.

Some citrate research conducted with people who have a history of kidney stones involves supplementation with a combination of **potassium citrate** (page 572) and **magnesium citrate** (page 551). In one double-blind trial, the recurrence rate of kidney stones dropped from 64% to 13% for those receiving high amounts of both supplements.[26] In that trial, people were instructed to take six pills per day—enough potassium citrate to provide 1,600 mg of potassium and enough magnesium citrate to provide 500 mg of magnesium. Both placebo and citrate groups were also advised to restrict salt, sugar, animal protein, and foods rich in oxalate. Other trials have also shown that potassium and magnesium citrate supplementation reduces kidney stone recurrences.[27]

Citric acid (citrate) is found in many foods and may also protect against kidney stone formation.[28, 29] The best food source commonly available is citrus fruits, particularly lemons. One preliminary trial found that drinking 2 liters (approximately 2 quarts) of lemonade per day improved the quality of the urine in ways that are associated with kidney stone prevention.[30] Lemonade was far more effective in modifying these urinary parameters than orange juice. The lemonade was made by mixing 4 oz lemon juice with enough water to make 2 liters. The smallest amount of sweetener possible should be added to make the taste acceptable. Further study is necessary to determine if lemonade can prevent recurrence of kidney stones.

Drinking grapefruit juice has been linked to an increased risk of kidney stones in two large studies.[31, 32] Whether grapefruit juice actually causes kidney stone recurrence or is merely associated with something else that increases risks remains unclear; some doctors suggest that people with a history of stones should restrict grapefruit juice intake until more is known.

Bran, a rich source of insoluble **fiber** (page 512), reduces the absorption of **calcium** (page 483), which in turn causes urinary calcium to fall.[33] In one trial, risk of forming kidney stones was significantly reduced simply by adding one-half ounce of rice bran per day to the diet.[34] Oat and wheat bran are also good sources of insoluble fiber and are available in natural food stores and supermarkets. Before supplementing with bran, however, people should check with a doctor, because some people—even a few with kidney stones—don't absorb enough calcium. For those people, supplementing with bran might deprive them of much-needed calcium.

People who form kidney stones have been reported to process sugar abnormally.[35] Sugar has also been reported to increase urinary oxalate,[36] and in some reports, urinary calcium as well.[37] As a result, some doctors recommend that people who form stones avoid sugar.[38, 39] To what extent, if any, such a dietary change decreased the risk of stone recurrence has not been studied and remains unclear.

Drinking water increases the volume of urine. In the process, substances that form kidney stones are diluted, reducing the risk of kidney stone recurrence. For this reason, people with a history of kidney stones should drink at least two quarts per day. It is particularly important that people in hot climates increase their fluid intake to reduce their risk.[40]

Drinking coffee or other caffeine-containing beverages increases urinary calcium.[41] Long-term caffeine consumers are reported to have an increased risk of **osteoporosis** (page 333),[42] suggesting that the increase in urinary calcium caused by caffeine consumption may

be significant. However, coffee consists mostly of water, and increasing water consumption is known to reduce the risk of forming a kidney stone. While many doctors are concerned about the possible negative effects of caffeine consumption in people with a history of kidney stones, preliminary studies in both men[43, 44] and women[45] have found that coffee and tea consumption is actually associated with a *reduced* risk of forming a kidney stone. These reports suggest that the helpful effect of consuming more water by drinking coffee or tea may compensate for the theoretically harmful effect that caffeine has in elevating urinary calcium. Therefore, the bulk of current research suggests that it is not important for kidney stone formers to avoid coffee and tea.

The findings of some[46, 47] but not all[48] studies suggest that consumption of soft drinks may increase the risk of forming a kidney stone. The phosphoric acid found in these beverages is thought to affect calcium metabolism in ways that might increase kidney stone recurrence risk.

Nutritional supplements that may be helpful

IP-6 (page 539) (inositol hexaphosphate, also called phytic acid) reduces urinary calcium levels and may reduce the risk of forming a kidney stone.[49] In one trial, 120 mg per day of IP-6 for 15 days significantly reduced the formation of calcium oxalate crystals in the urine of people with a history of kidney stone formation.[50]

In the past, doctors have sometimes recommended that people with a history of kidney stones restrict **calcium** (page 483) intake because a higher calcium intake increases the amount of calcium in urine. However, calcium (from supplements or food) binds to oxalate in the gut before either can be absorbed, thus interfering with the absorption of oxalate. When oxalate is not absorbed, it cannot be excreted in urine. The resulting decrease in urinary oxalate actually *reduces* the risk of stone formation,[51] and the reduction in urinary oxalate appears to outweigh the increase in urinary calcium.[52] In clinical studies, people who consumed more calcium in the diet were reported to have a lower risk of forming kidney stones than people who consume less calcium.[53, 54, 55]

However, while *dietary* calcium has been linked to reduction in the risk of forming stones, calcium supplements have been associated with an *increased* risk in a large study of American nurses.[56] The researchers who conducted this trial speculate that the difference in effects between dietary and supplemental calcium resulted from differences in timing of calcium consumption. Dietary calcium is eaten with food, and so it can then block absorption of oxalates that may be present at the same meal. In the study of American nurses, however, most *supplemental* calcium was consumed apart from food.[57] Calcium taken without food will increase urinary calcium, thus increasing the risk of forming stones; but calcium taken without food cannot reduce the absorption of oxalate from food consumed at a different time. For this reason, these researchers speculate that calcium supplements were linked to *increased* risk because they were taken between meals. Thus, calcium supplements may be beneficial for many stone formers, as dietary calcium appears to be, but only if taken with meals.

When doctors recommend calcium supplements to stone formers, they often suggest 800 mg per day in the form of calcium citrate or calcium citrate malate, taken with meals. Citrate helps reduce the risk of forming a stone (see "Dietary changes that may be helpful" above).[58] Calcium citrate has been shown to increase urinary citrate in stone formers, which may act as protection against an increase in urinary calcium resulting from absorption of calcium from the supplement.[59]

Despite the fact that calcium supplementation taken with meals may be helpful for some, people with a history of kidney stone formation should not take calcium supplements without the supervision of a healthcare professional. Although the increase in urinary calcium caused by calcium supplements can be mild or even temporary,[60] some stone formers show a potentially dangerous increase in urinary calcium following calcium supplementation; this may, in turn, increase the risk of stone formation.[61] People who are "hyperabsorbers" of calcium should not take supplemental calcium until more is known. Using a protocol established years ago in the *Journal of Urology,* 24-hour urinary calcium studies conducted both with and without calcium supplementation determine which stone formers are calcium "hyperabsorbers."[62] Any healthcare practitioner can order this simple test.

Increased blood levels of vitamin D are found in some kidney stone formers, according to some,[63] but not all, research.[64] Until more is known, kidney stone formers should take **vitamin D** (page 607) supplements only after consulting a doctor.[65]

Both **magnesium** (page 551) and **vitamin B6** (page 600) are used by the body to convert oxalate into other substances. Vitamin B6 deficiency leads to an increase in kidney stones as a result of elevated urinary oxalate.[66]

Vitamin B6 is also known to reduce elevated urinary oxalate in some stone formers who are not necessarily B6 deficient.[67, 68]

Years ago, the *Merck Manual* recommended 100–200 mg of vitamin B6 and 200 mg of magnesium per day for some kidney stone formers with elevated urinary oxalate.[69] Most trials have shown that supplementing with magnesium[70, 71, 72] and/or vitamin B6[73, 74] significantly lowers the risk of forming kidney stones. Results have varied from only a slight reduction in recurrences[75] to a greater than 90% decrease in recurrences.[76]

Optimal supplemental levels of vitamin B6 and magnesium for people with kidney stones remain unknown. Some doctors advise 200–400 mg per day of magnesium. While the effective intake of vitamin B6 appears to be as low as 10–50 mg per day, certain people with elevated urinary oxalate may require much higher amounts, and therefore require medical supervision. In some cases, as much as 1,000 mg of vitamin B6 per day (a potentially toxic level) has been used successfully.[77]

Doctors who do advocate use of magnesium for people with a history of stone formation generally suggest the use of magnesium citrate because citrate itself reduces kidney stone recurrences. As with calcium supplementation, it appears important to take magnesium with meals in order for it to reduce kidney stone risks by lowering urinary oxalate.[78]

It has been suggested that people who form kidney stones should avoid **vitamin C** (page 604) supplements, because vitamin C can convert into oxalate and increase urinary oxalate.[79, 80] Initially, these concerns were questioned because the vitamin C was converted to oxalate *after* urine had left the body.[81, 82] However, newer trials have shown that as little as 1 gram of vitamin C per day can increase urinary oxalate levels in some people, even those without a history of kidney stones.[83, 84] In one case report, a young man who ingested 8 grams per day of vitamin C had a dramatic increase in urinary oxalate excretion, resulting in calcium-oxalate crystal formation and blood in the urine.[85] On the other hand, in preliminary studies performed on large populations, high intake of vitamin C was associated with no change in the risk of forming a kidney stone in women,[86] and with a reduced risk in men.[87] This research suggests that routine restriction of vitamin C to prevent stone formation is unwarranted. However, until more is known, people with a history of kidney stones should consult a doctor before taking large amounts (1 gram or more per day) of supplemental vitamin C.

Chondroitin sulfate (page 492) may play a role in reducing the risk of kidney stone formation. One trial found 60 mg per day of glycosamionoglycans significantly lowered urinary oxalate levels in stone formers.[88] Chondroitin sulfate is a type of glycosaminoglycan. A decrease in urinary oxalate levels should reduce the risk of stone formation.

In a double-blind trial, supplementation with 200 IU of synthetic **vitamin E** (page 609) per day was found to reduce several risk factors for kidney stone formation in people with elevated levels of urinary oxalate.[89]

Are there any side effects or interactions?
Refer to the individual supplement for information about any side effects or interactions.

Herbs that may be helpful

Two trials from Thailand reported that eating **pumpkin seeds** (page 733) reduces urinary risk factors for forming kidney stones.[90, 91] One of those trials, which studied the effects of pumpkin seeds on indicators of the risk of stone formation in children, used 60 mg per 2.2 pounds of body weight—the equivalent of only a fraction of an ounce per day for an adult.[92] The active constituents of pumpkin seeds responsible for this action have not been identified.

Are there any side effects or interactions?
Refer to the individual herb for information about any side effects or interactions.

LACTOSE INTOLERANCE

Lactose intolerance is the impaired ability to digest lactose (the naturally occurring sugar in milk). The enzyme **lactase** (page 545) is needed to digest lactose, and a few children and many adults do not produce sufficient lactase to digest the milk sugar. The condition is rare in infants.

Only one-third of the population worldwide retains the ability to digest lactose into adulthood. Most adults of Asian, African, Middle Eastern, and Native American descent are lactose intolerant. In addition, half of Hispanics and about 20% of Caucasians do not produce sufficient lactase as adults.[1]

A simple test for lactose intolerance is to drink at least two 8-ounce glasses of milk on an empty stomach and note any gastrointestinal symptoms that develop in the next four hours. The test should then be repeated using several ounces of cheese (which does not contain much lactose). If symptoms result from milk but not cheese, then the person probably has lactose intolerance. If symptoms occur with both milk and cheese, the person may be allergic to dairy products (very rarely can lactose intolerance be so severe that even eating cheese will cause symptoms). In addition to gastrointestinal problems, one study has reported a correlation in women between lactose intolerance and a higher risk of **depression** (page 145) and **PMS** (page 368).[2] However, this study is only preliminary and does not establish a cause-and-effect relationship.

CHECKLIST FOR LACTOSE INTOLERANCE		
Rating	**Nutritional Supplements**	**Herbs**
★★★	**Calcium** (page 483) (for preventing deficiency if dairy products are avoided only) **Lactase** (page 545)	

What are the symptoms of lactose intolerance?

In people with lactose intolerance, consuming foods containing lactose results in intestinal cramps, **gas** (page 195), and **diarrhea** (page 163).

Medical treatments

Over the counter **lactase** (page 545) (Lactaid, Dairy Ease), an enzyme that breaks down lactose, is used to either pre-treat milk or to be taken during the ingestion of dairy products.

A lactose-free diet is the most effective means of controlling the symptoms of lactose malabsorption in a person with lactase deficiency. However, some lactose-intolerant people can drink milk that has been predigested by the addition of lactase. Those individuals who must avoid dairy products should take supplemental **calcium** (page 483).

Dietary changes that may be helpful

Although symptoms of lactose intolerance are triggered by the lactose in some dairy products, few lactose-intolerant people need to avoid all dairy. Dairy products have varying levels of lactose, which affects how much lactase is required for proper digestion. Milk, ice cream, and yogurt contain significant amounts of lactose—although for complex reasons yogurt often does not trigger symptoms in lactose-intolerant people.

In addition, lactose-reduced milk is available in some supermarkets and may be used by lactose-intolerant people.

Many people with lactose maldigestion tolerate more lactose in experimental studies than in everyday life, in which their symptoms may result from other carbohydrates as well. Sucrose and the indigestible carbohydrates lactulose and fructooligosaccharides (FOS) have all been shown to produce symptoms in lactose-intolerant and milk-intolerant people.[3]

Nutritional supplements that may be helpful

Supplemental sources of the enzyme **lactase** (page 545) may be used to prevent symptoms of lactose intolerance when consuming lactose-containing dairy products. Lactase drops may be added to regular milk 24 hours before drinking to reduce lactose levels. Lactase drops, capsules, and tablets may also be taken orally, as needed, immediately before a meal that includes lactose-containing dairy products. The degree of lactose intolerance varies by individual, so a greater or lesser amount of oral lactase may be needed to eliminate symptoms of lactose intolerance.

Researchers have yet to clearly determine whether lactose-intolerant people absorb less **calcium** (page 483). As lactose-containing foods are among the best dietary sources of calcium, alternative sources of calcium (from food or supplements) are important for lactose-intolerant people. A typical amount of supplemental calcium is 1,000 mg per day.

Lactobacillus acidophilus (page 575) supplements do not appear to be effective in reducing the signs and symptoms of lactose intolerance. In a preliminary trial, people with lactose intolerance were given *Lactobacillus acidophilus* supplements twice daily for seven days, but failed to show any improvement in symptoms or laboratory measurements of lactose digestion.[4]

Are there any side effects or interactions?
Refer to the individual supplement for information about any side effects or interactions.

LEUKOPLAKIA

Leukoplakia is a common, potentially pre-cancerous disease of the mouth that involves the formation of white spots on the mucous membranes of the tongue and inside of the mouth.

Despite the increased risk associated with having leukoplakia, many people with this condition never get oral **cancer** (page 87). People with leukoplakia are typically middle-aged and older adults; men are more likely than women to develop the disease. The risk is much higher in smokers and users of smokeless tobacco than in people who do not use tobacco products of any kind. Betel nut chewers in Asia are also at high risk. People infected with **HIV** (page 239) or Epstein-Barr virus are at high risk for a particular form of this condition, called hairy leukoplakia, which requires treatment with antiviral medication. Another variation of this disease, proliferative verrucous leukoplakia, is much more likely to progress to cancer than are other forms. Genetic predisposition may be responsible for some cases of leukoplakia.[1]

CHECKLIST FOR LEUKOPLAKIA		
Rating	Nutritional Supplements	Herbs
★★★	**Beta-carotene** (page 469) **Vitamin A** (page 595)	
★★☆	**Vitamin E** (page 609)	**Green tea** (page 686)
★☆☆	**Vitamin C** (page 604)	

What are the symptoms of leukoplakia?

People with leukoplakia may notice a white patch on their tongue, gums, cheek, or roof of the mouth.

Medical treatments

Severe cases might require the use of prescription antiviral medication, such as oral acyclovir (Zovirax), famciclovir (Famvir), and zidovudine (Retrovir).

Treatment is usually directed at any underlying medical conditions.

Dietary changes that may be helpful

Some,[2, 3] but not all,[4] preliminary studies find that people who drink alcohol are more likely to have leukoplakia compared with nondrinkers. Even though it has not been proven that abstaining from alcohol aids in the healing of leukoplakia, people with this condition should, nonetheless, reduce their intake.

Preliminary reports have found that low dietary levels of **vitamin C** (page 604) and **fiber** (page 512),[5] **vitamin A** (page 595),[6] or, according to one study, many different nutrients,[7] are associated with an increased risk of leukoplakia. Except for vitamin A (see below), the effect of increasing intake of these nutrients in people with leukoplakia has not been studied.

Rare reports of leukoplakia triggered by **food allergies** (page 14) have appeared.[8] People with leukoplakia should discuss the issue of food allergies with a healthcare professional.

Lifestyle changes that may be helpful

Tobacco use of any kind greatly increases the risk of leukoplakia. People with leukoplakia must avoid all tobacco products.

Nutritional supplements that may be helpful

Beta-carotene (page 469) is the most widely used supplement in the treatment of leukoplakia. In a clinical trial of betel nut chewers with leukoplakia, supplementation with 150,000 IU of beta-carotene twice per week for six months significantly increased the remission rate compared with placebo (14.8% vs. 3.0%).[9] The effectiveness of beta-carotene for treating leukoplakia was also confirmed in a double-blind trial that used 100,000 IU per day for six months.[10] In one trial, supplementation with 33, 333 IU of beta-carotene per day, alone or combined with 50 IU of **vitamin E** (page 609), was reported not to reduce the incidence of leukoplakia.[11] These results have also been observed in smaller trials.[12, 13]

Drug therapy with a synthetic, prescription form of **vitamin A** (page 595) (known as Accutane, isotretinoin, and 13-*cis* retinoic acid) has been reported to be more effective than treatment with 50,000 IU per day of beta-carotene.[14] However, because of the potential toxicity of the vitamin A-like drug, it may be preferable to treat leukoplakia with beta-carotene, which is much safer.

Before the research on beta-carotene was published, vitamin A was used to treat leukoplakia.[15] One group of researchers reported that vitamin A (28,500 IU per day) was more effective than beta-carotene in treating people with leukoplakia.[16] Another trial found that the combination of 150,000 IU per week of beta-carotene plus 100,000 IU per week of vitamin A led to a significant increase in remission time compared to beta carotene alone in betel nut chewers.[17] Women who are or who could become pregnant should not take 100,000 IU of vitamin A per week without medical supervision.

According to a review of clinical trials, the combination of beta-carotene and **vitamin E** (page 609) has led to complete or partial remissions in six of eight trials studying people with leukoplakia.[18] In one trial, administration of 50,000 IU of beta-carotene, 1 gram of **vitamin C** (page 604), and 800 IU of vitamin E per day for nine months led to improvement in 56% of people with leukoplakia, with stronger effects in those who also stopped using tobacco and alcohol.[19] In a double-blind trial, a group of men with leukoplakia was given a combination of vitamin A (100,000 IU per week), beta-carotene approximately 67,000 IU per day), and vitamin E (80 IU per week).[20] A 38% decrease in the incidence of leukoplakia was observed after six months of treatment.

Although vitamin E has been used in successful trials in which patients are also given beta-carotene, few trials have investigated the effects of vitamin E when taken by itself. One trial used 400 IU of vitamin E two times per day.[21] After 24 weeks, 46% showed some improvement in signs or symptoms of leukoplakia or related conditions and 21% showed microscopic evidence of improvement.

Are there any side effects or interactions?

Refer to the individual supplement for information about any side effects or interactions.

Herbs that may be helpful

In a double-blind trial, people with leukoplakia took 3 grams per day of a mixture of whole **green tea** (page 686), green tea polyphenols, and green tea pigments orally and also painted the mixture of the tea on their lesions three times per day for six months.[22] Those in the green tea group had significant improvement in the healing of their lesions.

Are there any side effects or interactions?

Refer to the individual herb for information about any side effects or interactions.

LIVER CIRRHOSIS

Cirrhosis is a condition of severe damage to the liver that impairs its ability to function normally.

In the United States, the most common cause of liver cirrhosis is chronic **alcoholism** (page 12). Liver cirrhosis may also result from chronic viral infection of the liver (**hepatitis** [page 220] types B, C, and D) and a number of inherited diseases, such as **cystic fibrosis** (page 143), hemochromatosis, and **Wilson's disease** (page 453). If severe, liver cirrhosis may lead to liver

Leukoplakia

failure and death. In the Western world, liver cirrhosis is the third leading cause of death in people from ages 45 to 65 (after **cardiovascular disease** [page 98] and **cancer** [page 87]).[1] Liver cirrhosis may also cause a dangerous brain abnormality called portal-systemic encephalopathy (PSE), which may lead to coma. Another form of cirrhosis, primary biliary cirrhosis (PBC), damages the bile ducts in the liver, and occurs primarily in women over 35 years of age. The cause of PBC is not known.

CHECKLIST FOR LIVER CIRRHOSIS

Rating	Nutritional Supplements	Herbs
★★★	**SAMe** (page 583)	
★★☆	**Branched-chain amino acids** (page 479) **Fiber** (page 512) (combination of beta-glucan, inulin, pectin, and resistant starch) **L-ornithine-L-aspartate** (page 565) **Phosphatidylcholine** (page 546) **Zinc** (page 614) (for deficiency only)	**Bupleurum** (page 647) **Milk thistle** (page 710) (Silymarin) **Peony** (page 724) (white peony root)
★☆☆	Bile acids (for primary biliary cirrhosis only) **L-carnitine** (page 543) **Selenium** (page 584) **Vitamin E** (page 609)	

What are the symptoms of liver cirrhosis?

Many people with cirrhosis have no symptoms for years. Others may have weakness, loss of appetite, malaise, and weight loss. With blocked bile flow, it is common for people with cirrhosis to have jaundice, itching, and fatty yellow skin nodules. Later in the disease, there may be massive bleeding inside the throat, brain abnormalities due to accumulation of ammonia in the blood, liver failure, and death.

Medical treatments

Treatment is supportive, since cure is unlikely. Healthcare providers might recommend withdrawal of alcohol and other toxic agents, correction of nutritional deficiencies, and treatment of complications as they arise. A number of experimental drugs are being investigated for reversal of liver damage, but few have proven effec-

tive. Liver transplantation for patients with advanced disease has dramatically increased the life expectancy associated with cirrhosis.

Dietary changes that may be helpful

Adequate protein intake is essential for people with alcoholic liver cirrhosis, because this condition often results in significant protein, as well as calorie, deficiency.[2] However, people with liver cirrhosis may be unable to tolerate normal amounts of dietary protein because the cirrhotic liver is less able to detoxify ammonia, a major product of protein digestion. Ammonia toxicity contributes to PSE. The amount of protein that can be tolerated by people with cirrhosis varies considerably.[3] In these people, there is only a small margin of safety when treating protein deficiency. Extreme caution must be exercised when changing their protein intake. A doctor familiar with this disease should closely supervise any changes in dietary protein intake by people with cirrhosis.

Some people with cirrhosis and impaired bile flow (such as in **Wilson's disease** [page 453] or PBC) may have an excess amount of **copper** (page 499) accumulate in the liver.[4, 5] If laboratory tests confirm copper excess, most doctors would recommend avoiding foods rich in copper (such as chocolate, shellfish, and liver) along with medical treatment to reduce copper stores.[6]

Lifestyle changes that may be helpful

Alcoholism is the leading cause of liver cirrhosis in the Western world. Drinking too much alcohol also impairs the absorption and accelerates loss of several nutrients.[7, 8, 9] Therefore, avoidance of alcohol is strongly recommended for people with liver cirrhosis. Alcohol is directly toxic to the liver. In people with alcohol-induced liver cirrhosis, even moderate alcohol consumption increases the risk of portal hypertension, a dangerous blood pressure abnormality in the liver's circulation.[10]

Nutritional supplements that may be helpful

Large amounts of S-adenosylmethionine (**SAMe** [page 583]) may improve survival and liver function in alcoholic liver cirrhosis. A double-blind trial found that 1,200 mg of SAMe per day for two years significantly decreased the overall death rate and the need for liver transplantation in people with alcoholic liver cirrhosis, particularly in those with less advanced liver disease.[11] Preliminary trials suggest that lower amounts of SAMe (180 mg per day in one trial[12] and 800 mg per day in another[13]) may improve liver function in people with liver cirrhosis. SAMe supplementation has been shown to reverse the depletion of **glutathione** (page 531), an important antioxidant required for liver function.[14] It has also been shown to aid in the resolution of blocked bile flow (cholestasis), a common complication of liver cirrhosis.[15, 16]

In addition to protein deficiency as discussed above, liver cirrhosis is characterized by low blood levels of **branched-chain amino acids** (page 479) (BCAAs) in relation to other **amino acids** (page 465).[17] This imbalance may contribute to the development of PSE.[18] BCAA supplementation could be a way to correct this problem, as well as to provide a source of needed protein, but its effectiveness is unclear.[19] BCAAs (isoleucine, leucine, and valine) represent a good protein source for people with cirrhosis because they are less likely to induce PSE. A controlled study of protein-intolerant people with cirrhosis showed that BCAA supplementation corrected abnormal protein metabolism about as well as an equivalent amount of dietary protein without inducing PSE as frequently.[20] In a small double-blind trial, people with liver cirrhosis taking 5 grams per day of BCAAs had significant improvement in their ability to process protein.[21]

However, treatment trials using BCAAs alone or in solutions containing other amino acids in people with cirrhosis and PSE have reported conflicting results.[22, 23, 24] It may be that certain people with liver cirrhosis can benefit from supplementation with BCAAs while others cannot, for reasons that are unclear.[25] In a double-blind trial, people with liver cirrhosis and PSE received 0.24 grams per 2.2 pounds body weight (approximately 16–17 grams per day) of BCAAs for 15 days, after which most experienced significant improvement in brain function, mental status, and protein metabolism. Those who continued taking BCAAs for three months also had mild improvement in liver function tests.[26]

Therapeutic effects of oral BCAAs have also been shown in children with liver failure[27] and in adults with cirrhosis of the liver without PSE.[28] Overall, it appears that BCAA supplementation does not always help in cirrhosis, but some people with and without PSE may benefit. A qualified doctor must closely supervise such BCAA supplementation.

In a study of people with cirrhosis, supplementing with 10 grams of fermentable **fiber** (page 512) per day (containing equal parts of beta-glucan, inulin, pectin, and resistant starch) for 30 days resulted in an improve-

ment in liver function.[29] The impaired brain function that often accompanies cirrhosis of the liver (hepatic encephalopathy) also improved.

Phosphatidylcholine (page 546) (PC) breaks down scar tissue in the liver and may be able to reverse tissue changes that cause cirrhosis.[30] In animal studies, PC has been repeatedly shown to prevent or reverse the progression of alcohol-induced cirrhosis,[31, 32, 33] but this has not yet been demonstrated in humans. In a controlled trial, Czech researchers found that PC supplementation (900 mg per day for four months) improved liver function in people with cirrhosis.[34]

Alcoholic liver cirrhosis is associated with **zinc** (page 614) deficiency.[35, 36] In a double-blind trial, zinc acetate supplementation (200 mg three times daily, providing a total of 215 mg of elemental zinc per day), given to cirrhosis patients for seven days, significantly improved portal-systemic encephalopathy (PSE).[37] A second trial achieved similar results after three months of treatment.[38] People with cirrhosis sometimes have impaired taste function, and it has been suggested that zinc deficiency may be the cause of this abnormality. Although one study demonstrated that taste problems in cirrhosis are due to the disease process itself and not to zinc deficiency,[39] a double-blind trial showed that 200 mg three times per day of zinc sulfate (providing 135 mg of elemental zinc per day) for six weeks significantly improved taste function in people with alcoholic liver cirrhosis.[40] A doctor should supervise long-term supplementation of zinc in these amounts.

People with cirrhosis have decreased secretion of bile acids.[41] Supplementation with bile acids (such as ursodeoxycholic acid and tauroursodeoxycholic acid) may improve the composition of bile and delay disease progression in primary biliary cirrhosis (PBC). In one trial, people with PBC were followed for five to nine years. Those who took 13–15 mg per 2.2 pounds body weight of ursodeoxycholic acid (about 900–1200 mg) per day had improved liver function tests and significantly delayed progression to cirrhosis.[42] Several other trials have confirmed that bile acids improve liver function in people with PBC.[43, 44, 45, 46, 47] Commercial supplements of bile acids are available as ox bile concentrates. However, these ox bile preparations contain other types of bile acids than those used in PBC research. The effectiveness and appropriate amount of ox bile concentrates in the treatment of PBC is unknown.

L-ornithine-L-aspartate (page 565) (OA) is a nutritional supplement that has been investigated as a treatment for cirrhosis and hepatic encephalopathy. In a double-blind trial, participants taking 18 grams of OA for 14 days had significant improvements in liver function, mental status, and brain function.[48] Similar benefits have also been demonstrated using injections of OA.[49, 50]

L-carnitine (page 543) injections have been used to improve circulation to the liver in people with cirrhosis,[51] but trials of the oral supplement are lacking.

Vitamin E (page 609) has been shown to decrease damage in cirrhotic livers and may reduce immune abnormalities that contribute to the development of the disease.[52] However, a study reported that supplementation of 500 IU per day of vitamin E for one year failed to influence laboratory tests, liver function, survival or hospitalization rates in people with alcoholic cirrhosis.[53] Further clinical trials are needed to determine if any benefits may be expected from vitamin E supplementation in people with liver cirrhosis.

Selenium (page 584) levels have been found to be low in people with liver cirrhosis[54] and the need for **antioxidants** (page 467) has been found to be increased.[55] A small, preliminary trial suggested that 100 mcg per day of selenium may improve liver function in people with alcoholic cirrhosis.[56] Larger, double-blind trials of selenium in people with liver cirrhosis are needed.

People with primary biliary cirrhosis are at increased risk of bone loss. In a preliminary trial, supplementation with 0.5 micrograms of calcitriol (a prescription form of **vitamin D** [page 607]) twice daily for 12 months prevented a loss in bone mineral density.[57] Whether regular vitamin D might also prevent bone loss in people with PBC is unknown.

Are there any side effects or interactions?
Refer to the individual supplement for information about any side effects or interactions.

Herbs that may be helpful
The Chinese herb **bupleurum** (page 647) is an important component of the formula known as sho-saiko-to. Sho-saiko-to was shown in one preliminary trial to reduce the risk of liver cancer in people with liver cirrhosis.[58] The amount of this formula used was 2.5 grams three times daily.

One double-blind trial showed that the Chinese formula shakuyaku-kanzo-to (containing **white peony** [page 724] and licorice roots) effectively relieved muscle cramps due to cirrhosis of the liver.[59] This formula is approved by the Japanese Ministry of Health and Welfare for cirrhosis-induced muscle cramps.

An extract of **milk thistle** (page 710) *(Silybum marianum)* that is high in a flavonoid compound known as silymarin may improve liver function and increase survival in people with cirrhosis. Clinical trials have shown that silymarin (420–600 mg per day) improves liver function tests and protects liver cells against oxidative damage in people with alcohol-related liver disease.[60, 61, 62, 63] However, evidence is conflicting regarding the ability of silymarin to prolong survival of people with liver cirrhosis. In one double-blind trial, a significant increase in survival was found in people with cirrhosis who were given 140 mg of silymarin three times a day for approximately two years.[64] Positive results were also found in a 12-month controlled study of adults with diabetes and alcoholic liver cirrhosis taking the same daily amount of silymarin.[65] However, another double-blind trial found that 150 mg of silymarin three times a day for two years had no significant effect on survival among alcoholics with liver cirrhosis.[66]

For people with chronic liver disease, milk thistle extract may be taken long-term. Milk thistle extracts containing 80% silymarin are commercially available and may be taken in amounts that deliver 420 mg of silymarin per day.

Are there any side effects or interactions?
Refer to the individual herb for information about any side effects or interactions.

LOW BACK PAIN

What do I need to know?
Self-care for low back pain can be approached in a number of ways—but it can be hard to know just where to start. To make it easier, our doctors recommend trying these simple steps first:

Get a checkup
> See your healthcare provider to make sure your symptoms are not related to a medical problem

Take care of your back
> Practice good workplace and lifestyle habits, such as lifting and standing properly; learn proper exercises to reduce low back pain from a qualified instructor

See a chiropractor
> Work with a qualified practitioner to correct spinal problems that may lead to back pain and disability

Quit smoking

Smokers suffer more low back pain, probably due to reduced nutrition to spinal discs

Try proteolytic enzymes

Take 4 to 8 tablets a day of enzyme preparations containing trypsin, chymotrypsin, and/or bromelain to control inflammation

Try B vitamins

Take vitamins B$_1$ (150 mg a day), B$_6$ (150 mg a day), and B$_{12}$ (250 mcg a day) so you need less anti-inflammatory medication, and to help you prevent relapses of low back pain

Check out devil's claw

Take a concentrated extract providing 50 to 60 mg a day of harpagoside to reduce symptoms

About low back pain

The low back supports most of the body's weight, and as a result, is susceptible to pain caused by injury or other problems. Over 80% of adults experience low back pain (LBP) sometime during their life.[1] More than half will have a repeat episode.

It is often difficult to pinpoint the root of low back pain, though poor muscle tone, joint problems, and torn muscles or ligaments are common causes. A herniated or slipped disc may also cause low back pain as well as sciatica, a condition where pain travels down one or both buttocks and/or legs.

Standing or sitting for extended periods, wearing high heels, and being sedentary increase the risk of developing low back pain, as do **obesity** (page 446) and back strain due to improper lifting. Up to half of **pregnant** (page 363) women experience some low back pain.[2] Long hours spent driving a car may contribute to a herniated disc.[3] This is possibly due to the vibration caused by the car.[4]

Many people with low back pain recover without seeing a doctor or receiving treatment. Up to 90% recuperate within three to four weeks,[5] though recurrences are common,[6, 7, 8] and chronic low back pain develops in many people.[9] Low back pain is considered acute, or short-term, when it lasts for a few days up to many weeks. Chronic low back pain refers to any episode that lasts longer than three months.

While low back pain is rarely life threatening, it is still important to have chronic or recurring back pain assessed by a healthcare professional. Potentially serious causes include spinal tumor, **infection** (page 265), fracture, nerve damage, **osteoporosis** (page 333), arthritis, or pain caused by conditions found in internal organs such as the kidneys.

CHECKLIST FOR LOW BACK PAIN		
Rating	Nutritional Supplements	Herbs
★★★	**Enzymes** (page 506) (chymotrypsin, trypsin)	
★★☆	**D,L-phenylalanine** (page 568) (DLPA) **Vitamin B$_1$** (page 597), **Vitamin B$_6$** (page 600), **Vitamin B$_{12}$** (page 601) (in combination)	Colchicine (from autumn crocus) **Willow** (page 760)
★☆☆	**Bromelain** (page 481) **Enzymes** (page 506) (papain) **Vitamin C** (page 604)	**Cayenne** (page 654) (topical) **Devil's claw** (page 668) **Eucalyptus** (page 673) (topical) **Ginger** (page 680) **Peppermint** (page 726) (topical) **Turmeric** (page 753)

What are the symptoms of low back pain?

Low back pain may be a steady ache or a sharp, acute pain that is worse with movement.

Medical treatments

Over the counter nonsteroidal anti-inflammatory drugs (NSAIDs), such as aspirin (Bayer, Ecotrin, Bufferin), ibuprofen (Motrin, Advil), and naproxen (Aleve), may help provide pain relief in mild cases. Individuals with low back pain due to strained muscles might benefit from topical application of methylsalicylate (Ben-Gay, Icy Hot, Flexall Ultra Plus) or trolamine salicylate (Aspercreme, Myoflex).

Prescription strength NSAIDs, such as celecoxib (Celebrex), valdecoxib (Bextra), ibuprofen (Motrin), naproxen (Naprosyn, Anaprox), indomethacin (Indocin), diclofenac (Voltaren), and etodolac (Lodine), might be necessary. Moderate to severe pain might require the use of narcotics combined with acetaminophen, such as codeine (Tylenol with Codeine), hydrocodone (Vicodin, Lortab), and oxycodone (Percocet). Muscle relaxants, such as carisoprodol (Soma), cyclobenzaprine (Flexeril), and baclofen (Lioresal), might be prescribed.

Hot and cold application, rest, strengthening and

flexibility exercises, physical therapy, and instruction on good posture and body mechanics may be included in a conventional treatment plan. In some cases, back surgery may be recommended.

Lifestyle changes that may be helpful

Preliminary data indicate that smoking may contribute to low back pain.[10] One survey of over 29,000 people reported a significant association between smoking and low back pain.[11] Smaller people (children, women, those who weigh less) are most affected. A study involving people with herniated discs found that both current and ex-smokers are at much higher risk of developing disc disease than nonsmokers.[12] Other research reveals 18% greater disc degeneration in the lower spines of smokers compared with nonsmokers.[13] Smoking is thought to cause malnutrition of spinal discs, which in turn makes them more vulnerable to mechanical stress.[14]

One survey reported that people who drank wine healed more quickly after disc surgery in the lower back than those who abstained.[15] However, alcohol consumption may cause **cirrhosis of the liver** (page 290), **cancer** (page 87), **high blood pressure** (page 246), and **alcoholism** (page 12). As a result, many doctors never recommend alcohol even though moderate consumption has been linked to some health benefits. For those deciding whether light drinking might help with recovery from disc surgery, it is best to consult a doctor.

Regular exercise and proper lifting techniques help prevent low back problems from developing. Proper lifting involves keeping an object close to the body and avoiding bending forwarding, reaching, and twisting while lifting. Low back pain and disc degeneration are both more likely to develop among sedentary people than those who are physically active.[16] However, long-term participation in some competitive sports may contribute to spinal disc degeneration.[17]

Therapeutic exercise helps people recover from low back pain[18] and low back surgery.[19] Less clear are details about how this should be done for greatest benefit. In other words, the best type of exercise, frequency, duration, and timing of a program still need to be determined. One study reported therapeutic exercise significantly improved chronic low back pain compared to exercise performed at home without professional guidance.[20] Another trial discovered that women with chronic low back pain who began supervised back strengthening exercises at a fitness center were more consistent exercisers than those who started and continued therapeutic exercises at home.[21] Both groups experienced significant improvement in pain. However, the supervised group experienced better long-term improvement.

While heavy lifting and other strenuous labor may contribute to low back pain, one trial found that people with sedentary jobs gained more benefit from an exercise program than those who have physically hard or moderate occupations.[22] Motivational programs may also improve exercise consistency, which in turn decreases pain and disability.[23] People with low back pain who wish to embark on an exercise program should first consult with a physical therapist or other practitioner skilled in this area.

Supervised bed rest, for two to four days, coupled with appropriate physical therapy and therapeutic exercise, is often recommended by medical doctors for acute low back pain.[24] However, reviews of bed rest recommendations have concluded that bed rest is, at best, ineffective and may even delay recovery.[25, 26] It is better to try to stay active and maintain a normal daily schedule as much as possible.

General recommendations for people recuperating from low back pain include wearing low-heeled comfortable shoes, sitting in chairs with good lower back support, using work surfaces that are a comfortable height, resting one foot on a low stool if standing for long periods, and supporting the low back during long periods of driving.[27]

Nutritional supplements that may be helpful

Three double-blind trials have investigated the effects of supplementing a combination of the **enzymes** (page 506) trypsin and chymotrypsin for seven to ten days on severe low back pain with or without accompanying leg pain. Eight tablets per day were given initially in all trials, but in two trials the number of pills was reduced to four per day after two to three days. One of these trials reported small, though statistically significant improvements, for some measures in people with degenerative arthritis of the lower spine.[28] People with sciatica-type leg pain had significant improvement in several measures in one trial,[29] while another found the enzymes were not much more effective than a placebo.[30] These trials included chronic low back conditions, so their relevance to acute LBP alone may be limited.

Several animal studies and some research involving humans suggest that a synthetic version of the natural amino acid **phenylalanine** (page 568) called D-phenyl-alaline (DPA), reduces pain by decreasing the enzyme that breaks down endorphins.[31] It is less clear whether DPA may help people with LBP, though there are a small number of reports to that effect,[32] including one uncontrolled report of 27 of 37 people with LBP experiencing "good to excellent relief."[33] In a double-blind trial, University of Texas researchers found that 250 mg of DPA four times per day for four weeks was no more effective than placebo for 30 people with various types of chronic pain; 13 of these people had low back pain.[34] In a Japanese clinical trial, 4 grams of DPA per day was given to people with chronic low back pain half an hour before they received acupuncture.[35] Although not statistically significant, the results were good or excellent for 18 of the 30. The most common supplemental form of phenylalanine is **D,L-phenylalanine** (page 568) (DLPA). Doctors typically recommend 1,500–2,500 mg per day of DLPA.

A combination of **vitamin B$_1$** (page 597), **vitamin B$_6$** (page 600), and **vitamin B$_{12}$** (page 601) has proved useful for preventing a relapse of a common type of back pain linked to vertebral syndromes,[36] as well as reducing the amount of anti-inflammatory medications needed to control back pain, according to double-blind trials.[37] Typical amounts used have been 50–100 mg each of vitamins B$_1$ and B$_6$, and 250–500 mcg of vitamin B$_{12}$, all taken three times per day.[38, 39] Such high amounts of vitamin B$_6$ require supervision by a doctor.

Proteolytic enzymes (page 506), including **bromelain** (page 481), papain, trypsin, and chymotrypsin, may be helpful in healing minor injuries because they have anti-inflammatory activity and are capable of being absorbed from the gastrointestinal tract.[40, 41, 42] Several preliminary trials have reported reduced pain and swelling, and/or faster healing in people with a variety of conditions who use either bromelain[43, 44, 45] or papain.[46, 47, 48]

A preliminary report in 1964 suggested that 500–1,000 mg per day of **vitamin C** (page 604) helped many people avoid surgery for their disc-related low back pain.[49] No controlled research has been done to examine this claim further.

Are there any side effects or interactions?
Refer to the individual supplement for information about any side effects or interactions.

Herbs that may be helpful
Colchicine, a substance derived from autumn crocus, may be helpful for chronic back pain caused by a herniated disc. A review shows that colchicine has provided relief from pain, muscle spasm, and weakness associated with disc disease[50, 51] including several double-blind trials.[52] The author of these reports has suggested that 0.6 to 1.2 mg of colchicine per day leads to dramatic improvement in four out of ten cases of disc disease. In most clinical trials, colchicine is given intravenously.[53] However, the oral administration of this herb-based remedy also has had moderate effectiveness. People with low back pain should consult a physician skilled in herbal medicines before taking colchicine due to potentially severe side effects.

Willow (page 760) bark is traditionally used for pain and conditions of inflammation. According to one controlled clinical trial, use of high amounts of willow bark extract may help people with low back pain. One trial found 240 mg of salicin from a willow extract to be more effective than 120 mg of salicin or a placebo for treating exacerbations of low back pain.[54]

Topical **cayenne** (page 654) pepper has been used for centuries to reduce **pain** (page 338), and more recently, to diminish localized pain for a number of conditions,[55] including chronic pain,[56] although low back pain has not been specifically investigated. Cayenne creams typically contain 0.025–0.075% capsaicin.[57] While cayenne cream causes a burning sensation the first few times used, this decreases with each application. Pain relief is also enhanced with use as substance P, the compound that induces pain, is depleted.[58] To avoid contamination of the mouth, nose, or eyes, hands should be thoroughly washed after use or gloves should be worn. Do not apply cayenne cream to broken skin.

One double-blind trial found that **devil's claw** (page 668) capsules (containing 800 mg of a concentrated extract taken three times per day) were helpful in reducing acute low back pain in some people.[59] Another double-blind trial (using 200 mg or 400 mg of devil's claw extract three times daily) achieved similar results in some people with exacerbations of chronic low back pain.[60]

Herbalists often use **ginger** (page 680) to decrease inflammation and the pain associated with it, including for those with low back pain. They typically suggest 1.5 to 3 ml of ginger tincture three times per day, or 2 to 4 grams of the dried root powder two to three times per day. Some products contain a combination of curcumin and ginger. However, no research has investigated the effects of these herbs on low back pain.

A combination of **eucalyptus** (page 673) and **peppermint** (page 726) oil applied directly to a painful area may help. Preliminary research indicates that the counter-irritant quality of these essential oils may decrease pain and increase blood flow to afflicted regions.[61] Peppermint and eucalyptus, diluted in an oil base, are usually applied several times per day, or as needed, to control pain. Plant oils that may have similar properties are rosemary, juniper, and wintergreen.

Turmeric (page 753) is another herb known traditionally for its anti-inflammatory effects, a possible advantage for people suffering from low back pain. Several preliminary studies confirm that curcumin, one active ingredient in turmeric, may decrease inflammation in both humans[62] and animals.[63, 64] In one double-blind trial, a formula containing turmeric, other herbs, and **zinc** (page 614) significantly diminished pain for people with **osteoarthritis** (page 328).[65] Standardized extracts containing 400 to 600 mg of curcumin per tablet or capsule are typically taken three times per day. For tinctures of turmeric, 0.5 to 1.5 ml three times per day are the usual amount.

Are there any side effects or interactions?
Refer to the individual herb for information about any side effects or interactions.

Holistic approaches that may be helpful
Acupuncture may be helpful in the treatment of low back pain in some people. Case reports[66, 67] and numerous preliminary trials[68, 69, 70, 71, 72, 73, 74] have described significant improvement in both acute and chronic back pain following acupuncture (or acupuncture with electrical stimulation) treatment. In a single controlled study of acute back pain, both electroacupuncture and drug therapy (acetaminophen) led to statistically significant pain reduction and improved mobility.[75]

Several controlled clinical trials have evaluated acupuncture for chronic low back pain. A controlled trial found acupuncture was significantly superior to placebo (fake electrical stimulation through the skin) in four of five measures of pain and physical signs.[76] Controlled trials using electroacupuncture have reported either benefit[77] or no benefit[78] for chronic back pain. A double-blind trial compared acupuncture to injections of anesthetic just below the skin at non-acupuncture points, and found no difference in effect between the two treatments.[79] Controlled trials have compared acupuncture to transcutaneous nerve stimulation (TENS). Some,[80, 81] though not all,[82] demonstrated greater pain relief with acupuncture when compared to TENS, and one found improved spinal mobility only with acupuncture.[83]

In one preliminary trial, acupuncture relieved pain and diminished disability in the low back during **pregnancy** (page 363) better than physiotherapy.[84]

A recent analysis and review of studies reported acupuncture was effective for low back pain,[85] though another recent review concluded acupuncture could not be recommended due to the poor quality of the research.[86] A third review concluded that acupuncture was beneficial for people with slipped discs and sciatica and could be recommended at the very least as a supplementary therapy.[87] Since the vast majority of controlled acupuncture research addresses chronic low back pain, it remains unknown whether people with acute low back pain benefit significantly from acupuncture.[88]

The federally funded Agency for Health Care Policy and Research has deemed spinal manipulation effective for acute low back pain during the first month following injury.[89] This recommendation is supported by other research, though some has not been well controlled.[90, 91] People whose initial pain or disability is severe to moderate appear to benefit the most, though those with longer lasting or chronic pain may also be helped by spinal manipulation.[92, 93] One 12-month controlled study found no difference in benefit between manipulation and standard physical therapy.[94] Another controlled study found a series of eight treatments with spinal manipulation was as effective as conventional medical therapy, but the manipulation group needed less pain medication and physical therapy.[95] Practitioners who perform spinal manipulation include chiropractors, some osteopaths, and some physical therapists.

Some researchers suggest that spinal manipulation should not be performed on people with a herniated (slipped) disc, because it may lead to spinal cord injuries.[96] However, other preliminary trials report that spinal manipulation helps those with herniated discs,[97, 98, 99, 100] as did one controlled study comparing manipulation to standard physical therapy.[101] In one investigation of 59 people with slipped discs who received chiropractic treatment, including manipulation, 90% reported improvement.[102] Those with a history of low back surgery had poor outcomes. People with LBP due to herniated discs who wish to try this method should first consult with a chiropractor or other physician skilled in spinal manipulation. A recent controlled study compared manipulation, acupuncture, and medication for chronic spinal pain. Only manipulation significantly improved pain and disability scores.[103]

There is inconclusive evidence that massage alone helps people with low back pain, though preliminary research indicates it has potential.[104] Many practitioners use massage in combination with other physical therapies, such as spinal manipulation or therapeutic exercise. People with low back pain who want to try massage should consult with a qualified massage therapist.

Some controlled trials indicate that biofeedback benefits people with chronic low back pain,[105, 106] but other trials do not.[107, 108] One study found that biofeedback was more effective than behavioral therapy or conservative medical treatment for people with chronic back pain. The study also found biofeedback to be the only method where people experienced significant reduction in pain for up to the two years of follow-up.[109] People wishing to try biofeedback should discuss this method with a qualified practitioner.

Emotional distress has been associated with aggravating low back pain,[110] including that caused by a herniated disc.[111] The effects on back pain of counseling aimed at reducing emotional stress remain unknown, though it is used in some clinics employing multidisciplinary approaches to treating chronic lower back pain.

LUNG CANCER

See also: **Breast Cancer** (page 65), **Colon Cancer** (page 123), **Prostate Cancer** (page 371), **Cancer Prevention and Diet** (page 87)

Lung cancer is a malignancy of the lung. It is characterized by unregulated replication of cells creating tumors, with the possibility of some of the cells spreading to other sites (metastasis).

This article includes a discussion of studies that have assessed whether certain vitamins, minerals, herbs, or other dietary ingredients offered in dietary or herbal supplements may be beneficial in connection with the reduction of risk of developing lung cancer, or of signs and symptoms in people who have this condition.

This information is provided solely to aid consumers in discussing supplements with their healthcare providers. It is not advised, nor is this information intended to advocate, promote, or encourage self prescription of these supplements for cancer risk reduction or treatment. Furthermore, none of this information should be misconstrued to suggest that dietary or herbal supplements can or should be used in place of conventional anticancer approaches or treatments.

It should be noted that certain studies referenced below, indicating the potential usefulness of a particular

dietary ingredient or dietary or herbal supplement in connection with the reduction of risk of lung cancer, are preliminary evidence only. Some studies suggest an association between high blood or dietary levels of a particular dietary ingredient with a reduced risk of developing lung cancer. Even if such an association were established, this does not mean that dietary supplements containing large amounts of the dietary ingredient will necessarily have a cancer risk reduction effect.

Cancer of the lung is the leading cause of death from cancer in both men and women in the United States. Cigarette smoking is by far the most important risk factor for the development of lung cancer. Air pollution is another risk factor. A previous diagnosis of tuberculosis increases the risk of lung cancer by 5 to 10%.

CHECKLIST FOR LUNG CANCER		
Rating	**Nutritional Supplements**	**Herbs**
★★★	**Beta-carotene** (page 469) (reduces risk) **Warning:** Beta-Carotene *increases* the risk of lung cancer in smokers.	
★★☆	**Selenium** (page 584) (reduces risk) **Vitamin E** (page 609) (reduces risk)	*Coriolus versicolor*
★☆☆	**Coenzyme Q**$_{10}$ (page 496) **Folic acid** (page 520) (reduces risk) **Melatonin** (page 555) **Multivitamins** (page 559) **Vitamin A** (page 595) **Vitamin B**$_{12}$ (page 601) (reduces risk)	**Asian ginseng** (page 630) Black tea (reduces risk) Dr. Sun's soup **Green tea** (page 686) (reduces risk) Hoxsey Formula

What are the symptoms of lung cancer?

In its early stages, lung cancer usually causes no symptoms. As a result, lung cancer is generally not diagnosed until the disease is relatively advanced. At the time of diagnosis, common symptoms of lung cancer are similar to those of some other respiratory diseases: cough, blood stained sputum, wheezing, and shortness of breath. Lung cancer is sometimes diagnosed from a chest x-ray done for another condition. Pneumonia lasting more than two months may indicate the presence of lung cancer and should be followed-up with further testing. Later symptoms of lung cancer generally result from spread to other parts of the body (metastasis). These symptoms may include chest or shoulder pain, unexplained weight loss, bone pain, hoarseness, headaches, seizures and swelling of the face or neck. Lung cancer is usually a fatal disease, except for the minority of patients diagnosed at the early stages of the disease.

Medical treatments

The chemotherapeutic agents commonly used to treat lung cancer include cyclophosphamide (Cytoxan), doxorubicin (Adriamycin), and cisplatin (Platinol). Immune system therapies, including Bacillus Calmette-Guerin (BCG) and levamisole hydrochloride (Ergamisol), are also sometimes prescribed for lung cancer patients.

Early stage lung cancer is primarily treated with surgery, often accompanied by radiation and chemotherapy. In more advanced stages of the disease, chemotherapy and surgery may still be used, although the surgery is no longer likely to achieve a cure.

Dietary changes that may be helpful

The following dietary changes have been studied in connection with lung cancer.

Fruits and vegetables

Most studies suggest that as consumption of fruits and vegetables increases, risk of lung cancer decreases.[1] Several ingredients in fruits and vegetables may be responsible for this apparent protective effect.

Flavonoids (page 516) are found in virtually all fruits and vegetables. Onions and apples contain large amounts of a flavonoid called quercetin. Consumption of flavonoids in general, or quercetin-containing foods in particular, has been associated with a reduced risk of lung cancer in some preliminary reports,[2, 3] although not every study finds an association between flavonoid consumption and a reduced risk of cancer. [4]

Researchers agree that people who eat yellow and orange fruits and vegetables—good sources of alpha-carotene and **beta-carotene** (page 469)—are at lower risk for lung cancer. However, double-blind trials have shown that when nonsmokers supplement with (synthetic) beta-carotene, their risk of lung cancer is not reduced, and when smokers take (synthetic) beta-carotene supplements, their risk of lung cancer *increases*. These findings suggest that beta-carotene may not be the cause of the low lung cancer risk found in people who eat carotene-rich foods.

Tomatoes

Tomatoes contain **lycopene** (page 548)—an **antioxidant** (page 467) similar in structure to **beta-carotene** (page 469). Most lycopene in our diet comes from tomatoes, though traces of lycopene exist in other foods. Lycopene has been reported to inhibit the proliferation of cancer cells in test tube research.[5, 6]

A review of published research found that higher intake of tomatoes or higher blood levels of lycopene correlated with a reduced risk of cancer in 57 of 72 studies. Findings in 35 of these studies were statistically significant.[7] Evidence of a protective effect for tomato consumption was strongest for several cancers including lung cancer.

Avoidance of meat and saturated fat

Consumption of fried and well-done red meat was associated with an elevated risk of lung cancer in one report.[8] Consumption of red meat in general, as well as fried meat, correlated with a high risk of lung cancer in another study.[9] People who cook with fat taken from meat (such as bacon fat and lard) have also been reported to be at high risk of lung cancer according to preliminary research.[10]

Incidence of lung cancer correlates with dietary fat intake from country to country.[11] Some,[12] but not all,[13] preliminary studies report consumption of saturated fat in both meat and dairy fat correlates with the risk of lung cancer, even among nonsmokers.[14] Lung cancer risk appears directly related to consumption of foods containing saturated fat—not only from consumption of well-cooked meat.[15] In one trial that was unable to find an association between lung cancer risk and total saturated fat intake, people consuming skim milk nonetheless had a 50% reduction in risk compared with people drinking whole-fat milk.[16]

Avoidance of dietary **cholesterol** (page 239)

Dietary cholesterol comes primarily from the consumption of eggs. Most,[17, 18, 19] but not all,[20] studies have reported that as dietary cholesterol increases, so does the risk of lung cancer. No clear explanation has yet emerged to account for this association.

Fish

Fish eaters have been reported to have low risks of many cancers including lung cancer.[21] The **omega-3 fatty acids** (page 509) found in fish are thought by some researchers to be the components of fish responsible for protection against cancer.[22]

Lung Cancer

Avoidance of sugar

Preliminary studies have reported associations between an increasing intake of sugar or sugar-containing foods and an increased risk of several cancers including lung cancer.[23] Whether this association exists because sugar directly promotes cancer or because sugar consumption is only a marker for some other dietary or lifestyle factor remains unknown.

Lifestyle changes that may be helpful

The following lifestyle changes have been studied in connection with lung cancer.

Smoking

Cigarette smoking is universally acknowledged to be the leading cause of lung cancer, both in the United States and worldwide. By far the most important way to reduce the risk of lung cancer is to not smoke.[24]

Passive smoke

Many studies now show that exposure to passive smoke—the cigarette smoke from others' cigarettes—significantly increases the risk of lung cancer.[25] As non-smoking sections of restaurants have nearly the same level of smoke as do the smoking sections, it makes sense to seek restaurants that do not permit any smoking and to avoid bars unless they are also non-smoking establishments.

Other inhalant pollution

Inhalant exposure to diesel exhaust, pitch and tar, dioxin, arsenic, chromium, cadmium, and nickel compounds may also increase the risk of lung cancer.[26] Exposure to asbestos is associated with an increased risk of lung cancer.

Radon exposure has been reported to contribute to the risk of lung cancer in the general population.[27] Radon, a natural radioactive substance, can leak into basements from the surrounding soil. Radon exposure can also occur from the water system of houses, particularly when people take showers. Underground miners are also exposed to varying amounts of radioactivity from radon.

Nutritional supplements that may be helpful

The following nutritional supplements have been studied in connection with lung cancer.

Folic acid (page 520) and ***vitamin B₁₂*** (page 601)

Folic Acid and vitamin B_{12} work together in the body to help cells replicate normally. In a double-blind trial, smokers with *pre*cancerous changes in the lungs were given a placebo or the combination of 10,000 mcg of folic acid and 500 mcg of vitamin B_{12} per day for four months.[28] A significant reversal of precancerous changes occurred in those given vitamin supplements compared with those given the placebo.[29] No trials have investigated whether either vitamin given alone or the combination of both vitamins would help to treat people who already have lung cancer.

Beta-carotene (page 469)

In double-blind trials, synthetic beta-carotene supplementation has led to an increased risk of lung cancer in smokers,[30, 31] though not in groups consisting primarily of nonsmokers.[32] Smokers should avoid synthetic beta-carotene supplements, including the relatively small amounts found in many **multivitamins** (page 559).

The researchers who conducted the lung cancer trials have been criticized for not having used the natural form of beta-carotene.[33] Preliminary evidence suggests that natural beta-carotene supplementation results in better **antioxidant** (page 467) activity[34] and anticancer activity in humans[35] than does supplementation with synthetic beta-carotene. Nonetheless, much less is known about natural beta-carotene and questions remain about its potential efficacy.[36] The effect of natural beta-carotene supplementation on lung cancer risk has yet to be studied.

The strong association between increased intake of beta-carotene from food and a reduced risk of lung cancer[37] does not necessarily mean that supplementation with natural beta-carotene supplements would reduce the risk of lung cancer. Dietary beta-carotene may be a marker for diets high in certain fruits and vegetables that contain other anticancer substances that may be responsible for the protective effects. Until more is known, some doctors advise smokers to avoid all forms of beta-carotene supplementation—even natural beta-carotene.

Selenium (page 584)

Selenium has been reported to have diverse anticancer actions.[38, 39] Selenium inhibits cancer growth in animals.[40] Low soil levels of selenium (probably associated with low dietary intake), have been associated with increased cancer incidence in humans.[41] Blood levels of selenium have been reported to be low in patients with many cancers,[42, 43, 44, 45, 46, 47, 48, 49] including lung cancer.[50] In preliminary reports, people with the lowest blood levels of selenium had between 3.8 and 5.8 times the risk of dying from cancer compared with those who had the highest selenium levels.[51, 52]

The strongest evidence supporting the anticancer effects of selenium supplementation comes from a double-blind trial of 1,312 Americans with a history of skin cancer who were treated with 200 mcg of yeast-based selenium per day or a placebo for 4.5 years and then followed for an additional two years.[53] Although no decrease in *skin* cancers occurred, a 50% reduction in overall cancer deaths and a 37% reduction in total cancer incidence was observed. A 46% decrease in lung cancer incidence and a 53% drop in deaths from lung cancer also occurred. These findings were all statistically significant.

Vitamin E (page 609)

Relatively high blood levels[54, 55] and dietary levels[56] of vitamin E have been associated with a reduced risk of lung cancer. In a preliminary trial, nonsmokers who took vitamin E supplements had a 45% lower risk of lung cancer compared with nonsmokers who did not supplement with vitamin E.[57] While a double-blind trial reported that vitamin E supplementation had no effect on lung cancer risk,[58] the amount used—approximately 50 IU per day—may have been too low to have a significant effect.

Vitamin A (page 595)

In one trial, patients with very early stage lung cancer ("stage I") were all treated with surgery and then given either 300,000 IU of vitamin A per day or no vitamin A.[59] After one year, 63% of those taking vitamin A were free of cancer compared with 52% of those not assigned to vitamin A. The average time until the reoccurrence of cancer was significantly prolonged in the vitamin A group.

However, the vast majority of lung cancer patients are diagnosed when the disease is more advanced than stage I. In a trial studying patients with more advanced disease, supplementation with 300,000 IU per day for one year followed by 150,000 IU per day for another year did not reduce lung cancer recurrences.[60] Moreover, another trial that studied smokers and workers exposed to asbestos found that daily supplementation with 25,000 IU of vitamin A plus 50,000 IU of synthetic **beta-carotene** (page 469) (which can act as a vitamin A precursor in the body) for four years led to a slight *increase* in the risk of getting lung cancer compared to no treatment.[61]

These studies suggest that vitamin A supplementation is unlikely to either prevent lung cancer or effectively treat lung cancer patients.

Melatonin (page 555)

Years ago, a preliminary study suggested that melatonin may help stabilize the condition of some people with advanced cancers.[62] Since then, Italian researchers have been investigating the effects of melatonin in cancer patients, often with partial success.[63, 64, 65, 66, 67, 68, 69, 70, 71, 72, 73, 74]

In patients with advanced lung cancer who were given 10 mg of melatonin at night in cycles of three weeks on followed by one week off, survival time was almost twice as long as survival in those not given melatonin—a statistically significant increase.[75] Melatonin supplementation was not helpful to patients whose cancer had spread to the liver.[76]

Coenzyme Q_{10} (page 496) supplementation

In an unpublished report, 4 of 11 lung cancer patients were said to be alive following ten years of supplementation with 100 mg of CoQ_{10} per day.[77] Such undocumented case reports require confirmation from published research trials.

Zinc (page 614)

Some lung cancer patients have been reported to lose excessive amounts of zinc in urine. In one trial, supplementing such patients with zinc led to an improvement in some aspects of immunity.[78] However, no trial has yet explored whether zinc supplementation would help prevent lung cancer or improve survival in patients already diagnosed with this disease.

Vitamin supplement use in general

In a preliminary trial, lung cancer patients who reported using vitamin supplements survived almost four times as long as those who did not.[79] This report did not determine which specific supplements were associated with extended survival although it is probable that many patients were using **multivitamins** (page 559). Possibly, use of supplements may have been a marker for other dietary or lifestyle factors responsible for the outcome. Nonetheless, the advantage favoring use of supplements was highly statistically significant.[80]

Are there any side effects or interactions?

Refer to the individual supplement for information about any side effects or interactions.

Herbs that may be helpful

The following herbs have been studied in connection with lung cancer.

Cloud mushroom (Coriolus versicolor)
Polysaccharopeptide (PSP) and polysaccharide krestin (PSK), both cloud mushroom extracts, have been studied in preliminary and double-blind trials and shown to be beneficial in extending the life of patients with several cancers[81, 82, 83, 84, 85] including lung cancer.[86] PSK and PSP are not available in the United States. Whether the hot water-extracted Coriolus products available in the United States are equivalent to the products used extensively in Japanese cancer research remains unknown. The amount used in most research trials is 3 grams per day.

Asian ginseng (page 630) (Panax ginseng)
Many studies of animals with cancer suggest Asian ginseng may improve **immune function** (page 255) and increase lifespan.[87] Although little is known about the effects of Asian ginseng in people already diagnosed with cancer, preliminary Chinese trials have shown increased survival or improvement of immune function in people with lung cancer already treated with chemotherapy, radiation therapy, and/or surgery.[88]

Green tea (page 686) and black tea (Camellia sinensis)
Numerous preliminary studies have shown an association between drinking green tea and a reduced risk of several types of cancer[89, 90, 91, 92] including lung cancer.[93] In contrast, preliminary studies of *black* tea consumption have not found that it protected against any type of cancer.[94, 95, 96]

Dr. Sun's Soup
The soup, develop by Alexander Sun, PhD, is prepared by heating the ingredients in water, freeze-drying them, then mixing the powder back into hot water or soup. In a preliminary trial, lung cancer patients were given 30 grams per day of Dr. Sun's Soup.[97] Dr. Sun's Soup improved quality of life and survival compared with people with lung cancer not given Dr. Sun's Soup.[98] Everyone in the trial had previously been treated with conventional therapies, including chemotherapy. More research is needed to determine the efficacy of this mixture.

Hoxsey formula
Harry Hoxsey, the son of a veterinarian, claimed to have obtained his cancer formula from his father, who in turn obtained it from his father (Harry's grandfather).[99] In all likelihood, the formula was developed by others as evidenced by the earlier appearance of an almost identical formula under other names in various medical and semi-official publications.[100] The exact ingredients of the formula were changed over time. The following ingredients are listed on a bottle of the formula from 1954 and are likely to be very similar to the formula currently in use in what is frequently called the "Hoxsey Clinic" (the Bio-Medical Center in Tijuana, Mexico).

Ingredients are listed in order from most to least amount present:

- Potassium iodide
- **Licorice** (page 702) (*Glycyrrhiza glabra*)
- **Red clover** (page 735) (*Trifolium pratense*)
- **Alder buckthorn** (page 622) (*Rhamnus frangula*)
- **Burdock** (page 648) (*Actrium lappa*)
- Stillingia root (*Stillingia sylvatica*)
- **Barberry** (page 632) root (*Berberis vulgaris*)
- Poke root (*Phytolacca decandra*)
- Cascara amarga (*Picramnia antidesma*) or **Cascara sagrada** (page 652) (*Rhamnus purshina*)
- **Prickly ash** (page 731) (*Zanthoxylum fraxineum*)

Hoxsey also used externally-applied formulas, which are discussed below under cancer salves.

One small preliminary trial found that 6 of 15 people with a variety of mostly advanced cancers who attended the Bio-Medical Center and took the Hoxsey formula claimed to be disease-free after a follow-up period of five years, including two lung cancer patients.[101] Average survival was surprisingly long, even for those who did eventually succumb to their cancers.[102] Several of these patients appeared to have had a poor chance of survival before taking the Hoxsey formula. Larger, double-blind trials are needed to confirm or contradict these findings. Until it is confirmed in other trials, the Hoxsey formula should be considered unproven.

Limited evidence suggests that some of the components of the Hoxsey formula may have anticancer activity. In animal and/or test tube research, **burdock root** (page 648),[103, 104] berberine (a constituent of **barberry** [page 632]),[105, 106] a protein found in poke root,[107, 108, 109, 110] **licorice** (page 702),[111, 112] stillingia,[113] and **red clover** (page 735),[114] have all been found to have anticancer activity. Constituents of **alder buckthorn** (page 622), **cascara** (page 652), and **prickly ash** (page 731) bark have produced mixed results in preliminary testing investigating anticancer actions.[115, 116, 117, 118]

Besides the small trial of cancer patients discussed above, no other human trials have studied the Hoxsey formula. The assertion by the American Cancer Society that the Hoxsey formula has been "extensively tested" and "found to be . . . useless"[119] is therefore false.

The original Hoxsey formula is prepared as a water extract and is available only at the Bio-Medical Center in Tijuana, Mexico.[120] Other versions of Hoxsey-like formulas are available, primarily from herbal companies that supply physicians. However, most of these are alcohol extracts (tinctures). Although these products may contain extracts from the same herbs, it is unknown whether these products have the same effects as does the original Hoxsey formula.

Cancer patients who attend the Bio-Medical Center in Mexico also are told to make several dietary changes and to take several supplements.[121] No scientific evidence supports the use of these dietary changes or supplements in the treatment of people with cancer.

Are there any side effects or interactions?
Refer to the individual herb for information about any side effects or interactions.

MACULAR DEGENERATION

Macular degeneration is the degeneration of the macula retinae, also called the macula lutea, an oval disc on the retina in the back of the eye.

Degeneration of the macula retinae is the leading cause of blindness in elderly Americans.[1]

CHECKLIST FOR MACULAR DEGENERATION

Rating	Nutritional Supplements	Herbs
★★☆	**Lutein** (page 548) and zeaxanthin **Multivitamin-multimineral** (page 559) **Zinc** (page 614)	*Ginkgo biloba* (page 681)
★☆☆	**Beta-carotene** (page 469) **Carotenes** (page 488) (prevention) (**lutein** [page 548], zeaxanthin, **lycopene** [page 548]) **Selenium** (page 584) **Vitamin C** (page 604) **Vitamin E** (page 609)	Bilberry (page 634)

What are the symptoms of macular degeneration?

Macular degeneration is typically painless and includes symptoms of dark or blurry areas in the center of vision, seeing distortions of straight lines, and difficulty doing activities that require sharp vision (e.g., driving and reading). Peripheral (side) vision may remain clear.

Medical treatments

Eyeglasses are often prescribed that provide protection from the sun's ultraviolet rays. Underlying medical conditions, such as **diabetes** (page 152) and **high blood pressure** (page 246), are treated when present. In some cases, laser eye surgery may be recommended.

Dietary changes that may be helpful

In a preliminary study, high intake of saturated fat and **cholesterol** (page 223) was associated with an increased risk of developing macular degeneration.[2]

According to preliminary research, people who eat fish more than once per week have half the risk of developing age-related macular degeneration compared with people who eat fish less than once per month.[3]

Total alcohol consumption has not been linked to macular degeneration in most studies.[4, 5] However, one research group has linked beer consumption to macular degeneration,[6, 7] and in one of two trials, wine drinkers were found to have a significantly *lower* risk of macular degeneration compared with people not drinking wine.[8, 9] Most doctors consider these reports too preliminary to suggest either avoiding beer or increasing wine consumption.

Lifestyle changes that may be helpful

Smoking has been linked to macular degeneration. Quitting smoking may reduce the risk of developing macular degeneration.

Nutritional supplements that may be helpful

Lutein (page 548) and zeaxanthin are **antioxidants** (page 467) in the **carotenoid** (page 488) family. These carotenoids, found in high concentrations in spinach, collard greens, and kale, have an affinity for the part of the retina where macular degeneration occurs. Once there, they protect the retina from damage caused by sunlight.[10]

Harvard researchers reported that people eating the most lutein and zeaxanthin—an average of 5.8 mg per day—had a 57% decreased risk of macular degeneration, compared with people eating the least.[11] While spinach and kale eaters have a lower risk of macular degeneration, blood levels of lutein did not correlate with risk of macular degeneration in one trial.[12, 13] In a double-blind study of people with macular degeneration, supplementation with lutein (10 mg per day) for one year significantly improved vision, compared with a placebo.[14] Lutein was beneficial for people with both early and advanced stages of the disease. Lutein and zeaxanthin can be taken as supplements; 6 mg per day of lutein may be a useful amount.

Macular Degeneration

Sunlight triggers oxidative damage in the eye, which in turn can cause macular degeneration.[15] Animals given **antioxidants** (page 467)—which protect against oxidative damage—have a lower risk of this vision problem.[16] People with high blood levels of antioxidants also have a lower risk.[17] Those with the highest levels (top 20th percentile) of the antioxidants **selenium** (page 584), **vitamin C** (page 604), and **vitamin E** (page 609) may have a 70% lower risk of developing macular degeneration, compared with people with the lowest levels of these nutrients (bottom 20th percentile).[18] People who eat fruits and vegetables high in **beta-carotene** (page 469), another antioxidant, are also at low risk.[19] Some doctors recommend antioxidant supplements to reduce the risk of macular degeneration; reasonable adult levels include 200 mcg of selenium, 1,000 mg of vitamin C, 400 IU of vitamin E, and 25,000 IU of natural beta-carotene per day. However, a preliminary study found no association between age-related macular degeneration and intake of antioxidants, either from the diet, from supplements, or from both combined.[20] Moreover, in a double-blind study of male cigarette smokers, supplementing with vitamin E (50 IU per day), synthetic beta-carotene (about 33,000 IU per day), or both did not reduce the incidence of age-related macular degeneration.[21]

Two important enzymes in the retina that are needed for vision require **zinc** (page 614). In a double-blind trial, supplementation with 45 mg of zinc per day for one to two years significantly reduced the rate of visual loss in people with macular degeneration.[22] However, in another double-blind trial, supplementation with the same amount of zinc did not prevent vision loss among people with a particular type of macular degeneration (the exudative form).[23]

In a blinded six-month study of people with macular degeneration, vision was the same or better in 88% people who took a nutritional supplement, compared with 59% of those who refused to take the supplement (a statistically significant difference). The supplement used in this study contained **beta-carotene** (page 469), **vitamin C** (page 604), **vitamin E** (page 609), **zinc** (page 614), **copper** (page 499), **manganese** (page 553), **selenium** (page 584), and **riboflavin** (page 598).[24] People wishing to take all of these nutrients may supplement with a **multivitamin-multimineral formula** (page 559).

Are there any side effects or interactions?
Refer to the individual supplement for information about any side effects or interactions.

Herbs that may be helpful
Ginkgo biloba (page 681) may help treat early-stage macular degeneration, according to small, preliminary clinical trials.[25] Many healthcare professionals recommend 120 to 240 mg of standardized extract (24% ginkgo flavone glycosides and 6% terpene lactones) in capsules or tablets per day.

Bilberry's (page 634) active **flavonoid** (page 516) compounds, anthocyanosides, act as **antioxidants** (page 467) in the retina of the eye. Therefore, supplementing with bilberry would theoretically be of value for the prevention or treatment of early-stage macular degeneration.[26] Bilberry has also been shown to strengthen capillaries and to reduce bleeding in the retina.[27] A typical amount of bilberry used in studies was 480–600 mg per day of an extract standardized to contain 25% anthocyanosides, taken in capsules or tablets.

Are there any side effects or interactions?
Refer to the individual herb for information about any side effects or interactions.

MALABSORPTION

Malabsorption is a broad term used to describe the inability to absorb nutrients through the gut lining into the bloodstream.

Malabsorption is not a disease by itself, but rather the result of some other condition that is present. The small intestine (also called the small bowel) is typically involved in malabsorption, since the majority of nutrients are absorbed there. Malabsorption may affect one or more of the many nutrients present in the diet, including protein, fat, carbohydrate, vitamins, and minerals.

There are over 100 different conditions that can lead to problems in absorbing food, most of which are rare. The degree of malabsorption depends on the type of underlying condition and the extent to which it has affected the gut. Some of the more common malabsorption syndromes are due to bacterial or **parasitic infections** (page 343), **Crohn's disease** (page 141), **celiac disease** (page 102), **ulcerative colitis** (page 433), liver disease (including **cirrhosis** [page 290], **hepatitis** [page 220], and **gallstones** [page 193]), **cystic fibrosis** (page 143), **lactose intolerance** (page 288), chronic pancreatitis, specific medications that affect the intestines, or surgery of the stomach or bowels. The four conditions that most often lead to malabsorption in the United States are lactose intolerance, celiac disease, Crohn's disease, and chronic pancreatitis.[1]

Malabsorption may also occur when certain minerals present in the digestive tract in large amounts prevent adequate absorption of other minerals that are present in relatively small amounts. Minerals that may have this type of interaction include **calcium** (page 483), **copper** (page 499), **iron** (page 540), **magnesium** (page 551), **manganese** (page 553), and **zinc** (page 614).

What are the symptoms of malabsorption?

People with malabsorption may have symptoms of frequent, loose, watery stools; pale, foul-smelling, bulky stools; abdominal pain, gas, and bloating; weight loss; fatigue; **canker sores** (page 90); muscle cramps; delayed growth or short stature; bone and joint pain; seizures; painful skin rash; **night blindness** (page 326); easy **bruising** (page 84); and infertility. In addition to physical symptoms, there may be emotional disturbances, including feelings of **anxiety** (page 30) and **depression** (page 145).

Medical treatments

Immunosuppressive drugs such as mercaptopurine (Purinethol) and anti-inflammatory glucocorticoids such as prednisone (Deltasone, Orasone) are sometimes used as components of prescription drug therapy.

Treatments are directed at any underlying medical condition, including **celiac disease** (page 102), tropical sprue, Whipple's disease, **pancreatic insufficiency** (page 341), and short bowel syndrome. People with severe damage to the absorptive surface of their intestines might be prescribed intravenous nutritional supplements.

Dietary changes that may be helpful

Some popular health regimens claim that certain dietary practices, such as eating only raw food or avoiding certain food combinations, will prevent malabsorption of nutrients. There is no evidence to support these claims.

MALE INFERTILITY

See also: Female Infertility (page 187)

Infertility is defined by doctors as the failure of a couple to achieve **pregnancy** (page 363) after a year of unprotected intercourse.

In men, infertility is usually associated with a decrease in the number, quality, or motility (power of movement) of sperm. There are multiple possible underlying causes for male infertility, some of which readily respond to natural medicine, while others do not. The specific cause of infertility should always be diagnosed by a physician before considering possible solutions.

CHECKLIST FOR MALE INFERTILITY		
Rating	Nutritional Supplements	Herbs
★★★	Vitamin C (page 604) (for sperm agglutination only) Zinc (page 614) (for deficiency)	
★★☆	Arginine (page 467) L-carnitine (page 543) Selenium (page 584) Vitamin B₁₂ (page 601)	Asian ginseng (page 630)
★☆☆	Acety-L-carnitine (page 461) Coenzyme Q₁₀ (page 496) SAMe (page 583) Vitamin E (page 609)	

What are the symptoms of infertility?

The inability of a couple to become **pregnant** (page 363) after one year of regular, unprotected sex may indicate infertility of one or both sexual partners. Low sperm count in the semen, decreased sperm motility, or abnormal shape of the sperm are responsible for infertility in about 40% of these couples.

Medical treatments

Initial treatments may include timing sexual activity for ovulation (usually during the second week of the menstrual cycle), avoiding drugs that may reduce sperm count, and limiting intercourse to no more than once every three days, except during ovulation. Artificial insemination can also be used to place sperm directly in the cervix or uterus. Another more advanced procedure is called "in vitro fertilization" (IVF), wherein the man's sperm and the woman's egg (collected from the ovary in a surgical procedure) are combined under controlled conditions in a laboratory. The fertilized embryo is then implanted into the woman's uterus.

Dietary changes that may be helpful

In a study of men with poor sperm quality, excessive alcohol consumption was associated with a decrease in the percentage of normal sperm.[1] In a study of Danish greenhouse workers, an unexpectedly high sperm count was found among organic farmers, who grew their products without the use pesticides or chemical fertilizers. The sperm count was more than twice as high in these men as in a control group of blue-collar workers.[2] Although these findings are not definitive, they suggest that consuming organically grown foods may enhance fertility.

Lifestyle changes that may be helpful

Some conventional medications can interfere with fertility. If in doubt, men taking prescription drugs should consult their physician.

The optimal temperature of the testes for sperm production is slightly lower than body temperature, which is why the testes hang away from the body in the scrotum. Men with low sperm counts are frequently advised to minimize lifestyle factors that may overheat the testes, such as wearing tight (e.g., "bikini-style") underwear or frequently using spas and hot baths.

Environmental exposures (e.g., formaldehyde), smoking, and use of recreational drugs (e.g., marijuana, cocaine, hashish) may reduce sperm count or cause abnormal sperm morphology (shape).[3, 4] Smoking adversely affects the semen quality of infertile men.[5]

Nutritional supplements that may be helpful

Vitamin C (page 604) protects sperm from oxidative damage.[6] Supplementing vitamin C improves the quality of sperm in smokers.[7] When sperm stick together (a condition called agglutination), fertility is reduced. Vitamin C reduces sperm agglutination,[8] and supplementation with 200–1,000 mg per day increased the fertility of men with this condition in a controlled study.[9, 10] Many doctors recommend 1 gram of vitamin C per day for infertile men, particularly those diagnosed with sperm agglutination. However, a double-blind trial studying the effects of combined vitamin C and **vitamin E** (page 609) supplementation found no improvements in semen quality among men with low sperm motility.[11]

Zinc (page 614) deficiency leads to reduced numbers of sperm and impotence in men.[12] The correlation between blood levels of zinc and sperm quality remains controversial. Infertile men have been reported to have lower levels of zinc in their semen, than do men with normal fertility.[13] Similarly, men with normal sperm density tend to have higher amounts of zinc in their semen, than do men with low sperm counts.[14] However, other studies have found that a high concentration of zinc in the semen is related to decreased sperm motility in infertile men.[15, 16] A few studies have shown that oral zinc supplementation improves both sperm count[17, 18] motility,[19, 20] and the physical characteristics of sperm in some groups of infertile men.[21] For infertile men with low semen zinc levels, a preliminary trial found that zinc supplements (240 mg per day) increased sperm counts and possibly contributed to successful impregnation by 3 of the 11 men.[22] However, these studies all included small numbers of volunteers, and thus the impact of their conclusions is limited. In a controlled trial, 100 men with low sperm motility received either 57 mg of zinc twice daily or a placebo.[23] After three months, there was significant improvement in sperm quality, sperm count, sperm motility, and fertilizing capacity of the sperm. The ideal amount of supplemental zinc remains unknown, but some doctors recommend 30 mg two times per day. Long-term zinc supplementation requires 1–2 mg of **copper** (page 499) per day to prevent copper deficiency.

Arginine (page 467), an **amino acid** (page 465) found in many foods, is needed to produce sperm. Research, most of which is preliminary shows that several months of L-arginine supplementation increases sperm count, quality,[24, 25, 26] and fertility.[27, 28] However, when the initial sperm count was extremely low (such as less than 10 million per ml), L-arginine supplementation produced little or no benefit.[29, 30] While some **pregnancies** (page 363) have been attributed to arginine supplementation in preliminary reports,[31] no controlled research has confirmed these claims. For infertile men with sperm counts greater than 10 million per milliliter, many doctors recommend up to 4 grams of L-arginine per day for several months.

In a double-blind study of infertile men with reduced sperm motility, supplementation with **selenium** (page 584) (100 mcg per day for three months) significantly increased sperm motility, but had no effect on sperm count. Eleven percent of 46 men receiving selenium achieved paternity, compared with none of 18 men receiving a placebo.[32]

Vitamin B$_{12}$ (page 601) is needed to maintain fertility. Vitamin B$_{12}$ injections have increased sperm counts for men with low numbers of sperm.[33] These results have been duplicated in double-blind research.[34] In one study, a group of infertile men were given oral vitamin

B12 supplements (1,500 mcg per day of methylcobalamin) for 2 to 13 months. Approximately 60% of those taking the supplement experienced improved sperm counts.[35] However, controlled trials are needed to confirm these preliminary results. Men seeking vitamin B12 injections should consult a physician.

L-carnitine (page 543) is a substance made in the body and also found in supplements and some foods (such as meat). It appears to be necessary for normal functioning of sperm cells. In preliminary studies, supplementing with 3–4 grams per day for four months helped to normalize sperm motility in men with low sperm quality.[36, 37] While the majority of clinical trials have used L-carnitine, one preliminary trial found that **acetyl-L-carnitine** (page 461) (4 grams per day) may also prove useful for treatment of male infertility caused by low quantities of immobile sperm.[38]

Coenzyme Q10 (page 496) (CoQ10) is a nutrient used by the body in the production of energy. While its exact role in the formation of sperm is unknown, there is evidence that as little as 10 mg per day (over a two-week period) will increase sperm count and motility.[39] In one study, men with low sperm counts were given CoQ10 (60 mg per day for about three months). No significant change was noted in most sperm parameters, but a significant improvement was noted in *in-vitro* fertilization rates.[40]

Vitamin E (page 609) deficiency in animals leads to infertility.[41] In a preliminary human trial, 100–200 IU of vitamin E given daily to both partners of infertile couples led to a significant increase in fertility.[42] Vitamin E supplementation may enhance fertility by decreasing **free-radical** (page 467) damage to sperm cells. In another preliminary study, men with low fertilization rates in previous attempts at *in vitro* fertilization were given 200 IU of vitamin E per day for three months.[43] After one month of supplementation, fertilization rates increased significantly, and the amount of oxidative stress on sperm cells decreased. However, the evidence in favor of vitamin E remains preliminary. A review of research on vitamin E for male infertility concluded that there is no justification for its use in treating this condition.[44] Controlled trials are needed to validate these promising preliminary findings.

Preliminary research suggests that oral **SAMe** (page 583) (S-adenosyl-L-methionine), in amounts of 800 mg per day, may also increase sperm activity in infertile men.[45]

Calcium (page 483) is a key regulator of human sperm function.[46] The concentration of calcium in semen determines sperm motility (i.e., the ability of sperm to move spontaneously).[47, 48] However, calcium deficiency has not been confirmed as a cause of male infertility nor is there any evidence that calcium supplementation improves male infertility.

Are there any side effects or interactions?
Refer to the individual supplement for information about any side effects or interactions.

Herbs that may be helpful
Asian ginseng (page 630) may prove useful for male infertility. One preliminary study found that 4 grams of Asian ginseng per day for three months led to an improvement in sperm count and sperm motility.[49]

Are there any side effects or interactions?
Refer to the individual herb for information about any side effects or interactions.

Holistic approaches that may be helpful
Acupuncture may be helpful in the treatment of some cases of male infertility due to impairment of sperm function. A controlled study of men with reduced sperm function found that one measure of sperm function significantly improved in the men treated with acupuncture (two times per week for five weeks) compared to controls.[50] Similar results have been reported in other studies.[51, 52] Nevertheless, double-blind trials are needed to determine conclusively whether acupuncture is a useful treatment for male infertility.

MEASLES

Measles is a potentially serious, highly contagious infection caused by the measles virus.

Infection is easily transmitted by kissing or being coughed or sneezed upon by an infected person. The recent introduction of an effective vaccine against measles has greatly reduced the number of cases in many countries, though some developing nations continue to experience serious measles epidemics in children.

What are the symptoms of measles?
Symptoms of measles begin with a runny nose, **cough** (page 139), muscle aches, fatigue, and a slight fever, often accompanied by redness of the eyes and **sensitivity to light** (page 356). Later, the fever rises and a mildly itchy red rash develops on the face and spreads

Measles

to the lower body. In severe cases, there may be high fever, convulsions, pneumonia, or severe **diarrhea** (page 163), and some severe cases can result in death.

	CHECKLIST FOR MEASLES	
Rating	Nutritional Supplements	Herbs
★★★	**Vitamin A** (page 595) (if deficient)	
★★☆	**Vitamin A** (page 595) (for severe cases of measles)	
★☆☆	**Flavonoids** (page 516)	

Medical treatments

Over the counter drugs focus on the treatment of symptoms, such as pain and fever. The safest drug for this purpose is acetaminophen (Tylenol). Children with fever who are under the age of 18 are no longer given aspirin-containing products. Use in these circumstances has been linked to an increased risk of Reye's syndrome, a potentially serious illness that can affect the liver and brain. Individuals with measles might also benefit from supplemental **vitamin A** (page 595).

Prescription antibiotics such as amoxicillin (Amoxil), amoxicillin/clavulanate (Augmentin), and cephalexin (Keflex) might be used in some individuals to prevent or treat a bacterial infection.

People with measles are commonly advised to rest and drink plenty of fluids. Healthcare providers may also recommend limited contact with non-immunized people to prevent transmission of the disease.

Lifestyle changes that may be helpful

Treatment of measles is aimed at minimizing discomfort as the symptoms develop. Since people with measles tend to run a high fever, reducing the temperature with a lukewarm bath can reduce aches and other discomforts.[1] Adding mineral salts or oatmeal to the bath water may reduce the itchiness of the skin.[2, 3] Because of their **sensitivity to light** (page 356), being in a room with dimmed lights will be soothing to the person with measles.

Nutritional supplements that may be helpful

Measles appears to increase the body's need for **vitamin A** (page 595).[4, 5] Studies in developing countries have shown that measles infection is more frequent and severe in people with low vitamin A blood levels,[6, 7] and preliminary research suggests this may also be true in the developed world.[8, 9, 10] Repeatedly in controlled trials, preventive supplementation with vitamin A, at oral doses of up to 400,000 IU per day, reduced the risk of death in children with measles living in developing countries.[11, 12, 13] Whether vitamin A supplementation would help people with measles in developed countries, where deficiency is uncommon, is less clear.[14] However, the American Academy of Pediatrics recommends that all children with measles be given a short course of high-dose vitamin A. Two controlled studies of urban South African[15] and Japanese[16] children hospitalized with severe measles showed that supplementation with 100,000 to 400,000 IU of vitamin A resulted in faster recoveries, fewer complications, and fewer pneumonia-related deaths. An older study in England found one ounce per day of **cod liver oil** (page 514) (containing about 40,000 IU of vitamin A, plus **vitamin D** (page 607) and omega-3 fatty acids) reduced measles-related deaths in children hospitalized with severe cases of the disease.[17] Such large doses of vitamin A should only be taken under a doctor's supervision.

Flavonoids (page 516) are nutrients found in the white, pithy parts of fruits and vegetables. In preliminary laboratory research, certain flavonoids have been found to inhibit the infectivity of measles virus in the test tube.[18] Whether flavonoid supplements could be effective in preventing or treating measles is unknown.

Are there any side effects or interactions?

Refer to the individual supplement for information about any side effects or interactions.

MÉNIÈRE'S DISEASE

Ménière's disease (MD) is a disorder of the inner ear causing episodes of dizziness (**vertigo** [page 441]); ringing, buzzing, roaring, whistling, or hissing sounds in the ears (**tinnitus** [page 430]); fluctuating levels of hearing loss; and a sensation of fullness in the ear.

Head trauma and syphilis can cause MD, although in most cases the cause is unknown.

What are the symptoms of Ménière's disease?

People with Ménière's disease may have vertigo that may be associated with nausea and vomiting. Symptoms may also include a recurrent feeling of fullness or pressure in the affected ear and hearing difficulty. People with Ménière's disease may also have tinnitus, which may be intermittent or continuous. The symptoms of MD are associated with an underlying condition referred to as endolymphatic hydrops, an excess accumulation of the fluid of the inner ear.[1] When people have only one of the symptoms associated with Ménière's disease, such as **tinnitus** (page 430) or **vertigo** (page 441), the condition is not usually considered MD.

CHECKLIST FOR MÉNIÈRE'S DISEASE		
Rating	Nutritional Supplements	Herbs
★★☆	**Flavonoids** (page 516) (hydroxyethylrutosides)	
★☆☆		*Ginkgo biloba* (page 681)

Medical treatments

Over the counter antihistamines, such as dimenhydrinate (Dramamine), meclizine (Bonine), and cyclizine (Marezine), might be useful to treat dizziness.

Prescription anticholinergic drugs, such as scopolamine (Transderm-Scop), prochlorperazine (Compazine), and trimethobenzamide (Tigan), and sedatives such as diazepam (Valium), lorazepam (Ativan), and alprazolam (Xanax), are often used to treat symptoms associated with Ménière's.

People frequently affected by disabling **vertigo** (page 441) might require a surgical treatment (vestibular neurectomy or labyrinthectomy). Some people might benefit from a tinnitus masker, which is a hearing device that produces a sound that is more tolerable than the ringing in the ears. Healthcare providers may also suggest the use of earplugs in the presence of loud noises to prevent damage to the ear.

Dietary changes that may be helpful

A low-salt diet (no more than 800–1,000 mg sodium per day) combined with diuretic medication, is believed to reduce endolymphatic hydrops,[2] and is often recommended in MD.[3, 4, 5] While the benefits of a low salt diet and diuretics have not been scientifically proven for this condition,[6] clinics specializing in MD report a significant reduction or stabilization of symptoms with this regimen.[7] Preliminary human trials suggest a low-salt diet may reduce the progression of hearing loss associated with MD.[8]

MD is associated with allergies to airborne particles, mold, and food in some individuals, according to many preliminary reports.[9, 10, 11, 12, 13] In one preliminary study, 50% of participants with MD reported known food or inhalant allergies.[14] In a controlled study, participants with MD who underwent allergy treatment, including avoiding foods suspected of provoking allergic reactions, reported statistically significant improvement in **tinnitus** (page 430), **vertigo** (page 441), and hearing.[15] In this study, the most common **food allergies** (page 14) were to wheat and soy. Most participants also had allergies to milk, corn, egg, and yeast.

Some cases of MD are associated with high blood **triglycerides** (page 235) and **cholesterol** (page 223), and abnormalities in blood sugar regulation, such as **diabetes** (page 152) and **hypoglycemia** (page 251).[16, 17, 18, 19, 20] In one preliminary study,[21] a modified hypoglycemia diet with moderate to high intake of protein, moderate to low intake of fat, and restricted intake of complex carbohydrates was found to reduce MD symptoms in a large number of patients with blood sugar abnormalities. Participants with high cholesterol were put on low cholesterol diets, and those that were overweight were put on calorie-restricted diets. In addition, refined carbohydrates, alcohol, and caffeine were prohibited, and small frequent meals with between meal snacks were recommended. A majority of participants were also given supplements of **calcium** (page 483), **fluoride** (page 519), and **vitamin D** (page 607) as described below, so the importance of these dietary changes to the overall effectiveness of the program cannot be determined. This intriguing report needs confirmation from controlled trials.

Lifestyle changes that may be helpful

Lifestyle changes often recommended for MD include the elimination of caffeine, nicotine, and alcohol.[22] Although not scientifically proven, intake of these substances is believed to increase the frequency of MD attacks. In animal studies, both alcohol and caffeine have been reported to impair mechanisms in the inner ear that assist in maintaining balance.[23]

Nutritional supplements that may be helpful

Certain **flavonoids** (page 516), known as hydroxyethylrutosides (HR), have been reported to improve symptoms of MD in one double-blind study. In this study, 2 grams per day of HR for three months resulted in either stabilization of or improvement in hearing.[24] Other types of flavonoids have not been studied as treatments for MD.

Some cases of MD are associated with otosclerosis,[25, 26, 27, 28] a disease affecting the small bones of the inner ear. Otosclerosis often goes undiagnosed in people with MD, although the coexistence is well documented.[29] While preliminary reports suggest otosclerosis may be a cause of MD,[30, 31] the relationship between these two conditions remains unclear. Sodium fluoride, a mineral compound available only by prescription, is reported to improve otosclerosis.[32, 33, 34, 35] In a preliminary study,[36] people with MD and otosclerosis were given supplements of 50 mg of sodium fluoride, 200 mg calcium carbonate, and a **multiple vitamin** (page 559) supplying 400–800 IU of **vitamin D** (page 607) per day, for periods ranging from six months to over five years. Many participants also had blood sugar abnormalities, and were asked to follow a modified hypoglycemia diet as described above. Significant improvement in **vertigo** (page 441) was reported within six months, but improvements in hearing required one to two years. Because most participants used both diet and supplements, the importance of **fluoride** (page 519), **calcium** (page 483), and/or vitamin D to the overall results of this trial is unclear.

Are there any side effects or interactions?
Refer to the individual supplement for information about any side effects or interactions.

Herbs that may be helpful
Although *Ginkgo biloba* (page 604) extract (GBE) has not been studied specifically for its effects in MD, in preliminary studies it has been reported to reduce symptoms of **tinnitus** (page 430), **vertigo** (page 441), and hearing loss due to unspecified inner ear disorders.[37] Controlled research using GBE is needed to determine whether it is a treatment option specifically for MD.

Are there any side effects or interactions?
Refer to the individual herb for information about any side effects or interactions.

Holistic approaches that may be helpful
People with MD are frequently found to have musculoskeletal disorders of the head and neck,[38] including cervical spine disorders (CSD; disorders of the joints of the neck),[39] and disorders of the jaw (craniomandibular disorders or CMD).[40] Physical therapy to the cervical spine relieves MD-like symptoms in some cases, according to one preliminary report.[41] Although spinal manipulation has been shown to reduce vertigo in preliminary human studies,[42, 43, 44] controlled research with MD patients is lacking.

Some authorities recommend psychological counseling[45] to reduce both the significant emotional distress caused by living with this disorder[46, 47] and possible stress-related MD symptoms,[48, 49] however, the benefits of counseling have not been established by controlled research. MD is not caused by psychological factors,[50] and it is unclear whether stress increases the frequency or severity of attacks.[51] Preliminary human studies suggest that stress increases awareness of symptoms,[52] particularly **vertigo** (page 441).[53] In a controlled human study of **tinnitus** (page 430), which included three participants with MD, weekly one-hour sessions of relaxation and coping techniques for ten weeks significantly reduced both tinnitus and tinnitus annoyance.[54] Since very few of these participants had MD, it is not clear whether these techniques would be helpful for people with MD.

Vestibular rehabilitation exercises, used primarily to aid in recovery from vertigo, are also recommended by some authorities for MD,[55] although controlled research on these exercises for MD is lacking. According to these authorities, the exercises should be started only after symptoms have been stabilized with other treatments, and should not be done during active MD. A qualified musculoskeletal healthcare specialist should be consulted.

Transcutaneous electrical nerve stimulation (TENS), a form of physiotherapy used by musculoskeletal healthcare specialists, has been reported to reduce tinnitus in people with MD in preliminary studies.[56, 57, 58] TENS is thought to improve tinnitus by increasing circulation to the inner ear.[59] In one large preliminary trial, participants with tinnitus due to various causes, including MD, received two 25- to 30-minute treatments to the ear per week for three to five weeks.[60] Sixty percent of people with MD reported significant improvement of tinnitus after this treatment, and many reported a decrease in pressure in the treated ear. A controlled trial comparing the effectiveness of TENS and applied relaxation (AR; the use of an audiotape to guide the participant through a series of muscle relaxation exercises) in MD found either treatment produced similar positive results,[61] but these could have been due to placebo effects. In this study, participants treated themselves with three 30-minute TENS treatments to the hand per day for two weeks, with one participant continuing treatment for three months.

Acupuncture is reported to reduce symptoms of MD in preliminary studies.[62, 63] In one trial, vertigo was eliminated after one to three treatments in a group of

34 MD patients, and measurements of hearing also improved.[64] Controlled research is needed to confirm these results.

MENKES' DISEASE

Menkes' disease is a rare hereditary disorder caused by an abnormality of **copper** (page 499) utilization.[1]

Until recently, Menkes' disease was considered universally fatal.[2] However, it now appears that the severity of the disease varies from person to person.[3, 4] Medical doctors often use genetic analysis[5] to diagnose this disorder, even before birth.[6, 7] In cases where the genetic defect appears responsive to copper therapy, early treatment is needed to minimize the severity of the physical defects that will develop later.[8] Treatment can even begin before birth; while still pregnant, mothers of babies identified with Menkes' disease can receive injections of copper histidine under the skin. Healthcare professionals, including geneticists (specialists in hereditary diseases), should be consulted in the treatment of Menkes' disease.

CHECKLIST FOR MENKES' DISEASE		
Rating	Nutritional Supplements	Herbs
★★☆	**Copper** (page 499) (injectable)	

What are the symptoms of Menkes' disease?
Menkes' disease can lead to growth retardation, white hair that has a kinky texture, and mental deterioration.

Medical treatments
There is no effective common treatment known.

Nutritional supplements that may be helpful
Copper (page 499) injections are used to treat Menkes' disease. The success of this treatment often depends on the severity of the disease.

Some studies have shown favorable effects of injectable copper on brain and nerve development in people with Menkes' disease when the degree of genetic defect was mild and treatment was begun early.[9] However, copper therapy does not benefit Menkes' patients if the genetic defects are severe, or if therapy is begun after the physical defects manifest.[10] Some researchers

have observed that damaging levels of copper can build up in the tissues of some copper-treated people with Menkes' disease.[11] For example, in one study a boy developed low blood pressure in response to changing body position (called orthostatic hypotension), an enlarged spleen, and ballooning of an artery in his abdomen. However, whether these anomalies resulted from therapy or from the Menkes' disease itself remains unclear. As a result, copper therapy is still considered experimental[12] and potentially dangerous. People with Menkes' disease should consult a healthcare professional before supplementing with copper.

In 1989, one researcher suggested that Menkes' disease is caused by a defect in **zinc** (page 614) metabolism that reduces copper availability.[13] The possibility of this zinc-copper interaction in Menkes' disease has since been investigated in preliminary test tube research.[14, 15, 16, 17] These studies have shown that supplementation with zinc does not alter the way cells from people with Menkes' disease use copper. Therefore, zinc supplementation is unlikely to be beneficial in Menkes' disease.

Are there any side effects or interactions?
Refer to the individual supplement for information about any side effects or interactions.

MENOPAUSE

What do I need to know?
Self-care for menopause can be approached in a number of ways—but it can be hard to know just where to start. To make it easier, our doctors recommend trying these simple steps first:

Eat soy and flaxseed
Make foods high in phytoestrogens, such as flaxseed, tofu, soy milk, tempeh, and roasted soy nuts, a regular part of your diet

Control symptoms with isoflavones
Supplements containing at least 80 to 100 mg a day of isoflavones from soy or red clover may help control symptoms

Cool down with black cohosh
Take 20 mg of a concentrated extract twice a day for relief from hot flashes

Find relief with exercise
Even light aerobic activities can help reduce menopausal symptoms

Quit smoking

Smokers are more likely to experience hot flashes and other menopausal symptoms

About menopause

Menopause is the cessation of the monthly female menstrual cycle. Women who have not had a menstrual period for a year are considered postmenopausal.

Most commonly, menopause takes place when a woman is in her late forties or early fifties. Women who have gone through menopause are no longer fertile. Menopause is not a disease and cannot be prevented. Many hormonal changes occur during menopause. Postmenopausal women are at higher risk of **heart disease** (page 98) and **osteoporosis** (page 333), presumably because of a decrease in the production of estrogen or other hormones.

CHECKLIST FOR MENOPAUSE

Rating	Nutritional Supplements	Herbs
★★★	**Soy** (page 587)	**Black cohosh** (page 637)
★★☆	**Progesterone** (page 577)	**Red clover** (page 735) **Sage** (page 740) and **alfalfa** (page 623) (in combination)
★☆☆	**DHEA** (page 503) **Flavonoids** (page 516) (hesperidin) **Vitamin C** (page 604) **Vitamin E** (page 609)	**Alfalfa** (page 623) **Asian ginseng** (page 630) Blue vervain (*Verbena hastata*) **Burdock** (page 648) **Dong quai** (page 668) **Licorice** (page 702) **Motherwort** (page 712) **Sage** (page 740) **St. John's wort** (page 747) **Wild yam** (page 759)

What are the symptoms of menopause?

Several unpleasant symptoms may accompany menopause. Some, such as vaginal dryness, result from the lack of estrogen. Others, such as hot flashes and decreased sex drive, are caused by more complex hormonal changes. Some women experience **depression** (page 145), **anxiety** (page 30), or **insomnia** (page 270) during menopause.

Medical treatments

The most common prescription drug treatment for symptoms of menopause is hormone replacement therapy. This includes an estrogen, either conjugated estrogen (Premarin), estradiol (Estrace, Estraderm), or ethinyl estradiol (Alesse), and a progestin (Provera, Prometrium). Some prescriptions contain both estrogens and progestins in a single tablet (Prempro, Premphase). Some products add methyltestosterone to esterified estrogens (Estratest) to help enhance sex drive.

Dietary changes that may be helpful

Soybeans contain compounds called phytoestrogens that are related in structure to estrogen, though some reports show soy's estrogenic activity to be quite weak.[1] Soy is known to affect the menstrual cycle in premenopausal women.[2] Societies with high consumption of soy products have a low incidence of hot flashes during menopause.[3]

In one double-blind trial, supplementation with 60 grams of soy protein caused a 33% decrease in the number of hot flashes after four weeks and a 45% reduction after 12 weeks.[4] However, in further analysis of the data in this trial, researchers credit constituents in soybeans *other than* phytoestrogens for the therapeutic effect.[5] In one controlled clinical trial, high intake of phytoestrogens from soy and **flaxseed** (page 517) reduced both hot flashes and vaginal dryness; however, much (though not all) of the benefit was also seen in the control group.[6] In another double-blind study, 100 mg per day of isoflavones extracted from soy was effective in relieving hot flashes.[7]

As a result of these studies, doctors often recommend that women experiencing menopausal symptoms eat tofu, soy milk, tempeh, roasted soy nuts, and other soy-based sources of phytoestrogens. Soy sauce contains very little phytoestrogen content, and many processed foods made from soybean concentrates have insignificant levels of phytoestrogens. Supplements containing isoflavones extracted from soy are commercially available, and flaxseed (as opposed to flaxseed oil) is also a good source of phytoestrogens.

Lifestyle changes that may be helpful

Sedentary women are more likely to have moderate or severe hot flashes compared with women who exercise.[8, 9] In one trial, menopausal symptoms were reduced immediately after aerobic exercise.[10]

Cigarette smoking may be related to hot flashes in

menopausal women. Preliminary data have shown that women who experience hot flashes are more likely to be smokers.[11] Another preliminary study found that new users of hormone replacement therapy for the relief of menopausal symptoms were more likely to be current cigarette smokers than were those who had never smoked.[12]

Nutritional supplements that may be helpful

Many years ago, researchers studied the effects of **vitamin E** (page 609) supplementation in reducing symptoms of menopause. Most,[13, 14, 15, 16, 17] but not all,[18] studies found vitamin E to be helpful. Many doctors suggest that women going through menopause take 800 IU per day of vitamin E for a trial period of at least three months to see if symptoms are reduced. If helpful, this amount may be continued. Using lower amounts for less time has led to statistically significant changes, but only marginal clinical improvement.[19]

In 1964, a preliminary trial reported that 1,200 mg each of **vitamin C** (page 604) and the **flavonoid** (page 516) hesperidin taken over the course of the day helped relieve hot flashes.[20] Although placebo effects are strong in women with hot flashes, other treatments used in that trial failed to act as effectively as the flavonoid/vitamin C combination. Since then, researchers have not explored the effects of flavonoids or vitamin C in women with menopausal symptoms.

The mineral **boron** (page 477) is known to affect estrogen metabolism. In one double-blind trial using 2.5 mg of boron per day for two months, hot flashes and night sweats worsened in 21 of 43 women, but the same symptoms improved in ten others.[21] Women who are experiencing hot flashes or night sweats that have been diagnosed as menopausal symptoms and who are also supplementing boron (sometimes found in significant amounts in **osteoporosis** [page 333] formulas and **multivitamin-mineral supplements** [page 559]) should consider discontinuing use of boron-containing supplements to see if the severity of their symptoms is reduced.

Aging in women is characterized by a progressive decline in blood DHEA (dehydroepiandrosterone) and DHEA-sulfate (DHEAS) levels. These levels can be restored with **DHEA** (page 503) supplementation. This process also improves the response of some brain chemicals, called endorphins, to certain drugs.[22] These endorphins are involved in sensations of pleasure and **pain** (page 338); improving their response may explain why DHEA has an effect on mood symptoms associated with menopause. In one double-blind trial, however, menopausal women who took 50 mg of DHEA per day for three months had no improvement in symptoms compared with women taking placebo.[23] Further study is needed to validate a role for DHEA in the management of menopausal symptoms.

Natural **progesterone** (page 577) supplementation has been anecdotally linked to reduction in symptoms of menopause.[24, 25, 26] In one trial, natural progesterone was found to have no independent effect on symptoms, and synthetic progestins were found to increase breast tenderness.[27] However, a double-blind trial found that topical administration of natural progesterone cream led to a reduction in hot flashes in 83% of women, compared with improvement in only 19% of those given placebo.[28] Preliminary research has found that oral, micronized progesterone therapy is associated with improved quality of life among postmenopausal women. However, oral micronized progesterone is available only by prescription in the United States.[29] Hot flashes, **anxiety** (page 30), **depression** (page 145), sleep problems, and sexual functioning were among the symptoms improved in a majority of women surveyed. Synthetic progestins, also available only by prescription, have reduced symptoms of menopause.[30, 31, 32]

Progesterone is a hormone and, as such, concerns about its inappropriate use (i.e., as an over-the-counter supplement) have been raised. The amount of progesterone in commercially available creams varies widely, and the progesterone content is not listed on the label because the creams are legally regulated as cosmetics, not dietary supplements. Therefore, a physician should be consulted before using these hormone-containing creams as supplements. Although few side effects have been associated with topical progesterone creams, skin reactions may occur in some users. Effects of natural progesterone on **breast cancer** (page 65) risk remain unclear; research has suggested both increased and reduced risk.

Are there any side effects or interactions?
Refer to the individual supplement for information about any side effects or interactions.

Herbs that may be helpful

Double-blind trials support the usefulness of **black cohosh** (page 637) for women with hot flashes associated with menopause.[33] A review of eight trials concluded black cohosh to be both safe and effective.[34] Many doctors recommend 20 mg of a highly concentrated extract taken twice per day; 2–4 ml of tincture three times per day may also be used.

A variety of herbs with weak estrogen-like actions similar to the effects of soy have traditionally been used for women with menopausal symptoms.[35] These herbs include **licorice** (page 702), **alfalfa** (page 623), and **red clover** (page 735). In a double-blind trial, a formula containing tinctures of licorice, **burdock** (page 648), **dong quai** (page 668), **wild yam** (page 759), and **motherwort** (page 712) (30 drops three times daily) was found to reduce symptoms of menopause.[36] No effects on hormone levels were detected in this study. In a separate double-blind trial, supplementation with dong quai (4.5 grams three times daily in capsules) had no effect on menopausal symptoms or hormone levels.[37] A double-blind trial using a standardized extract of subterranean clover *(Trifolium subterraneum),* a relative of red clover, containing 40 mg isoflavones per tablet did not impact symptoms of menopause, such as hot flashes, though it did improve function of the arteries.[38] An extract of red clover, providing 82 mg of isoflavones per day, also was ineffective in a 12-week double-blind study.[39] In another double-blind study, however, administration of 80 mg of isoflavones per day from red clover reduced the frequency of hot flashes in postmenopausal women. The benefit was noticeable after 4 weeks of treatment and became more pronounced after a total of 12 weeks.[40]

Sage (page 740) may reduce excessive perspiration due to menopausal hot flashes during the day or at night.[41] It is believed this is because sage directly decreases production of sweat. In a preliminary study, supplementation with a product containing extracts of the leaves of sage and alfalfa resulted in complete elimination of hot flushes and night sweats in 20 of 30 women, with varying degrees of improvement in the other ten cases.[42]

Blue vervain *(Verbene hastata).* is a traditional herb for menopause; however, there is no research to validate this use. Tincture has been recommended at an amount of 5–10 ml three times per day.

Preliminary evidence suggests that supplementation with **St. John's wort** (page 747) extract (300 mg three times daily for 12 weeks) may improve psychological symptoms, including sexual well-being, in menopausal women.[43]

A double-blind trial found that **Asian ginseng** (page 630) (200 mg per day of standardized extract) helped alleviate psychological symptoms of menopause, such as **depression** (page 145) and **anxiety** (page 30), but did not decrease physical symptoms, such as hot flashes or sexual dysfunction, in postmenopausal women who had not been treated with hormones.[44]

Warning: Kava should only be taken with medical supervision. Kava is not for sale in certain parts of the world.

In a double-blind trial, a standardized **kava** (page 698) extract was found to be effective at reducing **anxiety** (page 30) and other symptoms associated with menopause.[45] The study used 100 mg of kava extract standardized to contain 70% kava-lactones, three times per day. Most commercially available kava extracts contain up to 35% kava-lactones. In another study, administration of kava enhanced the anti-anxiety effect of hormone replacement therapy in postmenopausal women.[46]

Are there any side effects or interactions?
Refer to the individual herb for information about any side effects or interactions.

Holistic approaches that may be helpful
Acupuncture may be helpful in the treatment of menopausal symptoms. Animal research suggests that acupuncture may help normalize some biochemical changes that are associated with menopausal disturbances of memory, mood, and other functions.[47] One preliminary trial in humans demonstrated a significant reduction (more than 50%) in hot flashes in menopausal women receiving either electroacupuncture (acupuncture with electrical stimulation) or superficial acupuncture (shallow needle insertion).[48] Other preliminary trials support these results[49, 50] and suggest additional menopausal symptoms may also respond to acupuncture.[51] However, no placebo-controlled trials have been done to conclusively prove the effectiveness of acupuncture for menopausal symptoms.

MENORRHAGIA

Menorrhagia is the medical term for excessive bleeding at the time of the menstrual period, either in number of days or amount of blood or both.

Excessive menstrual bleeding must be evaluated by a doctor in order to rule out potentially serious underlying conditions that can cause this problem.

What are the symptoms of menorrhagia?

Menorrhagia does not produce symptoms unless blood loss is significant, at which time symptoms of **anemia** (page 25), such as fatigue, may occur. Women with menorrhagia may have heavy menstrual bleeding (consistently changing pads or tampons more frequently than every hour) or a period that lasts more than eight days.

Rating	Nutritional Supplements	Herbs
CHECKLIST FOR HEAVY MENSTRUATION (MENORRHAGIA)		
★★★	**Iron** (page 540) (for deficiency)	
★★☆	**Vitamin A** (page 595)	
★☆☆	**Flavonoids** (page 516) **Vitamin C** (page 604) **Vitamin E** (page 609)	**Black horehound** (page 638) **Cinnamon** (page 659) **Cranesbill** (page 665) **Oak** (page 716) **Periwinkle** (page 727) Shepherd's purse **Vitex** (page 757) **Witch hazel** (page 760)

Medical treatments

Prescription drug therapy includes birth control pills (Ortho-Novum, Loestrin, Mircette, Triphasil) and gonadotropin-releasing hormones, such asleuprolide (Lupron) and nafarelin (Synarel).

Therapy is also directed at treating any underlying medical conditions, such as **pregnancy** (page 363), **iron deficiency** (page 278) anemia, thyroid dysfunction, and tumor. Severe cases might require surgical treatments.

Nutritional supplements that may be helpful

Since blood is rich in **iron** (page 540), excessive blood loss can lead to iron depletion. **Iron deficiency** (page 278) can be identified with simple blood tests. If an iron deficiency is diagnosed, many doctors recommend 100–200 mg of iron per day, although recommendations vary widely.

The relationship between iron deficiency and menorrhagia is complicated. Not only can the condition lead to iron deficiency, but iron deficiency can lead to or aggravate menorrhagia by reducing the capacity of the uterus to stop the bleeding. Supplementing with iron decreases excess menstrual blood loss in iron-deficient women who have no other underlying cause for their condition.[1, 2] However, iron supplements should be taken only by people who have, or are at risk of developing, iron deficiency.

In a study of women with menorrhagia who took 25,000 IU of **vitamin A** (page 595) twice per day for 15 days, 93% showed significant improvement and 58% had a complete normalization of menstrual blood loss.[3] However, women who are or could become **pregnant** (page 363) should not supplement with more than 10,000 IU (3,000 mcg) per day of vitamin A.

In a study of women with menorrhagia associated with the use of an intrauterine device (IUD) for birth control, supplementing with 100 IU of **vitamin E** (page 609) every other day corrected the problem in all cases within ten weeks (63% responded within four weeks).[4] The cause of IUD-induced menstrual blood loss is different from that of other types of menorrhagia; therefore, it's possible that vitamin E supplements might not help with menorrhagia not associated with IUD use.

Both **vitamin C** (page 604) and **flavonoids** (page 516) protect capillaries (small blood vessels) from damage. In so doing, they might protect against the blood loss of menorrhagia. In one small study, 88% of women with menorrhagia improved when given 200 mg vitamin C and 200 mg flavonoids three times per day.[5]

Are there any side effects or interactions?

Refer to the individual supplement for information about any side effects or interactions.

Herbs that may be helpful

Among women taking **vitex** (page 757), menorrhagia has reportedly improved after taking the herb for several months.[6] With its emphasis on long-term balancing of a woman's hormonal system, vitex is not a fast-acting herb. For frequent or heavy periods, vitex can be used continuously for six to nine months. Forty drops of the concentrated liquid herbal extract of vitex can be added to a glass of water and drunk in the morning. Vitex is also available in powdered form in tablets and capsules. Thirty-five to forty milligrams may be taken in the morning.

Cinnamon (page 659) has been used historically for the treatment of various menstrual disorders, including heavy menstruation.[7] This is also the case with shepherd's purse (*Capsella bursa-pastoris*).[8] Other herbs known as astringents (tannin-containing plants that tend to decrease discharges), such as **cranesbill** (page

665), **periwinkle** (page 727), **witch hazel** (page 760), and **oak** (page 716), were traditionally used for heavy menstruation. Human trials are lacking, so the usefulness of these herbs is unknown. **Black horehound** (page 638) was sometimes used traditionally for heavy periods, though this approach has not been investigated by modern research.

Are there any side effects or interactions?
Refer to the individual herb for information about any side effects or interactions.

MIGRAINE HEADACHE

See also: Cluster Headache (page 117), **Tension Headache** (page 428)

What do I need to know?
Self-care for migraine headache can be approached in a number of ways—but it can be hard to know just where to start. To make it easier, our doctors recommend trying these simple steps first:

Find your migraine triggers
> A knowledgeable healthcare professional can help you learn if your diet, environment, or lifestyle helps trigger your migraines

Try magnesium
> Taking 200 mg of a well-absorbed magnesium supplement two or three times a day may help you have fewer migraines

Check out feverfew
> Take a standardized extract providing 250 mcg of parthenolide a day to help reduce the frequency, severity, and length of migraine attacks

See a chiropractor
> A qualified practitioner may be able to correct spinal problems that may cause some migraines

Try acupuncture
> See a qualified acupuncturist for help with stopping a migraine in its early stages or preventing future attacks

About migraine
Migraines are very painful headaches that usually begin on only one side of the head and may become worse with exposure to light.

What are the symptoms of migraine?
Migraines are commonly preceded by warning symptoms (prodrome), that may include **depression** (page 145), irritability, restlessness, loss of appetite, and a characteristic "aura"—usually a visual disturbance such as flashing lights or a localized area of blindness that follows the appearance of brilliantly colored shimmering lights. Migraines may also involve nausea, vomiting, and changes in vision.

CHECKLIST FOR MIGRAINE HEADACHE		
Rating	Nutritional Supplements	Herbs
★★★	**Magnesium** (page 551) **Vitamin B$_2$** (page 598)	**Feverfew** (page 677)
★★☆	**5-HTP** (page 459) **Coenzyme Q$_{10}$** (page 496) **Vitamin B$_{12}$** (page 601)	Butterbur
★☆☆	**Calcium** (page 481) **Fish oil** (page 514) (EPA/ DHA [page 509]) **Melatonin** (page 555) **SAMe** (page 583) **Vitamin D** (page 607)	**Cayenne** (page 654) **Ginger** (page 680) *Ginkgo biloba* (page 681)

Medical treatments
Over the counter nonsteroidal anti-inflammatory drugs (NSAIDs), such as aspirin (Bayer, Ecotrin, Bufferin), ibuprofen (Motrin, Advil), and naproxen (Aleve), may help provide pain relief in mild cases. Excedrin Migraine, which contains acetaminophen, aspirin, and caffeine, might also help with migraine pain.

The most commonly used prescription drugs are the serotonin receptor agonists, such as sumatriptan (Imitrex), naratriptan (Amerge), rizatriptan (Maxalt), and zolmitriptan (Zomig). Less frequently used agents include isometheptene-acetaminophen-dichloralphenazone (Midrin), dihydroergotamine (DHE), and ergotamine-caffeine (Cafergot). Many different drugs have been prescribed for migraine prevention, such as propranolol (Inderal), verapamil (Calan, Isoptin), and amitriptyline (Elavil).

Treatment might also include avoidance of certain triggers, such as alcohol and specific foods. Some individuals might benefit from the correction of vision, while others might benefit from biofeedback.

Dietary changes that may be helpful
Some migraine sufferers have an abnormality of blood-sugar regulation known as reactive **hypoglycemia** (page 251). In these people, improvement in the frequency and/or severity of migraines resulted from dietary

changes designed to control the blood sugar.[1, 2] For the treatment of reactive hypoglycemia, many healthcare practitioners recommend strict avoidance of refined sugar, caffeine, and alcohol, and eating small, frequent meals (such as six times per day).

Migraines can be triggered by **allergies** (page 14) and may be relieved by identifying and avoiding the problem foods.[3, 4, 5, 6] Uncovering these food allergies with the help of a doctor is often a useful way to prevent migraines. In children suffering migraines who also have **epilepsy** (page 183), there is evidence that eliminating offending foods will also reduce the frequency of seizures.[7]

Some people who suffer from migraines also react to salt, and reducing intake of salt is helpful for some of these people.[8] Some people with migraines have been reported to improve after removing all cows' milk protein from their diet. The presence of **lactose intolerance** (page 288) was found to be a strong predictor of improvement in that study.[9] In addition, some migraine sufferers have an impaired capacity to break down tyramine, a substance found in many foods[10] that is known to trigger migraines in some people.[11] People with this defect are presumably more sensitive than others to the effects of tyramine.[12] Ingestion of the artificial sweetener, aspartame, has also been reported to trigger migraines in a small proportion of people.[13, 14]

L-tryptophan, an **amino acid** (page 465) found in protein-rich foods, is converted to serotonin, a substance that might worsen some migraines. For that reason, two studies have investigated the effect of a low-protein diet on migraines; in these studies some people experienced a reduction in migraine symptoms.[15, 16] However, in a small double-blind trial, four of eight people had marked improvement in their migraine symptoms while receiving L-tryptophan (500 mg every six hours).[17] Moreover, some preliminary evidence discussed below suggests that **5-hydroxytryptophan** (page 459), a supplement related to L-tryptophan, may reduce symptoms in some migraine sufferers. Therefore, the idea that a low-protein diet would help migraine patients due to its low L-tryptophan content appears doubtful.

Lifestyle changes that may be helpful

Some doctors have found that reactions to smoking and birth control pills can be additional contributing factors in migraines.

Infection (page 265) with *Helicobacter pylori* (*H. pylori,* an organism that causes **peptic ulcers** [page 349]) may predispose people to migraine headaches. In a pre-

liminary trial, 40% of migraine sufferers were found to have *H. pylori* infection. Intensity, duration, and frequency of attacks of migraine were significantly reduced in all participants in whom the *H. pylori* was eradicated.[18] Controlled clinical trials are needed to confirm these preliminary results.

Nutritional supplements that may be helpful

Compared with healthy people, people with migraines have been found to have lower blood and brain levels of **magnesium** (page 551).[19, 20, 21, 22] Preliminary research in a group of women (mostly premenopausal) showed that supplementing with magnesium (usually 200 mg per day) reduced the frequency of migraines in 80% of those treated.[23] In a double-blind trial of 81 people with migraines, 600 mg of magnesium per day was significantly more effective than placebo at reducing the frequency of migraines.[24] Another double-blind trial found that taking 360 mg of magnesium per day decreased the number of days on which premenstrual migraines occurred.[25] One double-blind trial found no benefit from 486 mg of magnesium per day for three months. However, that study defined improvement according to extremely strict criteria, and even some known anti-migraine drugs have failed to show benefit when tested using those criteria.[26] Intravenous magnesium has been reported to produce marked and sometimes complete symptom relief during acute migraines, usually within 15 minutes or less.[27]

One group of researchers treated 49 migraine patients with large amounts of **vitamin B$_2$** (page 598) (400 mg per day). Both the frequency and severity of migraines decreased by more than two-thirds.[28] In a follow-up three-month, double-blind trial, the same researchers reported that 59% of patients assigned to receive vitamin B$_2$ had at least a 50% reduction in the number of headache days, whereas only 15% of those assigned to receive a placebo experienced that degree of improvement.[29] The effects of vitamin B$_2$ were most pronounced during the final month of the trial.[30]

In a preliminary trial, administration of 1 mg of vitamin B$_{12}$ per day (by the intranasal route) for 3 months reduced the frequency of migraine attacks by at least 50% in 10 of 19 people with recurrent migraines.[31] A placebo-controlled study is needed to determine how much of this improvement was due to a placebo effect.

The cause of migraine headache is believed to be related to abnormal serotonin function in blood vessels,[32] and 5-hydroxytryptophan (**5-HTP** [page 459], which is converted by the body into serotonin) may affect this abnormality. In one study, 40 people with recurrent migraines received either 5-HTP (200 mg per day) or methysergide (a drug used to prevent migraines) for 40 days. Both compounds reduced the frequency of migraines by about 50%.[33] Larger amounts of 5-HTP (600 mg per day) were also found to be as effective as medications for reducing migraine headache attacks in adults in two double-blind trials.[34, 35] Migraine attacks were reduced in frequency, severity, and duration in 90% of those taking 400 mg per day of 5-HTP in a double-blind placebo-controlled trial,[36] though another trial found no benefit of 5-HTP.[37] In another controlled study, 400 mg of dl-5-HTP (another form of 5-HTP) led to reduced consumption of pain-killing drugs and **pain** (page 338) scores after one to two months.[38] Children who suffered from migraines and had **problems sleeping** (page 270) responded well to a daily amount of 5-HTP equal to 20 mg for every 10 pounds of body weight in a controlled trial,[39] though an earlier study showed 5-HTP had no better effect than placebo for children with migraines.[40]

Fish oil (page 514) containing EPA and **DHA** (page 509) has been reported to reduce the symptoms of migraine headache in a double-blind trial using 1 gram of fish oil per 10 pounds of body weight.[41, 42] Fish oil may help because of its effects in modifying prostaglandins (hormone-like substances made by the body).

Taking large amounts of the combination of **calcium** (page 481) (1,000 to 2,000 mg per day) and **vitamin D** (page 607) has been reported to produce a marked reduction in the incidence of migraines in several women.[43, 44] However, the amount of vitamin D given to these women (usually 50,000 IU once a week), can cause adverse reactions, particularly when used in combination with calcium. This amount of vitamin D should be used only under medical supervision. Doctors often recommend that people take 800 to 1,200 mg of calcium and 400 IU of vitamin D per day. However, it is not known whether these amounts would have an effect on migraines.

In a preliminary trial, supplementation of migraine sufferers with 150 mg per day of coenzyme Q_{10} for three months reduced the average number of days with migraine headaches by 60%.[45] A placebo-controlled trial is needed to rule out the possibility that this improvement was due to a placebo effect.

Preliminary research also suggests that oral supplements of **SAMe** (page 583) (S-adenosyl-L-methionine) may reduce symptoms for some migraine sufferers.[46]

The function of the pineal gland and its cyclic secretion of **melatonin** (page 555) may be disturbed in people with migraine headaches.[47] Preliminary evidence suggests that 5 mg per day of melatonin, taken 30 minutes before bedtime, may reduce symptoms of migraine headache.[48]

Are there any side effects or interactions?
Refer to the individual supplement for information about any side effects or interactions.

Herbs that may be helpful
The most frequently used herb for the long-term prevention of migraines is **feverfew** (page 677).[49] Three double-blind trials have reported that continuous use of feverfew leads to a reduction in the severity, duration, and frequency of migraine headaches,[50, 51, 52] although one double-blind trial found feverfew to be ineffective.[53]

Studies suggest that taking standardized feverfew leaf extracts that supply a minimum of 250 mcg of parthenolide per day is most effective. Results may not be evident for at least four to six weeks. Although there has been recent debate about the relevance of parthenolide as an active constituent,[54] it is best to use standardized extracts of feverfew until research proves otherwise.

Anecdotal evidence suggests **ginger** (page 680) may be used for migraines and the accompanying nausea.[55] *Ginkgo biloba* (page 681) extract may also help because it inhibits the action of a substance known as platelet-activating factor,[56] which may contribute to migraines. No clinical trials have examined its effectiveness in treating migraines, however.

In a double-blind trial, supplementing with an extract of butterbur *(Petasites hybridus)* for four months was significantly more effective than a placebo at reducing the frequency of migraine attacks.[57] The amount of butterbur found to be effective was 75 mg twice a day of an extract standardized to contain at least 15% petasins. A smaller amount (50 mg twice a day) was ineffective. The most common side effect was burping.

There is preliminary evidence that capsaicin, the active constituent of **cayenne** (page 654), can be applied inside the nose as a treatment for acute migraine.[58] However, as intranasal application of capsaicin produces a burning sensation, it should be used only under the supervision of a doctor familiar with its use.

Are there any side effects or interactions?
Refer to the individual herb for information about any side effects or interactions.

Holistic approaches that may be helpful

Many reports have shown acupuncture to be useful in the treatment of migraines. In a preliminary trial, 18 of 26 people suffering from migraine headaches demonstrated an improvement in symptoms following therapy with acupuncture; they also had a 50% reduction in the use of pain medication.[59] Previous preliminary trials have demonstrated similar results,[60, 61, 62] which have also been confirmed in placebo-controlled trials.[63, 64] Improvement has been maintained at one[65] and three[66] years of follow-up. In preliminary research, patients suffering from chronic headaches of various types (including migraine, **cluster** [page 117], or **tension headaches** [page 428]) have also experienced an improvement in symptoms following acupuncture treatment.[67] In a trial comparing acupuncture to traditional drug therapy, a significantly greater cure rate was achieved in the acupuncture group relative to the drug treatment group (75% vs. 34%).[68]

Dry needling is a form of acupuncture that does not utilize traditional Chinese medicine diagnosis or traditional acupuncture points for treatment. Instead, acupuncture needles are inserted into painful muscle areas (trigger points). A study of 85 patients comparing dry needle acupuncture to conventional drug therapy found a similar reduction in frequency and duration of migraine attacks in both treatment groups.[69]

Percutaneous Electrical Nerve Stimulation (PENS) is an electrical nerve stimulation technique that has become increasingly popular in the complementary and alternative management of **pain** (page 338) syndromes. PENS involves insertion of needle probes, similar to acupuncture, at specific therapeutic points and then applying low levels of electrical current. In one study, PENS was significantly more effective than needles alone at relieving pain in migraine headaches (tension headaches and post-traumatic headaches were also improved).[70]

Practitioners of manipulation report success in treating migraine with manipulation.[71] Migraine sufferers are reported to often have neck pain, tenderness of the spinal joints of the neck,[72] and limited ability to move the neck,[73] all of which suggest the presence of neck problems that could respond to manipulation. Two preliminary trials reported significant benefit to 75–80% of migraine patients treated with manipulation,[74, 75] while a third preliminary trial reported reductions in headache frequency and duration, nausea, and **sensitivity to light** (page 356) one year after the completion of a two-month course of manipulation.[76] A controlled trial compared three types of manipulation and found all three provided significant improvement in headache frequency, severity, and duration.[77, 78] Another controlled trial compared two months of manipulation to sham (fake) manipulation and to placebo treatment with a non-functioning electrical unit. People in the manipulation group had significantly more improvement of headache frequency and duration, and of ability to function in daily life; they also used less medication.[79] The largest controlled trial to date compared eight weeks of manipulation, drug therapy, or both treatments in combination. Manipulation was as effective as the medication in reducing an overall score of migraine suffering, but had fewer reported side effects.[80]

MINOR INJURIES

Minor injuries include such injuries as bruises, sprains, strains, and skin wounds.

The healing of minor injuries requires the involvement of several body systems, including the circulatory system, the immune system, and the cellular mechanisms to repair and grow new tissues.

For more information about specific minor injuries, please refer to the following articles:

- **Bruising** (page 84)
- **Burns** (page 85)
- **Low back pain** (page 293)
- **Pain** (page 338)
- **Sprains and strains** (page 412)

MITRAL VALVE PROLAPSE

The mitral valve is one of the four valves separating chambers of the heart. Mitral valve prolapse (MVP) is a common and occasionally serious condition in which the cusp or cusps of the mitral valve bulge into one of the heart chambers during the heart's contraction. This bulging is caused by abnormalities in the valve's structure. When serious, mitral valve prolapse may progress to mitral regurgitation, where the incompetent valve can no longer keep blood from leaking backwards into the wrong chamber of the heart.

What are the symptoms of mitral valve prolapse?

Most people with MVP experience no symptoms. Some may experience difficulty breathing during exertion or when lying down, tremor, fatigue, lightheadedness, dizziness, and fainting. Some develop dull chest pain, palpitations (awareness of the heartbeat), **anxiety** (page 30), and other symptoms associated with the "fight or flight" response. When MVP causes these symptoms, it is referred to as dysautonomia syndrome.

CHECKLIST FOR MITRAL VALVE PROLAPSE		
Rating	**Nutritional Supplements**	**Herbs**
★★★	**Magnesium** (page 551)	
★☆☆	**L-carnitine** (page 543)	

Medical treatments

The prescription medications used do not cure mitral valve prolapse, but they can control symptoms associated with the condition. The beta-blockers, such as atenolol (Tenormin), propranolol (Inderal), and metoprolol (Lopressor, Toprol XL); blood thinners, including aspirin (Bayer Low Adult Strength, Ecotrin Adult Low Strength) and warfarin (Coumadin); and antibiotics to prevent infection and inflammation of the heart's inner lining may be prescribed.

Serious cases might require surgery to repair the affected heart valve.

Dietary changes that may be helpful

In people who have dysautonomia, low salt intake may be part of the problem. Therefore, unless there is another health problem (such as **high blood pressure** [page 246]) that is worsened by high salt intake, people with MVP should not restrict the amount of salt in the diet.[1]

Lifestyle changes that may be helpful

People with dysautonomia symptoms should avoid stressful situations and should work on techniques for coping with stress.

Nutritional supplements that may be helpful

Magnesium (page 551) deficiency has been proposed as one cause of the symptoms that occur in association with MVP.[2] In a study of people with severe MVP symptoms, blood levels of magnesium were low in 60% of cases. Those people with low magnesium levels participated in a double-blind trial, in which they received a placebo or magnesium (500 mg per day for one week,

then about 335 mg per day for four weeks). People receiving magnesium experienced a significant reduction in symptoms of weakness, chest pain, **anxiety** (page 30), shortness of breath, and palpitations.[3]

In one report, deficient levels of **L-carnitine** (page 543) were found in five consecutive people with MVP.[4] One of these people was given L-carnitine (1 gram three times per day for four months) and experienced a complete resolution of the symptoms associated with MVP.

Are there any side effects or interactions?
Refer to the individual supplement for information about any side effects or interactions.

MORNING SICKNESS

Morning sickness is the common but poorly understood nausea that frequently accompanies early **pregnancy** (page 363).

It is generally not serious, although it can be quite unpleasant. Hyperemesis gravidarum is uncontrollable nausea and vomiting during pregnancy that results in severe dehydration and pH imbalances in the blood. It is distinct from morning sickness with nausea and vomiting. The former condition requires treatment by a healthcare professional and, sometimes, hospitalization. Hyperemesis gravidarum can sometimes result from hyperthyroidism,[1] liver disease, kidney infection, pancreatitis, intestinal obstruction, or other causes—conditions that will not respond to any of the natural substances discussed in this article.

CHECKLIST FOR MORNING SICKNESS		
Rating	**Nutritional Supplements**	**Herbs**
★★★	**Vitamin B$_6$** (page 600)	
★★☆		**Ginger** (page 680)
★☆☆	**Adrenal extracts** (page 462) **Vitamin C** (page 604) **Vitamin K** (page 612)	

What are the symptoms of morning sickness?

Symptoms include nausea, vomiting, fatigue, lightheadedness, and dizziness during the early stages of pregnancy. Women with morning sickness may be particularly sensitive to certain odors and foods. However, eating small amounts of a particular food may relieve their symptoms.

Medical treatments

No over the counter drugs are FDA-approved for the treatment of morning sickness. However, drugs such as dimenhydrinate (Dramamine), diphenhydramine (Benadryl), and meclizine (Bonine) have been used.

Prescription medications used include prochlorperazine (Compazine), ondansetron (Zofran), meclizine (Antivert), promethazine (Phenergan), and metoclopramide (Reglan).

Healthcare practitioners typically recommend that women with morning sickness drink plenty of fluids and try to eat whatever they can, regardless of its nutritional value.

Dietary changes that may be helpful

Some doctors recommend that women with morning sickness eat dry crackers upon waking. Drinking liquids and eating solid foods at separate times may be helpful as well.

In a Harvard University study, women with a high intake of saturated fat (found mainly in meat and dairy) during the year prior to pregnancy had a much higher risk of severe morning sickness than did women eating less saturated fat. An increase in saturated fat intake of 15 grams per day (the equivalent of a four-ounce cheeseburger or three cups of whole milk) was associated with a greater than threefold increase in the risk of developing morning sickness.[2]

Nutritional supplements that may be helpful

In two double-blind trials, supplementation with **vitamin B6** (page 600) (10 or 25 mg three times per day) significantly reduced the severity of morning sickness.[3, 4]

Vitamin K (page 612) and **vitamin C** (page 604), taken together, may provide relief of symptoms for some women. In one study, 91% of women who took 5 mg of vitamin K and 25 mg of vitamin C per day reported the complete disappearance of morning sickness within three days.[5] Menadione was removed from the market a number of years ago because of concerns about potential toxicity. Although some doctors still use a combination of vitamin K1 (the most prevalent form of vitamin K in food) and vitamin C for morning sickness, no studies on this treatment have been done.

In a preliminary study done in the 1930s, eight women suffering from nausea and vomiting during the first trimester (13 weeks) of **pregnancy** (page 363) received large amounts of oral **adrenal cortex extract** (page 462). In most cases, vomiting stopped after three to four days.[6] In a follow-up study, women with nausea and vomiting of pregnancy received adrenal cortex extract, usually by injection at first, followed by oral administration. More than 85% of the women were completely relieved of the problem or showed definite improvement.[7] Since no safety data exist for use during pregnancy, adrenal extract should not be used in these situations unless supervised by a doctor.

Are there any side effects or interactions?
Refer to the individual supplement for information about any side effects or interactions.

Herbs that may be helpful

Ginger (page 680) is well-known for alleviating nausea and improving digestion. One gram of encapsulated ginger powder was used in one study to reduce the severe nausea and vomiting associated with hyperemesis gravidarum.[8] This condition is potentially life-threatening and should only be treated by a qualified healthcare professional.

Because ginger contains some compounds that cause chromosomal mutation in the test tube, some doctors are concerned about the safety of using ginger during **pregnancy** (page 363). However, the available clinical research, combined with the fact that ginger is widely used in the diets of many cultures, suggests that prudent use of ginger for morning sickness is probably safe in amounts up to 1 gram per day.[9]

Are there any side effects or interactions?
Refer to the individual herb for information about any side effects or interactions.

Holistic approaches that may be helpful

A controlled trial found that acupuncture significantly reduced symptoms in women with hyperemesis gravidarum, a severe form of nausea and vomiting of pregnancy that usually requires hospitalization.[10] Treatment consisted of acupuncture at a single point on the forearm three times daily for two consecutive days. Acupressure (in which pressure, rather than needles, is used to stimulate acupuncture points) has also been found in several preliminary trials to be mildly effective in the treatment of nausea and vomiting of pregnancy.[11, 12, 13]

MOTION SICKNESS

Motion sickness is nausea, vomiting, and related symptoms caused by repetitive angular and linear acceleration and deceleration.

CHECKLIST FOR MOTION SICKNESS		
Rating	Nutritional Supplements	Herbs
★★★		Ginger (page 680)
★☆☆		Black horehound (page 638)

What are the symptoms of motion sickness?

Motion sickness is characterized by cycles of nausea and vomiting. These episodes may be preceded by yawning, salivation, pallor, cold sweat, and sleepiness. Dizziness, headache, fatigue, and general discomfort are also common. Once nausea and vomiting develop, a person with motion sickness is typically weak and unable to concentrate.

Medical treatments

Treatment includes over the counter anti-nausea medication, such as dimenhydrinate (Dramamine), meclizine (Bonine), and cyclizine (Marezine).

Prescription medications are taken orally, inserted rectally, or worn as a patch. Commonly prescribed drugs for motion sickness include scopolamine (Transderm Scop), promethazine (Phenergan), prochlorperazine (Compazine), and trimethobenzamide (Tigan).

Individuals with motion sickness should get fresh air and close their eyes. People who frequently experiece motion sickness should avoid drinking alcohol prior to travel.

Herbs that may be helpful

Ginger (page 680) may be useful for the prevention and treatment of mild to moderate cases of motion sickness. A double-blind trial examined the effects of ginger supplements in people who were susceptible to motion sickness. Researchers found that those taking 940 mg of powdered ginger in capsules experienced less motion sickness than those who took dimenhydrate (Dramamine).[1] Another double-blind trial reported that 1 gram of powdered ginger root, compared with placebo, lessened seasickness by 38% and vomiting by

72% in a group of naval cadets sailing in heavy seas.[2] Two clinical trials, one with adults and one with children, found that ginger was as effective in treating seasickness as dimenhydrinate but with fewer side effects.[3, 4] In one controlled trial, though, neither powdered ginger (500 to 1,000 mg) nor fresh ginger (1,000 mg) provided any protection against motion sickness.[5] Doctors prescribing ginger for motion sickness recommend 500 mg one hour before travel and then 500 mg every two to four hours as necessary. The study with children used one-half the adult amount.

Ginger's beneficial effect on motion sickness appears to be related to its action on the gastrointestinal tract rather than on the central nervous system.[6, 7]

Black horehound (page 638) (Ballotta nigra, Marrubium nigrum) is sometimes used by herbalists to treat nausea associated with motion sickness.[8] However, there are no clinical trials to confirm its effectiveness for treating this condition.

Are there any side effects or interactions?
Refer to the individual herb for information about any side effects or interactions.

Holistic approaches that may be helpful

Acupuncture, acupressure, and electroacupuncture to specific points have been found to successfully prevent and treat motion sickness in some,[9, 10, 11] but not all,[12, 13] clinical trials.

MSG SENSITIVITY

MSG sensitivity (sometimes known as "Chinese Restaurant Syndrome") is a set of symptoms that may occur in some people after they consume monosodium glutamate (MSG). The syndrome was first described in 1968 as a triad of symptoms: "numbness at the back of the neck radiating to both arms and the back, general weakness and palpitations."[1] Although some Chinese (and other) restaurants now avoid the use of MSG, many still use significant amounts.

MSG is used worldwide as a flavor enhancer. The average person living in an industrialized country consumes about 0.3 to 1.0 gram of MSG per day. MSG is classified by the Food and Drug Administration as "generally recognized as safe." Indeed, many researchers have questioned the very existence of a true MSG-sensitivity reaction. Most clinical trials, including some double-blind trials, have failed to find any symptoms arising from consumption of MSG, even large amounts, when taken with food.[2, 3, 4, 5, 6] However, clinical trials have found that MSG taken *without* food may cause symptoms, though rarely the classic "triad" described above.[7, 8, 9] A large trial and a review of studies on MSG both suggested that large amounts of MSG given without food may elicit more symptoms than a placebo in people who believe they react adversely to MSG. However, persistent and serious effects from MSG consumption have not been consistently demonstrated.[10, 11, 12]

People sensitive to MSG may also react to aspartame (NutraSweet).[13]

CHECKLIST FOR MSG SENSITIVITY		
Rating	Nutritional Supplements	Herbs
★★☆	Vitamin B₆ (page 600)	

What are the symptoms of MSG sensitivity?
The symptoms of MSG sensitivity have commonly been described as headache, flushing, tingling, weakness, and stomachache. After eating meals prepared with MSG, people with MSG sensitivity may have **migraine** (page 316) headache, visual disturbance, nausea, vomiting, **diarrhea** (page 163), weakness, tightness of the chest, skin rash, or **sensitivity to light** (page 356), noise, or smells.

Medical treatments
Over the counter antihistamines, such as diphenhydramine (Benedryl), might help reduce the symptoms of MSG sensitivity.

Severe reactions may be treated with prescription antihistamines such as hydroxyzine (Atarax).

MSG sensitivity is not a universally accepted medical condition. Other than avoidance of foods containing MSG, there is no common treatment for this condition.

Dietary changes that may be helpful
Simply avoiding MSG will prevent MSG-sensitive reactions. MSG is found in some Chinese and Japanese food and is also contained in some flavor enhancers, such as Accent and the Japanese seasoning AJI-NO-MOTO. MSG may be difficult to avoid completely, as it also occurs in hydrolyzed vegetable protein, textured vegetable protein, gelatin, yeast extracts, calcium and sodium caseinate, vegetable broth, **whey** (page 613), smoke flavoring, malt extracts, and several other food ingredients—including "flavoring" and "natural flavoring"—without otherwise appearing on the label.

Nutritional supplements that may be helpful
Years ago, researchers discovered that animals who were deficient in **vitamin B₆** (page 600) could not properly process MSG.[14] Typical reactions to MSG have also been linked to vitamin B₆ deficiency in people.[15] In one study, eight out of nine such people stopped reacting to MSG when given 50 mg of vitamin B₆ per day for at least 12 weeks.

The actual percentage of people with MSG sensitivity who are deficient in vitamin B₆ and who respond to B₆ supplementation is unknown. Nonetheless, many doctors suggest that people having MSG-sensitivity symptoms try supplementing with vitamin B₆ for three months as a trial.

Are there any side effects or interactions?
Refer to the individual supplement for information about any side effects or interactions.

MULTIPLE SCLEROSIS

Multiple sclerosis (MS) is a slowly progressive, degenerative condition in which the myelin sheaths surrounding nerves in the brain and spinal cord are lost. Myelin sheaths are a type of connective tissue, composed of fats and proteins, that insulate nerve fibers. They protect nerves and are required for effective transmission of nerve impulses.

Indirect evidence suggests that MS may be an autoimmune disease, wherein the immune system attacks myelin in the central nervous system. MS is more common among people who live in temperate climates compared with those who live in tropical climates and receive greater exposure to the sun. Possible causes for MS may include genetic susceptibility, diet, environmental toxins, viral infections, and exposure to dogs, cats, or caged birds.[1] Epstein-Barr virus has also been named as a risk factor,[2] though the real cause or causes of MS are unknown.

What are the symptoms of multiple sclerosis?
MS is characterized by various neurological symptoms, with remissions and recurrent exacerbations. The most

common symptoms are paresthesia (numbness and tingling) in the extremities, trunk, or on one side of the face. Muscle weakness, loss of coordination of a leg or hand, and visual disturbances (such as partial blindness in one eye, dim vision, or double vision) are common in MS. Limbs that fatigue easily, difficulty in walking, difficulty with bladder control, **vertigo** (page 441), and mood disturbances may appear years before MS is diagnosed. The course of the disease is highly varied and unpredictable. In most people, the disease remits for varying periods of time. However, symptoms usually recur, and the progression is often relentless.

CHECKLIST FOR MULTIPLE SCLEROSIS		
Rating	Nutritional Supplements	Herbs
★★☆		Padma 28
★☆☆	**Calcium** (page 483) **Evening primrose oil** (page 511) **Fish oil** (page 514) **Inosine** (page 537) Linoleic acid **Magnesium** (page 551) **Niacin** (page 598) **Thiamine** (page 597) **Vitamin D** (page 607)	*Ginkgo biloba* (page 681) (injections)

Medical treatments

Corticosteroids, such as prednisone (Deltasone, Orasone), are the most common prescription drugs used. Though they may shorten the duration of flare-ups, they have little or no effect on long-term disability. Interferon-beta (Avonex, Betaseron) may reduce the frequency of relapses and delay long-term disability. Intravenous gamma globulins (Gamimune N, Sandoglobulin) given monthly may also control relapses. A variety of immunosuppressive drugs are also used, such as methotrexate (Rheumatrex), azathioprine (Imuran), cyclophosphamide (Cytoxan), and cladribine (Leustatin). However, these drugs are reserved for more severe forms of MS, have limited potential benefits, and are highly toxic. A large variety of drugs, including antispasmodics, antidepressants, and pain relievers, are also used to manage the various symptoms of MS.

Dietary changes that may be helpful

The amount and type of fat eaten may affect both the likelihood of healthy people getting the disease and the outcome of the disease for those already diagnosed with MS. For many years, the leading researcher linking dietary fat to MS risk and progression has been Dr. Roy Swank.

In one of Dr. Swank's reports, a low-fat diet was recommended to 150 people with MS.[3] Although hydrogenated oils, peanut butter, and animal fat (including fat from dairy) were dramatically reduced or eliminated, 5 grams per day of **cod liver oil** (page 514) were added, and linoleic acid from vegetable oil was used. After 34 years, the mortality rate among people consuming an average of 17 grams of saturated fat per day was only 31%, compared with 79% among those who consumed a higher average of 25 grams of saturated fat per day. People who began to follow the low-fat diet early in the disease did better than those who changed their eating habits after the disease had progressed.

A survey of people in 36 different countries also suggests that the types of fat people eat may impact MS.[4] In that report, people with MS who ate foods high in polyunsaturated and monounsaturated fatty acids were likely to live longer than those who ate more saturated fats. In another survey, researchers gathered information from nearly 400 people (half with MS) over three years.[5] They found that people who ate more fish were less likely to develop MS, while those who ate pork, hot dogs, and other foods high in animal (saturated) fats were at greater risk. This same report found consumption of vegetable protein, fruit juice, and foods rich in **vitamin C** (page 604), **thiamine** (page 597), **riboflavin** (page 598), **calcium** (page 483), and **potassium** (page 572) correlated with a decreased MS risk. Eating sweets was linked to an increased risk.

Despite research showing improvement with a low-fat diet in some people with MS, the link between foods containing animal fat and MS risk may not necessarily be due to the fat itself. Preliminary evidence from one report revealed an association between eating dairy foods (cows' milk, butter, and cream) and an increased prevalence of MS, yet no link was found between (high fat) cheese and MS in that same report.[6]

MS has been associated with a variety of dietary components apparently unrelated to fat intake,[7] and the link between MS and diet remains poorly understood. Nonetheless, the most consistent links to date appear to involve certain foods containing animal fat. People with MS wishing to pursue a nutritional approach that incorporates an understanding of this research should consult with a doctor familiar with the "Swank diet."

Some people with MS avoid gluten (a protein found

in wheat, rye, and barley) in hopes of diminishing symptoms, because a preliminary study reported that consumption of grain (bread and pasta) was linked to development of MS.[8] However, another trial found an association between eating cereals and breads and reduced MS risk.[9] Other researchers have found gluten sensitivity to be no more common among people with MS than among healthy people.[10] Thus, the idea that avoiding gluten will help MS remains speculative.

Lifestyle changes that may be helpful

While some studies dispute it,[11, 12] there is preliminary evidence that exposure to organic solvents,[13] insecticides,[14] and X-rays[15] may cause or aggravate MS. This may explain why clusters of multiple sclerosis cases occasionally occur in certain geographical areas or even in work sites.[16]

Swiss researchers found that nicotine temporarily impairs arm movement in people with MS.[17] In one study, when people with MS smoked cigarettes, movement capacity was diminished for 10 minutes in 76% of them. Although this evidence is preliminary, there are many other adverse health effects of smoking. Smokers with MS should quit smoking.

While the outcome of some research disputes the connection between MS and mercury exposure,[18] other investigations have reported an association between dental amalgams and this disease. One study found that mercury levels in the hair of people with MS are higher than in the hair of healthy people.[19] This same report found that people with MS who had their amalgam fillings removed experienced one-third fewer relapses than people who kept their fillings. Another preliminary study found that people having a large number of fillings that had been in place for a long time appeared to be at increased risk for MS compared with those having fewer fillings.[20] Preliminary evidence has also identified an association between **tooth decay** (page 431)—as opposed to fillings—and MS.[21] The importance of the reported links between mercury, tooth decay, and risk of MS has not been clearly established.

Nutritional supplements that may be helpful

Although some doctors recommend **fish oil** (page 514) capsules for people with MS, few investigations have explored the effects of this supplement. In one small trial, people with MS were given approximately 20 grams of fish oil in capsules per day.[22] After one to four months, 42% of these people received slight but significant benefits, including reduced urinary incontinence

and improved eyesight. However, a longer double-blind trial involving over 300 people with MS found that half this amount of fish oil given per day did not help.[23] A preliminary, two-year intervention trial tested the effects of fish oil supplements (5 ml of fish oil per day, providing 400 mg of EPA and 500 mg of **DHA** [page 509]) combined with other dietary supplements and dietary changes in people with newly diagnosed, relapsing-remitting MS.[24] The other supplements included 3,333 IU of **vitamin A** (page 595) per day, 400 IU of **vitamin D** (page 607) per day, and approximately 5.5 IU of **vitamin E** (page 609) per day. The dietary recommendations included reducing intake of sugar, coffee, tea, saturated fat from meat and dairy products, and alcohol, while increasing intake of fish, fruit, vegetables, and whole-grain bread. Sixty-nine percent of those following the regimen improved, 25% remained the same, and 6 % (one person) deteriorated. The many interventions used in this trial make it impossible to determine what was responsible for the positive outcomes. Given the lack of other effective treatments for MS, though, this approach is worth trying while awaiting further evidence.

In a small preliminary trial, people with MS were given 20 grams of **cod liver oil** (page 514), as well as approximately 680 mg of **magnesium** (page 551) and 1,100 mg of **calcium** (page 483) per day in the form of dolomite tablets.[25] After one year, the average number of MS attacks decreased significantly for each person. Unlike fish oil capsules, the cod liver oil in this trial contained not only eicosapentaenoic acid (EPA) and docosahexaenoic acid (DHA), but 5,000 IU of **vitamin D** (page 607). Therefore, it is not known whether the vitamin D or fatty acids were responsible for the cod liver oil's effects. (One preliminary study found that giving vitamin D-like drugs to animals with MS was helpful.)[26] It is also possible that the magnesium and/or calcium given to these people reduced MS attacks. Magnesium[27] and calcium[28] levels have been reported to be lower in the nerve tissue of people with MS compared with healthy people.

Animal studies have demonstrated that vitamin D can prevent an experimental form of multiple sclerosis. In humans, striking geographical differences in the prevalence of multiple sclerosis suggest that sun exposure (which promotes the synthesis of vitamin D) may protect against the development of the disease. While some scientists have theorized that vitamin D may help prevent MS, clinical trials are needed to validate that hypothesis.[29]

The omega-6 fatty acids, found in such oils as **evening primrose oil** (page 511) (EPO) and sunflower seed oil, also may be beneficial. When people with MS were given 4 grams of EPO for three weeks, their hand grip improved.[30] In a review of three double-blind trials, two of the trials reported that linoleic acid reduced the severity and length of relapses.[31] When the data were re-examined, it was found that taking linoleic acid decreased disability due to MS in all three trials. According to these researchers, taking linoleic acid while following a diet low in animal fat and high in polyunsaturated fat may be even more beneficial. Amounts used in these trials were approximately 17 to 23 grams of linoleic acid per day, provided by 26 to 35 grams of sunflower seed oil.

Deficiency of **thiamine** (page 597) (vitamin B₁) may contribute to nerve damage.[32] Many years ago, researchers found that injecting thiamine[33] into the spinal cord or using intravenous thiamine combined with **niacin** (page 598)[34] in people with MS led to a reduction in symptoms. Using injectable vitamins requires medical supervision. No research has yet studied the effects of oral supplementation with B vitamins in people with MS.

Inosine is a precursor to uric acid, a compound that occurs naturally in the body. Uric acid is believed to block the effect of a toxic free-radical compound (peroxynitrite) that may play a role in the development of multiple sclerosis.[35] In an attempt to raise uric acid levels, ten patients with MS were treated with inosine in amounts up to 3 grams per day for 46 weeks. Three of the ten treated patients showed some evidence of improved function and the others remained stable.[36] Controlled studies are needed to confirm these preliminary results.

Are there any side effects or interactions?
Refer to the individual supplement for information about any side effects or interactions.

Herbs that may be helpful
A commercial herbal product called Padma 28 was given to 100 people with MS.[37] After taking two pills three times per day, 44% of these people experienced increased muscle strength and general overall improvement. The composition of Padma 28 is based on a traditional Tibetan herbal formula.

Inflammation of nerve tissue is partly responsible for the breakdown of myelin in people with MS. When intravenous injections of a constituent of ***Ginkgo biloba***

(page 681), known as ginkgolide B, were given to people with MS for five days, 80% of them reportedly improved.[38] This specialized treatment is experimental, and it is not known whether oral use of ginkgo extracts would have a similar effect.

Are there any side effects or interactions?
Refer to the individual herb for information about any side effects or interactions.

NIGHT BLINDNESS

People with night blindness (also called impaired dark adaptation) see poorly in the darkness but see normally when adequate amounts of light are present. The condition does not actually involve true blindness, even at night.

CHECKLIST FOR NIGHT BLINDNESS		
Rating	Nutritional Supplements	Herbs
★★★	**Beta-carotene** (page 469) **Vitamin A** (page 595) **Zinc** (page 614) (for deficiency)	
★☆☆		**Bilberry** (page 634)

What are the symptoms of night blindness?
Symptoms include difficulty seeing when driving in the evening or at night, poor vision in reduced light, and feeling that the eyes take longer to "adjust" to seeing in the dark.

Medical treatments
Over the counter treatment typically consists of oral supplementation with **vitamin A** (page 595).

Therapy includes management of any underlying medical condition.

Nutritional supplements that may be helpful
Night blindness may be an early sign of **vitamin A** (page 595) deficiency. Such a deficiency may result from diets low in animal foods (the main source of vitamin A), such as eggs, dairy products, organ meats, and some fish. Low intake of fruits and vegetables containing **beta-carotene** (page 469), which the body converts into vitamin A, may also contribute to a vitamin A de-

ficiency. Doctors often recommend 10,000 to 25,000 IU of vitamin A per day to correct a deficiency. Beta-carotene is less effective at correcting vitamin A deficiency than is vitamin A itself, because it is not absorbed as well and is only slowly converted by the body into vitamin A.

Dietary **zinc** (page 614) deficiency is common, and a lack of zinc may reduce the activity of retinol dehydrogenase, an enzyme needed to help vitamin A work in the eye. Zinc helps night blindness in people who are zinc-deficient;[1] therefore, many physicians suggest 15 to 30 mg of zinc per day to support healthy vision. Because long-term zinc supplementation may reduce **copper** (page 499) levels, 1 to 2 mg of copper per day (depending on the amount of zinc used) is usually recommended for people who are supplementing with zinc for more than a few weeks.

Are there any side effects or interactions?
Refer to the individual supplement for information about any side effects or interactions.

Herbs that may be helpful
Bilberry (page 634), a close relative of the blueberry, is high in **flavonoids** (page 516) known as anthocyanosides. Anthocyanosides speed the regeneration of rhodopsin, the purple pigment that is used by the rods in the eye for night vision.[2] Supplementation with bilberry has been shown in early studies to improve dark adaptation in people with poor night vision.[3, 4] However, two newer studies found no effect of bilberry on night vision in healthy people.[5, 6] Bilberry extract standardized to contain 25% anthocyanosides may be taken in capsule or tablet form. Doctors typically recommend 240 to 480 mg per day.

Are there any side effects or interactions?
Refer to the individual herb for information about any side effects or interactions.

OSGOOD-SCHLATTER DISEASE

Osgood-Schlatter disease is a form of osteochondrosis, a disease of the growth center at the end of long bones. The disease occurs in adolescence, most commonly among 10- to 15-year-old boys, and is often the result of rapid growth combined with competitive sports that overstress the knee joint. The patellar tendon, which at-

taches the kneecap to the tibia, is sometimes strained and partially torn from the bone by the powerful quadriceps muscles. This tearing, called avulsion, may be extremely painful and is sometimes disabling. It may occur in one or both knees. The knee is usually tender to pressure at the point where the large tendon from the kneecap attaches to the prominence below.

CHECKLIST FOR OSGOOD-SCHLATTER DISEASE		
Rating	Nutritional Supplements	Herbs
★☆☆	**Manganese** (page 553), **Vitamin B₆** (page 600), and **Zinc** (page 614) (in combination) **Selenium** (page 584) **Vitamin E** (page 609)	

What are the symptoms of Osgood-Schlatter disease?
People with Osgood-Schlatter disease experience tenderness, swelling, and pain just below one knee that usually worsens with activity, such as going up or down stairs, and is relieved by rest. Symptoms may also include the appearance of a bony bump below the knee cap that is especially painful when pressed.

Medical treatments
In most cases, symptoms disappear without treatment when a child's growth is completed. Healthcare providers may recommend applying ice to the knee when pain first appears in order to help relieve inflammation. Participation in sports and excessive exercise might be limited. Severe cases might require immobilization of the leg in a cast or surgical treatment.

Nutritional supplements that may be helpful
Based on the personal experience of a doctor who reported his findings,[1] some physicians recommend **vitamin E** (page 609) (400 IU per day) and **selenium** (page 584) (50 mcg three times per day). One well-known, nutritionally oriented doctor reports anecdotally that he has had considerable success with this regimen and often sees results in two to six weeks.[2]

Another group of doctors has reported good results using a combination of **zinc** (page 614), **manganese** (page 553), and **vitamin B₆** (page 600) for people with Osgood-Schlatter disease; however, the amounts of these supplements were not mentioned in the report.[3] Most physicians would consider reasonable daily amounts of these nutrients for adolescents to be 15 mg of zinc, 5 to 10 mg of manganese, and 25 mg of vitamin B_6. Larger amounts might be used with medical supervision.

Are there any side effects or interactions?
Refer to the individual supplement for information about any side effects or interactions.

OSTEOARTHRITIS

What do I need to know?

Self-care for osteoarthritis can be approached in a number of ways—but it can be hard to know just where to start. To make it easier, our doctors recommend trying these simple steps first:

Help prevent joint damage with GS and CS
Take 1,500 mg a day of glucosamine sulfate, 800 to 1,200 mg a day of chondroitin sulfate, or a combination of the two, for pain and to protect joints

Use topical capsaicin
Treat discomfort with an ointment or cream containing 0.025 to 0.075% capsaicin four times a day over painful joints

Add antioxidants
Eat more fruits and vegetables and take 400 to 1,600 IU a day of vitamin E to put antioxidants to work protecting your joints

Get moving
Start a gentle program of walking and strengthening exercise to reduce pain and improve joint function

About osteoarthritis

Osteoarthritis (OA) is a chronic disease of the joints, especially the weight-bearing joints that develops when the linings of joints degenerate, leading to lipping and spurring of bone, **pain** (page 338), and decreased mobility and function.

OA is a universal consequence of aging among animals with a bony skeleton. Many factors contribute to the development of OA; the disease is primarily associated with aging and injury and was once called "wear-and-tear" arthritis. OA may occur secondary to many other conditions. However, in most cases, the true cause of OA is unknown.

CHECKLIST FOR OSTEOARTHRITIS

Rating	Nutritional Supplements	Herbs
★★★	**Chondroitin sulfate** (page 492) **Glucosamine sulfate** (page 529) **SAMe** (page 583) **Vitamin B₃** (page 598) (niacinamide)	**Boswellia** (page 644) (also in combination with **ashwagandha** [page 629], **turmeric** [page 753], and **zinc** [page 614]) **Cat's claw** (page 653) **Cayenne** (page 654) (topical, for pain only) **Ginger** (page 680)
★★☆	**Cartilage** (page 490) **Cetyl myristoleate** (page 490) **Collagen** (page 490) **DMSO** (page 508) (topical) **Enzymes** (page 506) (bromelain, trypsin, rutosid combination) **Green-lipped mussel** (page 533) **Vitamin E** (page 609)	**Devil's claw** (page 668) **Guggul** (page 688) **Nettle** (page 714) **Willow** (page 760)
★☆☆	**Boron** (page 477) **Bovine cartilage** (page 490) **D-phenylalanine** (page 568) (DPA) **Fish oil** (page 514) (EPA/ **DHA** [page 509]) **Glucosamine hydrochloride** (page 528) **Methylsulfonyl-methane** (page 558) (MSM)	Colchicine **Horsetail** (page 693) **Meadowsweet** (page 709) Yucca

What are the symptoms of osteoarthritis?

The onset of osteoarthritis is gradual and most often affects the hips, knees, fingers, and spine, although other joints also may be involved. **Pain** (page 338) is the main symptom, which usually worsens with exercise and is relieved by rest. Morning stiffness is also common and diminishes with movement. As osteoarthritis progresses, joint motion is lost, and tenderness and grating sensations may develop. Osteoarthritis of the spine may lead to shooting pains down the arms or legs.

Medical treatments

Over the counter nonsteroidal anti-inflammatory drugs (NSAIDs), such as aspirin (Bayer, Ecotrin, Bufferin), ibuprofen (Motrin, Advil), and naproxen (Aleve), as well as acetaminophen (Tylenol), may help provide pain relief in mild cases. Topical creams containing **capsaicin** (page 654) (Zostrix) may also be used for local pain relief.

Prescription medications for pain relief include NSAIDs, such as celecoxib (Celebrex), valdecoxib (Bextra), diclofenac (Voltaren), etodolac (Lodine), ibuprofen (Motrin), and indomethacin (Indocin).

Treatment designed to relieve osteoarthritis symptoms includes the use of hot soaks, warm paraffin applications, heating pads, and joint support devices.

Dietary changes that may be helpful

In the 1950s through the 1970s, Dr. Max Warmbrand used a diet free of meat, poultry, dairy, chemicals, sugar, eggs, and processed foods for people with **rheumatoid arthritis** (page 387) and OA, anecdotally claiming significant success.[1] He reported that clinical results took at least six months to develop. The Warmbrand diet has never been properly tested in clinical research. Moreover, although the diet is healthful and might reduce the risk of being diagnosed with many other diseases, it is difficult for most people to follow. This difficulty, plus the lack of published research, leads many doctors who are aware of the Warmbrand diet to use it only if other approaches have failed.

Solanine is a substance found in nightshade plants, including tomatoes, white potatoes, all peppers (except black pepper), and eggplant. In theory, if not destroyed in the intestine, solanine may be toxic. One horticulturist hypothesized that some people might not be able to destroy solanine in the gut, leading to solanine absorption and resulting in OA. This theory has not been proven. However, eliminating solanine from the diet *has* been reported to bring relief to some arthritis sufferers in preliminary research.[2, 3] In a survey of people avoiding nightshade plants, 28% claimed to have a "marked positive response" and another 44% a "positive response." Researchers have never put this diet to a strict clinical test; however, the treatment continues to be used by some doctors with patients who have OA. As with the Warmbrand diet, proponents claim exclusion of solanine requires up to six months before potential effects may be seen. Totally eliminating tomatoes and peppers requires complex dietary changes for most

people. In addition, even proponents of the diet acknowledge that many arthritis sufferers are not helped by using this approach. Therefore, long-term trial avoidance of solanine-containing foods may be appropriate only for people with osteoarthritis who have not responded to other natural treatments.

Most of the studies linking **allergies** (page 14) to joint disease have focused on **rheumatoid arthritis** (page 387), although mention of what was called "rheumatism" in older reports (some of which may have been OA) suggests a possible link between food reactions and aggravations of osteoarthritis symptoms.[4] If other therapies are unsuccessful in relieving symptoms, people with osteoarthritis might choose to discuss food allergy identification and elimination with a physician.

Lifestyle changes that may be helpful

Obesity increases the risk of osteoarthritis developing in weight-bearing joints, and **weight loss** (page 446) in women is associated with reduced risk for developing OA.[5, 6] Weight loss is also thought to reduce the **pain** (page 338) of existing OA.[7]

Nutritional supplements that may be helpful

Glucosamine sulfate (page 000) (GS), a nutrient derived from seashells, is a building block needed for the synthesis and repair of joint cartilage. GS supplementation has significantly reduced symptoms of osteoarthritis in uncontrolled[8, 9] and single-blind trials.[10, 11] Many double-blind trials have also reported efficacy.[12, 13, 14, 15, 16] Only one published trial[17] has reported no effect of GS on osteoarthritis symptoms. While most research trials use 500 mg GS taken three times per day, results of a three-year, double-blind trial indicate that 1,500 mg taken once per day produces significant reduction of symptoms and halts degenerative changes seen by X-ray examination.[18] GS does not *cure* people with osteoarthritis, and they may need to take the supplement for the rest of their lives in order to maintain benefits. Fortunately, GS appears to be virtually free of side effects, even after three or more years of supplementation. Benefits from GS generally become evident after three to eight weeks of treatment.

Only one trial has evaluated another form of glucosamine as a single remedy for OA.[19] This trial found only minor benefits from 1,500 mg per day of glucosamine hydrochloride (GH) for eight weeks in people with osteoarthritis of the knee; these people were also taking up to 4,000 mg per day of acetaminophen for pain relief. To more fairly evaluate the effects of GH, future research should exclude people taking pain-relieving medication. Another form of glucosamine sometimes found in combination formulas, **N-acetyl-glucosamine** (page 564) (NAG), has not been studied in people with osteoarthritis.

Chondroitin sulfate (page 492) (CS) is a major component of the lining of joints. The structure of CS includes molecules related to glucosamine sulfate. CS levels have been reported to be reduced in joint cartilage affected by OA. Possibly as a result, CS supplementation may help restore joint function in people with OA.[20] On the basis of preliminary evidence, researchers had believed that oral CS was not absorbed in humans;[21] as a result, early double-blind CS research was done mostly by giving injections.[22, 23] This research documented clinical benefits from CS injections. It now appears, however, that a significant amount of CS is absorbable in humans,[24] though dissolving CS in water leads to better absorption than swallowing whole pills.[25]

Strong clinical evidence now supports the use of oral CS supplements for OA. Many double-blind trials have shown that CS supplementation consistently reduces pain, increases joint mobility, and/or shows evidence (including X-ray changes) of healing within joints of people with OA.[26, 27, 28, 29, 30, 31, 32, 33, 34, 35] Most trials have used 400 mg of CS taken two to three times per day. One trial found that taking the full daily amount (1,200 mg) at one time was as effective as taking 400 mg three times per day.[36] Reduction in symptoms typically occurs within several months.

S-adenosyl methionine (**SAMe** [page 583]) possesses anti-inflammatory, **pain** (page 338)-relieving, and tissue-healing properties that may help protect the health of joints,[37, 38] though the primary way in which SAMe reduces osteoarthritis symptoms is not known. A very large, though uncontrolled, trial (meaning that there was no comparison with placebo) demonstrated "very good" or "good" clinical effect of SAMe in 71% of over 20,000 OA sufferers.[39] In addition to this preliminary research, many double-blind trials have shown that SAMe reduces pain, stiffness, and swelling better than placebo and equal to drugs such as ibuprofen and naproxen in people with OA.[40, 41, 42, 43, 44, 45, 46, 47] These double-blind trials all used 1,200 mg of SAMe per day.

Lower amounts of oral SAMe have also produced reductions in the severity of osteoarthritis symptoms in preliminary clinical trials. A two-year, uncontrolled trial showed significant improvement of symptoms

after two weeks at 600 mg SAMe daily, followed by 400 mg daily thereafter.[48] This amount was also used in a double-blind trial, but participants first received five days of intravenous SAMe.[49] A review of the clinical trials on SAMe concluded that its efficacy against osteoarthritis was similar to that of conventional drugs but that patients tolerated it better.[50]

People who have osteoarthritis and eat large amounts of **antioxidants** (page 467) in food have been reported to exhibit a much slower rate of joint deterioration, particularly in the knees, compared with people eating foods containing lower amounts of antioxidants.[51] Of the individual antioxidants, only **vitamin E** (page 609) has been studied as a supplement in controlled trials. Vitamin E supplementation has reduced symptoms of osteoarthritis in both single-blind[52] and double-blind research.[53, 54] In these trials, 400 to 1,600 IU of vitamin E per day was used. Clinical effects were obtained within several weeks. However, in a six-month double-blind study of patients with osteoarthritis of the knee, 500 IU per day of vitamin E was no more effective than a placebo.[55]

In the 1940s and 1950s, one doctor reported that supplemental **niacinamide** (page 598) (a form of vitamin B_3) increased joint mobility, improved muscle strength, and decreased fatigue in people with OA.[56, 57, 58] In the 1990s, a double-blind trial confirmed a reduction in symptoms from niacinamide within 12 weeks of beginning supplementation.[59] Although amounts used have varied from trial to trial, many doctors recommend 250 to 500 mg of niacinamide four or more times per day (with the higher amounts reserved for people with more advanced arthritis). The mechanism by which niacinamide reduces symptoms is not known.

The effects of New Zealand **green-lipped mussel** (page 533) supplements have been studied in people with OA. In a preliminary trial, either a lipid extract (210 mg per day) or a freeze-dried powder (1,150 mg per day) of green-lipped mussel reduced joint tenderness and morning stiffness, as well as improving overall function in most participants.[60] In a double-blind trial, 45% of people with osteoarthritis who took a green-lipped mussel extract (350 mg three times per day for three months) reportedly had improvements in pain and stiffness.[61] Another double-blind trial reported excellent results from green-lipped mussel extract (2,100 mg per day for six months) for pain associated with arthritis of the knee.[62] Side effects, such as **stomach upset** (page 260), **gout** (page 208), skin rashes, and one case of **hepatitis** (page 220) have been reported in people taking certain New Zealand green-lipped mussel extracts.[63]

The therapeutic use of **DMSO** (page 508) (dimethyl sulfoxide) is controversial because of safety concerns, but some preliminary research shows that diluted preparations of DMSO, applied directly to the skin, are anti-inflammatory and alleviate **pain** (page 338), including pain associated with OA.[64, 65] A recent double-blind trial found that a 25% concentration of DMSO in gel form relieved osteoarthritis pain significantly better than a placebo after three weeks.[66] DMSO appears to reduce pain by inhibiting the transmission of pain messages by nerves[67] rather than through a process of healing damaged joints. DMSO comes in different strengths and different degrees of purity; in addition, certain precautions must be taken when applying DMSO. For these reasons, DMSO should be used only with the supervision of a doctor.

According to a small double-blind trial, 2,250 mg per day of oral **methylsulfonylmethane** (page 558) (MSM), a variant of DMSO, reduced osteoarthritis pain after six weeks.[68]

In a double-blind study, a group of people with painful osteoarthritis of the knee received an oral **enzyme** (page 506)-flavonoid preparation or a nonsteroidal anti-inflammatory (NSAID) for six weeks. While both treatments relieved pain and improved joint function, the enzyme-flavonoid product appeared to be slightly more effective than the NSAID. No serious side effects were seen.[69] The enzyme-flavonoid product used in this study was Phlogenzym (Mucos Pharma, Geretsried, Germany). Each enteric-coated tablet contained 90 mg of bromelain, 48 mg of trypsin, and 100 mg of rutosid (a derivative of the flavonoid rutin); one tablet was given three times a day.

Cetyl myristoleate (page 490) (CMO) has been proposed to act as a joint "lubricant" and anti-inflammatory agent. In a double-blind trial, people with various types of arthritis who had failed to respond to nonsteroidal anti-inflammatory drugs (NSAIDs) received CMO (540 mg per day orally for 30 days), while others received a placebo.[70] These people also applied CMO or placebo topically, according to their perceived need. A statistically significant 63.5% of those using CMO improved, compared with only 14.5% of those using placebo.

Boron (page 477) affects **calcium** (page 483) metabolism, and a link between boron deficiency and arthritis has been suggested.[71] Although people with os-

teoarthritis have been reported to have lower stores of boron in their bones than people without the disease, other minerals also are deficient in the bones of people with OA.[72] One double-blind trial found that 6 mg of boron per day, taken for two months, relieved symptoms of osteoarthritis in five of ten people, compared with improvement in only one of the ten people assigned to placebo.[73] This promising finding needs confirmation from larger trials.

The omega-3 fatty acids present in **fish oil** (page 514), EPA and **DHA** (page 509), have anti-inflammatory effects and have been studied primarily for **rheumatoid arthritis** (page 387), which involves significant inflammation. However, osteoarthritis also includes some inflammation.[74] In a 24-week controlled but preliminary trial studying people with OA, people taking EPA had "strikingly lower" pain scores than people who took placebo.[75] However, in a double-blind trial by the same research group, supplementation with 10 ml of **cod liver oil** (page 514) per day was no more effective than a placebo.[76]

Supplementation with **D-phenylalanine** (page 568) (DPA), a synthetic variation of the **amino acid** (page 465), **L-phenylalanine** (page 568) (LPA), has reduced chronic **pain** (page 338) due to osteoarthritis in a preliminary trial.[77] In that study, participants took 250 mg three to four times per day, with pain relief beginning in four to five weeks. Other preliminary trials have confirmed the effect of DPA in chronic pain control,[78] but a double-blind trial found no benefit.[79] DPA inhibits the **enzyme** (page 506) that breaks down some of the body's natural painkillers, substances called enkephalins, which are similar to endorphins. An increase in the amount of enkephalins may explain the reported pain-relieving effect of DPA. If DPA is not available, a related product, **D,L-phenylalanine** (page 568) (DLPA), may be substituted (1,500 to 2,000 mg per day). Phenylalanine should be taken between meals, because protein found in food may compete for uptake of phenylalanine into the brain, potentially reducing its effect.[80]

Several trials have suggested that people with osteoarthritis may benefit from supplementation with bovine **cartilage** (page 490), which contains a mixture of protein and molecules related to **chondroitin sulfate** (page 492). In one preliminary trial, use of injected and topical bovine cartilage led to symptom relief in most people studied.[81] A ten-year study confirmed improvement with long-term use of bovine cartilage.[82] Optimal intake of bovine cartilage is not known.

Osteoarthritis

Are there any side effects or interactions?
Refer to the individual supplement for information about any side effects or interactions.

Herbs that may be helpful

Several double-blind trials have shown that topical use of **cayenne** (page 654) extract creams containing 0.025 to 0.075% capsaicin reduces **pain** (page 338) and tenderness caused by OA.[83, 84, 85, 86] These creams are typically applied four times daily for two to four weeks, after which twice daily application may be sufficient.[87] Products containing capsicum oleoresin rather than purified capsaicin may not be as effective.[88]

Willow (page 760) has anti-inflammatory and pain-relieving properties. Although pain relief from willow supplementation may be slow in coming, it may last longer than pain relief from aspirin. One double-blind trial found that a product containing willow along with **black cohosh** (page 637), guaiac *(Guaiacum officinale, G. sanctum)*, **sarsaparilla** (page 742), and aspen *(Populus* spp.) bark effectively reduced osteoarthritis pain compared to placebo.[89] Another trial found that 1,360 mg of willow bark extract per day (delivering 240 mg of salicin) was somewhat effective in treating pain associated with knee and/or hip OA.[90]

Stinging nettle (page 714) has historically been used for joint pain. Topical application with the intent of causing stings to relieve joint pain has been assessed in preliminary[91] and double-blind[92] trials. The results found intentional nettle stings to be safe and effective for relieving the pain of OA. The only reported adverse effect is a sometimes painful or numbing rash that lasts 6 to 24 hours.

Ginger (page 680) has historically been used for arthritis and rheumatism. A preliminary trial reported relief in pain and swelling among people with arthritis who used powdered ginger supplements[93] More recently, a double-blind trial found ginger extract (170 mg three times a day for three weeks) to be slightly more effective than placebo at relieving pain in people with osteoarthritis of the hip or knee.[94] In another double-blind study, a concentrated extract of ginger, taken in the amount of 255 mg twice daily for six weeks, was significantly more effective than a placebo, as determined by the degree of **pain** (page 338) relief and overall improvement.[95]

In a preliminary trial, supplementation with 500 mg of a concentrated extract (3.5% guggulsterones) of *Commiphora mukul* (guggul) three times per day for one month resulted in a significant improvement in symptoms in people with osteoarthritis of the knee.[96] Double-blind trials are needed to rule out the possibility of a placebo effect.

More recently, purified extracts of bovine **cartilage** (page 490) containing chondroitin sulfate have been found to benefit people with osteoarthritis.[97, 98]

In a double-blind study, **collagen** (page 490) hydrolysate was compared with gelatin and egg protein as a treatment for osteoarthritis of the hip and/or knee. When subjects took 10 grams per day either of gelatin or collagen hydrolysate for two months, they reported significantly more pain relief than when they took a similar amount of egg protein.[99] More research is needed to confirm the benefits of gelatin or collagen hydrolysate in osteoarthritis.

Devil's claw (page 668) extract was found in one clinical trial to reduce pain associated with osteoarthritis as effectively as the slow-acting analgesic/cartilage-protective drug diacerhein.[100] The amount of devil's claw used in the trial was 2,610 mg per day. The results of this trial are somewhat suspect, however, as both devil's claw and diacerhein are slow-acting and there was no placebo group included for comparison.

Boswellia (page 644) has anti-inflammatory properties that have been compared to those of the NSAIDs used by many for inflammatory conditions.[101] Clinical trials in humans using boswellia alone are lacking. However, one clinical trial found that a combination of boswellia, **ashwagandha** (page 629), **turmeric** (page 753), and **zinc** (page 614) effectively treated pain and stiffness associated with osteoarthritis but did not improve joint health, according to X-rays of the affected joint.[102] Unlike NSAIDs, however, long-term use of boswellia does not lead to irritation or ulceration of the stomach.

Horsetail (page 693) is rich in **silicon** (page 586), a trace mineral that plays a role in making and maintaining connective tissue. Practitioners of traditional herbal medicine believe that the anti-arthritis action of horsetail is due largely to its silicon content. The efficacy of this herb for osteoarthritis has not yet been evaluated in controlled clinical trials.

According to arthritis research, saponins found in the herb yucca appear to block the release of toxins from the intestines that inhibit normal formation of cartilage. A preliminary, double-blind trial found that yucca might reduce symptoms of OA.[103] Only limited evidence currently supports the use of yucca for people with OA.

Cat's claw (page 653) has been used traditionally for

OA. In a double-blind trial, 100 mg per day of a freeze-dried preparation of cat's claw taken for four weeks was significantly more effective than a placebo at relieving pain and improving the overall condition.[104]

Meadowsweet (page 693) was historically used for a wide variety of conditions, including treating complaints of the joints and muscles.[105] The herb contains salicylates, chemicals related to aspirin, that may account for its reputed ability to relieve the pain of OA.

Colchicine is a remedy derived from autumn crocus (*Colchicum autumnale*) that may be helpful for **chronic back pain** (page 293) caused by herniated discs. A review of research reports that colchicine can relieve **pain** (page 338), muscle spasm, and weakness associated with disc disease.[106] The author of this study suggests that colchicine produces dramatic improvement in about 40% of cases of disc disease. In most studies, colchicine has been given intravenously.[107] However, oral colchicine may also be moderately effective for OA. A physician expert in the use of herbal medicine should be consulted for the administration of colchicine.

Are there any side effects or interactions?
Refer to the individual herb for information about any side effects or interactions.

Holistic approaches that may be helpful
Several clinical trials have examined the efficacy of acupuncture for OA, with mixed results. Some trials found acupuncture treatment to be no more effective than either placebo[108] or sham acupuncture[109] at relieving osteoarthritis pain. Other trials have demonstrated a significant effect of acupuncture on the relief of osteoarthritis pain compared to placebo.[110, 111] A well-designed trial found that acupuncture treatments (twice weekly for eight weeks) significantly improved **pain** (page 338) and disability in people with osteoarthritis of the knee compared to no treatment.[112] When the group receiving no treatment was switched to acupuncture treatments, they experienced similar improvements.

In a controlled trial, a combination of manual physical therapy (by a qualified physical therapist) and supervised exercise significantly improved walking distance and pain in a group of people with osteoarthritis of the knee.[113] The therapeutic regimen consisted of manual therapy to the knee, low back, hip, and ankle as necessary, as well as a standardized knee-exercise program performed at home and in the clinic. The treatments were given twice weekly at the clinic for four weeks.

OSTEOPOROSIS

Osteoporosis is a condition in which the normal amount of bone mass has decreased.

People with osteoporosis have brittle bones, which increases the risk of bone fracture, particularly in the hip, spine, and wrist. Osteoporosis is most common in postmenopausal Asian and Caucasian women. Premenopausal women are partially protected against bone loss by the hormone called estrogen. Black women often have slightly greater bone mass than do other women, which helps protect against bone fractures. In men, testosterone partially protects against bone loss even after middle age. Beyond issues of race, age, and gender, incidence varies widely from society to society, suggesting that osteoporosis is largely preventable.

What are the symptoms of osteoporosis?
Osteoporosis is a silent disease that may not be noticed until a broken bone occurs. Signs may include diminished height, rounded shoulders, dowager's hump, and evidence of bone loss from diagnostic tests. Symptoms may include neck or back pain.

Medical treatments
The most commonly used prescription medications are the bisphosphonates, including alendronate (Fosamax), risedronate (Actonel), and etidronate (Didronel). Another less commonly prescribed drug is calcitonin (Miacalcin). The drug raloxifene (Evista), as well as those that provide hormone replacement therapy, such as estradiol (Estrace, Estraderm), conjugated estrogens (Premarin), and conjugated estrogens with medroxyprogesterone acetate (Premphase, Prempro), are often prescribed for **postmenopausal** (page 311) women.

Healthcare providers also recommend adequate dietary **calcium** (page 483) intake and weight-bearing exercise.

Dietary changes that may be helpful
Studies attempting to uncover the effects of high animal protein intake on the risk of osteoporosis have produced confusing and contradictory results.[1, 2, 3, 4, 5] The same is true of studies attempting to find out whether vegetarians are protected against osteoporosis.[6, 7, 8, 9, 10, 11, 12, 13] Moreover, while some studies report that protein supplementation lowers death rates and shortens hospital stays[14] or reduces bone loss among people with osteo-

Osteoporosis

	CHECKLIST FOR OSTEOPOROSIS	
Rating	Nutritional Supplements	Herbs
★★★	**Calcium** (page 483) **Strontium** (page 589) **Vitamin D** (page 607)	
★★☆	**Copper** (page 499) **Fish oil** (page 514) and **Evening primrose oil** (page 511) (in combination) **Ipriflavone** (page 539) Isoflavones (from **red clover** [page 735]) **Magnesium** (page 551) **Phosphorus** (page 570) (for elderly people taking calcium supplements) **Soy** (page 587) **Soy** (page 587) isoflavones (genistein) **Vitamin K** (page 612)	**Progesterone** (page 577)
★☆☆	**Boron** (page 477) **DHEA** (page 503) **Fish oil** (page 514) **Fluoride** (page 519) **Folic acid** (page 520) (to lower homocysteine) **Manganese** (page 553) **Silicon** (page 586) **Vitamin B-complex** (page 603) **Vitamin B$_6$** (page 600) (to lower homocysteine) **Vitamin B$_{12}$** (page 601) (to lower homocysteine) **Whey protein** (page 613) **Zinc** (page 614)	**Black cohosh** (page 637) **Horsetail** (page 693)

porosis,[15] others have found that such supplementation is of little value.[16]

These conflicting findings may occur in part because dietary protein produces opposing effects on bone. On one hand, dietary protein increases the loss of **calcium** (page 483) in urine,[17, 18] which should increase the risk of osteoporosis. On the other hand, normal bone formation requires adequate dietary protein, and low dietary protein intake has been associated with low bone mineral density.[19] Current research shows that finding the line between too much protein and too little protein remains elusive, though extremes in protein in-

take—either high or low—might possibly increase the risk of osteoporosis.

Short-term increases in dietary salt result in increased urinary calcium loss, which suggests that over time, salt intake may cause bone loss.[20] Increasing dietary salt has increased markers of bone loss in postmenopausal (though not premenopausal) women.[21, 22, 23] Although a definitive link between salt intake and osteoporosis has not yet been proven, many doctors recommend that people wishing to protect themselves against bone loss use less salt and eat fewer processed and restaurant foods, which tend to be highly salted.

Like salt, caffeine increases urinary loss of calcium.[24] Caffeine intake has been linked to increased risk of hip fractures[25] and to a lower bone mass in women who consumed inadequate calcium.[26] Many doctors recommend decreasing caffeinated coffee, black tea, and caffeine-containing soft drinks as a way to improve bone mass.

Curiously, while caffeine-containing tea consumption has been linked to osteoporosis in some studies,[27] others have reported that tea drinkers have a *lower* risk of osteoporosis than do people who do not drink tea.[28, 29] Possibly, the calcium-losing effect of caffeine in tea is overridden by other constituents of tea, such as **flavonoids** (page 516).

People who consume soft drinks have been reported to have an increased incidence of bone fractures,[30] although short-term consumption of carbonated beverages has not affected markers of bone health.[31] The problem, if one exists, may be linked to phosphoric acid, a substance found in many soft drinks. In one trial, children consuming at least six glasses (1.5 liters) of soft drinks containing phosphoric acid had more than five times the risk of developing low blood levels of calcium compared with other children.[32] Although a few studies have not linked soft drinks to bone loss,[33] the preponderance of evidence now suggests that a problem may exist.

Soy foods, such as tofu, soy milk, roasted soy beans, and soy protein powders, may be beneficial in preventing osteoporosis. Isoflavones from soy have protected against bone loss in animal studies.[34] In a double-blind trial, postmenopausal women who supplemented with 40 grams of soy protein powder (containing 90 mg of isoflavones) per day were protected against bone mineral loss in the spine, although lower amounts were not protective.[35] In a double-blind study, administration of the **soy** (page 587) isoflavone genistein (54 mg per day) to postmenopausal women for one year reduced bone breakdown, increased bone formation, and increased bone mineral density of the hip and spine.[36] The effect on bone density was similar to that of conventional hormone-replacement therapy.

The effect of dairy products on the risk of osteoporosis-related fractures is subject to controversy. According to a review of 46 studies,[37] different dairy products appear to have different effects on bone density and fracture rates. Milk, especially nonfat milk, probably does more good than harm because of its relatively lower protein and salt content, as well as its higher level of calcium. Cottage cheese and American cheese, on the other hand, probably do more harm than good. Cottage cheese is high in protein and salt but low in calcium, factors which could contribute to bone loss. American cheese is extremely high in salt and high in protein. These foods are not recommended as calcium sources for the prevention of osteoporotic fractures. Although there may be better ways of getting calcium, younger women who wish to prevent osteoporosis might consider nonfat milk and nonfat yogurt to be reasonable dietary calcium sources.

Lifestyle changes that may be helpful
Smoking leads to increased bone loss.[38] For this and many other health reasons, smoking should be avoided.

Exercise is known to help protect against bone loss.[39] The more weight-bearing exercise done by men and **postmenopausal** (page 311) women, the greater their bone mass and the lower their risk of osteoporosis. Walking is a perfect weight-bearing exercise. For premenopausal women, exercise is also important, but taken to extreme, it may lead to cessation of the menstrual cycle, which *contributes* to osteoporosis.[40]

Excess body mass helps protect against osteoporosis. As a result, researchers have been able to show that people who successfully **lose weight** (page 446) have greater bone *loss* compared with those who do not lose weight.[41] Therefore, people who lose weight need to be particularly vigilant about preventing osteoporotic fractures.

Nutritional supplements that may be helpful
Although insufficient when used as the only intervention, **calcium** (page 483) supplements help prevent osteoporosis.[42] Though some of the research remains controversial, the protective effect of calcium on bone mass is one of very few health claims permitted on supplement labels by the U.S. Food and Drug Administration.

In some studies, higher calcium intake has not correlated with a reduced risk of osteoporosis—for example, in women shortly after becoming **menopausal** (page 311)[43] or in men.[44] However, after about three years of menopause, calcium supplementation does appear to take on a protective effect for women.[45] Even the most positive trials using isolated calcium supplementation show only minor effects on bone mass. Nonetheless, a review of the research shows that calcium supplementation plus hormone replacement therapy is much more effective than hormone replacement therapy without calcium.[46] Double-blind research has found that increasing calcium intake results in greater bone mass in girls.[47] An analysis of many trials investigating the effects of calcium supplementation in premenopausal women has also shown a significant positive effect.[48] Most doctors recommend calcium supplementation as a way to partially reduce the risk of osteoporosis and to help people already diagnosed with the condition. In order to achieve the 1,500 mg per day calcium intake many researchers deem optimal, 800 to 1,000 mg of supplemental calcium are generally added to the 500 to 700 mg readily obtainable from the diet.

While phosphorus is essential for bone formation, most people do not require phosphorus supplementation, because the typical western diet provides ample or even excessive amounts of phosphorus. One study, however, has shown that taking calcium can interfere with the absorption of phosphorus, potentially leading to phosphorus deficiency in elderly people, whose diets may contain less phosphorus.[49] The authors of this study recommend that, for elderly people, at least some of the supplemental calcium be taken in the form of tricalcium phosphate or some other phosphorus-containing preparation.

Ipriflavone (page 539) is a synthetic **flavonoid** (page 516) derived from the **soy** (page 587) isoflavone called daidzein. It promotes the incorporation of calcium into bone and inhibits bone breakdown, thus preventing and reversing osteoporosis. Many clinical trials, including numerous double-blind trials, have consistently shown that long-term treatment with 600 mg of ipriflavone per day, along with 1,000 mg supplemental calcium, is both safe and effective in halting bone loss in postmenopausal women or in women who have had their ovaries removed. Ipriflavone has also been found to improve bone density in established cases of osteoporosis in most,[50, 51, 52, 53, 54, 55, 56, 57, 58, 59, 60] but not all,[61] clinical trials. Some studies have shown that ipriflavone therapy not only stops bone loss, it also actually increases bone density and significantly reduces the number of vertebral fractures and amount of bone pain.

However, one double-blind study has failed to confirm the beneficial effect of ipriflavone. In that study, ipriflavone was no more effective than a placebo for preventing bone loss in postmenopausal women with osteoporosis.[62] The women in this negative study were older (average age, 63.3 years) than those in most other ipriflavone studies and had relatively severe osteoporosis. It is possible that ipriflavone works only in younger women or in those with less severe osteoporosis.

Vitamin D (page 607) increases calcium absorption, and blood levels of vitamin D are directly related to the strength of bones.[63] Mild deficiency of vitamin D is common in the fit, active elderly population and leads to an acceleration of age-related loss of bone mass and an increased risk of fracture.[64] In double-blind research, vitamin D supplementation has reduced bone loss in women who consume insufficient vitamin D from food[65] and slowed bone loss in people with osteoporosis.[66] However, the effect of vitamin D supplementation on osteoporosis risk remains surprisingly unclear,[67, 68] with some trials reporting little if any benefit.[69] Moreover, trials reporting reduced risk of fracture have usually combined vitamin D with calcium supplementation,[70] making it difficult to assess how much benefit is caused by supplementation with vitamin D alone.[71]

Impaired balance and increased body sway are important causes of falls in elderly people with osteoporosis.[72] Vitamin D works with calcium to prevent some musculoskeletal causes of falls. In a double-blind trial, elderly women who were given 800 IU per day of vitamin D and 1,200 mg per day of calcium had a significantly lower rate of falls and subsequent fractures than did women given the same amount of calcium alone.[73]

Despite inconsistency in the research, many doctors recommend 400 to 800 IU per day of supplemental vitamin D, depending upon dietary intake and exposure to sunlight.

A preliminary trial found that elderly women with osteoporosis who were given 4 grams of **fish oil** (page 514) per day for four months had improved calcium absorption and evidence of new bone formation.[74] Fish oil combined with **evening primrose oil** (page 511) (EPO) may confer added benefits. In a controlled trial, women received 6 grams of a combination of EPO and fish oil, or a matching placebo, plus 600 mg of calcium per day for three years.[75] The EPO/fish oil group experienced no spinal bone loss in the first 18 months and a significant 3.1% increase in spinal bone mineral density during the last 18 months.

Vitamin K (page 612) is needed for bone formation. People with osteoporosis have been reported to have low blood levels[76, 77] and low dietary intake of vitamin K.[78, 79] One study found that postmenopausal (though not premenopausal) women may reduce urinary loss of calcium by taking 1 mg of vitamin K per day.[80] People with osteoporosis given large amounts of vitamin K_2 (45 mg per day) have shown an increase in bone density after six months[81] and decreased bone loss after one[82] or two[83] years.

Other preliminary studies have reported that vitamin K supplementation increases bone formation in some women[84] and that higher vitamin K intake correlates with greater bone mineral density.[85] Some doctors recommend 1 mg vitamin K_1 to postmenopausal women as a way to help maintain bone mass, though optimal intake remains unknown.

In a preliminary study, people with osteoporosis were reported to be at high risk for **magnesium** (page 551) malabsorption.[86] Both bone[87] and blood[88] levels of magnesium have been reported to be low in people with osteoporosis. Supplemental magnesium has reduced markers of bone loss in men.[89] Supplementing with 250 mg up to 750 mg per day of magnesium arrested bone loss or increased bone mass in 87% of people with osteoporosis in a two-year, controlled trial.[90] Some doctors recommend that people with osteoporosis supplement with 350 mg of magnesium per day.

One trial studying postmenopausal women combined hormone replacement therapy with magnesium (600 mg per day), calcium (500 mg per day), **vitamin C** (page 604), **B vitamins** (page 603), vitamin D, zinc, copper, manganese, **boron** (page 477), and other nutrients for an eight- to nine-month period.[91] In addition, participants were told to avoid processed foods, limit protein intake, emphasize vegetable over animal protein, and limit consumption of salt, sugar, alcohol, coffee, tea, chocolate, and tobacco. Bone density increased a remarkable 11%, compared to only 0.7% in women receiving hormone replacement alone.

Levels of **zinc** (page 614) in both blood and bone have been reported to be low in people with osteoporosis,[92] and urinary loss of zinc has been reported to be high.[93] In one trial, men consuming only 10 mg of zinc per day from food had almost twice the risk of osteoporotic fractures compared with those eating significantly higher levels of zinc in their diets.[94] Whether zinc supplementation protects against bone loss has not yet been proven, though in one trial, supplementation with several minerals including zinc and calcium was more effective than calcium by itself.[95] Many doctors recommend that people with osteoporosis, as well as those trying to protect themselves from this disease, supplement with 10 to 30 mg of zinc per day.

Copper (page 499) is needed for normal bone synthesis. Recently, a two-year, controlled trial reported that 3 mg of copper per day reduced bone loss.[96] When taken over a shorter period of time (six weeks), the same level of copper supplementation had no effect on biochemical markers of bone loss.[97] Some doctors recommend 2 to 3 mg of copper per day, particularly if zinc is also being taken, in order to prevent a deficiency. Supplemental zinc significantly depletes copper stores, so people taking zinc supplements for more than a few weeks generally need to supplement with copper also. All minerals discussed so far—calcium, magnesium, zinc, and copper—are sometimes found at appropriate levels in high-potency **multivitamin-mineral supplements** (page 559).

Boron (page 477) supplementation has been reported to reduce urinary loss of calcium and magnesium in some,[98] but not all,[99] preliminary research. However, those who are already supplementing with magnesium appear to achieve no additional calcium-sparing benefit when boron is added.[100] Finally, in the original report claiming that boron reduced loss of calcium,[101] the effect was achieved by significantly increasing estrogen and testosterone levels, hormones that have been linked to cancer risks. Therefore, it makes sense for people with osteoporosis to supplement with magnesium instead of, rather than in addition to, boron.

Interest in the effect of **manganese** (page 553) and bone health began when famed basketball player Bill Walton's repeated fractures were halted with manganese supplementation.[102] A subsequent, unpublished study reported manganese deficiency in a small group of osteoporotic women.[103] Since then, a combination of minerals including manganese was reported to halt bone loss.[104] However, no human trial has investigated the effect of manganese supplementation alone on bone mass. Nonetheless, some doctors recommend 10 to 20 mg of manganese per day to people concerned with maintenance of bone mass.

Silicon (page 586) is required in trace amounts for normal bone formation,[105] and supplementation with silicon has increased bone formation in animals.[106] In preliminary human research, supplementation with silicon increased bone mineral density in a small group of people with osteoporosis.[107] Optimal supplemental levels remain unknown, though some multivitamin-mineral supplements now contain small amounts of this trace mineral.

Strontium (page 589) may play a role in bone formation, and also may inhibit bone breakdown.[108] Preliminary evidence suggests that women with osteoporosis may have reduced absorption of strontium.[109] The first medical use of strontium was described in 1884. (Strontium supplements do not contain the radioactive form of strontium that is a component of nuclear fallout.) Years ago in a preliminary trial, people with osteoporosis were given 1.7 grams of strontium for a period of time ranging between three months and three years; afterward, they reported a significant reduction in bone pain, and there was evidence suggesting their bone mass had increased.[110] More recently, in a three-year double-blind study of postmenopausal women with osteoporosis, supplementing with strontium, in the form of strontium ranelate, significantly increased bone mineral density in the hip and spine, and significantly reduced the risk of vertebral fractures by 41%, compared with a placebo.[111] The amount of strontium used in that study was 680 mg per day, which is approximately 300 times the amount found in a typical diet. Increased bone formation and decreased bone pain were also reported in six people with osteoporosis given 600 to 700 mg of stable strontium per day.[112] Although the amounts of strontium used in these studies studies was very high, the optimal intake remains unknown. Some doctors recommend only 1 to 3 mg per day—less than many people currently consume from their diets, but an amount that has begun to appear in some mineral formulas geared toward bone health. Strontium preparations, providing 200 to 400 mg per day, were used for decades during the first half of the twentieth century without any apparent toxicity.[113] No significant side effects were observed in people taking large amounts of strontium; however, animal studies have demonstrated defects in bone mineralization, when strontium was administered in large amounts in combination with a low-calcium diet. People interested in taking large amounts of strontium should be supervised by a doctor, and should make sure to take adequate amounts of calcium. It should be noted that, although supplementing with strontium increases bone mineral density, only part of the increase is real. The rest is a laboratory error that results from the fact that strontium blocks X-rays to a greater extent than does calcium.[114] People taking large amounts of strontium should mention that fact to the radiologist when they are having their bone mineral density measured, so that the results will be interpreted correctly.

Folic acid (page 520), **vitamin B₆** (page 600), and **vitamin B₁₂** (page 601) are known to reduce blood levels of the **amino acid** (page 465) homocysteine, and homocystinuria, a condition associated with **high homocysteine** (page 234) levels, frequently causes osteoporosis. Therefore, some researchers have suggested that these vitamins might help prevent osteoporosis by lowering homocysteine levels.[115] In a double-blind study of people who had suffered a stroke and had high homocysteine levels, daily supplementation with 5 mg of folic acid and 1,500 mcg of vitamin B₁₂ for two years reduced the incidence of fractures by 78%, compared with a placebo.[116] The reduction in fracture risk appeared to be due to an improvement in bone quality, rather than to a change in bone mineral density. Whether these vitamins would be beneficial for people with normal homocysteine levels is not known. For the purpose of lowering homocysteine, amounts of folic acid and vitamins B₆ and B₁₂ found in high-potency **B-complex** (page 603) supplements and multivitamins should be adequate.

Preliminary evidence suggests that **progesterone** (page 577) might reduce the risk of osteoporosis.[117] A preliminary trial using topically applied natural progesterone cream in combination with dietary changes, exercise, vitamin and calcium supplementation, and estrogen therapy reported large gains in bone density over a three-year period in a small group of postmenopausal women, but no comparison was made to examine the effect of using the same protocol without progesterone.[118] Other trials have reported that adding natural progesterone to estrogen therapy did not improve the bone-sparing effects of estrogen when taken alone[119] and that progesterone applied topically every day for a year did not reduce bone loss.[120] In a more recent double-blind study, however, progesterone had a modest bone-sparing effect in post-menopausal women.[121]

In a preliminary trial, bone mineral density increased among healthy elderly women and men who were given 50 mg per day of **DHEA** (page 503) as a supplement.[122] It is not known if supplementation would have similar effects in people with established osteoporosis.

Some **whey proteins** (page 613) may reduce bone loss.[123] Milk basic protein (MBP) is a mixture of some of the proteins found in whey protein. A preliminary trial found that 300 mg per day of MBP improved blood measures of bone metabolism in men, suggesting more bone formation was occurring than bone loss.[124] A double-blind trial found that women taking 40 mg per day of MBP for six months had greater gains in bone density compared with those taking a placebo.[125] No osteoporosis-related research has been done using complete whey protein mixtures.

Are there any side effects or interactions?
Refer to the individual supplement for information about any side effects or interactions.

Herbs that may be helpful

In a double-blind study, supplementation with isoflavones from **red clover** (page 735) for one year reduced the amount of bone loss from the spine by 45%, compared with a placebo.[126] The supplement used provided daily 26 mg of biochanin A, 16 mg of formononetin, 1 mg of genistein, and 0.5 mg of daidzein.

Horsetail (page 693) is a rich source of **silicon** (page 586), and preliminary research suggests that this trace mineral may help maintain bone mass. Effects of horsetail supplementation on bone mass have not been studied.

Black cohosh (page 637) has been shown to improve bone mineral density in animals fed a low **calcium** (page 483) diet,[127] but it has not been studied for this purpose in humans.

Are there any side effects or interactions?
Refer to the individual herb for information about any side effects or interactions.

PAIN

Pain is a sensation that is transmitted from an area of tissue damage or stress along the sensory nerves to the brain. The brain interprets the information as the sensation of pain.

Substances that decrease pain either interfere with the ability of nerves to conduct messages, or alter the brain's capacity to receive sensations.

Pain may be a symptom of an underlying pathological condition, such as inflammation. It may also be due to other causes, such as **bruising** (page 84), **infection** (page 265), **burns** (page 85), headaches, and **sprains and strains** (page 412). Use caution when treating pain without understanding its cause—this may delay diagnosis of conditions that could continue to worsen without medical attention.

CHECKLIST FOR PAIN

Rating	Nutritional Supplements	Herbs
★★★		**Cayenne** (page 654) (capsaicin; topical use only)
★★☆	**D-phenylalanine** (page 568) (DPA)	**Corydalis** (page 663)
★☆☆	**Vitamin B$_{12}$** (page 601)	**American scullcap** (page 626) **Passion flower** (page 722) **Phyllanthus** (page 728) *Piscidia erythrina* **Valerian** (page 756) *Viburnum opulus* **Willow** (page 760)

What are the symptoms of pain?

Symptoms of pain include discomfort that is often worsened by movement or pressure and may be associated with irritability, problems sleeping, and fatigue. People with pain may have uncomfortable sensations described as burning, sharp, stabbing, aching, throbbing, tingling, shooting, dull, heavy, and tight.

Medical treatments

Over the counter nonsteroidal anti-inflammatory drugs (NSAIDs), including aspirin (Bayer, Ecotrin, Bufferin), ibuprofen (Advil, Motrin, Nuprin), and naproxen (Aleve), as well as acetaminophen (Tylenol), are commonly used for mild pain.

Prescription strength NSAIDs, including ibuprofen (Motrin), naproxen (Anaprox, Naprosyn), etodolac (Lodine), and indomethacin (Indocin), are prescribed when over the counter products are ineffective. Narcotic pain-relievers including codeine (Tylenol with Codeine) and hydrocodone (Vicodin, Lortab) are also used to treat moderate pain. Other narcotics, such as oxycodone (Oxycontin, Percocet, Percodan), hydromorphone (Dilaudid), morphine (MS Contin, Roxanol), fentanyl (Duragesic), methadone (Dolophine), and meperidine (Demerol), are usually reserved for treating severe pain. Oral corticosteroids such as prednisone (Deltasone) and methylprednisolone (Medrol) are often prescribed to reduce pain associated with inflammation.

Some severe painful conditions might require surgical treatments to disrupt the pain signal.

Lifestyle changes that may be helpful

Body weight may be related to pain tolerance. One study indicated women who are more than 30% above the ideal weight for their age experience pain more quickly and more intensely than do women of ideal weight.[1] No research has investigated the effect of **weight loss** (page 446) on pain tolerance.

Exercise increases pain tolerance in some situations,[2, 3] in part because exercise may raise levels of naturally occurring painkillers (endorphins and enkephalins).[4] Many types of chronic pain are helped by exercise,[5, 6, 7] though some types of physical activity may aggravate certain painful conditions.[8] People who want to initiate an exercise program for increasing pain tolerance should first consult a qualified health professional.

Nutritional supplements that may be helpful

Certain **amino acids** (page 465) have been found to raise pain thresholds and increase tolerance to pain. One of these, a synthetic amino acid called **D-phenylalanine** (page 568) (DPA), decreases pain by blocking the **enzymes** (page 506) that break down endorphins and enkephalins, the body's natural pain-killing chemicals.[9, 10] DPA may also produce pain relief by other mechanisms, which are not well understood.[11]

In animal studies, DPA decreased chronic pain within 15 minutes of administration and the effects lasted up to six days.[12] It also decreased responses to acute pain. These findings have been independently verified in at least five other studies.[13, 14] Clinical studies on humans suggest DPA may inhibit some types of chronic pain, but it has little effect on most types of acute pain.[15, 16]

Most human research has tested the pain-relieving effects of 750 to 1,000 mg per day of DPA taken for several weeks of continuous or intermittent use. The results of this research have been mixed, with some trials reporting efficacy,[17, 18, 19] others reporting no difference from placebo,[20] and some reporting equivocal results.[21] It appears that DPA may only work for some people, but a trial period of supplementation seems worthwhile for many types of chronic pain until more is known. If DPA is not available, a related product, **D,L-phenylalanine** (page 568) (DLPA), may be substituted at amounts of 1,500 to 2,000 mg per day.

As early as 1981, preliminary human research

Pain

showed that DPA made the pain-inhibiting effects of acupuncture stronger.[22] One controlled animal study[23] and two controlled trials in humans[24, 25] showed that DPA taken the day before acupuncture increased the effectiveness of acupuncture in reducing both acute dental and chronic **low back pain** (page 293).

Other **amino acids** (page 465) may be beneficial in reducing pain. In the central nervous system, L-tryptophan serves as a precursor to serotonin. Serotonin participates in the regulation of mood and may alter responses to pain. In a preliminary trial, 2,750 mg per day of L-tryptophan decreased pain sensitivity.[26] Another preliminary trial found that L-tryptophan (500 mg every four hours) taken the day before a dental procedure significantly decreased the postoperative pain experienced by patients.[27] In another preliminary trial, 3 grams of L-tryptophan taken daily for four weeks significantly decreased pain in a group of people with chronic jaw pain.[28] No research has been published investigating the pain control potential of **5-hydroxytryptophan** (page 459) (5-HTP), another serotonin precursor that, unlike L-tryptophan, is currently available without a prescription.

Vitamin B$_{12}$ (page 601) has exhibited pain-killing properties in animal studies.[29] In humans with vertebral pain syndromes, injections of massive amounts of vitamin B$_{12}$ (5,000 to 10,000 mcg per day) have reportedly provided pain relief.[30] Further studies are needed to confirm the efficacy of this treatment.

Are there any side effects or interactions?
Refer to the individual supplement for information about any side effects or interactions.

Herbs that may be helpful
Capsaicin is an extract of **cayenne** (page 654) pepper that may ease many types of chronic pain when applied regularly to the skin. In animal studies, capsaicin was consistently effective at reducing pain when given by mouth, by injection, or when applied topically.[31, 32] A controlled trial in humans found that application of a solution of capsaicin (0.075%) decreased sensitivity of skin to all noxious stimuli.[33] One review article deemed the research on capsaicin's pain-relieving properties "inconclusive."[34] However, in several uncontrolled and at least five controlled clinical trials, capsaicin has been consistently shown to decrease the pain of many disorders, including trigeminal neuralgia, **shingles** (page 401), **diabetic** (page 152) neuropathy, **osteoarthritis** (page 328), and **cluster headaches** (page 117).[35, 36, 37, 38, 39]

For treatment of chronic pain, capsaicin ointment or cream (standardized to 0.025 to 0.075% capsaicin) is typically applied to the painful area four times per day.[40] It is common to experience stinging and burning at the site of application, especially for the first week of treatment; avoid getting it in the eyes, mouth, or open sores.

Preliminary reports from Chinese researchers also note that 75 mg per day of THP (an alkaloid from the plant **corydalis** [page 663]) was effective in reducing nerve pain in 78% of of those tested.[41]

As early as 1763, use of **willow** (page 760) bark to decrease pain and inflammation was reported.[42] Its constituents are chemically related to aspirin. These constituents may decrease pain by two methods: by interfering with the process of inflammation, and by interfering with pain-producing nerves in the spinal cord.[43] No human studies have investigated the pain-relieving potential of willow bark, and questions have been raised as to the actual absorption of willow bark's pain-relieving constituents.[44] The potential pain-reducing action of willow is typically slower than that of aspirin.

In animal research, alcohol/water extracts of plants from the genus **phyllanthus** (page 728) (25 to 200 mg per 2.2 pounds body weight) have shown a marked ability to decrease pain.[45] This family includes the plants *Phyllanthus urinaria, P. caroliniensis, P. amarus,* and *P. niruri.* Like aspirin, phyllanthus extracts appear to reduce pain by decreasing inflammation.[46] Although they are six to seven times more potent than aspirin or acetaminophen[47] in test tube studies, extracts of these plants also demonstrate liver-protective properties,[48] suggesting they may be safer than drugs such as acetaminophen, which has well-documented toxicity to the liver. The usefulness of phyllanthus extracts for treating pain in humans is unknown.

Other herbs that have been historically used to relieve pain (although there are no modern scientific studies yet available) include **valerian** (page 756), **passion flower** (page 722), **American scullcap** (page 626), *Piscidia erythrina,* and crampbark (*Viburnum opulus*).

Are there any side effects or interactions?
Refer to the individual herb for information about any side effects or interactions.

Holistic approaches that may be helpful
Transcutaneous electrical nerve stimulation (TENS) is a form of electrical physical therapy that has been used

in the treatment of pain since the early 1970s. Pads are placed on the skin and a mild electrical current is sent through to block pain sensations. Many TENS units are small, portable, and may be hidden under clothing. A review of the first ten years of research on TENS described success rates in treating chronic pain varying from 12.5% to 92% after one year of treatment.[49] Variations in success rates were attributed to differences in the type of pain the TENS was treating. More current research identifies specific conditions that consistently respond well to TENS therapy:[50, 51] **rheumatoid arthritis** (page 387), **osteoarthritis** (page 328), **low back pain** (page 293), phantom limb pain, and post-herpetic nerve pain (**shingles** [page 401]). Pain caused by pinched nerves in the spine responds poorly to TENS therapy. While a small number of controlled trials have reported no benefit,[52, 53] most evidence suggests TENS is an effective form of therapy for many types of pain.[54, 55, 56]

Relaxation exercises may decrease the perception of pain. Pain increases as **anxiety** (page 30) increases; using methods to decrease anxiety may help reduce pain.[57] In one controlled hospital study, people who were taught mind-body relaxation techniques reported less pain, less difficulty sleeping, and fewer symptoms of **depression** (page 145) or anxiety than did people who were not taught the techniques.[58]

Acupuncture has been shown to decrease pain by acting on the enkephalin-based, pain-killing pathways.[59] In 1997, the National Institutes of Health (NIH) stated that acupuncture is useful for muscular, skeletal, and generalized pain, as well as for anesthesia and postoperative pain. The NIH statement was based on a critical review of over 67 controlled trials of acupuncture for pain control.

Practitioners of manipulation report that it often produces immediate pain relief either in the area manipulated or elsewhere.[60] Controlled trials have found that people given spinal manipulation may experience reduction in pain sensitivity of the skin in related areas,[61, 62] a reduction in joint and muscle tenderness in the area manipulated,[63] and a decrease in elbow tenderness when the neck was manipulated.[64] One study showed no effect of lower spine manipulation on sensitivity to deep pressure over low back muscles and ligaments.[65] Some researchers have speculated that joint manipulation affects pain by enhancing the effects of endorphins. However, only one[66] of three[67, 68] controlled studies has shown an effect of manipulation on endorphin levels.

Hypnosis has been shown to significantly reduce pain associated with office surgical procedures that are performed while the patient is conscious (i.e., without general anesthesia).[69] People undergoing office surgical procedures received standard care, structured attention or self-hypnotic relaxation in one study. Those using self-hypnosis had no increases in pain during the procedures, compared to those in the other groups. Hypnosis also appeared to stabilize bleeding, decrease the requirement for narcotic pain drugs during the procedure, and shorten procedure time.

PANCREATIC INSUFFICIENCY

Pancreatic insufficiency occurs when the pancreas does not secrete enough chemicals and digestive enzymes for normal digestion to occur.

When pancreatic insufficiency is severe, **malabsorption** (page 304) (impaired absorption of nutrients by the intestines) may result, leading to deficiencies of essential nutrients and the occurrence of loose stools containing unabsorbed fat (steatorrhea).

Severe pancreatic insufficiency occurs in **cystic fibrosis** (page 143), chronic pancreatitis, and surgeries of the gastrointestinal system in which portions of the stomach or pancreas are removed. Certain gastrointestinal diseases, such as stomach ulcers,[1] **celiac disease** (page 102),[2] and **Crohn's disease** (page 141),[3] and autoimmune disorders, such as **systemic lupus erythematosus** (page 421) (SLE),[4, 5, 6] may contribute to the development of pancreatic insufficiency. Mild forms of pancreatic insufficiency are often difficult to diagnose, and there is controversy among researchers regarding whether milder forms of pancreatic insufficiency need treatment.

Pancreatitis is an inflammation of the pancreas that reduces the function of the pancreas, causing pancreatic insufficiency, **malabsorption** (page 304), and **diabetes** (page 152).[7] Acute pancreatitis is usually a temporary condition and can be caused by **gallstones** (page 193), excessive alcohol consumption, **high blood triglycerides** (page 235), abdominal injury, and other diseases, and by certain medications and poisons.[8] Chronic pancreatitis is a slow, silent process that gradually destroys the pancreas and is most often caused by excessive alcohol consumption.

CHECKLIST FOR PANCREATIC INSUFFICIENCY

Rating	Nutritional Supplements	Herbs
★★★	**Digestive enzymes** (page 506)	
★★☆	**Beta-carotene** (page 469) **Methionine** (page 557) **Selenium** (page 584) **Vitamin C** (page 604) **Vitamin E** (page 609)	
★☆☆		Grape seed extract

What are the symptoms of pancreatic insufficiency?

People with pancreatic insufficiency may have symptoms of pale, foul-smelling, bulky stools that stick to the side of the toilet bowl or are difficult to flush, oil droplets floating in the toilet bowl after bowel movements, and abdominal discomfort, gas, and bloating. People with pancreatic insufficiency may also have bone pain, muscle cramps, **night blindness** (page 326), and easy bruising.

Medical treatments

Prescription drug therapy involves taking pancreatic enzymes (Pancrease MT, Lipram, Viokase) with meals.

Some healthcare practitioners might also recommend intravenous nutritional supplements that replace unabsorbed fat-soluble vitamins (e.g., vitamins A, D, E, K).

Dietary changes that may be helpful

A low-fat diet (with no more than 30 to 40% of calories from fat) is often recommended to help prevent the steatorrhea that often accompanies pancreatic insufficiency.[9] In a controlled study of chronic pancreatitis patients, a very low-fat diet resulted in less than one-fourth as much steatorrhea compared to a more typical fat intake.[10] Since a very low-fat diet may not be appropriate for a person with malnutrition, this recommendation should only be followed after consulting a healthcare professional.

A preliminary study of chronic pancreatitis patients reported that a high-fiber diet was associated with a small but significant increase in the amount of fat in the stool.[11] The patients all complained of increased flatu-

lence while using this diet, but an undesirable increase in the frequency of bowel movements did not occur. Increases in dietary fiber may not be well tolerated by people with pancreatitis, but more research is needed.

A few preliminary reports suggest that **food allergy** (page 14) may cause some cases of acute pancreatitis. Food allergies identified in these cases included beef, milk, potato, eggs,[12] fish and fish eggs,[13] and kiwi fruit.[14] No research has investigated the possible role of food allergy in other causes of pancreatic insufficiency.

Lifestyle changes that may be helpful

Since **alcoholism** (page 12) is one known cause of pancreatitis, total abstinence from alcohol is generally recommended to people with this disease.[15] In a study of alcoholic chronic pancreatitis patients, pancreatic function declined to a greater degree in those who continued to drink alcohol.[16] Another study found that abstinence from alcohol had a significant long-term beneficial effect on some of the problems associated with chronic pancreatitis.[17]

Cigarette smoking decreases pancreatic secretion[18] and increases the risk of pancreatitis[19] and pancreatic cancer,[20] providing yet another reason to quit smoking.

In a large international study, the major risk factors for early death in a group of patients with chronic alcoholic and nonalcoholic pancreatitis included smoking and drinking alcohol.[21]

Nutritional supplements that may be helpful

The mainstay of treatment for pancreatic insufficiency is replacement of **digestive enzymes** (page 506), using supplements prepared from pig pancreas (pancrelipase) or fungi.[22] Enzyme supplements have been shown to reduce steatorrhea[23, 24] associated with pancreatitis, while pain reduction has been demonstrated in some,[25, 26] though not all,[27, 28] double-blind studies. Digestive enzyme preparations that are resistant to the acidity of the stomach are effective at lower doses compared with conventional digestive enzyme preparations.[29] Some enzyme preparations are produced with higher lipase enzyme content for improved fat absorption, but one controlled study of chronic pancreatitis found no advantage of this preparation over one with standard lipase content.[30] People with more severe pancreatic insufficiency or who attempt to eat a higher-fat diet require more enzymes,[31] but large amounts of pancreatic digestive enzymes are known to damage the large intestine in some people with diseases causing pancreatic insufficiency.[32, 33, 34] Therefore, a qualified healthcare practitioner should be consulted about the appropriate and safe amount of enzymes to use.

Many, otherwise healthy people suffer from **indigestion** (page 260), and some doctors believe that mild pancreatic insufficiency can be a cause of indigestion. A preliminary study of people with indigestion reported significant improvement in almost all of those given pancreatic enzyme supplements.[35] One double-blind trial found that giving pancreatic enzymes to healthy people along with a high-fat meal reduced bloating, gas, and abdominal fullness following the meal.[36]

Stomach surgery patients often have decreased pancreatic function, **malabsorption** (page 304), and abdominal symptoms, including steatorrhea, but digestive enzyme supplementation had no effect on steatorrhea in two of three double-blind studies of stomach surgery patients,[37, 38, 39] although some other symptoms did improve.[40, 41] Patients who have surgery to remove part of the pancreas often have severe steatorrhea that is difficult to control with enzyme supplements.[42] In one double-blind study, neither high-dose nor standard-dose pancreatin was able to eliminate steatorrhea in over half of the pancreas surgery patients studied.[43]

Fat malabsorption in pancreatic insufficiency may result in deficiencies of fat-soluble vitamins, and these deficiencies may not always be prevented by enzyme supplementation.[44, 45, 46] One controlled study found that patients with chronic pancreatitis had vision abnormalities that are associated with vitamin A deficiency.[47] A controlled study of patients with steatorrhea found that a water-soluble form of **vitamin A** (page 595) was easier to absorb than conventional fat-soluble forms of vitamin A, resulting in vitamin A absorption equal to that of healthy people.[48] Two controlled studies of patients with chronic pancreatitis found evidence of vitamin E deficiency in their blood.[49, 50] People with more severe fat malabsorption tended to have the lowest vitamin E levels. Although doctors sometimes recommend supplementation with fat-soluble vitamins for people with pancreatitis,[51] no research has investigated the benefits of these supplements.

Pancreatic enzymes are also necessary for the absorption of **vitamin B$_{12}$** (page 601).[52] While people with pancreatic insufficiency have some malabsorption of this vitamin, true deficiency is considered rare.[53, 54, 55] No research has investigated whether long-term vitamin B$_{12}$ supplementation is beneficial for chronic pancreatitis.

Free radical damage has been linked to pancreatitis in animal and human studies,[56, 57, 58] suggesting that **antioxidants** (page 467) might be beneficial for this disease. One controlled study found that chronic pancreatitis patients consumed diets significantly lower in several antioxidants due to problems such as appetite loss and abdominal symptoms.[59] Several controlled studies found lower blood levels of antioxidants, such as selenium, vitamin A, vitamin E, vitamin C, **glutathione** (page 531), and several **carotenoids** (page 488), in patients with both acute and chronic pancreatitis.[60, 61, 62, 63, 64, 65]

There are few controlled trials of antioxidant supplementation to patients with pancreatitis. One small controlled study of acute pancreatitis patients found that sodium selenite at a dose of 500 micrograms (mcg) daily resulted in decreased levels of a marker of free radical activity, and no patient deaths occurred.[66] In a small double-blind trial including recurrent acute and chronic pancreatitis patients, supplements providing daily doses of 600 mcg **selenium** (page 584), 9,000 IU **beta-carotene** (page 469), 540 mg **vitamin C** (page 604), 270 IU **vitamin E** (page 609), and 2,000 mg **methionine** (page 557) significantly reduced pain, normalized several blood measures of antioxidant levels and free radical activity, and prevented acute recurrences of pancreatitis.[67] These researchers later reported that continuing antioxidant treatment in these patients for up to five years or more significantly reduced the total number of days spent in the hospital and resulted in 78% of patients becoming pain-free and 88% returning to work.[68]

In a preliminary report, three patients with chronic pancreatitis were treated with grape seed extract in the amount of 100 mg 2–3 times per day. The frequency and intensity of abdominal pain was reduced in all three patients, and there was a resolution of vomiting in one patient.[69]

Are there any side effects or interactions?
Refer to the individual supplement for information about any side effects or interactions.

PARASITES

Parasites are organisms larger than yeast or bacteria that can cause **infection** (page 265), usually in the intestines. The most common parasites to infect humans in the United States and Canada are giardia *(Giardia lamblia), Entamoeba histolytica,* cryptosporidium *(Cryptosporidium* spp.), roundworm *(Ascaris lumbricoides),* hookworm *(Ancylostoma duodenale* and *Necator americanus),* pinworm *(Enterobius vermicularis),* and tapeworm *(Taenia* spp.).

Infection with parasites can be life-threatening in people with severe impairment of **immune function** (page 255). People should consult a physician if they suspect a parasitic infection.

	CHECKLIST FOR PARASITES	
Rating	**Nutritional Supplements**	**Herbs**
★★☆	**Propolis** (page 579)	Berberine **Ipecac** (page 696) **Myrrh** (page 713) (for schistosomiasis)
★☆☆		**Anise** (page 627) **Barberry** (page 632) Black walnut **Chaparral** (page 657) Cloves Curled mint **Garlic** (page 679) **Goldenseal** (page 683) Goldthread Male fern **Oregon grape** (page 721) **Pumpkin seeds** (page 733) **Sweet Annie** (page 750) Tansy Wormseed **Wormwood** (page 762)

What are the symptoms of parasites?
Parasite infections can lead to a variety of symptoms, including **gas** (page 193), bloating, **diarrhea** (page 163), weight loss, abdominal cramping and pain, **constipation** (page 137), nausea, vomiting, loss of appetite, fever, rash, **cough** (page 139), itching anus, and bloody or foul-smelling stools.

Medical treatments
Over the counter antidiarrheal drugs, such as loperamide (Imodium A-D), bismuth subsalicylate (Pepto Bismol), and attapulgite (Kaopectate), might be helpful. Supportive care with the replacement of fluids and electrolytes, sometimes with the use of oral rehydration solutions (Pedialyte, Ceralyte, Infalyte), is often recommended.

Prescription medication, such as mebendazole (Vermox), thiabendazole (Mintezol), metronidazole (Flagyl), and praziquantel (Biltricide), may be prescribed based on the type of parasite found. Medicines to stop diarrhea, such as diphenoxylate (Lomotil, Lonox, Motofen), and opiates (codeine), may be prescribed for some individuals.

Severe **diarrhea** (page 163) may require hospitalization for urgent fluid and electrolyte replacement, especially in children and the elderly.

Dietary changes that may be helpful
When traveling in developing countries, people should avoid drinking tap water and eating uncooked foods, foods prepared by street vendors, ice, and fruits that cannot be peeled. All of these are potential sources of parasitic infection. People should not drink untreated stream water while camping, as it is frequently almost invariably contaminated with giardia, even in the United States. Undercooked fish, meat and poultry can also contain parasites.

Nutritional supplements that may be helpful
Propolis (page 579) is a resinous substance collected by bees from the leaf buds and bark of trees, especially poplar and conifer trees. The antimicrobial properties of propolis may help protect against parasitic **infections** (page 265) in the gastrointestinal tract. One preliminary trial of propolis extract for children and adults with giardiasis showed a 52% rate of successful parasite elimination in children and a 60% elimination rate in adults (amount not stated).[1] These results are not as impressive as those achieved with conventional drugs for giardiasis, though, so propolis should not be used as the sole therapy for parasites without first consulting a physician about available medical treatment.

Are there any side effects or interactions?
Refer to the individual supplement for information about any side effects or interactions.

Herbs that may be helpful
Berberine is derived from several plants, including **barberry** (page 632), **Oregon grape** (page 721), **goldenseal** (page 683), and goldthread *(Coptis chinensis).* Preliminary trials have shown that berberine can be used successfully to treat giardia **infections** (page

265).[2, 3] In addition, test tube studies show that berberine kills amoebae, although it is not known whether this effect occurs in humans.[4] The amount required is approximately 200 mg three times per day for an adult—a level high enough to potentially cause side effects. Therefore, berberine should not be used without consulting a healthcare provider.

Emetine and other alkaloids in **ipecac** (page 696) kill several types of parasites, including amoeba, pinworms, and tapeworms.[5, 6] Generally the amounts of ipecac needed to produce these effects in people are high and can lead to severe side effects. Emetine or its somewhat safer form, dihydroemetine, are reserved for rare cases of people infected with amoebae who are not cured by using anti-amoeba drugs.[7] Because of the danger involved, ipecac and emetine should never be used without first consulting a physician.

In a preliminary trial, patients with schistosomiasis (a parasitic infection) were treated with a combination of resin and volatile oil of **myrrh** (page 713), in the amount of 10 mg per 2.2 pounds of body weight per day for three days. The cure rate was 91.7% and, of those who did not respond, 76.5% were cured by a second six-day course of treatment, increasing the overall cure rate to 98.1%.[8]

Garlic (page 679) has been demonstrated to kill parasites, including amoeba[9] and hookworm,[10] in test tubes and in animals. Older studies in humans support the use of garlic to treat roundworm, pinworm, and hookworm.[11] However, due to a lack of clinical trials, the amount of garlic needed to treat intestinal parasites in humans is not known.

Wormseed *(Chenopodium ambrosioides)* is a traditional remedy for infections with worms. However, a study in Mexico found that the powdered herb was not effective at eradicating hookworm, roundworm, or whipworm.[12]

Pumpkin seeds (page 733) *(Cucurbita pepo)* have purported effects against tapeworms. Given their safety, they are often recommended as an addition to other, more reliable therapies. In Germany, 200–400 grams are commonly ground and taken with milk and honey, followed by castor oil two hours later.[13] Tapeworms can cause severe illness and should be treated only with medical supervision. In China, pumpkin seeds have been shown to effectively treat acute schistosomiasis, a severe parasitic disease occurring primarily in Asia and Africa that is transmitted by snails.[14] The assistance of a physician is required to help diagnose and treat any suspected intestinal parasite infection.

Several other herbs are traditionally used for treatment of parasites, including male fern *(Dryopteris filix mas)* root, tansy *(Tanacetum vulgare)* leaf, **wormwood** (page 762), **sweet Annie** (page 750), black walnut *(Juglans nigra)* fruit, and cloves *(Syzygium aromaticum)*. Numerous case reports and preliminary studies from the late 1800s and early 1900s have suggested some of these herbs can be helpful for some parasitic infections.[15]

In some cultures, it was customary to bathe in **chaparral** (page 657) once per year to eliminate skin parasites and to detoxify; however, there is no modern research demonstrating the effectiveness of this use of chaparral.

Anise (page 627) may have modest antiparasitic actions and has been recommended by some practitioners as a treatment for mild intestinal parasite infections.[16]

Curled mint *(Mentha crispa)* leaf, a close relative of **peppermint** (page 726), has been shown in a preliminary trial to help relieve the symptoms of giardia and amoeba infections in children and adults, as well as to eliminate these parasites in many cases.[17] This study used a tincture of curled mint in the amount of 2 ml three times per day for five days, or 1 ml three times per day for five days for children. Given their close relationship, peppermint could probably be substituted for curled mint when curled mint is unavailable.

Caution: Any herb potent enough to kill parasites could potentially harm the person taking it. Although some of these herbs have antiparasitic actions in test tubes,[18] none has been adequately tested in modern trials for efficacy or safety in humans. Safe and proper use requires the skills of an experienced practitioner.

Are there any side effects or interactions?
Refer to the individual herb for information about any side effects or interactions.

PARKINSON'S DISEASE

Parkinson's disease results from progressive damage to the nerves in the area of the brain responsible for controlling muscle tone and movement. The damaged cells are those needed to produce a neurotransmitter (chemical messenger in the brain) called dopamine, so people with Parkinson's disease manufacture inadequate amounts of dopamine.

Parkinson's disease occurs primarily, but not exclusively, in the elderly. Parkinson-like symptoms can also be caused by prescription and illicit drugs.

Parkinson's Disease

CHECKLIST FOR PARKINSON'S DISEASE

Rating	Nutritional Supplements	Herbs
★★☆	**Coenzyme Q₁₀** (page 496) **D-phenylalanine** (page 568) **Methionine** (page 557) **NADH** (page 564) **Vitamin B₂** (page 598) **Vitamin C** (page 604) and **vitamin E** (page 609) (in combination)	
★☆☆	**5-HTP** (page 459) (with Sinemet) **L-tyrosine** (page 544) **Phosphatidylserine** (page 569) **Vitamin B₆** (page 600) (with Sinemet or selegiline) **Vitamin D** (page 607)	*Mucuna prurient* **Psyllium husks** (page 732) (for constipation)

What are the symptoms of Parkinson's disease?

Symptoms include a fixed facial expression, wide-eyed stare with infrequent blinking, fluttering of the eyelids, drooling, illegible handwriting, monotone voice, and rhythmic movement of the fingers, hand, foot, or arm when at rest. People with Parkinson's disease often have difficulty getting out of bed or a soft chair, and may tend to stand stooped over and walk leaning forward with limited arm-swing and small, shuffling steps. **Depression** (page 145) and decreased mental functioning are also common symptoms in advanced stages.

Medical treatments

Prescription drug therapy does not cure Parkinson's, but symptoms are often improved with medications. The most commonly used drug is Sinemet, which contains both levodopa and carbidopa. Other drugs used include selegiline (Eldepryl), bromocriptine (Parlodel), amantadine (Symmetrel), pergolide (Permax), pramipexole (Mirapex), and ropinirole (Requip).

Surgery that destroys specific areas of the brain is recommended for individuals with severe symptoms that don't respond to drug therapy. Physical therapy, speech therapy, and aids to daily living, such as railings, non-

slip mats, and special chairs, may also be suggested in advanced cases.

Dietary changes that may be helpful

Clinical studies have shown that one can enhance the action of L-dopa and improve the symptoms of Parkinson's disease by consuming nearly all of the day's protein intake at dinner, while keeping the protein content of breakfast and lunch extremely low.[1, 2, 3] This dietary approach is now well-accepted, but must be carefully monitored by a qualified healthcare professional in order to avoid deficiencies of protein and certain vitamins and minerals.

Consumption of large amounts of fava beans *(Vicia faba),* also known as broad beans, might increase the action of L-dopa and possibly lead to L-dopa overdose. Parkinson's disease patients should, therefore, talk with a doctor before adding broad beans to their diet.

A preliminary study found that higher coffee and caffeine intake is associated with a significantly lower incidence of Parkinson's disease in older persons.[4] These findings do not mean that coffee or caffeinated beverages can be used as a treatment for Parkinson's disease, but simply that caffeine may in some way help to prevent the development of the disease in its early stages. Until more is known, increasing caffeine consumption is not recommended, even in people with a family history of Parkinson's disease.

Doctors recommend that people with Parkinson's disease supplement with **fiber** (page 512) and maintain adequate fluid intake to reduce **constipation** (page 137) associated with this disease.[5] See the discussion about **psyllium** (page 732) seed below in "Herbs that may be helpful."

Lifestyle changes that may be helpful

People with Parkinson's disease are at higher than normal risk for **osteoporosis** (page 333) and **vitamin D** (page 607) deficiency. Regular weight-bearing exercise, exposure to sunlight, and a variety of supplements and dietary changes may be helpful in preventing osteoporosis.

A twice-weekly, 14-week program of intensive exercise has been shown to significantly improve the signs and symptoms of Parkinson's Disease.[6] **Athletic training** (page 43) included resistance exercises in water to increase strength, as well as exercises increasing flexibility and balance.

There is substantial preliminary evidence that exposure to certain organochlorine insecticides (e.g., lindane [Kwell, Kildane, Scabene] and dieldrin [Dieldrite]) may contribute to the development of Parkinson's disease.[7, 8, 9] In California, death from Parkinson's disease increased by about 40% in all Californian counties reporting use of restricted agricultural pesticides since the 1970s compared with those reporting none.[10] Avoiding contact with pesticides and pesticide residues may be an important preventive measure for Parkinson's and other diseases. Interestingly, consumption of the fat substitute olestra appears to increase elimination of certain organochlorine pesticides in the feces.[11, 12] However, no scientific studies have tested olestra as a possible treatment or preventive measure against Parkinson's disease. Moreover, since olestra consumption may be associated with other health risks, such as depletion of **beta-carotene** (page 469), people with Parkinson's should consult with their doctor before consuming products containing olestra.

Nutritional supplements that may be helpful

In a double-blind trial, administration of 1,200 mg of coenzyme Q_{10} per day for 16 months to people with early Parkinson's disease significantly slowed the progression of the disease, compared with a placebo.[13] Smaller amounts of CoQ_{10} were slightly more effective than placebo, but the difference was not statistically significant.

Some preliminary studies have indicated that high dietary intakes of **antioxidant** (page 467) nutrients, especially **vitamin E** (page 607), are associated with a low risk of Parkinson's disease,[14, 15] even though Parkinson's patients are not deficient in vitamin E.[16, 17] The correlation between protection from Parkinson's and dietary vitamin E may be not be due to the vitamin E itself, however. Legumes (beans and peas) contain relatively high amounts of vitamin E. Independent of their vitamin E content, consumption of legumes has been associated with low risk of Parkinson's disease.[18] In other words, high vitamin E intake may be a marker for diets high in legumes, and legumes may protect against Parkinson's disease for reasons unrelated to their vitamin E content.

Interest in the relationship between antioxidants and Parkinson's disease led to a preliminary trial using high amounts of **vitamin C** (page 604) and vitamin E in early Parkinson's disease[19] and to a large ten-year controlled trial of high amounts of vitamin E combined with the drug deprenyl.[20] In the trial combining vita-

mins C and E, people with early Parkinson's disease given 750 mg of vitamin C and 800 IU of vitamin E four times each day (totaling 3,000 mg of vitamin C and 3,200 IU of vitamin E per day) were able to delay the need for drug therapy (i.e., L-dopa or selegiline) by an average of about two and a half years, compared with those not taking the vitamins.[21] The ten-year controlled trial used 2,000 IU of vitamin E per day found no benefit in slowing or improving the disease.[22] The difference in the outcomes between these two trials might be due to the inclusion of vitamin C and/or the higher amount of vitamin E used in the successful trial. However, the difference might also be due to a better study design in the trial that found vitamin E to be ineffective.

The amounts of vitamin E used in the above trials were very high, because raising **antioxidant** (page 467) levels in brain tissue is quite difficult to achieve.[23] In fact, some researchers have found that even extremely high intakes of vitamin E (4,000 IU per day) failed to increase brain vitamin E levels.[24] The difficulty in increasing brain vitamin E levels may explain the poor results of the large, controlled trial.

Although **vitamin B$_6$** (page 600) was reported many years ago in preliminary research to improve symptoms of Parkinson's disease,[25] it must not be used by people taking L-dopa alone. Taking vitamin B$_6$ with L-dopa increases the conversion of L-dopa to dopamine outside the brain, thereby reducing delivery of dopamine to the brain.[26, 27] However, vitamin B$_6$ can be used in conjunction with L-dopa plus carbidopa (Sinemet) or selegiline (Eldepryl, Atapryl).[28]

Preliminary trials have suggested that the **amino acid** (page 467), **methionine** (page 557) (5 grams per day), may effectively treat some symptoms of Parkinson's disease.[29]

Drug therapy for Parkinson's disease has been reported to deplete **vitamin B$_3$** (page 598) in humans.[30] Vitamin B$_3$ may be needed to decrease **SAMe** (page 583) levels, and in so doing, may possibly help people with Parkinson's disease. However, the two main forms of vitamin B$_3$, niacin and niacinamide, when taken in combination with L-dopa, have demonstrated no benefit for people with Parkinson's disease.[31] Nicotinamide adenine dinucleotide (**NADH** [page 564])—the active form of vitamin B$_3$ in the body—effectively raises the level of dopamine in the brain, making it potentially useful in the treatment of people with Parkinson's disease. In preliminary research, NADH supplementation reduced symptoms and improved brain function in people with Parkinson's disease.[32, 33] One researcher has recommended 5 mg taken twice per day for people with Parkinson's disease.[34] However, one small, double-blind, short-term trial using injections of NADH found no significant effects.[35]

In a preliminary study of 31 Brazilian individuals with Parkinson's disease, all had laboratory evidence of **vitamin B₂** (page 598) (riboflavin) deficiency. Nineteen of these individuals received 30 mg of supplemental riboflavin three times a day for six months. After three months, all participants treated with riboflavin demonstrated an improvement in motor capacity, and this improvement was either maintained or greater at six months.[36] The participants in this study also eliminated red meat from their diet, but it is not clear whether that dietary change played any role in the observed improvement.

In a preliminary report, 5-hydroxytryptophan (**5-HTP** [page 459]) used in combination with Sinemet improved the emotional **depression** (page 145) that is often associated with Parkinson's disease.[37] While 5-HTP may be helpful as a supplement to Sinemet treatment for Parkinson's, 5-HTP should never be used alone in Parkinson's disease.[38, 39, 40] 5-HTP is converted to serotonin in the brain, and increasing serotonin without increasing dopamine can cause Parkinson's symptoms, especially rigidity, to get worse.[41] People taking selegiline should not take 5-HTP without a physician's supervision, as this combination might raise serotonin to excessively high levels.[42]

L-tyrosine (page 544) is the direct precursor to L-dopa. Theoretically, supplementing L-tyrosine could be an alternative to L-dopa therapy; however, L-tyrosine should not be taken *with* L-dopa as it may interfere with the transport of L-dopa to the brain.[43] One small preliminary trial demonstrated that some people with Parkinson's disease who supplemented with L-tyrosine (45 mg per pound of body weight) for three years had better clinical results and fewer side effects than did patients using L-dopa.[44] Until these findings are confirmed, L-tyrosine should not be used as a replacement for, or in addition to, L-dopa.

In a small, four-week trial, **D-phenylalanine** (page 568) (DPA) supplementation improved motor control and tremors in people with Parkinson's disease.[45] Additional research is needed before the benefits of this treatment can be considered proven. DPA should not be taken with L-dopa as it may interfere with the transport of L-dopa to the brain.[46] People with Parkinson's

disease should consult with a physician before using DPA. Some commercially available phenylalanine products contain a 50:50 mixture of DPA and LPA, the form of phenylalanine that occurs naturally in food (these products are known as DLPA). People with Parkinson's disease should consult a physician before using DPA or DLPA.

People with Parkinson's disease treated with L-dopa have been reported to have reduced levels of the neurotransmitter **phosphatidylserine** (page 569).[47] In one trial, supplementing with phosphatidylserine (100 mg three times daily) improved the mood and mental function in patients with Parkinson's disease, but exerted no beneficial effects on muscle control.[48] The phosphatidylserine used in this trial was obtained from cow brain. That product is not available in the United States, because of concern that an extract of cow brain could cause Creutzfeld-Jakob disease, the human variant of "mad cow" disease. The phosphatidylserine sold in the United States is manufactured from plant sources and cow-brain phosphatidylserine.[49]

Vitamin D (page 607) deficiency is common in Parkinson's disease. People with Parkinson's often get insufficient sun exposure and have reduced levels of activity that adversely affect **calcium** (page 483) metabolism.[50] Low vitamin D levels in Parkinson's disease have been reported to increase the risk of hip fracture due to **osteoporosis** (page 333).[51] This risk has been significantly reduced with the use of synthetic, activated vitamin D—a prescription drug.[52] Whether the same effect could be achieved with supplemental vitamin D remains unknown, though some doctors recommend 400–1,000 IU vitamin D per day. People with Parkinson's disease may wish to discuss the use of synthetic activated vitamin D with a healthcare professional.

People with Parkinson's disease have shown both decreased and increased levels of **zinc** (page 614) and **copper** (page 499).[53, 54, 55, 56] Both nutrients function in the antioxidant **enzyme** (page 467) superoxide dismutase (SOD). SOD tends to be low in the area of the brain involved in Parkinson's disease. In theory, therefore, low levels of zinc and copper could leave the brain susceptible to **free radical** (page 467) damage. However, copper and zinc (as well as **iron** [page 540]) taken in excess can also act as *pro*-oxidants, and all have been associated with an *increased* risk of developing Parkinson's disease in preliminary research.[57, 58] Insufficient evidence currently exists for either recommending or avoiding supplementation with zinc and copper.

Are there any side effects or interactions?
Refer to the individual supplement for information about any side effects or interactions.

Herbs that may be helpful

In preliminary research, an extract of *Mucuna prurient* (HP-200) was studied in people with Parkinson's disease, 43% of whom were taking Sinemet before HP-200 treatment; the remaining 57% were not medicated.[59] Statistically significant reductions in symptom scores were seen from the beginning to the end of the 12-week trial. The amount used in the trial was 7.5 grams of the extract (dissolved in water) three to six times daily.

Other preliminary research has shown that **psyllium** (page 732) seed husks improve **constipation** (page 137) and bowel function in people with Parkinson's disease and constipation.[60] A typical recommendation for psyllium seed husks is 3 to 5 grams taken at night with a one to two glasses of fluid.

Are there any side effects or interactions?
Refer to the individual herb for information about any side effects or interactions.

PEPTIC ULCER

Peptic ulcers are erosions or open sores in the mucous lining of the stomach or duodenum (the first part of the small intestine). The term "peptic" distinguishes peptic ulcers from ulcerations that affect other parts of the body (e.g., diabetic leg ulcers).

Peptic ulcer should never be treated without proper diagnosis. They are usually caused by infection from *Helicobacter pylori (H. pylori)*. People with peptic ulcer due to infection should discuss conventional treatment directed toward eradicating the organism—various combinations of antibiotics, acid blockers, and bismuth—with a medical doctor. Ulcers can also be caused or aggravated by stress, alcohol, smoking, and dietary factors.

What are the symptoms of peptic ulcer?

Peptic ulcers are occasionally painless. However, the most common symptom is a dull ache in the upper abdomen that usually occurs two to three hours after a meal; the ache is relieved by eating. Other common symptoms include weight loss, bloating, belching, and

nausea. Untreated, peptic ulcers often bleed and may cause sharp burning pain in the area of the stomach or just below it.

CHECKLIST FOR PEPTIC ULCER		
Rating	Nutritional Supplements	Herbs
★★★		**Deglycyrrhizinated licorice** (page 702) (chewable) Mastic
★★☆	**Vitamin A** (page 595) **Zinc** (page 614) Zinc-L-Carnosine	Banana powder Neem
★☆☆	**Carnosine** (page 487) **DMSO** (page 508) **Fiber** (page 512) (for duodenal ulcer) **Flavonoids** (page 516) (**quercetin** [page 580], catechin, apigenin) **Glutamine** (page 530) **Vitamin C** (page 604)	**Calendula** (page 650) **Chamomile** (page 656) **Comfrey** (page 662) **Corydalis** (page 663) **Garlic** (page 679) **Marshmallow** (page 708) **Plantain** (page 729)

Medical treatments

Over the counter antacids, such as magnesium hydroxide (Phillips' Milk of Magnesia), aluminum hydroxide (Amphojel), calcium carbonate (Tums), and the combination magnesium-aluminum hydroxide (Mylanta, Maalox), help relieve the symptoms associated with peptic ulcers. The histamine H2 antagonists, such as cimetidine (Tagamet), ranitidine (Zantac), and famotidine (Pepcid), as well as the proton pump inhibitor omeprazole (Prilosec-OTC), are also beneficial.

Prescription drug therapy might involve antibiotics that eliminate *H. pylori* infection, such as amoxicillin (Amoxil), clarithromycin (Biaxin), metronidazole (Flagyl), and tetracycline (Sumycin), in combination with the proton pump inhibitors lansoprazole (Prevacid) and omeprazole (Prilosec). Bismuth subsalicylate (Pepto Bismol) may be added as well. Other medications may be prescribed to control stomach acidity, including prescription strength histamine H2 inhibitors, such as cimetidine (Tagamet), ranitidine (Zantac), and famotidine (Pepcid), as well as the prescription strength proton pump inhibitors omeprazole (Prilosec), lansoprazole (Prevacid), pantoprazole (Protonix), and rabeprazole (Aciphex).

Dietary changes that may be helpful

People with ulcers have been reported to eat more sugar than people without ulcers,[1] though this link may only occur in those with a genetic susceptibility toward ulcer formation.[2] Sugar has also been reported to increase stomach acidity,[3] which could aggravate ulcer symptoms.

Salt is a stomach and intestinal irritant. Higher intakes of salt have been linked to higher risk of stomach (though not duodenal) ulcer.[4] As a result of these reports, some doctors suggest that people with ulcers should restrict the use of both sugar and salt, although the benefit of such dietary changes remains unknown.

Many years ago, researchers reported that cabbage juice accelerated healing of peptic ulcers.[5, 6, 7, 8] Drinking a quart of cabbage juice per day was necessary for symptom relief in some reports. Although only preliminary modern research supports this approach,[9] many doctors claim considerable success using one quart per day for 10 to 14 days, with ulcer symptoms frequently decreasing in only a few days. Carrot juice may be added to improve the flavor.

Fiber (page 512) slows the movement of food and acidic fluid from the stomach to the intestines, which should help those with duodenal, though not stomach, ulcers.[10] When people with recently healed duodenal ulcers were put on a long-term (six-month), high-fiber diet, the rate of ulcer recurrence was dramatically reduced in one controlled study,[11] though short-term (four-week) use of fiber in people with active duodenal ulcers led to only negligible improvement.[12]

The relationship between **food allergies** (page 14) and peptic ulcers has been reported at least as far back as the 1930s.[13] Exposing the lining of the stomach to foods to which a person is allergic has been reported to cause bleeding in the stomach.[14] Although additional research is needed, avoiding food allergens may be helpful for people with peptic ulcers. Consult with a doctor to determine food sensitivities.

Lifestyle changes that may be helpful

Aspirin and related drugs (non-steroidal anti-inflammatory drugs),[15] alcohol,[16] coffee[17] (including decaf),[18] and tea[19] can aggravate or interfere with the healing of peptic ulcers. Smoking is also known to slow ulcer healing.[20] Whether or not an ulcer is caused by **infection** (page 265), people with peptic ulcer should avoid use of these substances.

Nutritional supplements that may be helpful

Vitamin A (page 595) is needed to heal the linings (called mucous membranes) of the stomach and intestines. In one controlled trial, vitamin A supplementation facilitated healing in a small group of people with stomach ulcer.[21] The amount used in that study (150,000 IU per day) can be toxic and may also cause birth defects. Such a high dose should not be taken by a pregnant woman, by a woman who could become **pregnant** (page 363), or by anyone else without careful supervision from a doctor. Objective evidence of ulcer healing from taking vitamin A has been reported by the same research group.[22] The effect of lower amounts of vitamin A has not been studied in people with peptic ulcer.

Zinc (page 614) is also needed for the repair of damaged tissue and has protected against stomach ulceration in animal studies.[23] In Europe, zinc combined with acexamic acid, an anti-inflammatory substance, is used as a drug in the treatment of peptic ulcers.[24] In a small controlled trial, high amounts of zinc accelerated the healing of gastric ulcers compared with placebo.[25] Some doctors suspect that such an exceptionally high intake of zinc may be unnecessary, suggesting instead that people with ulcers wishing to take zinc supplements use only 25 to 50 mg of zinc per day. Even at these lower levels, 1 to 3 mg of **copper** (page 499) per day must be taken to avoid copper deficiency that would otherwise be induced by the zinc supplementation.

Experimental animal studies have shown that a zinc salt of the amino acid **carnosine** (page 487) exerts significant protection against ulcer formation and promotes the healing of existing ulcers.[26, 27] However, because zinc by itself has been shown to be helpful against peptic ulcer, it is not known how much of the beneficial effect was due to the carnosine.[28, 29] Clinical studies in humans demonstrated that this compound can help eradicate *H. pylori,* an organism that has been linked to peptic ulcer and stomach cancer.[30] The amount of the zinc carnosine complex used in research studies for eradication of *H. pylori* is 150 mg twice daily.

Glutamine (page 530), an **amino acid** (page 465), is the principal source of energy for cells that line the small intestine and stomach. More than 40 years ago, glutamine was reported to help people with peptic ulcer in a preliminary trial.[31] Glutamine has also prevented stress ulcers triggered by severe burns in another preliminary study.[32] Despite the limited amount of published research, some doctors suggest 500 to 1,000 mg of glutamine taken two to three times per day to help people overcome peptic ulcers.

Oral supplementation with dimethyl sulfoxide (**DMSO** [page 508]) reduced relapse rates for peptic ulcer significantly better than did placebo or the ulcer drug cimetidine (Tagamet) in one study.[33] Previous research showed that DMSO in combination with cimetidine was more effective than cimetidine alone.[34] These trials used 500 mg of DMSO taken four times per day. The authors of these trials believe the antioxidant activity of DMSO may have a protective effect. Oral supplementation with DMSO should not be attempted without the supervision of a doctor.

Little is known about the effects of **vitamin C** (page 604) supplementation for people with peptic ulcer. People with **gastritis** (page 193), a related condition, have been found to have low levels of vitamin C in their stomach juice. Vitamin C may also help eradicate *H. pylori* in people with gastritis. Vitamin C may one day prove to have a therapeutic effect for people with peptic ulcer; however, further research in this area is needed.

Are there any side effects or interactions?
Refer to the individual supplement for information about any side effects or interactions.

Herbs that may be helpful
Licorice (page 702) root has a long history of use for soothing inflamed and injured mucous membranes in the digestive tract. Licorice may protect the stomach and duodenum by increasing production of mucin, a substance that protects the lining of these organs against stomach acid and other harmful substances.[35] According to laboratory research, **flavonoids** (page 516) in licorice may also inhibit growth of *H. pylori*.[36]

For people with peptic ulcer, many doctors who use herbal medicine use the deglycyrrhizinated form of licorice (DGL). In making DGL, the portion of licorice root that can increase blood pressure and cause water retention is almost completely removed, while the mucous-membrane-healing part of the root is retained. In some reports, DGL has compared favorably to the popular drug cimetidine (Tagamet) for treatment of peptic ulcer,[37] while in other trials cimetidine has appeared initially more effective.[38] After DGL and cimetidine were discontinued, though, one study reported fewer recurrences in the DGL group than in the cimetidine group.[39]

Though not every trial has reported efficacy,[40] most studies find DGL to facilitate healing of peptic ulcer. A review of the DGL research shows that the studies not reporting efficacy used capsules, and the trials finding DGL to be helpful used chewable tablets.[41] Doctors typically suggest taking one to two chewable tablets of DGL (250 to 500 mg) 15 minutes before meals and one to two hours before bedtime.

The gummy extract of *Pistachia lentiscus,* also known as mastic or gum mastic, has been shown in one preliminary study and one double-blind study to heal peptic ulcers.[42, 43] This may be related to its ability to kill *H. pylori* in test tubes.[44]

Ayurvedic doctors in India have traditionally used dried banana powder *(Musa paradisiaca)* to treat ulcers. In animal studies, banana powder protects the lining of the stomach from acid.[45] A human trial has also found dried banana helpful in those with peptic ulcer. In that report, two capsules of dried raw banana powder taken four times per day for eight weeks led to significant improvement.[46] Bananas and unsweetened banana chips may be good substitutes, although ideal intake remains unknown.

Administration of 30 to 60 mg of freeze-dried neem bark extract twice per day led to a significant reduction in stomach acid levels and near complete healing of all people with duodenal ulcers over ten weeks time in a preliminary clinical trial.[47]

Chamomile (page 656) has a soothing effect on inflamed and irritated mucous membranes. It is also high in the **flavonoid** (page 516) apigenin—another flavonoid that has inhibited growth of *H. pylori* in test tubes.[48] Many doctors recommend drinking two to three cups of strong chamomile tea each day. The tea can be made by combining 3 to 5 ml of chamomile tincture with hot water or by steeping 2 to 3 tsp of chamomile flowers in the water, covered, for 10 to 15 minutes. Chamomile is also available in capsules; two may be taken three times per day.

Calendula (page 650) is another plant with anti-inflammatory and healing activities that can be used as part of a traditional medicine approach to peptic ulcers. The same amount as chamomile can be used.

Marshmallow (page 708) is high in mucilage. High-mucilage-containing herbs have a long history of use for irritated or inflamed mucous membranes in the digestive system, though no clinical research has yet investigated effects in people with peptic ulcer.

Garlic (page 679) has been reported to have anti-

Helicobacter activity in test-tube studies.[49, 50] In a preliminary trial, garlic supplementation (300 mg in tablets three times daily for eight weeks) failed to eradicate *H. pylori* in participants with active infections.[51] In another preliminary trial, participants with active *H. pylori* infections added 10 sliced cloves of garlic to a meal.[52] The addition of garlic failed to inhibit the growth of the organism. Further trials using garlic extracts are needed to validate the anti-Helicobacter activity of garlic observed in test tubes. Until then, evidence to support the use of garlic for *H. pylori*-related peptic ulcers remains weak.

Extracts of the herb **corydalis** (page 663) are not only helpful as pain-relief agents but also may be useful in the treatment of stomach ulcers. In a study of people with stomach and intestinal ulcers or chronic inflammation of the stomach lining, 90 to 120 mg of corydalis extract per day (equal to 5 to 10 grams of the crude herb) was found to be effective in 76% of the participants.[53]

Comfrey (page 662) has a long tradition of use as a topical agent for improving healing of **wounds** (page 319) and **skin ulcers** (page 409).[54, 55] It is also used for people with gastrointestinal problems, including stomach ulcers, though these traditional uses have yet to be tested in scientific studies. People should only use comfrey preparations made from the leaves and avoid those made from the root.

Because of the anti-inflammatory and healing effects of **plantain** (page 729), it may be beneficial in some people with peptic ulcer. Clinical trials have not been done to confirm this possibility.

Are there any side effects or interactions?
Refer to the individual herb for information about any side effects or interactions.

Holistic approaches that may be helpful

Emotional stress has been shown to increase acid production in the stomach.[56] The reported association between stress and peptic ulcer might be attributable to a stress-induced increase in gastric acidity.[57, 58] During the air raids of London in World War II, British physicians observed an increase of more than 50% in the incidence of ruptured peptic ulcers.[59, 60] More recently, an increased incidence of bleeding stomach ulcers was seen in survivors of the Hanshin-Awaji earthquake in Japan.[61] Whether stress reduction techniques or psychological counseling helps prevent ulcers or ulcer recurrence has not been adequately studied in medical trials.

PERIPHERAL VASCULAR DISEASE

Peripheral vascular disease (PVD) refers to a variety of conditions that primarily affect the arteries of the body, with the exception of the coronary arteries that supply blood to the heart. (Those are covered in the article on **cardiovascular disease** [page 98].) The most common areas for PVD are the arteries of the legs and upper arms, the carotid (neck) arteries, the abdominal aorta and its branches, and the renal (kidney) arteries.

The cause of most types of PVD is hardening of the arteries (**atherosclerosis** [page 38]), which itself has many causes. Conditions affecting the veins, such as **chronic venous insufficiency** (page 116), **varicose veins** (page 440), and **hemorrhoids** (page 219), are not usually included in PVD.

PVD of the carotid arteries is a major cause of **stroke** (page 419). **Intermittent claudication** (page 276) refers to pain in the lower legs after walking short distances and is caused by PVD of the leg arteries. One cause of **erectile dysfunction** (page 185) may be PVD of the penis. **Raynaud's disease** (page 382) is a painful condition caused by spasms of arteries after exposure to cold. Thromboangiitis obliterans (TAO), also known as Buerger's disease, is an uncommon PVD that occurs in both arteries and veins. This condition causes tender areas of inflammation in the arms or legs, followed by cold hands or feet.

Aneurysm is a ballooning of an artery due to weakening of the blood vessel walls. Aneurysms may be an inherited disorder or may be due to **atherosclerosis** (page 38).[1, 2] The most common aneurysm is abdominal aortic aneurysm (AAA), which occurs in the large artery that carries blood from the heart to the lower body. AAA is much more common in men, and risk increases with age. Large AAAs are usually surgically repaired because they can undergo life-threatening ruptures.

What are the symptoms of peripheral vascular disease?

People with peripheral vascular disease may have symptoms of pain, aching, cramping, or fatigue of the muscles in the affected leg that are relieved by rest and worsened by elevation. Other people with peripheral vascular disease may have swollen feet and ankles accompanied by a dull ache made worse with prolonged standing and relieved by elevation. People with chronic peripheral vascular disease may have darkened areas of skin, leg ulcers, and varicose veins.

CHECKLIST FOR PERIPHERAL VASCULAR DISEASE

Rating	Nutritional Supplements	Herbs
★★☆	Inositol hexaniacinate (page 537)	
★☆☆	Copper (page 499) (for abdominal aortic aneurysm) Folic acid (page 520) (for thromboangiitis obliterans)	

Medical treatments

Over the counter aspirin (Bayer Low Adult Strength, Ecotrin Adult Low Strength) may be recommended to prevent platelet aggregation and clotting.

Prescription drug treatment may include antiplatelet medications, such as clopidogrel (Plavix), ticlopidine (Ticlid), dipyridamole (Persantine) and dipyridamol with aspirin (Aggrenox), and cholesterol lowering drugs in combination with anti-claudication medications, such as cilostazol (Pletal) and pentoxifylline (Trental).

Exercise rehabilitation therapy, **weight loss** (page 446), and smoking cessation is often recommended. Healthcare providers might advise individuals to elevate their legs frequently, avoid prolonged standing or sitting, and wear graduated compression stockings with supportive shoes. Surgical options to restore blood supply (revascularization procedures, such as, angioplasty, atherectomy, stent placement, and bypass) are usually reserved for those with progressive or disabling symptoms. Any ulcers that develop are treated with compressive bandages that contain antibiotic solutions. Recurrent ulceration may be surgically treated with skin grafts and repair or bypass of the affected veins.

Lifestyle changes that may be helpful

People with TAO are usually heavy smokers, and this is considered a major cause of the disease.[3] It is important for people with TAO to quit smoking.

Nutritional supplements that may be helpful

As with other vascular diseases, people with TAO are more likely to have high levels of **homocysteine** (page 234) and low levels of **folic acid** (page 520).[4] However, no research has tested folic acid as prevention or treatment for this disease.

One controlled study compared a type of niacin (vitamin B$_3$) known as **inositol hexaniacinate** (page 537) to the drug pyridinolcarbamate for the treatment of **skin ulcers** (page 409) caused by PVD.[5] A placebo was not included in this trial, and both 1.2 grams daily of inositol hexaniacinate and 1.5 grams daily of the drug produced beneficial results in about half of the patients.

As in many vascular diseases, people with AAA often have abnormal **cholesterol** (page 223) and **triglyceride** (page 235) levels,[6] and their blood vessel walls contain evidence of **free radical** (page 467) damage.[7, 8] However, it is not known whether lowering blood fats or taking free radical-destroying **antioxidants** (page 467) will reduce the risk of AAA. The arterial walls of AAA are depleted of large molecules related to cartilage, including **chondroitin sulfate** (page 492),[9, 10] but no research has investigated whether supplements of chondroitin sulfate might help prevent problems with AAA. **Copper** (page 499) is required for normal artery structure.[11] Animal studies have shown that copper deficiency leads to weak aortic walls[12] and rupture of the aorta.[13] Combating deficiency with copper supplements prevented rupture in an animal study.[14] Copper deficiency in humans with AAA has been suggested in some studies,[15, 16] but not in others.[17, 18, 19] No studies have been done using copper supplements to prevent or manage aneurysms.

Are there any side effects or interactions?

Refer to the individual supplement for information about any side effects or interactions.

Holistic approaches that may be helpful

Intravenous chelation therapy has been reported to be an effective treatment for PVD.[20, 21] A partially controlled study reported improvements after ten chelation treatments.[22] However, two double-blind studies found no difference between chelation therapy and a placebo in patients with **intermittent claudication** (page 276).[23, 24]

Preliminary reports suggest acupuncture may reduce pain and improve blood flow in TAO,[25, 26] but controlled studies are needed to better evaluate these claims.

PHENYLKETONURIA

Phenylketonuria (PKU) is a rare genetic disorder that results in excessive accumulation of the **amino acid** (page 465), **phenylalanine** (page 568), and reduced levels of the amino acid, **L-tyrosine** (page 544), in the blood.[1]

If untreated, high levels of phenylalanine can cause severe mental retardation, behavioral disturbances, and other brain and nerve problems. Fortunately, newborn screening programs now identify most cases of PKU in the United States and other countries. Early diagnosis and treatment is the key to reducing or preventing PKU-related conditions.[2] Gene therapy is currently being researched as a possible cure.[3, 4] Research is also being conducted on methods to decrease levels of phenylalanine in the blood through the use of certain enzymes[5] and amino acids.[6]

Rating	Nutritional Supplements	Herbs
★★☆	**Branched-chain amino acids** (page 479) (BCAA) **Fish oil** (page 514) (if PUFA deficient) **L-tyrosine** (page 544) (if deficient) **Selenium** (page 584) (if deficient)	
★☆☆	**Vitamin B₁₂** (page 601) (if deficient) **Vitamin K** (page 612) (if deficient)	

CHECKLIST FOR PHENYLKETONURIA

What are the symptoms of phenylketonuria?

Infants with PKU may be lethargic, feed poorly, and have a "mousy" odor from their sweat and urine. **Eczema** (page 117), **sensitivity to sunlight** (page 356), and light skin are also characteristic of PKU. Symptoms of children with untreated PKU include significantly diminished mental capacity, hyperactivity, and seizures.

Medical treatments

Over the counter supplementation with the amino acid **L-tyrosine** (page 544) is recommended.

Other treatment consists of strict adherence to a diet low in phenylalanine, in order to prevent a buildup of phenylalanine in the body.

Dietary changes that may be helpful

PKU can be controlled by a diet low in **phenylalanine** (page 568).[7] The greatest benefits are achieved when the diet is started in the first few days of life,[8] although later treatment will still help to reduce the severity of PKU-related conditions.[9, 10, 11] Maintaining low phenylalanine levels through dietary control improves muscle control and behavioral and intellectual function.[12, 13]

The effects of elevated phenylalanine appear to be less severe in older children and adults than in newborns and young children, in whom the nervous system is still developing. This, combined with the difficulties inherent in following a strict lifelong diet, have caused researchers to examine whether the dietary regimen may be relaxed as children get older. While some research suggests that relaxation of dietary measures may not be harmful,[14, 15, 16] this has not been found to be true in all studies.[17] Therefore, more research is needed to resolve this issue.[18, 19] In a survey of 111 PKU treatment centers, 87% favored lifelong dietary restriction of phenylalanine.[20] The PKU diet is strict, and should be undertaken with the help of a nutritionist and a physician.

Breast-feeding, as opposed to formula feeding, appears to confer some benefits in children born with PKU who were not treated until 20–40 days of age. In a preliminary study, children with PKU who had been breast-fed rather than formula fed prior to receiving dietary treatment scored significantly higher on IQ testing.[21] Infants with PKU tend to retain abnormal amounts of the trace mineral **molybdenum** (page 559). Since infant formulas are supplemented with amounts of molybdenum that far exceed amounts found in breast milk, infants with PKU who are also fed formula run the risk of accumulating excessive molybdenum.[22]

A PKU diet is low in protein, providing no more than the minimum amount of **phenylalanine** (page 568) needed by the body. All high-protein foods, such as dairy products, eggs, fish, meats, poultry, legumes, and nuts, are usually eliminated.[23] Lower protein foods, such as fruits, vegetables and some grain products, are allowed in measured amounts, along with specially prepared phenylalanine-free or nearly phenylalanine-free foods. This diet is supplemented with an **amino acid** (page 465) formula to increase protein intake without adding more phenylalanine than is nutritionally required.

Phenylalanine levels fluctuate as a consequence of changes in diet, health, and growth; therefore, levels must be checked regularly.[24] A nutrition specialist can also provide information on homemade and specially prepared foods for people with PKU, including infant formulas, low protein pastas, breads, crackers, and other foods.

People with PKU who are not following the PKU diet can become deficient in **biotin** (page 473), a water-soluble B vitamin. This is because **phenylalanine** (page 568) blocks biotin metabolism. In a controlled study of children with PKU, elevated phenylalanine levels resulted in **seborrheic dermatitis** (page 400) caused by biotin deficiency, which was corrected by a return to the phenylalanine-restricted diet.[25]

There is debate about whether it is safe for people with PKU to consume aspartame, a low-calorie sweetener that contains about 50% phenylalanine. In one study, blood levels of phenylalanine increased only slightly after people with PKU ingested a 12-ounce soft drink sweetened with aspartame.[26] However, that study did not address long-term effects of regular aspartame consumption. Until more is known, it is prudent for people with PKU to completely avoid aspartame-containing beverages and foods.

Lifestyle changes that may be helpful
Access to PKU resource/support groups, and education of family members may help simplify the complex dietary restrictions and improve one's ability to follow them.[27, 28, 29]

PKU during **pregnancy** (page 363) (maternal PKU) is of particular concern. Excessively high or low levels of phenylalanine may occur during pregnancy, both of which may adversely affect the fetus.[30] Maternal PKU can lead to fetal malformations, including small head size (microcephaly), heart abnormalities, failure to grow properly in the uterus (called intrauterine growth retardation), and mental retardation.[31] Adverse effects on the offspring can be reduced and by careful dietary control both prior to and during pregnancy.[32, 33, 34] Consultation and follow-up visits with medical and nutritional specialists are necessary for effective monitoring and dietary guidance in people with PKU.

Nutritional supplements that may be helpful
Because of the importance of strict dietary control, nutritional supplementation should be supervised by a specialist.

In a double-blind trial, regular use of **branched-chain amino acids** (page 479) (BCAAs) (i.e., valine, isoleucine, and leucine) by adolescents and young adults with PKU improved performance on some tests

of mental functioning.[35] Participants received either placebo, or 150 mg per 2.2 pounds of body weight each of valine and isoleucine, and 200 mg per 2.2 pounds of body of leucine, taken with meals and at bedtime. Participants received one mixture or the other for four three-month periods, for a total of six months' supplementation of each regimen over the course of a year.

PKU results from a deficiency or malfunction of the enzyme, phenylalanine hydroxylase, which converts phenylalanine to **L-tyrosine** (page 544).[36] People with PKU have elevated concentrations of phenylalanine and low levels of L-tyrosine,[37] which may contribute to behavior problems.[38, 39] In addition, low L-tyrosine levels in **pregnant** (page 363) women with PKU may contribute to fetal damage.[40] In some,[41] but not all,[42] double-blind studies, keeping L-tyrosine levels in the normal range by adding supplemental L-tyrosine to the diet improved behavior. In a preliminary study, blood L-tyrosine levels fluctuated significantly in people with PKU, suggesting a need for careful laboratory monitoring of people supplementing with L-tyrosine.[43]

The PKU diet is low in fatty acids, some of which are essential for proper brain development.[44] In one controlled study of children with PKU who were deficient in fatty acids, supplementation with **fish oil** (page 514) (but not with black currant seed oil) for six months improved the deficiency. The children received 500 mg of oil per 8.8 pounds of body weight each day for 6 months. The amount varied from 5–8 capsules (each containing 500 mg) per day for each child.[45]

People with PKU may be deficient in several nutrients, due to the restricted diet which is low in protein and animal fat. Deficiencies of long-chain polyunsaturated fatty acids (LC-PUFAs),[46, 47, 48] **selenium** (page 584),[49, 50, 51, 52] **vitamin B$_{12}$** (page 601),[53] and **vitamin K** (page 612) may develop on this diet.[54]

Selenium is important for normal **antioxidant** (page 467) function. Research suggests that selenium deficiency and decreased antioxidant activity may contribute to the brain and nerve disorders associated with PKU.[55] In two preliminary studies involving selenium-deficient people with PKU, supplementation with selenium in the form of sodium selenite corrected the deficiency,[56] whereas supplementation with selenium in the form of selenomethionine did not.[57]

Vitamin B$_{12}$ (page 601) is found almost exclusively in foods of animal origin, which are restricted on the PKU diet. People on the PKU diet who are inconsistent in their use of a vitamin B$_{12}$ supplement may become deficient in this vitamin. In a survey of young adults with PKU, 32% were found to have low or low-normal blood levels of vitamin B_{12}.[58] **Vitamin B_{12} deficiency** (page 601) can cause **anemia** (page 25) and nerve problems.

Because the PKU diet is low in animal products, fat intake is also significantly reduced. The results of a preliminary study of children with PKU suggested that the low-fat PKU diet intake may impair the absorption of **vitamin K** (page 612), a fat-soluble vitamin, from the diet, possibly resulting in a vitamin K deficiency. In that study, children with PKU on a strict diet had low levels of certain vitamin K-dependent proteins needed for normal blood clotting.[59]

Are there any side effects or interactions?
Refer to the individual supplement for information about any side effects or interactions.

PHOTOSENSITIVITY

People with photosensitivity have an immunological response to light, usually sunlight. They typically break out in a rash when exposed to sunlight; how much exposure it takes to cause a reaction varies from person to person. Several conditions, such as erythropoietic protoporphyria and polymorphous light eruption, share the common symptom of hypersensitivity to light—also typically sunlight.

People taking certain prescription drugs (sulfonamides, tetracycline, and thiazide diuretics) or herbs (**St. John's wort** [page 747], for example) and those with **systemic lupus erythematosus** (page 421) have increased susceptibility to adverse effects from sun exposure.

CHECKLIST FOR PHOTOSENSITIVITY		
Rating	Nutritional Supplements	Herbs
★★★	Beta-carotene (page 469)	
★☆☆	Adenosine monophosphate (page 461) Fish oil (page 514) Vitamin B_3 (page 598) (niacinamide) Vitamin B_6 (page 600) Vitamin E (page 609)	

What are the symptoms of photosensitivity?
Symptoms may include a pink or red skin rash with blotchy blisters, scaly patches, or raised spots on areas directly exposed to the sun. The affected area may itch or burn, and the rash may last for several days. In some people, the reaction to sunlight gradually becomes less with subsequent exposures.

Medical treatments
Over the counter supplementation with **beta-carotene** (page 469) may reduce the severity of reactions.

The prescription drug hydroxychloroquine (Plaquenil) might help to reduce the severity of reactions. Oral corticosteroids such as triamcinolone (Aristocort, Kenalog), betamethasone (Valisone, Diprosone), and fluocinonide (Lidex) are often prescribed to clear up the skin rash once it has appeared. In some cases, psoralens, such as trioxsalen (Trisoralen), plus ultraviolet therapy (PUVA) is administered over the course of several weeks to prevent photosensitivity.

Other treatment includes the avoidance of direct sunlight and the use of sunscreen. In addition, individuals should avoid medications and substances that are known to cause photosensitivity.

Dietary changes that may be helpful
One of the conditions that may trigger photosensitivity—porphyria cutanea tarda—has been linked to alcohol consumption.[1] People with this form of porphyria should avoid alcohol. Some people have been reported to develop a photosensitivity reaction to the artificial sweetener, saccharin.[2]

Lifestyle changes that may be helpful
People with photosensitivity need to protect themselves from the sun by using sunscreen, wearing protective clothing (such as long-sleeved shirts), and avoiding excess exposure to the sun.

Nutritional supplements that may be helpful
Years ago, researchers theorized that **beta-carotene** (page 469) in skin might help protect against sensitivity to ultraviolet light from the sun. Large amounts of beta-carotene (up to 300,000 IU per day for at least several months) have allowed people with photosensitivity to stay out in the sun several times longer than they otherwise could tolerate.[3, 4, 5] The protective effect appears to result from beta-carotene's ability to protect against **free-radical** (page 467) damage caused by sunlight.[6]

Adenosine monophosphate (page 461) (AMP) is a substance made in the body that is also distributed as a supplement, although it is not widely available. According to one report, 90% of people with porphyria cutanea tarda responded well to 160 to 200 mg of AMP per day taken for at least one month.[7] Complete alleviation of photosensitivity occurred in about half of the people who took AMP.

In a small preliminary trial, supplementation with fish oil (page 514) (10 grams per day for three months) reduced photosensitivity in 90% of people suffering from polymorphous light eruptions.[8]

Less is known about the effects of supplementation with other antioxidants (page 467) on photosensitivity. Research with vitamin E (page 609) has been limited and has not yielded consistent results.[9, 10]

Cases have been reported of people with photosensitivity who responded to vitamin B6 (page 600) supplementation.[11, 12] Amounts of vitamin B6 used to successfully reduce reactions to sunlight have varied considerably. Some doctors suggest a trial of 100 to 200 mg per day for three months. People wishing to take more than 200 mg of vitamin B6 per day should do so only under medical supervision.

Niacinamide (page 598), a form of vitamin B3, can reduce the formation of a kynurenic acid—a substance that has been linked to photosensitivity. One trial studied the effects of niacinamide in people who had polymorphous light eruption.[13] While taking one gram three times per day, most people remained free of problems, despite exposure to the sun. Because of the potential for adverse effects, people taking this much niacinamide should do so only under medical supervision.

Are there any side effects or interactions?
Refer to the individual supplement for information about any side effects or interactions.

PRE- AND POST-SURGERY HEALTH

Major surgery causes serious stress to the body. The body's immune system (page 255) is weakened and gastrointestinal function is changed after major surgery, leaving the body vulnerable to infection (page 265) and in a state of nutritional insufficiency.[1] Steps can be taken using natural approaches to strengthen the body before and after surgery, enhance defenses, prevent complications, and speed recovery.

Rating	Nutritional Supplements	Herbs
★★★	**Glutamine** (page 530) Nutritional formulas supplemented with nutrients, taken after surgery	
★★☆	**Arginine** (page 467) **Fish oil** (page 514) **Iron** (page 540) (if deficient or for major surgery) Ribonucleic acid (RNA) **Taurine** (page 590) **Vitamin C** (page 604) (if deficient)	**Ginger** (page 680)
★☆☆	**Fructo-oligosaccharides** (page 522) (FOS) **Selenium** (page 584) **Vitamin A** (page 595) **Vitamin B₁** (page 597) **Vitamin B₆** (page 600) **Vitamin B₁₂** (page 601) **Vitamin E** (page 609) **Zinc** (page 614)	Curcumin (from **turmeric** [page 753])

CHECKLIST FOR PRE- AND POST-SURGERY HEALTH

Medical treatments

Over the counter nonsteroidal anti-inflammatory drugs (NSAIDs), including aspirin (Bayer, Ecotrin, Bufferin), ibuprofen (Advil, Motrin, Nuprin), and naproxen (Aleve), as well as acetaminophen (Tylenol), are commonly used for mild pain following surgery.

Prescription strength NSAIDs, including ibuprofen (Motrin), naproxen (Anaprox, Naprosyn), etodolac (Lodine), and indomethacin (Indocin), are prescribed when over the counter products are ineffective. Narcotic pain-relievers including codeine (Tylenol with Codeine) and hydrocodone (Vicodin, Lortab) are also used to treat moderate pain. Other narcotics, such as oxycodone (Oxycontin, Percocet, Percodan), hydromorphone (Dilaudid), morphine (MS Contin, Roxanol), fentanyl (Duragesic), methadone (Dolophine), and meperidine (Demerol), are usually reserved for treating severe pain. Oral corticosteroids such as prednisone (Deltasone) and methylprednisolone (Medrol) are often prescribed to reduce pain and inflammation. Antibiotics may be used after surgery to treat bacterial infections.

Other treatment includes adequate rest, nutrition, fluid intake, and proper care of the surgical wounds.

Dietary changes that may be helpful

Malnutrition, either before or after surgery, has a negative effect on recovery from surgery.[2, 3, 4, 5, 6] Malnutrition is common among the elderly and chronically ill even in developed countries, and one study found that half of older general surgery patients had moderate to severe malnutrition from protein deficiency.[7]

Being malnourished prior to surgery was associated with increased post-operative inflammation in one recent preliminary study.[8] A study of patients requiring lung surgery found that those who were better nourished prior to surgery had shorter hospital stays and required less intensive post-surgery care.[9] Dietary restriction and even fasting is often required prior to certain types of surgery. However, one study found that a four- to eight-day calorie-restricted diet lowered nutritional health and caused decreased immune system activity in pre-surgery patients, but adding a nutritional formula providing extra calories and protein reduced this negative effect of the restricted diet.[10] In another study, the clear liquid diet commonly recommended to patients before colon surgery was compared with a liquid diet providing protein, calories, and other nutrients; the patients who received extra nutrition prior to surgery had shorter hospital stays than those who received only clear liquids.[11] After reviewing animal and human studies comparing fasting and clear liquid pre-surgery diets to pre-surgery diets including liquid carbohydrate formulas, some authorities recommend a carbohydrate formula rather than fasting in preparation for surgery.[12]

Liquid diets using specially prepared nutritional formulas containing all necessary nutrients are frequently used around the time of surgery, especially in patients who cannot eat solid food. Studies have also shown that use of nutritional formulas soon after surgery has a positive effect on recovery time after cesarean section[13] and reduces rates of infection after abdominal surgeries.[14] Reviews of nutrition research on all types of surgery patients have concluded that undernourished patients will have better results if they receive supplemental nutrition before and after surgery, and that supplemental nutrition is more helpful when given orally rather than directly to the bloodstream (intravenously).[15, 16, 17]

Whether people who are not malnourished benefit from these diet supplements is unknown.

After major surgery, it is sometimes necessary to supply nourishment by a route that bypasses the digestive tract, such as intravenously, rather than by mouth. This form of nutrition is known as "parenteral," while food taken into the digestive tract is known as "enteral." While there is debate about whether parenteral nutrition is less healthful than enteral nutrition,[18] the decision to use one or the other is a complicated one, and should be discussed in individual cases with the treating physician.

Lifestyle changes that may be helpful

Smoking compromises overall health and is associated with poorer outcomes of many types of surgery.[19, 20, 21] Smoking may lessen the nausea and vomiting commonly experienced after surgery due to effects of anesthesia, according to a preliminary study,[22] but the disadvantages far outweigh this single possible benefit.

Nutritional supplements that may be helpful

Vitamin A (page 595) plays an important role in **wound healing** (page 319),[23] and one animal study suggests that vitamin A deficiency might contribute to poor recovery after surgery.[24] Vitamin A may be particularly beneficial to post-surgical patients who are using corticosteroid medications. These medications typically slow wound healing, and a number of animal studies have found that both topical and oral vitamin A reverse this effect; however, vitamin A does not change healing time in animals not given corticosteroids.[25, 26, 27] Similar results have been reported for topical vitamin A in some human cases, and these researchers suggest a topical preparation containing 200,000 IU of vitamin A per ounce for improved surgical wound healing in patients using corticosteroids after surgery.[28] Topical vitamin A may also reduce scarring in patients taking corticosteroids.[29]

Selenium (page 584) is a mineral nutrient with an important role in **immune function** (page 255) and **infection** (page 265) prevention,[30, 31, 32] and selenium deficiency has been reported in patients after intestinal surgery.[33] A controlled trial of critically ill patients, including some with recent major surgery, found that those receiving daily intravenous selenium injections for three weeks showed less biochemical signs of body stress compared with unsupplemented patients. The amount used in this trial was 500 mcg twice daily for the first week, 500 mcg once daily for the second week, and 100 mcg three times daily for the third week.[34]

Zinc (page 614) is another mineral nutrient important for proper immune system function and wound healing.[35] One study found most surgery patients recovering at home had low dietary intakes of zinc.[36] Low blood levels of zinc have been reported in patients after lung surgery.[37, 38] In one study this deficiency lasted for up to seven days after surgery and was associated with higher risk of pneumonia,[39] while another study found an association between post-operative zinc deficiency and fatigue.[40] Poor post-operative wound healing is also more common in people with zinc deficiency.[41] Zinc supplements given to patients before surgery prevented zinc deficiency in one study, but the effect of these supplements on post-surgical health was not evaluated.[42]

One preliminary study found **iron** (page 540) levels to be reduced after both minor and major surgeries, and iron supplementation prior to surgery was not able to prevent this reduction.[43] A controlled trial found that intravenous iron was more effective than oral iron for restoring normal iron levels after spinal surgery in children.[44] One animal study reported that supplementation with **fructo-oligosaccharides** (page 522) (FOS) improved the absorption of iron and prevented **anemia** (page 25) after surgery,[45] but no human trials have been done to confirm this finding. Some researchers speculate that iron deficiency after a trauma such as surgery is an important mechanism for avoiding infection, and they suggest that iron supplements should not be given after surgery.[46]

Patients who have undergone major surgery frequently need blood transfusions to replace blood lost during the procedure. Studies have found that 18 to 21% of surgery patients were anemic prior to surgery,[47, 48] and these anemic patients required more blood after surgery than did non-anemic surgery patients. Supplementation with iron prior to surgery was found in a controlled trial to reduce the need for blood transfusions, whether or not iron deficiency was present.[49] **Iron** (page 540) supplements (99 mg per day) given before and for two months after joint surgery in another controlled trial improved blood values but did not change the length of hospitalization or the risk of post-operative fever.[50] Pre-operative iron supplementation in combination with a medication that stimulates red blood cell production in the bone marrow is considered by some doctors to be an effective way to minimize the need for post-operative blood transfusions.[51]

Vitamin C (page 604) deficiency can be detrimental to **immune function** (page 255) in hospitalized patients,[52] and one study found that half of surgery patients recovering at home had low dietary intakes of vitamin C.[53] Vitamin C is also a critical nutrient for **wound healing** (page 319),[54, 55] but studies of vitamin C supplementation have shown only minor effects on the healing of surgical wounds.[56, 57] Vitamin C deficiency also can increase the risk of excessive bleeding in the surgical setting.[58]

Some studies of surgery patients,[59, 60] though not all,[61] have found that blood levels of **vitamin E** (page 609) decrease during and after surgery. Animal research suggests that vitamin E may prevent skin scarring when used topically after surgery,[62] but a human study reported disappointing results.[63] Vitamin E taken by mouth may interfere with blood clotting[64]; therefore, use of vitamin E before surgery should be discussed with the surgeon. No research on either the usefulness or hazards of vitamin E supplementation around surgery has been done.

Vitamin B$_1$ (page 597), given as intramuscular injections of 120 mg daily for several days before surgery, resulted in less reduction of immune system activity after surgery in a preliminary trial.[65] In a controlled trial, an oral B vitamin combination providing 100 mg of B$_1$, 200 mg of **vitamin B$_6$** (page 600), and 200 mcg of **vitamin B$_{12}$** (page 601) daily given for five weeks before surgery and for two weeks following surgery also prevented post-surgical reductions in immune activity.[66] However, no research has explored any other benefits of B vitamin supplementation in surgery patients.

Glutamine (page 530), one of the most abundant **amino acids** (page 465) in the body, supports the health of the cells lining the gastrointestinal tract and is important for immune function.[67] Glutamine is depleted when the body is under stress, including the stress of surgery.[68] Blood levels of glutamine decrease following surgery, and as they return to normal, their increase parallels the increase in immune cells.[69] Two controlled trials have shown that the use of glutamine-enriched intravenous formulas, providing approximately 20 grams of glutamine per day, resulted in increased immune cell activity and shorter hospital stays.[70, 71] Double-blind studies report that patients receiving intravenous formulas supplemented with glutamine after surgery had better nutritional status and better health outcomes, including fewer infections and other complications, compared with patients receiving regular formulas.[72, 73]

The amino acid **arginine** (page 467) has a role in immune function, **infection** (page 265) prevention, and tissue repair after injury, including surgery.[74] Animal research suggests that supplemental arginine may improve the outcomes in cardiovascular[75] and colon surgeries.[76] Other animal studies suggest a possible role for arginine in prevention of adhesions, a painful type of internal scarring that can occur with surgery.[77] Human trials of formulas including arginine are discussed below, but the benefits of supplemental arginine alone have not been studied in surgery patients.

Taurine (page 590) is an amino acid abundantly present in the body that also appears to have an important role in immune cell functions.[78] A preliminary trial found that patients receiving an oral formula enriched with taurine (1 gram per liter) beginning two days before surgery and continuing until five days after surgery had less inflammation after surgery compared with those receiving a standard formula.[79]

Omega-3 fatty acids (page 509) have anti-inflammatory properties,[80] and animal studies suggest that supplementation with omega-3 fatty acids may improve recovery and prevent infection after surgery.[81, 82] A controlled human trial found that intravenous nutritional formulas containing omega-3 fatty acids given postoperatively lowered the production of inflammatory chemicals compared with standard nutritional formulas.[83] Other human studies of omega-3 fatty acid-supplemented nutritional formulas used in surgery patients have included other supplemental nutrients as well and are discussed below.[84]

Ribonucleic acid (RNA) is a member of the nucleotide family of biomolecules and supports protein synthesis and cell growth. During times of physical stress, RNA helps stimulate immune cell division and activity,[85, 86] and is needed in greater amounts. Animal studies show that nucleotides given in the diet support the immune response and decrease death rates in infected animals.[87, 88, 89] In human infants, those fed nucleotide-enriched formulas have healthier gastrointestinal systems and better immune function than do those fed ordinary formulas.[90, 91, 92] RNA is included in some oral and intravenous nutritional formulas used for surgery patients, and these formulas are discussed below.

Research on post-surgical recovery has explored the usefulness of liquid nutritional formulas supplemented with several nutrients believed to improve immune function and to speed the healing process. The most common of these supplemental nutrients are certain amino acids, essential fatty acids, and nucleotides.[93] Several controlled trials, some of which were double-blind, showed that giving an oral formula containing **arginine** (page 467), RNA, and omega-3 fatty acids

from **fish oil** (page 514) either after surgery[94, 95] or before and after surgery[96, 97, 98, 99] resulted in decreased inflammation, less reduction of immune cell function, fewer complications of surgery, and shorter hospital stays. The formula most commonly used in these studies contains 12.5 grams of arginine, 3.3 grams of omega-3 fatty acids, and 1.2 grams of RNA per liter, as well as additional **iron** (page 540), **zinc** (page 614), **selenium** (page 584), **copper** (page 499), and **vitamin C** (page 604). Typically, 1 to 1.5 liters per day was consumed by the surgery patients. One controlled trial, however, found that this enriched formula was no better than a standard formula when they were given only before surgery.[100] An analysis of 12 studies comparing traditional formulas with immune-enhancing formulas concluded that surgery patients receiving the supplemented formulas had the same risk of death, but that they had fewer infections and shorter hospital stays.[101]

Are there any side effects or interactions?
Refer to the individual supplement for information about any side effects or interactions.

Herbs that may be helpful
A recent study found that 24% of surgery patients had taken herbal supplements before their surgeries, and 50 different herbs had been used among these patients.[102] Little research exists, however, on the safety or efficacy of herbs before surgery. Some researchers and healthcare providers are concerned about possible harmful interactions between herbs and medications used around or during surgery, or the possibility that some herbs may increase bleeding during and after surgery.[103, 104] The use of herbs around the time of surgery should be discussed with a knowledgeable healthcare practitioner.

Nausea and vomiting can be experienced post-operatively as a result of anesthesia. **Ginger** (page 680) (*Zingiber officinale*) has antinausea properties and has been examined for its ability to prevent post-operative nausea and vomiting in several controlled trials. In two of these controlled trials, ginger was found more effective than placebo and equal to an antinausea medication;[105, 106] however, in two other controlled trials ginger was not found to have any benefit.[107, 108] A review considering the results of these trials concluded that 1 gram of ginger taken before surgery prevents nausea and vomiting slightly better than placebo, but this difference is not significant.[109]

Turmeric (page 753) (*Curcuma longa*) is an herb with anti-inflammatory effects.[110] One trial found curcumin (from turmeric) at 400 mg three times daily was more effective than either placebo or anti-inflammatory medication for relieving post-surgical inflammation. However, as the different treatment groups had different degrees of inflammation at the start of the study, firm conclusions cannot be drawn from this study.[111]

Are there any side effects or interactions?
Refer to the individual herb for information about any side effects or interactions.

Holistic approaches that may be helpful
Acupressure can be used to prevent nausea and vomiting. Wristbands designed to apply pressure to acupuncture points on the forearm were shown to effectively prevent post-operative nausea and vomiting in seven controlled trials[112, 113, 114, 115, 116, 117] and were as effective as an antinausea medication in another.[118] One controlled trial found no benefit from acupressure wristbands.[119] Acupuncture[120] and transcutaneous electrical nerve stimulation (TENS) of a wrist acupuncture point[121] have also been shown to be effective for post-operative nausea and vomiting in controlled trials. A controlled comparison study found that electro-acupuncture of the wrist points controlled post-operative nausea and vomiting as well as antinausea medication and better than TENS, but both electro-acupuncture and TENS helped more than no treatment.[122] A comprehensive review of research on acupuncture, electroacupuncture, TENS, acupoint stimulation, and acupressure for post-operative nausea and vomiting found these techniques to be more effective than placebo and as effective as commonly prescribed medications in adults but not in children.[123] However, laser stimulation of the acupuncture points on the wrists both before and after surgery was effective for children in one controlled trial.[124]

PREECLAMPSIA

See also: Gestational Hypertension (page 202) (Nonproteinuric)

Preeclampsia is defined as the combination of high blood pressure (**hypertension** [page 246]), swelling (**edema** [page 180]), and protein in the urine (albuminuria, proteinuria) developing after the 20th week of **pregnancy** (page 363).[1] Preeclampsia ranges in severity from mild to severe; the mild form is sometimes called proteinuric pregnancy-induced hypertension[2] or proteinuric gestational hypertension.[3]

Women with even mild preeclampsia must be monitored carefully by a healthcare professional. Hospitalization may be necessary to enable close observation.[4]

The cause of preeclampsia is unknown, although several factors have been shown to contribute.[5, 6] Preeclampsia is more common in women during their first pregnancy,[7] as well as in women who are **obese** (page 446),[8, 9] who have diabetes,[10] or who have **gestational hypertension** (page 202).[11, 12, 13] Women who have had preeclampsia during a previous pregnancy are also at increased risk.[14] Preeclampsia has also been associated with **calcium** (page 483) deficiencies,[15] **antioxidant** (page 467) deficiencies,[16, 17, 18] older maternal age,[19] and job stress.[20, 21, 22]

CHECKLIST FOR PREECLAMPSIA		
Rating	Nutritional Supplements	Herbs
★★★	**Calcium** (page 483) (for high-risk only)	
★★☆	**Folic acid** (page 524) **Vitamin C** (page 604) and **Vitamin E** (page 609) (in combination; for high-risk only)	**Lycopene** (page 548)
★☆☆	**Fish oil** (page 514) **Magnesium** (page 551) **Vitamin B$_2$** (page 598) **Vitamin B$_6$** (page 600) **Vitamin B$_{12}$** (page 601) **Zinc** (page 614)	

What are the symptoms of preeclampsia?
Symptoms, which typically appear after the 20th week of **pregnancy** (page 363), include swelling of the face and hands, visual disturbances, headache, and **high blood pressure** (page 246). In severe preeclampsia, symptoms are more pronounced. Jaundice may also be present. Severe preeclampsia may lead to seizures (eclampsia) and may cause death to both mother and fetus if left untreated.[23] Like eclampsia, severe preeclampsia is a medical emergency requiring hospitalization.[24, 25]

Medical treatments
Prescription medications to reduce high blood pressure (hypertension) may be used. The category of prescription drugs known as diuretics are commonly used to treat hypertension. Agents often used include the thiazide diuretics, such as hydrochlorothiazide (HydroDIURIL), indapamide (Lozol), and metolazone (Zaroxolyn); loop diuretics including furosemide (Lasix), bumetanide

(Bumex), and torsemide (Demadex); and potassium-sparing diuretics, such as spironolactone (Aldactone), triamterene (Dyazide, Maxzide), and amiloride (Midamor). Diuretics are usually combined with beta-blockers, such as propranolol (Inderal), metoprolol (Lopressor, Toprol XL), atenolol (Tenormin), and bisoprolol (Zebeta), or ACE inhibitors, including captopril (Capoten), benazepril (Lotensin), lisinopril (Zestril, Prinivil), enalapril (Vasotec), and quinapril (Accupril). The Angiotensin II receptor antagonists, such as losartan (Cozaar), valsartan (Diovan), irbesartan (Avapro), candesartan (Atacand), and telmisartan (Micardis), are commonly used either alone or in combination with other agents. Calcium channel blockers, such as amlodipine (Norvasc), verapamil (Calan SR, Verelan PM), and diltiazem (Cardizem CD), may also be used either alone or in combination with other drugs to treat **high blood pressure** (page 246). Another group of commonly used antihypertensive drugs, sympatholytic agents, includes prazosin (Minipress), doxazosin (Cardura), terazosin (Hytrin), and methyldopa (Aldomet).

Other treatment for preeclampsia includes strict bed rest, maintenance of normal salt intake, intravenous **magnesium** (page 551) sulfate, and possibly hospitalization for observation. The definitive conventional treatment of preeclampsia is induced delivery or cesarean section.

Dietary changes that may be helpful

Unlike other conditions that cause **high blood pressure** (page 246), salt restriction and use of diuretics can worsen preeclampsia by reducing blood flow to the kidneys and placenta.[26] In preeclampsia, unrestricted use of salt and an increased consumption of water are needed to maintain normal blood volume and circulation to the placenta.[27]

Data from one preliminary study suggest diets high in trans fatty acids are associated with an increased risk of preeclampsia.[28] Trans fatty acids are found in foods that contain partially hydrogenated vegetable oils, such as margarine. Foods that have been deep-fried (e.g., French fries) are also rich sources of trans fatty acids.

Lifestyle changes that may be helpful

Regular prenatal care is essential for the prevention and early detection of preeclampsia.

Job stress (lack of control over work pace and the timing and frequency of breaks) may be detrimental, and reducing job stress may be beneficial in the prevention of preeclampsia.[29] In a preliminary study, women exposed to high job stress were found to be at greater risk of developing preeclampsia and, to a lesser extent, **gestational hypertension** (page 202) than were women exposed to low job stress. In this study, evaluation of job stress was based on scores assessing on-the-job psychological demand and decision-making latitude. High stress was defined as high psychological demand with low decision latitude, and low stress was defined as low-demand, high-latitude.[30]

For women with preeclampsia, obstetricians and midwives often recommend bed rest and lying on the left side; this position helps reduce **edema** (page 180) and lower **blood pressure** (page 246) by increasing urinary output.[31] However, a review of clinical trials concluded that bed rest can significantly *worsen* pregnancy-induced hypertension.[32] Women with preeclampsia should discuss the pros and cons of bed rest with their doctors.

Nutritional supplements that may be helpful

Calcium (page 483) deficiency has been associated with preeclampsia.[33] In numerous controlled trials, oral calcium supplementation has been studied as a possible preventive measure.[34, 35, 36, 37] While most trials have found a significant reduction in the incidence of preeclampsia with calcium supplementation,[38, 39, 40, 41, 42, 43] some have reported no change.[44]

An analysis of double-blind trials[45] found calcium supplementation to be highly effective in preventing preeclampsia. However, a large and well-designed double-blind trial[46] and a critical analysis[47] of six double-blind trials[48, 49, 50, 51, 52, 53] concluded that calcium supplementation did *not* reduce the risk of preeclampsia in healthy women at low risk for preeclampsia. For healthy, *high-risk* (i.e., calcium deficient) women, however, the data show a clear and statistically significant beneficial effect of calcium supplementation in reducing the risk of preeclampsia.[54, 55, 56]

The National Institutes of Health recommends an intake of 1,200 to 1,500 mg of elemental **calcium** (page 483) daily during normal **pregnancy** (page 363).[57] In women at risk of preeclampsia, most trials showing reduced incidence have used 2,000 mg of supplemental calcium per day.[58] Nonetheless, many doctors continue to suggest amounts no higher than 1,500 mg per day.

Women with preeclampsia have been shown to have elevated blood levels of **homocysteine** (page 234).[59, 60, 61, 62] Research indicates elevated homocysteine occurs prior to the onset of preeclampsia.[63] Elevated homocysteine damages the lining of blood vessels,[64, 65, 66, 67, 68, 69, 70] which can lead to the preeclamptic signs of **elevated blood pressure** (page 246), swelling, and protein in the urine.[71]

In one preliminary trial, women with a previous pregnancy complicated by preeclampsia and high homocysteine supplemented with 5 mg of **folic acid** (page 520) and 250 mg of **vitamin B$_6$** (page 600) per day, successfully lowering homocysteine levels.[72] In another trial studying the effect of vitamin B$_6$ on preeclampsia incidence, supplementation with 5 mg of vitamin B$_6$ twice per day significantly reduced the incidence of preeclampsia. Women in that study were not, however, evaluated for homocysteine levels.[73] In fact, no studies have yet determined whether lowering elevated homocysteine reduces the incidence or severity of preeclampsia. Nevertheless, despite a lack of proof that elevated homocysteine levels cause preeclampsia, many doctors believe that pregnant women with elevated homocysteine should attempt to reduce those levels to normal.

Lycopene (page 548) is a carotenoid found in tomatoes, watermelon, and several other foods. The concentration of lycopene in the blood has been found to be significantly lower in women with preeclampsia than in healthy pregnant women. In a double-blind trial, supplementation of pregnant women with lycopene significantly reduced the incidence of preeclampsia by 51.4%, compared with a placebo.[74] The amount of lycopene used was 2 mg twice a day; treatment was begun between the sixteenth and twentieth week of pregnancy and was continued until delivery.

A marginal **zinc** (page 614) deficiency has been reported in some women with preeclampsia.[75, 76] The common practice of prescribing **iron** (page 540) and folic acid supplements to pregnant women can lead to reduced zinc absorption.[77] Trials studying the relationship between zinc supplementation and preeclampsia incidence have produced conflicting results. In one double-blind trial, the incidence of preeclampsia was significantly lower in women receiving a **multivitamin-mineral** (page 559) supplement, which provided 20 mg of zinc per day, than in women who received the same supplement without zinc.[78] However, in another double-blind trial, a *higher* incidence of preeclampsia was reported in pregnant women given 20 mg of zinc per day than was reported in women given a placebo.[79] In yet another trial, zinc supplementation failed to prevent preeclampsia.[80] Therefore, current evidence does not sufficiently support the use of zinc as a way to protect against preeclampsia.

Fish oil (page 514) supplementation has been proposed to lower the incidence of preeclampsia.[81, 82] However, controlled clinical trials suggest that fish oil does not reduce symptoms[83] or protect against preeclampsia.[84, 85]

Women with preeclampsia have been found to be depleted in **antioxidants** (page 467).[86, 87] Some[88, 89] but not all studies[90] have reported deficiencies in **vitamin C** (page 604), **vitamin E** (page 609), and **beta-carotene** (page 469) in preeclampsia patients. In a double-blind trial, supplementation of vitamin C (one gram per day) and vitamin E (400 IU per day) reduced the incidence of preeclampsia by 76% in women at high risk.[91] However, for those already suffering from this condition, supplementation with these same vitamins has led to only insignificant effects.[92]

Magnesium (page 551) deficiency has been implicated as a possible cause of preeclampsia.[93, 94, 95, 96, 97] Magnesium supplementation has been shown to reduce the incidence of preeclampsia in high-risk women in one trial,[98] but not in another double-blind trial.[99]

Women who are deficient in **vitamin B$_2$** (page 598) (riboflavin) are more likely to develop preeclampsia than women with normal vitamin B$_2$ levels.[100] These results were observed in a developing country, where vitamin B$_2$ deficiencies are more common than in the United States. Nevertheless, insufficient vitamin B$_2$ may contribute to the abnormalities underlying the disease process.

Are there any side effects or interactions?
Refer to the individual supplement for information about any side effects or interactions.

PREGNANCY AND POSTPARTUM SUPPORT

See also: Birth Defects Prevention (page 63), **Breast-feeding Support** (page 74)

What do I need to know?
Self-care for pregnancy can be approached in a number of ways—but it can be hard to know just where to start. To make it easier, our doctors recommend trying these simple steps first:

Eat well
   A well-balanced and varied diet that includes fresh fruits and vegetables, whole grains, legumes, and fish will provide the nutrients you and your baby need

Avoid harmful habits
   Give up alcohol, caffeine, smoking, and recreational drugs to reduce the risk of birth defects and pregnancy complications

Gain the right amount of weight
> Follow the advice of your healthcare provider to prevent problems associated with inadequate or excessive weight gain

Prenatal supplement
> Starting *before* you become pregnant, if possible, take a multivitamin-mineral supplement high in folic acid, iron, and calcium to prevent complications due to vitamin or mineral deficiencies

About pregnancy and postpartum support

Pregnancy, the period during which a woman's fertilized egg (embryo) gestates and becomes a fetus, lasts an average of 40 weeks from the date of the last menstrual period to delivery of the infant.

In the first trimester (13 weeks), many pregnant women experience nausea. Usually these women report that they feel best during the second trimester. During the third (final) trimester, the increasing size of the fetus begins to place mechanical strains on the expectant mother, often causing **back pain** (page 293), leg swelling, and other health problems.

CHECKLIST FOR PREGNANCY AND POSTPARTUM SUPPORT

Rating	Nutritional Supplements	Herbs
★★★	**Folic acid** (page 520)	
★★☆	**Biotin** (page 473) **Fish oil** (page 514) (to prevent premature delivery) **Iron** (page 540) (with medical supervision) **S-adenosylmethionine** (page 583) (SAMe) (for cholestasis only) **Vitamin B$_6$** (page 600) (if homocysteine levels are elevated) **Zinc** (page 614)	**Lavender** (page 701) (in bath, for perineal pain after childbirth)
★☆☆	**Calcium** (page 483)	**Dandelion** (page 666) (leaves and root) Goat's rue **Nettle** (page 714) **Red raspberry** (page 735) **Sage** (page 740) **Vitex** (page 757)

Medical treatments

Over the counter dimenhydrinate (Dramamine) may be used when nausea is severe enough to require medication.

With some health problems that develop during pregnancy (e.g., **preeclampsia** [page 361], eclampsia), bed rest, restriction of salt intake, and medication to lower blood pressure may be recommended. Women who are pregnant are advised to avoid caffeine, alcohol, nicotine, and other drugs (including over the counter medicines) that have not been prescribed by their doctor.

Dietary changes that may be helpful

Nearly all pregnant women can benefit from good nutritional habits prior to and during pregnancy. The increased number of **birth defects** (page 63) during times of famine attest to the adverse effects of poor nutrition during pregnancy.[1] For example, in a dietary survey of pregnant women, higher dietary intake of **niacin** (page 598) (a form of vitamin B$_3$) during the first trimester was correlated with higher birth weights, longer length, and larger head circumference (all signs of healthier infants).[2]

Women who consume a standard Western diet (high in fat and sugar and low in complex carbohydrates) during pregnancy and **breast-feeding** (page 74) may not be obtaining adequate amounts of essential vitamins and minerals; this can result in health problems for the newborn.[3] Pregnant women should choose a well-balanced and varied diet that includes fresh fruits and vegetables, whole grains, legumes, and fish. Refined sugars, white flour, fried foods, processed foods, and chemical additives should be avoided.

Consumption of moderate to large amounts of caffeine while pregnant has been associated with an increased risk of miscarriage.[4, 5, 6, 7] Although some studies suggest that only very large amounts of caffeine increase the risk of miscarriage,[8] an analysis of clinical trials found that women who consumed more than 150 mg of caffeine (roughly one to two cups of coffee) per day while pregnant had an increased risk of miscarriage or delivering a baby with a low birth weight.[9] The FDA has advised women to avoid drinking coffee and consuming other caffeine-containing foods and beverages during pregnancy.[10]

Lifestyle changes that may be helpful

A woman can reduce her risk of complications during pregnancy and delivery by avoiding harmful substances, such as alcohol, caffeine, nicotine, recreational drugs, and some prescription or over-the-counter drugs.

Even minimal alcohol consumption during pregnancy can increase the risk of **hyperactivity** (page 55), short attention span, and emotional problems in the child.[11] Pregnant women should, therefore, avoid alcohol completely.

Cigarette smoking during pregnancy causes lower birth weights and smaller-sized newborns. The rate of miscarriage in smokers is twice as high as that in non-smokers,[12] and babies born to mothers who smoke have more than twice the risk of dying from sudden infant death syndrome (SIDS).[13]

Weight Gain in Pregnancy
No single maternal weight gain target meets the needs of all women. The amount of weight a woman optimally gains varies with her height, age, plans to breast feed, and whether she is delivering twins. However, a few basic guidelines are generally accepted:[14] Women who enter pregnancy at more than 120% of standard weight still have an obligatory weight gain of 15–25 pounds at a rate of about 0.7 pounds per week. Women who are at ideal body weight and are *not* going to nurse have a target of gaining about 22 pounds overall at a rate of 0.8 pounds per week. Women who enter pregnancy between 90% and 110% of ideal body weight and plan to nurse have a target weight gain of 25–35 pounds overall at a rate of 0.9 pounds per week during the second and third trimesters. Physically immature adolescents and women less than 90% of ideal body weight have a target weight gain of 32 (28–40) pounds at a rate of 1.1 pounds per week. Women who know they are going to have twins have a target weight gain of 40 (35–45) pounds with a weekly rate of 1.4 pounds during the last 20 weeks of pregnancy.

Another way to determine the appropriate weight gain for pregnancy is by using the Body Mass Index (BMI). The BMI is calculated by dividing your body weight (in kilograms) by the square of your height (in meters). (A kilogram is equal to 2.2 pounds; a meter is equal to about 39 inches.) According to the standard set in 1990 by the Institute of Medicine (IOM) of the National Academy of Sciences,[15] a woman with a low BMI (less than 19.8) should gain a total of 12.5–18 kg (27.5–39.7 pounds) during pregnancy; a woman with a normal BMI (19.8–26) should gain a total of 11.5–16 kg (25.4–35.3 pounds) during pregnancy; a woman with a high BMI (greater than 26.0–29.0) should gain a total of 7–11.5 kg (15.4–25.4 pounds) during preg-

nancy. Adolescents and black women should strive for gains at the upper end of the recommended range. Short women (less than five feet) should strive for gains at the lower end of this range. Obese women (BMI greater than 29) have a separate recommended target weight gain of about 6 kg (13.2 pounds). Published studies suggest that only 30–40% of American women actually have weight gains within the IOM's recommended ranges.[16, 17, 18]

Although the IOM's national recommendations concerning pregnancy weight gain have been widely adopted, they have not been universally accepted.[19] The amount of weight gain during pregnancy varies considerably among women with good pregnancy outcomes.[20, 21] For that reason, weight gain alone is not likely to be a perfect screening tool for pregnancy complications. Nevertheless, weight gains outside the IOM's recommended ranges are associated with twice as many poor pregnancy outcomes than are weight gains within the ranges. A systematic review of all studies published between 1990 and 1997 that specifically examined fetal and maternal outcomes showed that weight gain within the IOM's recommended ranges is associated with the best outcome for both mothers and infants.[22]

Weight-loss (page 446) programs are not generally recommended during pregnancy. Nevertheless, it should be noted that being overweight while pregnant increases the incidence of various conditions in both the mother and the fetus, such as gestational diabetes and **blood pressure problems** (page 246). The risk is proportional to the amount of excess weight. Overweight women have a higher risk of cesarean deliveries and a higher incidence of anesthetic and post-operative complications in these deliveries. Poor responsiveness in the newborn, large head, and some birth defects are more frequent in infants of obese mothers. Maternal obesity increases the risk of newborn death. The average cost of hospital prenatal and postnatal care is higher for overweight mothers than for normal-weight mothers. Infants of overweight mothers require admission into intensive care units more often than do infants of normal-weight mothers.[23]

Some women will be concerned that the IOM's recommended weight gain will result in too much weight gain or more weight retention after the baby is born, but there is no evidence to support this concern. Although there are risks associated with being overweight during pregnancy, dieting during pregnancy can seriously endanger the health of the fetus. A low rate of pregnancy weight gain has been shown, in most studies, to increase the risk of premature delivery.[24] There is no evidence that restricting normal weight gain in pregnancy is either safe or beneficial.[25]

Nutritional supplements that may be helpful

Most doctors, many other healthcare professionals, and the March of Dimes recommend that *all women of childbearing age* supplement with 400 mcg per day of **folic acid** (page 520). Such supplementation could protect against the formation of neural tube defects (such as spina bifida) during the time between conception and when pregnancy is discovered.

The requirement for the B vitamin folic acid doubles during pregnancy, to 800 mcg per day from all sources.[26] Deficiencies of folic acid during pregnancy have been linked to low birth weight[27] and to an increased incidence of neural tube defects (e.g., spina bifida) in infants. In one study, women who were at high risk of giving birth to babies with neural tube defects were able to lower their risk by 72% by taking folic acid supplements prior to and during pregnancy.[28] Several preliminary studies have shown that a deficiency of folate in the blood may increase the risk of stunted growth of the fetus.[29, 30, 31, 32, 33, 34, 35, 36] This does not prove, however, that folic acid supplementation results in higher birth weights. Although some trials have found that folic acid and **iron** (page 540), when taken together, have improved birth weights,[37, 38, 39, 40] other trials have found supplementation with these nutrients to be ineffective.[41, 42, 43]

The relationship between folate status and the risk of miscarriage is also somewhat unclear. In some studies, women who have had habitual miscarriages were found to have elevated levels of **homocysteine** (page 234) (a marker of folate deficiency).[44, 45, 46, 47] In a preliminary study, 22 women with recurrent miscarriages who had elevated levels of homocysteine were treated with 15 mg per day of **folic acid** (page 520) and 750 mg per day of **vitamin B₆** (page 600), prior to and throughout their next pregnancy. This treatment reduced homocysteine levels to normal and was associated with 20 successful pregnancies.[48] It is not known whether supplementing with these vitamins would help prevent miscarriages in women with normal homocysteine levels. As the amounts of folic acid and vitamin B₆ used in this study were extremely large and potentially toxic, this treatment should be used only with the supervision of a doctor.

In other studies, however, folate levels did not correlate with the incidence of habitual miscarriages.[49, 50, 51]

Preliminary[52] and double-blind[53] evidence has shown that women who use a **multivitamin-mineral** (page 559) formula containing folic acid beginning three months before becoming pregnant and continuing through the first three months of pregnancy have a significantly lower risk of having babies with neural tube defects (e.g., spina bifida) and other congenital defects.

In addition to achieving significant protection against birth defects, women who take **folic acid** (page 520) supplements during pregnancy have been reported to have fewer infections, and to give birth to babies with higher birth weights and better Apgar scores.[54] (An Apgar score is an evaluation of the well-being of a newborn, based on his or her color, crying, muscle tone, and other signs.) However, if a woman waits until after discovering her pregnancy to begin taking folic acid supplements, it will probably be too late to prevent a neural tube defect.

Biotin (page 473) deficiency may occur in as many as 50% of pregnant women.[55] As biotin deficiency in pregnant animals results in birth defects, it seems reasonable to use a prenatal multiple vitamin and mineral formula that contains biotin.

In a preliminary study, pregnant women who used a **zinc** (page 614)-containing nutritional supplement in the three months before and after conception had a 36% decreased chance of having a baby with a neural tube defect, and women who had the highest dietary zinc intake (but took no vitamin supplement) had a 30% decreased risk.[56]

Iron (page 540) requirements increase during pregnancy, making iron deficiency in pregnancy quite common.[57] Iron supplement use in the United States is estimated at 85% during pregnancy, with most women taking supplements three or more times per week for three months.[58] Pregnant women with a documented iron deficiency need doctor-supervised treatment. In one study, 65% of women who were not given extra iron developed **iron deficiency** (page 278) during pregnancy, compared with none who received an iron supplement.[59] However, there is a clear increase in reported side effects with increasing supplement amounts of iron, especially iron sulfate.[60, 61] Supplementation with large amounts of iron has also been shown to reduce blood levels of zinc.[62] Although the significance of that finding is not clear, low blood levels of **zinc** (page 614) have been associated with an increased risk of complications in both the mother and fetus.[63]

Iron supplementation was associated in one study with an increased incidence of birth defects,[64] possibly as a result of an iron-induced deficiency of zinc. Although additional research needs to be done, the evidence suggests that women who are supplementing with iron during pregnancy should also take a **multivitamin-mineral** (page 559) formula that contains adequate amounts of zinc. To be on the safe side, pregnant women should discuss their supplement program with a doctor.

Supplementation with **fish oil** (page 514) (providing either 2.7 g or 6.1 g per day of the omega-3 fatty acids EPA and **DHA** [page 509]) significantly reduced recurrence of premature delivery, according to data culled from six clinical trials involving women with a high risk for such complications.[65] Fish oil supplementation did not prevent premature delivery of twin pregnancies, nor did it have any preventive effect against intrauterine growth retardation or pregnancy-induced hypertension. Fish oils should be free of contaminants, such as mercury and organochlorine pesticides. Women who eat substantial amounts of certain types of seafood (e.g., swordfish, tuna) may be consuming contaminants that can increase the risk of brain and nervous system abnormalities in their offspring. Exposure to mercury and polychlorinated biphenyls (PCBs) was found to be increased in relation to maternal intake of seafood. Higher exposure to these toxic contaminants has been linked to an increased risk of deficits in the developing brains and nervous systems of the children.[66]

S-adenosylmethionine (**SAMe** [page 583]) supplementation has been shown to aid in the resolution of blocked bile flow (cholestasis), an occasional complication of pregnancy.[67, 68]

Calcium (page 483) needs double during pregnancy.[69] Low dietary intake of this mineral is associated with increased risk of **preeclampsia** (page 361), a potentially dangerous (but preventable) condition characterized by high blood pressure and swelling. Supplementation with calcium may reduce the risk of pre-term delivery, which is often associated with preeclampsia. Calcium may reduce the risk of **pregnancy-induced hypertension** (page 202),[70] though these effects are more likely to occur in women who are calcium deficient.[71, 72] Supplementation with up to 2 grams of calcium per day by pregnant women with low dietary calcium intake has been shown to improve the bone strength of the fetuses.[73]

Pregnant women should consume 1,500 mg of **calcium** (page 483) per day from all sources—food plus supplements. Food sources of calcium include dairy products, dark green leafy vegetables, tofu, sardines (canned with edible bones), salmon (canned with edible bones), peas, and beans.

Are there any side effects or interactions?
Refer to the individual supplement for information about any side effects or interactions.

Herbs that may be helpful
Many tonic herbs, which are believed to strengthen or invigorate organ systems or the entire body, can be taken safely every day during pregnancy. Examples include **dandelion** (page 666) leaf and root, **red raspberry** (page 735) leaf, and **nettle** (page 714). Dandelion leaf and root are rich sources of vitamins and minerals, including **beta-carotene** (page 469), **calcium** (page 483), **potassium** (page 572), and **iron** (page 540). Dandelion leaf is mildly diuretic (promotes urine flow); it also stimulates bile flow and helps with the common digestive complaints of pregnancy. Dandelion root is traditionally used to strengthen and invigorate the liver.[74]

Red raspberry leaf is the most frequently mentioned, traditional herbal tonic for general support of pregnancy and **breast-feeding** (page 74). Rich in vitamins and minerals (especially iron), it is traditionally used to strengthen and invigorate the uterus, increase milk flow, and restore the mother's system after childbirth.[75]

Nettle leaf is rich in the minerals calcium and iron, is mildly diuretic, and is diuretic. Nettle leaf is rich in the minerals calcium and iron, is and mildly diuretic. Nettle enriches and increases the flow of breast milk and restores the mother's energy following childbirth.[76]

In one study, the addition of **lavender** (page 701) oil to a bath was more effective than a placebo in relieving perineal pain after childbirth (the perineum is the area between the vulva and the anus.)[77] The improvement was not statistically significant, however, so more research is needed to determine whether lavender oil is truly effective.

Numerous herbs, known as galactagogues, are used in traditional herbal medicine systems around the world to promote production of breast milk.[78] These are known as galactagogues. **Vitex** (page 757) is one of the best recognized herbs in Europe for promoting lactation. An older German clinical trial found that 15 drops of a vitex tincture three times per day could increase the amount of milk produced by mothers with or without pregnancy complications, as compared with mothers given **vitamin B₁** (page 597) or nothing.[79] However, *vitex should not be taken during pregnancy.*

Goat's rue *(Galega officinalis)* has a history of use in Europe for supporting breast-feeding. Taking 1 teaspoon of goat's rue tincture per day is considered by some European practitioners to be helpful in increasing milk volume.[80] Studies to support the use of goat's rue as a galactagogue are lacking.

Sage (page 740) has traditionally been used to dry up milk production when a woman no longer wishes to breast-feed.[81] It should not be taken during pregnancy.

Are there any side effects or interactions?
Refer to the individual herb for information about any side effects or interactions.

Holistic approaches that may be helpful

In one preliminary study, acupuncture relieved pain and diminished disability in the low back during pregnancy better than physiotherapy.[82]

A controlled trial found that acupuncture significantly reduced symptoms in women with hyperemesis gravidarum, a severe form of nausea and vomiting of pregnancy that usually requires hospitalization.[83] Treatment consisted of acupuncture at a single point on the forearm three times daily for two consecutive days. Acupressure (in which pressure, rather than needles, is used to stimulate acupuncture points) has also been found in several preliminary trials to be mildly effective in the treatment of nausea and vomiting of pregnancy.[84, 85, 86]

PREMENSTRUAL SYNDROME

Premenstrual syndrome (PMS) is a poorly understood complex of symptoms occurring a week to ten days before the start of each menstrual cycle.

PMS is believed to be triggered by changes in progesterone and estrogen levels.

CHECKLIST FOR PREMENSTRUAL SYNDROME (PMS)

Rating	Nutritional Supplements	Herbs
★★★	**Calcium** (page 483) **Vitamin B₆** (page 600)	**Vitex** (page 757)
★★☆	**Evening primrose oil** (page 511) **Magnesium** (page 551) **Multiple vitamin-mineral** (page 559) **Potassium gluconate** (page 572) **Vitamin E** (page 609)	
★☆☆	**Fiber** (page 512) **Progesterone** (page 577) **Vitamin A** (page 595) (see dosage warnings) **Vitamin B-complex** (page 603)	**Black cohosh** (page 637) **Dong quai** (page 668) *Ginkgo biloba* (page 681) **Peony** (page 724) **Yarrow** (page 763)

What are the symptoms of PMS?

Many **premenopausal** (page 311) women suffer from symptoms of PMS at different points in their menstrual cycle. Symptoms include cramping, bloating, mood changes, and breast tenderness tied to the menstrual cycle.

Medical treatments

Over the counter pain medications, such as ibuprofen (Motrin, Advil), naproxen (Aleve), aspirin (Bayer, Ecotrin, Bufferin), and acetaminophen (Tylenol), may provide relief from premenstrual pain.

Prescription drug treatment is directed primarily at relieving symptoms. Commonly prescribed drugs include birth control pills (Ortho-Novum, Loestrin, Mircette, Triphasil); pain relievers, such as ibuprofen (Motrin) and naproxen (Anaprox, Naprosyn); diuretics, such as hydrochlorothiazide (HydroDIURIL); antidepressants, such as fluoxetine (Prozac); and anti-anxiety drugs, such as lorazepam (Ativan) and alprazolam (Xanax).

Dietary changes that may be helpful

Women who eat more sugary foods have been reported to have an increased risk of PMS.[1] Some doctors recommend that women with PMS cut back on sugar consumption for several months to see if it reduces their symptoms. However, no trials have yet to study the isolated effects of sugar restriction in women with PMS.

Alcohol can affect hormone metabolism, and **alcoholic** (page 12) women are more likely to suffer PMS than are nonalcoholic women.[2] Some doctors recommend that women with PMS avoid alcohol for several months to evaluate whether such a change will reduce symptoms.

In a study of Chinese women, increasing tea consumption was associated with increasing prevalence of PMS.[3] Among a group of college students in the United States, consumption of caffeine-containing beverages was associated with increases in both the prevalence and severity of PMS.[4] Moreover, the more caffeine women consumed, the more likely they were to suffer from PMS.[5] A preliminary study showed that women with heavy caffeine consumption were more likely to have shorter menstrual periods and shorter cycle length compared with women who did not consume caffeine.[6] Some doctors recommend that women with PMS avoid caffeine.

Several studies suggest that diets low in fat or high in fiber may help to reduce symptoms of PMS.[7] Many doctors recommend diets very low in meat and dairy fat and high in fruit, vegetables, and whole grains.

Lifestyle changes that may be helpful

Women with PMS who jogged an average of about 12 miles a week for six months were reported to experience a reduction in **breast tenderness** (page 189), **fluid retention** (page 180), **depression** (page 145), and stress.[8] Doctors frequently recommend regular exercise as a way to reduce symptoms of PMS.

Nutritional supplements that may be helpful

Many,[9, 10, 11, 12, 13] though not all,[14] clinical trials show that taking 50–400 mg of **vitamin B$_6$** (page 600) per day for several months help relieve symptoms of PMS. A composite analysis of the best designed controlled trials shows that vitamin B$_6$ is more than twice as likely to reduce symptoms of PMS as is placebo.[15] Many doctors suggest 100–400 mg per day for at least three months. However, intakes greater than 200 mg per day can cause side effects and should never be taken without the supervision of a healthcare professional.

Women who consume more **calcium** (page 483) from their diets are less likely to suffer severe PMS.[16] A large double-blind trial found that women who took 1,200 mg per day of calcium for three menstrual cycles had a 48% reduction in PMS symptoms, compared to a 30% reduction in the placebo group.[17] Other double-blind trials have shown that supplementing 1,000 mg of calcium per day relieves premenstrual symptoms.[18, 19]

Women with PMS have been shown to have impaired conversion of linoleic acid (an essential fatty acid) to gamma linolenic acid (GLA).[20] Because a deficiency of GLA might, in theory, be a factor in PMS and because **evening primrose oil** (page 511) (EPO) contains significant amounts of GLA, researchers have studied EPO as a potential way to reduce symptoms of PMS. In several double-blind trials, EPO was found to be beneficial,[21, 22, 23, 24] whereas in other trials it was no more effective than placebo.[25, 26]

Despite these conflicting results, some doctors consider EPO to be worth a try; the amount usually recommended is 3–4 grams per day. EPO may work best when used over several menstrual cycles and may be more helpful in women with PMS who also experience breast tenderness or **fibrocystic breast disease** (page 189).[27]

Women with PMS have been reported to be at increased risk of magnesium deficiency.[28, 29] Supplementing with **magnesium** (page 551) may help reduce symptoms.[30, 31] In one double-blind trial using only 200 mg per day for two months, a significant reduction was reported for several symptoms related to PMS (**fluid retention** [page 180], weight gain, swelling of extremities, breast tenderness, and abdominal bloating).[32] Magnesium has also been reported to be effective in reducing the symptoms of menstrual migraine headaches.[33] While the ideal amount of magnesium has yet to be determined, some doctors recommend 400 mg per day.[34] Effects of magnesium may begin to appear after two to three months.

A preliminary, uncontrolled trial found that women with severe PMS who took **potassium** (page 572) supplements had complete resolution of PMS symptoms within four menstrual cycles.[35] Most participants took 400 mg of potassium per day as potassium gluconate plus 200 mg of potassium per day as potassium chloride for the first two cycles, then switched to solely the gluconate form (600 mg potassium per day) for the remainder of the year-long trial. Without exception, all of the women found their symptoms (i.e., bloating, fatigue, irritability, etc.) decreasing gradually over three cycles and disappearing completely by the fourth cycle.

Controlled trials are needed to confirm these preliminary observations.

The **amino acid** (page 465), L-tryptophan has been shown to help relieve PMS symptoms. In a double-blind trial, women with premenstrual discomfort received 6 grams per day of L-tryptophan or placebo for 17 days.[36] Those who took L-tryptophan had significant improvement of symptoms, including mood swings, tension, irritability, breast sensitivity, water retention, and headache. There was a slight reduction in premenstrual depression, but it was not statistically significant. L-tryptophan is available only by prescription. It has not been determined whether **5-hydroxytryptophan** (page 549) (5-HTP, a metabolic byproduct of L-tryptophan that is available without prescription) has similar effects.

Although women with PMS do not appear to be deficient in **vitamin E** (page 609),[37] a double-blind trial reported that 300 IU of vitamin E per day may decrease symptoms of PMS.[38]

Some of the nutrients mentioned above appear together in **multivitamin-mineral** (page 559) supplements. One double-blind trial used a multivitamin-mineral supplement containing **vitamin B$_6$** (page 600) (600 mg per day), **magnesium** (page 551) (500 mg per day), **vitamin E** (page 609) (200 IU per day), **vitamin A** (page 595) (25,000 IU per day), **B-complex** (page 603) vitamins, and various other vitamins and minerals.[39] This supplement was found to relieve each of four different categories of PMS symptoms. Related results have been reported in other clinical trials.[40, 41]

Most well-controlled trials have not found vaginally applied natural **progesterone** (page 577) to be effective against the symptoms of premenstrual syndrome.[42] Only anecdotal reports have claimed that orally or rectally administered progesterone may be effective.[43] Progesterone is a hormone, and as such, there are concerns about its inappropriate use. A physician should be consulted before using this or other hormones. Few side effects have been associated with use of topical progesterone creams, but skin reactions may occur. The effect of natural progesterone on **breast cancer** (page 65) risk remains unclear; some research suggests the possibility of increased risk, whereas other research points to a possible reduction in risk.

Very high amounts of vitamin A—100,000 IU per day or more—have reduced symptoms of PMS,[44, 45] but such an amount can cause serious side effects with long-term use. Women who are or who could become **pregnant** (page 363) should not supplement with more than 10,000 IU (3,000 mcg) per day of vitamin A. Other people should not take more than 25,000 IU per day without the supervision of their doctor. As yet, no trials have explored the effects of these safer amounts of vitamin A in women suffering from PMS.

Many years ago, research linked B vitamin deficiencies to PMS in preliminary research.[46, 47] Based on that early work, some doctors recommend B-complex vitamins for women with PMS.[48]

Are there any side effects or interactions?
Refer to the individual supplement for information about any side effects or interactions.

Herbs that may be helpful
Vitex (page 757) has been shown to help re-establish normal balance of estrogen and progesterone during the menstrual cycle. Vitex also blocks prolactin secretion in women with excessive levels of this hormone; excessive levels of prolactin can lead to breast tenderness and failure to ovulate. A double-blind trial has confirmed that vitex reduces mildly elevated levels of prolactin before a woman's period.[49] Studies have shown that using vitex once in the morning over a period of several months helps normalize hormone balance and thus alleviate the symptoms of PMS.[50] A preliminary trial[51] and a double-blind trial[52] have found that women taking 20 mg per day of a concentrated vitex extract for three menstrual cycles experience a significant reduction in symptoms of PMS.

Vitex has been shown to be as effective as 200 mg **vitamin B$_6$** (page 600) in a double-blind trial of women with PMS.[53] Two surveys examined 1,542 women with PMS who had taken a German liquid extract of vitex for their PMS symptoms for as long as 16 years.[54] With an average intake of 42 drops per day, 92% of the women surveyed reported the effectiveness of vitex as "very good," "good," or "satisfactory."

Some healthcare practitioners recommend 40 drops of a liquid, concentrated vitex extract or one capsule of the equivalent dried, powdered extract once per day in the morning with some liquid. Vitex should be taken for at least four cycles to determine efficacy.

A double-blind trial has shown that standardized *Ginkgo biloba* (page 681) extract, when taken daily from day 16 of one menstrual cycle to day 5 of the next menstrual cycle, alleviates congestive and psychological symptoms of PMS better than placebo.[55] The trial used 80 mg of a ginkgo extract two times per day.

In Traditional Chinese Medicine, **dong quai** (page

668) is rarely used alone and is typically used in combination with herbs such as **peony** (page 724) *(Paeonia officinalis)* and osha *(Ligusticum porteri)* for **menopausal** (page 311) symptoms as well as for menstrual cramps.[56] However, no clinical trials have been completed to determine the effectiveness of dong quai for PMS.

Black cohosh (page 637) is approved in Germany for use in women with PMS.[57] This approval appears to be based on historical use as there are no modern clinical trials to support the use of black cohosh for PMS.

Based on anecdotal evidence, **yarrow** (page 763) tea has been used by European doctors when the main symptom of PMS is spastic pain.[58] Combine 2–3 teaspoons of yarrow flowers with one cup of hot water, then cover and steep for 15 minutes. Drink three to five cups per day beginning two days before PMS symptoms usually commence. In addition, 1–3 cups of the tea added to hot or cold water can be used as a sitz bath.

Are there any side effects or interactions?
Refer to the individual herb for information about any side effects or interactions.

PROSTATE CANCER

See also: Breast Cancer (page 65), **Colon Cancer** (page 123), **Lung Cancer** (page 298), **Cancer Prevention and Diet** (page 87)

Prostate cancer is a malignancy of the prostate. It is characterized by unregulated replication of cells creating tumors, with the possibility of some of the cells spreading to other sites (metastasis).

This article includes a discussion of studies that have assessed whether certain vitamins, minerals, herbs, or other dietary ingredients offered in dietary or herbal supplements may be beneficial in connection with the reduction of risk of developing prostate cancer, or of signs and symptoms in people who have this condition.

This information is provided solely to aid consumers in discussing supplements with their healthcare providers. It is not advised, nor is this information intended to advocate, promote, or encourage self use of these supplements for cancer risk reduction or treatment. Furthermore, none of this information should be misconstrued to suggest that dietary or herbal supplements can or should be used in place of conventional anticancer approaches or treatments.

It should be noted that certain studies referenced below, indicating the potential usefulness of a particular dietary ingredient or dietary or herbal supplement in connection with the reduction of risk of prostate cancer, are preliminary evidence only. Some studies suggest an association between high blood or dietary levels of a particular dietary ingredient with a reduced risk of developing prostate cancer. Even if such an association were established, this does not mean that dietary supplements containing large amounts of the dietary ingredient will necessarily have a cancer risk reduction effect.

Prostate cancer is the most common cancer among men in the United States. Although the cause is not known, most researchers believe that alterations in testosterone metabolism and/or bodily responses to testosterone are involved.

Throughout the world, autopsy reports show that evidence of microscopic prostate cancer is extremely common in older men. However, most men who have such microscopic disease are never diagnosed with, nor do they die from, prostate cancer. Unlike this dormant form of the disease, the incidence of potentially life-threatening prostate cancer varies greatly in different parts of the world. Researchers believe that some factors, possibly involving diet or lifestyle issues, determine the risk of having potentially life-threatening prostate cancer.

American men are at high risk of being diagnosed with such prostate cancer, and African-American men are at particularly high risk, for reasons that are not completely clear. A family history of prostate cancer increases the risk to a limited extent. Farmers, mechanics, workers in tire and rubber manufacturing, sheet metal workers, and workers exposed to cadmium have also been reported to be at increased risk.

CHECKLIST FOR PROSTATE CANCER

Rating	Nutritional Supplements	Herbs
★★☆	**Lycopene** (page 548) **Selenium** (page 584) (reduces risk) **Vitamin D** (page 607) **Vitamin E** (page 609) (reduces risk)	PC-SPES (take only under medical supervision)
★☆☆	**Coenzyme Q$_{10}$** (page 496) **Melatonin** (page 555)	**Shiitake** (page 746)

What are the symptoms of prostate cancer?

Prostate cancer usually grows slowly, initially producing no symptoms. Later in the course of the disease, symptoms that overlap with symptoms of prostatic hyperplasia, a very common benign condition, may appear. Some of these symptoms include frequent urination (including having to urinate more frequently at night), pain on urination, a weak urinary stream, dribbling after urination, and a sensation of incomplete emptying. In addition, blood may appear in urine. None of these symptoms is specific to prostate cancer; the diagnosis of this disease requires the help of a doctor.

If prostate cancer spreads to a distant part of the body, it most often is found in bone, a condition that may cause bone pain. Late stages of the disease are associated with severe weight loss, untreatable fatigue-inducing anemia, and finally death.

Medical treatments

Prescription drug treatment for prostate cancer focuses on anti-hormone therapy, which interferes with the body's ability to make testosterone. Medications used include diethylstilbestrol (Stilphostrol), goserelin (Zoladex), leuprolide (Lupron), flutamide (Eulexin), bicalutamide (Casodex), and ketoconazole (Nizoral). Though the treatments cannot cure prostate cancer, they often slow the cancer's growth and reduce the tumor size.

Treatment of men with prostate cancer varies depending on the age and health of the patient, extent of the cancer, and to some degree, the views of the oncologist. Surgical removal of the prostate gland is often performed if the cancer appears to be contained within the prostate gland. Surgical removal of the testicles (orchiectomy) might be recommended to halt testosterone production. Radiation, with or without surgery, is also commonly used to treat men with prostate cancer. External beam radiation delivers radioactivity from a machine. With brachytherapy, radiation is emitted from tiny radioactive seeds that are inserted directly into the prostate. Men who are older and appear to have less aggressive disease might delay treatment until symptoms develop—a plan called "watchful waiting." Watchful waiting is sometimes considered a reasonable approach, because the side effects of treatment are usually significant, while their therapeutic benefits often appear to be relatively small and sometimes unclear. In addition, since prostate tumors often grow slowly, older men often die from diseases unrelated to the prostate cancer.

Dietary changes that may be helpful

The following dietary changes have been studied in connection with prostate cancer.

Avoidance of alcohol

Although the effect of drinking alcohol on prostate cancer risk appears weak, some association between beer drinking and an increased risk may exist, according to an analysis of most published reports.[1]

Tomatoes

Tomatoes contain **lycopene** (page 548)—an **antioxidant** (page 467) similar in structure to **beta-carotene** (page 469). Most lycopene in our diet comes from tomatoes, though traces of lycopene exist in other foods. Lycopene has been reported to inhibit the proliferation of cancer cells in test tube research.[2]

A review of published research found that higher intake of tomatoes or higher blood levels of lycopene correlated with a reduced risk of cancer in 57 of 72 studies. Findings in 35 of these studies were statistically significant.[3] Evidence of a protective effect for tomato consumption was stronger for prostate cancer than for most other cancers.

Cruciferous vegetables

Cabbage, Brussels sprouts, broccoli, and cauliflower belong to the *Brassica* family of vegetables, also known as "cruciferous" vegetables. In test tube and animal studies, these foods have shown to have anticancer activity,[4] possibly due to several substances found in them, such as **indole-3-carbinol** (page 536),[5] glucaric acid (**calcium D-glucarate** [page 486]),[6] and **sulforaphane** (page 589).[7] A recent preliminary study of men newly diagnosed with prostate cancer showed a 41% decreased risk of prostate cancer among men eating three or more servings of cruciferous vegetables per week, compared with those eating less than one serving per week.[8] Protective effects of cruciferous vegetables were thought to be due to their high concentration of the carotenoids **lutein** (page 548) and zeaxanthin, as well as their stimulatory effects on the breakdown of environmental carcinogens associated with prostate cancer.[9]

Meat and how it is cooked

Meat contains high amounts of arachidonic acid. Some by-products of arachidonic acid have promoted prostate cancer in animals.[10] Preliminary reports have suggested that frequently eating well-done steak[11] or cured meats[12] may also increase the risk of prostate cancer in men, though the association between prostate cancer and other meats has not been consistently reported.

Fish

Fish eaters have been reported to have low risk for prostate cancer.[13] The **omega-3 fatty acids** (page 509) found in fish are thought by some researchers to be the components of fish responsible for protection against cancer.[14]

Low-fat diet and prevention

When combined with a low-fiber diet, men consuming a high-fat diet have been reported to have higher levels of testosterone,[15] which might increase their risk of prostate cancer. The risk of prostate cancer correlates with dietary fat from country to country,[16] a finding supported in some,[17, 18] but not all,[19] preliminary trials. In one study, prostate cancer patients consuming the most saturated fat (from meat and dairy), and followed for over five years, had over three times the risk of dying from prostate cancer compared with men consuming the least amount of saturated fat.[20]

Avoidance of alpha-linolenic acid

Alpha-linolenic acid is a fatty acid found in many foods. Most,[21, 22, 23] but not all,[24] studies have found that high dietary or blood levels of alpha-linolenic acid correlate with an increased risk of prostate cancer. It is not clear, however, whether this association reflects a cause-effect relationship.

Concentrations of alpha-linolenic acid are much higher in **flaxseed oil** (page 517), canola oil, soybean oil, and certain nuts compared to the concentrations found in meat. However, because so much meat is consumed as part of many western diets, a significant portion of dietary alpha-linolenic acid often does come from meat. Therefore, at least in theory, alpha-linolenic may merely be a marker for meat consumption. When researchers have adjusted for the intake of meat or saturated fat, however, a correlation between alpha-linolenic acid and prostate cancer risk has remained.[25, 26] On the other hand, in a preliminary study of men with prostate cancer, supplementation with 30 grams of ground flaxseed per day for approximately one month appeared to decrease the rate of tumor growth.[27]

How alpha-linolenic acid might increase the risk of prostate cancer remains unclear. Alpha-linolenic acid has promoted the growth of prostate cancer cells in one test tube study,[28] but inhibited prostate cell growth in another.[29]

Soy (page 587)

Genistein is an isoflavone found in soybeans and many soy foods, such as tofu, soy milk, and some soy protein powders. Except for soy sauce and soy protein concentrates processed with alcohol, most soy-based foods contain significant amounts of isoflavones, such as genistein. Genistein inhibits growth of prostate cancer cells, helps kill these cells,[30] and has other known anticancer actions, according to test tube research findings.[31]

In preliminary research, men who consumed soy milk more than once per day were reported to have a significantly lower risk of prostate cancer compared with other men.[32] Some researchers are now saying that genistein may eventually be shown to have the potential to treat prostate cancer,[33] while others say only that enough evidence exists to recommend that future genistein research be devoted to the subject of prostate cancer prevention.[34]

Lifestyle changes that may be helpful

The following lifestyle change has been studied in connection with prostate cancer.

Maintaining healthful body weight

Several studies have reported that the risk of prostate cancer increases with increasing body **weight** (page 446).[35, 36]

Nutritional supplements that may be helpful

The following nutritional supplements have been studied in connection with prostate cancer.

Beta-carotene (page 469)

In a double-blind trial, supplementation with synthetic beta-carotene led to a 23% increase in the risk of prostate cancer in smokers, though this increase did not reach statistical significance.[37] However, in a double-blind study of mostly *non*smoking men, supplementation with synthetic beta-carotene led to a statistically significant 32% reduction in risk of prostate cancer in those who initially had the lowest blood levels of beta-carotene.[38] In the same report, supplementation with synthetic beta-carotene in men who had the highest blood levels of beta-carotene at the beginning of the trial led to a 33% increase in the risk of prostate cancer, though this finding may have been due to chance.[39]

No trials have investigated the effect of natural beta-carotene supplements on the risk of prostate cancer.

Selenium (page 584)

Selenium has been reported to have diverse anticancer actions.[40, 41] Selenium inhibits cancer in animals.[42] Low soil levels of selenium (probably associated with low dietary intake), have been associated with increased cancer incidence in humans.[43] Blood levels of selenium have been reported to be low in patients with prostate cancer.[44] In preliminary reports, people with the lowest blood levels of selenium had between 3.8 and 5.8 times the risk of dying from cancer compared with those who had the highest selenium levels.[45, 46]

The strongest evidence supporting the anti-cancer effects of selenium supplementation comes from a double-blind trial of 1,312 Americans with a history of skin cancer who were treated with 200 mcg of yeast-based selenium per day or placebo for 4.5 years and then followed for an additional two years.[47] Although no decrease in *skin* cancers occurred, a dramatic 50% reduction in overall cancer deaths and a 37% reduction in total cancer incidence were observed. A statistically significant 63% decrease in prostate cancer incidence was reported.[48]

Lycopene (page 548)

In a preliminary trial, 26 men with prostate cancer were randomly assigned to receive lycopene (15 mg twice a day) or no lycopene for three weeks before undergoing prostate surgery. Prostate tissue was then obtained during surgery and examined. Compared with the unsupplemented men, those receiving lycopene were found to have significantly less aggressive growth of cancer cells.[49] In addition, a case report has been published of a 62-year-old man with advanced prostate cancer who experienced a regression of his tumor after starting 10 mg of lycopene per day and 300 mg of **saw palmetto** (page 743) three times per day. As saw palmetto has not been previously associated with improvements in prostate cancer, the authors of the report attributed the response to the lycopene.[50] Long-term controlled studies are needed to confirm these promising initial reports.

Calcium (page 483)

> **Warning:** Calcium supplements should be avoided by prostate cancer patients.

Increasing calcium intake from food, water, and supplements has been associated with an *increased* risk of prostate cancer in some preliminary studies[51, 52] but not in others.[53, 54] A few researchers now believe that increasing calcium intake may increase the risk of prostate cancer by reducing the amount of vitamin D activated in the kidneys.[55] (Vitamin D may protect against prostate cancer. See the Vitamin D discussion in this article.) If the relationship between higher calcium intake and increased risk of prostate cancer were to be confirmed by future research, then the question would arise whether the negative effect of calcium from food and supplements could be overcome by taking **vitamin D** (page 607) supplements.

Vitamin E (page 609)

Relatively high blood levels of vitamin E have been associated with relatively low levels of hormones linked to prostate cancer.[56] While a relationship between higher blood levels of vitamin E and a reduced risk of prostate cancer has been reported only inconsistently,[57, 58] supplemental use of vitamin E[59] has been associated with a reduced risk of prostate cancer in smokers. In a double-blind trial studying smokers, vitamin E supplementation (50 IU of vitamin E per day for an average of six years) led to a 32% decrease in prostate cancer incidence and a 41% decrease in prostate cancer deaths.[60] Both findings were statistically significant.[61] The effects of vitamin E have yet to be studied in men already diagnosed with prostate cancer.

Vitamin D (page 607)

Where sun exposure is *low,* the rate of prostate cancer has been reported to be high.[62] In the body, vitamin D is changed into a hormone with great activity. This activated vitamin D causes "cellular differentiation"—essentially the opposite of cancer.

In a preliminary trial, 7 of 16 men who had prostate cancer that had spread to bone and who had been unresponsive to conventional treatment were found to have evidence of vitamin D deficiency.[63] All 16 were given 2,000 IU of vitamin D per day for 12 weeks, and levels of pain were recorded for 14 of these men. Vitamin D supplementation led to reduced pain in 4 of the 14 men, and 6 showed evidence of increased strength.[64] Those with vitamin D deficiency were more likely to respond, compared with those who were not deficient.[65]

In another preliminary study, men with prostate cancer that had relapsed after surgery or radiation therapy were treated with 2,000 IU of vitamin D per day for nine months. In approximately half of the men, the prostate-specific antigen (PSA) level decreased, suggesting that the progression of the disease had been halted or reversed; this decrease was sustained for 5 to 17 months.[66] In addition, the study was done in Toronto, Canada, where the amount of sunlight is limited and vitamin D status tends to be low. It is not known whether vitamin D supplementation would be as effective in geographical regions such as the Southern United States, where the amount of sunlight is greater.

Melatonin (page 555)

Years ago, a preliminary study suggested that melatonin may help stabilize the condition of some people with advanced cancers.[67] Since then, Italian researchers have been investigating the effects of melatonin in cancer patients, often with partial success.[68, 69, 70, 71, 72, 73, 74, 75, 76, 77, 78, 79]

Patients with advanced prostate cancer who had previously not responded to drug therapy (triptorelin) were given melatonin plus triptorelin in a preliminary trial.[80] PSA scores, a marker of disease progression, fell (i.e., improved) more than 50% in 8 of 14 patients.

Patients with advanced cancer have been reported to have improved survival and fewer side effects from taking chemotherapy when given melatonin plus chemotherapy vs. chemotherapy alone.[81]

Coenzyme Q₁₀ (page 496)

In an unpublished report, after one year, 10 of 15 prostate cancer patients experienced a 78% decrease in the level of PSA—a marker of cancer activity.[82] The amount of coenzyme Q_{10} given to these men was 600 mg per day; after four months, PSA scores began to decline.[83] Such undocumented case reports require confirmation from published research trials.

Shark cartilage (page 490)

Growth of cancerous tumors requires a large blood supply. Substances that interfere with the development of new vessels that supply blood to tumors are thought by many researchers to have potential anticancer effects. Such substances are called "antiangiogenic." Shark cartilage has been reported to have antiangiogenic activity.[84]

In a preliminary report, high amounts of shark cartilage were administered by enemas or suppositories to eight late-stage cancer patients.[85] After 7 to 11 weeks, 6 of the 8 were reported to show significant reductions in tumor size, though the long-term outcomes of these patients were not reported.[86]

In a telephone survey of cancer patients, 11 of 18 patients claimed a reduction in tumor size had resulted from the use of shark cartilage, 17 of 21 reported an improvement in their quality of life, and 7 of 7 prostate cancer patients reported a reduction in PSA scores—a marker of cancer progression.[87] However, a report limited to patients capable of responding by phone necessarily omits patients who have died while taking shark cartilage and includes no objective medical information. The meaning of these findings, supported by a company selling shark cartilage, remains unclear.

In a preliminary trial, 60 late-stage cancer patients were given 1 gram of shark cartilage for every 2.2 pounds of body weight per day in three divided doses and followed for 12 weeks or longer.[88] No evidence of a therapeutic effect was found.[89]

Because the evidence remains weak and mixed, shark cartilage remains unproven as a treatment for men with prostate cancer.

Zinc (page 614)

Prostate cancer patients have been reported to have subnormal levels of zinc within the prostate, which might facilitate the growth of cancer, according to some researchers.[90] Zinc has interfered with the growth of prostate cancer cells in test tube research.[91] However, no trials have directly explored whether zinc supplements help prevent prostate cancer or can effectively treat men who already have the disease.

Are there any side effects or interactions?

Refer to the individual supplement for information about any side effects or interactions.

Herbs that may be helpful

The following herbs have been studied in connection with prostate cancer.

PC-SPES

"PC" in this formula's name stands for prostate cancer, while "SPES" is the Latin word for hope. The complete formula consists of isatis (Isatis indigotica), **licorice** (page 702) (Glycyrrhiza glabra) and/or Gan cao (G. uralensis), **Chinese scullcap** (page 658) (Scutellaria baicalensis), **reishi** (page 737) (Ganoderma lucidum), **saw palmetto** (page 743) (Serenoa repens), **Asian ginseng** (page 630) (Panax ginseng) or sanqi ginseng (P. pseudoginseng), denodrantherm (Denodrantherma morifolium), and rabdosia (Rabdosia rubescens).

In several preliminary trials, this formula has been shown to reduce blood levels of prostate specific antigen (PSA, a marker for prostate cancer progression) in men with prostate cancer.[92, 93, 94, 95, 96] While such a reduction suggests a therapeutic effect, trials have yet to explore whether PC-SPES increases survival in people with prostate cancer.

One trial distinguished prostate cancer patients with androgen-dependent (an earlier, milder form of the cancer) and androgen-independent (a later, more severe form of the cancer) disease.[97] PSA scores began to decline in most people within two to six weeks after first receiving PC-SPES. Scores reached their lowest point in an average of 23 weeks in men with androgen-dependent prostate cancer and 16 weeks in men with androgen-independent prostate cancer. PSA scores declined an average of 80% and became undetectable in four out of every five men with androgen-dependent disease. In contrast, 54% of androgen-independent prostate cancer patients had a PSA decline of 50% or more. After an average of about one year, 31 of 32 androgen-dependent prostate cancer patients continued to have normal PSA scores. However, 28 of the 35 patients with androgen-independent prostate cancer ultimately developed PSA increases consistent with progression of their cancer, despite continued use of PC-SPES. Improvement or disappearance of cancer was seen in four patients who had previously had cancer spread to the bone, as well as in one patient who had previously had cancer spread to the bladder. Rarely, PSA levels have risen slightly (less than 20%) during PC-SPES use, according to other studies.[98] Testosterone levels are almost always decreased by PC-SPES therapy, according to most studies, which presumably accounts, in part, for the therapeutic effect.[99, 100]

Many men who take the formula have been reported to develop symptoms of estrogen excess, including breast tenderness, enlargement of the breasts, loss of libido, and the more serious problem of blood clots in the veins (venous thrombosis).[101, 102, 103] At least one person who took PC-SPES developed a potentially life-threatening blood clot in the lung. For this reason, some doctors recommend that people taking PC-SPES also take blood-thinning medication, such as heparin or warfarin (Coumadin).[104, 105] However, each of these drugs can cause excessive bleeding. Because of the potential side effects of PC-SPES and the complex medical issues involved with the use of blood-thinning drugs, people should never take PC-SPES without the close supervision of a doctor. The amount of PC-SPES used in most studies was 320 to 960 mg three times per day.[106, 107, 108]

In February 2002, the sole supplier of PC-SPES in the United States (BotanicLab) issued a recall of the product after the California Health Department reported it contained warfarin, a prescription drug that can cause severe bleeding. However, PC-SPES is known to contain compounds that, though distinct from warfarin, could potentially be mistakenly identified as warfarin using currently available laboratory methods.[109] There has been one case report of excessive bleeding occurring in a man who was taking PC-SPES.[110] However, the warfarin concentration in this patient's blood was not high enough to explain his abnormal bleeding. In addition, allegations have been made that PC-SPES contains small amounts of a synthetic estrogen (diethylstilbestrol; DES). That claim has been disputed by BotanicLab.

Although additional information is needed to determine whether PC-SPES has been adulterated with one or more prescription drugs, at the time of this writing (February 2003) the product is not available in the United States.

Warning: PC-SPES has been reported to cause serious side effects, including potentially life-threatening blood clots. PC-SPES should never be taken without the close supervision of a doctor. PC-SPES is not for sale is certain parts of the world.

Shiitake (page 746) (Lentinus edodes)
Several trials studying cancer patients have investigated the effects of lentinan, a carbohydrate found in shiitake mushrooms.[111, 112, 113, 114] Injection of lentinan repeatedly has been found to have beneficial effects on the **immune systems** (page 255) of cancer patients.[115, 116] Two trials reported that lentinan injections prolonged life in people with a variety of advanced cancers.[117, 118] Another trial found that intravenous lentinan increased five-year survival rates in prostate cancer patients compared with those not given lentinan.[119] It is unknown whether consumption of shiitake mushrooms or lentinan supplements would have the same effects reported in studies using injectable lentinan.

Other herbal therapies
No studies have investigated the effects of the Hoxsey herbal formula, Coriolus versicolor (PSK), the Essiac formula, or most other herbal therapies in men with prostate cancer.

Are there any side effects or interactions?
Refer to the individual herb for information about any side effects or interactions.

PROSTATITIS

Prostatitis is an inflammation of the prostate gland. It is a term that encompasses four disorders of the prostate: acute bacterial prostatitis, chronic bacterial prostatitis, chronic nonbacterial prostatitis, and prostadynia.

Chronic nonbacterial prostatitis (NBP), also called chronic abacterial prostatitis (CAP), is the most common form of prostatitis. NBP is usually caused by infectious agents such as fungi, mycoplasma, or viruses.[1] Prostadynia (PD), also called chronic pelvic pain syndrome, is a noninfectious form of prostatitis. Although the cause is unknown, it has been proposed that PD may be a neuromuscular condition, causing pain of the pelvic floor muscles.[2] Acute bacterial prostatitis (ABP) results from a **urinary tract infection** (page 436) (usually from *E. coli* bacteria) that has spread to the prostate. Chronic bacterial prostatitis (CBP) is usually the result of a partial blockage of the male urinary tract, such as occurs with **benign prostatic hyperplasia** (page 58) (BPH). Such blockages promote the harboring of bacteria from a previous infection and reduce circulation, thereby preventing both the body's natural **immune mechanisms** (page 255) and medication from getting to the site.

CHECKLIST FOR PROSTATITIS

Rating	Nutritional Supplements	Herbs
★★★	**Quercetin** (page 580) (NBP, PD)	
★★☆	**Bromelain** (page 481) (NBP, PD) **Flower Pollen** (page 571) (not bee pollen) (NBP, PD)	
★☆☆	**Vitamin C** (page 604) (ABP, CBP) **Zinc** (page 614) (CBP, NBP)	Pau d'arco (page 722) Pygeum (page 734) (CBP, NBP) Saw palmetto (page 743) (NBP)

What are the symptoms of prostatitis?

Men with prostatitis may have symptoms including pain or discomfort in the lower abdomen, testicles, and penis; discomfort during ejaculation or urination; or a weak urinary stream with dribbling. Advanced cases may also have fever, chills, frequent urge to urinate, burning urination, blood passed in the urine, and pain in the joints and muscles.

Medical treatments

Over the counter pain medications, such as aspirin (Bayer, Ecotrin, Bufferin), ibuprofen (Motrin, Advil), naproxen (Aleve), and acetaminophen (Tylenol), may be beneficial. Stool softeners, such as docusate (Colace, Surfak), might be recommended.

Prescription drug treatment primarily includes fluoroquinolone antibiotics, such as ciprofloxacin (Cipro), norfloxacin (Noroxin), oflaoxacin (Floxin), and levofloxacin (Levaquin), which are often taken for 4 to 12 weeks.

Health care practitioners may recommend bed rest and plenty of fluids.

Lifestyle changes that may be helpful

Urination and ejaculation may provide defense against prostatic infection by flushing the urethra. The prostate also secretes an antibacterial substance known as "prostatic antibacterial factor" into the seminal fluid (semen), which helps to fight infection.[3] In one preliminary study, unmarried men with NBP who had avoided sexual activity for personal or religious reasons and who had not responded to medication, were encouraged to masturbate at least twice a week for six months. Out of 18 men, 78% experienced moderate to complete relief of symptoms.[4]

Use of tobacco, especially by smoking, reduces the **zinc** (page 614) content of prostatic fluid, and may therefore reduce natural immunity to prostate infection.[5] No research, however, has investigated the effect of smoking cessation on the prevention of prostatitis.

Nutritional supplements that may be helpful

Quercetin (page 580), a **flavonoid** (page 516) with anti-inflammatory and **antioxidant** (page 467) effects, has recently been reported to improve symptoms of NBP and PD. An uncontrolled study reported that 500 mg of quercetin twice daily for at least two weeks significantly improved symptoms in 59% of men with chronic prostatitis.[6] These results were confirmed in a double-blind study, in which similar treatment with quercetin for one month improved symptoms in 67% of men with NBP or PD.[7] Another uncontrolled study combined 1,000 mg per day of quercetin with the enzymes **bromelain** (page 481) and papain, resulting in significant improvement of symptoms.[8] Bromelain and papain promote absorption of quercetin and have anti-inflammatory effects as well.[9]

An extract of flower **pollen** (page 571), derived primarily from rye, may improve symptoms of chronic prostatitis and prostadynia. In a small, uncontrolled trial, men with chronic NBP or prostadynia given two tablets of flower pollen extract twice daily for up to 18 months reported complete or marked improvement in symptoms.[10] In a larger, uncontrolled trial, one tablet three times daily for six months produced a favorable response in 80% of the men based on symptoms, laboratory tests, and doctor evaluations.[11] Men who did not respond in this study were found to have structural abnormalities of the urinary tract, suggesting that uncomplicated prostate conditions are more likely to respond to flower pollen. Additional uncontrolled studies support the effectiveness of flower pollen extract,[12, 13, 14] but no controlled research has been published.

In healthy men, prostatic secretions contain a significant amount of **zinc** (page 614), which has antibacterial activity and is a key factor in the natural resistance of the male **urinary tract infection** (page 436).[15, 16] In CBP[17, 18, 19, 20] and NBP[21] these zinc levels are significantly reduced; however, it is not clear whether this indicates a predisposition to, or is the result of, prostatic infection.[22, 23] Zinc supplements increased semen levels of zinc in men with NBP in one study,[24] but not in another.[25] While zinc supplements have been associated with improvement of **benign prostatic hyperplasia** (page 58) (BPH), according to one preliminary report,[26] no research has examined their effectiveness for prostatitis. Nonetheless, many doctors of natural medicine recommend zinc for this condition.

Test tube studies have shown that **vitamin C** (page 604) inhibits the growth of *E.coli*,[27] the most common cause of ABP and CBP. Results from preliminary human studies indicate vitamin C supplementation can cause changes in urine composition that may inhibit the growth of urinary *E. coli*.[28, 29] Although vitamin C has not been studied in bacterial prostatitis, the association of this condition with urinary tract infections leads many nutritionally oriented doctors to recommend its use, in the form of ascorbic acid, for bacterial prostatitis due to *E. coli* infection.

Are there any side effects or interactions?
Refer to the individual supplement for information about any side effects or interactions.

Herbs that may be helpful
Saw palmetto (page 743), known more for its use in **BPH** (page 58), has also been used historically for symptoms of prostatitis.[30] According to laboratory studies, saw palmetto contains constituents that act to reduce swelling and inflammation.[31] However, there is no scientific research evaluating the effects of saw palmetto in men with prostatitis.

In a small preliminary trial, men with chronic prostatitis or BPH were given 200 mg per day of **pygeum** (page 734) extract for 60 days, resulting in some improvement of symptoms and laboratory evaluation of the prostate and urinary tract.[32] The extract used in this study was standardized to contain 14% **beta-sitosterol** (page 471) and 0.5% n-docosanol. Other preliminary trials have also reported improvement of prostatitis symptoms with pygeum.[33]

Pau d'arco (page 722) extract has been used traditionally for prostatitis.[34] According to test tube studies, pau d'arco exerts antibacterial activity against *E.coli*,[35] which suggests a possible mechanism for this claim. However, no scientific studies of the effectiveness of pau d'arco for preventing or treating prostatitis have been done.

Are there any side effects or interactions?
Refer to the individual herb for information about any side effects or interactions.

Holistic approaches that may be helpful
Acupuncture may be helpful for chronic prostatitis according to one small, uncontrolled study.[36] Seventeen patients with chronic prostatitis that was unresponsive to conventional therapy were treated with electroacupuncture (acupuncture with electrical stimulation). The effectiveness of electroacupuncture therapy was reported to be moderate in 70% and excellent in 30% of the patients treated.

Prostatic massage through the rectum was once a common treatment for CBP and NBP, and is still prescribed by some practitioners. Prostatic massage is thought to promote circulation and drainage of infected areas.[37] While little scientific research has been done to evaluate the effectiveness of this treatment, some physicians and their patients have reported symptomatic improvement.[38] Prostatic massage should be conducted only by a trained specialist. Prostatic massage should be avoided in ABP because it is painful and could spread the infection.[39] Also avoid this therapy in the presence of prostatic calculi (stones), a condition common in elderly men in which small calcifications develop in the prostate.

Controlled studies indicate psychological factors, such as **anxiety** (page 30) and **depression** (page 145), occur more frequently in men with NBP and PD.[40, 41, 42] This may be because psychological factors contribute to the development of NBP and PD, or perhaps they occur as a result of prostatitis. Nonetheless, some practitioners believe psychotherapy may help reduce symptoms in these cases.[43]

Some researchers have reported that certain cases of chronic prostatitis are helped by biofeedback (using simple electronic devices to measure and report information about a person's biological system) and other treatments aimed at reducing chronic pain.[44] This suggests that some of the causes of PD, and possibly NBP, may be neuromuscular. In support of this idea, smooth muscle relaxing medications are reported to reduce symptoms in men with CBP, NBP, and PD, and to reduce the recurrence rate of CBP.[45] However, no controlled research has explored the effectiveness of biofeedback or alternative neuromuscular therapies for prostatitis.

A sitz bath is the immersion of the pelvic region (up to the navel) in water. Sitz baths are reported to provide temporary relief of symptoms in men with chronic prostatitis, although no controlled research has evaluated these claims.[46, 47] This therapy is not recommended in ABP, as it may worsen the infection.[48] In chronic prostatitis, doctors of natural medicine recommend "contrast sitz baths," a series of alternating hot and cold baths, requiring two tubs (or a bathtub and adequately sized basin), one for each temperature. The hot sitz bath is taken first with the water at a temperature of 105–115°F for 3 minutes. This is immediately followed by the cold sitz bath at 55–85° F for 30 seconds. This process is repeated two more times, for a total of six baths (three hot and three cold) per treatment.[49]

PSORIASIS

What do I need to know?

Self-care for psoriasis can be approached in a number of ways—but it can be hard to know just where to start. To make it easier, our doctors recommend trying these simple steps first:

Try topical creams
> Apply a cream containing 0.025 to 0.075% capsaicin four times a day to relieve itching and help heal sores

Address your stress
> Learn stress-reduction techniques such as meditation to improve healing of sores

Give aloe a go
> Improve skin-healing by applying a 0.5% extract to affected areas three times a day

Check out fish oil
> Capsules providing 1.8 to 3.6 grams of EPA (eicosapentaenoic acid) a day may improve symptoms

About psoriasis

Psoriasis is a common, poorly understood condition that affects primarily the skin but may also affect nails. A related condition, psoriatic arthritis, affects joints.

The fact that some people with psoriasis improve while taking prescription drugs that interfere with the **immune system** (page 255) suggests that the disease might result from a derangement of the immune system. A dermatologist should be consulted to confirm the diagnosis of psoriasis.

CHECKLIST FOR PSORIASIS		
Rating	Nutritional Supplements	Herbs
★★★	**Fumaric acid esters** (page 524)	**Capsaicin cream** (page 654) (topical)
★★☆	**Fish oil** (page 514) (EPA/**DHA** [page 509])	**Aloe** (page 624)
★☆☆	**Folic acid** (page 520) (only for people who are *not* taking prescription drugs such as methotrexate that interfere with folic acid metabolism)	**Barberry** (page 632) **Burdock** (page 648) **Coleus** (page 660) **Oregon grape** (page 721)

What are the symptoms of psoriasis?

The hallmark symptom of psoriasis is well-defined, red patches of skin covered by a silvery, flaky surface that has pinpoint spots of bleeding underneath if scraped. The patches typically appear during periodic flare-ups and are in the same area on both sides of the body. In some people with psoriasis, the fingernails and toenails may have white-colored pits, lengthwise ridges down the nail, or yellowish spots, or may be thickened or may separate at the cut end.

Medical treatments

Over the counter coal tar-containing products (Estar, P & S Plus, Balnetar, Tegrin for Psoriasis) might be beneficial. Individuals with mild cases might notice slight improvement using hydrocortisone (Cortaid, Lanacort).

Prescription strength topical corticosteroid creams or ointments are commonly prescribed. Drugs available include triamcinolone (Aristocort, Kenalog), fluocinonide (Lidex), betamethasone (Valisone, Diprosone, Diprolene), mometasone (Elocon), and clobetasol (Temovate). Topical calcipotriene (Dovonex) and anthralin (Drithocreme, Athra-Derm) are also prescribed. Severe cases of psoriasis may be treated with oral methotrexate (Rheumatrex), cyclosporine (Neoral, Sandimmune), hydroxyurea (Hydrea), sulfasalazine (Azulfidine), and thioguanine (Tabloid). Ultraviolet therapy using psoralens, such as methoxsalen (Oxsoralen-Ultra), is reserved for individuals who do not respond well to other therapies.

Dietary changes that may be helpful

Ingestion of alcohol has been reported to be a risk factor for psoriasis in men but not women.[1, 2] It would therefore be prudent for men with psoriasis to restrict their intake of alcohol or avoid it entirely.

Anecdotal evidence suggests that people with psoriasis may improve on a hypoallergenic diet.[3] Three trials have reported that eliminating gluten (found in wheat, rye, and barley) improved psoriasis for some people.[4, 5, 6] A doctor can help people with psoriasis determine whether gluten or other foods are contributing to their skin condition.

Nutritional supplements that may be helpful

Fumaric acid (page 524), in the chemically bound form known as fumaric acid esters, has been shown in case studies,[7] preliminary trials[8, 9, 10] and double-blind trials[11, 12, 13] to be effective against symptoms of psoriasis. However, because fumaric acid esters can cause significant side effects, they should be taken only under the supervision of a doctor familiar with their use. Nevertheless, these side effects have been reported to decrease in frequency over the course of treatment and, if they are closely monitored, rarely lead to significant toxicity.[14]

In a double-blind trial, **fish oil** (page 514) (10 grams per day) was found to improve the skin lesions of psoriasis.[15] In another trial, supplementing with 3.6 grams per day of purified eicosapentaenoic acid (EPA, one of the fatty acids found in fish oil) reduced the severity of psoriasis after two to three months.[16, 17] That amount of EPA is usually contained in 20 grams of fish oil, a level that generally requires 20 pills to achieve. However, when purified EPA was used in combination with purified docosahexaenoic acid (**DHA** [page 509], another fatty acid contained in fish oil), no improvement was observed.[18]

Additional research is needed to determine whether **fish oil** (page 514) itself or some of its components are more effective for people with psoriasis. One trial showed that applying a preparation containing 10% fish oil directly to psoriatic lesions twice daily resulted in improvement after seven weeks.[19] In addition, promising results were reported from a double-blind trial in which people with chronic plaque-type psoriasis received 4.2 g of EPA and 4.2 g of **DHA** (page 509) or placebo intravenously each day for two weeks. Thirty-seven percent of those receiving the essential fatty acid infusions experienced greater than 50% reduction in the severity of their symptoms.[20]

Supplementing with fish oil also may help prevent the increase in blood levels of **triglycerides** (page 235) that occurs as a side effect of certain drugs used to treat psoriasis (e.g., etretinate and acitretin).[21]

Folic acid (page 520) antagonist drugs have been used to treat psoriasis. In one preliminary report, extremely high amounts of folic acid (20 mg taken four times per day), combined with an unspecified amount of **vitamin C** (page 604), led to significant improvement within three to six months in people with psoriasis who had *not* been taking folic acid antagonists; those who had previously taken these drugs saw a worsening of their condition.[22]

Although some doctors have been impressed with the effectiveness of **flaxseed oil** (page 517) (usually 1 to 3 tbsp per day) against psoriasis, there have been no published trials to support that observation.

The **vitamin D** (page 607) that is present in food or manufactured by sunlight is converted in the body into a powerful hormone-like molecule called 1,25-dihydroxyvitamin D. That compound and a related naturally occurring molecule (1 alpha-hydroxyvitamin D3) have been found to reduce skin lesions when given orally to people with psoriasis.[23] Topical application of these compounds has also been effective in some,[24, 25, 26, 27] but not all,[28, 29] trials. These activated forms of vitamin

D are believed to help by preventing the excessive pro-liferation of cells that occurs in the skin of people with psoriasis. Because these potent forms of vitamin D can cause potentially dangerous increases in blood levels of calcium, they are available only by prescription. Toxic-ity is usually less of a problem with activated vitamin D applied topically than with activated vitamin D taken orally. The use of these compounds (under the supervi-sion of a qualified dermatologist) may be considered in difficult cases of psoriasis. The form of vitamin D that is available without a prescription is unlikely to be ef-fective against psoriasis.

Are there any side effects or interactions?
Refer to the individual supplement for information about any side effects or interactions.

Herbs that may be helpful

Cayenne (page 654) contains a resinous and pungent substance known as capsaicin. This chemical relieves **pain** (page 338) and itching by depleting certain neuro-transmitters from sensory nerves. In a double-blind trial, application of a capsaicin cream to the skin re-lieved both the itching and the skin lesions in people with psoriasis.[30] Creams containing 0.025 to 0.075% capsaicin are generally used. There may be a burning sensation the first several times the cream is applied, but this usually become less pronounced with each use. The hands must be carefully and thoroughly washed after use, or gloves should be worn, to prevent the cream from accidentally reaching the eyes, nose, or mouth and causing a burning sensation. The cream should not be applied to areas of broken skin.

A double-blind trial in Pakistan found that topical application of an **aloe** (page 624) extract (0.5%) in a cream was more effective than placebo in the treatment of adults with psoriasis.[31] The aloe cream was applied three times per day for four weeks.

In traditional herbal texts, **burdock root** (page 648) was believed to clear the bloodstream of toxins.[32] It was used both internally and externally for psoriasis. Tradi-tional herbalists recommend 2 to 4 ml of burdock root tincture per day. For the dried root preparation in tablet or capsule form, the common amount to take is 1 to 2 grams three times per day. Many herbal preparations will combine burdock root with other alterative herbs, such as **yellow dock** (page 763), **red clover** (page 735), or **cleavers** (page 660). Burdock root has not been stud-ied in clinical trials to evaluate its efficacy in helping people with psoriasis.

Although clinical trials are lacking, some herbalists use the herb, **coleus** (page 660), in treating people with psoriasis.[33] Coleus extracts standardized to 18% forskolin are available, and 50 to 100 mg can be taken two to three times per day. Fluid extract can be taken in the amount of 2 to 4 ml three times per day.

An ointment containing **Oregon grape** (page 721) (10% concentration) has been shown in a clinical trial to be mildly effective against moderate psoriasis but not more severe cases.[34] Whole Oregon grape extracts were shown in one laboratory study to reduce inflammation often associated with psoriasis.[35] In this study, isolated alkaloids from Oregon grape did not have this effect. This suggests that there are other active ingredients be-sides alkaloids in Oregon grape. **Barberry** (page 632), which is very similar to Oregon grape, is believed to have similar effects. An ointment, 10% of which con-tains Oregon grape or barberry extract, can be applied topically three times per day.

Are there any side effects or interactions?
Refer to the individual herb for information about any side effects or interactions.

Holistic approaches that may be helpful

A preliminary trial treated 61 psoriasis patients with acupuncture that did not respond to conventional med-ical therapies. After an average of nine acupuncture treatments, 30 (49%) of the patients demonstrated al-most complete clearance of the lesions, and 14 (23%) of the patients experienced a resolution for two-thirds of lesions.[36] A controlled trial of 56 patients with psori-asis found, however, that acupuncture and "fake" acupuncture resulted in similar, modest effects.[37] More controlled trials are necessary to determine the useful-ness of acupuncture in the treatment of psoriasis.

Stress reduction has been shown to accelerate healing of psoriatic plaques in a blinded trial.[38] Thirty-seven people with psoriasis about to undergo light therapy were randomly assigned to receive either topical ultravi-olet light treatment alone or in combination with a mindfulness meditation-based stress reduction tech-nique guided by audiotape. Those who received the stress-reduction intervention showed resolution of their psoriasis significantly faster than those who did not.

Hypnosis and suggestion have been shown in some cases to have a positive effect on psoriasis, further sup-porting the role of stress in the disorder.[39] In one case report, 75% resolution of psoriasis resulted from using a hypnotic sensory-imagery technique.[40] Hypnosis may be especially useful for psoriasis that appears to be activated by stress.

RAYNAUD'S DISEASE

Raynaud's disease is a condition caused by constriction and spasms of small arteries, primarily in the hands after exposure to cold. Frequently, white or bluish discoloration of the hands (and sometimes toes, cheeks, nose, or ears) will occur after exposure to cold or emotional stress.

The cause of Raynaud's disease is unknown. A condition called Raynaud's phenomenon causes similar symptoms, but it is the result of connective tissue disease or exposure to certain chemicals. The same natural remedies are used to treat both disorders.

CHECKLIST FOR RAYNAUD'S DISEASE

Rating	Nutritional Supplements	Herbs
★★☆	Fish oil (page 514) Inositol hexaniacinate (page 537) (vitamin B₃)	
★☆☆	Evening primrose oil (page 511) L-carnitine (page 543) Magnesium (page 551)	Ginkgo biloba (page 681)

What are the symptoms of Raynaud's disease?

Fingers (generally not the thumb) or other affected parts of the body may feel numb or cold during an episode, and later, after warming, may become bright red with a throbbing painful sensation.

Medical treatments

Prescription drug treatment includes calcium channel blockers, such as nifedipine (Adalat, Procardia), diltiazem (Cardizem), and verapamil (Calan, Isoptin), and sympatholytic agents, including reserpine, prazosin (Minipress), doxazosin (Cardura), terazosin (Hytrin), methyldopa (Aldomet), and guanethidine (Ismelin).

In severe cases, sympathectomy (surgical interruption of sympathetic nerve pathways) may be recommended. People with Raynaud's disease are commonly advised to dress warmly during the winter and to avoid tobacco use and unnecessary exposure to cold, especially of the affected parts.

Lifestyle changes that may be helpful

Dressing warmly and wearing gloves or mittens often help prevent attacks of Raynaud's disease. Individuals with Raynaud's disease should not smoke, because nicotine decreases blood flow to the extremities. Women with Raynaud's disease should not use birth control pills, as this method of contraception can adversely affect circulation.

Nutritional supplements that may be helpful

In a double-blind trial, supplementation with 12 large capsules of **fish oil** (page 514) per day (providing 4 grams of eicosapentaenoic acid [EPA] per day) for 6 or 12 weeks reduced the severity of blood-vessel spasm in 5 of 11 people with Raynaud's phenomenon.[1] Fish oil was effective in people with primary Raynaud's disease, but not in those whose symptoms were secondary to another disorder.

Inositol hexaniacinate (page 537)—a variation on the B vitamin niacin—has been used with some success for relieving symptoms of Raynaud's disease.[2] In one study, 30 people with Raynaud's disease taking 4 grams of inositol hexaniacinate each day for three months showed less spasm of their arteries.[3] Another study, involving six people taking 3 grams per day of inositol hexaniacinate, again showed that this supplement improved peripheral circulation.[4] People taking this supplement in these amounts should be under the care of a doctor.

Fatty acids in **evening primrose oil** (page 511) (EPO) inhibit the formation of biochemical messengers (prostaglandins) that promote blood vessel constriction. A double-blind trial of 21 people with Raynaud's disease found that, compared with placebo, supplementation with EPO reduced the number and severity of attacks despite the fact that blood flow did not appear to increase.[5] Researchers have used 3,000–6,000 mg of EPO per day.

In one study, 12 people with Raynaud's disease were given **L-carnitine** (page 543) (1 gram three times a day) for 20 days.[6] After receiving L-carnitine, these people showed less blood-vessel spasm in their fingers in response to cold exposure.

Abnormalities of **magnesium** (page 551) metabolism have been reported in people with Raynaud's disease.[7] Symptoms similar to those seen with Raynaud's disease occur in people with magnesium deficiency,[8] probably because a deficiency of this mineral results in spasm of blood vessels.[9] Some doctors recommend that people with Raynaud's disease supplement with 200–600 mg of magnesium per day, although no clinical trials support this treatment.

Are there any side effects or interactions?
Refer to the individual supplement for information about any side effects or interactions.

Herbs that may be helpful

Ginkgo biloba (page 681) has been reported to improve the circulation in small blood vessels.[10] For that reason, some doctors recommend ginkgo for people with Raynaud's disease. One preliminary trial found that 160 mg of standardized ginkgo extract per day reduced pain in people with Raynaud's disease.[11] Larger clinical trials are needed to confirm ginkgo's effectiveness for this condition. Ginkgo is often used as a standardized extract (containing 24% ginkgo flavone glycosides and 6% terpene lactones). Doctors who recommend use of ginkgo often suggest that people take 120–160 mg per day.

Are there any side effects or interactions?
Refer to the individual herb for information about any side effects or interactions.

RECURRENT EAR INFECTIONS

Many children suffer recurrent infections of the middle ear, a condition also known as otitis media (OM).

Rating	Nutritional Supplements	Herbs
★★★	**Xylitol** (page 614)	
★☆☆	**Vitamin C** (page 604) **Zinc** (page 614)	Echinacea (page 669) Garlic (page 679) Linden (page 704) Mullein (page 713) St. John's wort (page 747)

CHECKLIST FOR RECURRENT EAR INFECTIONS

What are the symptoms of recurrent ear infections?

Ear infections can cause irritability, difficulty sleeping, runny nose, fever, fluid draining from the ear, loss of balance, mild to severe ear pain, and hearing difficulty. Untreated infections can cause permanent hearing impairment and can also spread to other parts of the head, including the brain. Frequent or persistent ear infections in children can reduce their hearing when normal hearing is critical for speech and language development.

Medical treatments

Over the counter analgesics, such as acetaminophen (Tylenol) and ibuprofen (Motrin), may help relieve **pain** (page 338) associated with acute ear infections.

Prescription drug treatment for acute ear infections usually consists of antibiotics, such as amoxicillin/clavulanate (Augmentin), azithromycin (Zithromax), and cephalexin (Keflex). Serous otitis, which results from the accumulation of fluid in the tubes that drain the middle ear, may eventually lead to an acute ear infection. Though antibiotics are frequently used for serous otitis, the benefit is often small and side effects or drug resistance may result. [1, 2]

Chronic infections or persistent fluid in the ear may require myringotomy, an operation in which small "tympanostomy tubes" are inserted in the affected eardrums. The procedure equalizes ear pressure and allows drainage of fluid from the middle ear. Enlarged or infected adenoids may be removed (adenoidectomy) during the myringotomy procedure. Though frequently performed, myringotomy has not consistently demonstrated long-term efficacy for preventing recurrent ear infections. [3]

Dietary changes that may be helpful

The incidence of **allergy** (page 14) among children with recurrent ear infections is much higher than among the general public.[4] In one study, more than half of all children with recurrent ear infections were found to be allergic to foods. Removing those foods led to significant improvement in 86% of the allergic children tested.[5] Other reports show similar results.[6, 7] In one preliminary study, children who were allergic to cow's milk were almost twice as likely to have recurrent ear infections as were children without the allergy.[8] People with recurrent ear infections should discuss allergy diagnosis and elimination with a doctor.

Although sugar intake has not been studied in relation to recurrent ear infections, eating sugar is known to impair **immune function** (page 255).[9, 10] Therefore, some doctors recommend that children with recurrent ear infections reduce or eliminate sugar from their diets.

Lifestyle changes that may be helpful

When parents smoke, their children are more likely to have recurrent ear infections.[11] It is important that children are not exposed to passive smoke.

Humidifiers are sometimes used to help children with recurrent ear infections, and animal research has supported this approach.[12] Nonetheless, human research studying the effect of humidity on recurrent ear infections has yet to conclusively show that use of humidifiers is of significant benefit.

Use of pacifiers in infants increases the risk of ear infections.[13, 14, 15]

Nutritional supplements that may be helpful

Xylitol (page 614), a natural sugar found in some fruits, interferes with the growth of some bacteria that may cause ear infections.[16, 17, 18] In double-blind research, children who regularly chewed gum sweetened with xylitol had a reduced risk of ear infections.[19, 20] However, when they only chewed the gum while experiencing respiratory infections, no effect on preventing ear infections was found.[21]

Vitamin C (page 604) supplementation has been reported to stimulate **immune function** (page 255).[22, 23] As a result, some doctors recommend between 500 mg and 1,000 mg of vitamin C per day for people with ear infections. Nonetheless, vitamin C supplementation has not been studied by itself in people with ear infections.

Zinc (page 614) supplements have also been reported to increase immune function.[24, 25] As a result, some doctors recommend zinc supplements for people with recurrent ear infections, suggesting 25 mg per day for adults and lower amounts for children. For example, a 30-pound child might be given 5 mg of zinc per day while suffering from OM. Nonetheless, zinc supplementation has not been studied in people with ear infections.

Are there any side effects or interactions?

Refer to the individual supplement for information about any side effects or interactions.

Herbs that may be helpful

Echinacea (page 669) has been reported to support healthy short-term **immune response** (page 255). As a result, it has been suggested that some children with recurrent ear infections may benefit from [26] 1–2 ml (depending on age) of echinacea tincture taken three times per day or more.[27] Doctors who use echinacea suggest that supplementation be started as soon as symptoms start to appear and continued until a few days after they are gone. Nonetheless, research has not been done to determine whether echinacea supplementation either reduces symptoms or prevents recurrence of ear infections.

Ear drops with **mullein** (page 713), **St. John's wort** (page 747), and **garlic** (page 679) in an oil or glycerin base are traditional remedies used to alleviate symptoms, particularly pain, during acute ear infections. No clinical trials have investigated the effects of these herbs in people with ear infections. Moreover, oil preparations may obscure a physician's view of the ear drum and should only be used with a healthcare professional's directions.

An unpublished clinical trial of children with colds found that **linden** (page 704) tea, aspirin, and bed rest were more effective than antibiotics at speeding recovery and reducing complications such as ear infection.[28] (Aspirin is no longer given to children due to the threat of Reye's syndrome.) However, no research has yet confirmed the use of linden for preventing ear infections.

Are there any side effects or interactions?

Refer to the individual herb for information about any side effects or interactions.

RESTLESS LEGS SYNDROME

Restless Legs Syndrome (RLS) is a poorly understood condition that causes leg symptoms shortly before going to sleep—symptoms that are temporarily relieved by movement. Occasionally the condition may also involve the arms. It can cause sudden jerking motions of the legs and can lead to **insomnia** (page 270).

RLS is most common in middle-aged women, **pregnant** (page 363) women, and people with severe kidney disease, **rheumatoid arthritis** (page 387), and nerve diseases (neuropathy). Restless legs have also been reported to occur in people with **varicose veins** (page 440) and to be relieved when the varicose veins are treated.[1]

What are the symptoms of RLS?

RLS is characterized by an almost irresistible urge to move the affected limbs because of unpleasant sensations beneath the skin, which are described as creeping, crawling, itching, aching, tingling, drawing, searing, pulling, or **painful** (page 338). These symptoms occur primarily in the calf area but may be felt anywhere in the legs or arms. The sensations are typically worse during rest or decreased activity, such as lying down or sitting for prolonged periods.

CHECKLIST FOR RESTLESS LEGS SYNDROME

Rating	Nutritional Supplements	Herbs
★★☆	**Iron** (page 540) (Only in people who are iron-deficient)	
★☆☆	**Folic acid** (page 520) **Vitamin E** (page 609)	

Medical treatments

Severe symptoms are treated with dopaminergic agents, such as pramipexole (Mirapex), pergolide (Permax), ropinirole (Requip), bromocriptine (Parlodel), and levodopa with carbidopa (Sinemet); benzodiazepines, including diazepam (Valium) and clonazepam (Klonopin); and opiates (codeine, oxycodone). Unfortunately, these medications tend to lose their effectiveness with nightly use.

Symptoms may also respond to correction of an underlying medical condition, such as **iron-deficiency anemia** (page 278), kidney disease, **diabetic** (page 152) neuropathy, amyloidosis, **chronic venous insufficiency** (page 116), or malignancy.

Dietary changes that may be helpful

Preliminary studies of large groups of people with reactive **hypoglycemia** (page 251) have reported that 8% have restless legs. These symptoms have been reported to improve following dietary modifications designed to regulate blood-sugar levels;[2] changes included a sugar-free, high-protein diet along with frequent snacking and at least one night-time feeding.[3] For patients with reactive hypoglycemia, some doctors recommend elimination of sugar, refined flour, caffeine, and alcohol from the diet; eating small, frequent meals; and eating whole grains, nuts and seeds, fresh fruits and vegetables, and fish. One study found caffeine ingestion to be associated with increased symptom severity in people with RLS.[4]

Lifestyle changes that may be helpful

Anecdotal evidence suggests that RLS symptoms may decrease with a cessation of smoking.[5] Although additional research is needed to confirm such reports, a trial of smoking cessation seems prudent for people who suffer from restless legs.

Nutritional supplements that may be helpful

Mild iron deficiency is common, even in people who are not anemic. When iron deficiency is the cause of RLS, supplementation with **iron** (page 540) has been reported to reduce the severity of the symptoms. In one trial, 74 mg of iron taken three times a day for two months, reduced symptoms in people with RLS.[6] In people who are not deficient in iron, iron supplementation has been reported to not help reduce symptoms of RLS.[7] Most people are not iron deficient, and taking too much can lead to adverse effects. Therefore, iron supplements should only be taken by people who have a diagnosed deficiency.

In some people with RLS, the condition may be genetic. People with familial RLS appear to have inherited an unusually high requirement for **folic acid** (page 520). Although not all people with RLS suffer from uncomfortable sensations, folate-deficient people with this condition always do.[8] In one report, 45 people were identified to be from families with folic acid-responsive RLS. The amount of folic acid required to relieve their symptoms was extremely large, ranging from 5,000 to 30,000 mcg per day.[9] Such amounts should only be taken under the supervision of a healthcare professional.

In a group of nine people with RLS, 300 IU of **vitamin E** (page 609) per day produced complete relief in seven.[10] Doctors who give vitamin E to people with RLS generally recommend at least 400 IU of vitamin E per day, and the full benefits may not become apparent for three months.[11]

Are there any side effects or interactions?
Refer to the individual supplement for information about any side effects or interactions.

RETINOPATHY

The term retinopathy indicates damage to the retina at the back of the eye. Several conditions, such as **diabetes** (page 152) and **high blood pressure** (page 246), can lead to the development of retinopathy.

What are the symptoms of retinopathy?

Retinopathy often has no early warning signs. If retinopathy progresses, partial or total blindness may result.

Retinopathy

CHECKLIST FOR RETINOPATHY		
Rating	**Nutritional Supplements**	**Herbs**
★★☆	**Proanthocyanidins** (page 574) **Vitamin E** (page 609) (for prevention of retrolental fibroplasia in premature infants, and for prevention of diabetic retinopathy)	**Bilberry** (page 634)
★☆☆	**Flavonoids** (page 516) (**quercetin** [page 580], rutin) Following are associated with diabetic retinopathy: **Selenium** (page 584), **vitamin A** (page 595), **vitamin C** (page 604), and **vitamin E** (page 609) (combined) **Magnesium** (page 551) **Vinpocetine** (page 594) **Vitamin B$_{12}$** (page 601) **Vitamin E** (page 609) (associated with abetalipoproteinemia)	*Ginkgo biloba* (page 681)

Medical treatments

In treating advanced retinopathy, doctors may use laser surgery to shrink abnormal blood vessels at the back of the eye. This treatment results in a loss of some peripheral (side) vision, a sacrifice that preserves the remaining field of vision. Laser surgery for retinopathy may also reduce color and **night vision** (page 326). A surgical alternative to laser surgery, called vitrectomy, is sometimes used if the eye has become cloudy due to hemorrhage (bleeding). Vitrectomy replaces the vitreous humor (transparent fluid in the interior of the eyeball behind the lens) with a salt solution.

Dietary changes that may be helpful

Animal studies suggest that dietary fructose may contribute to the development of retinopathy.[1] Although such an association has not been demonstrated in humans, some doctors advise their diabetic patients to avoid foods containing added fructose or high-fructose corn syrup. Fructose that occurs naturally in fruit has not been found to be harmful.[2]

Lifestyle changes that may be helpful

In a study of people with **diabetes** (page 152), cigarette smoking was found to be a risk factor for the development of retinopathy.[3] In a study of people with type 1 (insulin-dependent) diabetes, those who maintained their blood sugar levels close to the normal range had less severe retinopathy, compared with those whose blood sugar levels were higher.[4] Tighter control of blood-sugar levels can be achieved with a medically supervised program of diet, exercise, and, when appropriate, medication.

Nutritional supplements that may be helpful

Free radicals (page 467) have been implicated in the development and progression of several forms of retinopathy.[5] Retrolental fibroplasia, a retinopathy that occurs in some premature infants who have been exposed to high levels of oxygen, is an example of free radical-induced damage to the retina. In an analysis of the best published trials, large amounts of **vitamin E** (page 609) were found to reduce the incidence of severe retinopathy in premature infants by over 50%.[6, 7] Some of the evidence supporting the use of vitamin E in the prevention of retrolental fibroplasia comes from trials that have used 100 IU of vitamin E per 2.2 pounds of body weight in the form of oral supplementation.[8] Use of large amounts of vitamin E in the prevention of retrolental fibroplasia requires the supervision of a pediatrician.

Vitamin E has also been found to prevent retinopathy in people with a rare genetic disease known as abetalipoproteinemia.[9] People with this disorder lack a protein that transports fat-soluble nutrients, and can therefore develop deficiencies of vitamin E and other nutrients.

In one trial, vitamin E failed to improve vision in people with diabetic retinopathy,[10] although in a double-blind trial, people with type 1 **diabetes** (page 152) given very high amounts of vitamin E were reported to show a normalization of blood flow to the retina.[11] This finding has made researchers hopeful that vitamin E might help prevent diabetic retinopathy. However, no long-term trials have yet been conducted with vitamin E in the actual prevention of diabetic retinopathy.

Because oxidation damage is believed to play a role in the development of retinopathy, **antioxidant** (page 467) nutrients might be protective. One doctor has administered a daily regimen of 500 mcg **selenium** (page 584), 800 IU **vitamin E** (page 609), 10,000 IU **vita-**

min A (page 595), and 1,000 mg **vitamin C** (page 604) for several years to 20 people with diabetic retinopathy. During that time, 19 of the 20 people showed either improvement or no progression of their retinopathy.[12] People who wish to supplement with more than 250 mcg of selenium per day should consult a healthcare practitioner.

Low blood levels of **magnesium** (page 551) have been found to be a risk factor for retinopathy in white people with **diabetes** (page 152),[13, 14] but not in black people with diabetes.[15] So far, no studies have determined whether supplementing with magnesium would help prevent the development of retinopathy.

One study investigated the effect of adding 100 mcg per day of **vitamin B$_{12}$** (page 601) to the insulin injections of 15 children with diabetic retinopathy.[16] After one year, signs of retinopathy disappeared in 7 of 15 cases; after two years, 8 of 15 were free of retinopathy. Adults with diabetic retinopathy did not benefit from vitamin B$_{12}$ injections. Consultation with a physician is necessary before adding injectable vitamin B$_{12}$ to insulin.

Quercetin (page 580) (a **flavonoid** [page 516]) has been shown to inhibit the enzyme, aldose reductase.[17] This enzyme appears to contribute to worsening of diabetic retinopathy. However, because the absorption of quercetin is limited, it is questionable whether supplementing with quercetin can produce the tissue levels that are needed to inhibit aldose reductase. Although human studies have not been done using quercetin to treat retinopathy, some doctors prescribe 400 mg of quercetin three times per day. Another flavonoid, rutin, has been used with success to treat retinopathy in preliminary research.[18]

Proanthocyanidins (page 574) (OPCs), a group of flavonoids found in pine bark, grape seed, and other plant sources have been reported in preliminary French trials to help limit the progression of retinopathy.[19, 20] In one controlled trial, 60% of people with diabetes taking 150 mg per day of OPCs from grape seed extract had no progression of retinopathy compared to 47% of those taking a placebo.[21]

Preliminary studies have reported improved vision in people with various diseases of the retina who took 45 mg per day of **vinpocetine** (page 594).[22]

Are there any side effects or interactions?
Refer to the individual supplement for information about any side effects or interactions.

Herbs that may be helpful
Bilberry (page 634) extracts standardized to contain 25% anthocyanosides have been suggested as a treatment for people with early-stage **diabetic** (page 152) or **hypertensive** (page 246) retinopathy. In a small preliminary trial, people with various types of retinopathy, including diabetic retinopathy and **macular degeneration** (page 303), were given 600 mg of bilberry extract per day for one month.[23] While researchers found that the tendency to hemorrhage in the eye was reduced and that blood vessels were strengthened, there were no reports of improved vision. A small double-blind trial found that 160 mg of bilberry extract taken twice per day for one month led to similar improvements in blood-vessel health in the eye and slightly improved vision in people with diabetic and/or hypertensive retinopathy.[24] Larger and longer clinical trials are needed to establish the effectiveness of bilberry for treating retinopathies.

The use of 160 mg per day of a standardized extract of ***Ginkgo biloba*** (page 681) for six months has been reported in a small double-blind trial[25] to improve impaired visual function in people with mild diabetic retinopathy.

Are there any side effects or interactions?
Refer to the individual herb for information about any side effects or interactions.

RHEUMATOID ARTHRITIS

What do I need to know?
Self-care for rheumatoid arthritis can be approached in a number of ways—but it can be hard to know just where to start. To make it easier, our doctors recommend trying these simple steps first:

Check for food allergies or sensitivities
> Your doctor can help you figure out if certain foods are making your arthritis worse

Choose good oils
> Animal fats may contribute to inflammation, but olive oil may make you feel better

Try fish oil
> 3,000 mg of omega-3 fatty acids a day helps many people reduce pain

Give vitamin E a try
> Large amounts of vitamin E (1,800 IU) a day can help ease symptoms

CHECKLIST FOR RHEUMATOID ARTHRITIS

Rating	Nutritional Supplements	Herbs
★★★	**Borage oil** (page 475) **Fish oil** (page 514) (EPA/ **DHA** [page 509]) **Vitamin E** (page 609)	*Tripterygium wilfordii* Hook F
★★☆	**Cetyl myristoleate** (page 490) **DMSO** (page 508) **Evening primrose oil** (page 511) **Green-lipped mussel** (page 533) **Pantothenic acid** (vitamin B$_5$) (page 568) **Propolis** (page 579) (topical) **Selenium** (page 584) **Zinc** (page 614)	**Boswellia** (page 644) **Cayenne** (page 654) (topical) **Devil's claw** (page 668) **Turmeric** (page 753)
★☆☆	**Betaine HCl** (page 473) **Boron** (page 477) **Bromelain** (page 481) **Copper** (page 499) **D-phenylalanine** (page 568) (DPA)	**Burdock** (page 648) Cajeput oil (topical) Camphor oil **Cat's claw** (page 653) **Chaparral** (page 657) (topical) **Eucalyptus** (page 673) oil (topical) Fir needle oil (topical) **Ginger** (page 680) **Meadowsweet** (page 709) **Nettle** (page 714) **Picrorhiza** (page 728) Pine needle oil (topical) **Rosemary** (page 739) oil (topical) **Willow** (page 760) Yucca

About rheumatoid arthritis

Rheumatoid arthritis (RA) is a chronic inflammatory disease in which the immune system attacks the joints and sometimes other parts of the body. The cause of RA remains unknown.

What are the symptoms of rheumatoid arthritis?

The most common symptom of RA is joint pain and morning joint stiffness. Several joints on both sides of the body are usually affected, especially those of the

hands, wrists, knees, and feet. Affected joints may feel warm or appear swollen. People with RA may have other symptoms, including weakness, fatigue, weight loss, and, occasionally, fever.

Medical treatments

Over the counter medications, such as aspirin (Bayer, Ecotrin, Bufferin), ibuprofen (Motrin, Advil), and naproxen (Aleve), may help alleviate mild RA pain.

Prescription strength nonsteroidal anti-inflammatory drugs (NSAIDs), such as celecoxib (Celebrex), valdecoxib (Bextra), indomethacin (Indocin), nabumetone (Relafen), naproxen sodium (Anaprox, Naprosyn), and oxaprozin (Daypro), are commonly used to treat RA. Individuals with more severe forms of RA are treated with hydroxychloroquine (Plaquenil), sulfasalazine (Azulfidine), oral corticosteroids, penicillamine (Cuprimine), azathioprine (Imuran), cyclosporine (Neoral, Sandimmune), methotrexate (Rheumatrex), and cyclophosphamide (Cytoxan).

Joint replacement surgery is sometimes used in cases of severe deformity or disability.

Dietary changes that may be helpful

Feeding a high-fat diet to animals who are susceptible to autoimmune disease has increased the severity of RA.[1] People with RA have been reported to eat more fat, particularly animal fat, than those without RA.[2] In short-term studies, diets completely free of fat have helped people with RA.[3] Since at least some dietary fat is essential for humans, though, the significance of this finding is not clear.

Strictly vegetarian diets that are also very low in fat have been reported to reduce RA symptoms.[4, 5] In the 1950s through the 1970s, Max Warmbrand, a naturopathic doctor, used a very low-fat diet to treat people with RA. He recommended a diet free of meat, dairy, chemicals, sugar, eggs, and processed foods.[6] A short-term (ten weeks) study employing a similar approach failed to produce beneficial effects.[7] Long before publication of that negative report, however, Dr. Warmbrand had claimed that his diet took at least six months to achieve noticeable results. In one trial lasting 14 weeks—still significantly less than six months—a pure vegetarian, gluten-free (no wheat, rye, or barley) diet was gradually changed to permit dairy, leading to improvement in both symptoms and objective laboratory measures of disease.[8] The extent to which a low-fat vegetarian diet (or one low in animal fat) would help people with RA remains unclear.

Preliminary evidence suggests that consumption of olive oil, rich in oleic acid, may *decrease* the risk of developing RA.[9] One trial in which people with RA received either fish oil or olive oil, found that olive oil capsules providing 6.8 grams of oleic acid per day for 24 weeks produced modest clinical improvement and beneficial changes in **immune function** (page 255). However, as there was no placebo group in that trial, the possibility of a placebo effect cannot be ruled out.[10]

Fasting has been shown to improve both signs and symptoms of RA, but most people have relapsed after the returning to a standard diet.[11, 12] When fasting was followed by a 12-month vegetarian diet, however, the benefits of fasting appeared to persist.[13, 14] It is not known why the combination of these dietary programs (i.e., fasting followed by a vegetarian diet) might be helpful, and the clinical trial that investigated this combination[15] has been criticized both for its design and interpretation.[16, 17, 18]

Food sensitivities develop when pieces of intact protein in food are able to cross through the intestinal barrier. Many patients with RA have been noted to have increased intestinal permeability, especially when experiencing symptoms,[19] and RA has been linked to **allergies and food sensitivities** (page 14).[20] In many people, RA worsens when they eat foods to which they are allergic or sensitive and improves by avoiding these foods.[21, 22, 23, 24] In one study, the vast majority of RA patients had elevated levels of antibodies to milk, wheat, or both, suggesting a high incidence of allergy to these substances.[25] English researchers have reported that one-third of people with RA may be able to control their disease completely through allergy elimination.[26] Identification and elimination of symptom-triggering foods should be done with the help of a physician.

Drinking four or more cups of coffee per day has been associated with an increased risk of developing rheumatoid arthritis in preliminary research.[27]

Lifestyle changes that may be helpful

Although exercise may initially increase **pain** (page 338), gentle exercises help people with RA.[28, 29] Women with RA taking low-dose steroid therapy can safely participate in a weight-bearing exercise program with many positive effects on physical function, activity and fitness levels, and bone mineral density, and with no aggravation of disease activity.[30] Many doctors recommend swimming, stretching, or walking to people with RA.

Nutritional supplements that may be helpful

People with RA have been reported to have an impaired **antioxidant** (page 467) system, making them more susceptible to free radical damage.[31] **Vitamin E** (page 609) is an important antioxidant, protecting many tissues, including joints, against oxidative damage. Low vitamin E levels in the joint fluid of people with RA have been reported.[32] In a double-blind trial, approximately 1,800 IU per day of vitamin E was found to reduce pain from RA.[33] Two other double-blind trials (using similar high levels of vitamin E) reported that vitamin E had approximately the same effectiveness in reducing symptoms of RA as anti-inflammatory drugs.[34, 35] In other double-blind trials, 600 IU of vitamin E taken twice daily was significantly more effective than placebo in reducing RA, although laboratory measures of inflammation remained unchanged.[36, 37]

Oils containing the omega-6 fatty acid gamma linolenic acid (GLA)—**borage** (page 475) oil,[38, 39, 40] black currant seed oil,[41] and **evening primrose oil** (page 511) (EPO)[42, 43]—have been reported to be effective in the treatment for people with RA. Although the best effects have been reported with use of borage oil, that may be because more GLA was used in borage oil trials (1.1–2.8 grams per day) compared with trials using black currant seed oil or EPO. The results with EPO have been mixed and confusing, possibly because the placebo used in those trials (olive oil) may have anti-inflammatory activity. In a double-blind trial, positive results were seen when EPO was used in combination with fish oil.[44] GLA appears to be effective because it is converted in part to prostaglandin E_1, a hormone-like substance known to have anti-inflammatory activity.

Many double-blind trials have proven that omega-3 fatty acids in **fish oil** (page 514), called EPA and **DHA** (page 509), partially relieve symptoms of RA.[45, 46, 47, 48, 49, 50] The effect results from the anti-inflammatory activity of fish oil.[51] Many doctors recommend 3 grams per day of EPA and DHA, an amount commonly found in 10 grams of fish oil. Positive results can take three months to become evident. In contrast, a double-blind trial found **flaxseed oil** (page 517) (source of another form of omega-3 fatty acid) not to be effective for RA patients.[52]

Cetyl myristoleate (page 490) (CMO) has been proposed to act as a joint "lubricant" and anti-inflammatory agent. In a double-blind trial, people with various types of arthritis that had failed to respond to nonsteroidal anti-inflammatory drugs received either CMO (540 mg per day orally for 30 days) or a placebo.[53] These people also applied CMO or placebo topically, according to their perceived need. Sixty-four percent of those receiving CMO improved, compared with 14% of those receiving placebo. More research is needed to determine whether CMO has a legitimate place in the treatment options offered RA patients.

The use of dimethyl sulfoxide (**DMSO** [page 508]) for therapeutic applications is controversial in part because some claims made by advocates appear to extend beyond current scientific evidence, and in part because topical use greatly increases the absorption of any substance that happens to be on the skin, including molecules that are toxic to the body. Nonetheless, there is some preliminary evidence that when applied to the skin, it has anti-inflammatory properties and alleviates pain, such as that associated with RA.[54, 55] DMSO appears to reduce pain by inhibiting the transmission of pain messages by nerves.[56] It comes in different strengths and degrees of purity, and certain precautions must be taken when applying DMSO. For these reasons, DMSO should be used only under the supervision of a doctor.

Research suggests that people with RA may be partially deficient in **pantothenic acid** (page 568) (vitamin B5).[57] In one placebo-controlled trial, those with RA had less morning stiffness, disability, and pain when they took 2,000 mg of pantothenic acid per day for two months.[58]

Supplementation with New Zealand **green-lipped mussel** (page 533) *(Perna canaliculus)* significantly improved RA symptoms in 68% of participants in a double-blind trial.[59] Other studies have been carried out, some of which have confirmed these findings, while others have not.[60, 61, 62, 63, 64] In a recent double-blind trial, use of green-lipped mussel as a lipid extract (210 mg per day) or a freeze-dried powder (1,150 mg per day) for three months led to a decrease in joint tenderness and morning stiffness, and to better overall function.[65] However, members of the Australian Rheumatism Association have reported side effects, such as **stomach upset** (page 260), **gout** (page 208), and skin rashes, occurring in people taking certain New Zealand green-lipped mussel extracts. One case of **hepatitis** (page 220) has been reported in association with the use of a New Zealand green-lipped mussel extract.[66]

Deficient **zinc** (page 614) levels have been reported in people with RA.[67] Some trials have found that zinc reduced RA symptoms,[68] but others have not.[69, 70] Some suggest that zinc might only help those who are zinc-deficient,[71] and, although there is no universally

accepted test for zinc deficiency, some doctors check white-blood-cell zinc levels.

People with RA have been found to have lower **selenium** (page 584) levels than healthy people.[72, 73] One[74] of two double-blind trials using at least 200 mcg of selenium per day for three to six months found that selenium supplementation led to a significant reduction in pain and joint inflammation in RA patients, but the other reported no beneficial effect.[75] More controlled trials are needed to determine whether selenium reduces symptoms in people with RA.

Copper (page 499) acts as an anti-inflammatory agent needed to activate superoxide dismutase (SOD), an enzyme that protects joints from inflammation. People with RA tend toward copper deficiency[76] and copper supplementation has been shown to increase SOD levels in humans.[77] The *Journal of the American Medical Association* quoted one researcher as saying that while "Regular aspirin had 6% the anti-inflammatory activity of [cortisone] . . . copper [when added to aspirin] had 130% the activity [of cortisone]."[78]

Several copper compounds have been used successfully in treating people with RA,[79] and a controlled trial using copper bracelets reported surprisingly effective results compared with the effect of placebo bracelets.[80] Under certain circumstances, however, copper can *increase* inflammation in rheumatoid joints.[81] Moreover, the form of copper most consistently reported to be effective, copper aspirinate (a combination of copper and aspirin), is not readily available. Nonetheless, some doctors suggest a trial of 1–3 mg of copper per day for at least several months.

Boron (page 477) supplementation at 3–9 mg per day may be beneficial, particularly in treating people with juvenile RA, according to very preliminary research.[82] The benefit of using boron to treat people with RA remains unproven.

D-phenylalanine (page 568) has been used with mixed results to treat chronic **pain** (page 338), including pain caused by RA.[83] No research has evaluated the effectiveness of DL-phenylalanine, a related supplement, in treating people with RA. The effect of either form of phenylalanine in the treatment of people with RA remains unproven.

Many years ago, two researchers reported that some individuals with RA had inadequate **stomach acid** (page 260).[84] Hydrochloric acid, called HCl by chemists, is known to help break down protein in the stomach before the protein can be absorbed in the intestines. Allergies generally occur when inadequately broken down protein is absorbed from the intestines. Therefore, some doctors believe that when stomach acid is low, supplementing with **betaine HCl** (page 473) can reduce food-allergy reactions by helping to break down protein before it is absorbed. In theory such supplementation might help some people with RA, but no research has investigated whether betaine HCl actually reduces symptoms of RA.

Supplementation with betaine HCl should be limited to people who have a proven deficit in stomach acid production. Of doctors who prescribe betaine HCl, the amount used varies with the size of the meal and with the amount of protein ingested. Although typical amounts recommended by doctors range from 600 to 2,400 mg of betaine HCl per meal, use of betaine HCl needs to be monitored by a healthcare practitioner and tailored to the needs of the individual.

Bromelain (page 481) has significant anti-inflammatory activity. Many years ago in a preliminary trial, people with RA who were given bromelain supplements experienced a decrease in joint swelling and improvement in joint mobility.[85] The amount of bromelain used in that trial was 20–40 mg, three or four times per day, in the form of enteric-coated tablets. The authors provided no information about the strength of activity in the bromelain supplements that were used. (Today, better quality bromelain supplements are listed in gelatin-dissolving units [GDU] or in milk-clotting units [MCU].) Enteric-coating protects bromelain from exposure to stomach acid. Most commercially available bromelain products today are not enteric-coated.

Propolis (page 579) is the resinous substance collected by bees from the leaf buds and bark of trees, especially poplar and conifer trees. Anti-inflammatory effects from topical application of propolis extract have been noted in one animal study,[86] and a preliminary controlled trial found that patients with RA treated with topical propolis extract (amount and duration not noted) had greater improvements in symptoms compared to placebo.[87]

Are there any side effects or interactions?
Refer to the individual supplement for information about any side effects or interactions.

Herbs that may be helpful
Boswellia (page 644) is an herb used in Ayurvedic medicine (the traditional medicine of India) to treat arthritis. Boswellia has reduced symptoms of RA in most reports.[88] While some double-blind trials[89] using

boswellia have produced positive results, some equivocal results[90] and negative findings have also been reported.[91] In some trials where boswellia has appeared ineffective, though, patients have been allowed to continue use of nonsteroidal anti-inflammatory drugs (NSAIDs). Such use of NSAIDs can confound experimental results, because boswellia and NSAIDs work in a similar fashion to reduce inflammation. Some doctors suggest using 400–800 mg of gum resin extract in capsules or tablets three times per day.

A cream containing small amounts of capsaicin, a substance found in **cayenne** (page 654) pepper, can help relieve pain when rubbed onto arthritic joints, according to the results of a double-blind trial.[92] Capsaicin achieves this effect by depleting nerves of a pain-mediating neurotransmitter called substance P. Although application of capsaicin cream initially causes a burning feeling, the burning lessens with each application and disappears for most people in a few days. Creams containing 0.025–0.075% of capsaicin are available and may be applied to the affected joints three to five times a day. A doctor should supervise this treatment.

Devil's claw (page 668) has anti-inflammatory and analgesic actions. Several open and double-blind trials have been conducted on the anti-arthritic effects of devil's claw.[93] The results of these trials have been mixed, so it is unclear whether devil's claw lives up to its reputation in traditional herbal medicine as a remedy for people with RA. A typical amount used is 800 mg of encapsulated extracts three times per day or powder in the amount of 4.5–10 grams per day.

Turmeric (page 753) is a yellow spice often used to make curry dishes. The active constituent, curcumin, is a potent anti-inflammatory compound that protects the body against **free radical** (page 467) damage.[94] A double-blind trial found curcumin to be an effective anti-inflammatory agent in RA patients.[95] The amount of curcumin usually used is 400 mg three times per day.

Ginger (page 680) is another Ayurvedic herb used to treat people with arthritis. A small number of case studies suggest that taking 6–50 grams of fresh or powdered ginger per day may reduce the symptoms of RA.[96] A combination formula containing ginger, turmeric, boswellia, and **ashwagandha** (page 629) has been shown in a double-blind trial to be slightly more effective than placebo for RA;[97] the amounts of herbs used in this trial are not provided by the investigators.

The historic practice of applying **nettle** (page 714) topically (with the intent of causing stings to relieve arthritis) has been assessed by a questionnaire study.[98]

The nettle stings were reported to be safe except for causing a sometimes painful, sometimes numbing rash lasting 6 to 24 hours. Further studies are required to determine whether this practice is therapeutically effective.

Yucca, a traditional remedy, is a desert plant that contains soap-like components known as saponins. Yucca tea (7 or 8 grams of the root simmered in a pint of water for 15 minutes) is often drunk for symptom relief three to five times per day. The effects of yucca in the treatment of people with RA has not been studied.

Burdock root (page 648) has been used historically both internally and externally to treat painful joints. Its use in the treatment of people with RA remains unproven.

Although **willow** (page 760) is slow acting as a pain reliever, the effect is thought to last longer than the effect of willow's synthetic cousin, aspirin. One double-blind trial found that willow bark combined with guaiac, **sarsaparilla** (page 742), **black cohosh** (page 637), and poplar (each tablet contained 100 mg of willow bark, 40 mg of guaiac, 35 mg of black cohosh, 25 mg of sarsaparilla, and 17 mg of poplar) relieved pain due to RA better than placebo over a two-month period.[99] The exact amount of the herbal combination used in the trial is not given, however, and patients were allowed to continue their other pain medications. Clinical trials on willow alone for RA are lacking. Some experts suggest that willow may be taken one to four weeks before results are noted.[100]

Topical applications of several botanical oils are approved by the German government for relieving symptoms of RA.[101] These include primarily cajeput (*Melaleuca leucodendra*) oil, camphor oil, **eucalyptus** (page 673) oil, fir (*Abies alba* and *Picea abies*) needle oil, pine (*Pinus* spp.) needle oil, and **rosemary** (page 739) oil. A few drops of oil or more can be applied to painful joints several times a day as needed. Most of these topical applications are based on historical use and are lacking modern clinical trials to support their effectiveness in treating RA.

Preliminary studies conducted in India with the herb **picrorhiza** (page 728) show a benefit for people with RA.[102] Currently, this therapeutic effect remains weakly supported and therefore unproven.

Southwestern Native American and Hispanic herbalists have long recommended topical use of **chaparral** (page 657) on joints affected by RA. The anti-inflammatory effects of chaparral found in test tube research suggests this practice might have value, though clinical trials have not yet investigated chaparral's usefulness in people with RA. Chaparral should not be used internally for this purpose.

Cat's claw (page 653) has been used traditionally for RA, but no human trials have investigated this practice.

Meadowsweet (page 709) was used historically for a wide variety of conditions, including treating rheumatic complaints of the joints and muscles.[103]

In a preliminary trial, an extract of the Chinese herbal remedy Tripterygium wilfordii Hook F, in the amount of 360 to 570 mg per day for 16 weeks, produced improvement in symptoms and laboratory tests in eight of nine patients with rheumatoid arthritis. However, one patient developed high blood pressure during the trial.[104] In a double-blind trial, an extract of this herb, given in the amount of 360 mg per day for 20 weeks was significantly more effective than a placebo at reducing disease activity.[105] A lower amount (160 mg/day) was also more effective than the placebo, but the difference was not statistically significant. No serious side effects were reported.

Are there any side effects or interactions?
Refer to the individual herb for information about any side effects or interactions.

Holistic approaches that may be helpful

The role of manipulation in managing RA has received little study. In one small controlled trial,[106] patients with RA were found to have more tenderness at certain body locations compared to healthy people. Six minutes of gentle spinal manipulation decreased this tenderness temporarily in the spinal areas but not in areas around the knees or ankles. The effect of manipulation on the symptoms or progression of RA has not been investigated.

RICKETS/OSTEOMALACIA

Rickets is an abnormal bone formation in children resulting from inadequate **calcium** (page 483) in their bones.

This lack of calcium can result from inadequate dietary calcium,[1] inadequate exposure to sunshine (needed to make vitamin D), or from not eating enough **vitamin D** (page 607)—a nutrient needed for calcium absorption. Vitamin D is found in animal foods, such as egg yolks and dairy products.

Rickets can also be caused by conditions that impair absorption of vitamin D and/or calcium, even when these nutrients are consumed in appropriate amounts. Activation of vitamin D in the body requires normal liver and kidney function. Damage to either organ can cause rickets. Some variations of rickets do not respond well to supplementation with vitamin D and calcium. Proper diagnosis must be made by a healthcare professional.

Osteomalacia is an adult version of rickets. This condition is treated with vitamin D, sometimes in combination with calcium supplements. Osteomalacia should be diagnosed, and its treatment monitored, by a doctor.

CHECKLIST FOR RICKETS		
Rating	Nutritional Supplements	Herbs
★★★	Calcium (page 483) Vitamin D (page 607)	

What are the symptoms of rickets and osteomalacia?

In children, symptoms of rickets include delayed sitting, crawling, and walking; pain when walking; and the development of bowlegs or knock-knees. Symptoms of osteomalacia include bowing of the legs and a decrease in height.

Medical treatments

Over the counter supplementation with oral vitamin D is recommended.

Treatment of rickets and osteomalacia sometimes include intravenous **calcium** (page 483). Some health care providers may recommend the use of artificial ultraviolet B radiation or increased exposure to sunlight.

Dietary changes that may be helpful

Dietary changes should only be considered if a medical professional has diagnosed rickets and determined the cause to be a simple nutritional deficiency. Rickets is more likely to occur in a child consuming a pure vegan diet (which does not include animal products and thus no vitamin D) than in a child consuming milk or other animal foods. Dark skin and/or a lack of sunlight exposure (which reduces the amount of vitamin D made in the skin) also increase the risk of developing rickets.

The few foods that contain **vitamin D** (page 607) include egg yolks, butter, vitamin D-fortified milk, fish liver oil, breast milk, and infant formula. **Calcium** (page 483), in addition to being present in breast milk and formula, is found in dairy products, sardines, salmon (canned with edible bones), green leafy vegetables, and tofu. Vegans may use supplements instead of eggs and dairy as sources for both calcium and vitamin D.

Lifestyle changes that may be helpful

Direct exposure of the skin (i.e., hands, face, arms, etc.) to sunlight stimulates the body to manufacture **vitamin D** (page 607). However, both clothing and use of a sunscreen prevent the ultraviolet light that triggers the formation of vitamin D from reaching the skin. Depending on latitude, sunlight during the winter may not provide enough ultraviolet light to promote adequate vitamin D production. At other times during the year, even 30 minutes of exposure per day will usually lead to large increases in the amount of vitamin D made. If it is difficult to get sunlight exposure, full-spectrum lighting can be used to stimulate vitamin D production.

Nutritional supplements that may be helpful

Vitamin D (page 607) and **calcium** (page 483) supplements should be used to treat rickets only if a medical professional has diagnosed rickets and has also determined the cause is a nutritional deficiency. Amounts needed to treat rickets should be determined by a doctor and will depend on the age, weight, and condition of the child. For *prevention* of rickets, 400 IU of vitamin D per day is considered reasonable. Doctors often suggest 1,600 IU per day for *treating* rickets caused by a lack of dietary vitamin D.

The National Institutes of Health has stated that the following amounts of total calcium intake per day are useful to *prevent* rickets:

- 400 mg until six months of age
- 600 mg from six to twelve months
- 800 mg from one year through age five
- 800–1,200 mg from age six until age ten

Are there any side effects or interactions?
Refer to the individual supplement for information about any side effects or interactions.

SCHIZOPHRENIA

Schizophrenia is a common and serious mental disorder characterized by loss of contact with reality.

The behaviors, described below, must be present for

six months or longer to establish a diagnosis. Approximately 1% of the world's population is affected by this condition. Schizophrenia is more common among lower socioeconomic classes in urban areas, perhaps because its disabling effects lead to unemployment and poverty. In the United States, 25% of all hospital beds are occupied by people with schizophrenia.

	CHECKLIST FOR SCHIZOPHRENIA	
Rating	**Nutritional Supplements**	**Herbs**
★★★	**Folic acid** (page 520) (if deficient) **Glycine** (page 532)	
★★☆	**Melatonin** (page 555) (for sleep disturbances only) **Niacin/niacinamide** (page 598) (vitamin B_3) **Omega-3 fatty acids** (page 509) (fish oil) **Vitamin B_6** (page 600) **Vitamin C** (page 604)	*Ginkgo biloba* (page 681) (in combination with haloperidol)
★☆☆	D-Serine **Vitamin B_{12}** (page 601)	

What are the symptoms of schizophrenia?

Symptoms and signs of schizophrenia include loss of contact with reality (psychosis), auditory and visual hallucinations (false perceptions), delusions (false beliefs), abnormal thinking, restricted range of emotions, diminished motivation, and disturbed work and social functioning. People with schizophrenia may also engage in speech that does not make sense, exhibit silly or childlike facial expressions, and experience poor memory or confusion.

Medical treatments

Antipsychotic medications, also known as major tranquilizers, are used to treat schizophrenia. Commonly prescribed drugs include olanzapine (Zyprexa), quetiapine (Seroquel), risperidone (Risperdal), and clozapine (Clozaril). Older agents, such as haloperidol (Haldol), chlorpromazine (Thorazine), and fluphenazine (Prolixin), are also prescribed. Other medications might be prescribed to control **depression** (page 145), **anxiety** (page 30), or hostility in schizophrenic individuals.

Psychological counseling or electroconvulsive therapy (electrical current applied to the brain) may also be recommended.

Dietary changes that may be helpful

For many years there has been speculation that certain dietary proteins may contribute to the symptoms of schizophrenia.[1, 2, 3] Gluten, a protein from wheat and some other grains, and to a lesser extent casein, a dairy protein, have been the targets of research on food sensitivities as contributors to schizophrenia.[4] People with schizophrenia have been shown to be more likely to have **immune** (page 255) reactions to these proteins, than the general population.[5] A preliminary trial of a gluten-free/dairy-free diet found that patients with schizophrenia improved on the diet and had shorter hospital stays than those eating normal diets.[6] The results of double-blind trials, however, have been inconsistent. The gluten-free/dairy-free diet improved responses to medications in one controlled trial.[7] These improvements were lost and symptoms of schizophrenia were aggravated when gluten was re-introduced in a "blinded" fashion. Another clinical trial found similar positive responses in only 8% of patients.[8] Other controlled trials have found no improvement when gluten and dairy were removed from the diet.[9, 10] In one clinical trial, blinded reintroduction of gluten appeared to cause *improvement* of symptoms.[11] These results suggest that some, but not all, people with schizophrenia may benefit from a gluten-free/dairy-free diet.

Lifestyle changes that may be helpful

Exercise has long been recognized for its benefits in treating mild to moderate **depression** (page 145) and there is some evidence that it may also be helpful in reducing **anxiety** (page 30).[12] In one reported case, physical activity improved the functioning of a man diagnosed with schizophrenia.[13] In another reported case, aggressive outbursts in a schizophrenic patient were reduced after he began exercising.[14] A preliminary trial of an exercise program for hospitalized psychiatric patients with varying diagnoses resulted in significantly reduced symptoms of depression and an insignificant trend towards reduced anxiety.[15] Additional research is needed to determine the specific benefits of exercise in people with schizophrenia.

Nutritional supplements that may be helpful

People with schizophrenia may have a greater tendency to be deficient in **folic acid** (page 520), than the general population[16] and they may show improvement when given supplements. A preliminary trial found that, among schizophrenic patients with folic acid deficiency, those given folic acid supplements had more improvement, and shorter hospital stays than those not given supplements.[17] In a double-blind trial, a very high amount of folic acid (15 mg daily) was given to schizophrenic patients being treated with psychiatric medications who had low or borderline folic acid levels. The patients receiving the folic acid supplements had significant improvement, which became more significant over the six-month course of the trial.[18] The symptoms of folic acid deficiency can be similar to those of schizophrenia, and two cases of wrong "schizophrenia" diagnoses have been reported.[19, 20] In one of these cases, an initial supplement of 20 mg daily of folic acid and a maintenance supplemental intake of 10 mg daily, led to resolution of symptoms.[21]

There have been several reports of **glycine** (page 532) reducing the symptoms of people with schizophrenia who were unresponsive to drug therapy.[22] Large amounts of glycine (0.8 gram per 2.2 pounds of body weight per day) have been shown to reduce negative symptoms of schizophrenia and improve psychiatric rating scores in one preliminary trial;[23] however, these results have not been repeated in later trials using similar (very high) amounts.[24, 25] Earlier double-blind trials found significant improvements in **depression** (page 145) and mental symptoms in people with schizophrenia who took glycine for six weeks.[26, 27] Most trials demonstrated a moderate improvement in schizophrenia symptoms in those taking glycine supplements.[28] Long-term supplementation with high amounts of glycine may be toxic to nerve tissue, however. Some preliminary successes have been reported using smaller amounts of glycine, such as 10 grams per day.[29] Long-term studies on the safety of glycine therapy are needed.

The term "orthomolecular psychiatry" was coined by Linus Pauling in 1968 to refer to the treatment of psychiatric illnesses with substances (such as vitamins) that are normally present in the body. In orthomolecular psychiatry, high amounts of vitamins are sometimes used, not to correct a deficiency *per se,* but to create a more optimal biochemical environment. The mainstay of the orthomolecular approach to schizophrenia is **niacin** (page 598) or **niacinamide** (page 598) (**vitamin B₃** [page 598]) in high amounts. In early double-blind trials, 3 grams of niacin daily resulted in a doubling of the recovery rate, a 50% reduction in hospitalization rates, and a dramatic reduction in suicide rates.[30] In a preliminary trial, some schizophrenic patients continued a course of vitamins (4 to 10 grams of niacin or niacinamide, 4 grams of **vitamin C** [page 604], and 50 mg or more of **vitamin B₆** [page 600]) after being dis-

charged from the hospital, while another group of patients discontinued the vitamins upon discharge. Both groups continued to take their psychiatric medications. Those who continued to take the vitamins had a 50% lower re-admission rate compared with those who did not.[31] Several later double-blind trials, including trials undertaken by the Canadian Mental Health Association, have been unable to reproduce these positive results.[32, 33] Early supporters of niacin therapy contend that many of these trials were poorly designed.[34] One clinical trial reported no greater improvement in a group of schizophrenic patients given 6 grams of niacin than in others given 3 mg of niacin; all patients were also being treated with psychiatric medications.[35]

There are potential side-effects of niacin therapy, including an uncomfortable flushing sensation, dermatitis (skin inflammation), **heartburn** (page 260), aggravation of **peptic ulcers** (page 349), increased blood sugar, increased panic and **anxiety** (page 30), and elevation of liver **enzymes** (page 506), which may indicate damage to liver cells. A positive side effect of niacin therapy is reduction of **cholesterol levels** (page 223). Some of these effects, such as flushing, gastric upset, and reduction of serum cholesterol, do not occur with the use of **niacinamide** (page 598).[36] Because of the seriousness of some of these side effects, high amounts of **niacin** (page 598) should not be used without the supervision of a healthcare practitioner.

Vitamin B₆ (page 600) has been used in combination with niacin in the orthomolecular approach to schizophrenia. Pioneers of orthomolecular medicine reported benefits from this combination. However, although two placebo-controlled trials found significant improvement when schizophrenic patients were given either 3 grams of niacin or 75 mg of pyridoxine along with their psychiatric medications, this improvement was lost when the two vitamins were combined.[37, 38] In a double-blind trial, schizophrenic patients were given either a vitamin program based on their individual laboratory tests or a placebo (25 mg of **vitamin C** [page 604]) in addition to their psychiatric medications. The vitamin program included large amounts of various B vitamins, as well as vitamin C and **vitamin E** (page 609). After five months, the number of patients who improved was not different in the vitamin group compared with the placebo group.[39]

Clinical trials of the effects of **vitamin B₆** (page 600) have yielded differing results. The results of supplementation with 100 mg daily in one schizophrenic patient included dramatic reduction in side effects from medication, as well as reduction in schizophrenic symptoms.[40] In a preliminary trial, 60 mg per day of vitamin B$_6$ resulted in symptomatic improvement in only 5% of schizophrenic patients after four weeks.[41] Another preliminary trial, however, found that a higher amount of vitamin B$_6$—50 mg three times daily given for eight to twelve weeks—in addition to psychiatric medications, did bring about significant improvements in schizophrenic patients. These patients experienced a better sense of well-being, increased motivation, and greater interest in their "personal habits and their environment."[42]

Up to 6 grams daily of **vitamin C** (page 604) has been reported to be beneficial for people with schizophrenia;[43, 44] in one case the addition of 400 IU daily of vitamin E enhanced this benefit.[45] A small preliminary trial using 8 grams daily of vitamin C showed decreases in hallucinations, suspiciousness, and unusual and disorganized thoughts in 77% of schizophrenic patients.[46] In all reported cases, patients were also being treated with sychiatric medications. Some early studies found no difference between blood and urine vitamin C levels in schizophrenics and non-schizophrenics, either before or after supplementation.[47, 48, 49] However, later studies found that blood and urine levels of vitamin C were lower in schizophrenics than in non-schizophrenics before and after a single 1,000 mg "load" of vitamin C was taken. After four weeks of daily supplementation with 1,000 mg of vitamin C, blood levels became the same, but urinary levels remained lower in the schizophrenic group, leading the researchers to conclude that the amount of vitamin C required by people with schizophrenia may be greater than that of the general population.[50, 51]

There are two different classes of essential fatty acids: omega-6 fatty acids and **omega-3 fatty acids** (page 509). There is considerable evidence these fatty acids are deficient, or are not used properly, in people with schizophrenia.[52, 53, 54, 55, 56, 57] Some investigators suggest this altered fatty acid metabolism may be involved in the increased need for **niacin** (page 598) seen in some schizophrenic patients.[58] A case has been reported in which a man with schizophrenia had dramatic and sustained improvement while being supplemented with 2 grams daily of omega-3 fatty acids.[59] In a preliminary trial, schizophrenic patients receiving omega-3 fatty acids showed improvement in symptoms, as well as a reduction in adverse effects from their anti-psychotic medications.[60] Another study found that people with schizophrenia had lower blood levels of both omega-3

and omega-6 fatty acids, compared with non-schizophrenic people, even though both groups were consuming similar amounts of these fatty acids.[61] In a separate preliminary study, higher intake of omega-3 fatty acids was associated with less severe disease, and supplementation with 10 grams of concentrated **fish oil** (page 514), a source of omega-3 fatty acids, led to significant improvement in symptoms over a six-week period.[62]

However, in a double-blind trial that included 87 patients with chronic schizophrenia or a related illness (schizoaffective disorder), supplementation with 3 grams per day of eicosapentaenoic acid (one of the omega-3 fatty acids found in fish oil) was ineffective.[63] The patients in this negative study were older and had been ill for longer, compared with patients in earlier studies who improved with omega-3 fatty acid supplementation.

Several clinical trials have examined the effects of supplementation with essential fatty acids in people with schizophrenia, with inconsistent results.[64, 65, 66, 67] While the results of trials using omega-3 fatty acids are promising, further double-blind trials are needed to establish whether fatty acid supplementation is an effective therapy for schizophrenia. Trials of omega-6 fatty acids (like GLA from **borage** [page 475] oil) have yielded predominantly negative results.[68]

The results of one double-blind trial indicate that **melatonin** (page 555) supplementation improves sleep quality in people with schizophrenia.[69] In one study, all patients with a diagnosis of schizophrenia were found to have low melatonin output. Replacement of melatonin with 2 mg of a controlled-release supplement per day for three weeks improved sleep duration and quality compared to placebo. When patients receiving placebo were crossed over to the melatonin group, they too experienced improved sleep quality.

L-tryptophan is the **amino acid** (page 465) precursor of serotonin, a neurotransmitter (chemical messenger in the brain). There is evidence that L-tryptophan levels in schizophrenic people are lower than in non-schizophrenics[70] and the way the body uses L-tryptophan is altered in people with schizophrenia.[71, 72] In a preliminary trial, patients with schizophrenia were given 2–8 grams of L-tryptophan and 100 mg of **vitamin B$_6$** (page 600) daily. This resulted in decreased agitation and less fear and **anxiety** (page 30), but these improvements were not as great as those achieved with psychiatric medications.[73] It is not clear whether the benefits seen in this trial were due to vitamin B$_6$,

L-tryptophan, or a combination of the two. No other clinical trials using L-tryptophan have been published. L-tryptophan is currently available by prescription only.

Vitamin B$_{12}$ (page 601) deficiency can cause symptoms that are similar to those of schizophrenia and one case has been reported in which such symptoms cleared after supplementation with vitamin B$_{12}$.[74] Some studies have reported finding lower levels of vitamin B$_{12}$ in people with schizophrenia than in the general population,[75] but others have found no difference.[76] No trials of vitamin B$_{12}$ supplementation in schizophrenic patients have been published.

Supplementation with the amino acid, D-serine, may improve mental symptoms in people with schizophrenia who are also taking antipsychotic medications. In a double-blind trial, D-serine or placebo was dissolved in orange juice and taken daily for six weeks by people with schizophrenia who were also taking antipsychotic medications.[77] The amount of D-serine used was 30 mg per 2.2 pounds of body weight per day. Those taking the D-serine experienced significant improvements in mental functioning and symptoms related to schizophrenia. Further trials are needed to determine if these effects can be produced in the absence of concurrent antipsychotic medications.

Are there any side effects or interactions?
Refer to the individual supplement for information about any side effects or interactions.

Herbs that may be helpful

In a double-blind trial, supplementation of schizophrenic patients with *Ginkgo biloba* (page 681) extract, in the amount of 250 mg per 2.2 pounds of body weight per day for 12 weeks, enhanced the effectiveness of the antipsychotic drug haloperidol (Haldol) and also reduced the side effects of the drug.[78]

Are there any side effects or interactions?
Refer to the individual herb for information about any side effects or interactions.

Holistic approaches that may be helpful

Magnetic stimulation to the skull and underlying motor cortex (the part of the brain that controls movement) significantly reduced auditory hallucinations in a group of people with schizophrenia in a small, controlled trial.[79] The procedure was performed by psychiatrists using sophisticated electromagnetic medical equipment, not a simple magnet.

SEASONAL AFFECTIVE DISORDER

Seasonal affective disorder (SAD) is an extreme form of common seasonal mood cycles, in which depression develops during the winter months.

How seasonal changes cause depression is unknown, but most of the research into mechanisms and treatment has focused on changes in levels of the brain chemicals **melatonin** (page 555) and serotonin in response to changing exposure to light and darkness.

CHECKLIST FOR SEASONAL AFFECTIVE DISORDER		
Rating	**Nutritional Supplements**	**Herbs**
★★☆	**Vitamin D** (page 607) (if blood levels are low)	**St. John's wort** (page 747)
★☆☆	**5-HTP** (page 459)	

What are the symptoms of seasonal affective disorder?

SAD is characterized by typical symptoms of **depression** (page 145), such as sadness, hopelessness, and thoughts of suicide (in some cases), and "atypical" depressive symptoms such as excessive sleep, lethargy, carbohydrate cravings, overeating, and **weight gain** (page 446). The symptoms usually occur the same time of year, typically fall and winter, and disappear with the onset of spring and summer.

Light exposure research and treatment measures in "lux" units. For example, the intensity of light on a high mountain at the equator at midday is greater than 100,000 lux, compared with less than 11 lux generated by a moonlit night. A well-lit kitchen or office may be around 500 lux.

Medical treatments

Some healthcare practitioners might prescribe antidepressants, such as fluoxetine (Prozac), paroxetine (Paxil), and sertraline (Zoloft).

Treatment includes daily exposure to bright light, often 2,500 lux administered in two-hour increments. Individuals with SAD should spend as much time as possible outside during the day. Use of a "dawn simulator," a light programmed to slowly increase in intensity in the morning, is also recommended. Some healthcare providers might also recommend aerobic exercise under bright lights.

Dietary changes that may be helpful

Cravings for simple carbohydrates are increased in SAD, and women diagnosed with this form of winter depression have been found to eat more carbohydrates, both sweets and starches, than do healthy women. These women also report eating in response to emotionally difficult conditions, **anxiety** (page 30), depression, and loneliness more frequently than healthy women, but eating patterns associated with SAD are distinct from those of women with **eating disorders** (page 174).[1]

People with SAD process sugar differently in winter compared with summer or after light therapy in winter.[2] Changes in neurotransmitters that may affect cravings also occur in women with SAD.[3] Because consumption of carbohydrates can influence neurotransmitter levels,[4] some authorities have speculated that eating simple carbohydrates may be a form of self-medication in people with SAD. A review of the research on diet and mood found that, while eating simple carbohydrates in reaction to depressed mood does bring about a temporary lift in mood, other evidence suggests that long-term control of negative moods is, for some people, best achieved by eliminating simple carbohydrates from the diet.[5] No research has yet been conducted, however, to evaluate the benefits of a diet low in simple carbohydrates (or any other dietary intervention) for people with SAD.

Lifestyle changes that may be helpful

Exercise can ease **depression** (page 145) and improve well being, in some cases as effectively as antidepressant medications.[6] One study found that both one hour of aerobic exercise three times per week and the same amount of anaerobic exercise were significantly and equally effective in reducing symptoms of depression.[7] In a preliminary study of women with SAD, exercise while exposed to light was more likely to be associated with fewer seasonal depressive symptoms than was exercise performed with little light exposure.[8] A controlled study of 120 indoor employees used relaxation training as the placebo in a study of fitness training, light exposure, and winter depressive symptoms. Fitness training was performed two to three times per week while exposed to either bright light (2,500–4,000 lux) or ordinary light (400–600 lux). Compared to relaxation,

exercise in bright light improved general mental health, social functioning, depressive symptoms, and vitality, while exercise in ordinary light improved vitality only.

Nutritional supplements that may be helpful

L-tryptophan is the **amino acid** (page 465) used by the body to manufacture serotonin. Several trials, some controlled, have shown that experimentally inducing a tryptophan deficiency in people with SAD who are in remission brings about a relapse of **depressive** (page 145) symptoms.[9, 10, 11, 12, 13] This suggests that supplemental L-tryptophan might be helpful in SAD. In small, preliminary trials, 4 to 6 grams of L-tryptophan given in divided amounts daily was as effective as light therapy[14, 15] and more effective than placebo.[16] L-tryptophan may be of particular use in people with winter depression who do not benefit from light therapy. In a preliminary trial, people with SAD who responded only partially or not at all to bright light therapy were given 1,000 mg of L-tryptophan three times daily in addition to 10,000 lux light therapy for 30 minutes every morning. Sixty-four percent of them had significant improvement in depressive symptoms while receiving both L-tryptophan and bright light therapy.[17] L-tryptophan is currently available by prescription only.

5-HTP (page 459) is a substance related to L-tryptophan that increases serotonin production and has shown antidepressant activity.[18] It may also be useful in the treatment of SAD, but there is currently no research testing this possibility.

Vitamin D (page 607) is well known for its effects on helping to maintain normal **calcium** (page 483) levels, but it also exerts influence on the brain, spinal cord, and hormone-producing tissues of the body that may be important in the regulation of mood.[19] A double-blind study found that mood improved in healthy people without SAD who received 400 or 800 IU per day of vitamin D for five days in late winter.[20]

In another study, people with SAD were randomly assigned to receive either 100,000 IU of vitamin D one time only or two hours of bright-light therapy every day for one month. After one month, researchers observed a significant improvement in depression in the group that received vitamin D, but not in the group given light therapy.[21] However, a one-year study of healthy postmenopausal women found that supplementation with 400 IU of vitamin D per day did not prevent the mood decline that often occurs in the winter.[22] Certain differences in these studies might account for the different results: In the study in which vitamin D was beneficial, the participants suffered from SAD and their pretreatment vitamin D blood levels tended to be low. In the negative study, the participants did not have SAD, and their pretreatment vitamin D blood levels were higher. Although additional research needs to be done, the available evidence suggests that people with SAD who have marginal or deficient vitamin D levels might benefit from supplementation. This treatment should be supervised by a doctor to assure that the amount of vitamin D used is high enough to be effective, but not so high as to cause adverse effects.

Depression (page 145) can be one of the first symptoms of **vitamin B$_{12}$** (page 601) deficiency.[23] Vitamin B$_{12}$, in the form of cyanocobalamin, given orally in the amount of 1,500 mcg three times daily to patients with seasonal depression, showed no superiority over placebo in a double-blind trial.[24] Vitamin B$_{12}$ cannot be recommended for the treatment of SAD.

Melatonin (page 555) is a hormone produced in the body in response to the rhythms of light and darkness. Changes in melatonin levels are believed to be an important factor in seasonal depression. Supplementation with melatonin, however, has been ineffective when taken at night or in the morning.[25] Melatonin may even reverse the benefits of light therapy in people with SAD.[26] A small, double-blind study, however, found that 125 mcg of melatonin taken both 8 and 12 hours after awakening was effective for reducing depression's symptoms.[27]

Are there any side effects or interactions?
Refer to the individual supplement for information about any side effects or interactions.

Herbs that may be helpful

St. John's wort (page 747), an herb well known for its antidepressant activity,[28] has been examined for its effectiveness in treating SAD. In a preliminary trial, patients with seasonal depression were given 900 mg per day of St. John's wort in addition to either bright light (3,000 lux for two hours) or a dim light (300 lux for two hours) placebo.[29] Both groups had significant improvement in **depressive** (page 145) symptoms, but there was no difference between the groups. The authors concluded that St. John's wort was beneficial with or without bright light therapy, but a placebo effect from the herb cannot be ruled out in this study. Another preliminary study asked 301 SAD patients to report the changes in their symptoms resulting from the use of St. John's wort at 300 mg three times daily.[30] Sig-

nificant overall improvement was reported by these patients. Some of the subjects used light therapy in addition to St. John's wort. They reported more improvement in sleep, but overall improvement was not significantly different from those using St. John's wort alone. Double-blind research is needed to confirm the usefulness of St. John's wort for treating SAD.

Are there any side effects or interactions?
Refer to the individual herb for information about any side effects or interactions.

Holistic approaches that may be helpful

Diminished sunlight exposure in winter contributes to changes in brain chemistry and plays a role in seasonal mood changes. Artificial lights have been widely used to increase light exposure during winter months. Many studies show the benefit of light therapy in the treatment of SAD.[31, 32, 33, 34] In a controlled trial, 96 patients with SAD were treated with light at 6,000 lux for 1.5 hours in either morning or evening, or with a sham negative ion generator, which was used as the placebo. After three weeks of treatment, morning light produced complete or near-complete remission for 61% of patients, while evening light helped 50%, and placebo helped 32%.[35] Another study similarly found morning light to have more antidepressant activity than evening light for people with SAD. This study also found that patterns of **melatonin** (page 555) production were altered in seasonal depression, and that morning light therapy shifted this pattern toward those of control subjects who did not have seasonal depression.[36] Blood flow to certain regions of the brain was measured after light therapy and was increased in seasonal depression patients who benefited from the light therapy. The increase in regional brain blood flow did not occur in those patients who did not respond to the light therapy.[37] Light therapy begun prior to the onset of winter depression appears to have a preventive effect in people susceptible to SAD.[38]

A review of clinical trials of light therapy for SAD concluded that the intensity of the light is related to the effectiveness of the treatmnent.[39] A higher response rate was seen in trials where light intensity was greater, compared with trials that used light therapy of lower intensity. Red and potentially harmful ultraviolet wavelengths are not necessary for a response to light therapy.[40]

A study of the adverse side effects from high-intensity light therapy found them to be common, mild and brief. Among people who underwent brief treatment with

10,000 lux, 45% experienced side effects such as headaches and eye and vision changes. Described as mild and temporary, they did not interfere with treatment.[41]

Dawn simulation is a form of light therapy involving gradually increasing bedside light in the morning. In a comparison study, dawn simulation using 100–300 lux for 60–90 minutes every morning improved symptoms of SAD similarly to bright light therapy using 1,500–2,500 lux for two hours every morning.[42]

A negative ionizer is a device that emits negatively charged particles into the air. Negative air ionization may be useful in treating SAD. One double-blind trial compared the benefits of high-density negative ionization, providing 2.7 million ions per cubic centimeter, and low-density negative ionization, providing 10,000 ions per cubic centimeter, for people with SAD. Atypical depressive symptoms improved by 50% or more for 58% of patients receiving the high-density ionization for 30 minutes daily, while only 15% of those receiving low-density ionization had 50% or greater improvement. There were no side effects, and all of the patients who responded to the therapy relapsed when ionization was discontinued.[43] In another controlled trial, high-density ionization was found equally as effective as light therapy, and both were significantly more effective than low-density ionization.[44]

SEBORRHEIC DERMATITIS

Seborrheic dermatitis is a common inflammatory condition of the skin. Cradle cap is a type of seborrheic dermatitis found in infants; it is usually self-limiting and subsides by the age of six months.

A qualified physician should diagnose these conditions. It is not clear whether research on cradle cap is applicable to the type of seborrheic dermatitis that occurs in adults.

What are the symptoms of seborrheic dermatitis?
A dry, flaky scalp is typical of mild cases of seborrheic dermatitis. More severe cases have itching, burning, greasy scales overlying red patches on the scalp. Seborrheic dermatitis may be confused with severe dandruff. However, seborrheic dermatitis may also be found on the eyebrows, eyelids, forehead, ears, chest, armpits, groin, and the skin folds beneath the breasts or between the buttocks.

CHECKLIST FOR SEBORRHEIC DERMATITIS		
Rating	Nutritional Supplements	Herbs
★★☆		*Aloe vera* (page 624) (topical)
★☆☆	**Biotin** (page 473) (cradle cap) **Borage oil** (page 475), topical (cradle cap) **Folic acid** (page 520) (seborrheic dermatitis) **Vitamin B$_6$** (page 600), topical (seborrheic dermatitis) **Vitamin B$_{12}$** (page 601), injection (seborrheic dermatitis)	

Medical treatments
Over the counter products commonly used to treat dandruff often contain selenium sulfide (Selsun Blue, Head & Shoulders), salicylic acid (Ionil Plus, P & S), or coal tar (Ionil T).

Prescription drug treatment includes the use of selenium (Selsun) and topical cortisone-like drugs, such as betamethasone (Diprosone Lotion) and fluocinonide (Lidex Solution), to control symptoms.

Dietary changes that may be helpful
An early study reported that nursing infants with cradle cap improved when high-**biotin** (page 473) foods, such as liver and egg yolk, were added to the mother's diet.[1]

A preliminary report suggested that an allergy elimination diet for an infant may be useful in the treatment of cradle cap. The most common offending foods identified were milk, wheat, and eggs.[2] More research is needed to confirm the value of this approach in the treatment of cradle cap.

Nutritional supplements that may be helpful
A group of researchers found that infants with cradle cap appeared to have an imbalance of essential fatty acids in their blood that returned to normal when their skin rashes eventually went away.[3] In a preliminary trial, these researchers later found that application of 0.5 ml of **borage oil** (page 475) twice daily to the affected skin resulted in clinical improvement of cradle cap within two weeks.[4]

Preliminary studies have found that injecting either the infant or the nursing mother with **biotin** (page 473) may be an effective treatment for cradle cap.[5, 6] Studies of oral biotin have yielded mixed results in infants. Older preliminary studies and case reports suggest that 4 mg per day of oral biotin might be sufficient for mild cases of cradle cap, but 10 mg per day was required for more severe cases.[7] Two more recent, controlled trials found that oral biotin (4 or 5 mg per day) produced no benefit.[8, 9] Thus, the scientific support for using oral biotin to treat cradle cap is weak. The role of biotin in adult seborrheic dermatitis has not been studied.

One physician reported that injections of **B-complex vitamins** (page 603) were useful in the treatment of seborrheic dermatitis in infants.[10] A preliminary trial found that 10 mg per day of **folic acid** (page 520) was helpful in 17 of 20 cases of adult seborrheic dermatitis.[11] However, this study also found that oral folic acid did not benefit infants with cradle cap. A preliminary study found that topical application of **vitamin B$_6$** (page 600) ointment (containing 10 mg B$_6$ per gram of ointment) to affected areas improved adult seborrheic dermatitis.[12] However, oral vitamin B$_6$ (up to 300 mg per day) was ineffective. Injections of **vitamin B$_{12}$** (page 601) were reported to improve in 86% of adults with seborrheic dermatitis in a preliminary trial.[13] Oral administration of vitamin B$_{12}$ for seborrheic dermatitis has not been studied.

Are there any side effects or interactions?
Refer to the individual supplement for information about any side effects or interactions.

Herbs that may be helpful

A crude extract of **Aloe vera** (page 624) (*Aloe barbadensis*) may help seborrheic dermatitis when applied topically. In a double-blind trial, people with seborrheic dermatitis applied either a 30% crude aloe emulsion or a similar placebo cream twice a day for four to six weeks.[14] Significantly more people responded to topical aloe vera than to placebo: 62% of those using the aloe vera reported improvements in scaling and itching, compared to only 25% in the placebo group.

Are there any side effects or interactions?
Refer to the individual herb for information about any side effects or interactions.

SHINGLES AND POSTHERPETIC NEURALGIA

Shingles is a disease caused by the same virus *(Varicella zoster)* that causes chicken pox. Acute, painful inflamed blisters form on one side of the trunk along a peripheral nerve.

Shingles usually affects the elderly or people with compromised **immune function** (page 255). Nerve pain that persists after other symptoms have cleared is called postherpetic neuralgia.

Rating	Nutritional Supplements	Herbs
★★★		**Cayenne** (page 654) (topical; for pain only)
★★☆		**Peppermint oil** (page 726) (topical; for postherpetic neuralgia)
★☆☆	**Adenosine monophosphate** (page 461) (injection) **Lysine** (page 550) **Vitamin B$_{12}$** (page 601) (injection) **Vitamin E** (page 609)	**Licorice** (page 702) (topical) **Wood betony** (page 761)

CHECKLIST FOR SHINGLES AND POSTHERPETIC NEURALGIA

What are the symptoms of shingles?

Symptoms include **pain** (page 338), itching, or a tingling sensation prior to the appearance of a severely painful skin rash of red, fluid-filled blisters that later crust over. The rash is typically located on the trunk or face and only affects one side of the body. Pain may resolve rapidly or persist in the area of the rash for months to years after the rash disappears.

Medical treatments

Over the counter treatment for shingles might include analgesics, such as aspirin (Bayer, Bufferin, Ecotrin), ibuprofen (Motrin, Advil), or acetaminophen (Tylenol). Anti-itch creams containing antihistamines (Caladryl) and hydrocortisone (Cortaid, Lanacort) might be useful. The oral antihistamine diphenhydramine (Benadryl) might help reduce inflammation and itching.

Topical capsaicin (Zostrix) may provide temporary relief from postherpetic neuralgia pain.

Prescription drug treatment might include analgesics for pain relief, such as ibuprofen (Motrin), naproxen (Naprosyn), and acetaminophen with codeine (Tylenol with Codeine). Oral antibiotics such as cephalexin (Keflex) and amoxicillin/clavulanate (Augmentin) might be used to treat infected blisters. Other drugs used for short-term relief might include the antihistamine hydroxyzine (Atarax); tranquilizers, such as lorazepam (Ativan) and alprazolam (Xanax); and oral corticosteroids, such as prednisone (Deltasone) and methylprednisolone (Medrol). Antiviral medicines such as oral acyclovir (Zovirax), famciclovir (Famvir), foscarnet (Foscavir), and valacyclovir (Valtrex) may also be prescribed.

Dietary changes that may be helpful

Varicella zoster, the virus that causes shingles, is a type of herpes virus. Another herpes virus, herpes simplex virus (HSV), has a high requirement for the amino acid **arginine** (page 467). On the other hand, **lysine** (page 550) inhibits HSV replication.[1] Therefore, a diet that is low in arginine and high in lysine may help prevent herpes viruses from replicating. For that reason, some doctors advise people with shingles to avoid foods with high arginine-to-lysine ratios, such as nuts, peanuts, and chocolate. Nonfat yogurt and other nonfat dairy can be a healthful way to increase lysine intake. This dietary advice for shingles has not been subjected to scientific study.

Lifestyle changes that may be helpful

Stress and **depression** (page 145) have been linked to outbreaks of shingles in some,[2, 3] but not all,[4] studies.[5] A small, preliminary study found that four children with shingles outbreaks, but who were otherwise healthy, all reported experiencing severe, chronic child abuse when the shingles first appeared.[6] Among adults, how a stressful event is perceived appears to be more important than the event itself. In one study, people with shingles experienced the same kinds of life events in the year preceding the illness as did people without the condition; however, recent events perceived as stressful were significantly more common among people with shingles.

Nutritional supplements that may be helpful

Adenosine monophosphate (page 461) (AMP), a compound that occurs naturally in the body, has been found to be effective against shingles outbreaks. In one double-blind trial, people with an outbreak of shingles were given injections of either 100 mg of AMP or placebo three times a week for four weeks. Compared with the placebo, AMP promoted faster healing and reduced the duration of pain of the shingles.[7] In addition, AMP appeared to prevent the development of postherpetic neuralgia.[8, 9]

Some doctors have observed that injections of **vitamin B₁₂** (page 601) appear to relieve the symptoms of postherpetic neuralgia.[10, 11] However, since these studies did not include a control group, the possibility of a placebo effect cannot be ruled out. Oral vitamin B₁₂ supplements have not been tested, but they are not likely to be effective against postherpetic neuralgia.

Some doctors have found **vitamin E** (page 609) to be effective for people with postherpetic neuralgia—even those who have had the problem for many years.[12, 13] The recommended amount of vitamin E by mouth is 1,200–1,600 IU per day. In addition, vitamin E oil (30 IU per gram) can be applied to the skin. Several months of continuous vitamin E use may be needed in order to see an improvement. Not all studies have found a beneficial effect of vitamin E;[14] however, in the study that produced negative results, vitamin E may not have been used for a long enough period of time.

Because shingles is caused by a herpes virus, some doctors believe that **lysine** (page 550) supplementation could help people with the condition, since lysine inhibits replication of herpes simplex, a related virus. However, lysine has not been shown to inhibit *Varicella zoster*, nor has it been shown to provide any benefit for people with shingles outbreaks. Therefore, its use in this condition remains speculative.

Are there any side effects or interactions?
Refer to the individual supplement for information about any side effects or interactions.

Herbs that may be helpful

The hot component of **cayenne** (page 654) pepper, known as capsaicin, is used to relieve the pain of postherpetic neuralgia. In a double-blind trial, a cream containing 0.075% capsaicin, applied three to four times per day to the painful area, greatly reduced pain.[15] In another study, a preparation containing a lower concentration of capsaicin (0.025%) was also effective.[16] Two or more weeks of treatment may be required to get the full benefit of the cream.

One case report has been published concerning an elderly woman with postherpetic neuralgia who experienced dramatic pain relief from topical application of 2 to 3 drops of peppermint oil to the affected area 3 or 4 times per day.[17] Each application produced almost complete pain relief, lasting approximately 6 hours. The woman began to experience redness at the site of application after four weeks of use. The oil was therefore diluted by 80% with almond oil; the diluted preparation did not cause redness, and continued to produce "adequate" though somewhat less-pronounced pain relief.

Licorice (page 702) has been used by doctors as a topical agent for shingles and postherpetic neuralgia; however, no clinical trials support its use for this purpose. Glycyrrhizin, one of the active components of licorice, has been shown to block the replication of *Varicella zoster*.[18] Licorice gel is usually applied three or more times per day. Licorice gel is not widely available but may be obtained through a doctor who practices herbal medicine.

Wood betony (page 761) *(Stachys betonica)* is a traditional remedy for various types of nerve pain. It has not been studied specifically as a remedy for postherpetic neuralgia.

Are there any side effects or interactions?
Refer to the individual herb for information about any side effects or interactions.

Holistic approaches that may be helpful

Acupuncture may be helpful in some cases of shingles and postherpetic neuralgia. Anecdotal case reports of people treated with electroacupuncture (acupuncture with applied electrical current) described improvement in seven of eight people.[19] A controlled trial, however, found no difference in response between acupuncture treatment and placebo.[20] The authors of this trial reported some difficulty in evaluating the results due to difficulty in assessing measures of pain in this study group. Large, controlled trials using well-designed pain evaluation methods are still needed to determine the value of acupuncture in the treatment of shingles and postherpetic neuralgia.

Hypnosis has improved or cured some cases of postherpetic neuralgia, as well as the acute pain of shingles.[21]

SICKLE CELL ANEMIA

Anemia is a deficiency of the oxygen-carrying capacity of red blood cells. Sickle cell anemia is an inherited chronic anemia in which the red blood cells become sickle or crescent-shaped. The symptoms of sickle cell anemia are caused by the clogging of small blood vessels by the sickle cells or by poor delivery of oxygen to the tissues due to the anemia itself.

A sickle cell crisis is a painful episode that occurs when the body becomes severely deprived of oxygen. The disease and the trait occur in people of African descent, as well as in people from Mediterranean countries, India, and the Middle East, but rarely in people of European descent.

CHECKLIST FOR SICKLE CELL ANEMIA

Rating	Nutritional Supplements	Herbs
★★☆	**Fish oil** (page 514) **Folic acid** (page 520) (for lowering homocysteine levels) **L-arginine** (page 467) (for pulmonary hypertension) **Vitamin B₁₂** (page 601) (for sickle cell patients with diagnosed B₁₂ deficiencies) **Zinc** (page 614)	
★☆☆	**Beta-carotene** (page 469) and other **carotenoids** (page 488) **Magnesium** (page 551) **Vitamin A** (page 595) **Vitamin B₂** (page 598) **Vitamin B₆** (page 600) **Vitamin C** (page 604) **Vitamin E** (page 609)	**Garlic** (page 679)

What are the symptoms of sickle cell anemia?

Symptoms include fatigue, joint and abdominal pain, irritability, yellow discoloration of the skin and eyes, leg sores, gum disease, frequent respiratory infections, blindness later in life, and periods of prolonged, sometimes painful erections in males. People with sickle cell anemia can have episodes of severe pain in the arms, legs, chest, and abdomen that may be accompanied by fever, nausea, and difficulty breathing. These symptoms occur only in people who inherit copies of the sickle cell gene from both parents. People who inherit a sickle cell gene from only one parent have what is known as sickle cell trait and are without symptoms.

Medical treatments

In some cases, the prescription drug hydroxyurea (Hydrea) is used to increase hemoglobin levels. Doctors might also recommend preventive antibiotics for common respiratory infections. Acute episodes may be treated with supplemental oxygen, intravenous antibiotics, prescription painkillers, and blood transfusions.

Healthcare practitioners typically advise people with sickle cell anemia to avoid high altitudes, to maintain an adequate fluid intake, and to receive vaccinations. Occasionally bone marrow transplants are recommended.

Dietary changes that may be helpful

People with sickle cell anemia suffer from many nutrient deficiencies, but preliminary research on dietary habits shows that food and nutrient intake by sickle cell patients in general meets or exceeds recommendations and is not significantly different from healthy controls.[1, 2, 3] This suggests the higher rate of nutrient deficiencies may be due to an increased need for many nutrients in sickle cell patients. The effectiveness of dietary interventions in supplying adequate nutrition to meet these higher demands has not been examined.

Nutritional supplements that may be helpful

In a preliminary study, individuals with pulmonary hypertension (a life-threatening complication of sickle cell anemia) received L-arginine in the amount of 100 mg per 2.2 pounds of body weight, three times per day for five days. L-arginine treatment resulted in a significant improvement in pulmonary hypertension, as determined by a 15% decline in the pulmonary artery systolic pressure.[4] Longer-term studies are needed to confirm these preliminary results.

Sickle cell anemia may result in **vitamin B$_{12}$** (page 601) deficiency. A study of children with sickle cell anemia found them to have a higher incidence of vitamin B$_{12}$ deficiency than children without the disease.[5] A study of 85 adults with sickle cell anemia showed more of them had vitamin B$_{12}$ deficiency than did a group of healthy people.[6] A subsequent preliminary trial demonstrated that for patients with low blood levels of vitamin B$_{12}$, intramuscular injections of 1 mg of vitamin B$_{12}$ weekly for 12 weeks led to a significant reduction in

symptoms.[7] Researchers do not know whether people with sickle cell anemia who are found to be deficient in vitamin B$_{12}$ would benefit equally from taking vitamin B$_{12}$ supplements orally.

In a preliminary trial, 20 patients with sickle cell anemia were given either 1 mg of **folic acid** (page 520) per day or folic acid plus 6 grams of aged **garlic** (page 679) extract, 6 grams of vitamin C, and 1,200 mg of vitamin E per day for six months.[8] Patients taking the combination had a significant improvement in their hematocrit (an index of anemia) and less painful crises than those taking just folic acid.

Preliminary research has found that patients with sickle cell anemia are more likely to have elevated blood levels of **homocysteine** (page 234) compared to healthy people.[9, 10] Elevated homocysteine is recognized as a risk factor for **cardiovascular disease** (page 98).[11] In particular, high levels of homocysteine in sickle cell anemia patients have been associated with a higher incidence of **stroke** (page 419).[12] Deficiencies of **vitamin B$_6$** (page 600), vitamin B$_{12}$, and folic acid occur more frequently in people with sickle cell anemia than in others[13, 14, 15] and are a cause of high homocysteine levels.[16] A controlled trial found homocysteine levels were reduced 53% in children with sickle cell anemia receiving a 2–4 mg supplement of folic acid per day, depending on age, but vitamin B$_6$ or B$_{12}$ had no effect on homocysteine levels.[17] A double-blind trial of children with sickle cell anemia found that children given 5 mg of folic acid per day had less painful swelling of the hands and feet compared with those receiving placebo, but blood abnormalities and impaired growth rate associated with sickle cell anemia were not improved.[18] In the treatment of sickle cell anemia, folic acid is typically supplemented in amounts of 1,000 mcg daily.[19] Anyone taking this amount of folic acid should have vitamin B$_{12}$ status assessed by a healthcare professional.

Iron deficiency (page 278) is relatively common in people with sickle cell anemia, especially in **pregnant** (page 363) women and in children.[20, 21] Iron deficiency in people with sickle cell anemia is best diagnosed with a laboratory test called serum ferritin.[22, 23] During sickle cell crises, however, serum ferritin is no longer useful as an indicator of iron deficiency.[24] The value of **iron** (page 540) supplementation for people with sickle cell anemia who are diagnosed with iron deficiency is unclear. Iron supplements have, in some reports, reduced the severity of anemia as measured by laboratory tests; however, some reports suggest they may increase the symptoms of sickle cell anemia.[25, 26] Moreover, a state of iron deficiency has been shown to reduce sickling of red blood cells in the blood of people with sickle cell anemia.[27] A small trial of iron *restriction* in patients with sickle cell anemia found improvement in anemia and clinical symptoms as well as decreased red blood cell breakdown during iron restriction.[28] A doctor should be consulted before deciding to supplement or restrict iron in sickle cell anemia.

Low concentrations of red blood cell magnesium have been noted in patients with sickle cell anemia.[29, 30] Low magnesium, in turn, is thought to contribute to red blood cell dehydration and a concomitant increase in symptoms. In a preliminary trial, administration of 540 mg of **magnesium** (page 551) per day for six months to sickle cell anemia patients reversed some of the characteristic red blood cell abnormalities and dramatically reduced the number of painful days for these patients.[31] The form of magnesium used in this trial, magnesium pidolate, is not supplied by most magnesium supplements; it is unknown whether other forms of magnesium would produce similar results.

In test tube studies, **vitamin B$_6$** (page 600) has been shown to have anti-sickling effects on the red blood cells of people with sickle cell anemia.[32, 33] Vitamin B$_6$ deficiency has been reported in some research to be more common in people with sickle cell anemia than in healthy people.[34, 35] In a controlled trial, five sickle cell anemia patients with evidence of vitamin B$_6$ deficiency were given 50 mg of vitamin B$_6$ twice daily. The deficiency was reversed with this supplement, but improvement in anemia was slight and considered insignificant.[36] Therefore, evidence in support of vitamin B$_6$ supplementation for people with sickle cell anemia remains weak.

Antioxidant (page 467) nutrients protect the body's cells from oxygen-related damage. Many studies show that sickle cell anemia patients tend to have low blood levels of antioxidants, including **carotenoids** (page 488), **vitamin A** (page 595), **vitamin E** (page 609), and **vitamin C** (page 604), despite adequate intake.[37, 38, 39, 40, 41, 42] Low blood levels of vitamin E in particular have been associated with higher numbers of diseased cells in children[43] and with greater frequency of symptoms in adults.[44] A small, preliminary trial reported a 44% decrease in the average number of diseased cells in six sickle cell anemia patients given 450 IU vitamin E per day for up to 35 weeks. This effect was maintained as long as supplementation continued.[45]

In another preliminary trial, 13 patients with sickle cell anemia were given two supplement combinations for seven to eight months each. The first combination included 109 mg **zinc** (page 614), 153 IU **vitamin E** (page 609), 600 mg **vitamin C** (page 604), and 400 ml (about 14 ounces) of soybean oil containing 11 grams of linoleic acid and 1.5 grams of alpha linolenic acid. The second combination included 140 IU vitamin E, 600 mg vitamin C, and 20 grams of **fish oil** (page 514) containing 6 grams of omega-3 fatty acids. Reduction in diseased cells was observed only during the administration of the first protocol. The authors concluded that zinc was the important difference between the two combinations and may be a protector of red blood cell membranes.[46]

Fish oil alone has also been studied. In a double-blind trial, supplementation with menhaden oil, in the amount of 250 mg per 2.2 pounds of body weight per day for one year, reduced the frequency of severe pain episodes by approximately 45%, compared with placebo.[47]

The zinc deficiency associated with sickle cell anemia appears to play a role in various aspects of the illness. For example, preliminary research has correlated low zinc levels with poor growth in children with sickle cell anemia.[48] In a preliminary trial, 12 people with sickle cell anemia received 25 mg of zinc every four hours for 3 to 18 months.[49] The number of damaged red blood cells fell from 28% to 18.6%. Addition of 2 mg of copper per day did not inhibit the effect of zinc. (Zinc supplementation in the absence of copper supplementation induces a copper deficiency.) Patients with the highest number of damaged red blood cells had a marked response to zinc, but those with lower levels of damaged cells (less than 20% irreversibly sickled cells) had little or no response. Chronic leg ulcers occur in about 75% of adults with sickle cell disease. In a controlled trial, sickle cell patients with low blood levels of zinc received 88 mg of zinc three times per day for 12 weeks.[50] Ulcer healing rate was more than three times faster in the zinc group than in the placebo group.

Are there any side effects or interactions?
Refer to the individual supplement for information about any side effects or interactions.

SINUS CONGESTION

Sinus congestion (also called nasal congestion or rhinitis) involves blockage of one or more of the four pairs of sinus passageways in the skull.

The blockage may result from inflammation and swelling of the nasal tissues, obstruction by one of the small bones of the nose (deviated septum), or from secretion of mucus. It may be acute or chronic. Acute sinus congestion is most often caused by the **common cold** (page 129). Sinus congestion caused by the common cold is not discussed here. Chronic sinus congestion often results from environmental irritants such as tobacco smoke, food allergens, inhaled **allergens** (page 14), or foreign bodies in the nose.

Sinus congestion leads to impaired flow of fluids in the sinuses, which predisposes people to bacterial **infections** (page 265) that can cause **sinusitis** (page 407). At least two serious disorders have been associated with chronic nasal congestion: chronic lymphocytic leukemia and **HIV** (page 239).[1, 2] For this reason, chronic nasal congestion lasting three months or more should be evaluated by a medical professional.

CHECKLIST FOR SINUS CONGESTION		
Rating	Nutritional Supplements	Herbs
★☆☆		**Eucalyptus** (page 673)

What are the symptoms of sinus congestion?

Sinus congestion typically causes symptoms of pressure, tenderness, or pain in the area above the eyebrows (frontal sinus) and above the upper, side teeth (maxillary sinus). Other symptoms include nasal stuffiness sometimes accompanied by a thick yellow or green discharge, postnasal drip, bad breath, and an irritating dry cough.

Medical treatments

Over the counter products may help to reduce the symptoms associated with sinus congestion. Analgesics, such as aspirin (Bayer, Ecotrin, Bufferin), ibuprofen (Motrin, Advil), and acetaminophen (Tylenol), reduce pain due to sinus pressure. Topical nasal decongestants such asoxymetazoline (Afrin) and phenylephrine (NeoSynephrine) may provide relief from nasal congestion, but they should only be used for a few days. The oral decongestant pseudoephedrine (Sudafed) may help relieve nasal congestion, while antihistamines such as diphenhydramine (Benadryl), brompheniramine (Dimetapp), and chlorpheniramine (Chlor-Trimeton) might help dry excess mucous. Guaifenesin (Robitussin) is an expectorant used to remove mucous in the sinuses, lungs, and ears.

Prescription strength **pain** (page 338) relievers, such as ibuprofen (Motrin), naproxen (Naprosyn), and acetaminophen with codeine (Tylenol with Codeine), may be prescribed. Oral antibiotics, such as amoxicillin/clavulanate (Augmentin), loracarbef (Lorabid), and cefprozil (Cefzil), are generally prescribed for sinus infection. Corticosteroid nasal sprays, such as flunisolide (Nasalide), fluticasone (Flonase), or triamcinolone (Nasacort), may also be used to reduce inflammation.

Surgery may be used to unblock the sinuses and drain thick secretions if drug therapy is ineffective or if structural abnormalities are involved.

Dietary changes that may be helpful

Food allergy (page 14) appears to play an important role in many cases of rhinitis, which is related to sinus congestion. In a study of children under one year of age with allergic rhinitis and/or **asthma** (page 32), 91% had a significant improvement in symptoms while following an allergy-elimination diet.[3] In the experience of one group of doctors, food allergy was the most common cause of chronic rhinitis.[4] Two other researchers have found food allergy to be a contributing factor to allergic rhinitis in 25%[5] and 39%[6] of cases, respectively. Food allergies are best identified by means of an allergy-elimination diet, which should be supervised by a doctor.

Lifestyle changes that may be helpful

The most common cause of nasal congestion is **allergy** (page 14) to inhalants, such as pollen, molds, dust mites, trees, or animal dander. Exposure to various chemicals in the home or workplace may also contribute to allergic rhinitis. Indoor and outdoor air pollution may also be a factor in susceptible people. Smoking and secondhand exposure to tobacco smoke have been implicated in chronic nasal congestion[7] and the prevalence of chronic rhinitis among men has been shown to increase with increasing cigarette consumption.[8] People exposed to chlorine, such as lifeguards and swimmers, may also be at risk of developing nasal congestion.[9]

Careful evaluation by an allergist or other healthcare professional may help identify factors contributing to nasal congestion. Sometimes strict avoidance of the triggering agents (e.g., thoroughly vacuuming house dust or using dust covers on the mattresses) may provide relief. Where complete avoidance of irritants is not possible, desensitization techniques (immunotherapy [allergy shots]) may be helpful.

Nasal irrigation with warm water or saline may be helpful for reducing symptoms of sinus congestion, although steam inhalations appear to be less useful. In a study of people suffering from the **common cold** (page 129), steam inhalation did not improve sinus congestion any better than placebo.[10] In a similar controlled study, irrigation of the nasal passages with heated water or saline, decreased nasal secretions, although inhalation of water vapor did not.[11]

Herbs that may be helpful

Eucalyptus (page 673) oil is often used in a steam inhalation to help clear nasal and sinus congestion. Eucalyptus oil is said to function in a fashion similar to that of menthol by acting on receptors in the nasal mucous membranes, leading to a reduction in the symptoms of nasal stuffiness.[12]

Are there any side effects or interactions?
Refer to the individual herb for information about any side effects or interactions.

Holistic approaches that may be helpful

Acupuncture may be useful for decreasing chronic sinus congestion. In one clinical study, most participants experienced at least temporary relief after acupuncture needles were inserted alongside the nose.[13]

SINUSITIS

Sinusitis is an inflammation of the sinus passages.

There are four pairs of sinuses in the human skull that help circulate moist air throughout the nasal passages. The **common cold** (page 129) is the most prevalent predisposing factor to sinusitis. **Hay fever** (page 209), other environmental triggers, **food allergens** (page 14), and dental **infections** (page 265) can also lead to sinusitis.

What are the symptoms of sinusitis?

Acute sinusitis typically causes symptoms of nasal congestion and a thick yellow or green discharge. Other symptoms include tenderness and **pain** (page 338) over the sinuses, frontal headaches, and sometimes chills, fever, and pressure in the area of the sinuses. Chronic sinusitis differs slightly, in that symptoms can be milder and may only include postnasal drip, bad breath, and an irritating dry cough.

CHECKLIST FOR SINUSITIS		
Rating	**Nutritional Supplements**	**Herbs**
★★★	**Bromelain** (page 481)	
★★☆		**Cineole** (page 673) (a component of eucalyptus)
★☆☆	**Vitamin C** (page 604)	**Eucalyptus** (page 673) **Gentian** (page 680) root, primrose flowers, sorrel herb, elder flowers, and European **vervain** (page 756) (in combination) **Horseradish** (page 693) **Wood betony** (page 761)

Medical treatments

Over the counter analgesics, such as aspirin (Bayer, Ecotrin, Bufferin), ibuprofen (Motrin, Advil), and acetaminophen (Tylenol), reduce pain due to sinus pressure. Topical nasal decongestants such as oxymetazoline (Afrin) and phenylephrine (NeoSynephrine) may provide relief from nasal congestion, but they should only be used for a few days. The oral decongestant pseudoephedrine (Sudafed) may also help relieve nasal congestion and sinus pressure. Guaifenesin (Robitussin) is an expectorant used to remove mucous in the sinuses, lungs, and ears.

Prescription drug therapy for sinus **infections** (page 265) usually includes antibiotics, such as amoxicillin/clavulanate (Augmentin), loracarbef (Lorabid), cefprozil (Cefzil), and levofloxacin (Levaquin). Corticosteroid nasal sprays, such as flunisolide (Nasalide), fluticasone (Flonase), or triamcinolone (Nasacort), may also be used to reduce inflammation.

Surgery may be used to unblock the sinuses and drain thick secretions if drug therapy is not effective, or if there are structural abnormalities.

Dietary changes that may be helpful

According to some studies, 25–70% of people with sinusitis have environmental **allergies** (page 14).[1] Although food allergies may also contribute to the problem, some researchers believe food allergies only rarely cause sinusitis.[2, 3] People with sinusitis may benefit by working with a doctor to evaluate what, if any, ef-

Sinusitis

fect the elimination of food and other allergens might have on reducing their symptoms.

Nutritional supplements that may be helpful
Bromelain (page 481), an **enzyme** (page 506) derived from pineapple, has been reported to relieve symptoms of acute sinusitis. In a double-blind trial, 87% of patients who took bromelain reported good to excellent results compared with 68% of those taking placebo.[4] Other double-blind research has shown that bromelain reduces symptoms of sinusitis.[5, 6] Research with bromelain for sinusitis generally uses the enteric-coated form. Enteric-coating prevents the stomach juices from partially destroying the bromelain. Most commercially available bromelain products today are not enteric-coated, and it is not known how the potency of these different products compares.

Studies conducted in the past have used bromelain compounds with therapeutic strengths measured in units called Rorer units (RU). Potency of contemporary bromelain compounds are quantified in either MCUs (milk clotting units) or GDUs (gelatin dissolving units); one GDU equals 1.5 MCU. One gram of bromelain standardized to 2,000 MCU would be approximately equal to 1 gram with 1,200 GDU of activity, or 8 grams with 100,000 RU of activity. Physicians sometimes recommend 3,000 MCU taken three times per day for several days, followed up by 2,000 MCU per day.[7] Much of the research conducted has used smaller amounts likely to be the equivalent (in modern units of activity) of approximately 500 MCU taken four times a day.

Histamine is associated with increased nasal and sinus congestion. In one study, **vitamin C** (page 604) supplementation (1,000 mg three times per day) reduced histamine levels in people with either high histamine levels or low blood levels of vitamin C.[8] Another study found that 2,000 mg of vitamin C helped protect people exposed to a histamine challenge test.[9] Not every study reported reductions in histamine.[10] Although preliminary evidence supports the use of vitamin C when injected into the sinuses of people suffering with acute sinusitis, the effect of oral vitamin C on symptoms of sinusitis has yet to be formally studied.[11]

Are there any side effects or interactions?
Refer to the individual supplement for information about any side effects or interactions.

Herbs that may be helpful
The main ingredient of **eucalyptus** (page 673) oil, cineole, has been studied as a treatment for sinusitis. In a double-blind study of people with acute sinusitis that did not require treatment with antibiotics, those given cineole orally in the amount of 200 mg 3 times per day recovered significantly faster than those given a placebo.[12] Eucalyptus oil is also often used in a steam inhalation to help clear nasal and sinus congestion. Eucalyptus oil is said to function in a fashion similar to menthol by acting on receptors in the nasal mucous membranes, leading to a reduction in the symptoms of nasal stuffiness.[13]

One of the most popular supportive treatments for both acute and chronic sinusitis in Germany is an herbal combination containing **gentian** (page 680) root, primrose flowers, sorrel herb, elder flowers, and European **vervain** (page 756).[14] The combination has been found to be useful in helping to promote mucus drainage ("mucolytic" action) from the sinuses.[15] The combination is typically used together with antibiotics for treating acute sinusitis.

Horseradish (page 693) is another herb used traditionally as a mucus-dissolver.[16] One half to one teaspoon (3–5 grams) of the freshly grated root can be eaten three times per day. Horseradish tincture is also available. One quarter to one half teaspoon (2 to 3 ml) can be taken three times per day.

Wood betony (page 761) (*Stachys betonica*) is used in traditional European herbal medicine as an anti-inflammatory remedy for people with sinusitis. Modern clinical trials have not been conducted to confirm this use of wood betony.

Are there any side effects or interactions?
Refer to the individual herb for information about any side effects or interactions.

Holistic approaches that may be helpful
A warm salt-water solution poured through the nose may offer some relief from both **allergic** (page 14) and **infectious** (page 265) sinusitis. A ceramic pot, known as a "neti lota" pot, makes this procedure easy. Alternatively, a small watering pot with a tapered spout may be used. Fill the pot with warm water and add enough salt so the solution tastes like tears. Stand over a sink, tilt your head far to one side so your ear is parallel to the floor, and pour the solution into the upper nostril, allowing it to drain through the lower nostril. Repeat on

the other side. This procedure may be performed two or three times a day.

Some practitioners may treat sinus problems using various manipulation techniques. A single case study described treatment of chronic sinusitis and sinus headaches with spinal manipulation, massage, and a technique called: "bilateral nasal specific" (BNS). The BNS procedure involves inflating small balloons within the nasal passages, creating a change of pressure and, theoretically, a realignment of nasal bones. Initial treatment of a 41-year-old woman with manipulation and massage for approximately one year had resulted in only temporary, mild relief. Her headaches resolved immediately following each treatment that included BNS, followed by increased amounts of postnasal discharge and an improved sense of smell. At the end of two additional months of care, her headaches were reduced significantly in intensity and frequency.[17]

SKIN ULCERS

Skin ulcers are open sores that are often accompanied by the sloughing-off of inflamed tissue.

Skin ulcers can be caused by a variety of events, such as trauma, exposure to heat or cold, problems with blood circulation, or irritation from exposure to corrosive material. Pressure ulcers, also known as decubitus ulcers or bedsores, are skin ulcers that develop on areas of the body where the blood supply has been reduced because of prolonged pressure; these may occur in people confined to bed or a chair, or in those who must wear a hard brace or plaster cast. Skin ulcers may become infected, with serious health consequences. Other health conditions that can cause skin ulcers include mouth ulcers (**canker sores** [page 90]), **chronic venous insufficiency** (page 116), **diabetes** (page 152), **infection** (page 265), and **peripheral vascular disease** (page 352).

What are the symptoms of skin ulcers?

People with a skin ulcer may have an area of reddened skin. In advanced cases, people may have areas where the skin is open and oozing fluid.

Medical treatments

Over the counter topical antibiotics, such as neosporin (Myciguent), bacitracin (Baciguent), and combinations of the two with polymyxin B (Neosporin, Polysporin), are used to treat skin infections.

Prescription strength topical antibiotics, such as metronidazole (MetroGel) and mupirocin (Bactroban), might be necessary to treat infection.

Healthcare providers recommend shifting position at least every two hours to avoid sustained pressure on the same area of the body. Some people might benefit from special mattresses or supports. For skin ulcers in general, wound dressings need to be changed frequently. Severe cases might require surgery to remove diseased tissue and to repair the wound.

CHECKLIST FOR SKIN ULCERS		
Rating	Nutritional Supplements	Herbs
★★☆	Essential fatty acids (topical, for prevention of pressure ulcers) **Evening primrose oil** (page 511) **Flavonoids** (page 516) (hydroxyethylrutosides) **Flavonoids** (page 516) (diosmin, hesperidin) **Folic acid** (page 520) **Vitamin C** (page 604) **Vitamin E** (page 609) (oral) **Zinc** (page 614) (oral and topical)	**Aloe vera** (page 624) **Gotu kola** (page 684) (topical and by intramuscular injection)
★☆☆	**Vitamin E** (page 609) (topical)	

Dietary changes that may be helpful

Dietary deficiencies may hinder the body's ability to heal pressure ulcers. A controlled study of 28 malnourished nursing home patients with skin ulcers found that ulcer healing was significantly enhanced by a high-protein diet (24% protein) compared with a lower protein (14%) diet.[1] A controlled study of critically ill older patients found that increasing calorie and protein intake with dietary supplements for 15 days reduced the risk of developing a skin ulcer.[2]

Nutritional supplements that may be helpful

Antioxidants (page 467) such as **vitamin C** (page 604), **vitamin E** (page 609), and **glutathione** (page 531) are depleted in healing skin tissue.[3] One animal study found that vitamin E (alpha-tocopherol) applied to the skin shortened the healing time of skin ulcers.[4] Another animal study reported that administration of oral vitamin E before skin lesions were introduced into the skin prevented some of the tissue damage associated with the development of pressure ulcers.[5] A controlled human trial found that 400 IU of vitamin E daily improved the results of skin graft surgery for chronic venous ulcers.[6] No further research has investigated the potential benefit of vitamin E for skin ulcers.

Animal research has suggested that vitamin C may help prevent skin ulcers,[7] and in a preliminary study,[8] elderly patients with pressure ulcers had lower blood levels of vitamin C than did ulcer-free patients. Supplementation with vitamin C (3 grams per day) increased the speed of healing of leg ulcers in patients with a blood disorder called **thalassemia** (page 25), according to a double-blind study.[9] And while a double-blind trial of surgical patients with pressure ulcers found that supplementation with 500 mg of vitamin C twice a day accelerated ulcer healing,[10] a similar double-blind trial found no difference in the effectiveness of either 20 mg per day or 1,000 mg per day of vitamin C.[11]

An older preliminary report suggested that large amounts of **folic acid** (page 520) given both orally and by injection could promote healing of chronic skin ulcers due to poor circulation.[12] No controlled research has further investigated this claim.

Zinc (page 614) plays an important role in tissue growth processes important for skin ulcer healing. One study reported that patients with pressure ulcers had lower blood levels of zinc and iron than did patients without pressure ulcers,[13] and preliminary reports suggested zinc supplements could help some types of skin ulcer.[14] Supplementation with 150 mg of zinc per day improved healing in a preliminary study of elderly patients suffering from chronic leg ulcers.[15] Double-blind trials using 135 to 150 mg of zinc daily have shown improvement[16] only in patients with low blood zinc levels,[17] and no improvement in leg ulcer healing.[18, 19] A double-blind trial of 150 mg zinc per day in people with skin ulcers due to sickle cell anemia found that the healing rate was almost three times faster in the zinc group than in the placebo group after six months.[20] Lastly, a preliminary study of patients with skin ulcers due to leprosy found that 50 mg of zinc per day in addition to anti-leprosy medication resulted in complete healing in most patients within 6 to 12 weeks.[21] Long-term zinc supplementation at these levels should be ac-

companied by supplements of copper and perhaps calcium, iron, and magnesium. Large amounts of zinc (over 50 mg per day) should only be taken under the supervision of a doctor.

Topically applied zinc using zinc-containing bandages has improved healing of leg ulcers in double-blind studies of both zinc-deficient[22] and elderly individuals.[23] Most controlled comparison studies have reported that these bandages are no more effective than other bandages used in the conventional treatment of skin ulcers,[24, 25] but one controlled trial found non-elastic zinc bandages superior to alginate dressings or zinc-containing elastic stockinettes.[26] Two controlled trials of zinc-containing tape for foot ulcers due to leprosy concluded that zinc tape was similarly effective, but more convenient than conventional dressings.[27, 28]

Pressure ulcers and diabetic ulcers frequently develop in malnourished and/or institutionalized people. A double-blind study[29] of malnourished people compared topical application of 20 ml of a solution containing essential fatty acids (EFAs) and linoleic acid extracted from sunflower oil with a control solution containing topical mineral oil. Each solution was applied to the skin three times per day. Compared with the control solution, the solution containing EFAs significantly reduced the incidence of pressure ulcers and improved the hydration and elasticity of the skin.

A preliminary report suggested that **evening primrose oil** (page 511) improves blood flow to the legs and heals or reduces the size of venous leg ulcers.[30] No controlled research has further investigated this claim.

A double-blind trial found that a combination of 900 mg per day of diosmin and 100 mg per day of hesperidin, two members of the **flavonoid** (page 516) family, resulted in significantly greater healing of venous leg ulcers after two months.[31, 32] Related flavonoids known as hydroxyethylrutosides have also been investigated for venous ulcer healing. While one controlled study reported significant additional benefit when 2,000 mg per day of hydroxyethylrutosides were added to compression stocking therapy,[33] another double-blind trial using 1,000 mg per day found no effect on ulcer healing;[34] a second double-blind trial found no effect of 1,000 mg per day hydroxyethylrutosides on the prevention of venous ulcer recurrences.[35]

Are there any side effects or interactions?
Refer to the individual supplement for information about any side effects or interactions.

Herbs that may be helpful

Gotu kola (page 684) *(Centella asiatica)* extracts are sometimes used topically to help speed wound healing. Test tube studies have found that extracts of gotu kola high in the active triterpene constituents asiaticosides, madecassoides, asiatic acids, and madecassic acids increase collagen synthesis.[36, 37] An animal study found that topical application of asiaticoside isolated from gotu kola, used in a 0.2% solution, improved healing in nonulcer skin wounds.[38] An overview of three small human clinical trials suggests that topical use of an ointment or powder containing a gotu kola extract high in the active triterpene compounds may speed wound healing in people with slow-healing skin ulcers.[39] These studies used either a topical ointment with a 1% extract concentration or a powder with a 2% extract concentration. People in these studies were typically treated with intramuscular injections of either isolated asiaticosides or the mixed triterpenes three times per week while using the topical ointment or powder.

Aloe vera (page 624) has been used historically to improve wound healing and contains several constituents that may be important for this effect. A group of three patients who had chronic skin ulcerations for 5, 7, and 15 years, respectively, had a rapid reduction in ulcer size after the application of aloe gel on gauze bandages to the ulcers, according to a preliminary report.[40] A controlled study found most patients with pressure ulcers had complete healing after applying an aloe hydrogel dressing to the ulcers every day for ten weeks.[41] However, this result was not significantly better than that achieved with a moist saline gauze dressing. The amorphous hydrogel dressing used in the above study and derived from the aloe plant (Carrasyn Gel Wound Dressing, Carrington Laboratories, Irving, TX) is approved by the U.S. Food and Drug Administration for the management of mild to moderate skin ulcers.

Are there any side effects or interactions?
Refer to the individual herb for information about any side effects or interactions.

Holistic approaches that may be helpful

A double-blind trial found systemic hyperbaric oxygen (HBO) treatments, in which the patient is placed in a chamber with highly concentrated oxygen, five days per week for six weeks significantly improved healing of nondiabetic chronic leg ulcers.[42] This trial confirms the results from several preliminary studies of systemic HBO therapy.[43, 44] While topical application of HBO (the affected body part is encased in a balloon-like chamber and exposed to concentrated oxygen) for skin ulcers has been reported effective in preliminary trials,[45] controlled trials have produced conflicting results.[46, 47] In controlled studies of diabetic patients with skin ulcers or gangrene, systemic HBO has been shown to prevent amputation of affected limbs.[48, 49]

Electrical stimulation applied to the skin is thought to have several biological effects that might accelerate skin ulcer healing.[50] A variety of techniques have been investigated, and controlled or double-blind trials have shown positive results for the use of low-voltage galvanic current, high-voltage pulsed current, transcutaneous electrical nerve stimulation (TENS), and pulsed high-frequency electromagnetic therapy.[51]

SNORING

Snoring is caused by the movement of air across the soft tissues in the mouth or throat, such as the uvula, soft palate, and sometimes the vocal cords.

Any restriction of airflow, as occurs with nasal congestion, asthma, or polyps, increases the likelihood of snoring. Simple snoring is usually without health consequences, but inadequate sleep quality and quantity, nighttime dips in the body's oxygen levels,[1] and headaches[2] sometimes accompany snoring. In addition, an association between snoring and **heart disease** (page 98) has been established.[3, 4] When the resistance to airflow in the airways becomes so great as to cause significant interruptions in breathing, it is known as sleep apnea. Sleep apnea represents a more serious health concern than simple snoring;[5] therefore, chronic snoring, which can be associated with sleep apnea, should be evaluated by a healthcare provider.

What are the symptoms of snoring?

People with snoring may make a rough, rattling, noisy sound while breathing in during sleep.

Medical treatments

Healthcare practitioners may recommend avoidance of alcoholic beverages, sleeping pills, antihistamines, and overeating before bedtime. Sleeping on one side, rather than on the back, or raising the head of the bed may provide benefit. Weight loss is helpful, especially for people who are obese. Allergies and nasal infections are treated when detected. Surgery may be recommended to correct structural problems with the airway, such as enlarged tonsils and adenoids or a deviated nasal septum.

Lifestyle changes that may be helpful

Allergies can inflame the nasal passages, sinuses, and airways of the lungs, and commonly cause or contribute to snoring. Data collected from people with **allergic rhinitis** (page 407) (stuffy nose)[6, 7] and **asthma** (page 32)[8, 9] show that these people are more likely to be snorers than are nonallergic people. In addition, two preliminary studies have found that when snoring is treated using a continuous positive airway pressure device, an instrument primarily used to treat sleep apnea, nighttime asthma attacks decrease.[10, 11] Children who snore are also more likely than other children to have **allergies** (page 14),[12] and one preliminary study found that more than half of children with allergies are snorers.[13] One researcher reported that children with allergy symptoms, including snoring, commonly have **food sensitivities** (page 14). Although little more is known about food sensitivities and snoring, it may be helpful to test for food sensitivities.[14] The possibility of asthma and allergies should therefore be considered in people who snore.

A number of studies have found an association between snoring and heart disease. **High blood pressure** (page 246) and **coronary artery disease** (page 98) have been correlated with snoring in both men and women, and the correlation is stronger in people with normal weight.[15, 16, 17, 18] In women, snoring is more common after **menopause** (page 311), and is strongly associated with high blood pressure in women around the age of menopause.[19, 20] Researchers suggest that, with such a strong correlation, it is important to screen for hypertension and heart disease in people who snore.[21]

Obesity (page 446) and lack of physical activity are commonly associated with heavy snoring.[22, 23] Even in children, obesity may be linked to snoring and sleep disorders.[24] One study found that obese men who snore were significantly more likely to develop **diabetes** (page 152) over a ten-year period than were obese men who did not snore.[25] Snoring is clearly a problem that should be addressed in obese men, and increasing physical activity and weight loss are widely recommended.[26, 27, 28] A preliminary trial found that weight loss was more important in reducing snoring than either changes in sleep position or use of a nasal decongestant spray.[29] In a report by the U.S. Army, weight

control and physical training was advised to reduce the severity of snoring and sleep apnea, and in one presented case, full recovery from severe snoring was achieved with weight loss and use of a continuous positive airway pressure device.[30] Two other cases have been reported in which combined weight loss and use of a continuous positive airway pressure device resulted in full recovery from snoring and sleep apnea.[31]

Smoking increases the likelihood of snoring because of its effects on the nasal passages and sinuses.[32] In addition, nicotine may cause sleep disturbances that result in more snoring.[33] Men are more likely to snore as they age, but one study found that smoking increases the likelihood of snoring particularly in men under the age of 60.[34] A sleep study found that heavy smokers are more likely to snore than are moderate and light smokers, and that people who have quit smoking are no more likely to snore than are people who have never smoked.[35] Teenagers who smoke have also been found to be more likely to snore than non-smoking teenagers, and that snoring was associated with frequent nighttime wakening and daytime sleepiness.[36] Exposure to environmental smoke, or "second-hand smoke," has been shown to increase the likelihood of snoring in children.[37, 38] Smoking cessation and elimination of environmental smoke exposure are therefore important in the treatment of snoring.

It has long been thought that consumption of **alcohol** (page 12) contributes to snoring, and at least one study has found this to be true,[39] but several studies have been unable to verify this link.[40, 41, 42]

SPRAINS AND STRAINS

What do I need to know?

Self-care for sprains and strains can be approached in a number of ways—but it can be hard to know just where to start. To make it easier, our doctors recommend trying these simple steps first:

Get professional help for serious injuries
> See a doctor if you cannot move or put weight on the body part, if the part looks crooked, if pain or tenderness is severe, if there is numbness or redness in the area, or if you have any other concerns about your injury

Control swelling and pain
> Use the R.I.C.E treatment: **R**est the body part, **I**ce it every hour, **C**ompress it with elastic band-

ages, tape, or a brace, and **E**levate it above your heart

Control inflammation with proteolytic enzymes
Take 4 to 8 tablets a day of enzyme preparations containing trypsin, chymotrypsin, and/or bromelain for inflammation

Try topical horse chestnut extract
Apply a product containing 2% aescin every two hours to control swelling

Take a multivitamin-mineral supplement
A multivitamin during recovery can help insure against deficiencies that slow the healing process

About sprains and strains

Sprains and strains are types of minor injuries to the soft tissues and connective tissues of the musculoskeletal system. Sprains usually refer to injuries to ligaments, but sometimes to other connective tissues, such as tendons and the capsules surrounding joints. Strains usually refer to injuries to muscles or to the areas where muscles become tendons.

Sprains and strains may occur together, and occasionally are quite severe, requiring immobilization of the body part in a rigid cast for weeks, long-term rehabilitation programs, and sometimes surgery.

What are the symptoms of sprains and strains?

The most common type of sprain is the ankle sprain. Ankle sprains have differing degrees of severity. Mild or minimal sprains with no tear of the ligament usually produce mild tenderness and some swelling. Moderate sprains, in which the ligament has been partially ruptured, produce obvious swelling, **bruising** (page 84), significant tenderness, and difficulty walking. Severe sprains, as when the ligament is completely torn from the bone (called avulsion), make walking impossible and produce marked swelling, internal bleeding and joint instability.

Symptoms of strains include muscle soreness, muscle spasm, pain, and possibly swelling or warmth over the involved muscle.

Medical treatments

Over the counter pain medications, such as aspirin (Bayer, Ecotrin, Bufferin), acetaminophen (Tylenol), and ibuprofen (Motrin, Advil), are routinely recommended to relieve minor pain and reduce inflammation. Topical methyl salicylate-menthol (Icy Hot,

Ben-Gay), trolamine salicylate (Aspercreme), and combination counterirritant products (Maximum Strength Flexall 454) may also help to relieve pain from muscle strain.

Prescription medications, such as acetaminophen with codeine (Tylenol with Codeine) or acetaminophen with hydrocodone (Vicodin), may be used for moderate pain. Strains may be treated with muscle relaxants, such as cyclobenzaprine (Flexeril), carisoprodol (Soma), and baclofen (Lioresal).

Treatment of minor sprains and strains includes resting the affected area, applying cold packs or ice, wrapping the area with a compression bandage (ACE), and keeping the affected area elevated as much as possible. Mild to moderate ankle sprains usually require strapping with elastic bandages or tape or immobilization with a brace. Health care providers recommend "RICE" for sprains and strains, which stands for rest, ice, compression, and elevation. A sprained ankle should always be X-rayed to rule out a fracture.

CHECKLIST FOR SPRAINS AND STRAINS		
Rating	**Nutritional Supplements**	**Herbs**
★★★	**Enzymes** (page 506) (chymotrypsin, trypsin)	
★★☆	**Bromelain** (page 481) **L-carnitine** (page 543) (for preventing exercise-related muscle injury) **Vitamin A** (page 595) (for deficiency only) **Vitamin C** (page 604) **Zinc** (page 614) (if deficient)	**Horse chestnut** (page 692) (topical)
★☆☆	**Chondroitin sulfate** (page 492) **Copper** (page 499) **DMSO** (page 508) (topical) **Enzymes** (page 506) (papain) **Glucosamine sulfate** (page 528) **Manganese** (page 553) **Multiple vitamin-mineral** (page 559) **Silicon** (page 586) **Vitamin E** (page 609) (for exercise-related muscle strain)	Arnica (topical) **Comfrey** (page 662) (topical)

Dietary changes that may be helpful

Adequate amounts of calories and protein are required for the body to repair damaged connective tissue. While major injuries requiring hospitalization raise protein and calorie requirements significantly, minor sprains and strains do *not* require changes from a typical, healthful diet.[1]

Nutritional supplements that may be helpful

Proteolytic enzymes (page 506), including bromelain, papain, trypsin, and chymotrypsin, may be helpful in healing minor injuries such as sprains and strains because they have anti-inflammatory activity and appear to promote tissue healing.[2, 3, 4]

Several preliminary trials have reported reduced pain and swelling, and/or faster healing in people with a variety of conditions using either bromelain,[5] papain from papaya,[6, 7] or a combination of trypsin and chymotrypsin.[8] Double-blind trials have reported faster recovery from athletic injuries, including sprains and strains, and earlier return to activity using eight tablets daily of trypsin/chymotrypsin,[9, 10, 11, 12] four to eight tablets daily of papain,[13] eight tablets of bromelain (single-blind only),[14] or a combination of these enzymes.[15] However, one double-blind trial using eight tablets per day of trypsin/chymotrypsin to treat sprained ankles found no significant effect on swelling, **bruising** (page 84), or overall function.[16]

Bromelain (page 481) is measured in MCUs (milk clotting units) or GDUs (gelatin dissolving units). One GDU equals 1.5 MCU. Strong products contain at least 2,000 MCU (1,333 GDU) per gram (1,000 mg). A supplement containing 500 mg labeled "2,000 MCU per gram" would have 1,000 MCU of activity, because 500 mg is half a gram. Some doctors recommend 3,000 MCU taken three times per day for several days, followed by 2,000 MCU three times per day. Some of the research, however, uses smaller amounts, such as 2,000 MCU taken in divided amounts in the course of a day (500 MCU taken four times per day). Other enzyme preparations, such as trypsin/chymotrypsin, have different measuring units. Recommended use is typically two tablets four times per day on an empty stomach, but as with bromelain, the strength of trypsin/chymotrypsin tablets can vary significantly from product to product.

One controlled trial showed that people who supplement with 3 grams per day **L-carnitine** (page 543) for three weeks before engaging in an exercise regimen are less likely to experience muscle soreness.[17]

Antioxidant (page 467) supplements, including **vitamin C** (page 604) and **vitamin E** (page 609), may help prevent exercise-related muscle injuries by neutralizing free radicals produced during strenuous activities.[18] Controlled research, some of it double-blind, has shown that 400–3,000 mg per day of vitamin C may reduce pain and speed up muscle strength recovery after intense exercise.[19, 20] Reductions in blood indicators of muscle damage and free radical activity have also been reported for supplementation with 400–1,200 IU per day of vitamin E in most studies,[21, 22, 23] but no measurable benefits in exercise recovery have been reported.[24] A combination of 90 mg per day of **coenzyme Q$_{10}$** (page 496) and a very small amount of vitamin E did not produce any protective effects in one double-blind trial.[25]

Vitamin C (page 604) is needed to make collagen, the "glue" that strengthens connective tissue. Injury, at least when severe, appears to increase vitamin C requirements,[26] and vitamin C deficiency causes delayed healing from injury.[27] Preliminary human studies have suggested that vitamin C supplementation in non-deficient people can speed healing of various types of trauma, including musculoskeletal injuries,[28, 29] but double-blind research has not confirmed these effects for athletic injuries, which included sprains and strains.[30]

Zinc (page 614) is a component of many enzymes, including some that are needed to repair wounds. Even a mild deficiency of zinc can interfere with optimal recovery from everyday tissue damage as well as from more serious trauma.[31] Trace minerals, such as **manganese** (page 553), **copper** (page 499), and **silicon** (page 586) are also known to be important in the biochemistry of tissue healing.[32, 33, 34, 35] However, there have been no controlled studies of people with sprains or strains to explore the effect of deficiency of these minerals, or of oral supplementation, on the rate of healing.

Many vitamins and minerals have essential roles in tissue repair, and deficiencies of one or more of these nutrients have been demonstrated in animal studies to impair the healing process.[36] This could argue for the use of **multiple vitamin-mineral** (page 559) supplements by people with minor injuries who might have deficiencies due to poor diets or other problems, but controlled human research is lacking to support this.

Glucosamine sulfate (page 528) and **chondroitin sulfate** (page 492) may both play a role in **wound healing** (page 319) by providing the raw material needed by the body to manufacture molecules called glycosaminoglycans found in skin, tendons, ligaments, and joints.[37] Test tube and animal studies have found that these substances, and others like them, can promote improved tissue healing.[38, 39, 40, 41] Injectable forms of chondroitin sulfate have been used in Europe for various types of sports-related injuries to tendons and joints,[42, 43, 44, 45] and one preliminary trial reported reduced pain and good healing in young athletes with chondromalacia patella (cartilage softening in the knee) who were given 750–1,500 mg per day of oral glucosamine sulfate.[46] However, specific human trials of glucosamine and chondroitin sulfate for healing sprains and strains are lacking.

The use of **DMSO** (page 508), a colorless, oily liquid primarily used as an industrial solvent, for therapeutic applications is controversial. However, some evidence indicates that dilutions, when applied directly to the skin, have anti-inflammatory properties and inhibit the transmission of pain messages by nerves, and in this way might ease the pain of minor injuries such as sprains and strains.[47, 48, 49] However no controlled research exists to confirm these effects in sprains and strains. DMSO comes in different strengths and different degrees of purity. In addition, certain precautions must be taken when applying DMSO. For those reasons, DMSO should be used only with the supervision of a doctor.

Are there any side effects or interactions?
Refer to the individual supplement for information about any side effects or interactions.

Herbs that may be helpful
Horse chestnut (page 692) contains a compound called aescin that acts as an anti-inflammatory and reduces **edema** (page 177) (swelling with fluid) following trauma, particularly sports injuries, surgery, and head injury.[50] A topical gel containing 2% of the compound aescin found in horse chestnut is widely used in Germany to treat minor sports injuries, including sprains and strains.[51] The gel is typically applied to affected area every two hours until swelling begins to subside.

Arnica is considered by some practitioners to be among the most effective **wound-healing** (page 319) herbs available.[52] As a homeopathic remedy, arnica is often recommended as both an internal and topical mean to treat minor injuries. Some healthcare practitioners recommend mixing 1 tablespoon of arnica tincture in 500 ml water, then soaking thin cloth or gauze in the liquid and applying it to the injured area for at least 15 minutes four to five times per day.

Comfrey (page 662) is also widely used in traditional medicine as a topical application to help heal wounds.[53]

Are there any side effects or interactions?
Refer to the individual herb for information about any side effects or interactions.

Holistic approaches that may be helpful
Spinal manipulation is used by chiropractors, licensed naturopathic doctors, and some osteopathic doctors to relieve pain and improve healing of sprains and strains. One preliminary trial tested a combination of chiropractic manipulation, muscle stretching, and special exercises known as "proprioceptive neurofacilitation" to people who had sprain/strain neck injuries that had not resolved with other treatment.[54] Treatment was reported to help the majority of people, and over one-third reported that their symptoms were completely gone or only mildly bothersome. In a larger preliminary trial,[55] people who were still suffering neck pain a year after whiplash-type accidents were treated with spinal manipulation for an average of four months. At the end of the treatments, 72% reported at least some benefit and nearly half reported significant benefit or complete recovery, but people with the most severe symptoms derived little benefit.

STRESS

About stress
The popular idea of stress in relation to human health is often described as an unpleasant mental or emotional experience, as when people say they are "stressed out." This expression relates primarily to the idea of prolonged or sudden and intense stress, which can have unpleasant effects on the body, impairing the ability to function, and even harming health.[1, 2, 3] However, the biological concept of stress is much more broadly defined as any challenge (physical or psychological) that requires an organism to adapt in a healthy manner. In other words, responses to stress can sometimes be of benefit when the organism is strengthened by the experience. The discussion below focuses on reducing the effects of excessive, unwanted stress.

Stress

CHECKLIST FOR STRESS

Rating	Nutritional Supplements	Herbs
★★★	**Tyrosine** (page 465) **Vitamin C** (page 604)	**Rhodiola** (page 738)
★★☆	**DHA** (page 509) (docosahexaenoic acid) **Flaxseed** (page 517) **Multivitamin-mineral supplement** (page 559)	**Asian ginseng** (page 630) **Eleuthero** (page 672)
★☆☆	**Probiotics** (page 575)	**Ashwagandha** (page 629)

What are the symptoms of stress?

Symptoms may include anxiety, fatigue, **insomnia** (page 270), stomach problems, sweating, racing heart, rapid breathing, shortness of breath, and irritability. Many health problems have been associated with various kinds of sudden or long-term stress, including **alcohol abuse** (page 12),[4] **asthma** (page 32),[5] **chronic fatigue** (page 111),[6, 7] **erectile dysfunction** (page 185) and **male infertility** (page 305),[8] **fibromyalgia** (page 191),[9] headaches,[10] heart disease,[11, 12, 13] **high blood pressure** (page 246),[14, 15] **immune system** (page 255) dysfunction,[16, 17, 18] **indigestion** (page 260), **irritable bowel syndrome** (page 280),[19] mood disorders such as **anxiety** (page 30) and **depression** (page 145),[20, 21] **peptic ulcers** (page 349),[22] **pregnancy** (page 363) complications,[23, 24, 25] **rheumatoid arthritis** (page 387),[26] skin diseases,[27] impaired **wound healing** (page 357),[28] and others.[29, 30, 31, 32, 33, 34] Problems with recovery from surgery and impaired workplace performance are also associated with excessive stress.[35, 36, 37, 38]

Medical treatments

Over-the-counter treatment is limited, but sleep aids containing diphenhydramine (Benadryl, Sominex, Nytol) and doxylamine (Unisom) might relieve stress-induced **insomnia** (page 270).

Prescription medications used to treat anxiety, a condition related to stress, include the benzodiazepines lorazepam (Ativan), alprazolam (Xanax), clonazepam (Klonapin), and diazepam (Valium), as well as buspirone (Buspar) and hydroxyzine pamoate (Vistaril). Other benzodiazepines, such as estazolam (ProSom) and flurazepam (Dalmane), as well as zolpidem (Ambien) might provide short term relief for stress-related insomnia. People with panic attacks and depression might benefit from the selective serotonin reuptake in-

hibitors paroxetine (Paxil), sertraline (Zoloft), and fluoxetine (Prozac).

Medical management of stress includes teaching people how to avoid or cope with stressful situations and encouraging a healthful diet, good exercise habits, and adequate sleep. Those unable to find relief on their own might benefit from professional counseling.

Dietary changes that may be helpful

Flaxseed (page 517) is a good source of **fiber** (page 512) and alpha-linolenic acid (an **omega-3 fatty acid** [page 509]) and is a major source of lignans that may influence hormone function. A controlled study found that adding 30 grams per day of freshly ground flaxseed to the diets of **postmenopausal women** (page 311) reduced the blood pressure–elevating effect of mental stress and reduced stress-related changes in fibrinogen, a blood component associated with increased risk of heart disease.[39] However, flaxseed had no significant effect on blood levels of an adrenal stress hormone.

Lifestyle changes that may be helpful

While cigarette smokers often describe their habit as relaxing, smoking is associated with increased stress levels,[40] and stopping the habit eventually results in reduced feelings of stress.[41]

Drinking alcohol can reduce feelings of stress,[42] but using **alcohol** (page 12) regularly in response to chronic or repetitive stress can lead to an unhealthy dependency.

Exercise has long been thought to have potential benefits to mental health and stress reduction;[43, 44] however, exercise can also be stressful when it is intense or competitive.[45, 46] Many preliminary studies have found that regular exercisers score higher on measures of psychological well-being and perceived stress,[47, 48, 49, 50, 51] and that people who improve their exercise habits develop changes in their mental attitudes that are associated with better resistance to stress.[52] A controlled trial found that a single session of aerobic exercise reduced the anxiety associated with a subsequent experience designed to be psychologically stressful.[53] However, studies of overall aerobic fitness have found that people with higher fitness levels are not different from those with lower fitness in their resistance to stress. One preliminary study gave aerobically fit and unfit women a mentally stressful test, and found no differences between them in physical or psychological measures of their stress reaction.[54] Another preliminary study found that while physical activity was associated with reduced stress symptoms, having high aerobic fitness had no influence.[55] This may mean that effects other than improved aerobic fitness, such as an improved self-image or the social support from belonging to an exercise group, are responsible for the benefits of exercise on controlling stress. A preliminary study in Thailand found that postmenopausal women who completed an aerobic exercise program consisting of 40- to 50-minute sessions twice weekly for 12 weeks had improved scores on a questionnaire designed to measure psychological stress.[56] In a controlled trial, cancer patients hospitalized for chemotherapy who exercised for 30 minutes daily until discharge had significant improvement in several measures of psychological distress, while a similar group who did not exercise showed no change in these measures.[57] In a controlled trial, 10 weeks of aerobic exercise resulted in healthier responses to acute mental stress in college students compared with students who did no exercise.[58]

Nutritional supplements that may be helpful
Tyrosine (page 465) is an **amino acid** (page 465) used by the body to produce certain adrenal stress hormones and chemical messengers in the nervous system (neurotransmitters). Animal research shows that brain levels of these substances decline with stress, and that giving animals tyrosine supplements reverses this decline and improves various tests of performance in stressed animals.[59] In a controlled study, a protein drink containing 10 grams per day of tyrosine was more effective than a carbohydrate drink for improving mental performance scores in a group of cadets taking a stressful six-day combat training course.[60] A double-blind trial in humans found that one-time administration of 150 mg of tyrosine per 2.2 pounds of body weight helped prevent a decline in mental performance for about three hours during a night of sleep deprivation.[61] Single administrations of tyrosine (100 to 150 mg per 2.2 pounds of body weight) have also helped preserve mental performance during physically stressful conditions such as noise or extreme cold in several controlled studies.[62, 63, 64, 65]

Animal studies suggest that supplementing with **vitamin C** (page 604) can reduce blood levels of stress-related hormones and other measures of stress.[66, 67, 68, 69] Controlled studies of athletes have shown that vitamin C supplementation (1,000 to 1,500 mg per day) can reduce stress hormone levels after intense exercise.[70, 71] Surgery patients given 2,000 mg per day of vitamin C during the week before and after surgery had a more

rapid return to normal of several stress-related hormones compared with patients not given vitamin C.[72] In a double-blind trial, young adults took 3,000 mg per day of vitamin C for two weeks, then were given a psychological stress test involving public speaking and mental arithmetic.[73] Compared with a placebo group, those taking vitamin C rated themselves less stressed, scored better on an **anxiety** (page 30) questionnaire, had smaller elevations of blood pressure, and returned sooner to lower levels of an adrenal stress hormone following the stress test.

Animal and human studies suggest that deficiencies of **omega-3 fatty acids** (page 509) may contribute to behaviors associated with unhealthy responses to stress.[74, 75] A double-blind study of students with a low dietary intake of **DHA** (page 509) (docosahexaenoic acid, an omega-3 fatty acid) reported that taking 1.5 to 1.8 grams of DHA per day for three months prevented an increase in aggressiveness in these students during a stressful final exam period.[76] This group of researchers reported in another double-blind study that 1.5 grams per day of DHA given to medical students during a stressful exam period resulted in changes in some, though not all, blood measurements indicating improved responses to stress.[77]

When asked why they are taking nutritional supplements, combating stress is one of the most common reasons given by people.[78, 79, 80] Despite this popular attitude, human research on the effects of supplements on stress is sparse and conflicting.[81] While there are animal studies and preliminary human reports suggesting that many vitamins are important for protecting the body from the consequences of physical stresses such as surgery,[82] evidence supporting the use of vitamins to combat everyday stress is somewhat limited.

Several studies have evaluated a daily supplement of **vitamin B₁** (page 597) (15 mg), **vitamin B₂** (page 598) (15 mg), **vitamin B₃** (page 598) (50 mg), **vitamin B₆** (page 600) (10 mg), **vitamin B₁₂** (page 601) (10 mcg), **vitamin C** (page 604) (500 mg), pantothenic acid (23 mg), **folic acid** (page 520) (400 mcg), **biotin** (page 473) (150 mcg), **calcium** (page 483) (100 mg), **magnesium** (page 551) (100 mg), and **zinc** (page 614) (10 mg) for combating stress effects. People participating in preliminary trials of this combination have reported some benefits that relate to the effects of chronic stress, including improved concentration, better mood, and less fatigue.[83, 84] A small double-blind study of this combination reported no significant psychological benefits relating to stress.[85] However, in a larger double-blind trial with healthy young men, this supplement resulted in significantly less anxiety and perceived stress according to some measurements after one month, though other stress-related symptoms did not improve.[86] Another large, double-blind study of people experiencing high stress levels found this combination significantly helpful after one month according to several measures of anxiety, well-being, and psychological stress.[87]

In a year-long double-blind trial, a one-a-day type **multivitamin-mineral supplement** (page 559) was no better than a supplement containing only **vitamin B₂** (page 598), **calcium** (page 483), and **magnesium** (page 551) for improving mental or physical measures of quality of life in a group of healthy adults.[88]

Stress is understood to have a detrimental effect on the balance of intestinal bacteria,[89, 90] but whether **probiotic** (page 575) supplements improve the ability to handle stress is unknown. In a six-month preliminary trial, a **multivitamin-mineral (MVM) supplement** (page 559) that also contained a blend of *Lactobacillus acidophilus*, *Bifidobacterium bifidum*, and *Bifidobacterium longum* was effective for improving scores on a stress questionnaire.[91] However, this improvement could have been a placebo effect or could have been due to the MVM component. Controlled research comparing MVM supplements with and without added probiotics is necessary to determine whether probiotics are helpful for treating stress.

Are there any side effects or interactions?
Refer to the individual supplement for information about any side effects or interactions.

Herbs that may be helpful

The herbs discussed here are considered members of a controversial category known as adaptogens, which are thought to increase the body's resistance to stress, and to generally enhance physical and mental functioning.[92, 93] Many animal studies have shown that various herbal adaptogens have protective effects against physically stressful experiences,[94, 95] but whether these findings are relevant to human stress experiences is debatable.

Animal studies have demonstrated protective effects of **rhodiola** (page 738) extracts against physical stresses.[96, 97, 98] A double-blind study of healthcare workers experiencing the stress of night duty found that taking 170 mg per day of a standardized rhodiola extract prevented some of the decline in a set of mental

performance measures during the first two weeks. However, when this regimen was repeated after a two-week period of not taking the extract, rhodiola did not provide protection from mental performance decline.[99] In another double-blind study, 100 mg per day of the same extract was given to medical students during a stressful exam period. Those taking the extract reported a better sense of general well-being, and performed better on tests of mental and psychomotor performance.[100] A third double-blind study of military cadets performing a 24-hour duty showed that 370 to 555 mg of rhodiola extract per day significantly reduced mental fatigue, as measured by several performance tasks.[101]

Animal studies support the idea that **Asian ginseng** (page 630) is an adaptogen.[102] Some studies have suggested that Asian ginseng can enhance feelings of well-being in elderly people with **age-associated memory impairment** (page 8),[103] nurses working night shifts,[104] or people with **diabetes** (page 152).[105] In a double-blind trial, people taking a daily combination of a **multivitamin-mineral supplement** (page 559) (MVM) with 40 mg of ginseng extract (standardized for 4% ginsenosides) for 12 weeks reported greater improvements in quality of life measured with a questionnaire compared with a group taking only MVM.[106] The same MVM-ginseng combination was tested in a double-blind study of night-shift healthcare workers.[107] Compared with a placebo group, the group receiving the MVM-ginseng combination improved on one out of four measures of mental performance, one out of three measures of mood (increased calmness, but no change in alertness or contentment), and a measure of reported fatigue. However, in another double-blind study, healthy adults given 200 or 400 mg per day of a standardized extract of Asian ginseng (equivalent to 1,000 or 2,000 mg of ginseng root) showed no significant improvement in any of several measures of psychological well-being after two months.[108]

Animal research has reported antistress effects of *Eleutherococcus senticosus* (page 672) (also known as Siberian ginseng),[109] and Russian research not available in the English language reportedly describes human studies showing similar effects in humans.[110, 111] A double-blind study of healthy elderly people reported that those who took 60 drops per day of a eleuthero liquid extract (concentration not specified) scored higher in some quality-of-life measures after four weeks, but not after eight weeks, compared with a group taking a placebo.[112] Athletes experiencing the stress of training who took an eleuthero extract equivalent to 4 grams per day had no changes in their blood levels of an adrenal stress hormone after six weeks.[113] More research is needed to clarify the value of eleuthero for treating stress.

Animal studies have suggested that **ashwagandha** (page 629) may be helpful for reducing the effects of stress,[114, 115, 116] including chronic psychological stress.[117] However, no controlled research has been done to explore these effects in humans.

An herbal formula from the Ayurvedic medicine tradition, containing extracts of **ashwagandha** (page 629), asparagus, pueraria, argyreia, dioscorea, mucuna, and piper, has been studied as an aid to coping with the stress of military combat. A double-blind study found that soldiers performed similarly in a set of mental and psychological tests after an eight-day combat mission whether they were given two capsules daily (exact content not revealed) of this formula or a placebo.[118] This suggests there was no real benefit of the herbal formula under these conditions.

Are there any side effects or interactions?
Refer to the individual herb for information about any side effects or interactions.

Holistic approaches that may be helpful

Mind-body medicine is a branch of healing that focuses on the role of thoughts and emotions on physical health. Many techniques used in this healing system, including biofeedback, relaxation training, tai chi, yoga, and meditation, affect the nervous system in ways that could theoretically help people cope with stress.[119] In a controlled trial, tai chi practice, meditation, walking exercise, and quiet reading all resulted in similar biochemical and psychological improvements in the response to a stressful experience.[120] Meditation, practiced for spiritual reasons, for relaxation, or as part of the treatment of a disease, has been reported helpful for stress reduction in preliminary studies.[121, 122, 123] A controlled study found 15 minutes of meditation twice a day reduced measures of stress in adolescents during two experiences designed to produce stress.[124] Other controlled studies have found reductions in reported stress and related psychological measures after a program of meditation.[125, 126]

Stress reduction programs involving combinations of group counseling, instruction in coping skills and problem-solving, relaxation training, meditation, or other methods are effective for reducing stress and helping to prevent or manage health problems relating

to stress, according to preliminary and controlled research.[127, 128, 129, 130, 131, 132]

STROKE

Stroke is a condition caused by a lack of blood supply to the brain or by hemorrhage (bleeding) within the brain.

Stroke is the third leading cause of death in the United States, but most strokes are not fatal. Depending on the area of the brain that is damaged, a stroke can cause coma, reversible or irreversible paralysis, speech problems, visual disturbances, and dementia. Factors that increase the risk of certain types of stroke include **hypertension** (page 246), **diabetes** (page 152), elevated levels of **high cholesterol** (page 223) or **homocysteine** (page 234), and **atherosclerosis** (page 38) (hardening of the arteries) of the blood vessels that supply the brain.

CHECKLIST FOR STROKE		
Rating	**Nutritional Supplements**	**Herbs**
★★☆	**Potassium** (page 572) **Vinpocetine** (page 594)	
★☆☆	**Folic acid** (page 520) (for high homocysteine only) **Magnesium** (page 551) **Tocotrienols** (page 593) **Vitamin B$_6$** (page 600) (for high homocysteine only) **Vitamin B$_{12}$** (page 601) (for high homocysteine only) **Vitamin E** (page 609)	

What are the symptoms of stroke?

Symptoms of stroke include weakness, numbness, or inability to move an arm or leg; sudden and intense headache; severe dizziness or loss of coordination and balance; difficulty with speaking or understanding; and blurred or decreased vision in one or both eyes. People with stroke may also have seizures, vomiting, drooling, and difficulty swallowing. Some people experience temporary warning episodes of neurologic symptoms called transient ischemic attacks (TIAs) before suffering a complete stroke. People experiencing symptoms suggestive of having suffered a stroke or a TIA require immediate (emergency room) medical attention.

Medical treatments

Over the counter aspirin (Bayer Low Adult Strength, Ecotrin Adult Low Strength) may help prevent future strokes in men.

Prescription anticoagulants, such as warfarin (Coumadin) are routinely given to individuals who have had strokes.

Individuals who experience a stroke caused by blockage of blood vessels (ischemic stroke) receive clot-dissolving (thrombolytic) medications, such as recombinant tissue plasminogen activator (Alteplase) and the anticoagulant heparin. Individuals who have a stroke due to bleeding in the brain (hemorrhagic stroke) usually receive a surgical procedure that stops bleeding and repairs blood vessels. After the acute treatment of stroke, doctors often recommend rehabilitation, including physical, speech, and occupational therapy.

Dietary changes that may be helpful

Researchers have found an association between diets low in **potassium** (page 572) and increased risk of stroke.[1, 2, 3] People who take potassium supplements have been reported to have a low risk of suffering a stroke.[4] However, the association of increasing dietary potassium intake and decreasing stroke mortality only occurred in black men and **hypertensive** (page 246) men in one study.[5] Others have found an association between increased risk of stroke and the combination of low dietary potassium plus high salt intake.[6] Increasing dietary potassium has lowered blood pressure in humans, which by itself should reduce the risk of stroke.[7] However, some of the protective effect of potassium appears to extend beyond its ability to **lower blood pressure** (page 246).[8] Maintaining a high potassium intake is best achieved by eating fruits and vegetables.

Diets high in fruit and/or vegetables are associated with a reduced risk of stroke, according to most studies.[9, 10] In a large preliminary study, cruciferous and green leafy vegetables, as well as citrus fruit and juice, conferred the highest degree of protection.[11] Because it is not clear which components of fruits and vegetables are most responsible for the protective effect against stroke, people wishing to reduce their risk of stroke should rely primarily on eating more fruits and vegetables themselves, rather than taking supplements.

A large study also found that women who eat higher amounts of whole grains are at lower risk of ischemic stroke.[12] Those women who ate more than one whole-grain food on an average day (twice the amount of **fiber** (page 512) eaten by the average American) had approx-

imately a 35% lower risk of suffering an ischemic stroke compared with women who ate virtually no whole-grain products on an average day. This study fits with previous research showing that women who consume more whole grains are also at reduced risk for **heart disease** (page 98) caused by **atherosclerosis** (page 38).

The influence of dietary fat on the risk of stroke is not as clear as it is for heart disease risk. Some recent reports suggest an association between increased fat intake, including saturated fat (primarily found in meat and dairy), and a *decreased* stroke risk.[13, 14] These unexpected findings may be due to unique dietary conditions in the country studied (Japan) or to flaws in study design.[15, 16, 17] Other evidence suggests the opposite relationship—that people consuming more saturated fat are at *higher* risk of stroke.[18]

Evidence regarding the role of unsaturated fats (primarily found in vegetable oils, cooked and processed foods made with vegetable oils, nuts, and seeds) is equally unclear,[19, 20, 21] suggesting that unsaturated fats may have varying effects on different types of stroke or that some unsaturated fats differ from others in their influence on stroke risk.

Evidence is accumulating in favor of fish consumption, a rich source of **omega-3 fatty acids** (page 509), as a way to help prevent stroke. Eating fish has been linked to reduced stroke risk in most,[22, 23, 24] but not all,[25, 26] studies.

High salt intake is associated with both stroke[27] and **hypertension** (page 246), a major risk factor for stroke.[28] Salt intake may increase stroke risk independent of its effect on blood pressure.[29] Among **overweight** (page 446) people, an increase in salt consumption of about 1/2 teaspoon (2.3 grams) per day was associated with a 32% increase in stroke incidence and an 89% increase in stroke mortality.[30] Reducing salt intake is recommended as a way to reduce the risk of stroke.[31]

Having one or two drinks per day has lowered stroke risk in most studies,[32, 33] though some researchers report no protection[34] and others find that even light drinking leads to an increased risk of stroke.[35] Regular heavy drinking or binge drinking, however, has consistently raised the risk of suffering a stroke by increasing **blood pressure** (page 246) and causing heart muscle abnormalities and other effects.[36, 37, 38]

Lifestyle changes that may be helpful

Smoking is associated with a significantly increased risk of stroke.[39, 40, 41] Even secondhand smoke puts non-smokers at increased risk.[42]

Exercise reduces the risk of stroke according to most,[43, 44, 45, 46] though not all,[47] studies. The benefits of exercise are probably due to its effects on body weight, **blood pressure** (page 246), and glucose tolerance.

Obesity (page 446) has been associated with an increased risk of stroke in most studies.[48, 49] Excess abdominal fat appears to be more directly linked to increased risk of stroke, compared with fat accumulation in the thighs and buttocks.[50, 51, 52] While losing weight and keeping it off is difficult for most people, normalizing weight with a healthful diet and exercise program is one of the best ways to reduce the risk of many diseases, including stroke.

Nutritional supplements that may be helpful

Vinpocetine (page 594) given by intravenous injection has been reported to improve some biochemical measures of brain function in stroke patients.[53, 54] A controlled trial found intravenous vinpocetine given within 72 hours of a stroke reduced some of the losses in brain function that typically follow a stroke.[55] However, the reliability of human stroke research using vinpocetine has been questioned,[56, 57] and more double-blind trials are needed. No studies using oral vinpocetine for treating acute strokes have been published.

Elevated blood levels of **homocysteine** (page 234), a toxic **amino acid** (page 645) byproduct, have been linked to risk of stroke in most studies.[58, 59, 60] What is not clear, however, is whether high homocysteine levels cause strokes or are simply a marker for some other causative factor. Supplementation with **folic acid** (page 520), **vitamin B₆** (page 600), and **vitamin B₁₂** (page 601) generally lowers homocysteine levels in humans.[61, 62, 63] Whether lowering homocysteine will result in a decrease in the risk of suffering a stroke, however, remains unknown.

Narrowing of the neck arteries (carotid stenosis) caused by **atherosclerosis** (page 38) is a risk factor for stroke. Preliminary diet studies have found that people who eat foods high in **antioxidants** (page 467) such as **vitamin C** (page 604) and **vitamin E** (page 609) have less carotid stenosis.[64, 65]

In a double-blind trial, people with atherosclerosis in the carotid arteries were given a palm oil extract containing 160–240 mg of **tocotrienols** (page 593) (a vitamin E-like supplement) and approximately 100–150 IU **vitamin E** (page 609) per day. After 18 months, they had significantly less atherosclerosis or less progression of atherosclerosis compared to a group receiving placebo.[66] Vitamin E plus aspirin, has been more

effective in reducing the risk of strokes and other related events than has aspirin, alone.[67] However, most preliminary trials have shown no protective effects from antioxidant supplementation.[68, 69, 70, 71, 72, 73] A large Finnish trial concluded that supplementation with either vitamin E or **beta-carotene** (page 469) conferred no protection against stroke in male smokers,[74] although a later review of the study found that those smokers who have either **hypertension** (page 246) (high blood pressure) or **diabetes** (page 152) *do* appear to have a reduced risk of stroke when taking vitamin E.[75]

People with high risk for stroke, such as those who have had TIAs or who have a heart condition known as atrial fibrillation,[76] are often given aspirin or anticoagulant medication to reduce blood clotting tendencies. Some natural inhibitors of blood clotting such as **garlic** (page 679, [78, 79] **fish oil** (page 514),[80] and **vitamin E** (page 609),[81, 82] may have protective effects, but even large amounts of fish oil are known to be less potent than aspirin.[83] Whether any of these substances is an adequate substitute to control risk of stroke in high-risk people is unknown, and anyone taking anticoagulant medication should advise their prescribing doctor before beginning use of these natural substances.

Researchers have found an association between diets low in **magnesium** (page 551) and increased risk of stroke, an effect explained partially, but not completely, by the ability of magnesium to reduce **high blood pressure** (page 246).[84] Protection from stroke associated with drinking water high in magnesium has also been reported.[85] Intravenous magnesium given immediately after a stroke has been proposed as a treatment for reducing stroke deaths,[86] but results so far have been inconclusive.[87]

Are there any side effects or interactions?
Refer to the individual supplement for information about any side effects or interactions.

SYSTEMIC LUPUS ERYTHEMATOSUS

Systemic lupus erythematosus (SLE) is an autoimmune illness that causes a characteristic butterfly-shaped rash on the face accompanied by inflammation of connective tissue, particularly joints, throughout the body. In autoimmune diseases, the **immune system** (page 255) attacks the body instead of protecting it. Kidney, lung, and vascular damage are potential problems resulting from SLE.

The cause of SLE is unknown, though 90% of cases occur in women of childbearing age. Several drugs, such as procainamide, hydralazine, methyldopa, and chlorpromazine, may create SLE-like symptoms. Environmental pollution and industrial emissions were associated with an increased risk of SLE in one study.[1] In one reported case, **zinc** (page 614) supplementation appears to have aggravated drug-induced SLE.[2] Ultraviolet radiation from sun exposure is a commonly recognized trigger of the skin manifestations of lupus.[3] Some environmental chemicals such as hydrazine[4] and food dyes such as tartrazine[5] may be environmental triggers of SLE in susceptible people.

Risk factors include a family history of SLE, other collagen diseases or **asthma** (page 30),[6] menstrual irregularity,[7] beginning menstruation at age 15 or later,[8] exposure to toxic chemicals,[9] and low blood levels of **antioxidant** (page 467) nutrients, such as **vitamin A** (page 595) and **vitamin E** (page 609), or **beta-carotene** (page 469).[10] Free radicals are thought to promote SLE.[11]

Discoid lupus erythematosus (DLE) is a milder form of lupus that affects the skin. Like SLE, it's not known what causes DLE, though sun exposure may trigger the first outbreak. DLE is most common among women in their thirties.

Rating	Nutritional Supplements	Herbs
★★☆	**DHEA** (page 503) **Fish oil** (page 514) (EPA/DHA [page 509])	*Tripterygium wilfordii*
★☆☆	**Pantothenic acid** (page 568) **Vitamin E** (page 609)	**Astragalus** (page 631)

CHECKLIST FOR SYSTEMIC LUPUS ERYTHEMATOSUS

What are the symptoms of SLE?

Symptoms include decreased energy, weakness, fever, nausea, **diarrhea** (page 163), muscle and joint pain, chest pain, **bruising** (page 84), loss of appetite, weight loss, and a red, butterfly-shaped rash across the nose and cheeks. In addition, people with SLE may have symptoms of mouth sores, joint swelling, hair loss, changes in personality, seizures, and a coin-shaped, red skin rash elsewhere on the body that is aggravated by sunlight. Kidney, lung, and blood-vessel damage are potentially life-threatening manifestations of SLE.

Medical treatments

Prescription drug treatment includes cortisone-like drugs, such as prednisone (Deltasone, Orasone), methylprednisolone (Medrol), and dexamethasone (Decadron); the hormone dehydroepiandrosterone (**DHEA** [page 503]); immunosuppressants, such as azathioprine (Imuran), chlorambucil (Leukeran), cyclosporine (Sandimmune), methotrexate (Rheumatrex), and cyclophosphamide (Cytoxan); and the antimalarial drugs hydroxychloroquine (Plaquenil) and chloroquine (Aralen). The goal of therapy is to suppress symptoms and relieve discomfort.

Dietary changes that may be helpful

An isolated case of someone with SLE improving significantly after the introduction of a vegetarian diet has been reported.[12] In Japan, women who frequently ate fatty meats, such as beef and pork, were reported to be at higher risk for SLE compared with women eating little of these foods.[13] Consuming fewer calories, less fat, and foods low in **phenylalanine** (page 568) and **tyrosine** (page 465) (prevalent in high protein foods, such as meat and dairy) might be helpful, according to animal and preliminary human studies.[14]

Foods high in omega-3 fatty acids, such as fish and **flaxseed** (page 517), may decrease lupus-induced inflammation. In one preliminary trial, nine people with kidney damage due to SLE were fed increasing amounts of flaxseed for a total of 12 weeks.[15] After examining the results, researchers concluded that 30 grams per day was the optimal intake for improving kidney function, decreasing inflammation, and reducing **atherosclerotic** (page 38) development. Flaxseeds also contain **antioxidants** (page 467), potentially helpful to those with SLE.[16]

To date, all studies on **fish oil** (page 514) have used supplements and not fish (see below). Nonetheless, many doctors recommend that SLE patients eat several servings of fatty fish each week.

Spanish researchers discovered that people with SLE tend to have more **allergies** (page 14), including food allergies, than do healthy people or even people with other autoimmune diseases.[17] While one study reported that drinking milk was associated with a decrease in SLE risk,[18] other investigations point to both beef[19] and dairy[20] as foods that might trigger allergic reactions in some people with SLE. Casein, the main protein in cow's milk, has immune-stimulating properties.[21] This might explain why some people with SLE have been reported to be intolerant of milk products. Although there are several published case reports of patients with SLE showing clinical improvement after avoiding allergenic foods, additional research is needed to determine the importance of allergies as a cause of SLE. People with SLE who wish to explore whether allergies are contributing to their condition should consult a doctor.

Alfalfa (page 623) seeds and sprouts contain the amino acid L-canavanine, which provokes a lupus-like condition in monkeys[22] and possibly humans.[23] For this reason, some doctors recommend that people with SLE should avoid these foods. Cooking alfalfa seeds has been reported to erase this effect.[24]

Lifestyle changes that may be helpful

In preliminary research, smoking has been linked to significantly increased risk of developing SLE, while drinking alcohol has been associated with a decrease in risk.[25] The importance of these associations remains unclear, though an increased risk for many other diseases has been definitively linked to excessive consumption of alcohol.

Nutritional supplements that may be helpful

Low blood levels of the hormone DHEA and the related compound DHEA-sulfate have been associated with more severe symptoms in people with SLE.[26] Preliminary trials have suggested that 50 to 200 mg per day DHEA improved symptoms in people with SLE.[27, 28] One double-blind trial of women with mild to moderate SLE found that 200 mg of **DHEA** (page 503) per day improved symptoms and allowed a greater decrease in prednisone use,[29] but a similar trial in women with severe SLE found only insignificant benefits.[30]

Experts have concerns about the use of **DHEA** (page 503), particularly because there are no long-term safety data. Side effects at high intakes (50 to 200 mg per day) in one 12-month trial included acne (in over 50% of people), increased facial hair (18%), and increased perspiration (8%). Less common problems reported with DHEA supplementation were breast tenderness, weight gain, mood alteration, headache, oily skin, and menstrual irregularity.[31]

High amounts of DHEA have caused cancer in animals.[32, 33] Although *anti*cancer effects of DHEA have also been reported,[34] they involve trials using animals that do not process DHEA the way humans do, so these positive effects may have no relevance for people.

Links have begun to appear between higher DHEA levels and risks of prostate cancer in humans.[35] At least one person with **prostate cancer** (page 371) has been reported to have had a worsening of his cancer despite feeling better while taking very high amounts (up to 700 mg per day) of DHEA.[36] While younger women with breast cancer may have low levels of DHEA, postmenopausal women with **breast cancer** (page 65) appear to have high levels of DHEA, which has researchers concerned.[37] These cancer concerns make sense because DHEA is a precursor to testosterone (linked to prostate cancer) and estrogen (linked to breast cancer). Until more is known, it would be prudent for people with breast or prostate cancer or a family history of these conditions to avoid supplementing with DHEA. Preliminary evidence has also linked higher DHEA levels to ovarian cancer in women.[38]

Some doctors recommend that people taking DHEA have liver enzymes measured routinely. Anecdotes of DHEA supplementation (of at least 25 mg per day) leading to **heart arrhythmias** (page 93) have appeared.[39] At only 25 mg per day, DHEA has lowered HDL cholesterol while increasing insulin-like growth factor (IGF).[40] Decreasing HDL could increase the risk of **heart disease** (page 98). Increasing IGF might increase the risk of breast cancer.

The omega-3 fatty acids in **fish oil** (page 514)—eicosapentaenoic acid (EPA) and docosahexaenoic acid (**DHA** [page 509])—decrease inflammation. Supplementation with EPA and DHA has prevented autoimmune lupus in animal research.[41] In a double-blind trial, 20 grams of fish oil daily combined with a low-fat diet led to improvement in 14 of 17 people with SLE in 12 weeks.[42] Smaller amounts of fish oil have led to only temporary improvement in another double-blind trial.[43] People wishing to take such a large amount of fish oil should first consult with a doctor.

Antioxidant (page 467) levels have been reported to be low in people with SLE, though this finding was not statistically significant in one trial.[44] When animals are fed antioxidant-deficient diets, they develop a condition similar to SLE; supplementation with antioxidants, such as **vitamin C** (page 604), **vitamin E** (page 609), **beta-carotene** (page 469), and **selenium** (page 584), has helped animals with existing SLE.[45] It remains unclear whether antioxidant supplementation would have a positive effect on people with SLE.

Some preliminary evidence suggests that **vitamin E** (page 609) might help people with discoid lupus erythematosus (DLE). Two doctors reported good to excellent results by giving 800–2,000 IU of vitamin E per day to eight people with DLE.[46, 47] According to these physicians, lower amounts of vitamin E did not work as well. In another small trial, vitamin E, also given in high amounts, had no effect.[48] Unlike with DLE, there appear to be no reports on the effects of vitamin E in people with SLE.

In one preliminary report, 250,000 IU beta-carotene per day cleared up all facial rashes in as little as one week for three people with DLE.[49] However, another study involving 26 people (19 with DLE and seven with SLE) found that using an even higher intake (400,000 IU per day) for an average of five and a half months was ineffective.[50] Research has not yet supported the use of beta-carotene for people with SLE.

Preliminary research suggests that **pantothenic acid** (page 568), when taken together with vitamin E, may help those with DLE. In one trial, taking 10 to 15 grams of pantothenic acid per day with 1,500 to 3,000 IU of vitamin E per day for as long as 19 months helped 67 people with DLE.[51] Pantothenic acid by itself for shorter periods of time in lower amounts has been reported to fail.[52] The amounts of pantothenic acid and vitamin E used in the first trial are very high and should not be taken without the supervision of a physician.

In a preliminary study, supplementation with pycnogenol was said to be beneficial in a small group of people with SLE.[53] However, in this study, the pycnogenol and placebo groups were not comparable; moreover, according to some criteria, the placebo group actually fared better than the treatment group. Until a better designed study is performed, pycnogenol cannot be recommended as a treatment for lupus.

Are there any side effects or interactions?
Refer to the individual supplement for information about any side effects or interactions.

Herbs that may be helpful
Preliminary evidence indicates that some Chinese herbs may help those with SLE. In one preliminary trial, a formula composed of 17 Chinese herbs was given to people with SLE.[54] Of the people who were also taking cortisone, 92% improved, but 85% of those taking the herbs alone also benefited. People with SLE-induced kidney damage given a combination of conventional drugs plus a Chinese herbal formula for six months did significantly better than those given the drugs alone.[55]

Various Chinese herbs have prolonged survival in animals with SLE.[56]

One of these Chinese herbs, *Tripterygium wilfordii,* is thought to benefit those with SLE or DLE by both suppressing **immune function** (page 255) and acting as an anti-inflammatory agent. When people with DLE took 30 to 45 grams of tripterygium per day for two weeks in a preliminary trial, most experienced some degree of improvement, including reduction or disappearance of skin rashes.[57] Skin rashes in eight people completely cleared up, while in ten people over 50% of the rash improved.

A preliminary trial gave the same dose of tripterygium to people with SLE. [58] After one month, 54% experienced relief from symptoms such as joint pain and malaise.

Use of the crude tripterygium herb is not recommended, and people interested in using it should work with their doctor to obtain the specially prepared and standardized extracts used in clinical studies. Because of potential side effects, people with SLE or DLE should consult with a doctor experienced in herbal medicine before using this herb. In the first two studies summarized, less than 8% of women with DLE and approximately one-third of women with SLE experienced **amenorrhea** (page 22) (cessation of menstruation) after taking tripterygium. Other side effects ranged from stomach upset or pain, to nausea, loss of appetite, dizziness, and increased facial coloring. Both studies found that these effects subsided with time once people stopped using the herb. However, some reports have found more serious side effects and even death with use of tripterygium.[59] **Pregnant** (page 363) women should not use the herb.

Finally, a report suggests that long-term use (over five years) of tripterygium significantly reduced bone density in women taking it to treat lupus.[60] While this loss of bone density was less severe than that found with long-term use of prednisone, lupus patients should have their bone density checked at yearly intervals by their doctor when using the herb.

One Chinese preliminary trial also found that **astragalus** (page 631) could decrease overactive immune function in people with systemic lupus erythematosus.[61] However, much more research is needed to know whether astragalus is safe in lupus or any other autoimmune disease.

Are there any side effects or interactions?
Refer to the individual herb for information about any side effects or interactions.

TARDIVE DYSKINESIA

Tardive Dyskinesia (TD) is a condition of abnormal, repetitive, uncontrollable movements that develop after a long-term use of so-called antipsychotic medications used to treat **schizophrenia** (page 393) and related psychiatric disorders. The term "tardive" (which means "late") is used because the condition appears only after long-term use of these drugs, which include chlorpromazine (Thorazine), thioridazine (Mellaril), and trifluoperazine (Stelazine). Dyskinesia means "abnormal movement."

The uncontrollable movements of TD can interfere greatly with a person's quality of life. TD may gradually diminish in severity after the medication is discontinued, but all too often the problem is permanent, persisting after withdrawal from the drugs that caused the condition. Conventional treatment for TD is unsatisfactory, so prevention is considered crucial. It is important that people requiring antipsychotic drugs be given the lowest effective dose and that treatment be discontinued as soon as it is feasible.

CHECKLIST FOR TARDIVE DYSKINESIA

Rating	Nutritional Supplements	Herbs
★★★	**Vitamin E** (page 609)	
★★☆	**Choline** (page 546) **Lecithin** (page 546) **Manganese** (page 553) **Melatonin** (page 555)	
★☆☆	**Branched-chain amino acids** (page 479) (BCAA) **DMAE** (page 508) **Evening primrose oil** (page 511) **Vitamin B-complex** (page 603) **Vitamin B₃** (page 598) (niacin or niacinamide) **Vitamin B₆** (page 600) **Vitamin C** (page 604)	

What are the symptoms of tardive dyskinesia?

Symptoms of TD include repetitive and involuntary movements (tics), most often of the facial muscles and tongue (such as lip smacking), although any muscle in the body can be affected (e.g., moving legs back and forth). Symptoms may be mild or severe and can interfere with eating and walking.

Medical treatments

Prescription drugs used to treat tardive dyskinesia include trihexyphenidyl (Artane, Trihexy), benztropine (Cogentin), and dopamine-depleting agents, such as reserpine.

Electroconvulsive therapy (electrical current applied to the brain) may be administered in severe cases. Healthcare providers may recommend discontinuing the use of antipsychotic drugs if possible.

Nutritional supplements that may be helpful

Vitamin E (page 609) has been found in a number of studies to reduce the severity of TD. In a double-blind trial, people with TD were randomly assigned to receive vitamin E (800 IU per day for two weeks and 1,600 IU per day thereafter) or a placebo. Vitamin E was significantly more effective than placebo in reducing involuntary movements.[1] An uncontrolled study of 20 people with TD reported that 1,600 IU of vitamin E per day may be the optimal amount;[2] this large amount should be supervised by a healthcare practitioner. Other studies have also found that vitamin E supplements reduce the severity of TD.[3, 4, 5] Two studies failed to show a beneficial effect of vitamin E.[6, 7] However, the people in those studies had been receiving neuroleptics for at least ten years, and research has shown that vitamin E is most effective when started within the first five years of neuroleptic treatment.[8, 9]

Choline (page 546) and **lecithin** (page 546) have both been used for people with TD. While some studies have shown a beneficial effect,[10, 11, 12] others have reported variable improvement[13] or no improvement.[14] In a small, two-week, double-blind trial, people with TD were given 25 grams of lecithin twice a day, or a matching placebo. All participants experienced significant improvement of symptoms.[15]

Dimethylaminoethanol (page 508) (DMAE) is a natural choline precursor. Although some preliminary data suggested that DMAE could decrease TD symptoms,[16] most studies show that DMAE is no more effective than placebo for TD.[17]

One doctor has found that administering the trace mineral **manganese** (page 553) (15 mg per day) can prevent the development of TD and that higher amounts (up to 60 mg per day) can reverse TD that has already developed.[18] Other researchers have reported similar improvements with manganese.[19, 20]

Several people have experienced an improvement in TD while taking **evening primrose oil** (page 511) (EPO).[21] In a double-blind study, however, supplementing with EPO (12 capsules per day) resulted only in a minor, clinically insignificant improvement.[22]

Preliminary research has linked TD to the inability of the body to metabolize the amino acid **phenylalanine** (page 568). Supplementing with **branched-chain amino acids** (page 479) (BCAA), including valine, isoleucine, and leucine, could reduce excess phenylalanine in people with this disorder. In one trial, researchers examined the effects of BCAA supplementation in people with TD (from 150 mg per 2.2 pounds body weight, up to 209 mg per 2.2 pounds body weight) after breakfast and one hour before lunch and dinner for two weeks.[23] The BCAA mixture included equal parts valine and isoleucine plus 33% more leucine than either of the other two amino acids. Of nine people treated, six experienced at least a 58% reduction in symptoms, and all nine had a least a 38% decrease.

During a ten-year period, doctors at the North Nassau Mental Health Center in New York treated approximately 11,000 people with **schizophrenia** (page 393) with a megavitamin regimen that included **vitamin C** (page 604) (up to 4 grams per day), **vitamin B₃** (page 598)—either as niacin or niacinamide—(up to 4 grams per day), **vitamin B₆** (page 600) (up to 800 mg per day), and **vitamin E** (page 609) (up to 1,200 IU per day). During that time, not a single new case of TD was seen, even though many of the people were taking neuroleptic drugs.[24] Another psychiatrist who routinely used **niacinamide** (page 598), vitamin C, and **vitamin B-complex** (page 603) over a 28-year period rarely saw TD develop in her patients.[25] Further research is needed to determine which nutrients or combinations of nutrients were most important for preventing TD. The amounts of niacinamide and vitamin B₆ used in this research may cause significant side effects and may require monitoring by a doctor.

In a double-blind trial, supplementation with 10 mg of **melatonin** (page 555) each night for six weeks reduced abnormal movements by 23.8% in patients with TD, compared with 8.4% in the placebo group, a statistically significant difference.[26]

Are there any side effects or interactions?
Refer to the individual supplement for information about any side effects or interactions.

TENDINITIS

Tendinitis is a condition where a tendon or the connective tissue that surrounds the tendon becomes inflamed.

This is often due to overuse (e.g., repetitive work activities), acute injury, or excessive exercise. People who are at higher risk of developing tendinitis include athletes, manual laborers, and computer keyboard users. Occasionally, tendinitis may be due to diseases that affect the whole body, such as **rheumatoid arthritis** (page 387) or **gout** (page 208).

The most common sites of tendinitis are the shoulder, elbow, forearm, thumb, hip, hamstring muscles (in the back of the upper leg), and Achilles tendon (behind the ankle).[1]

CHECKLIST FOR TENDINITIS		
Rating	Nutritional Supplements	Herbs
★★★	**DMSO** (page 508) (topical)	
★★☆	**Bromelain** (page 481) **Proteolytic enzymes** (page 506)	

What are the symptoms of tendinitis?
People with tendinitis may have symptoms, which appear after injury or overuse, including swelling, redness, tenderness, and sharp pain in the affected area, which is worsened with movement or pressure.

Medical treatments
Over the counter pain medications, such as aspirin (Bayer, Ecotrin, Bufferin), acetaminophen (Tylenol), and ibuprofen (Motrin, Advil), are routinely recommended to relieve minor pain and reduce inflammation. Topical methyl salicylate (Icy Hot, Ben-Gay), trolamine salicylate (Aspercreme), and combination counterirritant products (Maximum Strength Flexall 454) may be beneficial to relieve pain.

Prescription strength nonsteroidal anti-inflammatory drugs (NSAIDs), such as celecoxib (Celebrex), valdecoxib (Bextra), ibuprofen (Motrin), naproxen (Anaprox, Naprosyn), and indomethacin (Indocin), may be necessary to treat inflammation and pain. Acetaminophen combined with codeine (Tylenol with Codeine) orhydrocodone (Vicodin) may be used to treat moderate pain.

Treatment may include local injections of steroids such as dexamethasone (Decadron-LA), methylprednisolone (Depo-Medrol), and hydrocortisone (Solu-Cortef), or anesthetics such as lidocaine (Xylocaine), as well as immobilization and controlled physical therapy.

Lifestyle changes that may be helpful

Many people suffer from tendinitis as a result of their work environment. Studies have shown that tendinitis of the wrist, hands, and fingers are often caused by repetitive work and physical stress.[2, 3, 4] Physical changes to the work environment, such as setting up the work station so that the body is in a balanced, untwisted position, minimizing the need to use excessive force, avoiding overuse of any one joint, changing positions frequently, and allowing for rest periods, have all been shown to diminish symptoms of lower arm tendinitis.[5] One study of computer workers with arm and wrist tendinitis found that using an ergonomic keyboard versus a standard keyboard reduced the severity of pain and improved hand function after six months of use.[6]

Nutritional supplements that may be helpful

DMSO (page 508), or dimethyl sulfoxide, has a long history as a topical anti-inflammatory agent. One double-blind trial used a 10% DMSO gel topically on patients with tendinitis of the elbow and shoulder and found that it significantly reduced pain and inflammation in each joint.[7] Other preliminary[8, 9] and double-blind[10, 11] trials found DMSO to be effective in treating tendinitis, but one double-blind trial found no difference between the effects of a 70% DMSO solution and a 5% DMSO placebo solution.[12] Certain precautions must be taken when applying DMSO, and it should only be used under the guidance of a qualified healthcare professional.

Alternative healthcare practitioners frequently recommend proteolytic enzymes (page 506) for various minor injuries. Research demonstrates that these enzymes are well absorbed when taken by mouth,[13, 14] and preliminary[15, 16, 17, 18] and double-blind[19, 20, 21, 22] trials have shown their effectiveness for reducing pain and swelling associated with various injuries and for speeding up the healing process. Unfortunately, many of these studies did not specifically identify the patients' injury, so it is unclear whether the positive results included improvements in tendinitis.

Bromelain (page 481), a proteolytic enzyme, is an anti-inflammatory agent and for this reason is helpful in healing minor injuries, particularly sprains and strains (page 412), muscle injuries, and the pain (page 338), swelling, and tenderness that accompany sports injuries.[23, 24, 25]

Are there any side effects or interactions?
Refer to the individual supplement for information about any side effects or interactions.

Holistic approaches that may be helpful

Acupuncture may be helpful for treating tendinitis. A controlled trial compared acupuncture to sham (fake) acupuncture in people with shoulder tendinitis and found that acupuncture treatment produced significantly higher scores on a combined measurement of pain, ability to perform daily activities, ability to move shoulder without pain, and strength.[26] This study also reported that the beneficial effects of acupuncture continued for at least three months following treatment. Another controlled study found traditional "deep" acupuncture more effective than superficial acupuncture for tennis elbow immediately after a series of ten treatments, but at 3 to 12 months' follow up, both treatment groups had improved similarly.[27] A third controlled study found no benefit from ten treatments of laser acupuncture for tennis elbow.[28]

Certain treatments used by physicians and other healthcare practitioners have been shown to be effective for tendinitis. In a controlled trial, patients with tendinitis of the shoulder received 24 treatments over six weeks of either ultrasound or a sham treatment.[29] Ultrasound resulted in considerable improvement in pain level and overall quality of life, but many of the patients had their original symptoms return after nine months. The use of ultrasound for tennis elbow has not been validated, according to a systematic review of controlled studies.[30] One controlled trial compared the effects of ultrasound alone to ultrasound plus a topical steroid medication (a process known as phonophoresis, where ultrasound is used to drive a substance into the skin).[31] Both of these treatments were given three times per week for three weeks and both produced similar reductions in pain and tenderness.

Preliminary studies have suggested that daily use of TENS (transcutaneous electrical nerve stimulation) for one to two weeks reduces or eliminates pain in patients with tendinitis.[32, 33] Controlled studies are needed to confirm these findings.

Tendinitis

TENSION HEADACHE

A tension-type headache is common and typically experienced as a dull, non-throbbing pain in the back of the neck or in a "headband" distribution.[1] It may be associated with tender nodules in the neck called triggerpoints,[2] or with tenderness in the muscles around the head.[3]

Rating	Nutritional Supplements	Herbs
CHECKLIST FOR TENSION HEADACHE		
★★☆	L-5-hydroxytryptophan (page 459) (5-HTP)	Peppermint (page 726) oil (topical)

What are the symptoms of tension headaches?
People with a headache may have symptoms including uncomfortable sensations described as pain, throbbing, aching, dullness, heaviness, and tightness in the head. People with a headache may also experience discomfort that is often worsened by movement or pressure and may be associated with irritability, problems sleeping, and fatigue.

Medical treatments
Over the counter pain medications, such as aspirin (Bayer, Ecotrin, Bufferin), acetaminophen (Tylenol), and ibuprofen (Motrin, Advil), are routinely recommended to relieve minor pain from tension headaches.

Healthcare practitioners might recommend application of moist heat to tight neck muscles and light massage.

Lifestyle changes that may be helpful
Tension-type headaches often occur more frequently and may become more severe during or following times of mental or emotional stress.[4, 5, 6] Several controlled studies have found tension-type headache sufferers to report higher levels of stress,[7, 8, 9] and to have significantly higher levels of **depression** (page 145) or **anxiety** (page 30),[10, 11, 12] significantly greater levels of suppressed anger,[13] or significantly greater muscle tension[14, 15] than those without headaches. Minimizing stress and getting enough sleep and regular exercise are often recommended to people with tension-type headaches. However, no research has investigated the effectiveness of these lifestyle changes.

One controlled study that included patients with muscle-contraction headache as well as other types of headache, revealed that smokers had significantly more severe headache episodes than nonsmokers.[16] Although other studies have not found an association between smoking and headaches, stopping smoking is always a good idea for many health reasons.

Nutritional supplements that may be helpful
L-5-hydroxytryptophan (page 459) (5-HTP) may be helpful for tension-type headaches. A recent double-blind study of adults with chronic tension-type headaches found 300 mg per day of 5-HTP reduced the number of headache days by 36%, but this was not significantly different from the 29% reduction in the placebo group.[17] (Headaches often improve significantly even when an inactive [placebo] treatment is given).[18] Headache severity was also similarly reduced by either 5-HTP or placebo. In this study, 5-HTP was significantly superior to placebo only in reducing the need for pain-relieving medications during headaches. Previous double-blind research studied 5-HTP in groups of patients suffering from many different types of headache, including some with tension-type headaches. Results from these studies also found substantial, but nonsignificant benefits of 5-HTP compared with placebo using either 400 mg per day in adults[19] or 100 mg per day in children.[20]

Are there any side effects or interactions?
Refer to the individual supplement for information about any side effects or interactions.

Herbs that may be helpful
A preliminary report suggested that **peppermint** (page 726) oil has relaxing and pain relieving effects, and may be useful as a topical remedy for tension-type headache.[21] In a double-blind study, spreading a 10% peppermint oil solution across the temples three times over a 30-minute period was significantly better than placebo and as effective as acetaminophen in reducing headache pain.[22] Similar use of an ointment combining menthol and other oils related to peppermint oil was also as effective as pain relieving medication and superior to placebo in another double-blind study.[23]

Are there any side effects or interactions?
Refer to the individual herb for information about any side effects or interactions.

Holistic approaches that may be helpful

Studies treating tension-type headache with acupuncture have had mixed results.[24] Two controlled trials of acupuncture compared to "fake" acupuncture found either significantly more pain reduction from real acupuncture[25] or no difference between the two treatments.[26] Two trials comparing acupuncture to traditional physical therapy (relaxation techniques, self-massage, cold therapy, transcutaneous electrical nerve stimulation [TENS], stretching, and/or preventive education) in tension-type headache patients found similar improvements from either treatment.[27, 28] Three controlled acupuncture trials treated patients with various types of headaches, including tension headache. Two of these studies,[29, 30] but not the third,[31] found acupuncture significantly more effective.

Two preliminary studies[32, 33] reported benefits from using finger pressure on specific acupuncture points (acupressure) to relieve tension-type headache pain in some patients. However, no controlled research on this approach has been done.

Spinal manipulation may also help some tension-type headache sufferers. Several preliminary studies report reduction in frequency and severity of tension-type headaches with spinal manipulation.[34, 35, 36, 37, 38, 39] A controlled trial compared spinal manipulation to drug therapy for tension-type headaches.[40] During the treatment period, both groups improved at similar significant rates, although the manipulation group complained of far fewer side effects. After a month following the end of treatment, only the manipulation group showed continued improvement. In another controlled trial, spinal manipulation resulted in fewer headache hours each day, decreased use of analgesics, and less intense pain per episode compared with massage.[41] A third controlled study reported that spinal manipulation with muscle massage was equally as effective as massage plus a "fake" laser treatment, suggesting that manipulation did not provide additional benefit.[42]

As mentioned above, two controlled studies found physical therapy (relaxation techniques, self-massage, cold therapy, TENS, stretching, and/or preventive education) as useful as acupuncture in significantly reducing headache pain and frequency.[43, 44] A preliminary study also found that physical therapy, consisting of posture education, home exercises, massage, and stretching of the neck muscles, significantly improved tension headaches up to 12 months after treatment ended.[45] Another preliminary study of massage, including deep penetrating techniques, reported significantly decreased pain in patients with chronic tension headache and neck pain.[46] A controlled study of headache patients with muscle spasm in the neck and shoulders found that adding TENS to physical therapy (consisting of heat packs, massage, and ultrasound) brought a significantly faster and greater decline in headaches than physical therapy alone.[47]

Several controlled trials utilizing electromyogram (EMG)-biofeedback (which teaches people how to mentally relax their neck or head muscles) have shown this treatment to be helpful in about 50% of tension-type headache sufferers, both in adults[48, 49, 50, 51, 52] and in children and adolescents.[53, 54] Progressive muscle relaxation is another muscle relaxation technique that has significantly reduced tension-type headache in controlled studies of adults,[55, 56] and children and adolescents.[57, 58]

Relaxation with techniques for stress management was found to be significantly better than drug therapy in a controlled trial of chronic tension-type headache sufferers,[59] although about half of all subjects continued to have headaches three to four days per week after the end of treatment.

Hypnotherapy was found to significantly reduce headache intensity and duration in chronic tension-type headache sufferers in one controlled trial.[60]

A large controlled study of tension headache patients compared relaxation therapies (including progressive muscle relaxation, hypnosis, and cognitive psychotherapy) with EMG-biofeedback, and found biofeedback to be significantly more effective than relaxation in decreasing headache pain and frequency.[61]

In a controlled trial, therapeutic touch, a type of hands-on healing, was found to significantly reduce tension headache pain for four hours following treatment.[62] No further research has been done on this approach.

Reflexology, a specific treatment involving massage of various reflex zones on the feet, has only been investigated as a treatment for tension-type headache in one preliminary trial.[63] A majority of people treated in this study reported being helped by this technique.

A controlled trial of homeopathy in headache patients, including tension-type headache, found no significant benefit of homeopathy compared to a placebo group.[64]

TINNITUS

Rarely, tinnitus is due to an actual sound, such as blood rushing through an enlarged vein—a problem that requires medical treatment. More commonly the problem is due to nerve irritation from an unknown source or an underlying ear problem often induced by noise damage. The cause of tinnitus should be diagnosed by a doctor.

Rating	Nutritional Supplements	Herbs
CHECKLIST FOR TINNITUS (RINGING IN THE EARS)		
★★☆	**Melatonin** (page 555) (insomnia-associated) **Zinc** (page 614) (for deficiency only)	
★☆☆	**Vitamin B**$_{12}$ (page 601) (injection)	*Ginkgo biloba* (page 681) *Periwinkle* (page 727)

What are the symptoms of tinnitus?

Symptoms may include hearing buzzing, roaring, ringing, whistling, or hissing sounds. These sounds may be intermittent, continuous, or pulsing. Tinnitus may interfere with normal activities and sleep, and there may be an associated decrease in the ability to hear conversation or other sounds in the environment.

Medical treatments

Treatment is typically directed at any underlying medical condition. In some cases, doctors recommend the use of a tinnitus masker, which is a hearing device that produces a sound that is more tolerable than the tinnitus. In addition, doctors may suggest the use of earplugs in the presence of loud noises to prevent damage to the ear.

Dietary changes that may be helpful

Ménière's disease (page 308) (a condition characterized by tinnitus, **vertigo** [page 441], and hearing loss) is reportedly associated with various metabolic abnormalities, including elevations of serum **cholesterol** (page 223) and/or **triglycerides** (page 235) and abnormal regulation of blood sugar. In one trial, people with Ménière's disease who replaced refined carbohydrates in their diet with foods high in **fiber** (page 512) and complex carbohydrates frequently experienced an improvement or disappearance of their tinnitus.[1]

Nutritional supplements that may be helpful

Zinc (page 614) supplements have been used to treat people who had both tinnitus and hearing loss (usually age-related). Of those who had initially low blood levels of zinc, about 25% experienced an improvement in tinnitus after taking zinc (90–150 mg per day for three to six months).[2] Such large amounts of zinc should be monitored by a doctor. Two controlled clinical trials[3, 4] found no benefit from zinc supplementation (66 mg per day in one double-blind trial) in people with tinnitus. However, participants in these studies were not zinc deficient. Preliminary research suggests that zinc supplementation is only helpful for tinnitus in people who are zinc deficient.[5] A doctor can measure blood levels of zinc.

In a double-blind trial, **melatonin** (page 555) supplementation (3 mg taken nightly) improved the symptoms of tinnitus.[6] Although improvement did not reach statistical significance for all participants, the results were significant in those who reported more severe symptoms (such as two-sided vs. one-sided tinnitus). Among participants who had difficulty sleeping due to tinnitus, 47% of those who took melatonin reported sleep improvement after one month, compared with only 20% of those who took placebo.

People exposed to loud noise on the job who develop tinnitus are commonly deficient in **Vitamin B**$_{12}$ (page 601).[7] Intramuscular injections of vitamin B$_{12}$ reduced the severity of tinnitus in some of these people. Injectable vitamin B$_{12}$ is available only by prescription. The effect of oral vitamin B$_{12}$ on tinnitus has not been studied.

Are there any side effects or interactions?
Refer to the individual supplement for information about any side effects or interactions.

Herbs that may be helpful

Lesser **periwinkle** (page 727) *(Vinca minor)* contains a compound known as vincamine. Extracts containing vincamine have been used in Germany to help decrease tinnitus.[8] Preliminary clinical trial data show that vinpocetine, a semi-synthetic version of vincamine, can help reduce symptoms in people whose tinnitus is due to poor blood flow.[9] Because these extracts are not widely available outside of Germany, consult with a doctor knowledgeable in botanical medicine about obtaining them.

Ginkgo biloba (page 681) has been used to treat tinnitus, with mixed results.[10] The largest placebo-controlled trial to date failed to find any effect of 150 mg per day of ginkgo extract in people with tinnitus.[11] Two smaller, controlled trials have found that standardized ginkgo extract (120 mg per day, containing 24% flavone glycosides and 6% terpene lactones), was effective at relieving the symptoms of tinnitus.[12, 13] One trial failed to find ginkgo beneficial, but used less than 30 mg of ginkgo extract per day, an amount unlikely to have any therapeutic effect.[14]

Are there any side effects or interactions?
Refer to the individual herb for information about any side effects or interactions.

Holistic approaches that may be helpful
Acupuncture has been studied as a treatment for tinnitus in several controlled trials. Preliminary trials have reported improvement in symptoms of tinnitus following acupuncture treatment, but this relief was either not permanent or did not reach statistical significance.[15] Most trials have shown no advantage of acupuncture treatment over placebo for the treatment of tinnitus.[16, 17, 18, 19, 20, 21, 22] A review of clinical trials concluded that acupuncture is not an effective treatment for tinnitus.[23]

TOOTH DECAY

Tooth decay is the gradual breakdown of the tooth, beginning with the enamel surface and eventually progressing to the inner pulp.

Tooth decay is caused by acids produced by certain mouth bacteria in dental plaque. Factors that affect this process include oral hygiene, diet, meal frequency, saliva production, and heredity. Teeth with significant decay are said to have caries, or cavities.

What are the symptoms of tooth decay?
People with tooth decay may have tooth pain, including sensitivity to cold food and drinks.

Medical treatments
Over the counter products containing fluoride (Gel Kam, ACT) may help prevent tooth decay.

Prescription strength fluoride toothpaste (Prevident) may be prescribed. Individuals living in communities without fluoridated water might be prescribed oral fluoride tablets or drops (Luride).

Treatment includes daily brushing of teeth with toothpaste (especially after meals), flossing, limiting sugar in the diet, and regular professional teeth cleanings by a dental hygienist. Dentists commonly apply fillings to dental cavities. Topical fluoride applications or sealants (plastic coatings that form a barrier between bacteria and the chewing surfaces of the teeth) may be recommended.

CHECKLIST FOR TOOTH DECAY		
Rating	**Nutritional Supplements**	**Herbs**
★★★	**Fluoride** (page 519) *Lactobacillus* **GG** (page 575) **Xylitol** (page 614)	
★★☆	**Cod liver oil** (page 514) **Vitamin B$_6$** (page 600)	Black tea **Green tea** (page 686) *(Camellia sinensis)* Neem
★☆☆	Sorbitol **Strontium** (page 589)	

Dietary changes that may be helpful
It has been noted for over 50 years that the incidence of tooth decay is low in people of traditional rural societies, such as Eskimos and African Bantus. However, the incidence of cavities increases as their diets begin to include more "westernized" processed foods.[1] Although many different factors have been implicated in this observation, including refined flours,[2, 3] inactivation of vitamins by heating foods,[4] and sugar intake,[5] no single agent has been found responsible. Nevertheless, a diet high in whole grains and low in processed foods is a healthful choice that probably helps defend against tooth decay.

Sugar, especially sucrose (table sugar), appears to be required by the oral bacteria for the production of tooth decay. This finding has caused sugar to be widely blamed in the popular press as the primary cause of dental caries. However, caries incidence has recently declined in a time of increasing sugar intake.[6] This has led to a reevaluation of caries causation, and sugar is now understood to be only one of the factors in the development of tooth decay.[7] Nearly as important as the total amount of sugar intake seems to be the consistency of the sugary foods and the length of time they are in contact with the teeth. Dry and sticky foods tend to stay in contact longer, causing more plaque formation.[8] Still, reduction of total dietary sugar is probably the most accepted dietary recommendation for the prevention of dental caries.[9]

Drinking fluoridated water (1 mg **fluoride** [page 519] per liter) has led to an estimated 40% to 60% reduction in dental caries in many cities in the United States and worldwide.[10, 11] While most experts believe water fluoridation to be associated with minimal risk,[12] others disagree. A minority of scientists believes fluoridation to be associated with an unacceptable risk of skeletal damage, including osteoporotic fractures and bone tumors, in exchange for a modest dental benefit.[13] Fluoride has topical action as well as whole-body effects,[14] suggesting that those who do not have access to fluoridated water can achieve some benefit with fluoride-containing toothpastes and mouthwashes. In areas without fluoridated water, a number of controlled trials have found oral use of chewable fluoride tablets (1 to 2 mg per day of fluoride)[15, 16] or fluoride mouthrinses (0.05% to 0.2% fluoride content)[17, 18] also reduce caries risk in children. Fluoride tablets[19] and mouthwash[20] have been found to be effective for caries prevention in young adults and the elderly. Tablets are slightly more effective than a mouthrinse for caries protection.[21] These products should not be used by young children (under three years of age), who might accidentally swallow dangerous amounts of fluoride.[22] The American Dental Association (ADA) recommends supplementing children in areas without fluoridated water with liquid fluoride drops,[23] but this should be done with the guidance of a dentist.

Lifestyle changes that may be helpful
The ADA recommends regular tooth brushing—daily brushing, ideally after each meal.[24] Although thorough brushing varies from person to person, five to ten strokes in each area should be adequate.[25] Toothpastes containing 1,000 to 2,500 ppm (1 to 2.5 mg per gram) of fluoride have been shown to reduce caries risk.[26]

A recent population survey found blood lead levels were associated with the amount of dental caries in children and adults. The authors estimated that lead exposure is responsible for roughly 10% of dental caries in young Americans.[27] For this and other health reasons, known and potential sources of lead exposure should be avoided. Common sources of lead exposure may in-

clude paint, foods grown near roadways, and water from lead pipes.[28]

Nutritional supplements that may be helpful
Test tube studies show that **vitamin B$_6$** (page 600) increases growth of beneficial mouth bacteria and decreases growth of cavity-causing bacteria.[29] A double-blind study found that pregnant women who supplemented with 20 mg per day of vitamin B$_6$ had significantly fewer new caries and fillings during pregnancy.[30] Lozenges containing vitamin B$_6$ were more effective than capsules in this study, suggesting an important topical effect. Another double-blind study gave children oral lozenges containing 3 mg of vitamin B$_6$ three times per day for eight months, but reported only insignificant reductions in new cavities.[31]

In a double-blind study of children aged 1 to 6 years, supplementation with *Lactobacillus GG* five days a week in milk for seven months reduced the incidence of cavities by 49%, compared with unsupplemented milk.[32] The amount of *Lactobacillus* added to the milk was 5 to 10 x 10e5 CFU per ml.

Certain sugar substitutes appear to have anti-caries benefits beyond that of reducing sugar intake. Children chewing gum containing either **xylitol** (page 614) or sorbitol for five minutes five times daily for two years had large reductions in caries risk compared with those not chewing gum. Sorbitol is only slowly used by oral bacteria, and it produces less caries than sucrose.[33] Xylitol gum was associated with a slightly greater risk reduction than sorbitol gum.[34] Bacteria in the mouth do not ferment xylitol, so they cannot produce the acids that cause tooth decay from xylitol.[35] A double-blind study found 100% xylitol-sweetened gum was superior to gum containing lesser amounts or no xylitol.[36] Another study found xylitol-containing gums gave long-term protection against caries while sorbitol-only gum did not.[37] Other research has confirmed the anti-caries benefits of xylitol in various forms, including gum,[38] chewable lozenges, toothpastes, mouthwashes, and syrups.[39] Mothers typically transmit one of the decay-causing bacteria to their infant children, but a double-blind trial found that the children of mothers who regularly chewed xylitol-containing gum for 21 months, starting 3 months after delivery, had a greatly reduced risk of acquiring these bacteria,[40, 41] and also had 70% less tooth decay.[42]

One older controlled trial found that children given 3 teaspoons of **cod liver oil** (page 514) per day (containing roughly 800 IU of **vitamin D** [page 607]) for an entire school year had over 50% fewer cavities.[43] These promising results have not been followed up with modern placebo-controlled trials.

Levels of **strontium** (page 589) in the water supply have been shown to correlate with the risk of dental caries in communities with similar fluoride levels.[44] Compared with children with fewer cavities, enamel samples from children with high numbers of caries have been found to contain significantly less strontium.[45] However, supplementation with strontium has not yet been studied as tooth decay prevention.

Are there any side effects or interactions?
Refer to the individual supplement for information about any side effects or interactions.

Herbs that may be helpful

Compounds present in both **green tea** (page 686) and black tea have been shown to inhibit the growth and activity of bacteria associated with tooth decay.[46, 47] Animals given tea compounds in their drinking water develop fewer dental caries than do those drinking plain water.[48, 49, 50] Human volunteers rinsing with an alcohol extract of tea leaves before bed each night for four days had significantly less plaque formation but similar amounts of plaque-causing bacteria compared with those with no treatment.[51] Tea drinking has not yet been tested as a tooth decay preventative in humans.

In a double-blind trial, 1 gram of neem leaf extract in gel twice per day was more effective than chlorhexidine or placebo gel at reducing plaque and bacteria levels in the mouth in 36 Indian adults.[52] A similar trial found neem gel superior to placebo and equally effective as chlorhexidine at reducing plaque and bacteria levels in the mouth.[53] These promising early studies should be followed by studies regarding prevention of cavities and relief from gingivitis or periodontal disease.

Are there any side effects or interactions?
Refer to the individual herb for information about any side effects or interactions.

ULCERATIVE COLITIS

Ulcerative colitis (UC) is a chronic inflammatory disease of the colon, which is relatively common but remains poorly understood.

Diagnosis must be made by a healthcare practitioner—typically a gastroenterologist. **Irritable bowel syndrome** (page 280), a completely unrelated and less serious condition, was sometimes called mucous colitis in the past. As a result, the general term "colitis" is still sometimes used inappropriately to refer to irritable bowel syndrome. It is critical that people who are diagnosed with "colitis" find out whether they have irritable bowel syndrome or UC.

What are the symptoms of UC?
UC is characterized by frequent abdominal pain and bloody **diarrhea** (page 163). Other symptoms may include fatigue, weight loss, decreased appetite, and nausea.

Medical treatments
The over the counter antidiarrheal drug loperamide (Imodium A-D) may be used in ulcerative colitis patients with **diarrhea** (page 163). Anal irritation and loose stools may sometimes be improved by giving bulk-forming laxative such as methylcellulose (Citrucel) or psyllium (Fiberall, Konsyl, Metamucil, Perdiem).

Diphenoxylate with atropine (Lomotil) is the prescription drug most often used to control diarrhea. Cramps may be treated with anticholinergic drugs, such as L-hyoscyamine (Levsin, Levbid) and belladonna (Belladonna Tincture). These drugs must be used with extreme caution to prevent toxic dilation of the colon. Sulfasalazine (Azulfidine) is used in individuals with mild to moderate colitis. Oral corticosteroids, such as prednisone (Deltasone), may be used during acute flare-ups however, long-term corticosteroid therapy may be more harmful than good. Therapy with corticosteroids, such as hydrocortisone enema (Cortenema) is commonly recommended. Mesalamine (Asacol, Pentasa, Rowasa) may be prescribed in some cases, as an enema, orally, or in suppository form. Certain immunosuppressive drugs may also be effective, including azathioprine (Imuran), cyclosporine (Sandimmune), and 6-mercaptopurine (Purinethol). Secondary bacterial **infections** (page 265) are managed with antibiotics.

Other treatment of UC includes avoiding raw fruits and vegetables. Sometimes a milk-free diet is suggested. Toxic colitis, a grave medical emergency complication of UC, is treated intensively in emergency departments with antibiotics, such as tobramycin (Nebcin), amikacin (Amikin), and gentamicin (Garamycin), intravenous fluid replacement, and either corticosteroids or adrenocorticotropic hormone (ACTH). Emergency surgical removal of the colon is sometimes necessary in the most severe cases. Elective surgery may be recommended for milder cases.

CHECKLIST FOR ULCERATIVE COLITIS		
Rating	Nutritional Supplements	Herbs
★★☆	Butyrate (enema) **Fish oil** (page 514) **Folic acid** (page 520) **Probiotics** (page 575)	**Aloe** (page 624) **Boswellia** (page 644) **DHEA** (page 503) **Psyllium** (page 732) Wheat grass (juice)
★☆☆		**Calendula** (page 650) **Chamomile** (page 656) **Flaxseed** (page 517) **Licorice** (page 702) **Marshmallow** (page 708) **Myrrh** (page 713) **St. John's wort** (page 747) (oil, taken as an enema) **Yarrow** (page 763)

Dietary changes that may be helpful

Some studies have shown that high sugar intake is associated with an increase in risk for UC.[1, 2] Other research has failed to find any association between UC and sugar intake.[3, 4] Until more is known, persons with inflammatory bowel diseases, including UC, should consider limiting their intake of sugar.

In two studies, people with a high intake of animal fat, **cholesterol** (page 223), or margarine had a significantly increased risk of UC, compared with people who consumed less of these fats.[5, 6] Although these associations do not prove cause-and-effect, reducing one's intake of animal fats and margarine is a means of improving overall health and possibly UC as well.

There is preliminary evidence that people who eat fast food at least twice a week have nearly four times the risk of developing UC than people who do not eat fast food.[7]

More than a half-century ago, several doctors reported that **food allergies** (page 14) play an important role in some cases of UC.[8, 9] Since that time, many doctors have observed that avoidance of allergenic foods will often reduce the severity of UC and can sometimes completely control the condition. In other old studies, milk has been reported to trigger UC,[10] and people with UC were found to have antibodies to milk in their blood, a possible sign of allergy.[11] Today the relation-

ship between food allergies and UC remains controversial[12] and is not generally accepted by the conventional medical community. People who wish to explore the possibility that food sensitivities may trigger their symptoms may wish to consult with an appropriate healthcare provider.

In a preliminary study, 39 patients with mild to moderate ulcerative colitis experienced significant improvement after receiving 30 grams (about 1 oz) per day of a germinated barley product for four weeks.[13] Controlled trials are needed to confirm this report.

Lifestyle changes that may be helpful

For unknown reasons, smokers have a lower risk of UC. The nicotine patch has actually been used to induce remissions in people with UC,[14] although this treatment has been ineffective in preventing relapses.[15] On the other hand, **Crohn's disease** (page 141), which is in many ways similar to UC, is made *worse* by smoking.[16] Despite the possible protective effect of smoking in people with UC, a strong case can be made that risks of smoking outweigh the benefits; even the use of nicotine patches carries its own side effects and remains experimental.

Nutritional supplements that may be helpful

UC is linked to an increased risk of **colon cancer** (page 000). Studies have found that people with UC who take **folic acid** (page 520) supplements or who have high blood levels of folic acid have a reduced risk of colon cancer compared with people who have UC and do not take folic acid supplements.[17, 18, 19] Although these associations do not prove that folic acid was responsible for the reduction in risk, this vitamin has been shown to prevent experimentally induced colon cancer in animals.[20] Moreover, low blood folic acid levels have been found in more than half of all people with UC.[21] People with UC who are taking the drug sulfasalazine, which inhibits the absorption of folic acid,[22] are at a particularly high risk of developing folic acid deficiency. Folic acid supplementation may therefore be important for many people with UC. Since taking folic acid may mask a **vitamin B_{12}** (page 601) deficiency, however, people with UC who wish to take folic acid over the long term should have their vitamin B_{12} status assessed by a physician.

Alcohol consumption is known to promote folic acid deficiency and has also been linked to an increased risk of colon cancer.[23] People with UC should, therefore, keep alcohol intake to a minimum.

Preliminary[24] and double-blind trials[25, 26, 27] have found that **fish oil** (page 514) supplementation reduces inflammation, decreases the need for anti-inflammatory drugs, and promotes normal weight gain in people with UC. However, fish oil has not always been effective in clinical trials for UC.[28] Amounts used in successful clinical trials provided 3.2 grams of EPA and 2.2 grams of **DHA** (page 509) per day—the two important fatty acids found in fish oil.

A fatty acid called butyrate, which is synthesized by intestinal bacteria, serves as fuel for the cells that line the small intestine. Administration of butyrate by enema has produced marked improvement in people with UC in most,[29, 30, 31, 32, 33, 34] but not all,[35] preliminary trials. Butyrate taken by mouth is not likely to be beneficial, as sufficient quantities do not reach the colon by this route. Although butyrate enemas are not widely available, they can be obtained by prescription through a compounding pharmacy, which prepares customized prescription medications to meet individual patient needs.

In a preliminary trial, 6 of 13 people with ulcerative colitis went into remission after taking 200 mg per day of **DHEA** (page 503) for eight weeks.[36] This large amount of DHEA has the potential to cause adverse side effects and should only be used under the supervision of a doctor.

In preliminary[37] and double-blind[38] trials, a **probiotic** (page 575) supplement (in this case, a non-disease-causing strain of *Escherichia coli*) was effective at maintaining remission in people with UC. In a double-blind trial, a combination probiotic supplement containing Lactobacilli, Bifidobacteria, and a beneficial strain of Streptococcus has been shown to prevent pouchitis, a common complication of surgery for UC.[39] People with chronic relapsing pouchitis received either 3 grams per day of the supplement or placebo for nine months. Eighty-five percent of those who took the supplement had no further episodes of pouchitis during the nine-month trial, whereas 100% of those receiving placebo had relapses within four months. Preliminary evidence suggests that combination probiotic supplements may be effective at preventing UC relapses as well.[40]

In a preliminary trial, people with UC significantly improved on a sugar-free, low-allergen diet with additional nutritional supplementation that included a **multivitamin-mineral** (page 559) supplement (2–6 tablets per day); a **fish oil** (page 514) supplement (400 mg per day); **borage oil** (page 475) (400 mg per day);

flaxseed oil (page 517) (400 mg per day); and a probiotic formula containing *Lactobacillus acidophilus* (page 575) and other species of beneficial bacteria.[41] Some participants received slight variations of this regimen. Since so many different supplements were given and since the trial was not controlled, it is not possible to say which, if any, of the nutrients was responsible for the improvement observed by the researchers.

Are there any side effects or interactions?
Refer to the individual supplement for information about any side effects or interactions.

Herbs that may be helpful
A small clinical study found that people with UC taking 550 mg of **boswellia** (page 644) gum resin three times daily for six weeks had similar improvement in symptoms and the severity of their disease as people with UC taking the drug sulfasalazine.[42] Overall, 82% of patients receiving boswellia, along with 75% of patients taking sulfasalazine, went into remission.

In a preliminary trial, people with UC remained in remission just as long when they took 20 grams of ground **psyllium** (page 732) seeds twice daily with water as when they took the drug mesalamine.[43] The combination of the two was slightly more effective than either alone. Controlled trials are now needed to confirm a therapeutic effect of psyllium for UC.

In a controlled trial, supplementation with wheat grass juice for one month resulted in clinical improvement in 78% of people with ulcerative colitis, compared with 30% of those receiving a placebo.[44] The amount of wheat grass used was 20 ml per day initially; this was increased by 20 ml per day to a maximum of 100 ml per day (approximately 3.5 ounces).

German doctors practicing herbal medicine often recommend **chamomile** (page 656) for people with colitis.[45] A cup of strong tea drunk three times per day is standard, along with enemas using the tea when it reaches body temperature.

Enemas of oil of **St. John's wort** (page 747) may also be beneficial.[46] Consult with a doctor before using St. John's wort oil enemas.

Aloe vera (page 624) juice has anti-inflammatory activity and been used by some doctors for people with UC. In a double-blind study of people with mildly to moderately active ulcerative colitis, supplementation with aloe resulted in a complete remission or an improvement in symptoms in 47% of cases, compared with 14% of those given a placebo (a statistically significant difference).[47] No significant side effects were seen. The amount of aloe used was 100 ml (approximately 3.5 ounces) twice a day for four weeks. Other traditional anti-inflammatory and soothing herbs, including **calendula** (page 650), **flaxseed** (page 517), **licorice** (page 702), **marshmallow** (page 708), **myrrh** (page 713), and **yarrow** (page 763). Many of these herbs are most effective, according to clinical experience, if taken internally as well as in enema form.[48] Enemas should be avoided during acute flare-ups but are useful for mild and chronic inflammation. It is best to consult with a doctor experienced with botanical medicine to learn more about herbal enemas before using them. More research needs to be done to determine the effectiveness of these herbs.

Are there any side effects or interactions?
Refer to the individual herb for information about any side effects or interactions.

URINARY TRACT INFECTION

What do I need to know?
Self-care for urinary tract infection can be approached in a number of ways—but it can be hard to know just where to start. To make it easier, our doctors recommend trying these simple steps first:

If you have a UTI, see a doctor
> Existing infections may require treatment with antibiotics

Check out cranberry
> To treat and to prevent recurrences, drink 4 to 10 ounces a day of cranberry juice or take 400 mg of powdered cranberry concentrate twice a day

Try proteolytic enzymes
> To enhance antibotic effectiveness, take 400 mg a day of enzymes such as bromelain and trypsin

Avoid allergic foods
> Work with a knowledgeable health practitioner to find out if you have allergies to foods that increase your susceptibility to urinary tract infections

Aim for a strong immune system with a multivitamin-mineral supplement
> Take one daily to avoid deficiencies and better resist infections

About UTIs
Urinary tract infections (UTIs) are **infections** (page 265) of the kidney, bladder, and urethra.

UTIs are generally triggered by bacteria and are more common when there is partial blockage of the urinary tract. In some people, UTIs tend to recur.

CHECKLIST FOR URINARY TRACT INFECTION (UTI)		
Rating	**Nutritional Supplements**	**Herbs**
★★☆	**Bromelain** (page 481)	**Cranberry** (page 664)
★☆☆	**D-mannose** (page 503) **Multivitamin-mineral** (page 559) **Vitamin A** (page 595) **Vitamin C** (page 604)	Asparagus Birch **Blueberry** (page 641) **Buchu** (page 645) Couch grass Goldenrod **Goldenseal** (page 683) **Horseradish** (page 693) **Horsetail** (page 693) Java tea **Juniper** (page 698) Lovage **Nettle** (page 714) **Oregon grape** (page 721) Parsley **Plantain** (page 729) **Sassafras** (page 742) Spiny restharrow **Uva ursi** (page 755)

What are the symptoms of UTIs?
Symptoms of a UTI usually begin suddenly and include frequent urination that is irritating or burning, a persistent urge to urinate even after the bladder has been emptied, and cramping or pressure in the lower abdomen. The urine often has a strong or unusual smell and may appear cloudy. In more serious **infections** (page 265), fever, chills, **pain** (page 338) in the back below the ribs, nausea, vomiting, and **diarrhea** (page 163) may also be present.

Medical treatments
Over the counter products containing phenazopyridine (Azo-Standard, Prodium) may be used to relieve pain, burning, and urgency, but they do not treat the infection.

Oral antibiotics are typically used to treat uncomplicated **infections** (page 265); the most commonly prescribed are the combination drug trimethoprim/sulfamethoxazole (Bactrim, Septra) and the fluoroquinolones, such as levofloxacin (Levaquin), ciprofloxacin (Cipro), and ofloxacin (Floxin). One of the third-generation cephalosporins, cefixime (Suprax) and the tetracyclinedoxycycline (Vibramycin) may be used as well.

Intravenous antibiotics, such as the aminoglycosides gentamicin (Garamycin) and tobramycin (Nebicin, Tobrex), may be used for more serious infections.

Dietary changes that may be helpful

When healthy volunteers consumed a large amount (100 grams) of refined sugar, the ability of their white blood cells to destroy bacteria was impaired for at least five hours.[1] Consumption of excessive amounts of alcohol has also been shown to suppress **immune function** (page 255).[2] Reduced intake of dietary fat has been shown to stimulate immunity.[3] For these reasons, many doctors recommend a reduced intake of sugar, alcohol, and fat during an acute **infection** (page 265) and for prevention of recurrences.

People who have recurrent or chronic infections should discuss the possible role of **allergies** (page 14) with a doctor, since chronic infections have been linked to allergies in many reports.[4, 5, 6, 7] Identifying and eliminating foods that trigger problems may help reduce the number of infections.

Nutritional supplements that may be helpful

The proteolytic **enzymes** (page 506), **bromelain** (page 481) (from pineapple) and trypsin may enhance the effectiveness of antibiotics in people with a UTI. In a double-blind trial, people with UTIs received antibiotics plus either bromelain/trypsin in combination (400 mg per day for two days) or a placebo. One hundred percent of those who received the enzymes had a resolution of their **infection** (page 265), compared with only 46% of those given the placebo.[8] This study used enteric-coated tablets. Enteric-coating prevents stomach acid from partially destroying the bromelain. Most commercially available bromelain products today are not enteric-coated, and it is not known if non-enteric coated preparations would be as effective.

Some bacteria that typically cause urinary tract infections can attach themselves to the lining of the urinary tract by binding to molecules of **mannose** (page 503) that naturally occur there.[9] Theoretically, if enough D-mannose is present in the urine, it would bind to the bacteria and prevent them from attaching to the urinary tract lining.[10] One animal study has demonstrated this protective effect,[11] but whether it would occur in humans is unknown, and no human research has investigated the effectiveness of oral D-mannose for the prevention or treatment of urinary tract infections.

Many doctors recommend 5,000 mg or more of **vitamin C** (page 604) per day for an acute UTI, as well as long-term supplementation for people who are prone to recurrent UTIs. Although no controlled clinical trials have demonstrated the effectiveness of vitamin C for this purpose, vitamin C has been shown to inhibit the growth of *E. coli,* the most common bacterial cause of UTIs.[12] In addition, supplementation with 4,000 mg or more of vitamin C per day, results in a slight increase in the acidity of the urine,[13] creating an "unfriendly" environment for some infection-causing bacteria.

Vitamin A (page 595) deficiency increases the risk of many infections. Although much of the promising research with vitamin A supplements and infections has focused on measles,[14] vitamin A is also thought to be helpful in other infections. Some doctors recommend that people with urinary tract infections take vitamin A. A typical amount recommended to correct a deficiency is 10,000 to 25,000 IU per day.

Since the **immune system** (page 255) requires many nutrients in order to function properly, many people take a **multivitamin-mineral** (page 559) supplement for "insurance." In one double-blind trial, healthy elderly people who used such a supplement for one year showed improvements in immune function, as well as a significant reduction in the total number of infections (including non-urinary-tract infections).[15]

Are there any side effects or interactions?

Refer to the individual supplement for information about any side effects or interactions.

Herbs that may be helpful

Modern research has suggested that **cranberry** (page 664) may prevent urinary tract infections. In a double-blind trial, elderly women who drank 10 ounces (300 ml) of cranberry juice per day had a decrease in the amount of bacteria in their urine.[16] In another study, elderly residents of a nursing home consumed either four ounces (120 ml) of cranberry juice or six capsules containing concentrated cranberry daily for 13 months. During that time, the number of UTIs decreased by 25%.[17] A small preliminary trial found that supplementation with encapsulated cranberry concentrate (400 mg twice per day for three months) significantly reduced the recurrence of UTIs in women (aged 18–45) with a history of recurrent infections.[18]

Research has suggested cranberry may be effective against UTIs because it prevents *E. coli,* the bacteria that causes most urinary tract **infections** (page 265), from attaching to the walls of the bladder.[19] Cranberry is not, however, a substitute for antibiotics in the treatment of acute UTIs. Moreover, in children whose UTIs are due to "neurogenic bladder" (a condition caused by spinal cord injury or myelomeningocele), cranberry juice supplementation did not reduce the rate of infection.[20] Drinking 10–16 ounces (300–500 ml) of unsweetened or lightly sweetened cranberry juice is recommended by many doctors for prevention, and as part of the treatment of UTIs. Alternatively, 400 mg of concentrated cranberry extracts twice per day can be used.

Blueberry (page 641) contains similar constituents as cranberry, and might also prevent bacteria from attaching to the lining of the urinary bladder.[21] However, studies have not yet been done to determine if blueberry can help prevent bladder infections.

Asparagus *(Asparagus officinalis),* birch *(Betula* spp.), couch grass *(Agropyron repens),* goldenrod *(Solidago virgaurea),* **horsetail** (page 693), Java tea *(Orthosiphon stamineus),* lovage *(Levisticum officinale),* parsley *(Petroselinum crispum),* spiny restharrow *(Ononis spinosa),* and **nettle** (page 714) are approved in Germany as part of the therapy of people with UTIs. These herbs appear to work by increasing urinary volume and supposedly helping to flush bacteria out of the urinary tract.[22] **Juniper** (page 698) is used in a similar fashion by many doctors. Generally, these plants are taken as tea.

Buchu (page 645) leaf preparations have a history of use in traditional herbal medicine as a urinary tract disinfectant and diuretic.[23] However, the German Commission E monograph on buchu concludes that insufficient evidence supports the modern use of buchu for the treatment of UTIs or inflammation.[24]

The volatile oil of **horseradish** (page 693) has been shown to kill bacteria that can cause urinary tract infections.[25] The concentration that is required to kill these bacteria can be attained in human urine after oral ingestion of the oil. One early study found that horseradish extract may help people with urinary tract infections.[26] Further studies are necessary to confirm the safety and effectiveness of horseradish in treating urinary tract infections.

Goldenseal (page 683) is reputed to help treat many types of **infections** (page 265). It contains berberine, an

alkaloid that may prevent UTIs by inhibiting bacteria from adhering to the wall of the urinary bladder.[27] Goldenseal and other plants containing berberine (such as **Oregon grape** [page 721]) may help in the treatment of UTIs. These herbs have not, however, been studied for the treatment of UTIs in humans.

Because of the anti-inflammatory effects of **plantain** (page 729), it may be beneficial in some people with UTIs. However, human trials have not been done to confirm this possibility or to confirm the traditional belief that plantain is diuretic.[28]

An extract of **uva ursi** (page 755) is used in Europe and in traditional herbal medicine in North America, as a treatment for UTI.[29] This herb is approved in Germany for treatment of bladder infections.[30] The active constituent in uva ursi is arbutin. In the alkaline environment of the urine, arbutin is converted into another chemical, called hydroquinone, which kills bacteria. A generally useful amount of uva ursi tincture is 3–5 ml three times per day. Otherwise, 100–250 mg of arbutin in herbal extract capsules or tablets three times per day can be used. Uva ursi should only be used to treat a UTI under the close supervision of a physician.

Are there any side effects or interactions?
Refer to the individual herb for information about any side effects or interactions.

Holistic approaches that may be helpful
Acupuncture might be of some benefit for women with recurrent UTIs. A controlled study compared acupuncture to sham ("fake") acupuncture or no treatment in a group of women with recurrent UTIs. After six months, the women receiving real acupuncture had half as many UTI episodes as the sham group and only one-third as many as the untreated group, a significant difference.[31]

VAGINITIS

Vaginitis is inflammation of the vagina.

Vaginitis is responsible for an estimated 10% of all visits by women to their healthcare practitioners. The three general causes of vaginitis are hormonal imbalance, irritation, and infection. Hormone-related vaginitis includes the atrophic vaginitis generally found in **postmenopausal** (page 311) or **postpartum** (page 363) women and, occasionally, in young girls before puberty. Irritant vaginitis can result from **allergies** (page 14) or irritating substances. Infectious vaginitis is most common in reproductive-age women and is generally caused by one of three types of infections: bacterial vaginosis (BV), candidiasis (**yeast infection** [page 454]), or trichomoniasis. A healthcare professional should be consulted for the diagnosis and treatment of any vaginal infection.

Although it is a type of vaginitis, yeast infection is not discussed on this page. For specific information on yeast infections (i.e., vaginitis caused by *Candida albicans*), see the **yeast infections** (page 454) article.

CHECKLIST FOR VAGINITIS

Rating	Nutritional Supplements	Herbs
★★★	*Lactobacillus acidophilus* (page 575)	
★☆☆	**Soy** (page 587) **Vitamin A** (page 595) **Vitamin E** (page 609)	**Barberry** (page 632) **Echinacea** (page 669) **Goldenseal** (page 683) **Tea tree** (page 751) Neem

What are the symptoms of vaginitis?

Hormone-related vaginitis is marked by dryness, irritation, thinning of the vaginal mucous membranes and painful intercourse. Irritant vaginitis is characterized by itching and soreness. Infectious vaginitis also itches and typically includes vaginal discharge that varies in color, consistency, and odor, depending upon the infectious organism. Discharge may range from scant to thick and white and may or may not be accompanied by a strong odor. Symptoms are often worse immediately after intercourse or the menstrual period.

Medical treatments

Over the counter drugs are available to treat vaginitis caused by candida. They include clotrimazole (Gyne-Lotrimin, Mycelex), miconazole (Monistat), and butoconazole (Femstat). Irritant vaginitis can be treated either by removal of the offending irritant or with an antihistamine agent, such as diphenhydramine (Benadryl).

Prescription drug therapy varies with the cause of the vaginitis. Hormone-related vaginitis is commonly treated with estrogen replacement therapy, including conjugated estrogens (Premarin), estradiol (Estrace), and ethinylestradiol (Estinyl). Bacterial vaginosis and trichomoniasis are each commonly treated with metronidazole (Flagyl).

Dietary changes that may be helpful

Food allergies (page 14) are believed to be a contributory factor in some cases of recurrent irritant vaginitis.

In a controlled trial, women with recurrent BV or vaginal candidiasis ate 5 ounces (150 grams) of yogurt containing live *Lactobacillus acidophilus* (page 575) daily.[1] They had more than a 50% reduction in recurrences, while women who consumed pasteurized yogurt that did not contain the bacteria had only a slight reduction.

In another study, women who ingested 45 grams of soy flour per day showed an improvement in the estrogen effect on their vaginal tissue.[2] That observation suggests that supplementing with soy may be helpful for preventing or reversing atrophic vaginitis.

Lifestyle changes that may be helpful

For irritant vaginitis, minimizing friction and reducing exposure to perfumes, chemicals, irritating lubricants, and spermicides can be beneficial.

Nutritional supplements that may be helpful

Lactobacillus acidophilus (page 575) is a strain of friendly bacteria that is an integral part of normal vaginal flora. Lactobacilli help maintain the vaginal microflora by preventing overgrowth of unfriendly bacteria and Candida. Lactobacilli produce lactic acid, which acts like a natural antibiotic. These friendly bacteria also compete with other organisms for the utilization of glucose. The production of lactic acid and hydrogen peroxide by lactobacilli also helps to maintain the acidic pH needed for healthy vaginal flora to thrive. Most of the research has used yogurt containing live cultures of *Lactobacillus acidophilus* or the topical application of such yogurt or *Lactobacillus acidophilus* into the vagina. The effective amount of acidophilus depends on the strain used, as well as on the concentration of viable organisms.

Vaginal application of a proprietary *Lactobacillus acidophilus* preparation may help nonspecific vaginitis. In one trial, 80% of women with nonspecific vaginitis who used the preparation were either cured or experienced marked improvement in symptoms.[3] In another trial, women who were predisposed to vaginal Candida **infection** (page 265) because they were **HIV-positive** (page 234) received either *Lactobacillus acidophilus* vaginal suppositories, the antifungal drug, clotrimazole (e.g., Gyne-Lotrimin), or placebo weekly for 21 months.[4] Compared to those receiving placebo, women receiving *Lactobacillus acidophilus* suppositories had only half the risk of experiencing an episode of Candida vaginitis—a result almost as good as that achieved with clotrimazole. In a preliminary trial, women with vaginal *Trichomonas* infection received vaginal *Lactobacillus acidophilus* suppositories for one year.[5] Over 90% of them were reported to be cured of their clinical symptoms in that time.

Some doctors recommend **vitamin E** (page 609) (taken orally, topically, or vaginally) for certain types of vaginitis. Vitamin E as a suppository in the vagina or vitamin E oil can be used once or twice per day for 3 to 14 days to soothe the mucous membranes of the vagina and vulva. Some doctors recommend vaginal administration of **vitamin A** (page 595) to improve the integrity of the vaginal tissue and to enhance the function of local immune cells. Vitamin A can be administered vaginally by inserting a vitamin A capsule or using a prepared vitamin A suppository. Vitamin A used this way can be irritating to local tissue, so it should not be used more than once per day for up to seven consecutive days.

Are there any side effects or interactions?
Refer to the individual supplement for information about any side effects or interactions.

Herbs that may be helpful
In a double-blind, placebo-controlled trial, a cream containing neem seed extract, saponins of *Sapindus mukerossi* (reetha), and quinine hydrochloride (5 ml applied vaginally once at bedtime) eliminated all symptoms in 10 of 14 women with chlamydia compared with none of 4 women given placebo cream.[6] Neither cream was effective in women with trichomoniasis or candidal vaginitis.

Topically applied **tea tree** (page 751) oil has been studied and used successfully as a topical treatment for *Trichomonas, Candida albicans,* and other vaginal **infections** (page 265).[7] Tea tree oil must be diluted when used as a vaginal douche, and should only be used for this purpose under the supervision of a healthcare practitioner. Some physicians suggest using tea tree oil by mixing the full-strength oil with **vitamin E** (page 609) oil in the proportion of 1/3 tea tree oil to 2/3 vitamin E oil. A tampon is saturated with this mixture or the mixture is put in a capsule to be inserted in the vagina each day for a maximum of six weeks.

Teas of **goldenseal** (page 683), **barberry** (page 632), and **echinacea** (page 669) are also sometimes used to treat infectious vaginitis. Although all three plants are known to be antibacterial in the test tube, the effectiveness of these herbs against vaginal infections has not been tested in humans. The usual approach is to douche with one of these teas twice each day, using 1–2 tablespoons (15–30 grams) of herb per pint of water. One to two pints (500–1,000 ml) are usually enough for each douching session. Echinacea is also known to improve **immune function** (page 255) in humans.[8] In order to increase resistance against infection, many doctors recommend oral use of the tincture or alcohol-preserved fresh juice of echinacea (1 teaspoon (5 ml) three or more times per day)—during all types of infection—to improve resistance.

Are there any side effects or interactions?
Refer to the individual herb for information about any side effects or interactions.

VARICOSE VEINS

Varicose veins are twisted, enlarged veins close to the surface. They can occur almost anywhere but most commonly occur in the esophagus and the legs.

Veins, which return blood to the heart, contain valves that keep blood from flowing backward as a result of gravity. When these valves become weak, blood pools in the veins of the legs and causes them to bulge. These enlarged vessels are called varicose veins. Standing and sitting for long periods of time, lack of exercise, **obesity** (page 446), and **pregnancy** (page 363) all tend to promote the formation of varicose veins. Sometimes varicose veins are painful, but elevating the affected leg usually brings significant relief.

CHECKLIST FOR VARICOSE VEINS

Rating	Nutritional Supplements	Herbs
★☆☆	**Flavonoids** (page 516) (hydroxyethylrutosides) **Proanthocyanidins** (page 574)	**Butcher's broom** (page 649) **Gotu kola** (page 684) **Horse chestnut** (page 692) **Witch hazel** (page 760)

What are the symptoms of varicose veins?

Symptoms of varicose veins may include a dull pain, itch, or heavy sensation in the legs. The sensation is worse after prolonged standing and better when the legs are elevated. Varicose veins typically appear on the legs as dilated, tortuous veins close to the surface of the skin, and may look blue. Advanced varicose veins may cause ankle and leg swelling or **skin ulcers** (page 409).

Medical treatments

Other treatment is to elevate the legs frequently, avoid prolonged standing or sitting, and wear compression stockings with supportive shoes. Other treatments include surgery to remove the vein, laser therapy, and sclerotherapy, which involves the injection of a chemical solution into the vein to cause it to close. Any skin ulcers that develop are treated with compressive bandages that contain antibiotic solutions.

Lifestyle changes that may be helpful

Keeping the legs elevated relieves pain. People with varicose veins should avoid sitting or standing for prolonged periods of time and should walk regularly.

Nutritional supplements that may be helpful

A controlled clinical trial found that oral supplementation with hydroxyethylrutosides (HR), a type of **flavonoid** (page 516) that is derived from rutin, improved varicose veins in a group of **pregnant** (page 363) women.[1] Further research is needed to confirm the benefits observed in this preliminary trial. A typical amount of HR is 1000 mg per day.

A small, preliminary trial found that supplementation with 150 mg of **proanthocyanidins** (page 574) per day improved the function of leg veins after a single application in people with widespread varicose veins.[2] Double-blind trials are needed to determine whether extended use of proanthocyanidins can substantially improve this condition.

Are there any side effects or interactions?
Refer to the individual supplement for information about any side effects or interactions.

Herbs that may be helpful

Although **witch hazel** (page 760) is known primarily for treating **hemorrhoids** (page 219), it may also be useful for varicose veins.[3] Topical use of witch hazel to treat venous conditions is approved by the German Commission E, authorities on herbal medicine.[4] Application of a witch hazel ointment three or more times per day for two or more weeks is necessary before results can be expected.

Horse chestnut (page 692) seed extract can be taken orally or used as an external application for disorders of venous circulation, including varicose veins.[5] Preliminary studies in humans have shown that 300 mg three times per day of a standardized extract of horse chestnut seed reduced the formation of enzymes thought to cause varicose veins.[6] Topical gel or creams containing 2% aescin can be applied topically three or four time per day to the affected limb(s).

Oral supplementation with **butcher's broom** (page 649)[7] or **gotu kola** (page 684)[8] may also be helpful for varicose veins.

Are there any side effects or interactions?
Refer to the individual herb for information about any side effects or interactions.

VERTIGO

Vertigo is a sensation of irregular or whirling motion, either of oneself or of external objects.

The word is sometimes incorrectly used as a general term to describe dizziness. The most common form of vertigo is benign positional paroxysmal vertigo (BPPV), in which brief attacks are brought on by certain changes in head position.[1] BPPV may be due to a previous head injury, viral **infection** (page 265), and certain drug therapies, although in about half the cases the cause is unknown.[2, 3] BPPV tends to resolve without treatment within weeks to months, but may persist for years in some cases.[4, 5]

People experiencing vertigo should have a complete medical evaluation to determine the cause. Common causes of non-BPPV vertigo include conditions in which there is decreased blood flow to certain areas of the brain, **Ménière's disease** (page 308), and infection of the inner ear.[6, 7] Vertigo may also be a symptom of numerous other conditions,[8, 9, 10] including **sinusitis** (page 407), **panic attacks** (page 30), **migraine headaches** (page 316), and problems with metabolism,[11, 12] such as **hypothyroidism** (page 252), **high blood triglycerides** (page 235), **diabetes** (page 152), and **hypoglycemia** (page 251).

What are the symptoms of vertigo?

People with vertigo may have sudden sensations of spinning or whirling motion that may be accompanied by lightheadedness and loss of balance, and less often by sweating, fatigue, nausea, and vomiting.[13, 14]

CHECKLIST FOR VERTIGO		
Rating	**Nutritional Supplements**	**Herbs**
★★☆	**Vinpocetine** (page 594) **Vitamin B₆** (page 600)	**Ginger** (page 680) *Ginkgo biloba* (page 681)

Medical treatments

Over the counter medication such as dimenhydrinate (Dramamine), meclizine (Bonine), and cyclizine (Marezine) may be helpful.

Prescription medications include anticholinergic drugs, such as scopolamine (Transderm Scop), prochlorperazine (Compazine), and meclizine (Antivert), as well as sedatives, including diazepam (Valium), lorazepam (Ativan), and alprazolam (Xanax).

Healthcare practitioners recommend getting fresh air, lying down, closing the eyes, and alcohol avoidance. People frequently affected by severe, disabling vertigo may require a surgical treatment, such as vestibular neurectomy or labyrinthectomy. These procedures involve surgical removal of either the nerves or labyrinthine structures that control balance and position senses.

Dietary changes that may be helpful

In preliminary studies, vertigo associated with **high triglycerides** (page 235), **diabetes mellitus** (page 152), and **hypoglycemia** (page 251) responded to dietary management of the underlying disorder.[15, 16] In a preliminary study of people with **migraine headaches** (page 316), most of whom (83%) also experienced vertigo, a multifaceted approach including dietary changes was investigated. Dietary changes involved the elimination of foods and food additives suspected of causing migraine attacks. This approach resulted in complete or substantial improvement of symptoms in a significant number of participants.[17] No other research has investigated the effects of diet on vertigo.

Lifestyle changes that may be helpful

Head positions that bring on sudden, acute attacks of vertigo, particularly bending the neck back while looking up, should be avoided. In one report, for example, the head position used in salons for shampooing hair was associated with the onset of vertigo.[18] According to

one authority,[19] certain chronic or repetitive body positions may produce painful nodules, called trigger points, in the muscles of the head and neck, which can lead to dizziness and possibly vertigo. These positions include forward bending of the neck as when sleeping on two pillows, backward neck bending as when painting a ceiling, and turning the neck to one side as in some reading positions.[20] A healthcare practitioner knowledgeable in postural education can give advice on avoiding such positions. Trigger point therapy is discussed below in "Other integrative approaches that may be helpful."

Nutritional supplements that may be helpful

A preliminary trial showed that 15 mg per day of **vinpocetine** (page 594) had a moderate or greater effect on reducing the signs and symptoms of vertigo in 77% of patients with this condition.[21] Other preliminary reports exist describing benefits of vinpocetine for vertigo and other symptoms of inner ear disorders,[22] but controlled research is needed to evaluate these claims.

Two preliminary human studies reported that **vitamin B₆** (page 600) supplementation reduced symptoms of vertigo produced with drugs in a laboratory setting.[23] Vitamin B₆ supplementation has not been studied in BPPV or other forms of vertigo and may not share the same causative mechanism as experimentally induced vertigo.

Are there any side effects or interactions?
Refer to the individual supplement for information about any side effects or interactions.

Herbs that may be helpful

In a preliminary clinical trial, a standardized extract of ***Ginkgo biloba*** (page 681) (GBE) significantly reduced symptoms of vertigo in a group of elderly people with mild cognitive impairment.[24] Participants were given 40 mg three times per day for one year. GBE has also been reported to significantly reduce vertigo of unknown cause in preliminary[25] and double-blind[26] trials. The amounts given were 120 mg and 160 mg per day, respectively, for three months.

One gram of powdered **ginger** (page 680) (*Zingiber officinale*) root in a single application has been reported to significantly reduce symptoms of artificially induced vertigo in one double-blind trial.[27] In a double-blind trial, 1 gram of powdered ginger root was found to have very little effect in reducing vertigo related to **seasickness** (page 322).[28]

Are there any side effects or interactions?
Refer to the individual herb for information about any side effects or interactions.

Holistic approaches that may be helpful

Other integrative approaches that may be helpful: Numerous preliminary reports suggest certain "vestibular rehabilitation" exercises may help some cases of vertigo.[29, 30, 31, 32, 33, 34] These exercises were also found to be effective in relieving vertigo in two controlled studies,[35] including one on BPPV.[36] While vestibular rehabilitation exercises may be done at home, initial guidance by a qualified practitioner is necessary.

BPPV appears to be caused by an accumulation of free-floating cell fragments in the fluid of the inner ear.[37, 38] Certain manipulation therapy maneuvers, referred to as particle repositioning maneuvers (PRMs), are intended to relocate this debris to a harmless location,[39, 40, 41] in order to improve symptoms. Both preliminary[42, 43, 44, 45, 46] and controlled[47, 48, 49] trials achieved significant improvement in, or elimination of, BPPV using these maneuvers. Most studies report that over 90% of people with BPPV treated one or two times with PRM respond to this treatment, although up to 45% may develop BPPV again within a few years, requiring further treatments.[50, 51, 52]

Research indicates some cases of vertigo are related to spinal disorders affecting the head and neck.[53, 54, 55, 56, 57, 58, 59] Preliminary studies report that certain treatments, such as spinal manipulation,[60, 61, 62, 63] physical therapy,[64] and combined approaches including manipulation and specific exercise programs,[65, 66] result in significant improvement of vertigo symptoms.

Trigger points are thought by most,[67, 68, 69] though not all,[70] authorities to potentially cause pain and abnormal function in other parts of the body. Trigger points appear to develop as the result of injury, poor posture, structural abnormalities of the leg or pelvis, emotional tension, and other body stressors.[71, 72] Also known as myofascial pain dysfunction (MPD), this condition, when it affects certain muscles of the head and neck, has been associated with vertigo in preliminary research.[73, 74, 75] Musculoskeletal healthcare specialists and other practitioners can often treat MPD with a variety of natural therapies, including deep pressure massage,[76, 77, 78, 79, 80] transcutaneous electrical nerve stimulation (TENS),[81, 82] and other approaches,[83] but no controlled studies have investigated the effectiveness of these treatments specifically for vertigo.

In a preliminary study of people with migraine headaches, most of whom (83%) also experienced vertigo, a combined and individualized approach using dietary changes, medication, physical therapy, lifestyle changes, and acupuncture resulted in complete or substantial improvement of symptoms in a significant number of participants.[84] In addition, a large number of case studies presented in two preliminary reports suggest acupuncture may help to reduce symptoms of vertigo.[85, 86] These preliminary studies have yet to be confirmed by controlled clinical trials.

VITILIGO

Vitiligo is a type of skin discoloration characterized by progressively widening areas of depigmented (very white) skin.

The depigmentation that occurs with this condition is associated with the local destruction of melanocytes, the cells that produce the pigment that darkens the skin, called melanin. Vitiligo affects 1–4% of the world's population.[1]

Rating	Nutritional Supplements	Herbs
★★☆	**L-phenylalanine** (page 568)	*Ginkgo biloba* (page 681) Khella **Picrorhiza** (page 728)
★☆☆	**Betaine HCl** (page 473) **Folic acid** (page 520) **PABA** (page 567) **Vitamin B-complex** (page 603) **Vitamin B₁₂** (page 601) **Vitamin C** (page 604) **Vitamin D** (page 607) (topical calcipotriol only)	

CHECKLIST FOR VITILIGO

What are the symptoms of vitiligo?
Symptoms of vitiligo include decreased or absent pigmentation in localized or diffuse areas of the skin. Hair in these areas is typically white, and the skin tends to sunburn more easily.

Medical treatments
Prescription topical corticosteroids, such as triamcinolone (Kenalog, Aristocort), betamethasone (Valisone,

Diprosone), and fluocinonide (Lidex), might help in some situations. Oral and topical psoralens, including methoxsalen (Oxsoralen) and trioxsalen (Trisoralen) with ultraviolet A irradiation (PUVA), are occasionally used.

Other treatment includes cosmetic creams and tanning solutions. Treatment may also involve the management of any underlying medical condition, such as Vogt-Koyanagi-Harada syndrome, scleroderma, melanoma-associated leukoderma, chronic mucocutaneous candidiasis, and autoimmune disorders (including Grave's disease, **diabetes mellitus** (page 152), **pernicious anemia** (page 601), and Addison's disease). Rarely, skin transplants may be necessary.

Nutritional supplements that may be helpful

Supplementation with the amino acid **L-phenylalanine** (page 568) (LPA) may have value when combined with ultraviolet (UVA) light therapy. Several clinical trials, including one double-blind trial, indicated that LPA (50 mg per 2.2 pounds of body weight per day— 3,500 mg per day for a 154-pound person—or less) increased the extent of repigmentation induced by UVA therapy. LPA alone also produced a more modest repigmentation in some people.[2] A study of vitiligo in children reported that LPA plus UVA was an effective treatment in a majority of the children.[3]

A group of Spanish doctors reported on their experience using LPA over a six-year period. Some of the 171 people with vitiligo received LPA (50 or 100 mg per 2.2 pounds body weight per day) for up to three years. Between April and October of each year, participants also applied a 10% LPA gel, prior to exposing their skin to the sun for 30 minutes. Some improvement was seen in 83% of participants, and the results were rated as good in 57% (75% improvement or better).[4]

A clinical report describes the use of vitamin supplements in the treatment of vitiligo.[5] **Folic acid** (page 520) and/or **vitamin B**$_{12}$ (page 601) and **vitamin C** (page 604) levels were abnormally low in most of the 15 people studied. Supplementation with large amounts of folic acid (1–10 mg per day), along with vitamin C (1 gram per day) and intramuscular vitamin B$_{12}$ injections (1,000 mcg every two weeks), produced marked repigmentation in eight people. These improvements became apparent after three months, but complete repigmentation required one to two years of continuous supplementation. In another study of people with vitiligo, oral supplementation with folic acid (10 mg per day) and vitamin B$_{12}$ (2,000 mcg per day), combined with sun exposure, resulted in some repigmentation

after three to six months in about half of the participants.[6] This combined regimen was more effective than either vitamin supplementation or sun exposure alone.

When used topically in combination with sun exposure, a pharmaceutical form of **vitamin D** (page 607), called calcipotriol, may be effective in stimulating repigmentation in children with vitiligo. In a preliminary study, children applied a cream containing calcipotriol daily and exposed themselves to sunlight for 10–15 minutes the following morning.[7] After 11 months, marked to complete repigmentation occurred in 55% of the children, moderate repigmentation occurred in 22%, and little or no improvement was seen in 22%. None of the children developed new areas of vitiligo. The first evidence of repigmentation occurred within 6 to 12 weeks in the majority of the children. All participants tolerated the cream well, with approximately 17% complaining of mild, transient skin irritation. Calcipotriol is a prescription medication to be used only under the supervision of a doctor. It is not known whether vitamin D as a dietary supplement has any effect on vitiligo.

In one early report, lack of stomach acid (achlorhydria) was associated with vitiligo. Supplementation with dilute hydrochloric acid after meals resulted in gradual repigmentation of the skin (after one year or more).[8] Hydrochloric acid, or its more modern counterpart **betaine HCl** (page 473), should be taken only under the supervision of a doctor.

Another early report described the use of **PABA** (page 567) (para-aminobenzoic acid)—a compound commonly found in **B-complex vitamins** (page 603)—for vitiligo. Consistent use of 100 mg of PABA three or four times per day, along with an injectable form of PABA and a variety of hormones tailored to individual needs, resulted, in many cases, in repigmentation of areas affected by vitiligo.[9]

Are there any side effects or interactions?
Refer to the individual supplement for information about any side effects or interactions.

Herbs that may be helpful
In a double-blind study of 52 people with slowly spreading vitiligo, supplementation with *Ginkgo biloba* extract (standardized to contain 24% ginkgoflavonglycosides), in the amount of 40 mg three times per day for up to six months, resulted in marked to complete repigmentation in 40% of cases, compared with only 9% among those receiving a placebo.[10]

An extract from khella (*Ammi visnaga*) may be useful in repigmenting the skin of people with vitiligo. Khellin, the active constituent, appears to work like psoralen drugs—it stimulates repigmentation of the skin by increasing sensitivity of remaining melanocytes to sunlight. Studies have used 120–160 mg of khellin per day.[11]

In preliminary trial, **Picrorhiza** (page 728), in combination with the drug methoxsalen and sun exposure, was reported to hasten recovery in people with vitiligo compared with use of methoxsalen and sun exposure alone.[12] Between 400 and 1,500 mg of powdered, encapsulated picrorhiza per day has been used in a variety of studies.

Are there any side effects or interactions?
Refer to the individual herb for information about any side effects or interactions.

Holistic approaches that may be helpful

People with vitiligo have occasionally improved using hypnosis along with other treatments.[13]

WARTS

Warts are a common abnormal skin growths caused by one of many types of human papilloma virus, which infects the outer layer of skin.

Common warts (verruca vulgaris) can appear on any part of the body but are more common on the fingers, hands, and arms. They are most common in people 30 years old or younger, but can occur at any age and are almost universal in the population. Other types of warts also exist, including flat warts, genital warts, laryngeal papillomas, and others.

CHECKLIST FOR WARTS		
Rating	Nutritional Supplements	Herbs
★★☆	Zinc (page 614) (oral)	Garlic (page 679) (topical application)
★☆☆		Greater celandine (page 684)

What are the symptoms of warts?

Appearance and size of warts depend on the location and the amount of irritation and trauma. Common warts are sharply demarcated, rough-surfaced, round or irregular in shape, firm, and either light gray, yellow, brown, or gray-black in color. They are small nodules ranging in size from 2–10 mm in diameter. Plantar warts (on the bottoms of the feet) are flattened and may be exquisitely tender. Flat warts, more common in children and young adults, are smooth, flat-topped yellow-brown elevations, most often seen on the face and along scratch marks. Genital warts (also called condyloma acuminata or venereal warts) are soft, moist, small pink or gray polyps that enlarge and are usually found in clusters on the anus and the warmer, moister areas of the female and male genitalia. Genital warts caused by HPV are considered a major cause of **cervical dysplasia** (page 3) and cervical cancer. All warts are contagious.

Medical treatments

Over the counter drugs used to treat common warts contain salicylic acid (Compound W, Dr Scholl's Wart Remover Kit, Mosco) and are applied topically on a daily basis.

Prescription medications are available to treat genital warts. They include podofilox (Condylox) and podophyllum resin (Podocon-25). The latter drug is only to be applied by a physician.

A protective pad may be worn to relieve the pain of plantar warts. In some cases, doctors may recommend removal of the wart using various procedures such as freezing with liquid nitrogen (cryotherapy), conventional surgery, laser surgery, or applying an electrical current to dry the wart (electrodesiccation with curettage).

Dietary changes that may be helpful

A preliminary study reported that the weekly consumption of two to four alcoholic drinks nearly doubled the risk of developing genital warts.[1] Those who consumed more than five alcoholic drinks had a more than doubled risk of developing genital warts. A case report of a 19-year-old with a urinary-tract wart found that abstinence from a high intake of pork led to a regression of the wart.[2]

Lifestyle changes that may be helpful

Warts can be spread by contact, and the transmission can occur between two people as well as between different parts of the body of the same person. To prevent the spread of the virus, warts should not be scratched. Genital warts are spread by sexual contact.

A study of **HIV** (page 239)-infected and HIV-negative women found that current smokers were over five times more likely to develop genital warts than non-smokers.[3]

Nutritional supplements that may be helpful

In a double-blind study, supplementation with oral **zinc** (page 614), in the form of zinc sulfate, for two months resulted in complete disappearance of warts in 87% of people treated, whereas none of those receiving a placebo improved.[4] The amount of zinc used was based on body weight, with a maximum of 135 mg per day. These large amounts of zinc should be used under the supervision of a doctor. Side effects included nausea, vomiting, and mild abdominal pain.

Are there any side effects or interactions?
Refer to the individual supplement for information about any side effects or interactions.

Herbs that may be helpful

In a preliminary trial, topical application of garlic cloves was used successfully to treat warts in a group of children. A clove was cut in half each night and the flat edge of the clove was rubbed onto each of the warts, carefully cleaning the surrounding areas, so as not to spread any garlic juice. The areas were covered overnight with Band-Aids or waterproof tape and were washed in the morning. In all cases, the warts cleared completely after an average of nine weeks.[5]

Herbalists have sometimes recommended the use of **greater celandine** (page 684) *(Chelidonium majus)* for the topical treatment of warts.[6] The milky juice from the fresh plant is typically applied to the wart once daily and allowed to dry.

Are there any side effects or interactions?
Refer to the individual herb for information about any side effects or interactions.

Holistic approaches that may be helpful

Distant healing is a conscious, dedicated act of mental activity that attempts to benefit another person's physical or emotional well-being at a distance. A controlled study found that distant healing by an experienced healer for six weeks had no effect on the number or size of warts.[7]

A controlled study found that the application of 122°F heat from a heat pad for 30 seconds led to regression in 25 warts.[8] After 15 weeks, none of the regressed warts had regrown.

Hypnosis is a widely recognized treatment for warts. One controlled trial found that twice-weekly hypnosis sessions resulted in greater wart disappearance than did medication, placebo, or no treatment after six weeks of therapy.[9]

WEIGHT LOSS AND OBESITY

See also: Childhood Obesity (page 107)

What do I need to know?

Self-care for weight loss and obesity can be approached in a number of ways—but it can be hard to know just where to start. To make it easier, our doctors recommend trying these simple steps first:

Find a diet that fits
> For long-term success, choose a healthy diet that you can stay with

Find support
> Improve your chances for long-term weight loss by joining a group while you adjust to new diet and exercise habits

Create a custom exercise plan
> Exercise you truly enjoy is that much easier to stick to, so find activities that fit your personal style, fitness level, and work-out opportunities

Get a boost from pyruvate
> Combining exercise with 6 to 10 grams a day of pyruvate may help speed up your metabolism

Try 5-HTP (5-hydroxytryptophan)
> Taking 600 to 900 mg a day may help curb your appetite

Aim for total nutrition with a multivitamin-mineral supplement
> Extra vitamins and minerals will help ensure your body gets the nutrition it needs, especially if you are avoiding certain foods

About weight loss and obesity

About two-thirds of the adult U.S. population is overweight.[1] Almost one-third not only exceeds ideal weight, but also meets the clinical criteria for obesity. In the 1990s, rates of obesity more than doubled, and are currently rising by over 5% per year.[2, 3] Excess body weight is implicated as a risk factor for many different disorders, including **heart disease** (page 98), **diabetes** (page 152), several **cancers** (page 87) (such as **breast cancer** [page 65] in postmenopausal women, and cancers of the uterus, **colon** [page 123], and kidney), prostate enlargement (**BPH** [page 58]), **female infertility** (page 187), uterine fibroids, and **gallstones** (page 193), as well as several disorders of pregnancy, including gestational diabetes, preeclampsia, and gestational hypertension.[4] The location of excess body fat may affect the amount of health risk associated with overweight. Increased abdominal fat, which can be estimated by waist size, may be especially hazardous to long-term health.[5, 6]

For overweight women, weight loss can significantly improve physical health. A four-year study of over 40,000 women found that weight loss in overweight women was associated with improved physical function and vitality as well as decreased bodily pain.[7] The risk of death from all causes, cardiovascular disease, cancer, or other diseases increases in overweight men and women in all age groups.[8] Losing weight and keeping it off is, unfortunately, very difficult for most people.[9, 10] However, repeated weight loss followed by weight regain may be unhealthy, as it has been associated with increased heart disease risk factors and bone loss in some studies.[11, 12] Rather than focusing on weight loss as the most important health outcome of a change in diet or lifestyle, some doctors advocate paying more attention to overall fitness and reduction in known risk factors for heart disease and other health hazards.[13]

Excess body mass has the one advantage of increasing bone mass—a protection against **osteoporosis** (page 333). Probably because of this, researchers have been able to show that people who successfully lose weight have greater loss of bone compared with those who do not lose weight.[14] People who lose weight should, therefore, pay more attention to preventing osteoporosis.

Medical treatments

Over-the-counter products such as Dexatrim Natural No Caffeine and Dexatrim Natural No Ephedrine are available to assist with weight loss.

Prescription medications commonly prescribed for weight loss include sibutramine (Meridia), orlistat (Xenical), and phentermine (Fastin, Ionamin). Stimulants, such as dextroamphetamine (Dexedrine) and methamphetamine (Desoxyn), are occasionally used.

Other treatment typically includes dietary changes to limit fat and calorie intake, increased exercise, and changes in eating habits or patterns. Severe cases might require surgical options to reduce the size of the stomach or to bypass a portion of the stomach and intestines.

Rating	Nutritional Supplements	Herbs
★★★	**Multivitamin-mineral** (page 559) (for very-low-calorie diets) **Pyruvate** (page 580)	
★★☆	**Beta-hydroxy beta-methylbutyrate (HMB)** (page 534) (for improving body composition only) **Calcium** (page 483) **Conjugated linoleic acid (CLA)** (page 499) **5-HTP** (page 459) **Fiber** (page 512) **Glucomannan** (page 526) **7-KETO** (page 460)	**Cayenne** (page 654) **Green tea** (page 686) **Yohimbe** (page 764)
★☆☆	**Amylase inhibitors** (page 466) **Blue-green algae (Spirulina)** (page 474) **Chitosan** (page 491) **Chromium** (page 493) **DHEA** (page 503) Guar gum **(-)-Hydroxycitric acid** (page 535) (HCA) **L-carnitine** (page 543) **Soy** (page 586) **Whey protein** (page 613)	**Bitter orange** (page 635) **Coleus** (page 660) **Guaraná** (page 687) **Guggul** (page 688) **Psyllium** (page 731)

CHECKLIST FOR WEIGHT LOSS AND OBESITY

Dietary changes that may be helpful

Breast-feeding (page 74)

In a preliminary study, breast-feeding during infancy was associated with a reduced risk of developing obesity during early childhood (ages three to four years).[15]

In a preliminary study, overweight individuals who adhered to a very-low-carbohydrate diet (25 grams per day initially, increased to 50 grams per day after a certain weight-loss target was achieved), with no limit on total calorie intake, lost on average more than 10% of their body weight over a six-month period.[16] The participants also engaged in aerobic exercise at least three times a week, so it is not clear how much of the weight loss was due to the diet. Blood tests taken during the study suggested that the low-carbohydrate diet induced a condition called mild metabolic acidosis, indicating that long-term consumption of this diet may not be entirely safe. Individuals wishing to consume a very-low-carbohydrate diet for weight loss or for other reasons should be monitored by a doctor.

Calorie restriction

Calories in the diet come from fat, carbohydrate, protein, or alcohol. Weight-loss diets are typically designed to limit calories either by restricting certain foods that are thought to result in increased calorie intake, and/or by emphasizing foods that are believed to result in reduced calorie intake. Some currently popular diets restrict fat while emphasizing fiber and a balanced intake of healthful foods. Others restrict carbohydrates, either to extremely low amounts as in the Atkins diet, or to a lesser degree, emphasizing foods low in the glycemic index or high in protein. Discussions of the research on these diets follow; however, it should be remembered that no diet has been proven effective for long-term weight loss, and many people find it difficult to stay on most diets.[17, 18]

Low-fat, low-calorie, high-fiber, balanced diets are recommended by many doctors for weight loss.[19] According to controlled studies, when people are allowed to eat as much food as they desire on a low-fat diet, they tend to lose more weight than people eating a regular diet.[20] However, low-fat diets have not been shown to be more effective than other weight-loss diets that restrict calories.[21] Nonetheless, a low-fat, high-fiber, balanced diet has additional potential benefits, such as reducing the risk of chronic diseases including heart disease and cancer.[22, 23]

Preliminary research indicates that people who successfully lost weight got fewer of their total calories from fat and more of them from protein foods. They also ate fewer snacks of low nutritional quality and got more of their calories from "hot meals of good quality."[24] Other preliminary studies find that dieters who maintain long-term weight loss report using fat restriction and eating a regular breakfast as key strategies in their success.[25, 26]

Low-carbohydrate, high-protein diets

Low-carbohydrate, high-fat diets such as the Atkins diet are very popular among people trying to lose weight. In a preliminary study, overweight individuals who adhered to a very-low-carbohydrate diet (25 grams per day initially, increased to 50 grams per day after a certain weight loss target was achieved), with no limit on total calorie intake, lost on average more than 10% of their body weight over a six-month period.[27] The participants also engaged in aerobic exercise at least

three times a week, so it is not clear how much of the weight loss was due to the diet. An analysis of other preliminary studies of this type of diet concluded that its effectiveness is primarily due to reduced calorie intake.[28] Recently, three controlled trials found people using low-carbohydrate, high-fat diets lost more weight in six months than those using diets low in fat and calories.[29, 30, 31] However, 20% to 40% of these dieters did not stay on their diets, and were not counted in the results. In addition, one of these trials continued for an additional six months, at the end of which there was no longer a significant difference in weight loss between the two diet groups. A recent 12-week controlled trial found that overweight adolescents also lost more weight with a low-carbohydrate diet than with a low-fat diet, even though they consumed 50% more calories than did the children on the low-fat diet.[32] That study suggests that the weight loss occurring on the Atkins diet is not due entirely to calorie restriction. Blood tests suggest that low-carbohydrate diets induce a condition called mild metabolic acidosis, which might increase the risk of osteoporosis and kidney stones.

The effect of low-carbohydrate diets on cardiovascular risk is also an unresolved issue. The short-term studies discussed above found that blood cholesterol levels did not worsen with these diets. Other heart-disease risk factors (triglyceride levels and insulin sensitivity) actually improved with a low-carbohydrate diet. Some studies, however, have shown a worsening of certain cardiovascular risk factors in people using a low-carbohydrate, high-fat diet for up to one year. Adverse changes included increases in blood levels of homocysteine, lipoprotein(a), and fibrinogen,[33] and a decrease in blood flow to the heart.[34] Individuals wishing to consume a very-low-carbohydrate diet for weight loss or for other reasons should be monitored by a doctor.

Some research has investigated weight-loss diets that are high in protein, but moderate in fat and not as low in carbohydrate content as the diets discussed above. While this type of diet does not usually lead to greater weight loss than other diets when calorie intakes are kept equal,[35] one controlled trial found greater body fat loss in women eating a diet almost equal in calories and fat but approximately twice as high in protein and lower in carbohydrate compared with a control group's diet.[36] Another controlled trial compared two diets similar in fat content but different in protein and carbohydrate content. People allowed to eat freely from the higher protein diet (25% of calories from protein, 45% calories from carbohydrate) consumed fewer calories and lost more weight compared with people eating the lower protein diet (12% of calories from protein, 59% calories from carbohydrate).[37]

Low glycemic index foods

Diets that emphasize choosing foods with a low glycemic index have been show to help control appetite in some,[38, 39, 40] though not all,[41] controlled studies. A controlled study in two phases found no difference in weight loss between a low and a high glycemic index diet in the first 12-week phase, but when the diets were switched for a second 12-week phase, the low glycemic index diet was significantly more effective for weight loss.[42] A preliminary study reported that obese children using a low glycemic index diet lost more weight compared with a similar group using a low-fat diet.[43]

Fiber

Adequate amounts of dietary fiber are believed to be important for people wishing to lose weight. Fiber adds bulk to the diet and tends to produce a sense of fullness, helping people consume fewer calories.[44] While research on the effect of fiber intake on weight loss has not produced consistent results,[45] a recent review of weight-loss trials that did not restrict calories concluded that higher fiber diets improved weight-loss results, especially in people who were overweight.[46]

Stabilizing food sensitivities

Although the relationship between **food sensitivities** (page 14) and body weight remains uncertain, according to one researcher, chronic food allergy may lead to overeating and obesity.[47]

Long-term changes

People who go on and off diets frequently complain that it takes fewer calories to produce weight gain with each weight fluctuation. Evidence now clearly demonstrates that the body gets "stingier" in its use of calories after each diet.[48] This means it becomes easier to gain weight and harder to lose it the next time. Dietary changes need to be long term.

Lifestyle changes that may be helpful

Support

Many doctors give overweight patients a pill, a pep talk, and a pamphlet about diet and exercise, but that combination leads only to minor weight loss.[49] When overweight people attend group sessions aimed at changing eating and exercise patterns, keep daily records of food intake and exercise, and eat a specific low-calorie diet the outcome is much more successful. Group sessions where participants are given information and help on how to make lifestyle changes appear to improve the chances of losing weight and keeping it off. Such changes may include shopping from a list, storing foods out of sight, keeping portion sizes under control, and avoiding fast-food restaurants.

Exercise

According to most short-term studies, the effect of exercise alone (without dietary restriction) on weight loss is small,[50, 51] partly because muscle mass often increases even while fat tissue is reduced,[52] and perhaps because some exercising people will experience increased appetites. The long-term effect of regular exercise on weight loss is much better, and exercise appears to help people maintain weight loss.[53, 54] People who have successfully maintained weight loss for over two years report continuing high levels of physical activity.[55] Combining exercise with healthier eating habits results in the best short- and long-term effects on weight loss,[56, 57] and should reduce the risk of many serious diseases.[58, 59, 60]

Avoid weight cycling

People who experience "weight cycling" (repetitive weight loss and gain) have a tendency toward **binge eating** (page 174) (periods of compulsive overeating, but without the self-induced vomiting seen in **bulimia** [page 174]), according to a review of numerous studies focusing on weight loss.[61] The researchers also found an association between weight cycling and **depression** (page 145) or poor body image. The most successful weight-loss programs (in which weight stays off, mood stays even, and no binge eating occurs) appear to use a combination of moderate caloric restriction, moderate exercise, and behavior modification, including examination and adjustment of eating habits.

Nutritional supplements that may be helpful

Multiple vitamin minerals (page 559)

Diets that are low in total calories may not contain adequate amounts of various vitamins and minerals. For that reason, taking a multiple vitamin-mineral supplement is advocated by proponents of many types of weight-loss programs, and is essential when calorie intake will be less than 1,100 calories per day.[62]

Pyruvate (page 580)

Pyruvate, a compound that occurs naturally in the body, might aid weight-loss efforts.[63] A controlled trial found that pyruvate supplements (22 to 44 grams per day) enhanced weight loss and resulted in a greater reduction of body fat in overweight adults consuming a low-fat diet.[64] Three controlled trials combining 6 to

10 grams per day of pyruvate with an exercise program reported greater effects on weight loss and body fat than that seen with a placebo plus the exercise program.[65, 66, 67] Animal studies suggest that pyruvate supplementation leads to weight loss by increasing the resting metabolic rate.[68]

5-HTP (page 459)

5-hydroxytryptophan (5-HTP), the precursor to the chemical messenger (neurotransmitter) serotonin, has been shown in three short-term controlled trials to reduce appetite and to promote weight loss.[69, 70, 71] In one of these trials (a 12-week double-blind trial), overweight women who took 600 to 900 mg of 5-HTP per day lost significantly more weight than did women who received a placebo.[72] In a double-blind trial with no dietary restrictions, obese people with type 2 (non-insulin-dependent) **diabetes** (page 152) who took 750 mg per day of 5-HTP for two weeks significantly reduced their carbohydrate and fat intake. Average weight loss in two weeks was 4.6 pounds, compared with 0.2 pounds in the placebo group.[73]

7-KETO (page 460)

The ability of 7-KETO (3-acetyl-7-oxo-dehydroepiandrosterone), a substance related to **DHEA** (page 503), to promote weight loss in overweight people has been investigated in one double-blind trial.[74] Participants in the trial were advised to exercise three times per week for 45 minutes and to eat an 1,800-calorie-per-day diet. Each person was given either a placebo or 100 mg of 7-KETO twice daily. After eight weeks, those receiving 7-KETO had lost more weight and lowered their percentage of body fat further compared to those taking a placebo. These results may have been due to increases in levels of a thyroid hormone (T3) that plays a major role in determining a person's metabolic rate, although the levels of T3 did not exceed the normal range.

HMB (page 534)

Biochemical and animal research show that HMB has a role in protein synthesis and might, therefore, improve muscle growth and overall body composition when given as a supplement. However, double-blind human research suggests that HMB may only be effective when combined with an exercise program in people who are not already highly trained athletes. Double-blind trials found no effect of 3 to 6 grams per day of HMB on body weight, body fat, or overall body composition in weight-training football players or other trained athletes.[75, 76, 77, 78, 79] However, one double-blind study found that 3 grams per day of HMB increased the amount of body fat lost by 70-year-old adults who were participating in a strength-training program for the first time.[80] A double-blind study of young men with no strength-training experience reported greater improvements in muscle mass (but not in percentage body fat) when HMB was used in the amount of 17 mg per pound of body weight per day.[81] However, another group of men in the same study given twice as much HMB did not experience any changes in body composition.

Calcium (page 483)

In a study of obese people consuming a low-calorie diet for 24 weeks, those receiving a calcium supplement (800 mg per day) lost significantly more weight than those given a placebo.[82] Calcium was effective when provided either as a supplement, or in the form of dairy products. In a second study, however, the amount of weight loss resulting from calcium supplementation (1,000 mg per day) was small and not statistically significant.[83] In that study, participants' typical diets contained more calcium than in the study in which calcium supplementation was more effective. Thus, it is possible that calcium supplementation enhances weight loss only when the diet is low in calcium.

CLA (page 499)

A double-blind trial found that exercising individuals taking 1,800 mg per day of conjugated linoleic acid (CLA) lost more body fat after 12 weeks than did a similar group taking a placebo.[84] However, two other studies found that amounts of CLA from 0.7 to 3.0 grams per day did not affect body composition.[85, 86] Most double-blind trials have found that larger amounts of CLA, 3.4 to 4.2 grams per day, do reduce body fat;[87, 88, 89] however, one double-blind study of experienced strength-training athletes reported no effect of 6 grams per day of CLA on body fat, muscle mass, or strength improvement.[90]

Fiber (page 512)

Fiber supplements are one way to add fiber to a weight-loss diet. Several trials have shown that supplementation with fiber from a variety of sources accelerated weight loss in people who were following a low-calorie diet.[91, 92, 93, 94] Other researchers found, however, that fiber supplements had no effect on body weight, even though it resulted in a reduction in food intake.[95]

Glucomannan (page 526)

Supplementation with 3 to 4 grams per day of a bulking agent called glucomannan, with or without a low-calorie diet, has promoted weight loss in overweight adults,[96, 97, 98] while 2 to 3 grams per day was effective in a group of obese adolescents in another controlled trial.[99]

HCA *(page 535)*

(-)-Hydroxycitric acid (HCA), extracted from the rind of the *Garcinia cambogia* fruit grown in Southeast Asia, has a chemicalcomposition similar to that of citric acid (the primary acid in oranges and other citrus fruits). Preliminary studies in animals suggest that HCA may be a useful weight-loss aid.[100, 101] HCA has been demonstrated in the laboratory (but not yet in clinical trials with people) to reduce the conversion of carbohydrates into stored fat by inhibiting certain enzyme processes.[102, 103] Animal research indicates that HCA suppresses appetite and induces weight loss.[104, 105, 106, 107] However, a double-blind trial found that people who took 1,500 mg per day of HCA while eating a low-calorie diet for 12 weeks lost no more weight than those taking a placebo.[108] A double-blind trial of *Garcinia cambogia* (2.4 grams of dry extract, containing 50% hydroxycitric acid) found that the extract did not increase energy expenditure; it was therefore concluded that this extract showed little potential for the treatment of obesity at this amount.[109] Nonetheless, another double-blind trial found that using the same amount of *Garcinia cambogia* extract significantly improved the results of a weight-loss diet, even though the amount of food intake was not affected.[110]

Amylase inhibitors *(page 466)*

Amylase inhibitors are also known as starch blockers because they contain substances that prevent dietary starches from being absorbed by the body. Starches are complex carbohydrates that cannot be absorbed unless they are first broken down by the digestive enzyme amylase and other, secondary, enzymes.[111, 112] When starch blockers were first developed years ago, they were found not to be potent enough to prevent the absorption of a significant amount of carbohydrate.[113, 114, 115, 116] Recently, highly concentrated starch blockers have been shown to be more effective,[117, 118, 119] but no published human studies exist investigating their usefulness for weight loss.

Blue-green algae *(page 474)*

Blue-green algae, or spirulina, is a rich source of protein, vitamins, minerals, and essential fatty acids. In one double-blind trial, overweight people who took 2.8 grams of spirulina three times per day for four weeks experienced only small and statistically nonsignificant weight loss.[120] Thus, although spirulina has been promoted as a weight-loss aid, the scientific evidence supporting its use for this purpose is weak.

Chitosan *(page 491)*

Chitosan is a fiber-like substance extracted from the shells of crustaceans such as shrimp and crab. Animal studies suggested that chitosan supplementation reduces fat absorption, but controlled human trials have found no impairment of fat absorption from supplementation with 2,700 mg of chitosan per day for seven days or 5,250 mg per day for four days.[121, 122] A double-blind study in Poland found that people taking 1,500 mg of chitosan three times per day during a weight-loss program lost significantly more weight than did people taking a placebo with the same program.[123] Other studies using smaller amounts of chitosan have reported no effects on weight loss.[124, 125, 126]

Chromium *(page 493)*

The mineral chromium plays an essential role in the metabolism of carbohydrates and fats and in the action of insulin. Chromium, usually in a form called chromium picolinate, has been studied for its potential role in altering body composition. Chromium has primarily been studied in body builders, with conflicting results.[127] In people trying to lose weight, a double-blind study found that 600 mcg per day of niacin-bound chromium helped some participants lose more fat and less muscle.[128] However, three other double-blind trials have found no effect of chromium picolinate on weight loss,[129, 130, 131] though in one of these trials lean body mass that was lost during a weight-loss diet was restored by continuing to supplement chromium after the diet. A recent comprehensive review combining the results of ten published and unpublished double-blind studies concluded that chromium picolinate supplementation may have a small beneficial effect on weight loss.[132]

DHEA *(page 503)*

One double-blind trial found 100 mg per day of DHEA was effective for decreasing body fat in older men,[133] and another double-blind trial found 1,600 mg per day decreased body fat and increased muscle mass in younger men.[134] However, DHEA has not been effective for improving body composition in women or in other studies of men.[135, 136, 137, 138, 139, 140, 141, 142]

Guar gum

Guar gum, another type of fiber supplement, has not been effective in controlled studies for weight loss or weight maintenance.[143, 144, 145]

L-carnitine *(page 543)*

The amino acid L-carnitine is thought to be potentially helpful for weight loss because of its role in fat metabolism. In a preliminary study of overweight adolescents participating in a diet and exercise program, those who took 1,000 mg of L-carnitine per day for three months lost significantly more weight than those who took a placebo.[146] A weakness of this trial, however, was the fact that the average starting body weight differed considerably between the two groups. A double-blind trial found that adding 4,000 mg of L-carnitine per day to an exercise program did not result in weight loss in overweight women.[147]

Soy (page 586)

Animal and human studies have suggested that when soy is used as a source of dietary protein, it may have several biological effects on the body that might help with weight loss.[148] A preliminary study found that people trying to lose weight using a meal-replacement formula containing soy protein lost more weight than a group not using any formula.[149] However, controlled studies comparing soy protein with other protein sources in weight-loss diets have not found any advantage of soy.[150, 151, 152] When soy protein is used for other health benefits, typical daily intake is 20 grams per day or more.

Whey protein (page 613)

Whey protein may aid weight loss due to its effect on appetite. In a preliminary study, people were given 48 grams of either whey protein or milk protein (casein). Whey consumption resulted in more hunger satisfaction and reduced the amount of food eaten 90 minutes later compared with casein consumption.[153] However, a double-blind study found that men taking 1.5 grams per 2.2 lbs body weight per day of whey protein for 12 weeks along with a low-calorie diet and a strength training exercise program lost the same amount of weight and body fat as did a control group that followed a similar program, but took a casein supplement instead of whey protein.[154]

Are there any side effects or interactions?

Refer to the individual supplement for information about any side effects or interactions.

Herbs that may be helpful

Cayenne (page 634)

Research has suggested that incorporating cayenne pepper into the diet may help people lose weight. Controlled studies report that adding 6 to 10 grams of cayenne to a meal or 28 grams to an entire day's diet reduces hunger after meals and reduces calories consumed during subsequent meals.[155, 156] Other controlled studies have reported that calorie burning by the body increases slightly when 10 grams of cayenne is added to a meal or 28 grams is added to an entire day's diet[157, 158, 159] However, no studies have been done to see if regularly adding cayenne to the diet has any effect on weight loss.

Green tea (page 686)

Green tea extract rich in polyphenols (epigallocatechin gallate, or EGCG) may support a weight-loss program by increasing energy expenditure or by inhibiting the digestion of fat in the intestine.[160, 161] Healthy young men who took two green tea capsules (containing a total of 50 mg of caffeine and 90 mg of EGCG) three times a day had a significantly greater energy expenditure and fat oxidation than those who took caffeine alone or a placebo.[162] In a preliminary study of moderately obese individuals, administration of a specific green tea extract (AR25) resulted in a 4.6% reduction in average body weight after 12 weeks.[163] The amount of green tea extract used in this study supplied daily 270 mg of EGCG and 150 mg of caffeine. While caffeine is known to stimulate metabolism, it appears that other substances besides caffeine were responsible for at least part of the weight loss. Although the extract produced few side effects, one individual had abnormal liver function tests during the study. In another study, consuming approximately 12 ounces of oolong tea (a semifermented version of green tea) daily for 12 weeks reduced waist circumference and the amount of body fat in a group of normal-weight to overweight men.[164] Additional studies are needed to confirm the safety and effectiveness of green tea extracts for promoting weight loss.

Yohimbine (page 764)

The ability of yohimbine, a chemical found in yohimbe bark, to stimulate the nervous system,[165, 166] and to promote the release of fat from fat cells,[167, 168] has led to claims that it might help weight loss by raising metabolic rate, reducing appetite, or increase fat burning. Although a preliminary trial found yohimbine ineffective for weight loss, a double-blind study found that women taking 5 mg of yohimbine four times per day along with a weight-loss diet lost significantly more weight than those taking a placebo with the same diet after three weeks.[169] However, a similar study using 18 mg per day of yohimbine for eight weeks reported no benefit to weight loss compared with a placebo.[170] A double-blind study of men who were not dieting reported no effect of up to 43 mg per day of yohimbine on weight or body composition after six months.[171] All of these studies used pure yohimbine; no study has tested the effects of yohimbe herb on weight loss.

Bitter orange (page 635)

Although historically used to stimulate appetite, bitter orange is frequently found in modern weight-loss formulas because synephrine is similar to the compound ephedrine, which is known to promote weight loss. In one study of 23 overweight adults, participants taking a daily intake of bitter orange (975 mg) combined with caffeine (525 mg) and St. John's wort (*Hypericum perforatum*, 900 mg) for six weeks lost significantly more body weight and fat than the control group.[172] No adverse effects on heart rate or blood pressure were found. Bitter orange standardized to contain 4% to 6% synephrine had an anti-obesity effect in rats. However, the amount used to achieve this effect was accompanied by cardiovascular toxicity and mortality.[173]

Coleus (page 660)

Although no clinical trials have been done, there are modern references to use of the herb coleus for weight loss.[174] Coleus extracts standardized to 18% forskolin are available, and 50 to 100 mg can be taken two to three times per day. Fluid extract can be taken in the amount of 2 to 4 ml three times per day.

Guaraná (page 687)

The herb guaraná contains caffeine and the closely related alkaloids theobromine and theophylline; these compounds may curb appetite and increase weight loss. Caffeine's effects are well known and include central nervous system stimulation, increased metabolic rate, and a mild diuretic effect.[175] In a double-blind trial, 200 mg per day of caffeine was, however, no more effective than a placebo in promoting weight loss.[176] Because of concerns about potential adverse effects, many doctors do not advocate using caffeine or caffeine-like substances to reduce weight.

Guggul (page 688)

Coupled with exercise in a double-blind trial, a combination of guggul, phosphate salts, hydroxycitrate, and **tyrosine** (page 465) has been shown to improve mood with a slight tendency to improve weight loss in overweight adults.[177] Daily recommendations for guggul are typically based on the amount of guggulsterones in the extract. A common intake of guggulsterones is 25 mg three times per day. Most guggul extracts contain 5% to 10% guggulsterones and can be taken daily for 12 to 24 weeks.

Are there any side effects or interactions?
Refer to the individual herb for information about any side effects or interactions.

WILSON'S DISEASE

Wilson's disease is a genetic disorder that results in excessive accumulation of **copper** (page 499) in many parts of the body, particularly the liver.

This condition is readily treatable, but if Wilson's disease is left untreated, it can be fatal.

Rating	Nutritional Supplements	Herbs
CHECKLIST FOR WILSON'S DISEASE		
★★★	Zinc (page 614)	

What are the symptoms of Wilson's disease?

Wilson's disease is initially silent and may first be noticed as fatigue, absent menstrual periods in premenopausal women, or repeated and unexplained spontaneous abortions. In more advanced stages, there may be headaches, tremors, uncoordinated limb movements, unsteady gait, drooling, difficulty swallowing, and joint pain. There also may also be strange thought patterns with unusual behaviors.

Medical treatments

Over the counter **zinc** (page 614) supplements are sometimes used, but not in combination with the prescription medications used to treat Wilson's disease, due to interactions.

The prescription drug trientine (Syprine) is commonly used to remove excess copper. Oral penicillamine (Depen), given with vitamin B_6 to avoid depletion of the vitamin, is also used.

Healthcare providers also recommend a low copper diet.

Dietary changes that may be helpful

Most foods contain at least some copper, so it is not possible to avoid the metal completely. Foods high in copper, such as organ meats and oysters, should be eliminated from the diet. Some foods are relatively high in copper but are quite nutritious (e.g., nuts and legumes)—these foods should be eaten in moderation by people with Wilson's disease. Grains contain significant amounts of copper but are important components of a healthful diet, and dietary restriction may be neither wise nor necessary, particularly if zinc is supplemented.

Nutritional supplements that may be helpful

Zinc (page 614) is known for its ability to reduce copper absorption and has been used successfully in patients with Wilson's disease,[1] with some trials lasting for years.[2, 3] Researchers have called zinc a "remarkably effective and nontoxic therapy for Wilson's disease."[4] The U.S. Food and Drug Administration has approved the use of zinc to treat Wilson's disease for maintenance therapy following drug therapy, although some scientists recommend that it be considered for initial therapy as well.[5]

Zinc has also been used to keep normal **copper** (page 499) levels from rising in people with Wilson's disease who had previously been treated successfully with prescription drugs.[6] Zinc (50 mg taken three times per day) has been used for such maintenance therapy,[7] though some researchers have used the same amount of zinc to successfully treat people with Wilson's disease who had not received drug therapy.[8]

Zinc is so effective in lessening the body's burden of copper that a copper deficiency was reported in someone with Wilson's disease who took too much (480 mg per day) zinc.[9] Nonetheless, zinc may not help everyone with Wilson's disease. Sometimes increased copper levels can occur in the liver after zinc supplementation;[10] however, leading researchers believe this increase is temporary and may not be not harmful.[11]

Zinc supplementation (25 mg or 50 mg three times daily) has also been used to successfully treat pregnant women with Wilson's disease.[12] Management of Wilson's disease with zinc should only be undertaken with the close supervision of a doctor.

Copper (page 499) is present in several dietary supplements, especially multimineral and **multivitamin-mineral** (page 559) preparations. Supplements containing even small amounts of copper should be avoided by virtually all Wilson's disease patients.

Are there any side effects or interactions?

Refer to the individual supplement for information about any side effects or interactions.

YEAST INFECTION

See also: Chronic Candidiasis (page 109)

What do I need to know?

Self-care for yeast infection can be approached in a number of ways—but it can be hard to know just where to start. To make it easier, our doctors recommend trying these simple steps first:

Ask your doctor about problem medicines
  Find out whether you can avoid taking antibiotics, oral contraceptives, or adrenal corticosteroids (such as prednisone) that may lead to yeast infection

Switch to cotton underwear
  Avoid the increased risks of yeast infection associated with nylon underwear and tights

Try beneficial bacteria
  To prevent the overgrowth of yeast organisms, eat yogurt containing live acidophilus cultures daily, and use acidophilus topically as vaginal suppositories or a douche

About yeast infection

Yeast infections usually result from an overgrowth of a species of fungus called *Candida albicans*. They can occur on the skin, under nails or mucous membranes of the mouth, vagina, bronchi, and lungs.

Vaginal yeast infections are one of the most common reasons that women consult healthcare professionals.

	CHECKLIST FOR YEAST INFECTION	
Rating	**Nutritional Supplements**	**Herbs**
★★★	*Lactobacillus acidophilus* (page 575)	
★★☆	**Boric acid** (page 476)	
★☆☆		**Cinnamon** (page 659)
		Echinacea (page 669)
		Oregano (page 719)
		Tea tree oil (page 751)

What are the symptoms of yeast infection?

Yeast infections are a type of **vaginitis** (page 438). The hallmark symptom of a yeast infection is itching of the external and internal genitalia, which is often associated with a white discharge that can be thick and/or curdy (like cottage cheese). Severe infections lead to inflammation of the tissue and subsequent redness, swelling, and even pinpoint bleeding.

Medical treatments

Over the counter drugs available to treat yeast infection caused by candida include clotrimazole (Gyne-Lotrimin, Mycelex), miconazole (Monistat), and butoconazole (Femstat).

Prescription drugs include oral fluconazole (Diflucan), nystatin (Mycostatin) vaginal tablets, terconazole (Terazol) vaginal cream, and butoconazole (Gynazole) vaginal cream. The antifungal creams may also be applied topically to the vulva (external genitalia) to help relieve itching.

Dietary changes that may be helpful

Some doctors believe that a well-balanced diet low in fats, sugars, and refined foods is important for preventing vaginal infections caused by Candida. In one preliminary trial, avoidance of sugar, dairy products, and artificial sweeteners resulted in a sharp reduction in the incidence and severity of Candida vaginitis.[1] Many doctors advise women who have a yeast infection (or are predisposed to such infections), to limit their intake of sugar, fruit juices, and refined carbohydrates. For persistent or recurrent infections, some doctors recommend that fruit also be avoided.

Another trial found that dramatic increases in intake of several sugars in healthy people partially increased stool sample levels of Candida, but only in 12 out of 28 people.[2]

Lifestyle changes that may be helpful

According to one study, yeast infections are three times more common in women who wear nylon underwear or tights, than in those who wear cotton underwear.[3] Additional predisposing factors for Candida infection include the use of antibiotics, oral contraceptives, or adrenal corticosteroids (such as prednisone).

Underlying health conditions that may predispose someone to Candida overgrowth include **pregnancy** (page 363), **diabetes** (page 152), and **HIV** (page 239) infection. **Allergies** (page 14) have also been reported to promote the development of recurrent yeast vaginitis. In a preliminary trial, when the allergens were

avoided and the allergies treated, the chronic recurrent yeast infections frequently resolved.[4] In most cases, sexual transmission does not play a role in yeast infection. However, in persistent cases, sexual transmission should be considered, and the sexual partner should be examined and treated.

Nutritional supplements that may be helpful

Lactobacillus acidophilus (page 575) is a species of friendly bacteria that is an integral part of normal vaginal flora. Lactobacilli help to maintain the vaginal ecosystem by preventing the overgrowth of unfriendly bacteria and Candida. Lactobacilli produce lactic acid, which acts like a natural antibiotic.

Lactobacillus acidophilus can be taken orally in the form of acidophilus yogurt, or in capsules or powder. It can also be administered vaginally. In a controlled trial, women who consumed 8 ounces of *Lactobacillus acidophilus*-containing yogurt per day had a threefold decrease in the incidence of vaginal yeast infections and a reduction in the frequency of Candida colonization in the vagina.[5] In another trial, women who were predisposed to vaginal Candida infection because they were **HIV** (page 239)-positive received either *Lactobacillus acidophilus* vaginal suppositories, the antifungal drug, clotrimazole (e.g., Gyne-Lotrimin), or placebo weekly for 21 months.[6] Compared to those receiving placebo, women receiving *Lactobacillus acidophilus* suppositories had only half the risk of experiencing an episode of Candida vaginitis—a result almost as good as that achieved with clotrimazole.

Many women find relief using an acidophilus-containing yogurt douche daily for a few days or weeks, depending on the severity of the infection.[7] Three capsules of acidophilus or one-quarter teaspoon of powder can be taken orally one to three times daily. Acidophilus can also be taken preventively during antibiotic use to reduce the risk of Candida vaginitis.[8, 9]

Boric acid (page 476) capsules inserted in the vagina have been used successfully as a treatment for vaginal yeast infections. One study demonstrated that 85% of women who used boric acid vaginal suppositories were cured of chronic recurring yeast vaginitis.[10] These women had all previously failed to respond to treatment with conventional antifungal medicines. The suppositories, which contained 600 mg of boric acid, were inserted vaginally twice a day for two weeks, then continued for an additional two weeks if necessary. Boric acid should never be swallowed.

Are there any side effects or interactions?
Refer to the individual supplement for information about any side effects or interactions.

Herbs that may be helpful

A small, preliminary trial found that a mouthwash with diluted **tea tree oil** (page 751) was effective in decreasing the growth of *Candida albicans* and in improving symptoms in **AIDS** (page 239) patients with oral Candida infections (thrush) that had not responded to drug therapy.[11] People in the study took 15 ml of the oral solution (dilution of tea tree oil was not given) four times per day and were instructed to swish it in their mouth for 30 to 60 seconds and then spit it out. For use of tea tree oil as a mouthwash, one should not exceed a 5% dilution and should be extremely careful not to swallow the solution.

Many doctors recommend that people with recurrent yeast infections take measures to support their **immune system** (page 255). **Echinacea** (page 669), which has the capacity to enhance immune function, is often used by people who suffer from recurrent **infections** (page 265). In one study, women who took echinacea experienced a 43% decline in the recurrence rate of yeast infections.[12]

The essential oil of **cinnamon** (page 659) contains various chemicals that are believed to be responsible for cinnamon's medicinal effects. Important among these compounds are eugenol and cinnamaldehyde. Cinnamaldehyde and cinnamon oil vapors exhibit extremely potent antifungal properties in test tubes.[13] In a preliminary study in people with **AIDS** (page 239), topical application of cinnamon oil was effective against oral thrush.[14]

A test tube study demonstrated that oil of **oregano** (page 719), and an extract in the oil called carvacrol in particular, inhibited the growth of *Candida albicans* far more effectively than a commonly employed antifungal agent called calcium magnesium caprylate.[15] However, clinical studies are needed to confirm these actions in humans.

Are there any side effects or interactions?
Refer to the individual herb for information about any side effects or interactions.

YELLOW NAIL SYNDROME

Yellow nail syndrome is believed to be caused by congenital abnormalities in the lymphatic system.

Although it primarily affects the nails and lymphatic tissue, it frequently is associated with lung disease.

CHECKLIST FOR YELLOW NAIL SYNDROME		
Rating	Nutritional Supplements	Herbs
★★☆	Vitamin E (page 609)	

What are the symptoms of yellow nail syndrome?

People with yellow nail syndrome may have symptoms including thickened, curved, slow-growing, yellow-to-greenish nails; and swelling of the lymph system in various parts of the body. Additional symptoms relating to the lungs may also occur.

Medical treatments

Prescription drug therapy might include oral antibiotics to control infection in the airway, such as amoxicillin/clavulanate (Augmentin), cephalexin (Keflex), clarithromycin (Biaxin), and azithromycin (Zithromax). Bronchodilators, such as albuterol (Proventil, Ventolin), salmeterol (Serevent), and ipratropium bromide (Atrovent), may be used to open airways.

Treatment may include physical therapy, such as postural drainage, clapping, and vibration. Healthcare practitioners typically recommend avoiding cigarette smoke and other respiratory irritants, cough suppressants, and sleeping pills.

Nutritional supplements that may be helpful

Supplementation with **vitamin E** (page 609) has been used successfully with people who have yellow nail syndrome in several preliminary reports.[1, 2, 3] Although topical use of the vitamin has also been reported to be effective,[4] taking vitamin E supplements is much easier and less messy. A typical amount is 800 IU per day, with results beginning to appear after several months.

Are there any side effects or interactions?
Refer to the individual supplement for information about any side effects or interactions.

PART TWO

Nutritional Supplements

5-HYDROXYTRYPTOPHAN

What is it?

5-HTP is used by the human body to make serotonin, an important substance for normal nerve and brain function. Serotonin appears to play significant roles in sleep, emotional moods, pain control, inflammation, intestinal peristalsis, and other body functions.[1]

Where is it found?

5-HTP is not present in significant amounts in a typical diet. The human body manufactures 5-HTP from L-tryptophan, a natural **amino acid** (page 465) found in most dietary proteins. However, eating food that contains L-tryptophan does not significantly increase 5-HTP levels. Supplemental 5-HTP is naturally derived from the seeds of *Griffonia simplicifolia,* a West African medicinal plant.

5-HTP has been used in connection with the following conditions (refer to the individual health concern for complete information):

Rating	Health Concerns
★★☆	**Depression** (page 145) **Fibromyalgia** (page 191) **Insomnia** (page 270) **Migraine headaches** (page 316) Sleep terrors **Tension headache** (page 428) **Weight loss and obesity** (page 446)
★☆☆	**Bipolar disorder/manic depression** (page 61) **Eating disorders** (page 174) **Parkinson's disease** (page 345) (with Sinemet) **Seasonal affective disorder** (page 397)

Who is likely to be deficient?

Disruptions in emotional well-being, including **depression** (page 145) and **anxiety** (page 30), have been linked to serotonin imbalances in the brain.[2] People with **fibromyalgia** (page 191) often have low serotonin levels in their blood.[3, 4, 5] Supplements of 5-HTP may increase serotonin synthesis in these cases. The cause of **migraine headaches** (page 316) is related to abnormal serotonin function in blood vessels,[6] and 5-HTP may help correct this abnormality. **Insomnia** (page 270) has been associated with tryptophan deficiency in the tissues of the brain;[7] therefore, 5-HTP may provide a remedy for this condition.

How much is usually taken?

In a controlled trial, 5-HTP (300 mg per day) was shown to be effective in reducing many symptoms of **fibromyalgia** (page 191), including **pain** (page 338), morning stiffness, sleep disturbances, and **anxiety** (page 30).[8]

For **depression** (page 145), 300 mg per day is often effective, though much of the research used 5-HTP in combination with drugs or was uncontrolled.[9, 10, 11] For **insomnia** (page 270), a single 100-mg nighttime dose of 5-HTP was sufficient to improve the duration and depth of sleep in one placebo-controlled trial.[12] For **migraine headaches** (page 316), amounts ranging from 400–600 mg per day have been shown to be effective at reducing the frequency and severity of attacks in most clinical trials.[13, 14, 15, 16, 17] For **tension headaches** (page 428), 100 mg of 5-HTP taken three times per day led to a significant decrease in consumption of pain-relievers, but no significant change in headache duration or intensity.[18]

Appetite reduction and **weight loss** (page 446) (averaging 11 pounds in 12 weeks) has occurred with amounts of 600–900 mg daily.[19, 20] In another clinical trial, 750 mg per day has been shown to be effective at decreasing carbohydrate and fat intake, and promoting weight loss.[21]

Are there any side effects or interactions?
During the clinical trials described above, some people taking large amounts of 5-HTP experienced gastrointestinal upset (e.g. nausea) or, less often, headache, sleepiness, muscle pain, or **anxiety** (page 30).

A substance known as "Peak X" has been found in low concentrations in several over-the-counter 5-HTP preparations. Some researchers think this substance may be linked[22, 23, 24] to toxicity previously reported[25, 26, 27] in a 1989 L-tryptophan contamination incident. However, there is serious question about whether Peak X is actually the toxic agent and it may be unrelated to the problems previously associated with L-tryptophan.[28, 29, 30, 31, 32, 33, 34, 35] Although two articles reported possible associations between 5-HTP consumption and toxicity symptoms similar to those attributed to contaminated L-tryprophan,[36, 37] evidence linking 5-HTP or Peak X with any toxicity symptoms remains speculative. Although the structure of Peak X has recently been identified, there is no firm evidence that this substance has caused or contributed to any toxicity or disease.[38]

Very high intakes of 5-HTP have caused muscle jerks in guinea pigs[39] and both muscle jerks[40] and diarrhea in mice.[41] Injected 5-HTP has also caused kidney damage in rats.[42] To date, these problems have not been reported in humans. "Serotonin syndrome," a serious but uncommon condition caused by excessive amounts of serotonin, has not been reported to result from supplementation with 5-HTP; in theory it could be triggered by the supplement.[43] However, the level of intake at which this toxic effect might potentially occur remains unknown.

5-HTP should not be taken with antidepressants, weight-control drugs, other serotonin-modifying agents, or substances known to cause liver damage, because in these cases 5-HTP may have excessive effects. People with liver disease may not be able to regulate 5-HTP adequately and those suffering from autoimmune diseases such as scleroderma may be more sensitive than others, to 5-HTP.[44] These people should not take 5-HTP without consulting a knowledgeable healthcare professional. The safety of taking 5-HTP during **pregnancy** (page 363) and breast-feeding is not known at this time.

7-KETO

What is it?
7-KETO (3-acetyl-7-oxo-dehydroepiandrosterone) is a naturally occurring metabolite (breakdown product) of the hormone dehydroepiandrosterone (**DHEA** [page 503]).[1] DHEA is the most abundant of the adrenal steroid hormones and serves as a precursor for sex hormones, such as estrogen and testosterone.

7-KETO was developed by researchers who were looking for biologically active metabolites of DHEA that could not be converted to the potentially cancer-causing sex steroids (e.g., estrogen and testosterone).

Tests in animals and test tubes were performed in the areas of immune modulation, memory enhancement, and thermogenesis (the process the body uses to convert stored calories into energy). In all cases, the effects of 7-KETO were stronger than those produced by DHEA.[2, 3, 4, 5]

The capacity of 7-KETO to promote **weight loss** (page 446) in overweight people been investigated in a double-blind study.[6] Participants in the study were advised to exercise three times per week for 45 minutes and to eat an 1,800-calorie per day diet. Each person was given either a placebo or 100 mg of 7-KETO twice daily. After eight weeks, those receiving 7-KETO had lost an average of 6.34 pounds, compared with 2.13 pounds in the placebo group (a statistically significant difference). In addition, the percentage of body fat decreased by 1.8% in the 7-KETO group, compared with only 0.57% in the placebo group. The increased weight loss in the 7-KETO group was associated with a significant increase in levels of T3 (a thyroid hormone that plays a major role in determining a person's metabolic rate), although the levels of T3 did not exceed the normal range.

Where is it found?
7-KETO is available as a dietary supplement.

7-KETO has been used in connection with the following conditions (refer to the individual health concern for complete information):

Rating	Health Concerns
★★☆	**Weight loss** (page 446)

Who is likely to be deficient?

Since the level of 7-KETO is directly related to the level of **DHEA** (page 503) in the body,[7] people with lower DHEA levels likely have low 7-KETO levels as well. Low DHEA levels are primarily associated with aging.

How much is usually taken?

The manufacturer of 7-KETO recommends 100 mg twice daily for **weight loss** (page 446).

Are there any side effects or interactions?

A safety study in humans has shown that 7-KETO did not raise estrogen or testosterone levels or produce any other negative effects at levels up to 200 mg per day for eight weeks.[8] Short-term animal studies also revealed no adverse effects with large amounts of 7-KETO.[9, 10, 11] However, the long-term safety of 7-KETO for humans has not been demonstrated, and, because it is chemically related to steroid hormones, the potential for adverse effects must be considered. In addition, the increase in T3 levels resulting from taking 7-KETO could, in theory, produce adverse effects on the heart or promote bone loss. For these reasons, people wishing to take 7-KETO, particularly those who have a thyroid disorder or are taking thyroid hormone, should consult a physician.

ACETYL-L-CARNITINE

What is it?

Acetyl-L-carnitine is similar in form to the amino acid **L-carnitine** (page 543) and also has some similar functions, such as being involved in the metabolism of food into energy. The acetyl group that is part of acetyl-L-carnitine contributes to the production of the neurotransmitter acetylcholine, which is required for mental function.

Where is it found?

Acetyl-L-carnitine is a molecule that occurs naturally in the brain, liver, and kidney. It is also available as a dietary supplement.

Acetyl-L-carnitine has been used in connection with the following conditions (refer to the individual health concern for complete information):

Rating	Health Concerns
★★★	Age-related cognitive decline (page 8)
★★☆	Alzheimer's disease (page 19) Cerebellar ataxia, degenerative Depression (page 145) (for elderly people) Type 1 diabetes Type 2 diabetes (page 152) Down's syndrome (page 169)
★☆☆	Amenorrhea (page 22) Male infertility (page 305) Peripheral neuropathy

Who is likely to be deficient?

Acetyl-L-carnitine levels may decrease with advancing age. However, because it is not an essential nutrient, true deficiencies do not occur.

How much is usually taken?

Most research involving acetyl-L-carnitine has used 500 mg three times per day, though some research has used double this amount.[1]

Are there any side effects or interactions?

Side effects from taking acetyl-L-carnitine are uncommon, although skin rash, increased appetite, nausea, vomiting, agitation, and body odor have been reported in people taking acetyl-L-carnitine.[2, 3]

ADENOSINE MONOPHOSPHATE

What is it?

Adenosine monophosphate (AMP) is an intermediary substance formed during the body's process of creating energy in the form of adenosine triphosphate (ATP) from food.

AMP may play a role in limiting postherpetic neuralgia, which is the pain that sometimes lingers after a bout of **shingles** (page 401) (herpes zoster). One double-blind study involving 32 adults with shingles found that injections of AMP given three times per week for a month following a flare-up of shingles relieved the pain more quickly than placebo.[1] Whether oral supplementation would have the same effect remains unclear. AMP also helps heal the lesions and prevents recurrence of pain or lesions.

Nineteen out of twenty-one people with porphyria cutanea tarda (a disease that develops in adulthood and causes **photosensitivity** (page 356), among other

Adenosine Monophosphate

symptoms) responded well to 160-200 mg of AMP per day taken for at least one month, according to one group of researchers.[2] Partial and even complete alleviation of photosensitivity associated with this condition occurred in several people.

A closely related molecule to AMP, adenosine, affects electrical signaling in the heart. Intravenous adenosine has been used successfully to treat children with tachycardia, a condition in which the heart beats too quickly.[3] Intravenous adenosine has also been reported to help most elderly people with tachycardia.[4]

Adenosine is formed by heart muscle when the oxygen supply is low,[5] and it improves the efficiency of the heart.[6] Adenosine has also been reported to improve the heart's ability to use blood sugar for energy during stress.[7]

Where is it found?

The body creates AMP within cells during normal metabolic processes. AMP is also found as a supplement, although it is not widely available.

Adenosine monophosphate (AMP) has been used in connection with the following conditions (refer to the individual health concern for complete information):

Rating	Health Concerns
★☆☆	**Photosensitivity** (page 356) **Shingles** (page 401)

Who is likely to be deficient?

Preliminary research suggests that people with herpes simplex or herpes zoster (**shingles** [page 401]) infections may have low levels of AMP; however, the clinical significance of this finding is unclear.[8]

How much is usually taken?

The trials using AMP for **photosensitivity** (page 356) have used 160–200 mg of AMP per day; however, the ideal intake of this supplement has not been determined. Research with **shingles** (page 401) has used a special gel form of AMP injected into muscle; a doctor should be consulted for this form of AMP.

Are there any side effects or interactions?

The limited number of human studies involving oral AMP have not indicated any side effects. However, some researchers have expressed concern that supple-

mental intake of AMP could, in theory, increase levels of adenosine, a substance related to AMP that may interfere with **immune function** (page 255).[9] Doctors using AMP injections report that too-rapid intravenous administration or inadvertent administration of an intramuscular injection into a vein could cause life-threatening arrhythmias of the heart.[10]

ADRENAL EXTRACT

What is it?

Adrenal extracts are derived from the adrenal glands of bovine (beef) sources. Commercially available adrenal extracts are made using the whole gland (whole or total adrenal extracts) or just the cortex or outer portion of the gland (adrenal cortex extracts). The adrenal glands are a pair of small glands that lie just above the kidneys.

The possible benefits of adrenal extract are thought to be the result of a combination of supplying small amounts of adrenal hormones and promoting improved adrenal function. The adrenal medulla secretes the hormones epinephrine (adrenaline) and norepinephrine (noradrenaline), while the adrenal cortex secretes an entirely different group of hormones called corticosteroids. Although all corticosteroids have similar chemical formulas, they differ in function. The three major types of corticosteroids are mineralocorticoids (e.g., aldosterone), glucocorticoids (cortisol or cortisone), and 17-ketosteroids (e.g., dehydroepiandrosterone [**DHEA** (page 503)]).

Adrenal extracts have been used in modern medicine since 1931, primarily in the injectable form along with **vitamin B$_6$** (page 600), **vitamin B$_{12}$** (page 601), or **vitamin C** (page 604). Although there is little in the area of scientific documentation for oral administration, a series of animal studies demonstrated that oral administration of adrenal extract to mice, rats, and dogs who had their adrenal glands removed produced the same activity as injectable adrenal extract.[1, 2, 3]

Whole adrenal extracts (usually in combination with essential nutrients required for proper adrenal function) are most often used in cases of low adrenal function presenting as fatigue, inability to cope with stress, and reduced resistance to infection. Because extracts made from the adrenal cortex contain small amounts of corticosteroids, they are typically used as "natural" cortisone in cases of **allergy** (page 14) and inflammation (**asthma** [page 32], **eczema** [page 177], **psoriasis** [page 379], **rheumatoid arthritis** [page 387], etc.). The effectiveness of adrenal extracts in these applications is unknown at this time. People taking prescribed corticosteroids should never substitute these drugs with an adrenal extract and should consult their physician before adding an adrenal extract to their steroid treatment.

In a preliminary study done in the 1930s, 8 women suffering from nausea and vomiting during the first trimester of **pregnancy** (page 363) received large amounts of oral adrenal cortex extract. In most cases, vomiting stopped after 3 to 4 days.[4] In a follow-up study, 202 women with nausea and vomiting due to pregnancy received adrenal cortex extract, usually by injection at first, followed by oral administration. More than 85% of the women were completely relieved of the problem or showed definite improvement.[5]

Where is it found?
Adrenal extracts are available in capsules or tablets. Adrenal extracts prepared for injection were commonly used at one time, but currently are unavailable.

Adrenal extract has been used in connection with the following conditions (refer to the individual health concern for complete information):

Rating	Health Concerns
★☆☆	Fatigue **Morning sickness** (page 320)

Who is likely to be deficient?
As adrenal extract is not an essential nutrient, no nutritional deficiency state exists. However, some people sub-optimal adrenal function or frank adrenal insufficiency. The diagnosis of adrenal problems should be made by a physician.

How much is usually taken?
The amount of adrenal extract taken will depend upon the quality and potency of the product. Follow the recommendations given on the product label or those given by your healthcare provider.

Are there any side effects or interactions?
Stomach irritation and/or nausea is a common side effect, especially with higher potency products. Other possible side effects include a general stimulatory effect that may manifest as **anxiety** (page 30), irritability, and/or **insomnia** (page 270). Since no safety data exist for use during **pregnancy** (page 363) or breast-feeding, adrenal extract should not be used in these situations unless supervised by a doctor.

Consumption of excessive amounts may produce signs and symptoms of corticosteroid excess similar to those experienced with the drug prednisone. However, serious side effects are not likely to result from taking a large amount of an adrenal extract for a short period of time or from excessive intake on a single occasion, but rather from long-term use of high amounts. With prednisone (a synthetic cortisone-like drug) at lower doses (less than 10 mg per day), the most notable side effects are usually increased appetite, weight gain, retention of salt and water, and increased susceptibility to **infection** (page 265).

ALANINE

What is it?
Alanine is a nonessential **amino acid** (page 465) used by the body to build proteins.

Alanine is present in prostate fluid, and it may play a role in supporting prostate health. One study, involving 45 men with benign prostatic hyperplasia (**BPH** [page 58]), found that 780 mg of alanine per day for two weeks and then 390 mg for the next two and a half months, taken in combination with equal amounts of the amino acids **glycine** (page 532) and **glutamic acid** (page 529), reduced symptoms of BPH;[1] this work has been independently confirmed.[2]

Where is it found?
As with the other **amino acids** (page 465), excellent sources of alanine include meat and poultry, fish, eggs, and dairy products. Some protein-rich plant foods also supply alanine.

Alanine has been used in connection with the following condition (refer to the individual health concern for complete information):

Rating	Health Concerns
★★☆	**Benign prostatic hyperplasia** (page 58) (in combination with glycine and glutamic acid)

Alanine

Who is likely to be deficient?
Since alanine is synthesized in the body and is also provided by most foods that are sources of protein, deficiencies are unlikely to occur.[3]

How much is usually taken?
Most people do not need to supplement with alanine; for those who do use this **amino acid** (page 465) as a supplement, appropriate amounts should be determined with the consultation of a physician.

Are there any side effects or interactions?
Alanine is free of side effects for the vast majority of people who take it; however, people with kidney or liver disease should not consume high intakes of **amino acids** (page 465) without consulting a healthcare professional.

ALPHA LIPOIC ACID

What is it?
Alpha lipoic acid (ALA) is a vitamin-like **antioxidant** (page 467), sometimes referred to as the "universal antioxidant" because it is soluble in both fat and water.[1] ALA is manufactured in the body and is found in some foods, particularly liver and yeast.

ALA is capable of regenerating several other antioxidants back to their active states, including **vitamin C** (page 604),[2] **vitamin E** (page 609),[3] **glutathione** (page 531),[4] and **coenzyme Q$_{10}$** (page 496).[5]

ALA has several potential benefits for people with diabetes. It enhances glucose uptake in type 2 (adult onset or non-insulin-dependent) **diabetes** (page 152), inhibits glycosylation (the abnormal attachment of sugar to protein), and has been used to improve diabetic nerve damage and reduce pain associated with that nerve damage.[6] Most studies have used intravenous alpha lipoic acid, but oral supplementation has nonetheless proved partially helpful in treating at least one form of diabetic neuropathy, using 800 mg per day.[7]

Preliminary evidence indicates that 150 mg of alpha lipoic acid, taken daily for one month, improves visual function in people with **glaucoma** (page 205).[8]

ALA has been shown to inhibit the replication of the **HIV** (page 239) virus in the test tube; however, it is not known whether supplementing with ALA would benefit HIV-infected people.[9]

Intravenous administration of ALA has significantly increased the survival rate of people who have eaten poisonous mushrooms.[10] Such a treatment should be prescribed by a doctor and should not be attempted on one's own.

Where is it found?
The body makes small amounts of alpha lipoic acid. There is only limited knowledge about the food sources of this nutrient. However, foods that contain mitochondria (a specialized component of cells), such as red meats, are believed to provide the most alpha lipoic acid. Supplements are also available.

Alpha lipoic acid has been used in connection with the following conditions (refer to the individual health concern for complete information):

Rating	Health Concerns
★★★	**Diabetes** (page 152)
★☆☆	**Glaucoma** (page 205)
	Hepatitis (page 220)

Who is likely to be deficient?
Although alpha lipoic acid was thought to be a vitamin when it was first discovered, subsequent research determined that it is created in the human body—and thus is not an essential nutrient. For this reason, deficiencies of alpha lipoic acid are not known to occur in humans.

How much is usually taken?
The amount of alpha lipoic acid used in research to improve diabetic neuropathies is 800 mg per day and 150 mg per day for **glaucoma** (page 205). However, much lower amounts, such as 20–50 mg per day, are recommended by some doctors for general **antioxidant** (page 467) protection, although there is no clear evidence that such general use has any benefit.

Are there any side effects or interactions?
Side effects with alpha lipoic acid are rare but can include skin rash and the potential of **hypoglycemia** (page 251) in diabetic patients. People who may be deficient in **vitamin B$_1$** (page 597) (such as alcoholics) should take vitamin B$_1$ along with alpha lipoic acid supplements. Chronic administration of alpha lipoic acid in animals has interfered with the actions of the vi-

tamin, **biotin** (page 473). Whether this has significance for humans remains unknown.[11]

AMINO ACIDS OVERVIEW

What are they?

Amino acids are the building blocks of protein. Twenty amino acids are needed to build the various proteins used in the growth, repair, and maintenance of body tissues. Eleven of these amino acids can be made by the body itself, while the other nine (called essential amino acids) must come from the diet. The essential amino acids are **isoleucine** (page 479), **leucine** (page 479), **lysine** (page 550), **methionine** (page 557), **phenylalanine** (page 568), threonine, tryptophan, and **valine** (page 479). Another amino acid, **histidine** (page 534), is considered semi-essential because the body does not always require dietary sources of it. The nonessential amino acids are **arginine** (page 467), **alanine** (page 463), asparagine, aspartic acid, **cysteine** (page 502), **glutamine** (page 530), **glutamic acid** (page 529), **glycine** (page 532), proline, serine, and **tyrosine** (page 544). Other amino acids, such as carnitine, are used by the body in ways other than protein-building and are often used therapeutically.

The classification of an amino acid as essential or nonessential does not reflect its importance, because all 20 amino acids are necessary for health. Instead, this classification system simply reflects whether or not the body is capable of manufacturing a particular amino acid.

Where are they found?

Foods of animal origin, such as meat and poultry, fish, eggs, and dairy products, are the richest dietary sources of the essential amino acids. Plant sources of protein are often deficient in one or more essential amino acids. However, these deficiencies can be overcome by consuming a wide variety of plant foods. For example, grains are low in **lysine** (page 550), whereas beans provide an excess of lysine. It was previously believed that, in order for vegetarians to obtain adequate amounts of protein, all of the essential amino acids had to be "balanced" at each meal. For example, a grain and a bean had to be consumed at the same meal. However, more recent research has indicated that, while consuming a proper mix of amino acids is important, it is not necessary to consume them all at the same meal.[1]

Amino acids have been used in connection with the following conditions (refer to the individual health concern for complete information)**:**

Rating	Health Concerns
★★★	**Angina** (page 27) (**carnitine** [page 543]) **Bronchitis** (page 80) (**N-acetyl cysteine** [page 562]) **Chronic obstructive pulmonary disease** (page 114) (**N-acetyl cysteine** [page 562]) **Cold sores** (page 119) (**lysine** [page 550]) **Congestive heart failure** (page 134) (**propionyl-L-carnitine** [page 543], **taurine** [page 590])
★★☆	**Alzheimer's disease** (page 19) (**acetyl-L-carnitine** [page 461]) **Angina** (page 27) (**arginine** [page 467]) **Athletic performance** (page 43) (**creatine** [page 501]) **Benign prostatic hyperplasia** (page 58) (**alanine** [page 463], **glutamic acid** [page 529], **glycine** [page 532]) **Chronic fatigue syndrome** (page 111) (**carnitine** [page 543]) **Congestive heart failure** (page 134) (**arginine** [page 467]) **Depression** (page 145) (**5-HTP** [page 459], **DLPA** [page 568], **L-phenylalanine** [page 568], **tyrosine** [page 544]) **Diabetes** (page 152) (**carnitine** [page 543]) **Fibromyalgia** (page 191) (**5-HTP** [page 459]) **High triglycerides** (page 235) (**carnitine** [page 543]) **HIV support** (page 239) (**N-acetyl cysteine** [page 562]) **Infertility (male)** (page 305) (**arginine** [page 467], **carnitine** [page 543]) **Insomnia** (page 270) (**5-HTP** [page 459]) **Intermittent claudication** (page 276) (**carnitine** [page 543]) **Liver support** (**taurine** [page 590]) **Migraine headaches** (page 316) (**5-HTP** [page 459]) **Pain** (page 338) (**DPA** [page 568]) **Phenylketonuria** (page 354) (**tyrosine** [page 544]) **Vitiligo** (page 443) (**L-phenylalanine** [page 568]) **Weight loss and obesity** (page 446) (**5-HTP** [page 459])

Amino Acids Overview

Amino Acids Overview

Rating	Health Concerns
★☆☆	**Alcohol withdrawal** (page 12) (**DLPA** [page 568], **glutamine** [page 530], **tyrosine** [page 544])
	Athletic performance (page 43) (**arginine** [page 467]/**ornithine** [page 565], **carnitine** [page 543])
	Diabetes (page 152) (**taurine** [page 590])
	Epilepsy (page 183) (**taurine** [page 590])
	High blood pressure (page 246) (**arginine** [page 467], **taurine** [page 590])
	HIV support (page 239) (**glutamine** [page 530], **methionine** [page 557])
	Liver support (**methionine** [page 557])
	Osteoarthritis (page 328) (**DPA** [page 568])
	Peptic ulcer (page 349) (**glutamine** [page 530])
	Rheumatoid arthritis (page 387) (**DPA** [page 568])

Who is likely to be deficient?

The vast majority of Americans eat more than enough protein and also more than enough of each essential amino acid for normal purposes. Dieters, some strict vegetarian body builders, and anyone consuming an inadequate number of calories may not be consuming adequate amounts of amino acids. In these cases, the body will break down the protein in muscle tissue and use those amino acids to meet the needs of more important organs or will simply not build more muscle mass despite increasing exercise.

How much is usually taken?

Nutrition experts recommend that protein, as a source of amino acids, should account for 10–12% of the calories in a balanced diet. However, requirements for protein are affected by age, weight, state of health, and other factors. On average, a normal adult requires approximately 0.36 grams of protein per pound of body weight. Using this formula, a 140-pound person would need 50 grams (or less than 2 ounces) of protein per day. An appropriate range of protein intake for healthy adults may be as low as 45–65 grams daily. Some athletes have higher amino acid requirements.[2] Most American adults eat about 100 grams of protein per day, or about twice what their bodies need and at least as much as any athlete requires.

Supplements of individual amino acids are recommended by doctors for specific purposes, such as **lysine** (page 550) for **herpes** (page 200) or **phenylalanine** (page 568) for **pain** (page 238).

Are there any side effects or interactions?

Most diets provide more protein than the body needs, causing excess nitrogen to be excreted as urea in urine. The excess nitrogen has been linked in some studies with reduced kidney function in old age. Most, but not all studies have found that when people have impaired kidney function, restricting dietary intake of protein slows the rate of decline of kidney function.[3]

Excessive protein intake also can increase excretion of **calcium** (page 483), and some evidence has linked high-protein diets with **osteoporosis** (page 333),[4] particularly regarding animal protein.[5] On the other hand, some protein is needed for bone formation. A double-blind study showed that elderly people whose diets provided slightly less than the recommended amount of protein suffered less bone loss if they consumed an additional 20 grams of protein per day.[6] A doctor can help people assess their protein intake.

AMYLASE INHIBITORS

What are they?

Amylase inhibitors are also known as starch blockers because they contain substances that prevent dietary starches from being absorbed by the body. Starches are complex carbohydrates that cannot be absorbed unless they are first broken down by the digestive enzyme amylase and other, secondary, enzymes.[1, 2] They are claimed to be useful for **weight loss** (page 446), but when they were first developed years ago, research did not find them very effective for limiting carbohydrate absorption.[3, 4, 5, 6] Later, however, highly concentrated versions of amylase inhibitors did show potential for reducing carbohydrate absorption in humans.[7, 8, 9]

Purified starch blocker extracts, when given with a starchy meal, have also been shown to reduce the subsequent rise in blood sugar levels of both healthy people and **diabetics** (page 152).[10, 11, 12, 13] This effect could be helpful in the treatment of blood sugar disorders.

Where are they found?

Amylase inhibitors can be extracted from several types of plants, especially those in the legume family. Currently available Amylase inhibitors are extracted from either white kidney bean or wheat.

Amylase inhibitors have been used in connection with the following conditions (refer to the individual health concern for complete information):

Rating	Health Concerns
★☆☆	Diabetes (page 152)
	Weight loss and obesity (page 446)

Who is likely to be deficient?

Amylase inhibitors are not essential nutrients and are not normally produced in the body, so no deficiency is possible.

How much is usually taken?

Depending on the potency of the amylase inhibitors, typical intake is 1,500 to 6,000 mg before meals.

Are there any side effects or interactions?

High amounts of amylase inhibitors may cause **diarrhea** (page 163) due to the effects of undigested starch in the colon.[14, 15] Diabetics taking medications to lower their blood sugar should not take amylase inhibitors without first consulting a doctor.

ANTIOXIDANTS AND FREE RADICALS

Free radicals are highly reactive compounds that are created in the body during normal metabolic functions or introduced from the environment. Free radicals are inherently unstable, since they contain "extra" energy. To reduce their energy load, free radicals react with certain chemicals in the body, and in the process, interfere with the cells' ability to function normally. Antioxidants work in several ways: they may reduce the energy of the free radical, stop the free radical from forming in the first place, or interrupt an oxidizing chain reaction to minimize the damage caused by free radicals.

Free radicals are believed to play a role in more than sixty different health conditions, including the aging process, **cancer** (page 87), and **atherosclerosis** (page 38).[1] Reducing exposure to free radicals and increasing intake of antioxidant nutrients has the potential to reduce the risk of free radical-related health problems.

Oxygen, although essential to life, is the source of the potentially damaging free radicals. Free radicals are also found in the environment. Environmental sources of free radicals include exposure to ionizing radiation (from industry, sun exposure, cosmic rays, and medical X-rays), ozone and nitrous oxide (primarily from automobile exhaust), heavy metals (such as mercury, cadmium, and lead), cigarette smoke (both active and passive), alcohol, unsaturated fat, and other chemicals and compounds from food, water, and air.

The body produces several antioxidant enzymes, including superoxide dismutase (SOD), catalase, and glutathione peroxidase, that neutralize many types of free radicals. Supplements of these enzymes are available for oral administration. However, their absorption is probably minimal at best. Supplementing with the "building blocks" the body requires to make SOD, catalase, and glutathione peroxidase may be more effective. These building block nutrients include the minerals **manganese** (page 553), **zinc** (page 614), and **copper** (page 499) for SOD and **selenium** (page 584) for glutathione peroxidase.

In addition to enzymes, many vitamins and minerals act as antioxidants in their own right, such as **vitamin C** (page 604), **vitamin E** (page 609), **beta-carotene** (page 469), **lutein** (page 548), **lycopene** (page 548), **vitamin B₂** (page 598), **coenzyme Q₁₀** (page 496), and **cysteine** (page 502) (an amino acid). Herbs, such as **bilberry** (page 634), **turmeric** (page 753) (curcumin), grape seed or pine bark extracts, and **ginkgo** (page 681) can also provide powerful antioxidant protection for the body.

Consuming a wide variety of antioxidant enzymes, vitamins, minerals, and herbs may be the best way to provide the body with the most complete protection against free radical damage.

ARGININE

What is it?

The **amino acid** (page 465) arginine has several roles in the body, such as assisting in **wound healing** (page 319), helping remove excess ammonia from the body, stimulating **immune function** (page 255), and promoting secretion of several hormones, including glucagon, insulin, and growth hormone.

The effect of arginine on growth hormone levels[1] has interested body builders. In a controlled trial, when arginine and **ornithine** (page 565) (500 mg of each, twice per day, five times per week) were combined with weight training, a greater decrease in body fat was obtained after only five weeks than when the same exercise was combined with a placebo.[2] In another study, however, 5 grams of arginine powder, taken orally 30 minutes prior to exercise, failed to affect growth hormone release and may have even impaired the release of growth hormone in younger adults.[3]

Arginine is also needed to increase protein synthesis, which can in turn increase cellular replication. Therefore, arginine may help people with inadequate numbers of certain cells. For example, some,[4] though not all,[5] studies have found that men with low sperm counts experienced an increase in the number of sperm when they supplemented with arginine.

Arginine's effect on increasing protein synthesis improves **wound healing** (page 319). This effect has been shown in both animals[6] and people (at 17 grams per day).[7]

Arginine is also a precursor to nitric oxide, which the body uses to keep blood vessels dilated, allowing the heart to receive adequate oxygen. Researchers have begun to use arginine in people with **angina** (page 27) and **congestive heart failure** (page 134).

Nitric oxide metabolism is also altered in people with interstitial cystitis, a condition of the bladder. Preliminary research found that supplementation with 1.5 grams of arginine per day for six months led to a significant decrease in most symptoms, including pain,[8] though short-term supplementation (five weeks) has not been effective, even at higher intakes (3-10 grams per day).[9] In 1999, a double-blind study using 1.5 grams of arginine for three months in a group of women with interstitial cystitis, reported considerable improvement compared with the effect of a placebo in a variety of indices. Perhaps due to the small size of the study, some of these changes did not quite reach statistical significance.[10]

Preliminary evidence suggests that arginine may help regulate **cholesterol levels** (page 223).[11] Arginine also appears to act as a natural blood thinner by reducing platelet aggregation.[12]

Where is it found?

Dairy, meat and poultry, and fish are good sources of arginine. Nuts and chocolate also contain significant amounts of this **amino acid** (page 465).

Arginine has been used in connection with the following conditions (refer to the individual health concern for complete information):

Rating	Health Concerns
★★☆	**Angina** (page 27)
	Congestive heart failure (page 134)
	Erectile dysfunction (page 185)
	HIV support (page 239) (in combination with **glutamine** [page 530] and **HMB** [page 534])
	Infertility (male) (page 305)
	Intermittent claudication (page 276) (I.V. only)
	Interstitial cystitis
	Pre- and post-surgery health (page 357)
	Sickle cell anemia (page 403) (for pulmonary hypertension)
★☆☆	**Athletic performance** (page 43) (for body composition and strength)
	Female infertility (page 187) (for in vitro fertilization)
	Gastritis (page 195)
	High blood pressure (page 246)
	Wound healing (page 357)

Who is likely to be deficient?

Normally, the body makes enough arginine, even when it is lacking in the diet. However, during times of unusual stress (including **infection** [page 265], **burns** [page 85], and **injury** [page 319]), the body may not be able to keep up with increased requirements.

How much is usually taken?

Most people do not need to take extra arginine. While some people with serious **infections** (page 265), **burns** (page 85), or other trauma should take arginine, appropriate amounts must be determined by a doctor. Levels used in research vary considerably (2–30 grams per day). Most research on **cardiovascular disease** (page 98) has used between 6 and 20 grams per day. Optimal intakes remain unknown and are likely to vary depending upon the individual.

Are there any side effects or interactions?

Arginine has so far appeared to be free of obvious side effects. However, longer-term studies are needed to confirm its safety.

There have been two case reports of severe allergic reactions following intravenous administration of L-arginine;[13] however, allergic reactions have not been reported after oral administration.

People with kidney or liver disease should consult their doctor before supplementing with arginine. Some doctors believe that people with herpes (either **cold sores** [page 119] or **genital herpes** [page 200]) should not take arginine supplements, because of the possibility that arginine might stimulate replication of the virus.

Administration of large amounts of arginine to animals has been found both to promote[14] and to interfere with **cancer** (page 87) growth.[15] In preliminary research, high intake (30 grams per day) of arginine has increased cancer cell growth in humans.[16] On the other hand, in people with cancer, arginine has been found to stimulate the **immune system** (page 255).[17] At this time it remains unclear whether arginine is dangerous or helpful for people with cancer.

Arginine works with **ornithine** (page 565) in the synthesis of growth hormone.

BETA-CAROTENE

What is it?
Beta-carotene is a substance from plants that the body converts into **vitamin A** (page 595). It also acts as an **antioxidant** (page 467) and an **immune system** (page 255) booster.

Other members of the antioxidant carotenoid family include cryptoxanthin, alpha-carotene, zeaxanthin, **lutein** (page 548), and **lycopene** (page 548). However, unlike beta-carotene, most of these nutrients are not converted to vitamin A in significant amounts.

Where is it found?
Dark green and orange-yellow vegetables are good sources of beta-carotene. It is also available in supplements.

Beta-carotene has been used in connection with the following conditions (refer to the individual health concern for complete information):

Rating	Health Concerns
★★★	**Leukoplakia** (page 289) **Lung cancer** (page 298) (**Warning:** Beta-carotene *increases* the risk of lung cancer in smokers.) **Night blindness** (page 326) **Photosensitivity** (page 356)
★★☆	**Immune function** (page 255) **Pancreatic insufficiency** (page 341)
★☆☆	**Alcohol withdrawal support** (page 12) **Asthma** (page 32) **Cataracts** (page 101) **Gastritis** (page 195) **Heart attack** (page 212) **HIV support** (page 239) **Macular degeneration** (page 303) **Sickle cell anemia** (page 403)

Who is likely to be deficient?
People who limit their consumption of beta-carotene-containing vegetables could be at higher risk of developing a **vitamin A** (page 595) deficiency. However, because beta-carotene is not an essential nutrient, true deficiencies do not occur. Nevertheless, very old persons with type 2 **diabetes** (page 152) have shown a significant age-related decline in blood levels of carotenoids, irrespective of their dietary intake.[1]

Which form is best?
Most beta-carotene in supplements is synthetic, consisting of only one molecule called all trans beta-carotene. Natural beta-carotene, found in food, is made of two molecules—all trans beta-carotene and 9-cis beta-carotene.

Researchers originally saw no meaningful difference between natural and synthetic beta-carotene. This view was questioned when the link between beta-carotene-containing foods (all natural) and **lung cancer** (page 298) prevention[2] was not duplicated in studies using synthetic pills.[3] In smokers, synthetic beta-carotene has apparently caused an increased risk of lung cancer[4, 5, 6] and disease of the blood vessels[7] in double-blind research. Animal research has begun to identify the ways in which synthetic beta-carotene might cause damage to lungs, particularly when animals are exposed to cigarette smoke.[8]

Much of natural beta-carotene is in the all trans molecule form—the same as synthetic beta-carotene. Moreover, much of the 9-cis molecule found only in natural beta-carotene is converted to the synthetic molecule before it reaches the bloodstream.[9] Also, absorption of 9-cis beta-carotene appears to be poor,[10] though some researchers question this finding.[11]

Despite the overlap between natural and synthetic forms, natural beta-carotene may possibly have activity that is distinct from the synthetic form. For example, studies in both animals[12] and humans[13] have shown that the natural form has **antioxidant** (page 467) activity that the synthetic form lacks. Also, in one trial, precancerous changes in people reverted to normal tissue with natural beta-carotene supplements, but not with synthetic supplements.[14] Israeli researchers have investigated whether the special antioxidant effects of natural beta-carotene might help people suffering from **asthma** (page 32) attacks triggered by exercise.[15] People with asthma triggered by exercise were given 64 mg per day of natural beta-carotene for one week. In that report, 20 of 38 patients receiving natural beta-carotene were protected against exercise-induced asthma. However, because synthetic beta-carotene was not tested, the difference between the activity of the two supplements cannot be deduced from this report.

Increasingly, doctors are recommending that people supplement only with natural beta-carotene. However, no studies have explored whether the adverse effect of synthetic beta-carotene in cigarette smokers would also occur with *natural* beta-carotene supplementation. Until more is known, smokers should avoid all beta-carotene supplements and others should avoid synthetic beta-carotene.

In supplements, the natural form can be identified by the phrases "from *D. salina,*" "from an algal source," "from a palm source," or as "natural beta-carotene" on the label. The synthetic form is identified as "beta-carotene."

How much is usually taken?

The most common beta-carotene supplement intake is probably 25,000 IU (15 mg) per day, though some people take as much as 100,000 IU (60 mg) per day. Whether the average person would benefit from supplementation with beta-carotene remains unclear.

Are there any side effects or interactions?

Beta-carotene supplementation, even in very large amounts, is not known to cause any serious side effects,[16, 17] however, excessive intake (more than 100,000 IU, or 60 mg per day) sometimes gives the skin a yellow-orange hue. People taking beta-carotene for long periods of time should also supplement with **vitamin E** (page 609), as beta-carotene may reduce vitamin E levels.[18] Beta carotene supplementation may also decrease blood levels of **lutein** (page 548), another carotenoid.[19]

Warning: Synthetic beta-carotene has now been linked to increased risk of **lung cancer** (page 298) in smokers. Until more is known, smokers should avoid all beta-carotene supplements.

Preliminary studies in animals indicate that beta-carotene supplementation, when combined with heavy **alcohol** (page 12) consumption, may enhance liver toxicity.[20] Until more is known, alcoholics and persons who consume alcohol on a daily basis should avoid supplementing with beta-carotene.

One study showed a slightly increased risk of vascular surgery among people with **intermittent claudication** (page 276) who took beta-carotene supplements.[21] Until more is known, persons wishing to use beta-carotene supplements should first consult with their doctor.

BETA-GLUCAN

What is it?

Beta-glucan is a fiber-type complex sugar (polysaccharide) derived from the cell wall of baker's yeast, **oat** (page 716) and barley fiber, and many medicinal mushrooms, such as **maitake** (page 707). In their natural states, yeast and mushrooms contain a mixture of beta-1,3-glucan and beta-1,6-glucan. Oats and barley contain a mixture of beta-1,3-glucan and beta-1,4-glucan. In addition to purified beta-1,3-glucan from these sources, you may see products listed as beta-1,3/1,6-glucan in the case of yeast-derived products and as beta-1,3/1,4-glucan when derived from oats. Similar (if not identical) properties have been shown for beta-glucan-rich extracts and purified beta-glucan derived from oats, baker's yeast, and mushrooms.

The two primary uses of beta-glucan are to enhance the **immune system** (page 255) and to lower blood **cholesterol** (page 223) levels. Numerous experimental studies in test tubes and animals have shown beta-glucan to activate white blood cells.[1, 2, 3, 4, 5] In fact, there have been hundreds of research papers on beta-glucan since the 1960s.[6] The research indicates that beta-1,3-glucan, in particular, is very effective at activating white blood cells known as macrophages and neutrophils. These cells provide one of the immune system's first lines of defense against foreign invaders. A beta-glucan-activated macrophage or neutrophil can recognize and kill tumor cells, remove cellular debris resulting from oxidative damage, speed up recovery of damaged tissue, and further activate other components of the immune system.[7, 8] Although the research in test tube and animal studies is promising, many questions remain about the effectiveness of beta-glucan as an oral supplement to enhance immune function in humans.

Beta-glucan is the key factor for the cholesterol-lowering effect of oat bran.[9, 10, 11, 12, 13] As with other soluble-fiber components, the binding of cholesterol (and bile acids) by beta-glucan and the resulting elimination of these molecules in the feces is very helpful for reducing blood cholesterol.[14, 15, 16] Results from a number of double-blind trials with either oat- or yeast-derived beta-glucan indicate typical reductions, after at least four weeks of use, of approximately 10% for total cholesterol and 8% for LDL ("bad") cholesterol, with elevations in HDL ("good") cholesterol ranging from zero to 16%.[17, 18, 19, 20, 21]

Like other sources of soluble **fiber** (page 512), beta-glucan is, according to preliminary studies, helpful in reducing the elevation in blood sugar levels that typically follow a meal.[22, 23, 24, 25] Beta-glucan produces this effect by delaying gastric emptying so that dietary sugar is absorbed more gradually, as well as by possibly increasing the tissue sensitivity to insulin. These effects suggest possible benefit in blood sugar control in people with **diabetes** (page 152).

Where is it found?
Beta-glucan is found in the cell walls of many yeast and cereal fibers, such as **oats** (page 716), wheat, and barley. As a dietary supplement, beta-glucan is available in liquid form as well as in capsules and tablets.

Beta-glucan has been used in connection with the following conditions (refer to the individual health concern for complete information):

Rating	Health Concerns
★★★	**High cholesterol** (page 223)
★☆☆	**Immune enhancement** (page 255)

Who is likely to be deficient?
Because beta-glucan is not an essential nutrient, deficiencies do not occur.

How much is usually taken?
For lowering **cholesterol** (page 223) levels, the amount of beta-glucan used in clinical trials has ranged from 2,900 to 15,000 mg per day. For enhancing **immune function** (page 255), an effective amount has not yet been determined due to the lack of studies in this application. However, manufacturers of beta-glucan products usually recommend between 50 and 1,000 mg daily (to be taken on an empty stomach), although some products contain as much as 500 mg per capsule.

Are there any side effects or interactions?
No side effects have been reported.

BETA-SITOSTEROL

What is it?
Beta-sitosterol is one of a group of organic compounds found in plants that, alone and in combination with similar plant sterols, reduces blood levels of **cholesterol** (page 223).[1, 2, 3]

The reduction of cholesterol levels appears to be because beta-sitosterol blocks absorption of cholesterol.[4] It has also been effective in reducing symptoms of **benign prostatic hyperplasia** (page 58).[5] Although molecules quite similar to beta-sitosterol inhibit **cancer** (page 87) cells in test tubes, the relevance of this information for people remains unknown.[6]

Where is it found?
Beta-sitosterol is one of several plant sterols (cholesterol is the main animal sterol) found in almost all plants. High levels are found in rice bran, wheat germ, corn oil, and soybeans. Peanuts and its products, such as peanut oil, peanut butter, and peanut flour, are good sources of plant sterols, particularly beta-sitosterol.[7]

Beta-sitosterol has been used in connection with the following conditions (refer to the individual health concern for complete information):

Rating	Health Concerns
★★★	**Benign prostatic hyperplasia** (page 58)
★★☆	**High cholesterol** (page 223)
★☆☆	**Athletic performance** (page 43) (in combination with beta-sitosterol glucoside for reducing the risk of post-exercise infection)

Who is likely to be deficient?
Because beta-sitosterol is not an essential nutrient, deficiencies do not occur.

How much is usually taken?
Between 500 mg and 10 grams of beta-sitosterol per day have been used in clinical research to reduce elevated blood **cholesterol** (page 223) levels. Between 60 (20 mg three times per day) and 130 mg per day have been used in trials reporting a reduction in **prostatic hyperplasia** (page 377)-related symptoms.[8, 9]

Beta-Sitosterol

Are there any side effects or interactions?

Ingesting plant sterols interferes with **beta-carotene** (page 469) and **vitamin E** (page 609) absorption, resulting in lower blood levels of these nutrients.[10]

BETAINE (TRIMETHYLGLYCINE)

What is it?

Betaine (trimethylglycine) functions very closely with **choline** (page 546), **folic acid** (page 520), **vitamin B₁₂** (page 598), and a form of the amino acid **methionine** (page 557) known as S-adenosylmethionine (**SAMe** [page 583]).[1, 2] All of these compounds function as "methyl donors." They carry and donate methyl molecules to facilitate necessary chemical processes. The donation of methyl groups by betaine is very important to proper liver function, cellular replication, and detoxification reactions. Betaine also plays a role in the manufacture of **carnitine** (page 543) and serves to protect the kidneys from damage.[3] Betaine is closely related to choline. The difference is that choline (tetramethylglycine) has four methyl groups attached to it. When choline donates one of these groups to another molecule, it becomes betaine (trimethylglycine). If betaine donates one of its methyl groups, then it becomes dimethylglycine.

Betaine has been reported to play a role in reducing blood levels of **homocysteine** (page 234), a toxic breakdown product of amino-acid metabolism that is believed to promote **atherosclerosis** (page 38) and **osteoporosis** (page 333). While the main nutrients involved in controlling homocysteine levels are folic acid, **vitamin B₆** (page 600), and **vitamin B₁₂** (page 601), betaine has been reported to be helpful in some people whose elevated homocysteine levels did not improve with these other nutrients. Betaine has also been shown to be helpful in certain rare genetic disorders involving **cysteine** (page 502) metabolism.[4, 5, 6, 7, 8] However, in normal situations or with supplementation of the other methyl donors, betaine is not likely to produce any lowering effect on homocysteine levels.[9, 10] Its primary use as a nutritional supplement is in supporting proper liver function.

Betaine is often referred to as a "lipotropic factor" because of its ability to help the liver process fats (lipids). In animal studies, betaine supplementation has been shown to protect against chemical damage to the liver.[11, 12, 13, 14] The first stage of liver damage that results

from drinking **alcohol** (page 12) is the accumulation of fat in the liver (alcohol-induced fatty liver disease). Betaine, because of its lipotropic effects, has been shown to produce significant improvements in this condition in several human clinical studies.[15, 16] Betaine has been studied in clinical trials conducted in Germany, Italy, and France in the treatment of **alcohol-related liver disease** (page 290).[17, 18, 19, 20, 21, 22, 23, 24] Some success was noted in these studies, but the popularity of betaine for alcohol-related liver disease has been supplanted by **SAMe** (page 583) and **milk thistle** (page 710) extract. However, it has recently been suggested that betaine may be a more cost-effective method as a first-step therapy for alcohol-induced fatty liver disease.[25]

Betaine is also showing promise as a toothpaste ingredient, as it has been shown to produce significant relief of dry mouth.[26]

Where is it found?

Dietary sources of betaine include fish, beets, and legumes. Betaine is most widely available as **betaine hydrochloride** (page 473) (betaine-HCl), but that form is used primarily as a source of hydrochloric acid for people with **hypochlorhydria** (page 260) (low stomach acid). The forms used specifically to provide betaine are betaine citrate and betaine aspartate. These forms have also been used to improve liver function.

Betaine has been used in connection with the following conditions (refer to the individual health concern for complete information):

Rating	Health Concerns
★★☆	Alcohol-induced fatty liver **Hepatitis** (page 220) (nonalcoholic steatohepatitis) **Homocysteine (high)** (page 234)
★☆☆	**Atherosclerosis** (page 38)

Who is likely to be deficient?

Betaine is not an essential nutrient, and thus no deficiency state exists.

How much is usually taken?

For people with alcohol-induced fatty liver, the recommended amount for betaine citrate or betaine aspartate supplementation is 1,000 to 2,000 mg three times daily. Lower amounts are often used as nutritional support for general liver health, although use of betaine in this manner has not undergone clinical research.

Are there any side effects or interactions?

No side effects with betaine at recommended levels have been noted.

BETAINE HYDROCHLORIDE

What is it?

Betaine hydrochloride is an acidic form of betaine, a vitamin-like substance found in grains and other foods. Betaine hydrochloride is recommended by some doctors as a supplemental source of hydrochloric acid for people who have a deficiency of stomach acid production (hypochlorhydria).

A deficiency of gastric acid secretion increases the likelihood and severity of certain bacterial and parasitic intestinal infections. A normal stomach's level of gastric acid is sufficient to destroy bacteria.[1] In one study, most fasting people who had normal acidity in the stomach had virtually no bacteria in the small intestine. Some bacterial colonization of the stomach occurred in people who had low levels of hydrochloric acid.[2]

Where is it found?

Gastric acid is produced by the parietal cells of the stomach. The acidity is quite strong in a normal stomach. In fact, the stomach can be between 100,000 and almost 1,000,000 times more acidic than water.

Betaine hydrochloride (HCl) has been used in connection with the following conditions (refer to the individual health concern for complete information):

Rating	Health Concerns
★☆☆	**Acne Rosacea** (page 4)
	Asthma (page 32)
	Chronic candidiasis (page 109)
	Dermatitis herpetiformis (page 151)
	Food allergies (page 14)
	Gallstones (page 193)
	Gastroesophageal reflux disease (page 198) (GERD)
	Hives (page 245)
	Indigestion (page 260)
	Iron-deficiency anemia (page 278) (as an adjunct to supplemental iron)
	Rheumatoid arthritis (page 387)
	Tic douloureux
	Vitiligo (page 445)

Who is likely to be deficient?

Some research suggests that people with a wide variety of chronic disorders, such as **allergies** (page 14),[3] **asthma** (page 32),[4] and **gallstones** (page 193),[5] do not produce adequate amounts of stomach acid.

How much is usually taken?

Betaine HCl is the most common hydrochloric acid-containing supplement. Normally it comes in tablets or capsules measured in grains or milligrams. Only people who have reduced levels of stomach acid ("hypochlorhydria") should take betaine HCl; this condition can be diagnosed by a doctor. When appropriate, some doctors recommend taking one or more tablets or capsules, each 5–10 grains (325–650 mg), with a meal that contains protein. Occasionally, **betaine (trimethylglycine)** (page 472) is recommended to reduce blood levels of a substance called **homocysteine** (page 234), which is associated with **heart disease** (page 98). This form of betaine is different from betaine HCl.

Are there any side effects or interactions?

Large amounts of betaine HCl can burn the lining of the stomach. If a burning sensation is experienced, betaine HCl should be immediately discontinued. People should not take more than 10 grains (650 mg) of betaine HCl without the recommendation of a physician. All people with a history of **peptic ulcers** (page 349), **gastritis** (page 195), or gastrointestinal symptoms—particularly **heartburn** (page 260)—should see a doctor before taking betaine HCl. People taking nonsteroidal anti-inflammatory drugs (NSAIDs), cortisone-like drugs, or other medications that might cause a peptic ulcer should not take betaine HCl. Betaine HCl helps make some minerals and other nutrients more absorbable.[6, 7]

BIOTIN

What is it?

Biotin, a water-soluble B vitamin, acts as a coenzyme in the metabolism of protein, fats, and carbohydrates.

Where is it found?

Good dietary sources of biotin include organ meats, oatmeal, egg yolk, **soy** (page 587), mushrooms, bananas, peanuts, and **brewer's yeast** (page 480). Bacteria in the intestine also produce significant amounts of biotin, but evidence is conflicting as to whether biotin produced by intestinal bacteria is present at a location or is in a form that permits significant absorption by the body.[1]

Biotin has been used in connection with the following conditions (refer to the individual health concern for complete information):

Rating	Health Concerns
★★☆	**Brittle nails** (page 79) **Diabetes** (page 152) **Pregnancy** (page 363)
★☆☆	**Seborrheic dermatitis** (page 400) (cradle cap)

Who is likely to be deficient?

Certain rare inborn diseases can leave people with depletion of biotin due to the inability to metabolize the vitamin normally. A dietary deficiency of biotin, however, is quite uncommon, even in those consuming a diet low in this B vitamin. Nonetheless, if someone eats large quantities of raw egg whites, a biotin deficiency can develop, because a protein in the raw egg white inhibits the absorption of biotin. Cooked eggs do not present this problem. Long-term antibiotic use can interfere with biotin production in the intestine and increase the risk of deficiency symptoms, such as **dermatitis** (page 151), **depression** (page 145), hair loss,[2] **anemia** (page 25), and nausea. Long-term use of anti-seizure medications may also lead to biotin deficiency.[3] **Alcoholics** (page 12), people with **inflammatory bowel disease** (page 269), and those with diseases of the stomach have been reported to show evidence of poor biotin status. However, the usefulness of biotin supplementation for these people remains unclear.[4] In animals, and possibly in humans, biotin deficiency can cause **birth defects** (page 63).[5] As biotin deficiency may occur in as many as 50% of pregnant women,[6] it seems reasonable to use a prenatal multiple vitamin and mineral formula that contains biotin.

How much is usually taken?

The ideal intake of biotin is unknown. However, the amount of biotin found in most diets, combined with intestinal production, appears to be adequate for preventing deficiency symptoms. Researchers have estimated that 30 mcg per day appears to be an adequate intake for adults.[7] Typically, consumption from a Western diet has been estimated to be 30–70 mcg per day. Larger amounts of biotin (8–16 mg per day) may be

supportive for people with **diabetes** (page 152) by lowering blood glucose levels and by preventing diabetic neuropathy.[8, 9] Biotin in the amount of 2.5 mg per day strengthened the fingernails of two-thirds of a group of people with **brittle nails** (page 79), according to one clinical trial.[10]

Are there any side effects or interactions?

Excess intake of biotin is excreted in the urine; no toxicity symptoms have been reported.

Biotin works with some other B vitamins, such as **folic acid** (page 520), **pantothenic acid** (page 568) (vitamin B_5), and **vitamin B_{12}** (page 601). However, no solid evidence indicates that people supplementing with biotin also need to take these other vitamins. Symptoms of pantothenic acid or **zinc** (page 614) deficiency have been reported to be lessened with biotin,[11] though people with these deficiencies should supplement with the nutrients in which they are deficient. Researchers have speculated that biotin and **alpha lipoic acid** (page 464) may compete with each other for absorption or uptake into cells; but little is known about the importance of these interactions in humans.[12]

There is one report of a 76-year-old woman who developed a life-threatening condition (eosinophilic pleuropericardial effusion) while taking 10 mg of biotin per day and 300 mg of pantothenic acid per day.[13] However, it is not clear whether the vitamins caused the problem.

BLUE-GREEN ALGAE

What is it?

Blue-green algae, of which spirulina is a well-known example, is a group of 1,500 species of microscopic aquatic plants. The two most common species used for human consumption are *Spirulina maxima* and *Spirulina platensis.* Spirulina is particularly rich in protein and also contains **carotenoids** (page 488), vitamins, minerals, and essential fatty acids.[1]

Spirulina's **vitamin B_{12}** (page 601) content does not appear to be readily usable by people.[2] Most health benefits to humans claimed for spirulina and other blue-green algae supplementation are supported by anecdotes rather than scientific research. Test tube and animal studies have demonstrated several properties of large amounts of spirulina or spirulina extracts, including **antioxidant** (page 467),[3] antiviral,[4, 5] **anticancer** (page 87),[6, 7, 8, 9] **anti-allergy** (page 14),[10, 11] **immune-enhancing** (page 255),[12, 13, 14] liver-protecting,[15, 16, 17] blood vessel-relaxing,[18] and blood lipid-lowering[19, 20] effects.

A small, controlled study found that **overweight** (page 446) people taking 8.4 grams per day of spirulina lost an average of three pounds in four weeks compared with one and a half pounds when taking placebo, though this difference was not statistically significant and no effects on **blood pressure** (page 246) or serum cholesterol were observed.[21] A later, controlled trial found a small **cholesterol-lowering** (page 223) effect when 4.2 grams of spirulina per day were taken for eight weeks, but serum triglycerides, blood pressure, and body weight were unchanged.[22]

Where is it found?
Blue-green algae grow in some lakes, particularly those rich in salts, in Central and South America, and Africa. They are also grown in outdoor tanks specifically to be harvested for nutritional supplements.

Blue-green algae have been used in connection with the following conditions (refer to the individual health concern for complete information):

Rating	Health Concerns
★☆☆	**Weight loss and obesity** (page 446)

Who is likely to be deficient?
As it is not an essential nutrient, blue-green algae is not associated with a deficiency state. However, people who do not consume several servings of vegetables per day could benefit from the **carotenoids** (page 488) and other nutrients in blue-green algae. Since it is a complete protein, it can be used in place of some of the protein in a healthy diet. However, very large amounts are required to provide significant quantities of these nutrients from blue-green algae.

How much is usually taken?
Blue-green algae can be taken as a powder or as flakes, capsules, or tablets. The typical manufacturer's recommended intake is 2,000–3,000 mg per day divided throughout the day. However, typical amounts shown to have helpful properties in animal studies would be equivalent to 34 grams per day or more, for a 150-pound human.

Are there any side effects or interactions?
Few side effects have been reported from the ingestion of blue-green algae. However, as blue-green algae can accumulate heavy metals from contaminated water, consuming blue-green algae could increase the body's load of lead, mercury, and cadmium,[23] though noncontaminated blue-green algae have been identified.[24] Another popular species of blue-green algae, *Aphanizomenon flos-aquae,* has been found to produce toxins.[25] A few reports also describe allergic reactions to blue-green algae. Animal studies have found spirulina to be safe during **pregnancy** (page 363).[26, 27, 28]

There is one case report of a man who developed liver damage while taking spirulina.[29] As he was also talking three prescription medications, it is not clear whether the spirulina caused or contributed to the liver injury.

BORAGE OIL

What is it?
Borage oil is derived from the seeds of the borage *(Borago officinalis)* plant, a large plant with blue, star-shaped flowers found throughout Europe and North Africa and naturalized to North America.[1]

Borage oil, **evening primrose oil** (page 511), and black currant seed oil contain gamma linolenic acid (GLA), a fatty acid that the body converts to a hormone-like substance called prostaglandin E_1 (PGE_1). PGE_1 has anti-inflammatory properties and may also act as a blood thinner and blood vessel dilator. Linoleic acid, a common fatty acid found in nuts and seeds and most vegetable oils (including borage oil), should theoretically convert to PGE_1. Many things can interfere with this conversion, however, including disease; the aging process; saturated fat; hydrogenated oils; blood sugar problems; and inadequate **vitamin C** (page 604), **magnesium** (page 551), **zinc** (page 614), and **B vitamins** (page 603). Supplements that provide GLA circumvent these conversion problems, leading to more predictable formation of PGE_1.[2]

Borage seed oil is the richest source of GLA, containing 20 to 26%. While GLA from evening primrose oil has been widely researched, scientific evidence supporting the use of borage oil has been limited. Nonetheless, one preliminary trial[3] and two double-blind trials[4, 5] have shown that borage oil, 1.1–2.8 grams per day for at least three months, reduces symptoms of rheumatoid arthritis.

Borage oil has also been used to treat people with atopic dermatitis (**eczema** [page 177]) in preliminary trials, with reductions in skin inflammation, dryness, scaliness, and itch, without side effects being reported.[6] However, a controlled study using 360 mg daily of GLA from borage oil in patients with atopic dermatitis (3 to 17 years of age) was unable to reproduce these results.[7] In another preliminary study, a group of children with infantile seborrheic dermatitis were treated with borage oil (0.5 ml) applied to the diaper region twice daily.[8] Within 10 to 12 days, all of the children were free from skin lesions, even in the areas not treated with borage. Moreover, using the oil topically two to three times a week kept the seborrhea in remission until the patients were six to seven months old. There were no relapses after the oil was discontinued.

Where is it found?

Borage oil is found primarily in supplements. Its presumed active ingredient, GLA, can also be found in black currant seed oil and **evening primrose oil** (page 511) supplements. However, it is not known whether the effects of these three oils in the body, are the same.

Borage oil has been used in connection with the following conditions (refer to the individual health concern for complete information):

Rating	Health Concerns
★★★	**Rheumatoid arthritis** (page 387)
★★☆	**Eczema** (page 177)
★☆☆	**Infantile seborrheic dermatitis** (page 400) (topical)

Who is likely to be deficient?

Many people in Western societies may be at least partially GLA-deficient as a result of aging, glucose intolerance, dietary fat intake, and other problems, though the exact incidence of deficiency remains unknown. People with deficiencies benefit from supplemental GLA intake from borage oil, black currant seed oil, or **evening primrose oil** (page 511).

Those with **premenstrual syndrome** (page 368),[9] **diabetes** (page 152),[10] scleroderma,[11] Sjogren's syndrome,[12] **tardive dyskinesia** (page 425),[13] **eczema** (page 177),[14] and other skin conditions[15] may have a metabolic block that interferes with the body's ability to make GLA. However, most clinical trials supplement-

ing GLA for these conditions has used evening primrose oil, and not borage oil.

How much is usually taken?

For the treatment of **rheumatoid arthritis** (page 387), the amounts of GLA from borage used in successful double-blind trials were 1.4–2.8 grams daily for at least two months.[16, 17] Although 360 mg of GLA daily from borage oil has been used to treat people with **eczema** (page 177), controlled research has not supported its use for this condition.[18] Topically, 0.5 ml of borage oil may be applied to areas of **seborrhea** (page 400) daily for two weeks, and then three times a week until the condition is stable.[19]

Are there any side effects or interactions?

Borage *seeds* contain small amounts of liver toxins called pyrrolizidine alkaloids (PA). However, testing has not demonstrated the presence of the alkaloid in the seed oil.[20] Most commercially available borage seed oil is, therefore, likely to be PA-free and presents no risk of PA toxicity. Minor side effects from borage oil use can include bloating, nausea, **indigestion** (page 260), and headache.[21]

BORIC ACID

What is it?

Boric acid is a chemical substance with mild antiseptic, antifungal, and antiviral properties.

Boric acid is commonly used in the form of suppositories inserted in the vagina to treat **yeast infection** (page 454). In one study of 100 women with chronic yeast **vaginitis** (page 438) that had failed to respond to treatment with over-the-counter or prescription antifungal medicines, 98% of the women successfully treated their **infections** (page 265) with boric acid capsules inserted into the vagina twice per day for two to four weeks.[1] Several commercial douching products contain boric acid.

The antiseptic activity of boric acid is also used in commercial "artificial tears" and eyewash products.

Boric acid also has antiviral activity. Topical application of diluted boric acid, in the form of sodium borate ointment, has been found to shorten the duration of **cold sores** (page 119) in a double-blind trial.[2] The duration of cold sores was approximately four days in the group receiving boric acid, compared with six days in the placebo group.

Where is it found?
Boric acid is a white, odorless powder or crystalline substance that is available in many over-the-counter pharmaceutical products for topical use, alone as a topical antiseptic, and in suppository form.

Boric acid has been used in connection with the following conditions (refer to the individual health concern for complete information):

Rating	Health Concerns
★★☆	Yeast infection (page 454)
★☆☆	Cold sores (page 119)

Who is likely to be deficient?
Boric acid is not taken internally and is not a nutrient; no deficiency exists.

How much is usually taken?
Boric acid is available in powder form from a pharmacy, without a prescription. This powder can be packed into an empty gelatin capsule and used as a suppository. For women with **vaginitis** (page 438), some doctors recommend that one such capsule, containing 600 mg of boric acid, be inserted into the vagina each night for two weeks. Some health food stores have suppositories that contain a combination of boric acid and herbs.

In the trial studying **cold sores** (page 119), an ointment diluted to 4% boric acid was applied four times per day. Because of the potential toxicity of such a preparation, people should consult their doctors before using boric acid.

Are there any side effects or interactions?
Boric acid suppositories should not be used during **pregnancy** (page 363). Boric acid is very toxic when taken internally and should also never be used on open **wounds** (page 319). When boric acid enters the body, it can cause nausea, vomiting, **diarrhea** (page 163), dermatitis, kidney damage, acute failure of the circulatory system, and even death. In the past, boric acid was used as a topical treatment for infants with diaper rash. However, even in diluted (3%) form it caused significant toxicity and two deaths.[3] Therefore, boric acid should not be applied to the skin of infants and small children. In fact, experts in the field have stated, "The

minor therapeutic value of this compound, in comparison with its potential as a poison, has led to the general recommendation that it no longer be used as a therapeutic agent."[4] However, in more recent research, no serious side effects were reported when boric acid was used as a treatment for **vaginitis** (page 438).

BORON

What is it?
Boron is a nonmetallic element present in the diet and in the human body in trace amounts. Whether boron is an essential nutrient for humans remains in debate.

Boron appears to affect the metabolism of **calcium** (page 483), **magnesium** (page 551), **copper** (page 499), phosphorus, and **vitamin D** (page 607). Preliminary research suggests that boron might affect bone and joint health, but little specific information is known. The most promising research with boron has linked supplementation to reduced loss of calcium in urine. This effect might lead to a lower risk of **osteoporosis** (page 333), but decreased loss of calcium from boron supplementation occurs mostly when people are not getting enough magnesium in their diets.[1]

Where is it found?
Raisins, prunes, and nuts are generally excellent sources of boron. Fruit (other than citrus), vegetables, and legumes also typically contain significant amounts. Actual amounts vary widely, depending upon boron levels in soil where the food is grown.

Boron has been used in connection with the following conditions (refer to the individual health concern for complete information):

Rating	Health Concerns
★☆☆	Osteoarthritis (page 328)
	Osteoporosis (page 333)
	Rheumatoid arthritis (page 387)

Who is likely to be deficient?
As boron is not yet considered an essential nutrient for humans, it is not clear whether deficiencies occur. However, diets that are low in fruit, vegetables, legumes, and nuts provide less boron than diets that contain more of these foods.

Boron

How much is usually taken?

A leading boron expert has suggested 1 mg per day of boron is a reasonable amount to consume.[2] People who eat adequate amounts of produce, nuts, and legumes are likely already eating two to six times this amount.[3] Therefore, whether the average person would benefit by supplementing with this mineral remains unclear.

Are there any side effects or interactions?

Accidental acute exposure to high levels of boron can cause nausea, vomiting, abdominal pain, rash, convulsions, and other symptoms.[4] Although chronic exposures can cause related problems, the small (usually 1–3 mg per day) amounts found in supplements have not been linked with toxicity in most reports. Nonetheless, in one double-blind trial using 2.5 mg of boron per day for two months, hot flashes and night sweats worsened in 21 of 43 women, though the same symptoms improved in 10 others.[5] Women whose have hot flashes or night sweats have been diagnosed as **menopausal** (page 311) symptoms and who supplement with boron should consider discontinuing use of boron-containing supplements to see if the severity of their symptoms is reduced.

One study found that 3 mg per day resulted in increased estrogen and testosterone levels.[6] Increased estrogen has also been reported in several women taking 2.5 mg per day.[7] The increase in estrogen is of concern because it could theoretically increase the risk of several **cancers** (page 87). Although no increased risk of cancer has been reported in areas of the world where boron intake is high, some doctors recommend that supplemental boron intake be limited to a maximum of 1 mg per day.

The relationship between boron and other minerals is complex and remains poorly understood. Boron may conserve the body's use of **calcium** (page 483), **magnesium** (page 551), and **vitamin D** (page 607). In one study, the ability of boron to reduce urinary loss of calcium disappeared when subjects were also given magnesium.[8] Therefore, boron may provide no special benefit in maintaining bone mass in the presence of adequate amounts of dietary magnesium.

BOVINE COLOSTRUM

What is it?

Bovine colostrum is the pre-milk liquid produced from the mammary glands of cows during the first 24 to 48 hours after giving birth.

Bovine colostrum is rich in immunoglobulins (antibodies), growth factors, various proteins, and enzymes. The question is whether these factors, which are meant for the calf, exert any effects in humans. Bovine colostrum may turn out to be an important nutritional supplement, but for now there are no conclusive data to support manufacturers' claims. Although various components of bovine colostrum theoretically may produce some benefits, there are no studies where bovine colostrum—in the forms that are commercially available—has been given to humans and shown benefits.

It has been claimed that bovine colostrum can help fight certain **infections** (page 265). However, the research studies used to support that claim used colostrum derived from cows immunized in a way that caused them to produce unusually large amounts of a specific antibody in their colostrum. For example, in a double-blind study, children with **diarrhea** (page 163) caused by a rotavirus were treated with immunoglobulins extracted from colostrum derived from cows immunized with rotavirus. Compared with the placebo, administration of the immunoglobulins significantly reduced the amount of diarrhea and the amount of oral rehydration solution required. In addition, the rotavirus was eliminated from the stool significantly more rapidly in the immunoglobulin group than in the placebo group (1.5 days vs. 2.9 days).[1]

In addition to a positive effect against acute rotavirus diarrhea,[2, 3] there is also evidence that specific forms of colostrum (derived from specially immunized cows or those with confirmed presence of specific antibodies) are effective against diarrhea caused by *Cryptosporidium parvum, Helicobacter pylori, Escherichia coli,* and *Clostridium difficile*.[4, 5, 6, 7, 8] However, it is not known whether commercially available colostrum provides significant amounts of the specific immunoglobulins that are active against these organisms. Furthermore, unless the immunoglobulins are present in high enough concentrations, the preparation is not likely to be effective. There is evidence that the majority of the antimicrobial effect of both bovine colostrum and one of its chief antibiotic components (lactoferrin) are destroyed by gastric secretions and by the digestive enzyme, trypsin.[9]

Bovine colostrum contains bovine versions of many human growth factors, including insulin-like growth factor, transforming growth factor, epithelial growth factor, and even growth hormone, that are capable of stimulating muscle growth. The concentration of bovine insulin-like growth factor I (ILGF-I) in colostrum ranges from 200 to 2,000 mcg/L, compared with less than 10 mcg/L in normal cow's milk.[10] Thus, in theory, bovine colostrum might be able to stimulate muscle growth in humans. However, although bovine ILGF-I has been shown to be identical to human ILGF-I in some analytical studies[11] and to be absorbed and transported into the circulation in calves,[12] the effects of bovine ILGF-I and other bovine growth substances in humans after oral administration, has not been determined in clinical trials.

In a preliminary study of male athletes, supplementation with 125 ml of colostrum per day for eight days produced a statistically significant increase in the serum concentration of insulin-like growth factor.[13] However, the magnitude of the increase was small, and the clinical significance of that change is not clear. Thus, claims that bovine colostrum can help burn fat and promote muscle growth by raising the level of ILGF-I or other molecules must be considered premature.

Bovine colostrum may be helpful in protecting against **peptic ulcer** (page 349) formation caused by nonsteroidal anti-inflammatory drugs (NSAIDs) such as aspirin, ibuprofen, and indomethacin. In a study in rats, pretreatment with 0.5 or 1.0 ml of a colostrum preparation reduced indomethacin-induced gastric injury by 30% and 60%, respectively.[14] Whether bovine colostrum exerts this effect in humans has not been determined.

Claims that bovine colostrum elevates mood, that "colostrum is a natural and healthy means of stimulating the brain to release serotonin and dopamine and prolong their re-uptake," or that "colostrum also activates the release of other chemicals in the brain that affect alertness and concentration" are unsubstantiated.

Where is it found?

Bovine colostrum is available in capsules, tablets, powdered drink mixes, liquid preparations, food bars, and skin care products.

Bovine colostrum has been used in connection with the following conditions (refer to the individual health concern for complete information):

Rating	Health Concerns
★★☆	Certain types of infectious **diarrhea** (page 163)

Who is likely to be deficient?

As bovine colostrum is not an essential nutrient, no deficiency state exists.

How much is usually taken?

Most manufacturers recommend 1,000 to 4,000 mg per day of freeze-dried colostrum.

Are there any side effects or interactions?

None are known.

BRANCHED-CHAIN AMINO ACIDS

What are they?

The branched-chain **amino acids** (page 465) (BCAAs) are leucine, isoleucine, and valine. BCAAs are considered essential amino acids because human beings cannot survive unless these amino acids are present in the diet.

BCAAs are needed for the maintenance of muscle tissue and appear to preserve muscle stores of glycogen (a storage form of carbohydrate that can be converted into energy).[1] BCAAs also help prevent muscle protein breakdown during exercise.[2]

Some research has shown that BCAA supplementation (typically 10–20 grams per day) does not result in meaningful changes in body composition,[3] nor does it improve exercise performance[4, 5, 6, 7, 8] or enhance the effects of physical training.[9, 10] However, BCAA supplementation may be useful in special situations, such as preventing muscle loss at high altitudes[11] and prolonging endurance performance in the heat.[12] Studies by one group of researchers suggest that BCAA supplementation may also improve exercise-induced declines in some aspects of mental functioning.[13, 14, 15]

BCAAs can activate glutamate dehydrogenase—an **enzyme** (page 506) that is deficient in amyotrophic lateral sclerosis (ALS), also called Lou Gehrig's disease. In one double-blind trial, 26 grams per day of BCAA supplements helped those with ALS maintain muscle strength.[16] However, a larger study was ended early when people using BCAAs not only failed to improve, but experienced higher death rates than the placebo group.[17] Other studies have shown no benefit of BCAA supplementation for ALS or other neuromuscular diseases,[18, 19] though a small group of people suffering from diseases of the nervous system collectively called spinocerebellar degeneration did improve when given BCAAs in a preliminary study.[20]

One study investigating the advantages of BCAA

supplementation for people with **diabetes** (page 152) undergoing an intense exercise program found no additional benefit of BCAAs on reducing abdominal fat or improving glucose metabolism.[21]

Patients with liver diseases that lead to coma—called hepatic encephalopathy—have low concentrations of BCAAs and excess levels of certain other amino acids. Preliminary research suggested that people with this condition might be helped by BCAAs. Double-blind studies have produced somewhat inconsistent results,[22, 23, 24] but a reanalysis of these studies found an overall benefit for the symptoms of encephalopathy.[25] Therapeutic effects of BCAAs have also been shown in children with liver failure[26] and adults with **cirrhosis of the liver** (page 290).[27] Any treatment of people with liver failure requires the direction of a physician.

People with chronic kidney failure may also benefit from BCAA supplementation. A preliminary study found improved breathing and sleep quality in people given intravenous BCAAs during kidney dialysis.[28]

Phenylketonuria (page 354) (PKU) is a genetic disease that causes abnormally high amounts of **phenylalanine** (page 568) and its end products to accumulate in the blood, causing damage to the nervous system. A controlled trial demonstrated that regular use of BCAAs by adolescents and young adults with PKU, improved performance on some tests of mental functioning.[29] This outcome makes sense because BCAAs may compete with phenylalanine, reducing its toxic effects.

In **tardive dyskinesia** (page 425), phenylalanine levels have also been reported to be elevated. As a result, one group of researchers gave tardive dyskinesia patients BCAAs (from 150 mg per 2.2 pounds body weight up to 209 mg per 2.2 pounds body weight) after breakfast and one hour before lunch and dinner for two weeks.[30] The BCAA mixture included equal parts valine and isoleucine plus 33% more leucine than either of the other two amino acids. Of nine patients so treated, six had at least a 58% decrease in symptoms, and all people in the study had a decrease of at least 38% in symptoms.

Where are they found?

Dairy products and red meat contain the greatest amounts of BCAAs, although they are present in all protein-containing foods. **Whey** (page 613) protein and egg protein supplements are other sources of BCAAs. BCAA supplements provide the **amino acids** (page 465) leucine, isoleucine, and valine.

BCAAs have been used in connection with the following conditions (refer to the individual health concern for complete information):

Rating	Health Concerns
★★☆	Kidney failure (intravenous BCAAs) **Liver cirrhosis** (page 290) **Phenylketonuria** (page 354)
★☆☆	**Athletic performance** (page 43) (for high altitude and extreme temperature only) Hepatic encephalopathy Spinocerebellar degeneration **Tardive dyskinesia** (page 425)

Who is likely to be deficient?

Only a person deficient in protein would become deficient in BCAAs, because most foods that are sources of protein supply BCAAs. Few people in Western societies are protein deficient.

How much is usually taken?

Most diets provide an adequate amount of BCAAs for most people, which is about 25–65 mg per 2.2 pounds of body weight.[31, 32] Athletes involved in intense training often take 5 grams of leucine, 4 grams of valine, and 2 grams of isoleucine per day to prevent muscle loss and increase muscle gain, though most research does not support this use of BCAAs.

Are there any side effects or interactions?

Side effects have not been reported with the use of BCAAs. Until more research is conducted, people with ALS should avoid taking supplemental BCAAs. In one study, supplementation with a large amount of BCAAs (60 grams) caused alterations in the blood levels of tryptophan, phenylalanine, and tyrosine.[33] The changes in the blood levels of these amino acids could, in theory, cause depression in susceptible individuals. Until more is known, individuals with a history of depression should consult a doctor before supplementing with BCAAs. People with **kidney** (page 284) or **liver** (page 290) disease should not consume high amounts of amino acids without consulting their doctor.

BREWER'S YEAST

What is it?

Brewer's yeast is the dried, pulverized cells of *Saccharomyces cerevisiae,* a type of fungus, and is a rich source of **B-complex vitamins** (page 603), protein (providing all essential **amino acids** [page 465]), and minerals, including a biologically active form of **chromium** (page 493) known as glucose tolerance factor (GTF). Brewer's yeast is usually a by-product of the brewing industry and should not be confused with nutritional yeast or torula yeast, which are low in chromium.

Where is it found?

Brewer's yeast, which has a very bitter taste, is recovered after being used in the beer-brewing process. Brewer's yeast can also be grown specifically for harvest as a nutritional supplement. "De-bittered" yeast is also available, though most yeast sold in health food stores that does not taste bitter is not real brewer's yeast.

Brewer's yeast has been used in connection with the following conditions (refer to the individual health concern for complete information):

Rating	Health Concerns
★★★	Diabetes (page 152) High cholesterol (page 223)
★★☆	Diarrhea (page 163) (infectious)

Who is likely to be deficient?

Brewer's yeast is not an essential nutrient, but it can be used as a source of **B-complex** (page 603) vitamins and protein. It is by far the best source of **chromium** (page 493), both in terms of quantity and bio-availability.

How much is usually taken?

Brewer's yeast is often taken as a powder, or as tablets or capsules. High-quality brewer's yeast powder or flakes contain as much as 60 mcg of **chromium** (page 493) per tablespoon (15 grams). When doctors recommend brewer's yeast, they will often suggest 1–2 tablespoons (15–30 grams) of this high-potency bulk product per day. Remember, if it is not bitter, it is not likely to be real brewer's yeast and therefore will not contain biologically active chromium. In addition, "primary grown" yeast (i.e., that grown specifically for harvest, as opposed to that recovered in the brewing process) may not contain GTF.

Are there any side effects or interactions?

Side effects have not been reported from the use of brewer's yeast, although **allergies** (page 14) to it exist in some people. It is not related to *Candida albicans* fungus, which causes **yeast infection** (page 454).

Because it contains a highly biologically active form of **chromium** (page 493), supplementation with brewer's yeast could potentially enhance the effects of drugs for **diabetes** (page 163) (e.g., insulin or other blood sugar-lowering agents) and possibly lead to **hypoglycemia** (page 251). Therefore, people with diabetes taking these medications should supplement with chromium or brewer's yeast only under the supervision of a doctor.

Saccharomyces boulardii (page 575) is registered in Europe under the name *Saccharomyces cerevisiae*, though the manufacturer states that *S. boulardii* is not the same as brewer's yeast *(S. cerevisiae)*. There is a case report of a person with severely impaired **immune function** (page 255) who, after receiving treatment with *S. boulardii*, developed an invasive fungal **infection** (page 265) identified as *S. cerevisiae*.[1] People with severe impairment of the immune system should therefore not take brewer's yeast or *S. boulardii* unless supervised by a doctor.

BROMELAIN

What is it?

Bromelain, derived from the pineapple plant, is one of a group of proteolytic **enzymes** (page 506) (enzymes capable of digesting protein).

It is widely believed that most orally ingested enzymes are destroyed by the digestive juices prior to being absorbed. However, there is evidence that significant amounts of bromelain can be absorbed intact.[1] Proteolytic enzymes *other than* bromelain are often used with people who suffer from **malabsorption** (page 304). Although bromelain in combination with other enzymes and ox bile has been reported to help digest food,[2] it is generally not used for this purpose. However, bromelain does contribute to the digestion of protein, and may therefore be used as a digestive aid. Although many doctors assume that other proteolytic enzymes, such as those found in pancreatin, are more effective than bromelain in helping digestion and absorption, almost no research compares the relative effects of these enzymes.

Bromelain is an anti-inflammatory agent and for this reason is helpful in healing **minor injuries** (page 319), particularly **sprains and strains** (page 412), muscle injuries, and the **pain** (page 338), swelling, and tenderness that accompany sports injuries.[3, 4, 5] Topically

Bromelain

Bromelain

applied bromelain in the form of a cream may be beneficial for frostbite,[6] possibly enhancing the rate of healing.[7] and for cleaning debris from **burns** (page 85).[8] These uses of bromelain should be supervised by a doctor.

Also as a result of its anti-inflammatory effect, bromelain has been found to dramatically reduce postoperative swelling in controlled human research.[9] Double-blind research has found bromelain effective in reducing swelling, bruising,[10] and pain, for women having minor surgery in conjunction with giving birth (episiotomy).[11]

The anti-inflammatory effect of bromelain is the probable reason this enzyme has been found effective for people suffering from **sinusitis** (page 407).[12] Some of the evidence supporting bromelain in the treatment of sinusitis comes from double-blind research.[13]

Bromelain, in combination with trypsin (another enzyme), may enhance the effect of antibiotics in people with a urinary tract infection (**UTI** [page 436]). In a double-blind study, 100% of people who received bromelain/trypsin in combination with antibiotics had a resolution of their UTIs, compared to only 46% of those who received antibiotics alone.[14]

Again, probably due to its anti-inflammatory action, bromelain was reported to help patients with **rheumatoid arthritis** (page 387) in preliminary research.[15] In that trial, in which bromelain was given for varying (3-week to 13-month) periods, 73% had good to excellent results.

Bromelain is a natural blood thinner because it prevents excessive blood platelet stickiness.[16] This may explain, in part, the positive reports in a few clinical trials of bromelain to decrease symptoms of **angina** (page 27) and thrombophlebitis.[17, 18] In addition, bromelain reduces the thickness of mucus, which may benefit patients with **asthma** (page 32) or chronic **bronchitis** (page 80).[19]

Preliminary evidence in both animals and people suggests that bromelain may possess antitumor activity, though the true importance of this effect is poorly understood.[20]

Bromelain can induce beneficial changes in white blood cells with possible effects on **immune function** (page 255).[21, 22] However, whether these effects would help people with immune system problems remains unclear.

Where is it found?
Bromelain is found mostly in the stems of pineapples and is available as a dietary supplement.

Bromelain has been used in connection with the following conditions (refer to the individual health concern for complete information):

Rating	Health Concerns
★★★	**Sinusitis** (page 407) **Wound healing** (page 319)
★★☆	**Post-surgical healing** (page 357) **Prostatitis** (page 377) (NBP, PD) **Sprains and strains** (page 412) **Tendinitis** (page 426) **Urinary tract infection** (page 436)
★☆☆	**Angina** (page 27) **Asthma** (page 32) **Low back pain** (page 293) **Rheumatoid arthritis** (page 387) Thrombophlebitis

Who is likely to be deficient?
Since bromelain is not essential, deficiencies of this plant-based **enzyme** (page 506) do not exist.

How much is usually taken?
Assessing the right amount of bromelain to take is complicated. Most bromelain research was conducted years ago, when amounts used were listed in units of activity that no longer exist. These old units do not precisely convert to new ones. Today, bromelain is measured in MCUs (milk clotting units) or GDUs (gelatin dissolving units). One GDU equals approximately 1.5 MCU. Strong products contain at least 2,000 MCU (1,200–1,333 GDU) per gram (1,000 mg). A supplement containing 500 mg labeled "2,000 MCU per gram" would have 1,000 MCU of activity. Some doctors recommend as much as 3,000 MCU taken three times per day for several days, followed by 2,000 MCU three times per day.[23] Much of the research uses smaller amounts, more like the equivalent of approximately 500 MCU taken four times per day. However, most of the bromelain used in the studies was enteric-coated in order to prevent it from being destroyed by gastric juice. It is likely, therefore, that currently available bromelain preparations (which typically are not enteric-coated) are of lower potency than the bromelain used in most studies.

Are there any side effects or interactions?
Bromelain is generally safe and free of side effects when taken in moderate amounts. However, one preliminary

report indicates increased heart rate with the use of bromelain.[24] In addition, some people are allergic to bromelain. One woman reportedly developed a hives and severe swelling after taking bromelain, even though she had tolerated bromelain on two other occasions previously.[25] Because bromelain acts as a blood thinner and little is known about how bromelain interacts with blood-thinning drugs, people should avoid combining such drugs with bromelain in order to reduce the theoretical risk of excessive bleeding.

CALCIUM

See also: Calcium: Which Form Is Best? (page 485)

What is it?

Calcium is the most abundant, essential mineral in the human body. Of the two to three pounds of calcium contained in the average body, 99% is located in the bones and teeth. Calcium is needed to form bones and teeth and is also required for blood clotting, transmission of signals in nerve cells, and muscle contraction. The importance of calcium for preventing **osteoporosis** (page 333) is probably its most well-known role.

Although calcium plays at least some minor role in lowering **blood pressure** (page 246), the mechanisms involved appear complex and somewhat unclear.[1] The level of calcium in the blood is tightly regulated by parathyroid hormone (PTH), and low intake of calcium causes elevations in PTH, which in turn have been implicated in the development of **hypertension** (page 246).[2] High calcium intake has also been associated with a reduced risk of **cardiovascular disease** (page 98) in **postmenopausal** (page 311) women.[3]

By reducing absorption of oxalate,[4] a substance found in many foods, calcium may be able to indirectly reduce the risk of **kidney stones** (page 284).[5] However, people with a history of kidney stones must talk with a doctor before supplementing with calcium because such supplementation might actually *increase* the risk of forming stones for the small number of people who absorb too much calcium.

Calcium also appears to partially bind some fats and cholesterol in the gastrointestinal tract. Perhaps as a result, some research suggests that calcium supplementation may help lower **cholesterol** (page 223) levels.[6]

Animal studies have established a role of calcium in the development of female egg cells (oocytes).[7, 8] Although the precise role of calcium is unclear, some researchers speculate that future studies may identify important uses for calcium in conditions of the human ovary, such as polycystic ovary syndrome (PCOS).[9]

Through a variety of mechanisms, calcium may have **anticancer** (page 87) actions within the colon. Most preliminary studies have shown high calcium diets are associated with reduced **colon cancer** (page 123) risk.[10] Most,[11, 12, 13] but not all,[14] preliminary studies have found taking calcium supplements to also be associated with a reduced risk of colon cancer or precancerous conditions in the colon. One preliminary study reported that high dietary, but not supplemental, calcium intake was associated with a decreased risk of precancerous changes in the colon.[15] In double-blind studies, calcium supplementation has significantly protected against precancerous changes in the colon in some,[16, 17] but not all, studies.[18, 19]

Warning: Calcium supplements should be avoided by **prostate cancer** (page 371) patients.

Where is it found?

Most dietary calcium comes from dairy products. The myth that calcium from dairy products is not absorbed is not supported by scientific research.[20, 21] Other good sources include sardines, canned salmon, green leafy vegetables, and tofu.

Calcium has been used in connection with the following conditions (refer to the individual health concern for complete information):

Rating	Health Concerns
★★★	**Gestational hypertension** (page 202) **Lactose intolerance** (page 288) (for preventing deficiency if dairy products are avoided only) **Osteoporosis** (page 333) **Preeclampsia** (page 361) (for deficiency) **Premenstrual syndrome** (page 368) **Rickets** (page 392)
★★☆	**Celiac disease** (page 102) (for deficiency only) **High blood pressure** (page 246) **High cholesterol** (page 223) **High triglycerides** (page 235) **Weight loss** (page 446)

Calcium

Rating	Health Concerns
★☆☆	**Amenorrhea** (page 22) (calcium for preventing bone loss) **Colon cancer** (page 123) (reduces risk) **Depression** (page 145) **Dysmenorrhea** (page 171) (painful menstruation) **Gingivitis (periodontal disease)** (page 203) **Insulin resistance syndrome** (page 273) (Syndrome X) **Kidney stones** (page 284) **Migraine headaches** (page 316) **Multiple sclerosis** (page 323) **Pregnancy and postpartum support** (page 363)

Calcium

Who is likely to be deficient?

Severe deficiency of either calcium or **vitamin D** (page 607) leads to a condition called **rickets** (page 392) in children and **osteomalacia** (page 392) in adults. Since vitamin D is required for calcium absorption, people with conditions causing vitamin D deficiency (e.g., pancreatic insufficiency) may develop a deficiency of calcium as well. Vegans (pure vegetarians), people with dark skin, those who live in northern climates, and people who stay indoors almost all the time are more likely to be vitamin D deficient than are other people. Vegans often eat less calcium and vitamin D than do other people. Most people eat well below the recommended amount of calcium. This lack of dietary calcium is thought to contribute to the risk of **osteoporosis** (page 333), particularly in white and Asian women.

How much is usually taken?

The National Academy of Sciences has established guidelines for calcium that are 25–50% higher than previous recommendations. For ages 19 to 50, calcium intake is recommended to be 1,000 mg daily; for adults over age 51, the recommendation is 1,200 mg daily.[22] The most common supplemental amount for adults is 800–1,000 mg per day.[23] General recommendations for higher daily intakes (1,200–1,500 mg) usually include the calcium most people consume from their diets. Studies indicate the average daily amount of calcium consumed by Americans is about 500–1,000 mg.

Are there any side effects or interactions?

Constipation (page 137), bloating, and **gas** (page 195) are sometimes reported with the use of calcium supplements.[24] A very high intake of calcium from dairy products plus supplemental calcium carbonate was reported in the past to cause a condition called "milk alkali syndrome." This toxicity is rarely reported today because most medical doctors no longer tell people with **ulcers** (page 349) to use this approach as treatment for their condition.

People with hyperparathyroidism, chronic kidney disease, or **kidney stones** (page 284) should not supplement with calcium without consulting a physician. For other adults, the highest amount typically suggested by doctors (1,200 mg per day) is considered quite safe. People with **prostate cancer** (page 371) should avoid supplementing with calcium.

In the past, calcium supplements in the forms of bone meal (including MCHC), dolomite, and oyster shell have sometimes had higher lead levels than permitted by stringent California regulations, though generally less than the levels set by the federal government.[25] "Refined" forms (which would include CCM, calcium citrate, and most calcium carbonate) have low levels.[26] More recently, a survey of over-the-counter calcium supplements found low or undetectable levels of lead in most products,[27] representing a sharp decline in lead content of calcium supplements since 1993. People who decide to take bone meal, dolomite, oyster shell, or coral calcium for long periods of time can contact the supplying supplement company to request independent laboratory analysis showing minimal lead levels.

Some studies have shown that calcium competes for absorption with a number of other minerals, while other studies have found no such competition. To be on the safe side, some doctors recommend that people taking calcium for long periods of time should also take a multimineral supplement.

One study has shown that taking calcium can interfere with the absorption of phosphorus, which, like calcium, is important for bone health.[28] Although most western diets contain ample or even excessive amounts of phosphorus, older people who supplement with large amounts of calcium may be at risk of developing phosphorus deficiency. For this reason, the authors of this study recommend that, for elderly people, at least some of the supplemental calcium be taken in the form of tricalcium phosphate or some other phosphorus-containing preparation.

Vitamin D (page 607)'s most important role is maintaining blood levels of calcium. Therefore, many doctors recommend that those supplementing with calcium also supplement with 400 IU of vitamin D per day.

Animal studies have shown that essential fatty acids (EFAs) increase calcium absorption from the gut, in part by enhancing the effects of vitamin D and reducing loss of calcium in the urine.[29]

Lysine (page 550) supplementation increases the absorption of calcium and may reduce its excretion.[30] As a result, some researchers believe that lysine may eventually be shown to have a role in the prevention and treatment of **osteoporosis** (page 333).[31]

CALCIUM: WHICH FORM IS BEST?

See also: Calcium (page 483)

For adults, dairy products supply 72% of the calcium in the U.S. diet, grain products about 11% and fruits and vegetables about 6%.[1] Milk drinkers get 80% more **calcium** (page 483) in their diet compared to non-milk-drinkers.[2] Apart from total calcium content, foods and supplements should be evaluated in terms of the *bioavailability* of the calcium they contained (i.e., how much of it is actually absorbed and utilized by the body.) Calcium absorption from various dairy products is similar, at about 30%.[3] However, many people choose alternatives to milk and dairy products for health reasons, such as the prevention of **atherosclerosis** (page 38) or food **allergies** (page 14). A variety of calcium-fortified nondairy beverages are now available. However, the bioavailability of calcium in these beverages may differ from that of milk. A study of calcium-fortified soy milk found that the calcium in it was absorbed at only 75% of the efficiency of the calcium in cow's milk.[4] While cow's milk and fortified soy milk are therefore not equivalent as calcium sources, the difference can easily be overcome by either consuming more of the fortified soy beverage, or by consuming soy beverages fortified with proportionally higher amounts of calcium.

Dietary supplements may contain one of several different forms of calcium. One difference between the various calcium compounds is the percentage of elemental calcium present. A greater percentage of elemental calcium means that fewer tablets are needed to achieve the desired calcium intake. For instance, in the calcium carbonate form, calcium accounts for 40% of the compound, while the calcium citrate form provides 24% elemental calcium.

Many medical doctors recommend calcium carbonate because it requires the fewest pills to reach a given level of calcium and it is readily available and inexpensive. For people concerned about cost and only willing to swallow two to three calcium pills per day, calcium carbonate is a sensible choice. Even for these people, however, low-quality calcium carbonate supplements are less than ideal. Depending on how the tablet is manufactured, some calcium carbonate pills have been found to disintegrate and dissolve improperly, which could interfere with absorption.[5] The disintegration of calcium carbonate pills can be easily evaluated by putting a tablet in a half cup of vinegar and stirring occasionally. After half an hour, no undissolved chunks of tablet should remain at the bottom.[6]

Calcium carbonate may not always show optimal absorption, but it clearly has positive effects. For example, calcium carbonate appears to be as well absorbed as the calcium found in milk.[7] In fact, some studies indicate that calcium carbonate is absorbed as well as most other forms besides calcium citrate/malate (CCM).[8, 9] For example, a recent study found absorption of calcium from calcium carbonate to be virtually identical to absorption of calcium from calcium citrate.[10]

For people willing to take more pills to achieve a given amount of calcium (typically 800–1,000 mg), calcium carbonate does not appear to be the optimal choice, because other forms have been reported to be absorbed, absorb better (however, they do require more pills per day because each pill contains less calcium). For this reason, some doctors recommend other forms of calcium, particularly CCM. Research shows that CCM is absorbed better than most other forms.[11, 12, 13] CCM may also be more effective in maintaining bone mass, than some other forms of calcium supplements.[14] Because of their similarity in both name and structure, CCM can be confused with calcium citrate, but they are not the same.

CCM is not the only form of calcium that might be absorbed better than carbonate. For example, most,[15, 16] though not all,[17] studies suggest that calcium citrate might have some absorption advantage over calcium carbonate. However, no evidence suggests that calcium citrate is as well absorbed as CCM.

Microcrystalline hydroxyapatite (MCHC), a variation on bonemeal, has attracted attention because of studies reporting increases in bone mass in people with certain conditions[18] and better effects on bone than calcium carbonate.[19] Similar positive studies exist using CCM.[20] However, unlike CCM, MCHC has only occasionally been compared with other forms of calcium. In limited research that does make comparisons, MCHC fared poorly in terms of solubility, absorption, and effect on calcium metabolism.[21, 22]

Remarkably little is known about the relative efficacy of **amino acid** (page 465) chelates (pronounced "kee-lates") of calcium. In the only commonly cited trial, absorption was measured for an amino acid chelate called calcium bisglycinate and compared with absorption from citrate, carbonate, and MCHC.[23] In that trial, the amino acid chelate showed the best absorption and MCHC the worst. Although CCM was studied in that trial, it was taken under different circumstances than the chelate (with meals), so drawing definitive conclusions is not possible.

Recently, coral calcium has been claimed to be a vastly superior form of calcium, even though its calcium content is primarily calcium carbonate. One small, controlled human study reported that coral calcium was better absorbed than ordinary calcium carbonate.[24] However, the method used in this study to measure calcium absorption has been criticized as much less sensitive than other methods.[25] No research has compared coral calcium to calcium citrate or to CCM. There is little evidence at this time that coral calcium is superior to other forms of calcium.

Whatever the form, calcium supplements typically are absorbed better when eaten with meals.[26] Moreover, research indicates that taking calcium with meals may reduce the risk of **kidney stones** (page 284) and supplementing with calcium between meals might actually increase the risk.[27]

Besides *how* to take calcium supplements, scientists have also been studying *when* to take them. Supplementing calcium in the evening appears better for **osteoporosis** (page 333) prevention than taking calcium in the morning, based on the circadian rhythm of bone loss.[28] In order to not increase the risk of forming **kidney stones** (page 284), most doctors tell people to take calcium supplements only with food.

What is the relationship between calcium supplements and stomach acid?

Years ago, researchers reported that people who do not make **hydrochloric acid** (page 473) in their stomachs cannot absorb calcium adequately when the calcium is taken alone.[29] In that report, adding hydrochloric acid restored normal calcium absorption. Although researchers have subsequently confirmed these findings, they have also discovered that these same people absorb calcium normally if they take it with meals. In addition, researchers have noted that giving these people hydrochloric acid does not further improve absorption during meals.[30] Others have confirmed that hydrochloric acid, either from pills or from the stomach, is unnecessary for the absorption of calcium, as long as the calcium supplement is taken with meals.[31, 32, 33, 34]

Some doctors have expressed a concern that antacids that contain calcium (like Tums) or calcium supplements that also act as antacids, interfere with the body's absorption of calcium. However, this is not the case. Calcium carbonate, the principal ingredient in both Tums and many calcium supplements provides significant (though not optimal) absorbable calcium, as discussed above. Other forms of calcium that might be more bio-available, such as calcium citrate, also act as antacids. The form of calcium associated most consistently with best bio-availability, CCM, is itself, an antacid despite the fact it is used almost exclusively as a source of calcium.

Other concerns about the antacid effect of most calcium supplements (particularly when taken by people who do not need and are not seeking an antacid) are voiced by some doctors because stomach acid is needed to protect against bacterial **infection** (page 265) and also to help digest protein. In theory, calcium supplements with antacid activity could at least temporarily interfere with these processes. However, to date, these concerns remain hypothetical.

CALCIUM D-GLUCARATE

What is it?
Calcium D-glucarate is the **calcium** (page 483) salt of D-glucaric acid, a natural substance found in many fruits and vegetables.

Calcium D-glucarate has been shown to inhibit beta-glucuronidase, an enzyme found in certain bacteria that reside in the gut. One of the key ways in which the body eliminates toxic chemicals as well as hormones such as estrogen is by attaching glucuronic acid to them in the liver and then excreting this complex in the bile. Beta-glucuronidase is a bacterial enzyme that uncouples (breaks) the bond between the excreted compound and glucuronic acid. When beta-glucuronidase breaks the bond, the hormone or toxic chemical that is released is available to be reabsorbed into the body instead of being excreted. An elevated beta-glucuronidase activity is associated with an increased risk for various **cancers** (page 87), particularly hormone-dependent cancers like **breast** (page 65), **prostate** (page 371), and **colon** (page 123) cancers.[1]

Studies in animals have shown that supplementing with calcium D-glucarate prevents the development of experimentally induced cancers.[2, 3, 4, 5] The amount of calcium D-glucarate used in these studies, however, would be too much for humans to take. Researchers at M.D. Anderson Cancer Center, Memorial Sloan-Kettering Cancer Center, and other major cancer centers began conducting research with calcium D-glucarate for the prevention and treatment of breast cancer.[6, 7] No human studies showing the efficacy or safety of calcium D-glucarate have been published.

Where is it found?
Calcium D-glucarate is available in capsules and tablets. Foods high in glucaric acid (a form of calcium D-glucarate) include apples, Brussels sprouts, broccoli, cabbage, and bean sprouts.[8]

Calcium D-glucarate has been used in connection with the following conditions (refer to the individual health concern for complete information):

Rating	Health Concerns
★☆☆	**Cancer** (page 87)

Who is likely to be deficient?
Calcium D-glucarate is not an essential nutrient, and thus no deficiency state exists.

How much is usually taken?
Manufacturers of calcium D-glucarate recommend a daily intake of 200 to 400 mg.

Are there any side effects or interactions?
No side effects have been reported with calcium D-glucarate. Although there are no known drug interactions, many drugs (especially hormones) are metabolized in the liver by binding to glucuronic acid. It is therefore possible that taking calcium D-glucarate could increase the elimination of certain drugs or hormones from the body, thereby reducing their effectiveness. If you are taking any prescription medication, please consult your physician or pharmacist before taking calcium D-glucarate.

CARNOSINE

What is it?
Carnosine is a small molecule composed of the **amino acids** (page 465), **histidine** (page 534) and **alanine** (page 463). It is found in relatively high concentrations in several body tissues—most notably in skeletal muscle, heart muscle, and brain.[1, 2]

The exact biological role of carnosine is not completely understood, but numerous animal studies have demonstrated that it possesses strong and specific **antioxidant** (page 467) properties, protects against radiation damage, improves the function of the heart, and promotes **wound healing** (page 319).[3, 4, 5, 6, 7, 8] Carnosine has been suggested to be the water-soluble counterpart to **vitamin E** (page 609) in protecting cell membranes from oxidative damage. Other suggested roles for carnosine include actions as a neurotransmitter (chemical messenger in the nervous system), modulator of enzyme activities, and chelator of heavy metals (i.e., a substance that binds heavy metals, possibly reducing their toxicity).

Based primarily on preliminary research from Russia, carnosine has been claimed to lower **blood pressure** (page 246), improve the functioning of the **immune system** (page 255), promote **wound healing** (page 319), and exert **anticancer** (page 87) effects. However, additional research is needed before these claims can be considered scientifically well documented.

The best-documented application of carnosine is in **peptic ulcers** (page 349). Experimental animal studies have shown that a zinc salt of carnosine exerts significant protection against ulcer formation and promotes the healing of existing ulcers.[9, 10] However, because **zinc** (page 614) by itself has been shown to be helpful against peptic ulcer, it is not known how much of the beneficial effect was due to the carnosine.[11, 12] Clinical studies in humans demonstrated that this compound can help eradicate *Helicobacter pylori*, an organism that has been linked to peptic ulcer and stomach **cancer** (page 87).[13] When 60 patients suffering from dyspepsia with *H. pylori* **infection** (page 265) were given either antibiotics alone (lansoprazole, amoxicillin, and clarithromycin) or antibiotics plus zinc carnosine for seven days, better results were seen in the group receiving zinc carnosine (94% eradication rate vs. 77%). The zinc salt of carnosine (in combination with sodium alginate) has also shown to be effective in severe **gingivitis** (page 203) caused by cancer chemotherapy.[14]

Carnosine

In a preliminary trial, supplementation with a zinc salt of carnosine enhanced the response to interferon therapy in patients with chronic hepatitis C.[15] It is not known whether this benefit was due primarily to the zinc or the carnosine, or whether other forms of carnosine would have the same effect.

Where is it found?
Dietary sources of preformed carnosine include meat and poultry and fish.

Carnosine has been used in connection with the following conditions (refer to the individual health concern for complete information):

Rating	Health Concerns
★★☆	Hepatitis C (page 220) (zinc [page 614]-L-carnosine)
★☆☆	Peptic ulcers (page 349) Wound healing (page 357)

Who is likely to be deficient?
Carnosine deficiency may occur in severe protein deficiency and in certain severe genetic disorders characterized by inborn errors in **amino acid** (page 465) metabolism.

How much is usually taken?
For eradication of *H. pylori,* the amount of the **zinc** (page 614) carnosine complex used in research studies was 150 mg twice daily. Due to the lack of human clinical trials, recommended levels for other applications are not known at this time.

Are there any side effects or interactions?
Due to the lack of human studies, side effects and interactions are not known.

CAROTENOIDS

What are they?
Carotenoids are a highly colored (red, orange, and yellow) group of fat-soluble plant pigments. All organisms, whether bacteria or plants, that rely on the sun for energy contain carotenoids. Their **antioxidant** (page 467) effects enable these compounds to play a crucial role in protecting organisms against damage during photosynthesis—the process of converting sunlight into chemical energy.

In humans, carotenoids play two primary roles: All exert antioxidant activity, but some are also converted into **vitamin A** (page 595). Of the 600 carotenoids that have been identified, about 30 to 50 are believed to have vitamin A activity. Carotenoids the body converts to vitamin A are referred to as "provitamin A" carotenoids. The most well known of this group are **beta-carotene** (page 469) and alpha-carotene. Some of the better known carotenoids without provitamin A activity—but with very high antioxidant activity—are **lutein** (page 548), **lycopene** (page 548), and zeaxanthin.[1, 2]

Preliminary and experimental studies suggest that a higher dietary intake of carotenoids offers protection against developing certain **cancers** (page 87) (e.g., lung, skin, uterine, cervix, gastrointestinal tract), **macular degeneration** (page 303), **cataracts** (page 101), and other health conditions linked to oxidative or **free radical** (page 467) damage.[3, 4, 5, 6] However, two double-blind studies have shown that supplementation with isolated synthetic beta-carotene does not reduce the risk of **lung cancer** (page 298) and may even increase that risk in smokers.[7, 8] This finding suggests that foods that are high in carotenoids may protect against cancer in humans for reasons unrelated to their carotenoid content, that synthetic beta-carotene may have different effects from natural beta-carotene (which is somewhat structurally distinct), or that carotenoids may need to be taken together or with supportive antioxidants (e.g., **vitamin C** [page 604], **vitamin E** [page 609], **selenium** [page 584]) in order to reduce the risk of cancer. Researchers have yet to determine which of these possibilities is true.

A high intake of carotenoids from dietary sources has been shown to be protective against **heart disease** (page 98) in several population-based studies.[9, 10] However, a high level of these antioxidants might simply be a marker for diets high in fruits and vegetables known to contain protective substances other than carotenoids. Furthermore, a diet rich in carotenoids tends to be lower in saturated fat and **cholesterol** (page 223) and higher in **fiber** (page 512), which has also found to be protective against heart disease.

Because of their **antioxidant** (page 467) activity, it has been suggested that **beta-carotene** (page 469) and other carotenoids might protect against **atherosclerosis** (page 38) by preventing oxidative damage to serum cholesterol. However, research is conflicting in this area. One thing is clear—carotenoids are significantly less effective in protecting against damage to serum cholesterol than is **vitamin E** (page 609). While feeding people beta-carotene has been shown to prevent oxidative damage to cholesterol in some trials,[11] other studies have reported that beta-carotene does not protect cholesterol from oxidative damage.[12, 13]

Just as in the case of cancer prevention, while a high intake of carotenoid-rich foods appears to be protective against cardiovascular disease, the same is not true for supplementation with synthetic beta-carotene. Double-blind intervention trials wherein people are supplemented with beta-carotene alone or placebo have not found benefit for synthetic beta-carotene supplementation. In fact, three of four trials have reported a *higher* risk of **cardiovascular disease** (page 98) in the beta-carotene groups compared with those receiving placebo.[14, 15, 16, 17] While these outcomes prove that synthetic beta-carotene does not protect against heart disease, the effects of natural beta-carotene and other carotenoids have yet to be tested in intervention trials assessing effects on heart disease.

A potential problem with much of the research on carotenoids in cardiovascular disease has been the focus on beta-carotene. A preliminary study found a strong association between dietary sources of **lycopene** (page 548), not beta-carotene, and reduced risk of **heart attacks** (page 98).[18] Lycopene exerts greater antioxidant activity compared to beta-carotene, and lycopene has also been reported to protect cholesterol against oxidative damage.[19]

Where are they found?
Carotenoids are found in all plant foods. In general, the greater the intensity of color, the higher the level of carotenoids. In green leafy vegetables, **beta-carotene** (page 469) is the predominant carotenoid. In the orange colored fruits and vegetables—such as carrots, apricots, mangoes, yams, winter squash—beta-carotene concentrations are high, but other pro-vitamin A carotenoids typically predominate. Yellow vegetables have higher concentrations of yellow carotenoids (xanthophylls), hence a lowered pro-vitamin A activity; but some of these compounds, such as **lutein** (page 548), may have significant health benefits, potentially due to their **antioxidant** (page 467) effects. The red and purple vegetables and fruits—such as tomatoes, red cabbage, berries, and plums—contain a large portion of non-vitamin A–active carotenoids. Legumes, grains, and seeds are also significant sources of carotenoids.

Carotenoids are also found in various animal foods, such as salmon, egg yolks, shellfish, milk, and poultry. A variety of carotenoids is also found in carrot juice and "green drinks" made from vegetables, dehydrated barley greens, or wheat grass.

Synthetic beta-carotene is available as a supplement. Mixed carotenoids (including the natural form of beta-carotene) are also available in supplements derived from palm oil, algae, and carrot oil.

Carotenoids have been used in connection with the following conditions (refer to the individual health concern for complete information):

Rating	Health Concerns
★☆☆	**Cataracts** (page 101) (prevention)
	Heart disease (page 98) (prevention)
	Macular degeneration (page 303) (prevention) (lutein [page 548], zeaxanthin, **lycopene** [page 548])
	Sickle cell anemia (page 403)

Who is likely to be deficient?
Carotenoid deficiency is not considered a classic nutritional deficiency like scurvy or beri-beri (severe **vitamin C** [page 604] and **vitamin B₁** [page 597] deficiencies, respectively). However, given the possible health benefits of carotenoids, most doctors recommend adequate intake. People who do not frequently consume carotenoid-rich foods or take carotenoid supplements are likely to be taking in less than adequate amounts, though optimal levels remain unknown. Also, deficiency may be found in people with chronic **diarrhea** (page 163) or other disorders associated with impaired absorption.

How much is usually taken?
Whether people who already consume a diet high in fruits and vegetables would benefit further from supplementation with a mixture of carotenoids remains unknown. While smokers clearly should not supplement with isolated synthetic **beta-carotene** (page 469), the effect in smokers of taking either natural beta-carotene or mixed carotenoids is not clear.

Nonetheless, based on health-promoting effects associated with these levels in preliminary research, some doctors recommend that most people supplement with up to 25,000 IU (15 mg) per day of natural beta-carotene and approximately 6 mg each of alpha-carotene, **lutein** (page 548), and **lycopene** (page 548).

Carotenoids

Are there any side effects or interactions?

Carotenoids are generally regarded as safe, based primarily on studies with **beta-carotene** (page 469). Increased consumption of carotenoids may cause to the skin to turn orange or yellow—a condition known as "carotenodermia." This occurrence is completely benign and is unrelated to jaundice—the yellowing of the skin that can result from liver disease or other causes.

Until more is known, people especially smokers should not supplement with synthetic beta-carotene. Two double-blind studies have shown that supplementation with isolated synthetic beta-carotene may increase the risk of **lung cancer** (page 298) in people who smoke.[20, 21] Moreover, three of four studies have found small increases in the risk of **heart disease** (page 98) in people assigned to take synthetic beta-carotene compared with those assigned to take placebo.[22, 23, 24, 25]

CARTILAGE AND COLLAGEN

What is it?

Cartilage, derived from shark, bovine (cow), and other animal sources, is a type of connective tissue composed of mucopolysaccharides (including **chondroitin sulfate** [page 492]), protein substances, **calcium** (page 483), **sulfur** (page 590), and collagen. Collagen is one of the proteins found in most connective tissues, including cartilage, bone, and skin. Gelatin is a form of collagen commonly used in foods, and preliminary reports suggest that consuming gelatin can improve the structure and health of the hair and nails.[1, 2, 3, 4] Collagen hydrolysate is produced by enzymatically breaking down bovine gelatin to smaller protein fragments.

Where is it found?

Cartilage is derived from either sharks or cows. Collagen is derived from either cows or chickens.

Cartilage and collagen have been used in connection with the following conditions (refer to the individual health concern for complete information):

Rating	Health Concerns
★★☆	**Osteoarthritis** (page 328)
★☆☆	Karposi's sarcoma (skin cancer) **Prostate cancer** (page 371) (shark cartilage)

Who is likely to be deficient?

Since they are not essential nutrients, neither cartilage nor collagen are associated with deficiencies.

How much is usually taken?

Bovine cartilage is typically recommended at 3 grams three times per day. Shark cartilage is sometimes taken in much higher amounts (e.g., 60 to 100 grams per day orally or by enema). These amounts are based on animal and anecdotal evidence and their safety and efficacy have not been confirmed by controlled clinical trials. Not only is toxicity information on this amount of shark cartilage lacking, but the amount of calcium in this amount of shark cartilage exceeds the 2 to 2.5 grams per day that is commonly considered to be the upper limit of safe intake. Type II collagen, when used for its effects on the immune system in rheumatoid arthritis, is used in very small amounts, from 0.02 mg to 10 mg per day. Gelatin and collagen hydrolysate is recommended at 7 to 10 grams per day.

Are there any side effects or interactions?

Reports have suggested that some people should not use a cartilage supplement. This concern is based only on theory, not clinical evidence. This would include those people with **cardiovascular disease** (page 98), women who are planning to be or are **pregnant** (page 363), nursing mothers, anyone having or having had surgery within 30 days, and **athletes** (page 43) training intensely. None of these concerns have been proven in clinical trials, however. Because shark cartilage contains **calcium** (page 483), people who ingest large amounts of shark cartilage (60 to 100 grams per day) may be consuming excessive amounts of this mineral. However, no cases of calcium toxicity resulting from the ingestion of shark cartilage have been reported.

While use of gelatin, collagen hydrolysate, or type II collagen has not resulted in any reports of serious side effects, people with known sensitivities to chicken or beef should consult a doctor before using them.

CETYL MYRISTOLEATE

What is it?

Cetyl myristoleate (CMO) is the common name for cis-9-cetyl myristoleate. CMO was discovered in 1972 by Harry W. Diehl, Ph.D., a researcher at the National Institutes of Health. At the time, Dr. Diehl was responsible for testing anti-inflammatory drugs on lab animals. In order for him to test the drugs, he first had to artificially induce arthritis in the animals by injecting a heat-killed bacterium called Freund's adjuvant. Dr. Diehl discovered that Swiss albino mice did not get arthritis after injection of Freund's adjuvant. Eventually, he was able to determine that cetyl myristoleate was the factor present naturally in mice that was responsible for this protection. When CMO was injected into various strains of rats, it offered the same protection against arthritis.[1]

It has been proposed that CMO acts as a joint "lubricant" and anti-inflammatory agent. Patents were granted to Dr. Diehl for the use of CMO in both **osteoarthritis** (page 328) and **rheumatoid arthritis** (page 387), based upon the animal studies and several case histories.[2, 3, 4] In a double-blind study, 106 people with various types of arthritis who had failed to respond to nonsteroidal anti-inflammatory drugs (NSAIDs) received cetyl myristoleate (540 mg per day orally for 30 days), while 226 others received a placebo. These people also applied cetyl myristoleate or placebo topically, according to their perceived need. Some 63.5% of those receiving cetyl myristoleate improved, compared with only 14.5% of those receiving the placebo (a statistically significant difference).[5]

Where is it found?

Cetyl myristoleate is found in certain animals, including cows, whales, beavers, and mice. As a nutritional supplement it is found in a highly purified, refined form in capsules and tablets. CMO is also available in creams and lotions for topical application.

CMO has been used in connection with the following conditions (refer to the individual health concern for complete information):

Rating	Health Concerns
★★☆	**Osteoarthritis** (page 328) **Rheumatoid arthritis** (page 387)

Who is likely to be deficient?

As cetyl myristoleate is not an essential nutrient, no deficiency state exists.

How much is usually taken?

Generally, CMO is taken in the amount of 400 to 500 mg daily for 30 days.

Are there any side effects or interactions?

No side effects or drug interactions have been reported.

CHITOSAN

What is it?

Chitosan is a polysaccharide found in the shells of crustaceans.

Like dietary **fiber** (page 512), chitosan is not digestible but may have beneficial effects on the gastrointestinal tract. Chitosan may also have an effect on the type of bacteria living in the intestines or on the action of these bacteria.

Where is it found?

Chitosan is extracted from the shells of crustaceans, such as shrimp and crab.

Chitosan has been used in connection with the following conditions (refer to the individual health concern for complete information):

Rating	Health Concerns
★☆☆	**High cholesterol** (page 223) Kidney failure **Weight loss** (page 446)

Who is likely to be deficient?

Chitosan is not an essential nutrient, so deficiencies do not occur.

How much is usually taken?

Most human research has used 3–6 grams per day with meals.

Are there any side effects or interactions?

While no long-term studies of the effects of chitosan on human health have been done, animal studies suggest that this compound could inhibit the absorption of **minerals** (page 559) and fat-soluble **vitamins** (page 559). Adverse effects on the growth of children and on the outcome of **pregnancy** (page 363) are also possible.[1] In addition, although chitosan-included alterations in intestinal flora are believed to be beneficial, the possibility that these changes may have negative long-term consequences has not been ruled out. People with **intestinal malabsorption** (page 304) syndromes should not use chitosan.

CHLOROPHYLL

What is it?

Chlorophyll is the substance responsible for the green color in plants that accomplishes photosynthesis.

Chlorophyll has been used traditionally to improve bad breath, as well as to reduce the odors of urine, feces, and infected wounds. Chlorophyll has anti-inflammatory, **antioxidant** (page 467), and **wound-healing** (page 319) properties.[1, 2]

Historically, chlorophyll was used for gastrointestinal problems, such as **constipation** (page 137), and to stimulate blood cell formation in **anemia** (page 25). Some preliminary evidence suggests that chlorophyll might help detoxify **cancer** (page 87)-promoting substances.[3, 4]

Where is it found?

Good dietary sources of chlorophyll include dark green leafy vegetables, algae (including **spirulina** [page 474] and chlorella), wheat grass, and barley grass. Supplements of chlorophyll as powder, capsules, tablets, and drinks are also available.

Chlorophyll has been used in connection with the following conditions (refer to the individual health concern for complete information):

Rating	Health Concerns
★★☆	**Fibromyalgia** (page 191)
★☆☆	**Constipation** (page 137) **Halitosis** (page 209) (bad breath)

Who is likely to be deficient?

Because chlorophyll is not known to be an essential nutrient, a deficiency does not exist. People who do not eat plenty of green foods lack chlorophyll in their diets.

How much is usually taken?

Optimal levels remain unknown. Chlorophyll in the amount of 100 mg two or three times per day can be used to treat **bad breath** (page 209).

Are there any side effects or interactions?

No side effects have been reported with the use of chlorophyll.

CHONDROITIN SULFATE

What is it?

Chondroitin sulfate consists of repeating chains of molecules called glycosaminoglycans (GAGs). Chondroitin sulfate is a major constituent of **cartilage** (page 490), providing structure, holding water and nutrients, and allowing other molecules to move through cartilage— an important property, as there is no blood supply to cartilage.

In degenerative joint disease, such as **osteoarthritis** (page 328), there is a loss of chondroitin sulfate as the cartilage erodes. Animal studies indicate that chondroitin sulfate may promote healing of bone, which is consistent with the fact that the majority of glycosaminoglycans found in bone consist of chondroitin sulfate.[1] Chondroitin sulfate has been shown, in numerous double-blind trials,[2, 3, 4, 5, 6, 7, 8, 9] to relieve symptoms and possibly slow the progression of, or reverse, osteoarthritis.[10]

Chondroitin and similar compounds are present in the lining of blood vessels and the urinary bladder. They help prevent abnormal movement of blood, urine, or components across the barrier of the vessel or bladder wall. Part of chondroitin's role in blood vessels is to prevent excessive blood clotting. However, whether supplements of chondroitin are able to favorably affect blood clotting remains unclear. In addition, chondroitin sulfate may lower blood **cholesterol levels** (page 223).[11] Older preliminary research showed that chondroitin sulfate may prevent **atherosclerosis** (page 38) in animals and humans and may also prevent **heart attacks** (page 212) in people who already have atherosclerosis.[12, 13, 14]

Chondroitin sulfate can help form a coating on nasal passages. Perhaps as a result, researchers found that when chondroitin sulfate was sprayed into the nasal passages of a small group of people who snore, the amount of time people spent snoring was reduced about one-third in a double-blind trial.[15] No further studies have investigated the effects of oral chondroitin sulfate on snoring.

Chondroitin sulfate is rich in **sulfur** (page 590) and is related to **glucosamine** (page 528). GAGs affect how the body processes oxalate—a substance linked to **kidney stones** (page 284). In one study of 40 people with a history of kidney stones, 30 mg twice a day of mixed GAGs reduced urinary oxalate excretion in 15 days—a change that could drop the risk of stone formation.[16] However, studies on the effect of GAGs on stone formation in humans have produced inconsistent results.[17]

Where is it found?
The only significant food source of chondroitin sulfate is animal **cartilage** (page 490).

Chondroitin sulfate has been used in connection with the following conditions (refer to the individual health concern for complete information):

Rating	Health Concerns
★★★	**Osteoarthritis** (page 327)
★★☆	**Wound healing** (page 319) (topical)
★☆☆	**Atherosclerosis** (page 38)
	Heart attack (page 212)
	High cholesterol (page 223)
	Kidney stones (page 284)
	Sprains and strains (page 412)
	Wound healing (page 319) (oral)

Who is likely to be deficient?
Because the body makes chondroitin, the possibility of a dietary deficiency remains uncertain. Nevertheless, chondroitin sulfate may be reduced in joint **cartilage** (page 490) affected by **osteoarthritis** (page 328) and possibly other forms of arthritis.

How much is usually taken?
For **atherosclerosis** (page 38), researchers have sometimes started therapy using very high amounts, such as 5 grams twice per day with meals, lowering the amount to 500 mg three times per day after a few months. Before taking such high amounts, people should consult a doctor. For **osteoarthritis** (page 328), a typical level is 400 mg three times per day. Oral chondroitin sulfate is rapidly absorbed in humans when it is dissolved in water prior to ingestion. Approximately 12% of chondroitin sulfate taken by mouth becomes available to the joint tissues from the blood.[18]

Are there any side effects or interactions?
Nausea may occur at intakes greater than 10 grams per day. No other adverse effects have been reported.

One doctor has raised a concern that chondroitin sulfate should not be used by men with **prostate cancer** (page 371). This concern is based upon two studies. In one, the concentration of chondroitin sulfate was found to be higher in cancerous prostate tissue as compared to normal prostate tissue.[19] In the other study, it was shown that higher concentrations of chondroitin sulfate in the tissue surrounding a cancerous prostate tumor predict a higher rate of recurrence of the **cancer** (page 87) after surgery.[20] However, no studies to date have addressed the question of whether taking chondroitin sulfate supplements could promote the development of prostate cancer. Simply because a substance is present in or around cancerous tissue does not by itself suggest that that substance is causing the cancer. For example, **calcium** (page 483) is a component of atherosclerotic plaques that harden the arteries; however, there is no evidence that taking calcium supplements causes atherosclerosis. To provide meaningful information, further studies would need to track the incidence of prostate cancer in men taking chondroitin supplements. Until then, most nutritionally-oriented doctors remain unconcerned about this issue.

It is not known whether taking **glucosamine sulfate** (page 529) and chondroitin sulfate in combination is a more effective treatment for **osteoarthritis** (page 328) than taking either one by itself.

CHROMIUM

What is it?
Chromium is an essential trace mineral that helps the body maintain normal blood sugar levels.

In addition to its well-studied effects in **diabetes** (page 152), preliminary research has found that chromium supplementation also improves glucose tolerance in people with Turner's syndrome—a disease linked with glucose intolerance.[1]

Chromium may also play a role in increasing HDL ("good") cholesterol,[2] while lowering total **cholesterol levels** (page 223).[3]

Chromium, in a form called chromium picolinate, has been studied for its potential role in altering body composition. Preliminary research in animals[4] and humans[5, 6] suggested that chromium picolinate increases fat loss and promotes a gain in lean muscle tissue. Double-blind research has also reported a reduction in body fat[7] and body weight[8] in people given 400 mcg of

Chromium

chromium (as chromium picolinate) per day for three months. However, other studies have failed to show a significant effect of chromium picolinate on body composition.[9]

Where is it found?

The best source of chromium is true **brewer's yeast** (page 480). Nutritional yeast and torula yeast do not contain significant amounts of chromium and are not suitable substitutes for brewer's yeast. Chromium is also found in grains and cereals, though much of it is lost when these foods are refined. Some brands of beer contain significant amounts of chromium.

Chromium has been used in connection with the following conditions (refer to the individual health concern for complete information):

Rating	Health Concerns
★★★	**Diabetes** (page 152) **High cholesterol** (page 223) **Hypoglycemia** (page 251)
★★☆	**High triglycerides** (page 235) **Insulin resistance syndrome** (page 273) (Syndrome X)
★☆☆	**Athletic performance** (page 43) **Depression** (page 145) **Weight loss** (page 446)

Who is likely to be deficient?

Most people eat less than the U.S. National Academy of Science's recommended range of 50–200 mcg per day. The high incidence of adult-onset **diabetes** (page 152) suggests to some doctors that many people should be supplementing with small amounts of chromium.

How much is usually taken?

A daily intake of 200 mcg is recommended by many doctors.

Are there any side effects or interactions?

In supplemental amounts (typically 50–300 mcg per day), chromium has not been found to cause toxicity in humans. While there are a few reports of people developing medical problems while taking chromium, a cause-effect relationship was not proven. One study suggested that chromium in very high concentrations in a test tube could cause chromosomal mutations in

ovarian cells of hamsters.[10, 11] Chromium picolinate can be altered by **antioxidants** (page 467) or hydrogen peroxide in the body to a form that could itself create free radical damage.[12] In theory, these changes could increase the risk of **cancer** (page 87), but so far, chromium intake has not been linked to increased incidence of cancer in humans.[13]

Chromium supplementation may enhance the effects of drugs for **diabetes** (page 152) (e.g., insulin, blood sugar-lowering agents) and possibly lead to **hypoglycemia** (page 251). Therefore, people with diabetes taking these medications should supplement with chromium only under the supervision of a doctor.

One report of severe illness (including **liver** (page 290) and **kidney** (page 284) damage) occurring in a person who was taking 1,000 mcg of chromium per day has been reported.[14] However, chromium supplementation was not proven to be the cause of these problems. Another source claimed that there have been reports of mild **heart rhythm abnormalities** (page 93) with excessive chromium ingestion.[15] However, no published evidence supports this assertion.

Three single, unrelated cases of toxicity have been reported from use of chromium picolinate. A case of kidney failure appeared after taking 600 mcg per day for six weeks.[16] A case of anemia, liver dysfunction, and other problems appeared after four to five months of 1,200–2,400 mcg per day.[17] A case of a muscle disease known as rhabdomyolysis appeared in a body builder who took 1200 mcg over 48 hours.[18] Whether these problems were caused by chromium picolinate or, if so, whether other forms of chromium might have the same effects at these high amounts remains unclear. No one should take more than 300 mcg per day of chromium without the supervision of a doctor.

Preliminary research has found that **vitamin C** (page 604) increases the absorption of chromium.[19]

COCONUT OIL

What is it?

Coconut oil is a member of the family of tropical oils, which also include palm, palm kernel, cocoa, and shea nut oils. These oils have been used for centuries in the traditional diets of people living in tropical regions such as the Polynesian islands. Because these populations experience less of the diseases, such as **heart disease** (page 98), that are common in Western countries, some people believe that tropical oils such as coconut oil, especially in their natural state, can be part of a healthful diet.[1, 2] Currently, these oils are used in Western countries in small amounts, primarily in the production of processed foods.

Tropical oils are high in saturated fat, which has been associated with increased risk of **high blood cholesterol** (page 223), **atherosclerosis** (page 38), and heart disease.[3, 4, 5] However, saturated fat is not a single substance but rather a family of molecules having varying lengths, and coconut oil has more of the shorter-length type of saturated fat molecules (known as lauric acid and myristic acid) compared with most animal fats.[6] This has led to speculation that coconut oil might have different effects on cholesterol levels and heart disease risk compared with other sources of saturated fats. Most controlled human studies, however, find significant cholesterol-raising effects of diets high in either myristic acid,[7, 8, 9] lauric acid,[10, 11] or a combination of these two fatty acids,[12] although this increase is usually a combination of both higher low-density lipoprotein (LDL; "bad") and high-density lipoprotein (HDL; "good") cholesterol.

Whether consuming coconut oil will result in unhealthy changes to blood cholesterol levels is controversial. In a double-blind study of young men with normal cholesterol levels, coconut oil was used to create a diet higher in both myristic and lauric acids, and this diet was compared with a similar diet with longer-chain saturated fatty acids. The coconut oil diet resulted in higher levels of both total and LDL cholesterol, whereas HDL levels were not significantly different.[13] Most other controlled studies of healthy young adults have reported that coconut oil increases both LDL and HDL compared with either beef fat, palm oil, or vegetable oils high in unsaturated fats.[14, 15, 16, 17] A controlled study of Polynesians found that a diet with coconut oil resulted in lower LDL levels compared with butter, while HDL was not different between the two diets.[18] However, one trial found no difference in the effects on cholesterol levels of a diet containing small amounts (4% of total calorie intake) of coconut oil compared with similar diets containing other fat sources.[19] More research is needed to determine whether consuming coconut oil will affect the risk of atherosclerosis and heart disease.

Animal studies suggest that coconut oil can affect energy and fat metabolism in a way that could improve the results of a **weight-loss** (page 446) diet.[20] In a two-week double-blind trial investigating the effect of dietary fat on fat metabolism, a diet containing shorter-chain saturated fatty acids from coconut oil and butter was compared with one containing longer-chain saturated fatty acids from beef fat.[21] The coconut oil-butter diet led to changes in fat metabolism that suggested that eating these fats might result in better control of body weight. However, no studies have investigated whether consuming coconut oil actually affects body weight.

According to test tube studies, some of the fatty acids present in coconut oil have antibacterial,[22, 23, 24] antiviral,[25, 26, 27, 28] and **immune system** (page 255)-stimulating effects,[29] suggesting that coconut oil might be helpful in fighting infections. However, no research has investigated these possible effects in humans.

Synthetic fats resembling those found in coconut oil have been found to have anticancer effects in animals but whether these effects would be possible in humans consuming coconut oil is unknown.[30, 31]

Where is it found?

Coconut oil may be found in many types of processed foods, including fried foods, crackers, desserts, candies, whipped topping, and non-dairy creamers. It is also available in some grocery stores for use in cooking.

Who is likely to be deficient?

There is no human requirement for coconut oil or the shorter-length fatty acids it contains, so no deficiency is possible.

How much is usually taken?

The traditional diets of Pacific Islanders contains several grams per day or more of lauric acid from coconut products, which would require at least one tablespoon per day of coconut oil. Research has not established a recommended intake for coconut oil.

Are there any side effects or interactions?

Serious allergic reactions to coconut or coconut oil have been reported but are considered rare.[32, 33, 34]

People using large amounts of coconut oil in their diet should have their blood cholesterol levels checked regularly.

Coconut Oil

COENZYME Q$_{10}$

What is it?

Coenzyme Q$_{10}$ (CoQ$_{10}$) is also called ubiquinone, a name that signifies its ubiquitous (widespread) distribution in the human body. CoQ$_{10}$ is used by the body to transform food into adenosine triphosphate (ATP), the energy on which the body runs.

CoQ$_{10}$ is a powerful **antioxidant** (page 467) that protects the body from free radicals[1] and helps preserve **vitamin E** (page 609), the major antioxidant of cell membranes and blood cholesterol.[2]

CoQ$_{10}$ supplementation has been investigated as a way to improve physical endurance because of its effect on energy production; however, most research shows that CoQ$_{10}$ does not improve **athletic performance** (page 43).[3] In other research, investigators reported no differences in CoQ$_{10}$ in muscles or blood from patients with **fibromyalgia** (page 191) compared with healthy people.[4]

Synthesis of sperm requires considerable energy. Due to its role in energy production, CoQ$_{10}$ has been studied in **infertile men** (page 305). Preliminary research reports that supplementation of CoQ$_7$, a related molecule, increased sperm counts in a group of infertile men.[5]

Healing of the gums of the mouth (periodontal tissue) may require increased energy production; therefore, researchers have explored the effects of CoQ$_{10}$ supplementation in people with **periodontal disease** (page 203), which has been linked to CoQ$_{10}$ deficiency. Double-blind research shows that people with gum disease given CoQ$_{10}$ achieve better results than those given a placebo.[6]

The role of CoQ$_{10}$ in energy formation also relates to how the body uses carbohydrates. Preliminary research suggests that a close relative of this nutrient lowered blood sugar levels in a group of people with **diabetes** (page 152).[7] People with type 2 (adult onset) diabetes have been found to have significantly lower blood levels of CoQ$_{10}$ compared with healthy people.[8]

Virtually every cell of the human body contains CoQ$_{10}$. It is concentrated in the mitochondria, the area of cells where energy is produced. The heart and liver contain the greatest amount of CoQ$_{10}$. It has helped some people with **congestive heart failure** (page 134), (CHF)[9] an effect reported in an analysis of eight controlled trials[10] and found in some,[11] though not all, double-blind studies.[12, 13, 14] The beneficial effects of

CoQ$_{10}$ may not be seen until after several months of treatment. Discontinuation of CoQ$_{10}$ supplementation in people with CHF has resulted in severe relapses and should only be attempted under the supervision of a doctor.[15]

Similar improvements have been reported in people with **cardiomyopathies** (page 95)—a group of diseases affecting heart muscle. Research (including double-blind studies) in this area has been consistently positive.[16]

Also, due to its effect on heart muscle, researchers have studied CoQ$_{10}$ in people with **heart arrhythmias** (page 93). Preliminary research in this area reported improvement after approximately one month in people with premature ventricular beats (a form of arrhythmia) who also suffer from **diabetes** (page 152).[17]

Angina (page 27) patients taking 150 mg per day of CoQ$_{10}$ report a greater ability to exercise without experiencing chest pain.[18] This has been confirmed in independent investigations.[19]

CoQ$_{10}$ appears to increase the heart's tolerance to a lack of oxygen. Perhaps as a result, preliminary research has shown that problems resulting from heart surgery occurred less frequently in people given CoQ$_{10}$ compared with the control group.[20]

Muscle mitochondria lack adequate CoQ$_{10}$ in people with muscular dystrophy, a problem that could affect muscle function. In a double-blind three-month trial, four of eight people with muscular dystrophy had improvements in heart function and sense of well-being when supplementing CoQ$_{10}$.[21]

Mitochondrial function also appears to be impaired in people with **Alzheimer's disease** (page 19). Due to CoQ$_{10}$'s effects on mitochondrial functioning, one group of researchers has given CoQ$_{10}$ (along with **iron** [page 540] and **vitamin B$_6$** [page 601]) to several people with Alzheimer's disease and reported the progression of the disease appeared to have been prevented for one and a half to two years.[22]

CoQ$_{10}$ also modulates **immunity** (page 255).[23] Perhaps as a result, a few cases have been reported in which women with metastatic **breast cancer** (page 65) (cancer that had spread to other tissues) had a regression of their **cancer** (page 87) after treatment with a very large amount of CoQ$_{10}$ (390 mg per day).[24]

CoQ$_{10}$ appears to modulate blood pressure by reducing resistance to blood flow.[25] Several trials have reported that supplementation with CoQ$_{10}$ significantly reduced blood pressure in people with **hypertension** (page 246), usually after ten weeks to four or more months of treatment.[26]

In a double-blind study of 21 patients with chronic renal (kidney) failure, 15 of whom were on dialysis, supplementation with 60 mg of CoQ_{10} three times per day for four weeks improved certain measures of kidney function (BUN [blood urea nitrogen], serum creatinine, and creatinine clearance), compared with placebo, and eliminated the need for dialysis in some patients.[27] Because chronic renal failure is a serious and complicated disease, individuals with this condition should take CoQ_{10} only under strict medical supervision.

In a double-blind trial, administration of 1,200 mg of CoQ_{10} per day for 16 months to people with early Parkinson's disease significantly slowed the progression of the disease, compared with a placebo.[28] Smaller amount of CoQ_{10} were slightly more effective than placebo, but the difference was not statistically significant.

Where is it found?

CoQ_{10} is found primarily in fish and meat, but the amounts in food are far less than what can be obtained from supplements.

Coenzyme Q_{10} has been used in connection with the following conditions (refer to the individual health concern for complete information):

Rating	Health Concerns
★★★	**Angina** (page 27) **Heart attack** (page 212) **High blood pressure** (page 246)
★★☆	**Cardiomyopathy** (page 95) Cerebellar ataxia (familial) **Congestive heart failure** (page 134) **Diabetes** (page 152) **Gingivitis (periodontal disease)** (page 203) **Halitosis** (page 209) (if gum disease) **Migraine headaches** (page 316) **Parkinson's disease** (page 345) Renal (kidney) failure
★☆☆	**Alzheimer's disease** (page 19) **Athletic performance** (page 43) **Breast cancer** (page 65) **Chronic obstructive pulmonary disease** (page 114) (COPD) **HIV support** (page 239) **Infertility (male)** (page 305) **Insulin resistance syndrome** (page 273) (Syndrome X) **Lung cancer** (page 303) Muscular dystrophy **Prostate cancer** (page 371)

Who is likely to be deficient?

Deficiency is poorly understood, but it may be caused by synthesis problems in the body rather than an insufficiency in the diet. Low blood levels have been reported in people with **heart failure** (page 134), **cardiomyopathy** (page 95), **gingivitis** (page 203) (inflammation of the gums), morbid **obesity** (page 446), **hypertension** (page 246), muscular dystrophy, **diabetes** (page 152), **AIDS** (page 239), and in some people on **kidney** (page 284) dialysis. People with **phenylketonuria** (page 354) (PKU) may be deficient in CoQ_{10} because of dietary restrictions.[29] CoQ_{10} levels are also generally lower in older people. The test used to assess CoQ_{10} status is not routinely available from medical laboratories.

Which form of coenzyme Q_{10} is best?

Some,[30] but not all,[31] research suggests that a fat-soluble form of CoQ_{10} is absorbed better than CoQ_{10} in granular (powder) form.[32]

How much is usually taken?

Adult levels of supplementation are usually 30–90 mg per day, although people with specific health conditions may supplement with higher levels (with the involvement of a physician). Most of the research on heart conditions has used 90–150 mg of CoQ_{10} per day. People with **cancer** (page 87) who consider taking much higher amounts should discuss this issue with a doctor before supplementing. There are several anecdotal reports of large amounts of CoQ_{10} resulting in improvements in certain types of cancer. However, controlled trials are needed to confirm these preliminary observations. Most doctors recommend that CoQ_{10} be taken with meals to improve absorption.

Are there any side effects or interactions?

Congestive heart failure (page 134) patients who are taking CoQ_{10} should not discontinue taking CoQ_{10} supplements unless under the supervision of a doctor.

An isolated test tube study reported that the **anticancer** (page 87) effect of a certain cholesterol-lowering drug was blocked by addition of CoQ_{10}.[33] So far, experts in the field have put little stock in this report because its results have not yet been confirmed in animal, human, or even other test tube studies. The drug used in the test tube is not used to treat cancer, and preliminary information regarding the use of high amounts of CoQ_{10} in humans suggests the possibility of *anti*cancer activity.[34, 35, 36]

COLLOIDAL SILVER

What is it?

Colloidal silver is a suspension of the element silver in a solution usually water.

Silver, like mercury, was used as a medicine in the late 1800s and early 1900s. Its prime application was as a topical antiseptic. Use of silver, in the form of silver nitrate solution, is still required by law in most states to be used in newborns as a topical eye drop to prevent eye **infections** (page 265).

In the early 1990s colloidal silver began appearing in the marketplace as a "nutritional supplement." Although tremendous claims and testimonials have been made for colloidal silver, almost none of these are documented with scientific research. Silver is an effective antimicrobial agent; however, the effective concentrations required for any sort of systemic effect with colloidal silver are not likely to be obtained safely with oral administration.[1] Yet, colloidal silver is promoted by certain distributors as an alternative to antibiotics and as treatment for almost every infectious disease.

In response to the growing popularity and unsubstantiated claims, the U.S. Food and Drug Administration (FDA) issued a Final Rule on August 17, 1999, stating that all over-the-counter (OTC) products containing colloidal silver or silver salts are not recognized as safe nor effective.[2] Colloidal silver products are classified by the FDA as misbranded because adequate directions cannot be written so the general public can use these drugs safely for their intended purposes. The products are also misbranded when their labeling falsely suggests there is substantial scientific evidence to establish the drugs are safe and effective for their intended uses. According to the Final Rule, a colloidal silver product for any drug use will first have to be approved by the FDA under drug application procedures.

Despite this Final Ruling from the FDA, colloidal silver will likely continue to be sold as a trace **mineral supplement** (page 559) without medical claims or claims of specific benefits, even though its need in human nutrition is unsubstantiated.

Where is it found?

Colloidal silver is sold as a water-based solution.

Colloidal Silver has been used in connection with the following conditions (refer to the individual health concern for complete information):

Rating	Health Concerns
★☆☆	**Minor burns** (page 85) (topical antiseptic)

Who is likely to be deficient?

Silver is not an essential nutrient, and thus no deficiency state exists.

How much is usually taken?

The typical recommendation is 1 teaspoon per day, with each teaspoon (5 ml) containing 10 parts per million (ppm) of silver or 50 mcg of silver. This amount is in keeping with the average amount of silver consumed from food and water: roughly 350 mcg per day for most people. However, little in known about the relative absorption and toxicity of colloidal silver, compared with that of the silver naturally present in our diet. Because of the lack of long-term safety or efficacy data for colloidal silver, its use cannot be recommended.

Are there any side effects or interactions?

When taken in low amounts (e.g., 50 mcg daily), the body appears able to efficiently excrete silver. However, any silver the body is unable to excrete accumulates in body tissues and can result in argyria—the depositing of silver in the internal organs, tissues, and skin.[3] Argyria causes the skin to turn gray or bluish gray and to turn dark on exposure to strong sunlight. This discoloration is permanent and there is no known effective treatment for it. In addition to argyria, the intake of very large amounts (far in excess of the amount that causes discoloration of the skin) of silver can cause neurological and organ damage and **atherosclerosis** (page 38).

The estimated amount of silver accumulation over a one-year period that is required to produce argyria is 1 to 6 grams. This amount is very large compared to the 50 mcg typically recommended and consumed by people using OTC colloidal silver products. Using the most conservative figure, 1,000 mg (1 gram) of silver corresponds to the silver content in 100 liters of 10 ppm colloidal silver, 50 liters of 20 PPM colloidal silver, or 33.3 liters of 30 PPM colloidal silver.

Colloidal Silver

CONJUGATED LINOLEIC ACID

What is it?

Conjugated linoleic acid (CLA) is a slightly altered form of the essential fatty acid linoleic acid.

Preliminary animal and test tube research suggests that CLA might reduce the risk of **cancers** (page 87) at several sites, including **breast** (page 65), **prostate** (page 371), colorectal, **lung** (page 298), skin, and stomach.[1, 2, 3, 4] Whether CLA will have a similar protective effect for people has yet to be demonstrated in human research.

In a double-blind study, volunteers participating in an exercise program received 600 mg of CLA or a placebo three times per day for 12 weeks. Compared with placebo, CLA significantly reduced percent body fat, but did not significantly reduce body weight.[5] In a double-blind study of obese men, supplementation with 4.2 grams of CLA per day for four weeks produced a small but statistically significant reduction in waist size. However, compared with the placebo, CLA did not promote weight loss.[6] At present, there is not sufficient evidence to support the use of CLA as a treatment for obesity.

Animal research suggests an effect of CLA supplementation on reducing **body fat** (page 446).[7, 8] Limited controlled human research found 5.6-7.2 grams per day of CLA produced nonsignificant gains in muscle size and strength in experienced[9] and inexperienced[10] weight-training men.

Animal research also suggests an effect of CLA supplementation on limiting **food allergy** (page 14) reactions,[11] preventing **atherosclerosis** (page 38),[12, 13] and improving glucose tolerance.[14] As with the cancer research, the effects of CLA on these conditions in humans remains unclear.

Where is it found?

CLA is found mainly in dairy products and also in beef and poultry, eggs, and corn oil. Bacteria that live in the intestine of humans can produce CLA from linoleic acid, but supplementation of a rich source of linoleic acid did not produce increases in blood levels of CLA in one human study.[15] CLA is available as a supplement.

CLA has been used in connection with the following conditions (refer to the individual health concern for complete information):

Rating	Health Concerns
★☆☆	Athletic performance (page 43) (body composition and strength)

Who is likely to be deficient?

No deficiencies of CLA are reported or believed to occur, since it is not an essential nutrient.

How much is usually taken?

Animal research uses very large amounts, equivalent to several grams per day for humans. Until human research is conducted with CLA, the appropriate amount to take of this nutrient remains unclear.

Are there any side effects or interactions?

Overweight (page 446) volunteers who took 4.5 grams of CLA per day for one year had an increase in their blood levels of lipoprotein(a), a risk factor for heart disease.[16] While the significance of this change is not certain, it is possible that long-term use of CLA could increase the risk of developing **heart disease** (page 98).

In a double-blind study of people with **type 2 diabetes** (page 152), supplementing with 3 grams of CLA per day for eight weeks significantly increased blood glucose levels by 6.3% and decreased insulin sensitivity.[17] A reduction in insulin sensitivity was also seen in a study of overweight men without diabetes after treatment with 3 grams of CLA per day for three months,[18] although in a study of young sedentary men, 4 grams of CLA per day for eight weeks improved insulin sensitivity.[19] Thus, although the studies are conflicting, CLA may be harmful for some people who have, or are at risk of developing, diabetes. One unpublished human trial reported isolated cases of gastrointestinal upset.[20]

COPPER

What is it?

Copper is an essential trace element present in the diet and in the human body. It is needed to absorb and uti-

Copper

lize **iron** (page 540). It is also part of the **antioxidant** (page 467) **enzyme** (page 506), superoxide dismutase (SOD). Copper is needed to make adenosine triphosphate (ATP), the energy the body runs on. Synthesis of some hormones requires copper, as does the synthesis of collagen (the "glue" that holds connective tissue together). In addition, the enzyme, tyrosinase, which plays a role in the production of skin pigment, requires copper to function.

Copper supplementation has been shown to increase SOD levels in humans.[1]

Where is it found?

The best source of copper is oysters. Nuts, dried legumes, cereals, potatoes, vegetables, and meat also contain copper.

Copper has been used in connection with the following conditions (refer to the individual health concern for complete information):

Rating	Health Concerns
★★★	**Anemia** (page 25)
★★☆	**High cholesterol** (page 223) **Menkes' disease** (page 311) (injectable copper histidine) **Osteoporosis** (page 333) **Wound healing** (page 319)
★☆☆	**Athletic performance** (page 43) **Benign prostatic hyperplasia** (page 58) **Cardiac arrhythmia** (page 93) **Hypoglycemia** (page 251) **Peripheral vascular disease** (page 352) **Rheumatoid arthritis** (page 387) **Sprains and strains** (page 412)

Who is likely to be deficient?

Many people consume slightly less than the "safe and adequate range" of copper, 1.5–3.0 mg per day. Little is known about the clinical effects of these marginally adequate intakes, though frank copper deficiency is uncommon. Children with **Menkes' disease** (page 311) are unable to absorb copper normally and become severely deficient unless medically treated early in life. Deficiency can also occur in people who supplement with zinc without also increasing copper intake. **Zinc** (page 614) interferes with copper absorption.[2] Health consequences of zinc-induced copper deficiency can be quite serious.[3] In the absence of copper supplementation, **vitamin C** (page 604) supplementation has also

been reported to mildly impair copper metabolism.[4] Copper deficiency can result in anemia, lower levels of HDL ("good") **cholesterol** (page 223), or **cardiac arrhythmias** (page 93).

How much is usually taken?

Most people consume less than the recommended amount of this mineral. Some doctors recommend supplementing the average diet with 1–3 mg of copper per day. While the necessity of supplementing a normal diet with copper has not been proven, most people who take **zinc** (page 614) supplements, including the zinc found in **multivitamin-mineral supplements** (page 559), should probably take additional copper.

Cupric oxide (CuO) is a form of copper frequently used in vitamin-mineral supplements sold over-the-counter. However, animal studies have shown conclusively this form of copper is poorly absorbed from the gut; it should therefore not be used in supplements.[5, 6, 7, 8] Several other forms of copper (including copper sulfate, cupric acetate, and alkaline copper carbonate) are better absorbed, and are therefore preferable to cupric oxide.[9]

Are there any side effects or interactions?

The level at which copper causes problems is unclear. But in combination with **zinc** (page 614), up to 3 mg per day is considered safe. People drinking tap water from new copper pipes should consult their doctor before supplementing, since they might be getting enough (or even too much) copper from their water. People with **Wilson's disease** (page 453) should never take copper.

Zinc interferes with copper absorption. People taking zinc supplements for more than a few weeks should also take copper (unless they have Wilson's disease). In the absence of copper supplementation, **vitamin C** (page 604) may interfere with copper metabolism. Copper improves absorption and utilization of **iron** (page 540).

Preliminary evidence shows that the levels of copper in the blood were higher among people who died from coronary **heart disease** (page 98) than among those who did not.[10] However, animals studies and some human studies suggest that, if anything, copper may prevent the development of heart disease. Although it is not clear why people who died of heart disease had elevated copper levels, this finding could be due to chronic inflammation, which is known to be associated with increased copper levels.[11]

CREATINE MONOHYDRATE

What is it?

Creatine (creatine monohydrate) is a colorless, crystalline substance used in muscle tissue for the production of phosphocreatine, an important factor in the formation of adenosine triphosphate (ATP), the source of energy for muscle contraction and many other functions in the body.[1, 2]

Creatine monohydrate supplementation increases phosphocreatine levels in muscle in most people, especially when accompanied by exercise or carbohydrate intake.[3, 4] However, about 30% of people who take creatine supplements fail to retain significant quantities in the muscle,[5, 6] which may explain the inconsistent results reported in studies of the effects of creatine on **athletic performance** (page 43).

Creatine may increase exercise-related gains in lean body mass,[7, 8, 9] though how much of these gains represents more muscle and how much is simply water retention is unclear.[10] Most, though not all, controlled studies have shown that 20 grams per day of creatine monohydrate taken for five to six days by sedentary or moderately active people, improves performance and delays muscle fatigue during short-duration, high-intensity exercise such as sprinting or weight lifting.[11, 12, 13] However, elderly people appear to gain only minimal, if any, exercise performance benefits from creatine supplementation,[14, 15] and performance outcomes for trained athletes using creatine supplements in competitive situations have not been consistent.[16, 17, 18] Creatine supplementation does not appear to increase endurance performance and may impair it by contributing to weight gain.[19]

Very little research has been done to investigate the exercise performance effects of long-term (over one month) creatine supplementation. Two controlled long-term trials using untrained women[20] or trained men[21] found that creatine improved gains made in strength and lean body mass from weight-training programs. However, a third preliminary trial found only insignificant gains from creatine supplementation in weight-training football players.[22]

The amount of creatine within cells may be deficient in people with muscular dystrophy. This deficiency may contribute to the weakness and degeneration of muscle tissue seen in this condition. A case report described a 9-year old boy with muscular dystrophy who experienced improved muscle performance after creatine supplementation.[23] A double-blind trial found that creatine supplementation (10 grams per day for adults, 5 grams per day for children) slightly but significantly improved muscle strength and performance of daily activities in people with varying types of muscular dystrophy.[24] Creatine supplementation has also been reported to improve strength in certain rare diseases of muscle and energy metabolism.[25, 26, 27]

For people with **congestive heart failure** (page 134), intravenous creatine has been found to improve heart function, but oral supplementation has not been effective, though skeletal muscle function does improve.[28, 29]

A double-blind, study found that 20 grams per day of creatine taken for five days followed by 10 grams per day for 51 days significantly lowered serum total **cholesterol** (page 223) and **triglycerides** (page 235), but did not change either LDL or HDL cholesterol, in both men and women.[30] However, another double-blind trial found no change in any of these blood levels in trained athletes using creatine during a 12-week strength training program.[31] Creatine supplementation in this negative trial was lower—only 5 grams per day was taken for the last 11 weeks of the study.

Where is it found?

Creatine is produced naturally in the human liver, pancreas, and kidneys. It is concentrated primarily in muscle tissues, including the heart. Animal proteins, including fish, are the main source of the 1–2 grams per day of dietary creatine most people consume. Supplements in the form of creatine monohydrate are well absorbed and tolerated by the stomach.

Creatine monohydrate has been used in connection with the following conditions (refer to the individual health concern for complete information):

Rating	Health Concerns
★★★	**Athletic performance** (page 43) (for high-intensity, short duration exercise or sports with alternating low- and high-intensity efforts)
★★☆	**Athletic performance** (page 43) (for non-weight bearing endurance exercise)
★☆☆	**Congestive heart failure** (page 134) **High cholesterol** (page 223) **High triglycerides** (page 235) Muscular dystrophy

Creatine Monohydrate

Who is likely to be deficient?

People involved in intense physical activity, especially those limiting their intake of red meat, may have low muscle stores of creatine. Several muscle diseases, as well as **rheumatoid arthritis** (page 387), and chronic circulatory and respiratory diseases, are associated with lowered creatine levels.[32]

How much is usually taken?

Two methods are used for supplementing with creatine. In the loading method, 20 grams of creatine per day (in four divided amounts mixed well in warm liquid) are taken for five to six days.[33] Muscle creatine levels increase rapidly, which is beneficial if a short-term rise in force is needed, such as during a weight-lifting competition, football game, or sprinting. To maintain muscle creatine levels after this loading period, 2–10 grams per day may be effective.[34, 35]

In another method, 3 grams of creatine monohydrate per day are taken over an extended **training** (page 43) period of at least four weeks, during which muscle creatine levels rise more slowly, eventually reaching levels similar to those achieved with the loading method.[36] However, no trials testing exercise performance changes have been done using this method. Taking creatine with sugar appears to maximize muscle uptake.[37, 38]

Caffeine intake should not be excessive, as large amounts may counteract the benefits of creatine supplementation.[39]

Are there any side effects or interactions?

Little is known about long-term side effects of creatine, but no consistent toxicity has been reported in studies of creatine supplementation. In a study of side effects of creatine, **diarrhea** (page 163) was the most commonly reported adverse effect of creatine supplementation, followed by muscle cramping.[40] Some reports showed that kidney, liver, and blood functions were not affected by short-term higher amounts[41, 42] or long-term lower amounts [43, 44] of creatine supplementation in healthy young adults. In a small study of people taking 5–30 grams per day, no change in kidney function appeared after up to five years of supplementation.[45] However, interstitial nephritis, a serious kidney condition, developed in an otherwise healthy young man, supplementing with 20 grams of creatine per day.[46] Improvement in kidney function followed avoidance of creatine. Details of this case strongly suggest that creatine supplementation triggered this case of kidney disease. Creatine supplementation may also be dangerous for people with existing kidney disease. In one report, a patient with nephrotic syndrome (a kidney disorder) developed glomerulosclerosis (another serious kidney condition) while taking creatine. when the creatine was discontinued, the glomerulosclerosis resolved.[47]

Muscle cramping after creatine supplementation has been anecdotally reported in three studies.[48, 49, 50]

CYSTEINE

What is it?

Cysteine is a nonessential **amino acid** (page 465) (protein building block), meaning that cysteine can be made in the human body. Cysteine is one of the few amino acids that contains **sulfur** (page 590). This allows cysteine to bond in a special way and maintain the structure of proteins in the body. Cysteine is a component of the **antioxidant** (page 467) **glutathione** (page 531). The body also uses cysteine to produce **taurine** (page 590), another amino acid.

Cysteine can also be converted into glucose and used as a source of energy. Cysteine strengthens the protective lining of the stomach and intestines, which may help prevent damage caused by aspirin and similar drugs.[1] In addition, cysteine may play an important role in the communication between **immune system** (page 255) cells.[2] Cysteine is rarely used as a dietary supplement. **N-acetyl cysteine** (page 562) (NAC), which contains cysteine, is more commonly used as a supplement.

Where is it found?

The body can synthesize cysteine from **methionine** (page 557) and other building blocks. Cysteine, the **amino acid** (page 465) from which NAC is derived, is found in most high-protein foods.

Who is likely to be deficient?

According to several studies, blood levels of cysteine and **glutathione** (page 531) are low in people infected with **HIV** (page 239).[3, 4, 5] Cysteine has a role in the proper function of the **immune system** (page 255), so a deficiency of this **amino acid** (page 465) may either contribute to, or result from, immune suppression associated with HIV.

How much is usually taken?

Most people do not need to supplement with cysteine. Almost nothing is known about appropriate supplemental levels, in part because almost all clinical research has been done with **N-acetyl cysteine** (page 562) and not cysteine itself.

Are there any side effects or interactions?
No consistent adverse effects of **NAC** (page 562) have been reported in humans. One small study found that daily amounts of 1.2 grams or more could lead to oxidative damage.[6] Extremely large amounts of cysteine, the **amino acid** (page 465) NAC is derived from, may be toxic to nerve cells in rats.[7]

Adequate amounts of **methionine** (page 557) are needed in the diet, as the precursor to cysteine, to prevent cysteine deficiency.

D-MANNOSE

What is it?
D-mannose is a simple sugar structurally related to glucose. It is absorbed slowly from the gastrointestinal tract, and then a large proportion of it is excreted into the urine.[1]

Where is it found?
D-Mannose is in many fruits, including Peaches, apples, oranges, cranberries, and blueberries.

D-Mannose has been used in connection with the following conditions (refer to the individual health concern for complete information):

Rating	Health Concerns
★☆☆	**Urinary tract infections** (page 436)

Who is likely to be deficient?
As D-mannose is not an essential nutrient, except in certain rare genetic disorders people produce sufficient amounts to provide for the bodies' needs.

How much is usually taken
Some doctors report that D-mannose might help prevent or treat urinary tract infections caused by *E. coli* and recommend 1 teaspoon (5 ml) dissolved in water or juice every two to three hours while awake.[2]

Are there any side effects or interactions?
Test tube studies suggest that consuming large amounts of mannose might lead to birth defects,[3] although this is not considered a likely risk in humans consuming mannose from foods and naturally producing their own mannose.[4] Nonetheless, until more is known, pregnant women should use supplemental mannose with caution.

DHEA

What is it?
DHEA (dehydroepiandrosterone) is one of the hormones produced by the adrenal glands. After being secreted by the adrenal glands, it circulates in the bloodstream as DHEA-sulfate (DHEAS) and is converted as needed into other hormones.

Little is known about how DHEA works in the body.[1] Confusing the picture is the fact that DHEA often has different effects in men, premenopausal women, and postmenopausal women.[2] Supplementation with DHEA-S (a form of DHEA) has resulted in increased levels of testosterone and androstenedione, two steroid hormones.[3]

The conversion of DHEA into testosterone[4] may account for the fact that low blood levels of DHEA have been reported in some men with **erectile dysfunction** (page 185). The findings of a double-blind trial using 50 mg supplements of DHEA taken daily for six months suggests that DHEA may improve erectile function in some men.[5]

Some,[6, 7] but not all,[8, 9] clinical trials have found that DHEA supplementation lowers fat mass without reducing total **body weight** (page 446).[10] In one trial, the reduction in fat mass occurred in men but not in women.[11]

DHEA is believed to indirectly affect blood sugar levels, but information remains incomplete and contradictory. Attempts to affect blood sugar levels in humans have led to improvements,[12] no effect,[13] and, at very high amounts (1,600 mg DHEA per day), a worsening of tolerance to sugar.[14]

DHEA modulates **immunity** (page 255). A group of elderly men with low DHEA levels who were given 50 mg of DHEA per day for 20 weeks experienced a significant activation of immune function.[15] Postmenopausal women have also shown increased immune functioning in just three weeks when given DHEA in double-blind research.[16]

Some reports have suggested that DHEA might reduce the risk of **heart disease** (page 98), perhaps by lowering **cholesterol levels** (page 223). DHEA may

DHEA

also be a blood thinner, an effect that in theory should help protect against heart disease.[17] However, most research supports the idea that DHEA protects against heart disease only weakly for men, and not at all for women.[18, 19] In fact, higher levels of DHEA and DHEAS have been associated with cardiovascular risk factors in women, including **high blood pressure** (page 246) and smoking.[20] Moreover, DHEA has also been reported to lower HDL ("good" cholesterol).[21] Until more is known, DHEA should not be used to protect against heart disease.

Claims have appeared that DHEA is an anti-aging hormone. However, the fact that young people have higher levels of DHEA than older people does not necessarily mean that supplementing DHEA will make people appear younger. In some,[22] but not all,[23] double-blind trials, DHEA has improved the sense of well being in elderly individuals. In one double-blind trial, DHEA supplementation did appear to reduce some of the adverse effects of aging, though it did not create "supermen/superwomen."[24] In that trial, healthy elderly women and men were given either 50 mg of DHEA or a placebo daily for one year. In addition to a re-establishment of more youthful levels of DHEAS, slight increases were also observed in other hormones, such as testosterone and estrogens. In women over 70 years of age, bone mineral loss was improved. A significant increase in most measures of libido was also seen in these older women. Improvements of the skin were also observed in both women and men, but particularly in women, in terms of hydration, thickness, pigmentation and production of sebum (oily secretion that lubricates the skin and hair).

Systemic lupus erythematosus (page 421) (SLE), an autoimmune disease, has been linked to abnormalities in sex hormone metabolism.[25] Supplementation with very large amounts of DHEA (200 mg per day) improved clinical status and reduced the number of exacerbations of SLE in a double-blind trial.[26] A preliminary trial has confirmed the benefit of 50-200 mg per day of DHEA for people with SLE.[27]

DHEA may play some role in protecting against **depression** (page 145). Low DHEA levels have been reported in older women suffering from this condition, though at least one report has linked severe depression to *increased* DHEA levels. After six months using 50 mg DHEA per day, "a remarkable increase in perceived physical and psychological well-being" was reported in both men and women in one double-blind trial.[28] In another double-blind trial, after only six weeks of tak-

ing DHEA at levels up to 90 mg per day, at least a 50% reduction in depression was seen in 5 of 11 participants.[29] Other researchers have reported dramatic reductions in depression at extremely high amounts of DHEA (90-450 mg per day) given for six weeks to adults who first became depressed after age 40 (in men) or at the time of **menopause** (page 311) (in women) in a double-blind trial.[30] Limiting supplementation to only two weeks is inadequate in treating people with depression.[31]

Despite the dramatic results reported in trials lasting at least six weeks, some experts claim that in clinical practice, DHEA appears to be effective for only a minority of depressed people.[32] Moreover, due to fears of potential side effects, most healthcare professionals remain concerned about the use of DHEA. As with other uses of DHEA, depressed people should not take this hormone without supervision from a healthcare professional.

Where is it found?

DHEA is produced by the adrenal glands. A synthetic form of this hormone is also available as a supplement in tablet, capsule, liquid, and sublingual form. Some products claim to contain "natural" DHEA precursors from **wild yam** (page 759). However, the body cannot convert these substances into DHEA[33] (although a series of reactions in a laboratory can make the conversion).

Dehydroepiandrosterone (DHEA) has been used in connection with the following conditions (refer to the individual health concern for complete information):

Rating	Health Concerns
★★☆	Addison's Disease (to correct deficiency) **Crohn's disease** (page 141) **Depression** (page 145) **Erectile dysfunction** (page 185) **HIV support** (page 239) (for fatigue and depression) **Lupus** (page 421) **Schizophrenia** (page 393) **Ulcerative colitis** (page 433)
★☆☆	**Alzheimer's Disease** (page 19) **Chronic fatigue syndrome** (page 111) **Immune Function** (page 255) **Menopause** (page 311) Multi-infarct dementia **Osteoporosis** (page 333) **Weight loss** (page 446)

Who is likely to be deficient?

Meaningful levels of DHEA do not appear in food, and therefore *dietary* deficiency does not exist. Some people, however, may not synthesize enough DHEA. DHEA levels peak in early adulthood and then start a lifelong descent. By the age of 60, DHEA levels are only about 5–15% of what they were at their peak at younger ages.[34] Whether the lower level associated with age represents a deficiency or a normal part of aging that should not be tampered with remains unknown.

People with true adrenal insufficiency (i.e., Addison's Disease; *not* the hypothetical adrenal "fatigue" or "burnout" that is sometimes incorrectly referred to as "insufficiency") have below normal levels of DHEA. When women with adrenal insufficiency were treated with 50 mg of DHEA every morning for three or four months, their DHEA and DHEAS levels returned to normal, with a simultaneous improvement in well-being and sexuality.[35, 36]

Some studies have reported lower DHEA levels in groups of **depressed** (page 145) patients.[37, 38] However, in one trial, severely depressed people were reported to show *increases* in blood levels of DHEA.[39] Despite these contradictory findings, a few clinical trials suggest that at least some people who are depressed may benefit from DHEA supplementation. (See "What does it do?" above for more information about use of DHEA supplements in the treatment of depression.)

People with multi-infarct dementia (deterioration of mental functions resulting from multiple small strokes) may have lower than normal DHEAS levels, according to a preliminary trial.[40] In this trial, intravenous injection of 200 mg per day of DHEAS for four weeks increased DHEAS levels and improved some aspects of mental function and performance of daily activities.

People infected with **HIV** (page 239)[41] and those with insulin-dependent **diabetes** (page 152),[42] congestive heart failure,[43] **multiple sclerosis** (page 323),[44] **asthma** (page 32),[45, 46] **chronic fatigue syndrome** (page 111),[47, 48] **rheumatoid arthritis** (page 387),[49, 50, 51] **osteoporosis** (page 333), and a host of other conditions have been reported to have low levels of DHEA in most,[52] but not all, studies.[53, 54] In most cases, the meaning of this apparent deficiency is not well understood.

Men under 60 years of age with **erectile dysfunction** (page 185) have been found to have lower DHEAS levels than men without the condition.[55] (See "What does it do?" above for more information about use of DHEA supplements in the treatment of men with erectile dysfunction.)

Most,[56, 57, 58, 59] but not all,[60, 61] studies have found that people with **Alzheimer's disease** (page 19) have lower blood DHEAS levels than do people without the condition.

How much is usually taken?

Most people do not need to supplement DHEA. The question of who should take this hormone remains controversial. Some experts believe that daily intakes of 5–15 mg of DHEA for women and 10–30 mg for men are appropriate amounts for people with deficient blood levels of DHEA or DHEAS.[62] While a few researchers suggest supplementation with as much as 50 mg per day in postmenopausal women,[63] others consider this level excessive.[64] People should consult a doctor to have DHEA levels monitored before and during supplementation. Healthy people with normal blood levels of DHEA or DHEAS should not take this hormone until more is known about its effects. However, some doctors recommend DHEA supplementation for selected people with **depression** (page 145), autoimmune diseases, or other problems, even if their blood levels are normal.

People with **systemic lupus erythematosus** (page 421) (SLE) have been shown to improve after taking 100–200 mg per day of DHEA. Such large amounts should never be taken without medical supervision.

Discrepancies between label claims and actual DHEA content of DHEA supplements have been reported.[65] Regrettably, the authors of this report failed to identify which brands were properly labeled and which were not.

Are there any side effects or interactions?

Experts have concerns about the use of DHEA, particularly because long-term safety data do not exist.

Side effects at high intakes (50–200 mg per day) appear to be **acne** (page 4) (in over 50% of people), increased facial hair (18%), and increased perspiration (8%). In a preliminary trial, DHEA was also reported to induce less common side effects, including breast tenderness, weight gain, mood alteration, headache, oily skin, and menstrual irregularity in some people.[66] Since this trial was not controlled, some of these less common "side effects" might have occurred even with a placebo. A case of mania has been reported in an older man who took 200–300 mg of DHEA per day for six months.[67] However, in that case report, other causes of mania could not be ruled out.

Significant increases in testosterone levels in both

DHEA

men and women have been reported in some trials.[68, 69] Other reports have found this change in women but not in men.[70] An increase in testosterone might increase the risk of several **cancers** (page 87), and high amounts of DHEA have caused cancer in animals.[71, 72] Moreover, a possible link between higher DHEA levels and risks of **prostate cancer** (page 371) in humans has been reported.[73] At least one person with prostate cancer has been reported to have had a worsening of his cancer, despite feeling better, while taking very high amounts (up to 700 mg per day) of DHEA.[74]

While younger women with **breast cancer** (page 65) may have low levels of DHEA, postmenopausal women with breast cancer appear to have high levels of DHEA, which has researchers concerned.[75, 76] Most,[77, 78, 79, 80, 81] but not all, studies[82, 83, 84] have found that as DHEA blood levels increase, so does the risk of breast cancer.

Supplementation with high levels of DHEA (100 mg per day) has adversely affected other indicators of cancer risk in both women and men.[85, 86] Elevated DHEA levels have been reported to be associated with both higher,[87] and lower risk for ovarian cancer.[88] The reason for this discrepancy is unknown.

The lack of knowledge about how DHEA supplementation might affect cancer risks provides a reason for caution. Until more is known, people with **breast** (page 65) or **prostate cancer** (page 371) or a family history of these conditions should avoid supplementing with DHEA.

Although *anti*cancer effects of DHEA have also been reported,[89] they involve trials using animals that do not process DHEA the way humans do. Therefore, these positive effects may have no relevance for people.

Some doctors recommend that people taking DHEA have liver enzymes measured routinely. Anecdotes of DHEA supplementation (of at least 25 mg per day) leading to **heart arrhythmias** (page 93) have appeared.[90]

The relationship between DHEA, blood pressure, and heart disease is poorly understood. Increased blood levels of DHEAS have been associated with increased blood pressure[91] and other **cardiovascular risk factors** (page 98) in some,[92] but not all,[93] studies. One study found that people with hypertension had significantly *decreased* blood levels of DHEA.[94] Until clinical trials clear up these inconsistencies and confirm its safety, people with **hypertension** (page 246) should avoid using DHEA, except under the close supervision of a doctor.

At only 25 mg per day, DHEA has lowered HDL cholesterol while increasing insulin-like growth factor (IGF).[95] Decreasing HDL could increase the risk of heart disease. Increasing IGF might increase the risk of breast cancer.

Special United Kingdom considerations
DHEA is either not available or may require a prescription. People should check with their physician.

DIGESTIVE ENZYMES

See also: Bromelain (page 481)

What are they?
Digestive enzymes are complex proteins involved in digestion that stimulate chemical changes in other substances. They work optimally at specific temperature and pH. Digestive enzymes include pancreatic enzymes, plant-derived enzymes, and fungal-derived enzymes. There are three classes of digestive enzymes: proteolytic enzymes needed to digest protein, **lipases** (page 547) needed to digest fat, and amylases needed to digest carbohydrates.

In several conditions that cause **malabsorption** (page 304), such as **pancreatic insufficiency** (page 341) and **cystic fibrosis** (page 143), doctors sometimes prescribe digestive enzymes to improve absorption of food.

Doctors often tell people to try using pancreatic enzymes with meals when they have symptoms of **indigestion** (page 260) that cannot be attributed to a specific cause. In a double-blind study, microencapsulated pancreatic enzymes were shown to reduce **gas, bloating, and fullness** (page 260) after a high-fat meal.[1]

According to one theory, **allergies** (page 14) are triggered by partially undigested protein. Proteolytic enzymes may reduce allergy symptoms by further breaking down undigested protein to sizes that are too small to cause allergic reactions.[2] Limited scientific evidence supports this theory.[3] Proteolytic enzymes such as trypsin, chymotrypsin, and **bromelain** (page 481) are partially absorbed by the body.[4, 5, 6] Once absorbed, they have anti-inflammatory activity and may even demonstrate antitumor effects.[7, 8, 9, 10] In one preliminary study of a handful of pancreatic **cancer** (page 87) patients, the combination of proteolytic enzymes and other cancer treatments appeared to extend survival, despite the fact that most of the patients died.[11]

Proteolytic enzymes may also improve **immune system** (page 255) function, for example, in people with **shingles** (page 401) (herpes zoster), though this area of research has not been adequately explored.[12]

Where are they found?

Only small amounts of the animal-based proteolytic enzymes, trypsin and chymotrypsin, are found in the diet; however, the pancreas can synthesize these enzymes. The plant-based proteolytic enzyme **bromelain** (page 481) comes from the stems of pineapples and is useful in many conditions. Papain comes from unripe papayas. All of these enzymes are available as supplements.

Enzymes have been used in connection with the following conditions (refer to the individual health concern for complete information):

Rating	Health Concerns
★★★	**Low back pain** (page 293) (chymotrypsin, trypsin) **Pancreatic insufficiency** (page 341) (including pancreatitis) **Sprains and strains** (page 412) (chymotrypsin, trypsin)
★★☆	**Celiac disease** (page 102) **Indigestion** (page 260) (**Lipase** [page 547]) **Osteoarthritis** (page 328) (bromelain, trypsin, rutosid combination) **Tendinitis** (page 426) (proteolytic enzymes)
★☆☆	**Acne Rosacea** (page 4) **Chronic candidiasis** (page 109) **Crohn's disease** (page 141) **Food allergies** (page 14) **Gastroesophageal reflux disease** (page 198) (GERD) **Low back pain** (page 293) (papain) **Sprains and strains** (page 412) (papain)

Who is likely to be deficient?

People with **pancreatic insufficiency** (page 341) and **cystic fibrosis** (page 143) frequently require supplemental pancreatic enzymes (which include proteolytic enzymes, **lipases** [page 547], and amylases). In addition, those with **celiac disease** (page 102)[13] or **Crohn's disease** (page 141)[14] and perhaps some people suffering from **indigestion** (page 260)[15] may be deficient in pancreatic enzymes. As **bromelain** (page 481) and papain are not essential, deficiencies do not exist.

How much is usually taken?

The digestive enzymes—proteolytic enzymes, **lipases** (page 547), and amylases—are generally taken together. Pancreatin, which contains all three digestive enzymes, is rated against a standard established by the U.S. Pharmacopeia (USP). For example, "4X pancreatin" is four times stronger than the USP standard. Each "X" contains 25 USP units of amylase, 2 USP units of lipase, and 25 USP units of protease (or proteolytic enzymes). Three to four grams of 4X pancreatin (or a lower amount at higher potency) with each meal is likely to help digest food in some people with pancreatic insufficiency.

Those with chronic pancreatitis need to discuss enzyme intakes with their physician. Under medical supervision, seriously ill people with **pancreatic insufficiency** (page 341) caused by pancreatitis are given very high levels of enzymes to improve fat digestion. In one successful trial, enough pancreatin was used with each meal to supply slightly over 1,000,000 USP units of lipase.[16] Because pancreatin is rapidly emptied from the stomach during digestion, people taking these enzymes may obtain better results by spreading out supplementation throughout the meal.[17]

Supplemental enzymes that state only product weight, but not activity units, may lack potency.

Are there any side effects or interactions?

The most important digestive enzymes in **malabsorption** (page 304) diseases are usually fat-digesting enzymes called **lipases** (page 547). Proteolytic enzymes can digest, as well as destroy, lipases. Therefore, people with enzyme deficiencies may want to avoid proteolytic enzymes in order to spare lipases.[18] If this is not possible (as most enzyme products contain both), people with malabsorption syndromes should talk with their doctor to see if their condition warrants finding products that contain the most lipase and the least protease.

In theory, too much enzyme activity could be irritating because it could start to "digest" parts of the body as the enzymes travel through the digestive system. Fortunately, that does not happen with supplemental amounts. Research has not determined the level at which such problems might arise.

A serious condition involving damage to the large intestines called fibrosing colonopathy has resulted from the use of pancreatic enzymes in children with **cystic fibrosis** (page 143). In some cases, the problem was linked to the use of high supplemental amounts of enzymes.[19, 20, 21] However, the amount of enzymes used

Digestive Enzymes

has not been linked to the problem in all reports.[22] In some cases, lower amounts of enzymes have caused fibrosing colonopathy if the enzymes are enteric-coated.[23] Some researchers now believe that some unknown interaction between the enteric coating and the enzymes themselves may cause damage to the intestines of children with cystic fibrosis.[24] Until more is known, children with cystic fibrosis needing to take pancreatic enzymes should only do so under the careful supervision of a knowledgeable healthcare professional.

DMAE

What is it?

DMAE (2-dimethylaminoethanol) is a chemical produced in the brain.

Like choline, DMAE may increase levels of the brain neurotransmitter acetylcholine; however, not all studies confirm that DMAE serves as a precursor to acetylcholine.[1] Early preliminary research suggested that DMAE may relieve the symptoms of **tardive dyskinesia** (page 425) (a trembling disorder caused by long-term anti-psychotic medication),[2] but several controlled studies did not find the effects of DMAE better than placebo.[3] In fact, one case report suggested that DMAE can cause symptoms of tardive dyskinesia.[4]

One small, uncontrolled four-week trial of senile patients given DMAE supplements of 600 mg three times per day, failed to show any changes in memory but did produce positive behavior changes in some of the patients.[5] However, subsequent double-blind research did not find a significant benefit from the use of DMAE in people with Alzheimer's disease.[6]

Where is it found?

DMAE is found as a supplement, although it is not widely available.

DMAE has been used in connection with the following conditions (refer to the individual health concern for complete information):

Rating	Health Concerns
★☆☆	**Alzheimer's disease** (page 19) **Tardive dyskinesia** (page 425)

Who is likely to be deficient?

No deficiencies of DMAE are reported or believed to occur.

How much is usually taken?

DMAE supplementation is not recommended at this time.

Are there any side effects or interactions?

Clinical studies of DMAE have used up to 1,600 mg per day with no reports of side effects.[7] For this reason, DMAE is believed to be relatively nontoxic. However, one study using higher intakes for **Alzheimer's disease** (page 19) patients did report symptoms of drowsiness and confusion with the use of DMAE.[8] A possible side effect of lucid dreaming (in which the dreamer is conscious and in control of a dream) is suggested with DMAE use.[9] **Depression** (page 145) and hypomania (moderate symptoms of mania) have been reported as side effects of DMAE.[10]

DMSO

What is it?

DMSO (dimethyl sulfoxide) is a colorless, slightly oily liquid that is primarily used as an industrial solvent.

The use of DMSO for therapeutic applications is controversial, but some evidence indicates that DMSO has anti-inflammatory properties and alleviates **pain** (page 338) when applied to the skin. These effects have been reported particularly with connective tissue diseases (such as scleroderma, **osteoarthritis** [page 328], and **rheumatoid arthritis** [page 387]) and **muscle injuries** (page 412).[1, 2, 3] DMSO applied to the affected area appears to reduce pain by inhibiting transmission of pain messages by nerves and may also soften the abnormal connective tissue associated with disorders such as **Dupuytren's contracture** (page 171), keloids, Peyronie's disease, and scleroderma.[4]

Double-blind and other controlled studies have found a 25% DMSO gel effective for pain relief in osteoarthritis of the knee[5] and a 50% DMSO cream helpful for symptoms of acute reflex sympathetic dystrophy.[6] However, while a double-blind trial successfully used a 10% DMSO gel to reduce pain and improve movement in people with acute **tendinitis** (page 426) of the shoulder or elbow,[7] an older double-blind trial found no difference between the effects of a 70% DMSO solution and a 5% DMSO "placebo" solution.[8]

Preliminary research has suggested that DMSO may help relieve symptoms of amyloidosis of the skin.[9]

Some medical doctors have instilled DMSO into the bladder to treat interstitial cystitis.[10] A study from Malaysia reports that oral DMSO reduced relapse rates for **peptic ulcer** (page 349) significantly better than placebo or the ulcer drug, cimetidine.[11] DMSO is sometimes used by physicians as a vehicle to help absorb other therapeutic agents through the skin.

Where is it found?

DMSO is derived from trees as a manufacturing by-product from the processing of paper. Metabolites (breakdown products) of DMSO, such as the sulfide and sulfone forms, are naturally present in the human body. However, the role of these in the body is not clear.

DMSO has been used in connection with the following conditions (refer to the individual health concern for complete information):

Rating	Health Concerns
★★★	**Tendinitis** (page 426) (topical)
★★☆	**Osteoarthritis** (page 328) (topical)
	Rheumatoid arthritis (page 387) (topical)
★☆☆	Amyloidosis (topical)
	Dupuytren's contracture (page 171) (topical)
	Keloid scars (topical)
	Peptic ulcer (page 349)
	Peyronie's disease (topical)
	Reflex sympathetic dystrophy (topical)
	Scleroderma (topical)
	Sprains and strains (page 412) (topical)

Who is likely to be deficient?

DMSO is not an essential nutrient and it is not needed in the functions of a healthy body; therefore, deficiencies do not exist.

How much is usually taken?

DMSO is not indicated for healthy people. Those who do use this substance should consult a doctor familiar with its use. Some physicians do not recommend the use of DMSO due to concerns about safety and questions about efficacy. The potential for contamination exists in some DMSO products designed for industrial uses. DMSO used topically is rapidly absorbed through intact skin. Therefore, the area of skin (and

the hands applying DMSO) must be clean, bec anything on the skin will also be absorbed along with the DMSO.

Are there any side effects or interactions?

DMSO frequently causes a **garlic** (page 679)-like body odor and taste in the mouth. Other reported side effects include **stomach upset** (page 260), **sensitivity to light** (page 356), visual disturbances, and headache. Skin irritation can develop at the site where DMSO is applied topically. Only highly purified, properly diluted DMSO should be used and the skin site and applying hand should be thoroughly cleaned before application, because the solvent properties of DMSO allow contaminants to be absorbed through the skin and transported into the bloodstream. Improperly diluted DMSO can also burn the skin. Check with a healthcare professional for appropriate use.

DOCOSAHEXAENOIC ACID

What is it?

Docosahexaenoic acid (DHA), an omega-3 fatty acid, belongs to the class of nutrients called essential fatty acids.

DHA has been shown to reduce levels of blood triglycerides. **High triglycerides** (page 235) are linked with **heart disease** (page 98) in most, but not all, research. DHA alone appears to be just as effective as **fish oils** (page 514) (which contain both DHA and eicosapentaenoic acid [**EPA** (page 514)]) in beneficially lowering triglyceride levels in people at risk for heart disease.[1] In part, this may be because some DHA is converted to EPA in the body.[2] Unlike EPA, however, DHA may not reduce excessive blood clotting.[3]

DHA appears to be essential for normal visual and neurological (nervous system) development in infants.[4, 5] However, DHA supplementation did not affect the development of visual acuity in formula-fed infants in a double-blind trial.[6] Nevertheless, other double-blind research links DHA supplementation in premature infants to better brain functioning.[7] The effects of DHA on the nervous system may well extend beyond infancy. Young adults given 1.5–1.8 grams DHA per day showed less evidence of aggression in response to mental stress, compared with people in the control group in a double-blind trial.[8]

Docosahexaenoic Acid

DHA supplementation in healthy young men has been shown to decrease the activity of **immune** (page 255) cells, such as natural killer (NK) cells and the cells that regulate inflammation responses in the body.[9] The anti-inflammatory effects of DHA may be useful in the management of autoimmune disorders; however, such benefits need to be balanced with the potential for increased risk of **infections** (page 265).

DHA deficiency plays an important role in a group of congenital diseases called peroxisomal disorders, which damage the protective covering (myelin) around nerves. Although rare, the worst of these disorders (i.e., Zellweger's syndrome) is life-threatening within the first year of life. Daily oral supplementation of 100–600 mg of DHA has been shown to increase blood levels of DHA, to protect myelin, and to improve the signs and symptoms of these potentially devastating disorders.[10]

Where is it found?

Cold-water fish, such as mackerel, salmon, herring, sardines, black cod, anchovies, and albacore tuna, are rich sources of DHA and EPA. Similarly, **cod liver oil** (page 514) contains large amounts of DHA and EPA. Certain microalgae contain DHA and are used as a vegetarian source of this nutrient in some supplements. Most **fish oil** (page 514) supplements contain 12% DHA.

DHA has been used in connection with the following conditions (refer to the individual health concern for complete information):

Rating	Health Concerns
★★★	Childhood intelligence **High blood pressure** (page 246) **High triglycerides** (page 235) Peroxisomal disorders **Rheumatoid arthritis** (page 387)
★★☆	**Depression** (page 145) **Epilepsy** (page 183) (given in combination with EPA) **Lupus** (page 421) **Psoriasis** (page 379)
★☆☆	**Angina** (page 27) **Chronic obstructive pulmonary disease** (page 114) (COPD) **Diabetes** (page 152) **Dysmenorrhea** (page 171) (painful menstruation) **Migraine headaches** (page 316) **Osteoarthritis** (page 328)

Who is likely to be deficient?

Premature infants who are not breast-fed are often DHA-deficient.[11] A link has appeared between DHA deficiency and **Alzheimer's disease** (page 19); however, no evidence at this time indicates that supplementation with DHA will help Alzheimer's patients.[12] Similarly, preliminary evidence shows that children with **attention deficit disorder** (page 55) (ADD) have low DHA levels. However, no evidence demonstrates that DHA supplementation improves ADD.[13] Preliminary evidence suggests that people with a variety of rare but related congenital diseases (Zellweger's syndrome, neonatal adrenoleukodystrophy, and infantile Refsum's disease) may be DHA-deficient, and may even benefit from DHA supplementation.[14] Many doctors believe the diets of most people eating a Western diet do not provide optimal amounts of omega-3 fatty acids.

At least four studies have reported a reduced blood level of omega-3 fatty acids in people with **depression** (page 145).[15, 16, 17, 18]

How much is usually taken?

Most healthy people do not supplement with **fish oil** (page 514) containing DHA or vegetarian sources of DHA. The level of DHA given to premature infants who are not breast-fed should be determined by a pediatrician. Much of the research in adults has been based on 1–3 grams per day of DHA from fish oil, although higher levels have been taken when isolated DHA from microalgae sources is used.

Because **cod liver oil** (page 514) contains large amounts of **vitamin A** (page 595) and **vitamin D** (page 607), women who are or who could become **pregnant** (page 363) should consult a doctor before taking cod liver oil. Adults should make sure the total amount of vitamin A and vitamin D from cod liver oil and other supplements does not exceed 25,000 IU (7,500 mcg) per day for vitamin A (15,000 IU per day for those over age 65) and 800 IU per day for vitamin D, unless they are being supervised by a doctor.

Are there any side effects or interactions?

While those with **heart disease** (page 98) and **diabetes** (page 152) often benefit from **fish oil** (page 514) (the primary source of DHA in the diet),[19, 20] such people should check with their doctor before taking more than 3 or 4 grams of fish oil per day for several months. Elevations in blood sugar have sometimes been reported,[21] though this may simply be due to small increases in **weight** (page 446) resulting from high dietary fish oil.[22] While DHA combined with EPA from fish oil consistently lowers **triglycerides** (page 235), it occasionally increases LDL **cholesterol** (page 223).[23]

Fish oil is easily damaged by oxygen, so small amounts of **vitamin E** (page 609) are often included in fish oil supplements to prevent such oxidative damage.[24] Doctors often recommend that people who supplement with fish oil or DHA take vitamin E supplements to protect EPA and DHA within the body from oxidative damage. Some evidence indicates that vitamin E may be protective against oxidative damage caused by fish oil.[25] However, animal researchers have reported that the oxidative damage caused by DHA alone was not prevented with vitamin E supplementation.[26] The level of oxidative damage caused by DHA has not been shown to result in significant health problems.

Some evidence suggests that adding vitamin E to EPA/DHA may prevent the **fish oil** (page 514)-induced increase in serum glucose.[27] Similarly, the impairment of glucose tolerance sometimes caused by the omega-3 fatty acid has been prevented by the addition of half an hour of moderate exercise three times a week.[28] The effect of DHA by itself on glucose levels has not been adequately studied.

People who take fish oil containing EPA and DHA and who also take 15 grams of pectin per day have been reported to have reductions in LDL **cholesterol** (page 223).[29] This suggests that pectin may overcome the occasional problem of increased LDL cholesterol from fish oil supplementation. The LDL cholesterol-raising effect of EPA and DHA may also be successfully prevented by taking **garlic** (page 679) supplements (or presumably adding garlic to the diet) along with EPA and DHA.[30] Adding pectin or garlic when people supplement with DHA by itself has yet to be studied.

According to a report in a Japanese medical journal, three people at high risk for **colon cancer** (page 123) developed a variety of **cancers** (page 87) after one to two years of supplementation with DHA.[31] To date, this report has not been confirmed by other researchers. To the contrary, test tube studies report that DHA is toxic to cancer cells[32] and may someday be considered as an adjunct to conventional treatment for cancer.[33] Similarly, animal studies suggest that DHA may inhibit cancer.[34]

EVENING PRIMROSE OIL

What is it?

Evening primrose oil (EPO), comes from the seeds of the evening primrose plant. Like black currant seed oil and **borage** (page 475) oil, EPO contains gamma linolenic acid (GLA), a fatty acid that the body converts to a hormone-like substance called prostaglandin E_1 (PGE_1).

PGE_1 has anti-inflammatory properties and may also act as a blood thinner and blood vessel dilator. The anti-inflammatory properties of EPO have been studied in double-blind research with people suffering from **rheumatoid arthritis** (page 387). Some, but not all, studies have reported that EPO supplementation provides significant benefit to these people.[1]

GLA, the primary active ingredient in EPO, has anticancer activity in test tube studies[2] and in some,[3] but not all,[4] animal studies. Injecting GLA into tumors has caused regression of cancer in people in preliminary research.[5] Preliminary evidence in people with cancer suggested "marked subjective improvement,"[6] though not all studies find GLA helpful.[7]

EPO has been reported to lower **cholesterol levels** (page 223) in people in some,[8] but not all,[9] research.

EPO supplementation has been shown to improve skin itching, redness, and dryness associated with kidney dialysis.[10, 11]

Linoleic acid, a common fatty acid found in nuts and seeds and most vegetable oils (including EPO), should theoretically be converted to PGE_1; but many things can interfere with this conversion, including disease; the aging process; saturated fat; hydrogenated oils; blood sugar problems; and inadequate **vitamin C** (page 604), **magnesium** (page 551), **zinc** (page 614), and **B vitamins** (page 603). Supplements that provide GLA circumvent these conversion problems, leading to more predictable formation of PGE_1.[12]

Where is it found?

EPO is found primarily in supplements. Its presumed active ingredient, GLA, can also be found in black currant seed oil and **borage** (page 475) oil supplements. However, it is not known whether the effects of these three oils in the body are the same.

Evening Primrose Oil

Evening primrose oil has been used in connection with the following conditions (refer to the individual health concern for complete information):

Rating	Health Concerns
★★★	**Diabetes** (page 152)
★★☆	**Eczema** (page 177) **Fibrocystic breast disease** (page 189) **Osteoporosis** (page 333) (in combination with fish oil [page 514]) **Premenstrual syndrome (PMS)** (page 368) **Rheumatoid arthritis** (page 387) **Skin ulcers** (page 409)
★☆☆	**Alcohol withdrawal** (page 12) **Atherosclerosis** (page 38) **Attention deficit disorder** (page 55) **Intermittent claudication** (page 276) **Irritable bowel syndrome** (page 280) (IBS) **Multiple sclerosis** (page 323) **Raynaud's disease** (page 382) Scleroderma Sjogren's syndrome **Tardive dyskinesia** (page 425)

Who is likely to be deficient?

Those with **premenstrual syndrome** (page 368),[13] **diabetes** (page 152),[14] scleroderma,[15] Sjogren's syndrome,[16] **tardive dyskinesia** (page 425),[17] **eczema** (page 177),[18] and other skin conditions[19] can have a metabolic block that interferes with the body's ability to make GLA. In preliminary research, supplementation with EPO has helped people with these conditions.[20, 21, 22, 23, 24]

There is evidence that alcoholics may be deficient in GLA, and a double-blind study suggested that **alcohol withdrawal** (page 12) may be facilitated with EPO supplementation.[25] Many people in Western societies may be at least partially GLA-deficient as a result of aging, glucose intolerance, high dietary fat intake, and other problems. People with deficiencies would presumably benefit from supplemental GLA intake from EPO, black currant seed oil, or **borage** (page 475) oil.

How much is usually taken?

Although many people may have inadequate levels of GLA, the optimal intake for this nutrient remains unknown. Researchers often use 3,000–6,000 mg of EPO per day, which provides approximately 270–540 mg of GLA.

Are there any side effects or interactions?

EPO has been reported to exacerbate symptoms of temporal lobe **epilepsy** (page 183), which can sometimes be mistaken for **schizophrenia** (page 393).[26, 27]

Other nutrients are needed by the body, along with EPO, to make PGE_1. Consequently, some experts suggest that **magnesium** (page 551), **zinc** (page 614), **vitamin C** (page 604), **niacin** (page 598), and **vitamin B$_6$** (page 600) should be taken along with EPO.

FIBER

What is it?

Dietary fiber comes from the thick cell wall of plants. It is an indigestible complex carbohydrate. Fiber is divided into two general categories-water soluble and water insoluble.

Soluble fiber lowers **cholesterol** (page 223).[1] An analysis of many trials of soluble fiber reveals it has a cholesterol-lowering effect, but the degree of cholesterol reduction in many studies was quite modest.[2] For unknown reasons, diets higher in *in*soluble fiber (mostly unrelated to cholesterol levels) have been reported to correlate better with protection against **heart disease** (page 98) in both men and women.[3, 4]

Soluble fibers can also lower blood sugar levels in people with **diabetes** (page 152), and some researchers find that increasing fiber decreases the body's need for insulin—a good sign for diabetics.[5] However, a research review reveals that just how much moderate amounts of soluble fiber really help people with diabetes remains unclear.[6] As with **heart disease** (page 98), a clear mechanism to explain how *in*soluble fiber helps diabetics has not been identified. Nonetheless, diets high in insoluble fiber (from whole grains) associate with protection from adult-onset diabetes.[7]

Insoluble fiber softens stool, which helps move it through the intestinal tract in less time. For this reason, insoluble fiber is partially effective as a treatment for **constipation** (page 137).[8] The reduction in "transit time" has also been thought to partially explain the link between a high fiber diet and a reduced risk of **colon cancer** (page 123) as found in some studies,[9] though **anticancer** (page 87) effects unrelated to "transit time" have also been reported.[10]

The true relationship between fiber and colon cancer risk has recently been clouded by data coming from several directions. In animal research, wheat bran is proving to be more protective than other diets containing equal amounts of insoluble fiber, suggesting that fiber in wheat may not be the primary cause of protection sometimes associated with wheat.[11] In human research, a recent well respected study found no significant link between fiber and colon cancer prevention.[12] A trial from South Africa found that avoidance of meat and dairy, and not the presence of fiber, appears to be primarily responsible for a low risk of colon cancer.[13] As a result of these negative findings some researchers and doctors have begun to question the idea that insoluble fiber protects against colon cancer, a concept that had arisen from a large body of older research.

Fiber also fills the stomach, reducing appetite. In theory, fiber should therefore reduce eating, leading to **weight loss** (page 446). However, at least some research has found increased fiber to have no effect on body weight despite decreasing appetite.[14]

Lignan, a fiber-like substance, has mild antiestrogenic activity. Probably for this reason, high lignan levels in urine (and therefore dietary intake) have been linked to protection from **breast cancer** (page 65) in humans.[15]

Where is it found?

Whole grains are particularly high in insoluble fiber. **Oats** (page 716), barley, beans, fruit (but not fruit juice), **psyllium** (page 732), and some vegetables contain significant amounts of both forms of fiber and are the best sources of soluble fiber. The best source of lignan, by far, is **flaxseed** (page 517) (not flaxseed oil, regardless of packaging claims to the contrary).

Fiber has been used in connection with the following conditions (refer to the individual health concern for complete information):

Rating	Health Concerns
★★★	**Constipation** (page 137) **Diabetes** (page 152) **Diverticular disease** (page 168) **High cholesterol** (page 223)
★★☆	**Diarrhea** (page 163) **Hemorrhoids** (page 219) **High blood pressure** (page 246) **Weight loss** (page 446)
★☆☆	**Cirrhosis** (page 290) (combination of beta-glucan, inulin, pectin, and resistant starch) **High triglycerides** (page 235) **Irritable bowel syndrome** (page 280) (fiber other than wheat) **Kidney stones** (page 284) **Peptic ulcer** (page 349) **Premenstrual syndrome** (page 368)

Who is likely to be deficient?

Most people who consume a typical Western diet are fiber-deficient. Eating white flour, white rice, and fruit juice (as opposed to whole fruit) all contribute to this problem. Many so-called whole wheat products contain mostly white flour. Read labels and avoid "flour" and "unbleached flour," both of which are simply white flour. Junk food is also fiber depleted. The diseases listed above are more likely to occur with low-fiber diets.

The benefits of eating whole grains are largely derived from the beneficial constituents present in the outer layers of the grains, which are stripped away in making white flour and white rice. Preliminary research has found that women who ate mostly whole grain fiber had a lower mortality rate than women who ate a comparable amount of refined grains.[16]

How much is usually taken?

Western diets generally provide approximately 10 grams of fiber per day. So-called "primitive societies" consume 40–60 grams per day. Increasing fiber intake to the amounts found in primitive diets may be desirable.

Are there any side effects or interactions?

While people can be **allergic** (page 14) to certain high-fiber foods (most commonly wheat), high-fiber diets are more likely to improve health than cause any health problems. Beans, a good source of soluble fiber, also contain special sugars that are often poorly digested, leading to gas. Special **enzyme** (page 506) products are now available in supermarkets to reduce this problem by improving digestion of these sugars.

Fiber reduces the absorption of many minerals. However, high-fiber diets also tend to be high in minerals, so the consumption of a high-fiber diet does not appear to impair mineral status. However, logic suggests that **calcium** (page 483), **magnesium** (page 551) and **multimineral supplements** (page 559) should not be taken at the same time as a fiber supplement.

Fiber

Fiber

Bran, an insoluble fiber, reduces the absorption of calcium enough to cause urinary calcium to fall.[17] In one study, supplementation with 10 grams of rice bran twice a day reduced the recurrence rate of **kidney stones** (page 284) by nearly 90% in recurrent stone formers.[18] However, it is not known whether other types of bran would have the same effect. Before supplementing with bran, people should check with a doctor, because some people—even a few with kidney stones—do not absorb enough calcium. For those people, supplementing with bran might deprive them of much-needed calcium.

People with scleroderma (systemic sclerosis) should consult a doctor before taking fiber supplements or eating high-fiber diets. Although a gradual introduction of fiber in the diet may improve bowel symptoms in some cases, there have been several reports of people with scleroderma developing severe **constipation** (page 137) and even bowel obstruction requiring hospitalization after fiber supplementation.[19]

FISH OIL AND COD LIVER OIL (EPA AND DHA)

What is it?

Oil from fish contains eicosapentaenoic acid (EPA) and docosahexaenoic acid (**DHA** [page 509]); both are omega-3 fatty acids.

Most fish oil supplements are 18% EPA and 12% DHA, or a total of 30% omega-3. These omega-3 fatty acids, unlike the omega-3 fatty acid found in flaxseed oil and other vegetable oils (such as alpha linolenic acid), keep blood triglycerides in check (**high triglycerides** [page 235] are generally linked with increased risk of **heart disease** [page 98]) and may inhibit the progression of **atherosclerosis** (page 27).[1] EPA and DHA keep blood from clotting too quickly.

EPA and DHA also have anti-inflammatory activity. As a result, fish oil is used to help people with various inflammatory conditions, such as **Crohn's disease** (page 141)[2] and **rheumatoid arthritis** (page 387).[3] The anti-inflammatory effects of EPA and DHA may also account for the findings of some reports that show fish oil supplementation helps some people with **kidney** (page 284) diseases[4, 5, 6] and may help protect against **chronic obstructive pulmonary disease** (page 114).[7]

The omega-3 fatty acids in fish oil help to balance the omega-6 fatty acids, which are found mostly in vegetable oils. When these two groups of fatty acids are out of balance, the body releases chemicals that promote inflammation. People appear to produce more of these inflammatory chemicals when experiencing psychological stress (e.g., academic examinations). With a fatty acid imbalance, inflammatory response to stress appears to be amplified.[8]

Prostaglandins are hormone-like substances produced within the body that regulate dilation of blood vessels, inflammatory response, and other critical processes. Omega-3 fatty acids are needed for prostaglandin formation. Probably as a result of their effect on prostaglandins responsible for blood vessel dilation, a double-blind trial found that omega-3 fatty acids from fish oil helped to treat people with **Raynaud's disease** (page 382).[9]

Schizophrenia (page 393) is linked with abnormalities in fatty acid metabolism, and preliminary research suggests that fish oil supplementation may be helpful to people with schizophrenia.[10] However, a double-blind study that used 3 grams per day of eicosapentaenoic acid failed to demonstrate any benefit for patients with chronic schizophrenia.[11]

DHA is essential for vision in infants. Researchers are now studying this relationship to better understand how much DHA is needed.

EPA and DHA also modulate **immune function** (page 255),[12] probably as a result of their effect on prostaglandin production. Perhaps as a result of this effect, fish oil has helped prevent some types of **cancer** (page 87) in animals[13, 14, 15] and humans,[16] although this evidence remains preliminary.

Preliminary evidence also shows that omega-3 fatty acids from fish oil may help regulate the rhythm of the heart. EPA and DHA have been reported to help prevent **cardiac arrhythmias** (page 93).[17]

Where is it found?

EPA and **DHA** (page 509) are found in mackerel, salmon, herring, sardines, sablefish (black cod), anchovies, albacore tuna, and wild game. Cod liver oil contains large amounts of EPA and DHA. Fish oil supplements typically contain 18% EPA and 12% DHA, though more purified (i.e., higher in EPA and DHA) fish oil supplements are sometimes available. In addition, DHA is available in a supplement that does not contain significant amounts of EPA.

Fish oil has been used in connection with the following conditions (refer to the individual health concern for complete information):

Rating	Health Concerns
★★★	**Crohn's disease** (page 141) (enteric-coated, free-fatty-acid form of fish oil) **High blood pressure** (page 246) **High triglycerides** (page 235) **Rheumatoid arthritis** (page 387)
★★☆	**Asthma** (page 32) **Atherosclerosis** (page 38) **Bipolar disorder** (page 61) **Breast-feeding support** (page 74) **Cardiac arrhythmia** (page 93) (do not take, or take only with a doctor's supervision, if there is a history of sustained ventricular tachycardia or ventricular fibrillation) **Cystic fibrosis** (page 143) (EPA) **Depression** (page 145) **Eczema** (page 177) **Heart attack** (page 212) **Immune function** (page 255) (omega-3 fatty acids for critically ill and post surgery patients only) Kidney disease **Lupus** (page 421) **Osteoporosis** (page 333) (in combination with **evening primrose oil** [page 511]) **Phenylketonuria** (page 354) (if deficient in polyunsaturated fatty acids) **Pre- and post-surgery health** (page 357) **Pregnancy and postpartum support** (page 363) (to prevent premature delivery) **Psoriasis** (page 379) **Raynaud's disease** (page 382) **Schizophrenia** (page 393) **Sickle cell anemia** (page 403) **Ulcerative colitis** (page 433)
★☆☆	**Angina** (page 27) **Chronic fatigue syndrome** (page 111) **Chronic obstructive pulmonary disease** (page 114) (COPD) **Colon cancer** (page 123) (reduces risk) **Diabetes** (page 152) **Dysmenorrhea** (page 171) (painful menstruation) **Endometriosis** (page 182) **Glaucoma** (page 206) **Migraine headaches** (page 316) **Multiple sclerosis** (page 323) **Osteoarthritis** (page 328) **Osteoporosis** (page 333) **Photosensitivity** (page 356) **Preeclampsia** (page 361)

Who is likely to be deficient?

So-called "primitive" diets have much higher levels of EPA and **DHA** (page 509) than modern diets. As a result, some researchers and doctors believe that most people who eat a typical western diet are likely to be consuming less-than-optimal amounts of EPA and DHA. To a very limited extent, omega-3 fatty acids from vegetable sources, such as **flaxseed oil** (page 517), can convert to EPA.

At least four studies have reported a reduced blood level of omega-3 fatty acids in people with **depression** (page 145).[18, 19, 20, 21]

People with **rheumatoid arthritis** (page 387) have been found to have decreased levels of omega-3 fatty acids, such as are found in fish oil, in their joint fluid and blood.[22]

How much is usually taken?

Presumably, healthy people who frequently eat fatty fish (several times per week) have no need to supplement with fish oil. How much EPA and **DHA** (page 509), if any, should be supplemented by healthy people who do *not* eat much fatty fish, remains unclear.

Most researchers studying the effects of EPA and DHA in humans who have a variety of health conditions have given those people at least 3 grams of the total of EPA plus DHA—an amount that may require 10 grams of fish oil, because most fish oil contains only 18% EPA and 12% DHA.

The health benefits for people with **Crohn's disease** (page 141) have been reported with a special, enteric-coated preparation of purified EPA/DHA manufactured from fish oil. This preparation of purified fatty acids has also been reported to not cause the gastrointestinal symptoms that often result from taking regular fish oil supplements, again suggesting unique benefit.[23]

In one trial, the maximum amount of fish oil tolerated by people being treated for cancer-related weight loss was reported to be approximately 21 grams per day.[24] However, in people who do not have **cancer** (page 87), the maximum tolerated amount may be different.

Are there any side effects or interactions?

While those with **heart disease** (page 98) and **diabetes** (page 152) have often been reported to benefit from supplementation with fish oil,[25, 26] both groups should check with their doctor before taking more than 3 grams of fish oil per day for several months. Elevations in blood sugar and **cholesterol** (page 223) levels may occur in some people who take fish oil.[27]

The increase in blood sugar appears to be related in part to the amount of fish oil used.[28] Some evidence suggests that adding **vitamin E** (page 609) to fish oil may prevent the fish oil-induced increase in blood sugar levels.[29] In other research, the impairment of sugar metabolism sometimes caused by supplementation with fish oil has been prevented by the addition of half an hour of moderate exercise three times a week.[30]

While supplementation with fish oil consistently lowers **triglycerides** (page 235), the effect of fish oil on LDL ("bad") cholesterol varies, and in some people, fish oil supplementation has been reported to increase LDL levels.[31] People who took fish oil and who also took 15 grams of pectin per day were reported to have reductions in LDL **cholesterol** (page 223).[32] This suggests that pectin may overcome the occasional problem of increased LDL cholesterol reported in people who supplement with fish oil. The LDL-cholesterol raising effect of EPA and **DHA** (page 509) has also been reported to be prevented by taking **garlic** (page 679) supplements (or presumably including garlic in the diet) along with EPA and DHA.[33]

FLAVONOIDS

What are they?

Flavonoids are a class of water-soluble plant pigments. Flavonoids are broken down into categories, though the issue of how to divide them is not universally agreed upon. One system breaks flavonoids into isoflavones, anthocyanidins, flavans, flavonols, flavones, and flavanones.[1] Some of the best-known flavonoids, such as genistein in **soy** (page 587), and **quercetin** (page 580) in onions, can be considered subcategories of categories. Although they are all structurally related, their functions are different. Flavonoids also include hesperidin, rutin, citrus flavonoids, and a variety of other supplements.

While they are not considered essential nutrients, some flavonoids support health by strengthening capillaries and other connective tissue, and some function as anti-inflammatory, antihistaminic, and antiviral agents. Quercetin has been reported to block the "sorbitol pathway" that is linked to many problems associated with **diabetes** (page 152). Rutin and several other flavonoids may also protect blood vessels.

As **antioxidants** (page 467), some flavonoids, such as quercetin, protect LDL ("bad") **cholesterol** (page 223) from oxidative damage. Others, such as the anthocyanidins from **bilberry** (page 634), purple cabbage, and grapes, may help protect the lens of the eye from **cataracts** (page 101). Animal research suggests that naringenin, found in grapefruit, may have **anticancer** (page 87) activity.[2] Soy isoflavones are also currently being studied to see if they help fight cancer.

In a small, preliminary trial, rutoside (500 mg twice daily), a derivative of the flavonoid, rutin, combined with **vitamin C** (page 604) (500 mg twice daily) produced marked improvement in three women with progressive pigmented purpura (PPP), a mild skin condition.[3] Although not a serious medical condition, cosmetic concerns lead persons with PPP to seek treatment with a variety of drugs. The vitamin C/rutoside combination represents a promising, non-toxic alternative to these drug treatments, but larger, controlled trials are needed to confirm these preliminary results.

Where are they found?

Flavonoids are found in a wide range of foods. For example, flavanones are in citrus, isoflavones in soy products, anthocyanidins in wine and **bilberry** (page 634), and flavans in apples and tea.

Flavonoids have been used in connection with the following conditions (refer to the individual health concern for complete information):

Rating	Health Concerns
★★★	**Chronic venous insufficiency** (page 116) (rutin) **Edema** (page 180) (water retention) (coumarin, hydroxyethylrutosides) **Hepatitis** (page 220) (catechin)
★★☆	**Bruising** (page 84) **Cold sores** (page 119) **Diabetes** (page 152) (**bilberry** [page 634]) **Dysmenorrhea** (page 171) (rutin plus **vitamin B₃** [page 598] [niacin] and **vitamin C** [page 604]) **Edema** (page 180) (water retention) (diosmin and hesperidin combination) **Gingivitis** (page 203) (periodontal disease) (in combination with **vitamin C** [page 604]) **Hemorrhoids** (page 219) (hydroxyethylrutosides derived from rutin) **Ménière's disease** (page 308) (hydroxyethylrutosides) **Retinopathy** (page 385) (**bilberry** [page 634]) **Skin ulcers** (page 409) (diosmin, hesperidin)

★☆☆ **Allergies** (page 14)
Atherosclerosis (page 38) (**quercetin** [page 580], **bilberry** [page 634])
Cancer (page 87) (naringenin)
Capillary fragility (page 93) (hesperidin, **quercetin** [page 580], rutin)
Cataracts (page 101) (**quercetin** [page 580], **bilberry** [page 634])
Diabetes (page 152) (**quercetin** [page 580])
Edema (page 180) (water retention) (**quercetin** [page 580])
Gingivitis (page 203) (periodontal disease)
Glaucoma (page 205) (rutin)
Hay fever (page 211) (**quercetin** [page 580], hesperidin, rutin)
Macular degeneration (page 303) (**bilberry** [page 634])
Measles (page 307)
Menopause (page 311) (hesperidin)
Menorrhagia (page 314) (heavy menstruation)
Night blindness (page 326) (**bilberry** [page 634])
Peptic ulcer (page 349) (**quercetin** [page 580])
Progressive pigmented purpura (in combination with **vitamin C** [page 604])
Retinopathy (page 385) (**quercetin** [page 580], rutin)

Who is likely to be deficient?

Flavonoid deficiencies have not been reported.

How much is usually taken?

Flavonoid supplements are not required to prevent deficiencies in people eating a healthy diet. Healthcare practitioners commonly recommend 1,000 mg of citrus flavonoids taken one to three times per day. Alternatively, 240–600 mg of **bilberry** (page 634) (standardized to 25% anthcyanosides) may be taken per day.

Are there any side effects or interactions?

No consistent side effects have been linked to the flavonoids except for catechin, which can occasionally cause fever, anemia from breakdown of red blood cells, and **hives** (page 245).[4, 5] These side effects subsided when treatment was discontinued.

In 1980, **quercetin** (page 580) was reported to induce cancer in animals.[6] Most further research did not find this to be true, however.[7, 8] While quercetin is mutagenic in test tube studies, it does not appear to be mutagenic in animal studies.[9] In fact, quercetin has been found to inhibit both tumor promoters[10] and human cancer cells.[11] People who eat high levels of flavonoids have been found to have an overall *lower* risk of getting a wide variety of **cancers** (page 87),[12] though preliminary human research studying only foods high in quercetin has found no relation to cancer risk one way or the other.[13] Despite the confusion, in recent years experts have shifted their view of quercetin from concerns that it might cause cancer in test tube studies to guarded hope that quercetin has anticancer effects in humans.[14]

The flavonoids work in conjunction with **vitamin C** (page 604). Citrus flavonoids, in particular, improve the absorption of vitamin C.[15, 16]

FLAXSEED AND FLAXSEED OIL

What is it?

Flaxseed, called linseed in some countries, is a good source of dietary **fiber** (page 512), **omega-3 fatty acids** (page 509), and lignans. Each of these components may contribute to the health effects of eating flaxseed, but flaxseed oil contains no fiber and very little lignan.

Like most vegetable oils, flaxseed oil contains linoleic acid, an essential fatty acid needed for survival. But unlike most oils, it also contains significant amounts of another essential fatty acid, alpha linolenic acid (ALA).

ALA is an omega-3 fatty acid. To a limited extent, the body turns ALA into eicosapentaenoic acid (EPA)—an omega-3 fatty acid found in **fish oil** (page 514)—which in turn converts to beneficial prostaglandins. (Prostaglandins are hormone-like substances made in many parts of the body rather than coming from one organ, as most hormones do.)

While fish oil has been shown to have anti-inflammatory activity, an anti-inflammatory effect of flaxseed oil has not been demonstrated conclusively. Some doctors have argued that, because ALA can be converted to EPA and **DHA** (page 509) (the fatty acids found in **fish oil** [page 514]), flaxseed oil should be useful for the same conditions as fish oil. However, the conversion of ALA to EPA and DHA is limited, so that argument may turn out to be incorrect. For example, while numerous studies have shown that fish oils are beneficial for **rheumatoid arthritis** (page 387), flaxseed oil failed to work for this condition in the only known trial.[1] In 1994, a diet purportedly high in ALA was successful in preventing **heart disease** (page 98),[2] but this study altered many dietary factors, so ALA may not have been solely responsible for the outcome.[3] Flaxseed oil does not appear to be a good replacement for fish oil for people with elevated **triglycerides** (page 235).[4, 5] ALA does not reduce excess platelet aggregation ("sticky platelets"), another risk factor for heart disease, the way fish oil does.[6] However, flaxseed oil may help **lower cholesterol** (page 223),[7] and research specific to flaxseed oil indicates that it may also **lower blood pressure** (page 246).[8]

Flaxseed is the most abundant food source of lignans, a family of phytochemicals that is drawing the interest of many health researchers.[9, 10, 11] Lignans are not actually present in flaxseed; rather intestinal bacteria produce them from precursors in flaxseed.[12, 13] Lignans have antioxidant activity,[14] and test tube and animal research suggests they may also have significant effects on the metabolism and function of the hormone estrogen.[15, 16, 17]

Where is it found?

In addition to its presence in flaxseed oil, small amounts of ALA are also found in canola, **soy** (page 587), black currant, and walnut oils. Small amounts of lignans are present in a wide variety of foods of plant origin.

Flaxseed and flaxseed oil has been used in connection with the following conditions (refer to the individual health concern for complete information):

Rating	Health Concerns
★★★	**Constipation** (page 137) (flaxseed) **Systemic lupus erythematosus** (page 421) (flaxseed)
★★☆	**High cholesterol** (page 223) (flaxseed)
★☆☆	**Benign prostatic hyperplasia (BPH)** (page 58) (flaxseed oil) **Constipation** (page 137) (flaxseed oil) **Ulcerative colitis** (page 433) (flaxseed)

Who is likely to be deficient?

ALA deficiencies are possible but believed to be rare, except in infants who are fed formula that is omega-3 deficient. Lignan is not an essential nutrient, so deficiencies are not possible.

How much is usually taken?

For promoting bowel regularlity, 1 tablespoon (15 ml) of whole or ground flaxseed is taken one or two times per day, accompanied by a full glass of water. When used to treat other health conditions, it is used in amounts of 30 to 35 grams (1 to 2 ounces) per day.

Although it is not suitable for cooking, flaxseed oil (unlike **fish oil** [page 514]) can be used in salads. Some doctors recommend that people use 1 tablespoon (15 ml) of flaxseed oil per day as a supplement in salads or on vegetables to ensure a supply of essential fatty acids. Some conversion of ALA to EPA does occur,[18] and this conversion can be increased by restricting the intake of other vegetable oils.[19]

For those who wish to replace fish oil with flaxseed oil, research suggests taking up to ten times as much ALA as EPA.[20] Typically, this means 7.2 grams of flaxseed oil equals 1 gram of fish oil. However, even if taken in such high amounts, flaxseed oil may not have the same effects as fish oil. But, flaxseed oil will not cause a fishy-smelling burp (a possible side effect of fish oil).

Are there any side effects or interactions?

Flaxseed oil toxicity has not been reported. However, there is conflicting information about the effect of flaxseed oil and one of its major constituents, ALA, on **cancer** (page 87) risk.

While most test tube and animal studies suggest a possible protective role for ALA against **breast cancer** (page 65),[21, 22, 23, 24, 25] one animal study[26] and a preliminary human study[27] suggested increased breast cancer risk from high dietary ALA. Another preliminary human study reported that higher breast tissue levels of ALA are associated with less advanced breast cancer at the time of diagnosis.[28] For **prostate cancer** (page 371), a test tube study reported ALA promoted cancer cell growth,[29] but preliminary human studies have shown ALA to be associated with either an increased[30, 31] or decreased risk,[32] or no change[33] at all.

Advocates of flaxseed oil speculate that a potential association between ALA and cancer may be due to the fact that meat contains ALA, thus implicating ALA when the real culprits are probably other components of meat. In some studies, however, saturated fat (and therefore probably meat) were taken into consideration, and ALA still correlated with increased risk. The associations between ALA and cancer might eventually be shown to be caused by substances found in foods rich in ALA rather than by ALA itself. However, ALA has been reported to become mutagenic (able to cause precancerous changes) when heated,[34] which concerns some doctors.

The effect of ALA as an isolated substance, and of

flaxseed oil on the risk of cancer in humans remains unclear, with most animal and test tube studies suggesting protection, and some preliminary human trials suggesting cause for concern. It is premature to suggest that ALA and flaxseed oil will either cause or protect against human cancer at this time.

Flaxseed oil is not suitable for cooking and should be stored in an opaque, airtight container in the refrigerator or freezer. If the oil has a noticeable odor it is probably rancid and should be discarded.

As with any source of fiber, flaxseed should not be taken if there is possibility that the intestines are obstructed. People with scleroderma (systemic sclerosis) should consult a doctor before using flaxseed. Although a gradual introduction of fiber in the diet may improve bowel symptoms in some cases, there have been several reports of people with scleroderma developing severe constipation and even bowel obstruction requiring hospitalization after fiber supplementation.[35]

Animal research suggests that large amounts of flaxseed or lignans consumed during pregnancy might adversely affect the development of the reproductive system.[36] No studies have attempted to investigate whether this could be a problem in humans.

Allergic reactions to flaxseed have occasionally been reported, but are considered very uncommon.[37, 38]

FLUORIDE

What is it?

Fluoride is a binary compound of fluorine and tin.

Fluoride appears to have at least two separate mechanisms by which it prevents **tooth decay** (page 431). It affects the demineralization and remineralization of teeth in a way that makes teeth stronger.[1] Fluoride also reduces the production of acid by oral bacteria, protecting the teeth from damage.[2] Fluoride appears to have both topical and whole-body effects.[3]

Fluoride is one of few materials known to stimulate osteoblasts, the cells responsible for building new bone.[4] While exposure to fluoride clearly causes people to have denser bones, the bone that is formed may not be of optimal quality,[5] and may not reduce fracture risk significantly.

Where is it found?

Fluoride is a trace mineral found in varying concentrations in foods and in water. Foods high in fluoride include fish, tea, and many different vegetables. Fluoride is added into the municipal water supply of many cities in the United States. For those people without access to fluoridated water, fluoride supplements are available in the forms of tablets and drops. These supplements are not available without a prescription. Many non-prescription dental care products contain fluoride as well, including toothpastes and mouthwashes.

Fluoride has been used in connection with the following conditions (refer to the individual health concern for complete information):

Rating	Health Concerns
★★★	**Tooth decay** (page 431)
★☆☆	**Osteoporosis** (page 333)

Who is likely to be deficient?

As fluoride is not considered an essential mineral, it does not have an associated deficiency state. Regardless, people living in areas with low concentrations of fluoride in the drinking water do appear to be at a higher risk of significant **tooth decay** (page 431) than those living in areas with high amounts of natural or added fluoride.

How much is usually taken?

Drinking water containing 1 mg of fluoride per liter is considered to be roughly the optimal amount for the prevention of tooth decay. For those without access to fluoridated drinking water, chewable fluoride tablets containing 0.25 to 1 mg per day of fluoride or fluoride mouthrinses with 0.05% to 0.2% fluoride content can be used. Liquid fluoride drops are also available.

Are there any side effects or interactions?

The risks associated with fluoridation of the public water supply have been the subject of vigorous and often heated debate since fluoridation began in 1945. Although much research has been done regarding the safety of fluoridation, a recent review found all prior studies to be of sub-optimal quality and far from definitive.[6]

Some,[7, 8] but not all,[9, 10] studies have found a correlation between the amount of fluoride intake and increased risk of osteoporotic fractures. The validity of the studies that found increased risk of fracture in communities with fluoridated water has been questioned by some scientists.[11] A pooled analysis of 29 studies on this issue concluded that there did not appear to be an increased risk of fracture in areas of water fluoridation.[12]

Dental fluorosis, a brown staining of teeth due to fluoride exposure during childhood, is the best-documented adverse effect of fluoride. At a water fluoride level of 1 part per million (or 1 mg per liter), roughly 13% will have fluorosis to an aesthetically concerning degree.[13]

Some scientists have concluded that water fluoridation is associated with an increased risk of bone tumors,[14] although most others disagree.[15]

FOLIC ACID

What is it?
Folic acid is a B vitamin needed for cell replication and growth. Folic acid helps form building blocks of DNA, the body's genetic information, and building blocks of RNA, needed for protein synthesis in all cells. Therefore, rapidly growing tissues, such as those of a fetus, and rapidly regenerating cells, like red blood cells and **immune** (page 255) cells, have a high need for folic acid. Folic acid deficiency results in a form of anemia that responds quickly to folic acid supplementation.

The requirement for folic acid increases considerably during **pregnancy** (page 363).[1] Deficiencies of folic acid during pregnancy are associated with low birth weight and an increased incidence of **neural tube defects** (page 63) in infants.[2] In one study, women who were at high risk of giving birth to babies with neural tube defects were able to lower their risk by 72% by taking folic acid supplements prior to and during pregnancy.[3] Most doctors, many other healthcare professionals, and the March of Dimes recommend that all women of childbearing age supplement with 400 mcg per day of folic acid. Such supplementation would protect against the formation of neural tube defects during the time between conception and when pregnancy is discovered. If a woman waits until after pregnancy has been discovered to begin taking folic acid supplements, it will probably be too late to prevent a neural tube defect.

Other **birth defects** (page 63) may be prevented with folic acid supplementation as well. Women who take folic acid-containing **multivitamin supplements** (page 559) around the time they conceive may also reduce the risk of other congenital malformations, such as **heart defects** (page 63), defects of the upper lip and mouth,[4] **urinary tract defects** (page 63),[5, 6] and **limb-**

reduction defects (page 63).[7, 8] Rates of prevention of **cleft lip** (page 63) and cleft palate may be improved by using very large amounts of folic acid (6 mg per day).[9] A doctor should supervise anyone wishing to take this much folic acid.

Folic acid is needed to keep **homocysteine** (page 234) (an **amino acid** [page 465] by-product) levels in blood from rising. A growing body of evidence suggests that an elevated homocysteine level is a risk factor for **heart disease** (page 98)[10] and may also be linked to several other diseases. Folic acid and certain other B vitamins function as cofactors for **enzymes** (page 506) that can lower homocysteine levels. Research has shown that supplementing with folic acid reduces homocysteine levels.[11] Of the B vitamins with a role in homocysteine metabolism, folic acid appears to be the most important in lowering homocysteine levels for the average person.[12, 13] A deficiency of folic acid has also been associated with peripheral vascular disease and coronary artery disease even in people with normal homocysteine levels, suggesting that the vitamin may have protective effects that extend beyond its role in maintaining normal homocysteine levels.[14]

In 1996, the FDA began to require that all enriched flour, rice, pasta, cornmeal, and other grain products contain 140 mcg of folic acid per 100 grams.[15] Among people who do not take **vitamin supplements** (page 559), this amount of food fortification has been associated with increased folic acid levels in the blood and decreased blood levels of homocysteine.[16] Nevertheless, evidence is mounting that the FDA-mandated level of folic acid fortification in food is inadequate to fully prevent neural tube defects.[17] Until fortification rates are quadrupled, women who can possibly become pregnant are advised to take a folic acid supplement of 400 mcg per day.

A diet low in folic acid has been associated with a high incidence of pre-cancerous polyps in the colon, suggesting that folic acid may prevent the development of **colon cancer** (page 123).[18] Two studies have shown that reduced folic acid levels are associated with an increase in the incidence of **cancer** (page 87) in people with **ulcerative colitis** (page 433)[19, 20] and a third study showed the degree of abnormal cell growth decreases as folic acid intake increases.[21] Three large population studies showed that low folic acid intake is associated with an increased risk of colorectal cancer.[22, 23, 24]

In addition, decreased blood levels of folic acid are associated with an increased risk of colon cancer in women.[25] Long-term supplementation with folic acid from a **multivitamin** (page 559) has been found in one large population study to be associated with a reduced risk of colon cancer. However, 15 years of supplementation was necessary before a significant reduction in colon-cancer risk became apparent. In that study, folic acid from dietary sources alone was associated with a modest reduction in the risk of colon cancer.[26]

Total folic acid intake was not associated with overall risk of **breast cancer** (page 65) in preliminary studies.[27, 28] However, among women who consume at least one alcoholic beverage per day, the risk of breast cancer appears to be highest among those with low folic acid intake. Current use of a multivitamin supplement has also been associated with lower breast cancer risk among women who consume at least 1.5 alcoholic beverages per day, compared with those who never use a multivitamin supplement.

Where is it found?

Beans, leafy green vegetables, citrus fruits, beets, wheat germ, and meat are good sources of folic acid.

Folic acid has been used in connection with the following conditions (refer to the individual health concern for complete information):

Rating	Health Concerns
★★★	**Birth defects prevention** (page 63) **Depression** (page 145) **Gingivitis (periodontal disease)** (page 203) (rinse only) **High homocysteine** (page 235) (in combination with **vitamin B₆** [page 600] and **vitamin B₁₂** [page 601]) **Pap smear (abnormal)** (page 3) (in women taking oral contraceptives) **Pregnancy and postpartum support** (page 363) **Schizophrenia** (page 393) (for deficiency)
★★☆	**Anemia** (page 25) (for thalassemia if deficient) **Atherosclerosis** (page 38) **Breast cancer** (page 65) (reduces risk in women who consume alcohol) **Canker sores** (page 90) (for deficiency only) **Celiac disease** (page 102) (for deficiency only) **Colon cancer** (page 123) (prevention) **Heart attack** (page 212) **Preeclampsia** (page 361) **Sickle cell anemia** (page 403) (for lowering homocysteine (page 235) levels) **Skin ulcers** (page 409) **Ulcerative colitis** (page 433)

Rating	Health Concerns
★☆☆	**Alzheimer's disease** (page 19) **Bipolar disorder/Manic depression** (page 61) **Crohn's disease** (page 141) **Dermatitis herpetiformis** (page 151) (for deficiency) **Diarrhea** (page 163) **Down's syndrome** (page 169) **Epilepsy** (page 183) **Gingivitis (periodontal disease)** (page 203) (pill) **Gout** (page 208) **HIV support** (page 239) **Lung cancer** (page 298) (reduces risk) **Osteoporosis** (page 333) **Peripheral vascular disease** (page 352) **Psoriasis** (page 379) **Restless legs syndrome** (page 384) **Seborrheic dermatitis** (page 400) **Stroke** (page 419) (for high homocysteine only) **Vitiligo** (page 443)

Who is likely to be deficient?

Many people consume less than the recommended amount of folic acid. Scientists have found that people with **heart disease** (page 98) commonly have elevated blood levels of **homocysteine** (page 235), a laboratory test abnormality often controllable with folic acid supplements. This suggests that many people in Western societies have a mild folic acid deficiency. In fact, it has been suggested that increasing folic acid intake could prevent an estimated 13,500 deaths from cardiovascular diseases each year.[29]

Folic acid deficiency has also been common in **alcoholics** (page 12), people living at poverty level, those with **malabsorption disorders** (page 304) or liver disease (e.g., **cirrhosis** [page 290]), and women taking the birth control pill. Recently, elderly people with hearing loss have been reported to be much more likely to be folic acid deficient than healthy elderly people.[30] A variety of prescription drugs including cimetidine, antacids, some **anticancer** (page 87) drugs, triamterene, sulfasalazine, and anticonvulsants interfere with folic acid.

Deficiency of folic acid can be precipitated by situations wherein the body requires greater than normal amounts of the vitamin, such as **pregnancy** (page 363), infancy, leukemia, exfoliative dermatitis, and diseases that cause the destruction of blood cells.[31]

The relationship between folic acid and prevention of **neural tube defects** (page 63) is partly thought to result from the high incidence of folate deficiency in many societies. To protect against neural tube defects, the U.S. Food and Drug Administration has mandated that some grain products provide supplemental folic acid at a level expected to increase the dietary intake by an average of 100 mcg per day per person. As a result of folic acid added to the food supply, fewer Americans will be depleted compared with the past. In 1999, scientific evidence began to demonstrate that the folic acid added to the U.S. food supply was having positive effects, including a partial lowering of homocysteine levels.[32] In the same year, however, a report from the North Carolina Birth Defects Monitoring Program suggested the current level of folic acid fortification has not reduced the incidence of neural-tube defects.[33] Many doctors and the Centers for Disease Control in Atlanta[34] believe that optimal levels of folic acid intake may still be higher than the amount now being added to food by several hundred micrograms per day. A low blood level of folate has also been associated with an increased risk of miscarriage.[35]

People with kidney failure have an increased risk of folic acid deficiency.[36] Recipients of kidney transplants often have elevated homocysteine levels, which may respond to supplementation with folic acid.[37] The usual recommended amount of 400 mcg per day may not be enough for these people, however. Larger amounts (up to 2.4 mg per day) may produce a better outcome, according to one double-blind trial.[38]

Folate deficiency is more prevalent among elderly African American women than among elderly white women.[39]

Which form is best?

Folic acid naturally found in food is much less available to the body compared with synthetic folic acid found both in **supplements** (page 559) and added to grain products in the United States. Women with a recent history of giving birth to babies with **neural tube defects** (page 63) participated in a study to determine which form of folic acid is best absorbed—dietary folic acid or folic acid from supplements.[40] They received either orange juice containing 400 mcg of folic acid per day or a supplement containing the same amount. Overall, the supplement folic acid was better absorbed than the folic acid from orange juice.

How much is usually taken?

Many doctors recommend that all women who are or who could become **pregnant** (page 363) take 400 mcg

per day in order to reduce the risk of **birth defects** (page 63). Some doctors also extend this recommendation to other people in an attempt to reduce the risk of **heart disease** (page 98) by lowering **homocysteine** (page 235) levels. Since the FDA mandated addition of folic acid to grain products, many people who eat grains have followed the new recommendation of supplementing only 100 mcg of folic acid per day. However, studies have found that this amount of folic acid is inadequate to maintain normal folate levels in a significant percentage of the groups assessed.[41] It now appears that, for pregnant women, supplementing with at least 300 mcg (and optimally 400 mcg) of folic acid per day is sufficient to prevent a folate deficiency, even if dietary intake is low.

Are there any side effects or interactions?

Folic acid is not generally associated with side effects.[42] However, folic acid supplementation can interfere with the laboratory diagnosis of **vitamin B$_{12}$** (page 601) deficiency, possibly allowing the deficiency to progress undetected to the point of irreversible nerve damage.[43] Although vitamin B$_{12}$ deficiency is uncommon, no one should supplement with 1,000 mcg or more of folic acid without consulting a doctor.

Vitamin B$_{12}$ deficiencies often occur without anemia (even in people who do not take folic acid supplements). Some doctors do not know that the absence of anemia does not rule out a B$_{12}$ deficiency. If this confusion delays diagnosis of a vitamin B$_{12}$ deficiency, the patient could be injured, sometimes permanently. This problem is rare and should not happen with doctors knowledgeable in this area using correct testing procedures.

Folic acid is needed by the body to utilize vitamin B$_{12}$. **Proteolytic enzymes** (page 506) inhibit folic acid absorption.[44] People taking proteolytic enzymes are advised to supplement with folic acid.

FRUCTO-OLIGOSACCHARIDES (FOS) AND OTHER OLIGOSACCHARIDES

What is it?

The term "oligosaccharide" refers to a short chain of sugar molecules ("oligo" means "few" and "saccharide" means "sugar.") Fructo-oligosaccharides (FOS) and inulin, which are found in many vegetables, consist of short chains of fructose molecules. Galacto-oligosaccharides (GOS), which also occur naturally, consist of short chains of galactose molecules. These compounds can be only partially digested by humans.[1, 2, 3, 4] When oligosaccharides are consumed, the undigested portion serves as food for "friendly" bacteria, such as **Bifidobacteria** (page 575) and *Lactobacillus* (page 575) species.

Clinical studies have shown that administering FOS, GOS, or inulin can increase the number of these friendly bacteria in the colon while simultaneously reducing the population of harmful bacteria.[5, 6, 7, 8, 9] Other benefits noted with FOS, GOS, or inulin supplementation include increased production of beneficial short-chain fatty acids such as butyrate, increased absorption of **calcium** (page 483) and **magnesium** (page 551), and improved elimination of toxic compounds.[10, 11]

Because FOS, GOS, and inulin improve colon function and increase the number of friendly bacteria, one might expect these compounds would help relieve the symptoms of **irritable bowel syndrome** (page 280). However, a double-blind trial found no clear benefit with FOS supplementation (2 grams three times daily) in patients with this condition.[12] Experimental studies with FOS in animals suggest a possible benefit in lowering blood sugar levels in people with **diabetes** (page 152) and in reducing elevated blood **cholesterol** (page 223) and **triglyceride** (page 235) levels.[13]

In a double-blind trial of middle-aged men and women with elevated cholesterol and triglyceride levels, supplementation with inulin (10 grams per day for eight weeks) significantly reduced insulin concentrations (suggesting an improvement in blood-glucose control) and significantly lowered triglyceride levels.[14] In a preliminary trial, administration of FOS (8 grams per day for two weeks) significantly lowered fasting blood-sugar levels and serum total-cholesterol levels in patients with type 2 (non-insulin-dependent) diabetes.[15] However, in another trial, people with type 2 diabetes supplementing with FOS (15 grams per day) for 20 days found no effect on blood-glucose or lipid levels.[16] In addition, double-blind trials of healthy people showed that supplementing with FOS or GOS for eight weeks had no effect on blood-sugar levels, insulin secretion, or blood lipids.[17, 18] Because of these conflicting results, more research is needed to determine the effect of FOS and inulin on diabetes and lipid levels.

Several double-blind trials have looked at the ability of FOS or inulin to lower blood cholesterol and triglyc-

eride levels. These trials have shown that in people with elevated total **cholesterol** (page 223) or **triglyceride** (page 235) levels, including people with type 2 (adult onset) **diabetes** (page 152), FOS or inulin (in amounts ranging from 8 to 20 grams daily) produced significant reductions in triglyceride levels. However, the effect on cholesterol levels was inconsistent.[19, 20, 21, 22] In people with normal or low cholesterol or triglyceride levels, FOS or inulin produced little effect.[23, 24, 25]

Where is it found?

FOS and inulin are found naturally in Jerusalem artichoke, **burdock** (page 648), chicory, leeks, onions, and asparagus. FOS products derived from chicory root contain significant quantities of inulin,[26] a fiber widely distributed in fruits, vegetables and plants, which is classified as a food ingredient (not as an additive) and is considered to be safe to eat.[27] In fact, inulin is a significant part of the daily diet of most of the world's population.[28] FOS can also be synthesized by **enzymes** (page 506) of the fungus *Apergillus niger* acting on sucrose. GOS is naturally found in soybeans and can be synthesized from lactose (milk sugar). FOS, GOS, and inulin are available as nutritional supplements in capsules, tablets, and as a powder.

FOS, GOS, and inulin have been used in connection with the following conditions (refer to the individual health concern for complete information):

Rating	Health Concerns
★★☆	**Elevated triglyceride levels** (page 235)
★☆☆	**Diabetes** (page 152)
	Pre- and post-surgery health (page 357)

Who is likely to be deficient?

As FOS, GOS, and inulin are not essential nutrients, no deficiency state exists.

How much is usually taken?

The average daily intake of oligosaccharides by people in the United States is estimated to be about 800 to 1,000 mg. For the promotion of healthy bacterial flora, the usual recommendation for FOS, GOS, or inulin is 2,000 to 3,000 mg per day with meals. In the studies on **diabetes** (page 152) and high blood lipids (**cholesterol** [page 223] and **triglycerides** [page 235]), amounts ranged from 8 to 20 grams per day.

Fructo-oligosaccharides (FOS)

Are there any side effects or interactions?
Generally, oligosaccharides are well tolerated. Some people reported increased **flatulence** (page 260) in some of the studies. At higher levels of intake, that is, in excess of 40 grams per day, FOS and the other oligosaccharides may induce **diarrhea** (page 163).

There is a report of a 39-year old man having a life-threatening allergic reaction after consuming high amounts of inulin from multiple sources, including FOS.[29] **Allergy** (page 14) to inulin in this person was confirmed by laboratory tests. Such sensitivities are extremely rare. People with a confirmed sensitivity to inulin should probably avoid FOS.

FUMARIC ACID

What is it?
Fumaric acid is related to malic acid, and, like **malic acid** (page 552), it is involved in the production of energy (in the form of adenosine triphosphate [ATP]) from food.

Where is it found?
Fumaric acid is formed in the skin during exposure to sunlight, as well as being available as an oral supplement and as a preparation for topical use.

Fumaric acid has been used in connection with the following conditions (refer to the individual health concern for complete information):

Rating	Health Concerns
★★★	**Psoriasis** (page 379)

Who is likely to be deficient?
No deficiencies of fumaric acid have been reported. However, some doctors suggest that people with **psoriasis** (page 379) may have a biochemical defect that interferes with adequate fumaric acid production in the skin.

How much is usually taken?
Only the esterified forms of fumaric acid are used therapeutically, such as fumaric acid monoethylester or fumaric acid di-methylester. Healthy people do not need to supplement with fumaric acid. Those using this substance (either orally or topically) should work with a dermatologist, since determining the optimal intake should be done on an individual basis. Even under these circumstances, supplementing should be started with small amounts (60–100 mg per day) and increased gradually over several weeks until an effect is noted.

Are there any side effects or interactions?
Kidney disorders have been reported in people taking fumaric acid esters, possibly due to taking large amounts too quickly.[1, 2] Most studies have reported **gastrointestinal upset** (page 195) and skin flushing as common side effects; some have also found decreased white blood cell counts with prolonged use.[3, 4].

GABA (GAMMA-AMINO BUTYRIC ACID)

What is it?
GABA is a natural calming and anti-epileptic agent in the brain that is manufactured from the amino acid **glutamine** (page 530) and glucose.

Since GABA does not cross the blood-brain barrier very well (i.e., it cannot be transported efficiently into the brain from the bloodstream), virtually all of the GABA found in the brain is manufactured there.[1] For that reason, supplemental GABA would not be expected to increase levels of GABA in the brain. Two doctors have reported that GABA is beneficial in the treatment of a variety of brain disorders, including **epilepsy** (page 183) and **schizophrenia** (page 393).[2] However, those reports have not been substantiated with clinical trials. High intake of GABA was shown to produce a significant increase in plasma growth-hormone levels (single administration of 5,000 mg) and prolactin (daily administration of 18,000 mg for four days) in one human study[3] but the clinical significance of these observations is not clear.

Where is it found?
GABA is found as a nutritional supplement, primarily in capsules and tablets.

Who is likely to be deficient?
Some people with **anxiety** (page 30), panic disorders, and **depression** (page 145) may not manufacture sufficient levels of GABA.

How much is usually taken?
Some doctors recommend GABA in the amount of 200 mg four times daily.

Are there any side effects or interactions?
The safety of GABA supplementation has not been demonstrated in human trials.

GAMMA ORYZANOL

What is it?
Gamma oryzanol is a naturally occurring mixture of plant chemicals called sterols and ferulic acid esters.

Some evidence suggests that gamma oryzanol increases testosterone levels, stimulates the release of endorphins (pain-relieving substances made in the body), and promotes the growth of lean muscle tissue.[1] Supplementation with gamma oryzanol for nine weeks did not influence **exercise performance** (page 43) in male weight lifters.[2]

Where is it found?
Gamma oryzanol is a natural component of rice bran, corn, and barley oils. Gamma oryzanol is also available as a supplement.

Gamma oryzanol has been used in connection with the following condition (refer to the individual health concern for complete information):

Rating	Health Concerns
★★☆	**Gastritis** (page 195)
★☆☆	**Athletic performance** (page 43)

Who is likely to be deficient?
Since gamma oryzanol is not an essential nutrient, it is not associated with a deficiency state.

How much is usually taken?
Much of the human research with gamma oryzanol used 300 mg per day. Healthy people do not appear to need this supplement.

Are there any side effects or interactions?
Some research suggests that gamma oryzanol taken in moderately high amounts (up to 600 mg per day) for several months can cause dry mouth, sleepiness, hot flushes, irritability, and light headedness in some individuals.[3]

GLANDULAR EXTRACTS

See also: **Adrenal Extracts** (page 462), **Liver Extracts** (page 547), **Spleen Extracts** (page 588), **Thymus Extracts** (page 591), **Thyroid Extracts** (page 592)

What is it?
A gland is defined as a secretory organ (i.e., an organ that secretes substances into the bloodstream or elsewhere in the body). The internal secretory organs of the body are called endocrine glands. These ductless glands secrete hormones directly into the blood stream. The glands that are known to have endocrine function include the pineal, pituitary, thyroid, parathyroid, thymus, adrenal, pancreas, and gonads (testes and ovaries). Although not technically glands, other organs of the body are commonly also referred to as "glandulars" when they are taken as supplements. For example, tissue extracts of the heart, spleen, prostate, uterus, brain, and other tissues are often used in so-called "glandular therapy," along with extracts from pineal, pituitary, thyroid, parathyroid, thymus, adrenal, pancreas, and gonads. Glandular therapy refers to the use of animal tissues to try to enhance the function of, or mimic the effect of, the corresponding human tissue.

There are two basic concepts upon which glandular therapy is based. The first is that "like heals like." For example, feeding prostate tissue might, in theory, help the body's prostate gland heal or function better. The second concept is that ingestion of certain glandular tissues will provide the body with hormones or other biologically active substances that are normally secreted by that gland. For almost as long as historic records have been kept, glandular therapy has been an important form of medicine. While ancient glandular therapy usually involved the use of fresh, whole glands, modern glandular therapy primarily involves the use of concentrated glandular extracts.

While it is well established that some glandular preparations may be effective orally because of active hormone or enzyme content (e.g., thyroid and pancreatic-enzyme preparations), the effects of other commercially available glandular products are not known as they have not been sufficiently studied.

Glandular Extracts

Detractors of glandular therapy often claim that when a glandular product is consumed, its potentially active components are destroyed by **digestive enzymes** (page 506) in the gastrointestinal tract before they can be absorbed into the body. Therefore, orally administered glandular products cannot be effective. However, there is now much evidence that, under normal conditions, some proteins, enzymes, and other large molecules can and do pass intact from the human gut into the bloodstream.[1, 2, 3, 4]

Where is it found?

Most glandular products are derived from beef (bovine) sources, with the exception of pancreatic extracts, which are most often derived from pork (porcine). The four most widely known methods of processing are the azeotrophic method, salt precipitation, freeze-drying, and predigestion.

The azeotrophic method begins by quick-freezing the material at well below 0 degrees F, and then washing the material with a powerful solvent (ethylene dichloride) to remove the fatty tissue. The solvent is then distilled off and the material is dried and ground into a powder so that it can be placed in tablets or capsules. Although the azeotrophic method aids in the removal of fat-stored toxins (like pesticides) and toxic heavy metals, it also removes fat-soluble hormones, enzymes, essential fatty acids, and other potentially beneficial materials.

The salt precipitation method involves the maceration of fresh glandular material in a salt and water solution. Like the azeotrophic method, this process also allows the fat-soluble material to be separated out. The benefit of the salt precipitation method is that no toxic solvents are used to remove the fatty material. The down side is that the salt content can be very high, and that some of the potentially beneficial constituents may be removed.

The freeze-drying process involves quickly freezing the glandular material at temperatures 40 to 60 degrees below 0 degrees F and then placing the material into a vacuum chamber, which removes the water by direct vaporization from its frozen state—hence the term freeze-drying. The benefits of freeze-drying are that it preserves more of the unaltered protein and enzymes as well as all of the fat-soluble components. Since the fat is not removed, potentially harmful contaminants that accumulate in fat tissue may remain in the product. It is

therefore critical that the glands be derived from livestock that have grazed on open ranges that are not sprayed with pesticides or herbicides. The animals should also be free of antibiotics, synthetic hormones, and infection.

The predigestion method employs the aid of plant and animal enzymes to partially digest or hydrolyze the glandular material. The partially digested material is then passed through a series of filtrations to separate out fat-soluble and large molecules. The purified material is then freeze-dried. This method of extraction is thought to be ideal for certain glandulars, such as liver and thymus, where the polypeptide (small proteins) and other water-soluble fractions are desired.

Who is likely to be deficient?

As glandulars are not essential nutrients, no deficiency states exist.

How much is usually taken?

The recommended amount may vary according to the potency and method of preparation of the particular product. Please consult the label on the specific glandular product.

Are there any side effects or interactions?

Refer to the specific glandular product.

GLUCOMANNAN

What is it?

Glucomannan is a water-soluble dietary **fiber** (page 512) that is derived from konjac root (*Amorphophallus konjac*). Like other forms of dietary fiber, glucomannan is considered a "bulk-forming laxative." Glucomannan promotes a larger, bulkier stool that passes through the colon more easily and requires less pressure—and subsequently less straining—to expel.

Good results have been noted in preliminary[1] and double-blind studies[2, 3, 4, 5] of glucomannan for the treatment of **constipation** (page 137). In constipated individuals, glucomannan and other bulk-forming laxatives generally help produce a bowel movement within 12 to 24 hours.[6] The use of glucomannan for **diverticular disease** (page 168) of the colon has also been studied in preliminary research; about one-third to one-half of the subjects were found to benefit from glucomannan.[7]

Glucomannan delays stomach emptying, leading to a more gradual absorption of dietary sugar; this effect can reduce the elevation of blood sugar levels that is typical after a meal.[8] Controlled studies have found that after-meal blood sugar levels are lower in people with diabetes given glucomannan in their food,[9] and overall diabetic control is improved with glucomannan-enriched diets according to preliminary[10] and controlled[11, 12] trials. One preliminary report suggested that glucomannan may also be helpful in pregnancy-related diabetes.[13] One double-blind study reported that glucomannan (8-13 grams per day) stabilized blood sugar in people with the **insulin resistance syndrome** (page 273) (syndrome X).[14] In a preliminary study,[15] addition of either 2.6 or 5.2 grams of glucomannan to a meal prevented **hypoglycemia** (page 251) in adults with previous stomach surgery; a similar study of children produced inconsistent results.[16]

Like other soluble fibers, glucomannan can bind to bile acids in the gut and carry them out of the body in the feces, which requires the body to convert more cholesterol into bile acids.[17] This can result in the lowering of blood **cholesterol** (page 223) and other blood fats. Controlled[18, 19] and double-blind[20, 21] studies have shown that supplementation with several grams per day of glucomannan significantly reduced total blood cholesterol, LDL ("bad") cholesterol, and **triglycerides** (page 235), and in some cases raised HDL ("good") cholesterol. One double-blind study reported that glucomannan (8-13 grams per day) lowered total and LDL cholesterol in people with the insulin resistance syndrome.[22]

Glucomannan may help **weight loss** (page 446) by occupying space in the stomach, thereby making a person feel full. One double-blind study reported weight loss averaging 5.5 pounds in adults when one gram of glucomannan was taken with a cup of water one hour before each meal for eight weeks.[23] However, a similar study of overweight children found that glucomannan was not significantly more effective than a placebo.[24] Other controlled studies have found that glucomannan improves the results of weight loss diets in overweight adults[25] and children.[26]

Where is it found?

Glucomannan is a purified fiber from konjac root that is available as a bulk powder or in hard-gelatin capsules.

Whether any foods contain significant amounts of glucomannan is unclear.

Glucomannan has been used in connection with the following conditions (refer to the individual health concern for complete information):

Rating	Health Concerns
★★★	**Constipation** (page 157) **Diabetes** (page 152) **High blood cholesterol** (page 246) **Insulin resistance syndrome** (page 273) (Syndrome X)
★★☆	**Obesity** (page 446)
★☆☆	**Diverticular disease** (page 168) **Hypoglycemia** (page 251)

Who is likely to be deficient?

As glucomannan is not an essential nutrient, no deficiency state exists.

How much is usually taken?

The amount of glucomannan shown to be effective as a laxative is 3–4 grams per day.[27, 28] Effective amounts for lowering blood cholesterol have been 4–13 grams per day.[29, 30, 31] For controlling blood sugar, 500–700 mg of glucomannan per 100 calories in the diet has been used successfully in controlled research.[32, 33] For weight loss, 1 to 3 grams before each meal has been effective.[34, 35] When using glucomannan and other dietary fiber supplements, it is best to start out with a small amount and increase gradually. It is recommended to drink at least 8 ounces of water each time any bulk-forming laxative, including glucomannan, is taken.

Are there any side effects or interactions?

People with any disorder of the esophagus (the tube leading from the mouth to the stomach) should not take any fiber supplement in a pill form, as the supplement may expand in the esophagus and lead to obstruction.[36] Preliminary reports in humans, as well and animal research, suggest that some people may be sensitive to inhaled glucomannan powder.[37]

Since intestinal bacteria ferment water-soluble fibers, a great deal of intestinal gas may be produced in individuals not accustomed to a high fiber diet, leading to flatulence and abdominal discomfort.

Glucomannan

GLUCOSAMINE

What is it?

Glucosamine is an important building block needed by the body to manufacture specialized molecules called glycosaminoglycans, found in cartilage.

Glucosamine is almost exclusively researched and used for the treatment of **osteoarthritis** (page 328) (OA).

Where is it found?

Glucosamine is not present in significant amounts in most diets. Supplemental sources are derived from the shells of shrimp, lobster, and crab, or may be synthesized.

Glucosamine has been used in connection with the following conditions (refer to the individual health concern for complete information):

Rating	Health Concerns
★★★	**Osteoarthritis** (page 328) (glucosamine sulfate)
★★☆	Knee pain (glucosamine HCl)
★☆☆	**Minor injuries** (page 319) **Osteoarthritis** (page 328) (glucosamine HCl) **Sprains and strains** (page 412) **Wound healing** (page 319) (oral)

Who is likely to be deficient?

A glucosamine deficiency in humans has not been reported.

Which form is best?

Glucosamine is available in several forms. The glucosamine sulfate (GS) form (stabilized with a mineral salt) is the only form clearly shown in clinical trials to be effective for **osteoarthritis** (page 328). For this reason, it is the preferred form.

GS is stabilized with one of two mineral salts: sodium chloride (NaCl) or potassium chloride (KCl).[1, 2] Although they both appear to effectively stabilize GS, the use of KCl as a stabilizer seems preferable since the average Western diet already provides far too much salt (NaCl) and not enough **potassium** (page 572). However, most of the research has been done with the NaCl-stabilized form.

Glucosamine hydrochloride (GH) has been widely available as a dietary supplement for years, but only one trial has evaluated this form of glucosamine as a single remedy for OA.[3] This trial found only minor significant benefits from 1,500 mg per day of GH for eight weeks, in people with osteoarthritis of the knee who were also taking up to 4,000 mg/day of acetaminophen. To more fairly evaluate the effects of GH, future research should involve people not taking pain-relieving medication.

Another form of glucosamine, **N-acetyl-glucosamine (NAG)** (page 564), has not been studied in people with **osteoarthritis** (page 328).

How much is usually taken?

Healthy people do not need to routinely supplement with glucosamine. Most research with people who have **osteoarthritis** (page 328), uses 500 mg three times per day of GS. Appropriate amounts for other conditions are not known.

Are there any side effects or interactions?

At the amount most frequently taken by adults—500 mg three times per day of GS—adverse effects have been limited to mild reversible gastrointestinal side effects. In one trial, people with **peptic ulcers** (page 349) and those taking diuretic drugs were more likely to experience side effects.[4]

Animal research has raised the possibility that glucosamine could contribute to **insulin resistance** (page 273).[5, 6] This effect might theoretically result from the ability of glucosamine to interfere with an **enzyme** (page 506) needed to regulate blood sugar levels.[7] However, available evidence does not suggest that taking glucosamine supplements will trigger or aggravate insulin resistance or **high blood sugar** (page 251).[8] Two large, 3-year controlled trials found that people taking GS had either slightly *lower* blood glucose levels or no change in blood sugar levels, compared with people taking placebo.[9, 10] Until more is known, people taking glucosamine supplements for long periods may wish to have their blood sugar levels checked; people with **diabetes** (page 152) should consult with a doctor before taking glucosamine and should have blood sugar levels monitored if they are taking glucosamine.

In 1999 the first case of an **allergic reaction** (page 14) to oral GS was reported.[11] Allergic reactions to this supplement appear to be rare.

Some GS is processed with sodium chloride (table salt), which is restricted in some diets (particularly for people with **high blood pressure** [page 246]).

The theory that GS and **chondroitin sulfate** (page 492) work synergistically in the treatment of **osteoarthritis** (page 328) remains unproven.

GLUCOSAMINE/ CHONDROITIN

Glucosamine and chondroitin are building blocks of connective tissue and are key components of the joints.

For detailed discussions of these nutrients, please see the individual articles for **glucosamine sulfate** (page 528) and **chondroitin sulfate** (page 492).

Glucosamine is a simple molecule that is available as a supplement in several forms: glucosamine sulfate, glucosamine hydrochloride and N-acetyl-glucosamine (**NAG** [page 564]). The glucosamine sulfate (GS) form (stabilized with a mineral salt, such as sodium chloride or potassium chloride) is the only form consistently shown in clinical trials to be effective for people with **osteoarthritis** (OA [page 328]).

Chondroitin sulfate (CS [page 492]) is a much larger and more complex molecule than GS. Like glucosamine, it is a major constituent of cartilage and has been the subject of many clinical trials. CS supplementation has proven to be an effective treatment for people with OA.

When to take glucosamine, chondroitin sulfate, or both: The popular idea that GS is clinically "preferred" over CS, or that CS is "not necessary,"[1] has not been examined (let alone supported) by appropriate comparative research. An analysis of controlled clinical trials evaluated the independent effects of GS and CS in the treatment of OA.[2] The authors concluded that the overall efficacy in trials of CS for people with OA exceeded the overall efficacy of GS for people with that condition. However, more than one-third of CS supplements have been reported to contain less than 40% of the amount of CS listed on the label.[3] Moreover, no single clinical trial has compared the effects of the two supplements.

Many people with osteoarthritis take combinations of CS and GS or glucosamine HCl. This practice may be based on the suggestion, made in a best-selling book,[4] that GS and CS in combination have stronger effects than either supplement alone. Although this idea may sound appealing, and may be harmless, it is based only on anecdotes and hypotheses. The theory that GS and CS work synergistically in the treatment of osteoarthritis remains unproven. To date, no clinical trials have compared glucosamine/chondroitin combinations with either of the supplements taken individually.

One preliminary trial found that the combination of glucosamine HCl (1,600 mg per day), CS (1,200 mg per day), and calcium ascorbate (1,000 mg per day) was effective at reducing joint noise, **pain** (page 338), and swelling in people with osteoarthritis of the temporomandibular joint (TMJ, or jaw joint).[5] However, this study was not well controlled and the outcomes measured were highly subjective. Moreover, participants in this study were allowed to use aspirin and ibuprofen, so the exact effects of the nutrient combination cannot be accurately assessed.

Similarly, the combination of glucosamine HCl (1,500 mg per day), CS (1,200 mg per day), and manganese ascorbate (228 mg per day) was evaluated in a double-blind trial and was associated with significant symptom reduction and improvement on x-ray for osteoarthritis of the knee (less so for spine). However, subjects were allowed to use acetaminophen for pain, and comparative effects of a glucosamine HCl/chondroitin sulfate combination and the individual nutrients were not examined.[6]

GLUTAMIC ACID

What is it?

Glutamic acid (glutamate) is an **amino acid** (page 465) used by the body to build proteins. Glutamate is the most common excitatory (stimulating) neurotransmitter in the central nervous system.

Under normal circumstances, humans are able to meet bodily glutamate requirements either from the diet or by making it from precursor molecules. Although **glutamine** (page 530) and glutamic acid have similar names, they are structurally different.

The fluid produced by the prostate gland contains significant amounts of glutamic acid, and this amino acid may play a role in normal function of the prostate. In one study, symptoms of **benign prostatic hyperplasia** (BPH [page 58]) were improved in a group of 45 men taking 780 mg of glutamic acid per day for two weeks and then 390 mg for the next two and a half months in combination with equal amounts of the amino acids, **alanine** (page 463) and **glycine** (page 532),[1] an effect also reported by other researchers.[2]

Glutamic acid may have protective effects on the heart muscle in people with **heart disease** (page 98).

Intravenous injections of glutamic acid (as monosodium glutamate) have been shown to increase exercise tolerance and heart function in people with stable **angina pectoris** (page 27).[3]

Where is it found?

Sources of glutamic acid include high-protein foods, such as meat, poultry, fish, eggs, and dairy products. Some protein-rich plant foods also supply glutamic acid.

Glutamic acid has been used in connection with the following conditions (refer to the individual health concern for complete information):

Rating	Health Concerns
★★☆	**Benign prostatic hyperplasia** (page 58)
★☆☆	Heart surgery (support)

Who is likely to be deficient?

Most food sources of protein supply glutamic acid, so only a person deficient in protein would become deficient in glutamic acid.[4]

How much is usually taken?

Healthy people do not need to take glutamic acid as a supplement; for those who do use this **amino acid** (page 465), appropriate amounts should be determined with the consultation of a physician.

Are there any side effects or interactions?

Glutamic acid is generally free of side effects for the vast majority of people who take it; however, people with **kidney** (page 284) or liver disease should not consume high intakes of **amino acids** (page 465) without consulting a healthcare professional. Because over stimulation of glutamate receptors is thought to be a possible cause of certain neurological diseases (e.g., amyotrophic lateral sclerosis [Lou Gehrig's disease] and **epilepsy** [page 183]), people with a neurological disease should consult of physician before supplementing with glutamate.

Monosodium glutamate (MSG), the form of glutamic acid that is used as a flavor enhancer, has been reported in anecdotal studies to have a number of different adverse effects (including headache, fatigue, and **depression** [page 145]). However, controlled trials have failed to confirm that MSG causes these side effects, and the safety of this compound remains controversial.

GLUTAMINE

What is it?

Glutamine is the most abundant **amino acid** (page 465) (protein building block) in the body and is involved in more metabolic processes than any other amino acid. Glutamine is converted to glucose when more glucose is required by the body as an energy source. It serves as a source of fuel for cells lining the intestines. Without it, these cells waste away. It is also used by white blood cells and is important for **immune function** (page 255).

In animal research, glutamine has anti-inflammatory effects. Glutamine in combination with **N-acetyl cysteine** (page 562) promotes the synthesis of **glutathione** (page 531), a naturally occurring **antioxidant** (page 467) that is believed to be protective in people with **HIV infection** (page 239).[1] Evidence indicates that intravenous glutamine supplementation increases the survival rate of critically ill people.[2]

Where is it found?

Glutamine is found in many foods high in protein, such as fish, meat, beans, and dairy products.

Glutamine has been used in connection with the following conditions (refer to the individual health concern for complete information):

Rating	Health Concerns
★★★	**Pre- and post-surgery health** (page 357)
★★☆	**Athletic performance** (page 43) (for prevention of post exercise infection in performance athletes) **Diarrhea** (page 163) **HIV support** (page 239) (in combination with **arginine** [page 467] and **HMB** [page 534]) **Immune function** (page 255) (for post-exercise infection prevention in endurance athletes) **Infection** (page 265) (for prevention of post exercise infection in performance athletes)
★☆☆	**Alcohol withdrawal support** (page 12) **Gastritis** (page 195) **HIV support** (page 239) **Peptic ulcer** (page 349)

Who is likely to be deficient?

Few healthy people are glutamine deficient, in part because the body makes its own. During fasting, starvation, **cirrhosis** (page 290), critical illnesses in general, and weight loss associated with **AIDS** (page 239) and **cancer** (page 87), however, deficiencies often develop.

How much is usually taken?

Healthy people do not need to supplement with glutamine. A physician should be consulted for the supplemental use of glutamine for the support of serious health conditions.

Are there any side effects or interactions?

No significant side effects have been reported in glutamine studies.

GLUTATHIONE

What is it?

Glutathione is a small protein composed of three **amino acids** (page 465): **cysteine** (page 502), **glutamic acid** (page 529), and **glycine** (page 532).

Glutathione is involved in detoxification—it binds to toxins, such as heavy metals, solvents, and pesticides, and transforms them into a form that can be excreted in urine or bile. Glutathione is also an important antioxidant. In preliminary research, dietary glutathione intake from fruit and raw vegetables has been associated with protection against some forms of **cancer** (page 87).[1, 2] Glutathione has also inhibited cancer in test tube[3] and animal studies.[4] In preliminary research, higher glutathione levels have also been associated with good health in older adults.[5]

Glutathione supplements appear to be efficiently absorbed in rats.[6, 7] However, the same may not be true for glutathione supplements in humans. For example, when seven healthy people were given a single application of up to 3,000 mg of glutathione, there was no increase in blood glutathione levels.[8] The authors of the study concluded "it is not feasible to increase circulating glutathione to a clinically beneficial extent by the oral administrating of a single application of 3,000 mg of glutathione." Absorption of glutathione may be better in rats because unlike the gastrointestinal tract of rats, the human gastrointestinal tract contains significant amounts of an **enzyme** (page 506) (gamma-glutamyltranspeptidase) that breaks down glutathione.

Preliminary evidence has suggested that absorption of glutathione can occur in the mouth when glutathione tablets are placed between the teeth and the inner cheek.[9]

Some researchers believe that supplements other than oral glutathione may be more effective in raising blood levels of glutathione. For example, in one trial, blood glutathione levels rose nearly 50% in healthy people taking 500 mg of **vitamin C** (page 604) per day for only two weeks.[10] Vitamin C raises glutathione by helping the body manufacture it. In addition to vitamin C, other nutritional compounds that may, according to preliminary research, help increase glutathione levels include **alpha lipoic acid** (page 464),[11] **glutamine** (page 530),[12] **methionine** (page 557),[13] **S-adenosyl methionine (SAMe)** (page 583),[14] and **whey protein** (page 613).[15] **Vitamin B$_6$** (page 600), **riboflavin** (page 598), and **selenium** (page 584) are required in the manufacture of glutathione. The extent to which any of these nutrients effectively increases glutathione levels in humans remains unclear.

Studies using intravenous or intramuscular glutathione have found it to be useful for preventing clot formation during operations;[16] reducing the side effects and increasing the efficacy of chemotherapy drugs (particularly cisplatin in women with ovarian cancer);[17, 18] treating **Parkinson's disease** (page 343);[19] reducing blood pressure in people with **diabetes** (page 152) who had **high blood pressure** (page 246);[20] and increasing sperm counts in men with **low sperm counts** (page 305).[21, 22] A glutathione nasal spray has also reduced symptoms in people with chronic **rhinitis** (page 407).[23] Whether oral preparations are also effective is unknown at this time. A small study in eight patients with liver cancer using oral glutathione showed modest benefits in women, but not in men, when given in a daily amount of 5,000 mg.[24]

An unpublished preliminary study of eight colon cancer patients also found that oral glutathione appeared to have **anticancer** (page 87) activity.[25] Nonetheless, because questions exist about the extent to which oral glutathione can be absorbed, some doctors are concerned that oral preparations may be either less effective than other forms or not effective at all.

Where is it found?

Dietary glutathione is found in fresh and frozen fruits and vegetables, fish, and meat.[26] Asparagus, avocado, and walnuts are particularly rich dietary sources of glutathione.

Glutathione

Glutathione has been used in connection with the following conditions (refer to the individual health concern for complete information):

Rating	Health Concerns
★☆☆	Colon cancer (page 134)

Who is likely to be deficient?

A deficiency can be the result of diseases that increase the need for glutathione, deficiencies of the **amino acids** (page 465) needed for synthesis, or diseases that inhibit glutathione formation.[27] Examples of some health conditions that are associated with glutathione deficiency include **diabetes** (page 152), **low sperm counts** (page 304), liver disease, **cataracts** (page 101), and **HIV infection** (page 239), respiratory distress syndrome, **cancer** (page 87), and idiopathic pulmonary fibrosis. Cigarette smoking is also associated with low glutathione levels because it increases the rate of utilization of glutathione.

How much is usually taken?

There is very little evidence that taking glutathione supplements provides any benefit, despite promising evidence about the effects of aerosol, intravenous, and intramuscular glutathione, for people with a wide variety of conditions. People who have a proven glutathione deficiency, which may require administration of glutathione intravenously, intramuscularly, or by aerosol, should be treated by a healthcare professional. All ovarian cancer patients currently taking cisplatin (Platinol) should discuss using intravenous glutathione with a healthcare professional.

Are there any side effects or interactions?

No side effects or interactions are known with oral administration of glutathione.

GLYCINE

What is it?

Glycine is a nonessential **amino acid** (page 465) used by the body to build proteins. It is present in considerable amounts in prostate fluid.

Glycine may play a role in maintaining the health of the prostate, since a study of 45 men with **benign pro-** static hyperplasia (page 58) (BPH) found that 780 mg of glycine per day for two weeks and then 390 mg for the next two and a half months, taken in combination with equal amounts of the amino acids, **alanine** (page 463) and **glutamic acid** (page 529), reduced symptoms of the condition.[1] This effect has been reported by others.[2] Glycine also enhances the activity of chemical messengers (neurotransmitters) in the brain that are involved in memory and cognition.[3]

Where is it found?

Glycine is found in many foods high in protein, such as fish, meat, beans, and dairy.

Glycine has been used in connection with the following conditions (refer to the individual health concern for complete information):

Rating	Health Concerns
★★★	Schizophrenia (page 393)
★★☆	Benign prostatic hyperplasia (page 58)

Who is likely to be deficient?

Few people are glycine deficient, in part because the body makes its own supply of the nonessential **amino acids** (page 465).

How much is usually taken?

Healthy people do not need to supplement with glycine. A physician should be consulted before supplemental glycine is used for the support of serious health conditions.

Are there any side effects or interactions?

No clear toxicity has emerged from glycine studies. However, people with kidney or liver disease should not consume high intakes of **amino acids** (page 465) without consulting a healthcare professional.

GRAPEFRUIT SEED EXTRACT

What is it?

Grapefruit seed extract (GSE) is a substance extracted from grapefruit seeds.

GSE has been shown to exert significant antibiotic effects in test tube studies.[1, 2] However, one study concluded that these effects were due to the chemical preservatives used to stabilize the grapefruit seed extract rather than to any particular compound found in the extract.[3]

Human research using grapefruit seed extract is very limited. In one study, 25 patients with symptoms associated with **irritable bowel syndrome** (page 280) such as intermittent **diarrhea** (page 163), **constipation** (page 137), **flatulence** (page 137), **bloating** (page 137), and abdominal discomfort were treated with either 2 drops of a 0.5% oral solution of grapefruit seed extract twice daily or 150 mg of encapsulated grapefruit seed extract three times daily.[4] After one month, symptoms had improved in 20% of those taking the liquid, while all of the patients taking capsules noted definite improvement of constipation, flatulence, abdominal discomfort, and night rest. These results need confirmation in double-blind studies.

Where is it found?

Grapefruit seed extract is available in liquid concentrate and in capsules and tablets.

Grapefruit seed extract has been used in connection with the following conditions (refer to the individual health concern for complete information):

Rating	Health Concerns
★☆☆	Irritable bowel syndrome (page 280)

Who is likely to be deficient?

Grapefruit seed extract is not an essential nutrient and no deficiency states have been reported.

How much is usually taken?

The typical recommendation for the liquid concentrate is 10–12 drops in 6–7 ounces of water one to three times daily. For capsules and tablets containing dried grapefruit seed extract, the usual recommendation is 100–200 mg one to three times daily.

Are there any side effects or interactions?

No side effects are known. The effects of grapefruit seed extract during **pregnancy** (page 363) and breast-feeding have not been sufficiently evaluated.

GREEN-LIPPED MUSSEL

What is it?

Green-lipped mussel (*Perna canaliculus*) is a New Zealand shellfish, from which an extract has been shown to be useful in the treatment of **rheumatoid arthritis** (RA [page 387]) and **osteoarthritis** (OA [page 328]).

Green-lipped mussel inhibits inflammation in the body. Although inflammation is normal under certain conditions, consistent or excessive inflammation can result in **pain** (page 338) and damage to the body, including the joints. The human body makes several chemical mediators of inflammation. Levels of these chemicals in the body may be higher in people with RA who are experiencing symptoms than in symptom-free people with arthritis.[1] Evidence indicates that controlling the production of inflammatory mediators in the body may help improve conditions such as arthritis, **asthma** (page 32), **psoriasis** (page 379), and **inflammatory bowel disease** (page 269) (including **ulcerative colitis** [page 433] and Crohn's disease), all of which involve elements of inflammation.[2]

Research on green-lipped mussel has focused primarily on OA and RA. Although some studies have failed to demonstrate therapeutic benefit of green-lipped mussel in people with arthritis,[3, 4] the outcomes of other studies have been more positive.[5, 6, 7] In one trial, both freeze-dried powder and lipid extract of green-lipped mussel were effective at reducing symptoms in 70% of people with OA and 76% of people with RA.[8] A similar study of people with either OA or RA showed green-lipped mussel reduced pain in 50% and 67% of the patients, respectively, after three months of supplementation.[9]

In 1986, dried mussel extracts became available that were stabilized with a preservative. The earlier studies that found no beneficial effect of green-lipped mussel on arthritis all used preparations that had not been stabilized, a point that may help explain some of the discrepancies in the research. One recent animal study compared the two forms and found a stabilized lipid extract to be significantly more effective than a nonstabilized extract at inhibiting inflammation.[10] Because both forms are currently available on the market, it may be prudent to check on the form.

Nonsteriodal anti-inflammatories (NSAIDs), such as aspirin and ibuprofen, are often used for inflammatory conditions. However, most of these medications can produce the unfortunate side effect of stomach irritation, which may lead to stomach **ulcer** (page 349) if taken frequently. One animal study found that green-lipped mussel significantly reduced stomach ulcers resulting from taking NSAIDs.[11]

In a double-blind study of people with asthma, supplementation with a proprietary extract of New Zealand green-lipped mussel (Lyprinol) twice a day for 8 weeks significantly decreased daytime wheezing and improved airflow through the bronchi.[12] Each capsule of Lyprinol contains 50 mg of omega-3 fatty acids.

Where is it found?
Green-lipped mussels are found in the oceans off New Zealand. In supplement form, green-lipped mussel is available as a lipid extract or a freeze-dried powder.

Green-lipped mussel has been used in connection with the following conditions (refer to the individual health concern for complete information):

Rating	Health Concerns
★★☆	**Asthma** (page 32) (Lyprinol) **Osteoarthritis** (page 328) **Rheumatoid arthritis** (page 387)

Who is likely to be deficient?
Because green-lipped mussel is not an essential nutrient, deficiencies do not occur.

How much is usually taken?
The studies on green-lipped mussel have used 210 mg per day of the lipid extract or 1,050–1,150 mg per day of the freeze-dried powder.

Are there any side effects or interactions?
Not all studies have demonstrated side effects; however, members of the Australian Rheumatism Association have reported side effects, such as **stomach upset** (page 260), **gout** (page 208), and skin rashes, occurring in people taking certain New Zealand green-lipped mussel extracts.[13] Another researcher observed nausea, **flatulence** (page 137), and **fluid retention** (page 180) in some of the study participants,[14] and one case of **hepatitis** (page 220) has been reported in association with the use of the freeze-dried powder.[15]

People with shellfish **allergy** (page 14) should consult a doctor before taking green-lipped mussel. Compared to lipid preparations, freeze-dried preparations contain substantially more of the protein fraction responsible for allergic reactions.

HISTIDINE

What is it?
Histidine is called a semi-essential **amino acid** (page 465) (protein building block) because adults generally produce adequate amounts but children may not. Histidine is also a precursor of histamine, a compound released by immune system cells during an **allergic reaction** (page 14).

Where is it found?
Dairy, meat and poultry, and fish are good sources of histidine.

Who is likely to be deficient?
According to limited research, many people with **rheumatoid arthritis** (page 387) have low levels of histidine. Taking histidine supplements might improve arthritis symptoms in some people.[1]

How much is usually taken?
Most people do not need to supplement histidine. Optimal levels for others remain unknown. Human research has used between 1 gram and 8 grams per day.

Are there any side effects or interactions?
No side effects have been reported with histidine. However, people with kidney or liver disease should not consume large amounts of **amino acids** (page 465) without consulting a healthcare professional.

HMB

What is it?
HMB (beta hydroxy-beta-methylbutyrate) is a metabolite of the essential **amino acid** (page 465) leucine (one of the **branched-chain amino acids** [page 479]).

As with other amino acid-related substances, HMB appears to play a role in the synthesis of protein—including the protein that builds new muscle tissue.

Animal research suggests that HMB may improve the growth of lean muscle tissue,[1] but only preliminary and limited research in humans supports the potential link between HMB and enhanced muscle building[2] or endurance performance[3] in **athletes** (page 43). One study involving people involved in a regular weight-lifting program found that supplements of 3 grams per day of HMB, compared with no supplements, contributed to greater gains of muscle mass and strength over the seven-week study.[4] However, a double-blind, controlled trial found no effect of 3 grams per day of HMB for four weeks on body composition or exercise performance in 41 weight-training football players.[5, 6]

Where is it found?

Small amounts of HMB are present in many foods of animal and plant origin, especially **alfalfa** (page 623) and catfish. The **amino acid** (page 465) leucine is metabolized into a compound called alpha-ketoisocaproate (KIC), which is then turned into HMB by the body. Dietary supplements of HMB are also available.

HMB has been used in connection with the following conditions (refer to the individual health concern for complete information):

Rating	Health Concerns
★★★	**High cholesterol** (page 223)
★★☆	**Athletic performance** (page 43) (for improving body composition with strength training in untrained people only)
	HIV support (page 239) (in combination with **glutamine** [page 530] and **arginine** [page 467])

Who is likely to be deficient?

HMB is not an essential nutrient. The body creates HMB from leucine, so any diet containing sufficient amounts of leucine (most do) should lead to the adequate production of HMB. Limited evidence indicates that athletes may benefit from supplemental intake of HMB.

How much is usually taken?

Most people do not need to use HMB. For those involved in regular exercise who do choose to take this supplement, the research generally uses 3 grams of HMB per day in combination with resistive exercise, such as weight lifting.

Are there any side effects or interactions?

No safety issues have been reported in the limited number of studies currently available.

HYDROXYCITRIC ACID

What is it?

(-)-Hydroxycitric acid (HCA) is a compound found in *Garcinia cambogia,* a type of fruit. HCA has a chemical structure similar to that of citric acid (the primary acid in citrus fruits).

Preliminary research in the laboratory and in animal research, suggests that HCA may be a useful **weight loss** (page 446) aid.[1, 2] HCA has been demonstrated in the laboratory (but not yet in trials with people) to reduce the conversion of carbohydrates into stored fat by inhibiting certain **enzyme** (page 506) processes.[3, 4] Animal research indicates that HCA suppresses appetite and induces weight loss.[5, 6, 7, 8] One case report found that eating 1 gram of the fruit containing HCA before each meal resulted in the loss of 1 pound per day.[9]

A double-blind trial that provided either 1,500 mg of HCA or a placebo per day to 135 overweight men and women, who also were on a calorie-restricted diet, found after 12 weeks that the HCA supplementation did not produce a significant change in **weight loss** (page 446).[10] Uncontrolled and/or preliminary evidence from several other human trials suggests the possibility that weight loss might occur;[11] however, none of these studies is as methodologically strong as the negative trial previously mentioned. These less-rigorous studies used a similar calorie-restricted diet and a similar amount of HCA as the negative trial. However, the double-blind study used a high-fiber diet not used in the prior studies. It has been suggested that such a diet might limit absorption of HCA.[12] Future studies that measure blood levels of HCA (to check whether or not the supplement was absorbed) are necessary to resolve this issue. At the present time, the effectiveness of HCA for weight loss remains unclear and unproven.

Where is it found?

HCA is found in only a few plants, with one rich source being the rind of a little pumpkin-shaped fruit called *Garcinia cambogia,* which is native to Southeast Asia. This fruit (also called Malabar tamarind) is used as a condiment in dishes such as curry.

HCA has been used in connection with the following conditions (refer to it for complete information):

Rating	Health Concerns
★☆☆	**Weight loss** (page 446)

Who is likely to be deficient?

Since it is not an essential nutrient, HCA is not associated with a deficiency state.

How much is usually taken?

Optimal amounts of HCA remain unknown. Although dieters sometimes take 500 mg of HCA three times per day (before each meal), this amount is far below the levels used in animal research (figured on a per-pound body weight basis). The effect of HCA is enhanced when used in conjunction with a low-fat diet, because HCA does nothing to reduce the caloric effects of dietary fat. Since HCA's mechanism of action seems to be at least partially a blockade of conversion of simple sugars into fats,[13] it is likely to work best in conjunction with a high simple sugar diet. HCA may therefore be less useful if it only offsets the negative effects of an otherwise unhealthy diet. High-fiber diets may impair absorption of HCA as noted above. HCA supplements are available in many forms, including tablets, capsules, powders, snack bars, and chewing gum.

Are there any side effects or interactions?

HCA has not been linked to any adverse effects.

INDOLE-3-CARBINOL

What is it?

Indole-3-carbinol is one of the major **anticancer** (page 87) substances found in cruciferous (cabbage family) vegetables. It is a member of the class of sulfur-containing chemicals called glucosinolates.[1] It is formed from parent compounds whenever cruciferous vegetables are crushed or cooked.[2, 3]

Indole-3-carbinol and other glucosinolates (e.g., other indoles and isothiocyanates such as **sulforaphane** [page 589]) are **antioxidants** (page 467) and potent stimulators of natural detoxifying **enzymes** (page 506) in the body.[4, 5] Indole-3-carbinol and other glucosinolates are believed to be responsible for the lowered risk of cancer in humans that is associated with the consumption of broccoli and other cruciferous vegetables like cauliflower, cabbage, andkale.[6, 7, 8, 9, 10, 11, 12]

Feeding indole-3-carbinol or broccoli extracts rich in indole-3-carbinol has dramatically reduced the frequency, size, and number of tumors in laboratory rats exposed to a carcinogen. It appears to be especially protective against **breast** (page 65)[13, 14, 15, 16] and cervical[17, 18] cancers because of a number of actions, including an ability to increase the breakdown of estrogen. However, while most animal studies report protective effects, a few indicate that indole-3-carbinol may actually promote cancer formation in certain situations, depending upon the chemical initiator of cancer, method of exposure, and species of animal studied.[19, 20]

Until there is further research and more human clinical data to determine if indole-3-carbinol actually inhibits rather than stimulates cancer formation, some researchers have recommended proceeding with caution when using isolated indole-3-carbinol as a dietary supplement.[21] The areas where its use has currently been documented in humans are only preliminary, but the results are promising. Indole-3-carbinol reduced or halted the formation of precancerous lesions (papillomas) in 12 out of 18 people with recurrent respiratory tract papillomas.[22] In addition, in a small double-blind trial, supplementation with 200 or 400 mg of indole-3-carbinol per day for 12 weeks reversed early-stage cervical cancer in 8 of 17 women.[23] Preliminary studies have also shown indole-3-carbinol has significantly increased the conversion of estrogen from cancer-producing forms to nontoxic breakdown products.[24, 25]

Where is it found?

Indole-3-carbinol is found in highest concentrations in broccoli, but is also found in other cruciferous vegetables, such as cauliflower, cabbage, and kale.

Indole-3-carbinol has been used in connection with the following conditions (refer to the individual health concern for complete information):

Rating	Health Concerns
★★☆	**Cancer prevention** (page 87) (cervical cancer)

Who is likely to be deficient?

As indole-3-carbinol is not an essential nutrient, no deficiency state exists.

How much is usually taken?

Based upon preliminary studies it is estimated that the minimum amount required for the prevention of **breast cancer** (page 65) is 300 to 400 mg daily.[26]

Are there any side effects or interactions?

No side effects from indole-3-carbinol have been reported.

INOSINE

What is it?

Inosine is a nucleoside, one of the basic compounds comprising cells. It is a precursor to **adenosine** (page 461), an important energy molecule, and plays many supportive roles in the body.

Based upon anecdotal reports by Russian and Eastern European athletes, inosine has been investigated for exercise-boosting (ergogenic) effects. However, controlled studies have concluded that inosine does not improve **athletic performance** (page 43) and may even impair it.[1, 2]

Inosine is a precursor to uric acid, a compound that occurs naturally in the body. Uric acid is believed to block the effect of a toxic free-radical compound (peroxynitrite) that may play a role in the development of multiple sclerosis (MS).[3] In an attempt to raise uric acid levels, ten patients with MS were treated with inosine in amounts up to 3 grams per day for 46 weeks. Three of the ten treated patients showed some evidence of improved function and the others remained stable.[4] Controlled studies are needed to confirm these preliminary results.

Where is it found?

Inosine is found in **brewer's yeast** (page 480) and organ meats. It is also available as a supplement.

Inosine has been used in connection with the following conditions (refer to the individual health concern for complete information):

Rating	Health Concerns
★☆☆	**Multiple Sclerosis** (page 323)

Who is likely to be deficient?

Inosine is not an essential nutrient, so deficiencies do not occur.

How much is usually taken?

Although a common amount of inosine taken by athletes is 5,000–6,000 mg per day, little scientific evidence supports the use of this supplement in any amount.

Are there any side effects or interactions?

No side effects have been reported with the use of inosine for two to five days in the limited research available. However, unused inosine is converted by the body to uric acid, which may be hazardous to people at risk for **gout** (page 208).

INOSITOL

What is it?

Inositol is part of the **vitamin B-complex** (page 603). It is required for proper formation of cell membranes.

Inositol affects nerve transmission and helps in transporting fats within the body. Inositol differs from inositol hexaniacinate, a form of **vitamin B$_3$** (page 598).

Where is it found?

Nuts, beans, wheat and wheat bran, cantaloupe, and oranges are excellent sources of inositol. Most dietary inositol is in the form of phytate.

Inositol has been used in connection with the following conditions (refer to the individual health concern for complete information):

Rating	Health Concerns
★★☆	**Anxiety** (page 30) **Depression** (page 145) Obsessive-compulsive disorder
★☆☆	**Bipolar disorder/manic depression** (page 61) **Diabetes** (page 152)

Who is likely to be deficient?

Clear deficiency of inositol has not been reported, although people with **diabetes** (page 152) have increased excretion and may benefit from inositol supplementation.

How much is usually taken?

Most people do not need to take inositol. In addition, the small amounts commonly found in **multivitamin**

supplements (page 559) are probably unnecessary and ineffective. Doctors sometimes suggest 500 mg twice per day. For **depression** (page 145), **anxiety** (page 30), and obsessive-compulsive disorder, 12–18 grams per day has been shown to be effective in double-blind trials.[1, 2, 3, 4]

Are there any side effects or interactions?

Toxicity has not been reported, although people with chronic renal failure show elevated levels and should not take inositol, except under medical supervision.

Large amounts of phytate, the common dietary form of inositol, reduce the absorption of **calcium** (page 483), **iron** (page 540), and **zinc** (page 614). However, supplemental inositol does not have this effect.

One review article suggested that inositol may stimulate uterine contractions.[5] While no research has demonstrated that inositol actually has this effect, women who are or could become **pregnant** (page 363) should consult a doctor before taking inositol.

IODINE

What is it?

Iodine is a trace mineral needed to make thyroid hormones, which are necessary for maintaining normal metabolism in all cells of the body.

Reports suggest that iodine may have a number of other important functions in the body unrelated to thyroid function that might help people with a wide variety of conditions.[1] These other uses for iodine are only supported by minimal research.

Where is it found?

Seafood, iodized salt, and sea vegetables—for example, **kelp** (page 543)—are high in iodine. Processed food may contain added iodized salt. Iodine is frequently found in dairy products. Vegetables grown in iodine-rich soil also contain this mineral.

Iodine has been used in connection with the following conditions (refer to the individual health concern for complete information):

Rating	Health Concerns
★★★	Childhood intelligence in newborns (if deficient) **Goiter** (page 206) (iodine deficiency-induced)
★★☆	**Hypothyroidism** (page 252)
★☆☆	**Fibrocystic breast disease** (page 189)

Who is likely to be deficient?

People who avoid dairy, seafood, processed food, and iodized salt can become deficient. Iodine deficiency can cause **low thyroid function** (page 252), **goiter** (page 206), and cretinism. Although iodine deficiencies are now uncommon in Western societies, the U.S. population has shown a trend of significantly decreasing iodine intake from 1988–1994.[2] If this trend continues, iodine deficiency diseases may become more common.

How much is usually taken?

Since the introduction of iodized salt, iodine supplements are unnecessary and not recommended for most people. For strict vegetarians who avoid salt and sea vegetables, 150 mcg per day is commonly supplemented. This amount is adequate to prevent a deficiency and higher amounts are not necessary.

Are there any side effects or interactions?

High amounts (several milligrams per day) of iodine can interfere with normal thyroid function and should not be taken without consulting a doctor.[3] Although potassium iodide supplementation (prescribed for some skin disorders) is usually well-tolerated, it has been known to produce adverse reactions such as rashes, itching or lesions on the skin, gastrointestinal symptoms, or **hypothyroidism** (page 252), especially in people with a prior history of thyroid problems.[4] Because of such potential problems, the use of potassium iodide therapy should be supervised by a doctor. The average diet provides about four times the recommended amount of iodine. For susceptible people, that amount of iodine may be enough to cause health problems.[5] A possible link to thyroid **cancer** (page 87) has been observed in areas where an iodine-rich diet is consumed,[6, 7] and among populations that supplement with iodine.[8, 9] However, there is insufficient evidence to conclude that iodine supplementation is responsible for the increased incidence of thyroid cancer. Some people react to supplemental iodine, the first symptom of which is usually an acne-like rash.

When people with small, nontoxic goiter (living in areas not deficient in iodine) received iodine injections, they had a higher incidence of abnormal antibodies suggestive of the early stages of autoimmune thyroid disease.[10]

Children with iodine deficiency may also have **iron-deficiency anemia** (page 278), and this anemia may interfere with the therapeutic action of iodine supplementation.[11] Correcting iron deficiency in such children with iron supplements has been shown to improve the efficacy of oral iodine in treating goiter.[12]

IP-6

What is it?
IP-6 is a naturally occurring component of plant fiber.

IP-6 may possess **antioxidant** (page 467),[1] **anticancer** (page 87),[2] and other beneficial properties. For example, animal studies have shown that supplementation with large amounts of IP-6 provides substantial protection against **colon cancer** (page 123)[3] and possibly **breast cancer** (page 65).[4, 5] In one of these studies, the effect of pure IP-6 was significant, while an equivalent amount given as a wheat-bran breakfast cereal was not.[6] However, while some animals are able to digest and/or absorb IP-6, it is not known whether humans can.[7] This uncertainty limits the applicability of the animal research to humans, except possibly for colon cancer prevention, which may not depend on absorption. Unfortunately, human research to date has not found an association between higher levels of dietary IP-6 in the colon and reduced indicators of colon cancer risk.[8] Injections of IP-6 used to treat cancerous tumors in mice have been shown to cause partial regression of these tumors.[9]

IP-6 may have a beneficial effect on blood sugar control, similar to the effect of many dietary fibers.[10] However, no studies have been done to test this effect on people with blood sugar disorders.

Where is it found?
IP-6, also known as phytate, is associated with dietary **fiber** (page 512) and thus is naturally present in a wide variety of plant foods, especially wheat bran, whole grains, and legumes. Usual dietary intakes range from 1–1.5 grams phytate per day.

IP-6 has been used in connection with the following conditions (refer to the individual health concern for complete information):

Rating	Health Concerns
★★☆	Kidney stones (page 284)

Who is likely to be deficient?
While there is no dietary requirement for IP-6, people consuming diets low in dietary **fiber** (page 512) and nuts and seeds have the lowest intake.

How much is usually taken?
Virtually all research suggesting beneficial effects from taking IP-6 involve animals and not people. It is not known whether IP-6 would be useful for humans or if so, what would be the optimal amount.

Are there any side effects or interactions?
Phytate in foods has been associated with reduced mineral absorption.[11] In particular, significant interference with **iron** (page 540) absorption has been reported.[12] People who are **iron deficient** (page 278) should talk with a doctor before supplementing with IP-6. Even for those who are not iron deficient, if IP-6 supplements are taken for more than several months and fatigue —a possible symptom of iron deficiency develops, a doctor should be consulted. How much iron supplementation (if any) should be used to counteract the iron-depleting effect of IP-6 varies from person to person, though many people are likely to not require such supplementation.

IPRIFLAVONE

What is it?
Ipriflavone is a synthetic **flavonoid** (page 516) (iso-flavone) derived from the **soy** (page 587) compound daidzein.

Ipriflavone promotes the incorporation of **calcium** (page 483) into bone. It also inhibits bone breakdown. Many clinical studies, including numerous double-blind studies, have clearly shown that long-term treatment with ipriflavone (along with 1,000 mg supplemental calcium per day) is both safe and effective in halting bone loss in **postmenopausal** (page 311) women or in women who have had their ovaries removed. Ipriflavone has also been found to improve bone density in cases of **osteoporosis** (page 333).[1, 2, 3, 4, 5, 6]

In one study demonstrating that ipriflavone prevents bone loss, 56 recently post-menopausal women with low bone density were assigned to receive either ipriflavone (200 mg three times per day) or a placebo for two years.[7] Consistent with most other studies with ipriflavone, all women also received 1,000 mg of elemental calcium daily. While vertebral (spine) bone density declined by 4.9% after two years in women taking only calcium, there was no change in bone density among woman taking ipriflavone supplementation.

Double-blind studies in women with osteoporosis

have also shown positive effects. The most significant studies were performed in elderly women with a history of vertebral fractures due to osteoporosis.[8, 9, 10] Ipriflavone therapy not only stopped bone loss, it actually increased bone density and significantly eliminated or improved vertebral fractures and bone **pain** (page 338).

One double-blind study has failed to confirm the beneficial effect of ipriflavone. In that study, ipriflavone was no more effective than a placebo for preventing bone loss in postmenopausal women with osteoporosis.[11] The women in this negative study were older (average age, 63.3 years) than those in most other ipriflavone studies and had relatively severe osteoporosis. It is possible that ipriflavone works only in younger women or in those with less severe osteoporosis.

Where is it found?

Ipriflavone does occur naturally in food but only in trace amounts. It is available as a nutritional supplement.

Ipriflavone has been used in connection with the following conditions (refer to the individual health concern for complete information):

Rating	Health Concerns
★★☆	**Osteoporosis** (page 333)

Who is likely to be deficient?

As ipriflavone is not an essential nutrient, no deficiency state exists.

How much is usually taken?

The typical supplemental amount of ipriflavone is 200 mg three times daily. Taking 300 mg twice daily has been reported to be just as effective as 200 mg three times per day.[12]

Are there any side effects or interactions?

In a trial of ipriflavone for osteoporosis, 29 of the 132 women in the ipriflavone group completing the three-year trial developed a clinically significant drop in lymphocytes.[13] These cells, which make up approximately 22 to 28% of the white blood cells in the normal adult, are critical components of the immune system and its ability to respond to viral infections. In some of these women, a return to normal levels took almost two years after they had stopped the ipriflavone. Since this finding has been reported in one other smaller clinical trial,[14] it suggests that women choosing to take ipriflavone should have their lymphocytes measured regularly by their doctor.

In double-blind studies, the frequency of perceived side effects in ipriflavone-treated people (14.5%) was actually less than that observed in people receiving the placebo (16.1%).[15] Side effects were mainly mild **stomach upset** (page 260). Researchers recommend that patients with severe kidney disease take a lower amount of ipriflavone (200 to 400 mg daily).[16]

IRON

What is it?

Iron is an essential mineral. It is part of hemoglobin, the oxygen-carrying component of the blood. **Iron-deficient** (page 278) people tire easily in part because their bodies are starved for oxygen. Iron is also part of myoglobin, which helps muscle cells store oxygen. Without enough iron, adenosine triphosphate (ATP; the fuel the body runs on) cannot be properly synthesized. As a result, some iron-deficient people become fatigued even when their hemoglobin levels are normal (i.e., when they are not anemic).

Although iron is part of the **antioxidant enzyme** (page 467) catalase, iron is not generally considered an antioxidant, because too much iron can cause oxidative damage.

Where is it found?

The most absorbable form of iron, called "heme" iron, is found in oysters, meat and poultry, and fish. Non-heme iron is also found in these foods, as well as in dried fruit, molasses, leafy green vegetables, wine, and iron supplements. Acidic foods (such as tomato sauce) cooked in an iron pan can also be a source of dietary iron.

Iron has been used in connection with the following conditions (refer to the individual health concern for complete information):

Rating	Health Concerns
★★★	Childhood intelligence (for deficiency) **Depression** (page 145) (for deficiency) **Iron-deficiency anemia** (page 278) **Menorrhagia** (page 314) (heavy menstruation) (for treatment of iron-deficiency only)

Rating	Health Concerns
★★☆	**Athletic performance** (page 43) (for treatment of iron-deficiency only)
	Attention deficit–hyperactivity disorder (page 55) (for deficiency only)
	Breast-feeding support (page 74)
	Canker sores (page 90)
	Celiac disease (page 102) (for treatment of iron-deficiency only)
	Pre- and post-surgery health (page 357) (if deficient or for major surgery)
	Pregnancy and postpartum support (page 363) (with medical supervision)
	Restless legs syndrome (page 384) (only if iron-deficiency)
★☆☆	**Alzheimer's disease** (page 19) (in combination with **coenzyme Q₁₀** [page 496] and **vitamin B₆** [page 600])
	Dermatitis herpetiformis (page 151)
	HIV support (page 239)
	Infertility (female) (page 187) (for treatment of iron-deficiency only)

Who is likely to be deficient?

Vegetarians eat less iron than non-vegetarians, and the iron they eat is somewhat less absorbable. As a result, vegetarians are more likely to have reduced iron stores.[1] However, **iron deficiency** (page 278) is not usually caused by a lack of iron in the diet alone. An underlying cause, such as iron loss in menstrual blood, often exists.

Pregnant (page 363) women, **marathon runners** (page 43), people who take aspirin, and those who have **parasitic** (page 343) infections, **hemorrhoids** (page 219), **ulcers** (page 349), **ulcerative colitis** (page 433), **Crohn's disease** (page 141), gastrointestinal **cancers** (page 87), or other conditions that cause blood loss or **malabsorption** (page 304) are likely to become deficient.

Infants living in inner city areas may be at increased risk of **iron-deficiency anemia** (page 278)[2] and suffer more often from developmental delays as a result.[3, 4] Supplementation of infant formula with iron up to 18 months of age in inner city infants has been shown to prevent iron-deficiency anemia and to reduce the decline in mental development seen in such infants in some,[5] but not all,[6] studies.

Breath-holding spells are a common problem affecting about 27% of healthy children.[7] These spells have been associated with iron-deficiency anemia,[8] and several studies have reported improvement of breath-holding spells with iron supplementation.[9, 10, 11, 12]

People who fit into one of these groups, even **pregnant** (page 363) women, shouldn't automatically take iron supplements. Fatigue, the first symptom of iron deficiency, can be caused by many other things. A doctor should assess the need for iron supplements, since taking iron when it isn't needed does no good and may do some harm.

Which forms of supplemental iron are best?

All iron supplements are not the same. Ferrous iron (e.g. ferrous sulfate) is much better absorbed than ferric iron (e.g. ferric citrate).[13, 14] The most common form of iron supplement is ferrous sulfate, but it is known to produce intestinal side effects (such as **constipation** [page 137], nausea, and **bloating** [page 137]) in many users.[15] Some forms of ferrous sulfate are enteric-coated to delay tablet dissolving and prevent some side effects,[16] but enteric-coated iron may not absorb as well as iron from standard supplements.[17, 18, 19] Other forms of iron supplements, such as ferrous fumarate,[20, 21] ferrous gluconate,[22] heme iron concentrate,[23, 24, 25, 26] and iron glycine **amino acid** (page 465) chelate[27, 28] are readily absorbed and less likely to cause intestinal side effects.

How much is usually taken?

If a doctor diagnoses **iron deficiency** (page 278), iron supplementation is essential. To treat iron deficiency, a common recommended amount for an adult is 100 mg per day; that amount is usually reduced after the deficiency is corrected. When iron deficiency is diagnosed, the doctor must also determine the cause. Usually it's not serious (such as normal menstrual blood loss or blood donation). Occasionally, however, iron deficiency signals **ulcers** (page 349) or even **colon cancer** (page 123).

Some **premenopausal** (page 311) women become marginally iron deficient unless they supplement with iron. However, the 18 mg of iron present in many **multivitamin-mineral supplements** (page 559) is often adequate to prevent deficiency. A doctor should be consulted to determine the amount of iron that is needed.

Are there any side effects or interactions?

Iron (ferrous sulfate) is the leading cause of accidental poisonings in children.[29, 30, 31] The incidence of iron poisonings in young children increased dramatically in 1986. Many of these children obtained the iron from a child-resistant container opened by themselves or another child, or left open or improperly closed by an adult.[32] Deaths in children have occurred from ingesting as little as 200 mg to as much as 5.85 grams of iron.[33] Keep iron-containing supplements out of a child's reach.

Hemochromatosis, hemosiderosis, polycythemia, and iron-loading anemias (such as thalassemia and **sickle cell anemia** [page 403]) are conditions involving excessive storage of iron. Supplementing iron can be quite dangerous for people with these diseases.

Supplemental amounts required to overcome iron deficiency can cause **constipation** (page 137). Sometimes switching the form of iron (see "Which forms of supplemental iron are best?" above), getting more exercise, or treating the constipation with **fiber** (page 512) and fluids is helpful, though fiber can reduce iron absorption (see below). Sometimes the amount of iron must be reduced if constipation occurs.

Some researchers have linked excess iron levels to **diabetes** (page 152),[34] **cancer** (page 87),[35] increased risk of **infection** (page 265),[36] **systemic lupus erythematosus** (page 421) (SLE),[37] exacerbation of **rheumatoid arthritis** (page 387),[38] and Huntington's disease.[39] The greatest concern has surrounded the possibility that excess storage of iron in the body increases the risk of **heart disease** (page 98).[40, 41, 42] Two analyses of published studies came to different conclusions about whether iron could increase heart disease risk.[43, 44] One trial has suggested that such a link may exist, but only in some people (possibly smokers or those with elevated **cholesterol** (page 223) levels).[45] The link between excess iron and any of the diseases mentioned earlier in this paragraph has not been definitively proven. Nonetheless, too much iron causes **free radical damage** (page 467), which can, in theory, promote or exacerbate most of these diseases. People who are not iron deficient should generally not take iron supplements.

Patients on kidney dialysis who are given injections of iron frequently experience "oxidative stress". This is because iron is a pro-oxidant, meaning that it interacts with oxygen molecules in ways that can damage tissues. These adverse effects of iron therapy may be counteracted by supplementation with **vitamin E** (page 609).[46]

Supplementation with iron, or iron and zinc, has been found to improve **vitamin A** (page 595) status among children at high risk for deficiency of the three nutrients.[47]

People with **hepatitis** (page 220) C who have failed to respond to interferon therapy have been found to have higher amounts of iron within the liver. Moreover, reduction of iron levels by drawing blood has been shown to decrease liver injury caused by hepatitis C.[48] Therefore, people with hepatitis C should avoid iron supplements.

In some people, particularly those with **diabetes** (page 152), **insulin resistance syndrome** (page 273), or liver disease, a genetic susceptibility to iron overload has been reported.[49]

Many foods, beverages, and supplements have been shown to affect the absorption of iron.[50]

Foods, beverages and supplements that interfere with iron absorption include

- **Green tea's** (page 686) (*Camellia sinensis*)[51, 52, 53, 54] effect may be desirable for people with iron overload diseases, such as hemochromatosis; the inhibitory effect of green tea on iron absorption was 26% in one study[55]
- Coffee (*Coffea arabica, C. robusta*)[56, 57, 58]
- Red wine, particularly the polyphenol component (also found in tea);[59, 60] since wine is also a dietary source of iron, it is not clear whether drinking red wine would lead to a deficiency of iron
- Phytate (phytic acid), found in unleavened wheat products such as matzoh, pita, and some rye crackers; in wheat germ, **oats** (page 716), nuts, cacao powder, vanilla extract, beans, and many other foods, and in **IP-6** (page 539) supplements[61, 62, 63]
- Whole wheat bran, independent of its phytate content, has been shown to inhibit iron absorption[64]
- **Calcium** (page 483) from food and supplements interferes with heme-iron absorption[65, 66]
- Soy protein[67, 68]
- Eggs[69, 70]

Foods and supplements that increase iron absorption include

- Meat, poultry, and fish[71, 72, 73, 74, 75]

Although **vitamin C** (page 604) increases iron absorption,[76, 77, 78, 79] the effect is relatively minor.[80]

Taking **vitamin A** (page 595) with iron helps treat **iron deficiency** (page 278), since vitamin A improves the absorption and/or utilization of iron.[81, 82]

Although soy protein has been shown to decrease iron absorption (see above), certain soy-containing foods (e.g. tofu, miso, tempeh) have significantly improved iron absorption.[83] Some soy sauces may also enhance iron absorption.[84]

Alcohol, but not red wine, has been reported to increase the absorption of ferric, but not ferrous, iron.[85, 86]

Iron has been reported to potentially interfere with **manganese** (page 553) absorption. In one trial, women with high iron status had relatively poor absorption of manganese.[87] In another trial studying manganese/iron interactions in women, increased intake of "non-heme iron"—the kind of iron found in most supplements—decreased manganese status.[88] These interactions suggest that taking **multiminerals** (page 559) that include manganese may protect against manganese deficiencies that might otherwise be triggered by taking isolated iron supplements.

KELP

What is it?
Kelp is a sea vegetable that is a concentrated source of minerals, including **iodine** (page 538), **potassium** (page 572), **magnesium** (page 551), **calcium** (page 483), and **iron** (page 540). Kelp as a source of iodine assists in making thyroid hormones, which are necessary for maintaining normal metabolism in all cells of the body.

Where is it found?
Kelp can be one of several brown-colored seaweed species called *Laminaria*.

Kelp has been used in connection with the following condition (refer to the individual health concern for complete information):

Rating	Health Concerns
★☆☆	Iodine deficiency

Who is likely to be deficient?
People who avoid sea vegetables, as well as dairy, seafood, processed food, and the salt shaker, can become deficient in iodine. Iodine deficiency can cause **low thyroid function** (page 252), **goiter** (page 206), and cretinism. Although iodine deficiency is now uncommon in Western societies, the U.S. population has shown a trend of significantly decreasing iodine intake.

How much is usually taken?
Since the introduction of iodized salt, additional sources of **iodine** (page 538), such as kelp, are not necessary for most people. However, kelp can be consumed as a source of other minerals. A report from Great Britain indicated that the average kelp-based supplement contained 1,000 mcg of iodine (the adult RDA in the United States is 150 mcg per day). It has been suggested that intakes above 2,000 mcg per day should be regarded as excessive or potentially harmful.[1]

Are there any side effects or interactions?
There have been several case reports of high intakes of kelp providing too much **iodine** (page 538) and interfering with normal thyroid function.[2, 3, 4, 5, 6] People with thyroid disease should check with a doctor before taking supplements that contain kelp.

L-CARNITINE

What is it?
L-carnitine is made in the body from the **amino acids** (page 465) **lysine** (page 550) and **methionine** (page 557), and is needed to release energy from fat. It transports fatty acids into mitochondria, the powerhouses of cells. In infancy, and in situations of high energy needs, such as **pregnancy** (page 363) and breast-feeding, the need for L-carnitine can exceed production by the body. Therefore, L-carnitine is considered a "conditionally essential" nutrient.[1]

L-carnitine's actions appear to be particularly important in the heart. As an example, patients with **diabetes** (page 152) and **high blood pressure** (page 246) were given 4 grams of L-carnitine per day in an preliminary study.[2] After 45 weeks, **irregular heartbeat** (page 93) and abnormal heart functioning decreased significantly compared with nonsupplemented patients. For **congestive heart failure** (page 134), much of the research has used a modified form of carnitine called propionyl-L-carnitine (PC). In one double-blind trial, using 500 mg PC per day led to a 26% increase in exercise capacity after six months.[3] In other research, patients with congestive heart failure given 1.5 grams PC daily for 15 days had a 21% increase in exercise tolerance and a 45% increase in oxygen consumption.[4]

Research shows that people who supplement with L-carnitine while engaging in an exercise regimen are less likely to experience muscle soreness.[5] However, the belief that carnitine's effect on energy release will help build muscle or improve **athletic performance** (page 43) has, so far, not been supported by most research.[6, 7] In a double-blind study of trained athletes, supplementation with 2 grams of L-carnitine two hours before and after a 20 km run failed to improve physical performance or exercise recovery.[8]

L-carnitine has been given to people with chronic lung disease in trials investigating how the body responds to exercise, however.[9, 10] In these double-blind reports, 2 grams of L-carnitine taken twice per day for two to four weeks led to positive changes in lung function and metabolism during exercise.

Beta thalassemia major is an inherited, fatal form of anemia commonly seen in people of Mediterranean descent. People with beta thalassemia major invariably require blood transfusions, which can eventually result in **iron** (page 540) overload.[11] L-carnitine stabilizes red blood cells and supplementation may decrease the need for blood transfusions. In a preliminary study, children with beta thalassemia major who took 100 mg of L-carnitine per 2.2 pounds of body weight per day for three months had a significantly decreased need for blood transfusions.[12]

Where is it found?

Dairy and red meat contain the greatest amounts of carnitine. Therefore, people who have a limited intake of meat and dairy products tend to have lower L-carnitine intakes.

L-carnitine has been used in connection with the following conditions (refer to the individual health concern for complete information):

Rating	Health Concerns
★★★	**Angina** (page 27) **Congestive heart failure** (page 134) (propionyl-L-carnitine) **Heart attack** (page 212) **Intermittent claudication** (page 276) (propionyl-L-carnitine)
★★☆	**Anemia** (page 25) (for thalassemia) **Attention deficit–hyperactivity disorder** (page 55) **Chronic fatigue syndrome** (page 111) **Chronic obstructive pulmonary disease** (page 114) (COPD) **Diabetes** (page 152) **High triglycerides** (page 235) **Infertility (male)** (page 305) **Intermittent claudication** (page 276) (L-carnitine) **Sprains and strains** (page 412) (for preventing exercise-related muscle injury)
★☆☆	**Athletic performance** (page 43) (for ultra-endurance only) Beta thalassemia major **Cardiomyopathy** (page 95) (only for children with inherited cardiomyopathy) Chemotherapy-induced fatigue **High cholesterol** (page 223) **Liver cirrhosis** (page 290) **Mitral valve prolapse** (page 319) **Raynaud's disease** (page 382) **Weight loss** (page 446)

Who is likely to be deficient?

Carnitine deficiencies are rare, even in strict vegetarians, because the body produces carnitine relatively easily.

Rare genetic diseases can cause a carnitine deficiency. Also, deficiencies are occasionally associated with other diseases, such as **diabetes** (page 152) and **cirrhosis** (page 290).[13, 14] Among people with diabetes, carnitine deficiency is more likely to be found in persons experiencing complications of diabetes (such as **retinopathy** (page 385), hyperlipidemia, or neuropathy), suggesting that carnitine deficiency may play a role in the development of these complications.[15] A carnitine deficiency can also result from oxygen deprivation which can occur in some **heart conditions** (page 98). In Italy, L-carnitine is prescribed for **heart failure** (page 134), **heart arrhythmias** (page 93), **angina** (page 27), and lack of oxygen to the heart.[16]

How much is usually taken?

Most people do not need carnitine supplements. For therapeutic use, typical amounts are 1–3 grams per day.

It remains unclear whether the propionyl-L-carnitine form of carnitine used in **congestive heart failure** (page 134) research has greater benefits than the L-carnitine form, since limited research in both animals and humans with the more common L-carnitine has also shown very promising effects.[17]

Are there any side effects or interactions?

L-carnitine has not been consistently linked with any toxicity.

The body needs **lysine** (page 550), **methionine** (page 557), **vitamin C** (page 604), **iron** (page 540), **niacin** (page 598), and **vitamin B$_6$** (page 600) to produce carnitine.

L-TYROSINE

What is it?

L-tyrosine is a nonessential **amino acid** (page 465) (protein building block) that the body synthesizes from **phenylalanine** (page 568), another amino acid. Tyrosine is important to the structure of almost all proteins in the body. It is also the precursor of several neurotransmitters, including L-dopa, dopamine, norepinephrine, and epinephrine.

L-tyrosine, through its effect on neurotransmitters, may affect several health conditions, including **Parkinson's disease (page 345), **depression** (page 145), and other mood disorders. Studies have suggested that tyrosine may help people with depression.[1] Preliminary findings indicate a beneficial effect of tyrosine, along with other amino acids, in people affected by dementia, including **Alzheimer's disease** (page 19).[2] Due to its role as a precursor to norepinephrine and epinephrine (two of the body's main stress-related hormones) tyrosine may also ease the adverse effects of environmental, psychosocial, and physical stress.[3, 4, 5, 6, 7, 8, 9]

L-tyrosine is converted by skin cells into melanin, the dark pigment that protects against the harmful effects of ultraviolet light. Thyroid hormones, which have a role in almost every process in the body, also contain tyrosine as part of their structure.

People born with the genetic condition **phenylketonuria** (page 354) (PKU) are unable to metabolize the amino acid **phenylalanine** (page 568). Mental retardation and other severe disabilities can result. While dietary phenylalanine restriction prevents these problems, it also leads to low tyrosine levels in many (but not all) people with PKU. Tyrosine supplementation may be beneficial in some people with PKU, though the evidence is conflicting.[10]

Where is it found?

Dairy products, meats, fish, wheat, **oats** (page 716), and most other protein-containing foods contain tyrosine.

L-tyrosine has been used in connection with the following conditions (refer to the individual health concern for complete information):

Rating	Health Concerns
★★☆	**Depression** (page 145) **Phenylketonuria** (page 354) (for deficiency)
★☆☆	**Alcohol withdrawal support** (page 12) **Parkinson's disease** (page 345)

Who is likely to be deficient?

Some people affected by **PKU** (page 354) are deficient in tyrosine. Tyrosine levels are occasionally low in **depressed** (page 145) people.[11] Any person losing large amounts of protein, such as those with some kidney diseases, may be deficient in several **amino acids** (page 465), including tyrosine.[12]

How much is usually taken?

Most people should not supplement with L-tyrosine. Some human research with people suffering from a va-

riety of conditions used 100 mg per 2.2 pounds of body weight, equivalent to about 7 grams per day for an average-sized person. The appropriate amount to use in people with **PKU** (page 354) is not known, therefore, the monitoring of blood levels by a physician is recommended.

Are there any side effects or interactions?

L-tyrosine has not been reported to cause any serious side effects. However, it is not known whether long-term use of L-tyrosine, particularly in large amounts (such as more than 1,000 mg per day) is safe. For that reason, long-term use of L-tyrosine should be monitored by a doctor.

Vitamin B6 (page 600), **folic acid** (page 520), and **copper** (page 499) are necessary for conversion of L-tyrosine into neurotransmitters.

LACTASE

What is it?

Lactase is the enzyme in the small intestine that digests lactose (the naturally occurring sugar in milk).

A few children and many people after childhood do not produce sufficient lactase, resulting in impaired ability to digest milk. These people are **lactose intolerant** (page 288) and often suffer from symptoms including cramps, gas, and **diarrhea** (page 163). Lactose intolerance is best diagnosed by a doctor, However, a reasonably reliable home test for lactose intolerance is to drink two 8-ounce glasses of milk on an empty stomach and note any gastrointestinal symptoms that develop over the next four hours; repeat the test on another day using several ounces of cheese (which does not contain much lactose). If symptoms result from milk but not cheese, then the person probably has lactose intolerance. If symptoms occur with both milk and cheese, the person may be **allergic** (page 14) to dairy.

Where is it found?

Lactase is produced by the body. Dairy products have varying levels of lactose, which affects how much lactase is required for proper digestion. Milk, ice cream, and yogurt contain significant amounts of lactose—although for complex reasons yogurt often doesn't trigger symptoms in lactose-intolerant people.

Lactase has been used in connection with the following conditions (refer to the individual health concern for complete information):

Rating	Health Concerns
★★★	**Diarrhea** (page 163) (for lactose-intolerant people) **Indigestion and heartburn** (page 260) (for lactose-intolerant people) **Irritable bowel syndrome** (page 280) (for lactose-intolerant people) **Lactose intolerance** (page 288)

Who is likely to be deficient?

Only one-third of all people retain the ability to digest lactose into adulthood. Most individuals of Asian, African, and Native American descent are **lactose intolerant** (page 288). In addition, half of Hispanics and about 20 percent of Caucasians do not produce lactase as adults.[1]

How much is usually taken?

Lactose-reduced milk is available and can be used in the same quantities as regular milk. Lactase drops can be added to regular milk 24 hours before drinking to reduce lactose levels. Lactase drops, capsules, and tablets can also be taken directly, as needed, immediately before a meal that includes lactose-containing dairy products. The degree of lactose intolerance varies by individual, so a greater or lesser amount of lactase may be needed to eliminate symptoms of lactose intolerance.

Are there any side effects or interactions?

Lactase is safe and does not produce side effects.

Some, but not all, studies suggest that lactose-intolerant individuals absorb less **calcium** (page 483).[2]

LECITHIN/PHOSPHATIDYL CHOLINE

What is it?

When medical researchers use the term "lecithin," they are referring to a purified substance called phosphatidyl choline (PC) that belongs to a special category of fat-soluble substances called phospholipids.

Phospholipids are essential components of cell membranes. Supplements labeled as "lecithin" usually contain 10–20% PC. Relatively pure PC supplements are generally labeled as "phosphatidylcholine." PC best duplicates supplements used in medical research.

Choline by itself (without the "phosphatidyl" group) is also available in foods and supplements. In high amounts, however, pure choline can make people smell like fish, so it's rarely used, except in the small amounts found in **multivitamin supplements** (page 559).

What does it do?

PC acts as a supplier of choline, which is needed for cell membrane integrity and to facilitate the movement of fats in and out of cells. It is also a component of the neurotransmitter acetylcholine and is needed for normal brain functioning, particularly in infants. Although the human body can synthesize choline, additional amounts from the diet are considered essential under certain circumstances. For this reason, PC has been used in a number of preliminary studies for a wide variety of neurological and psychiatric disorders, though not every study suggests that supplemental choline is capable of reaching the brain.[1] Choline participates in many functions involving cellular components called phospholipids.

Where is it found?

Choline, the major constituent of PC, is found in soybeans, liver, oatmeal, cabbage, and cauliflower. Soybeans, egg yolks, meat, and some vegetables contain PC. Lecithin (containing 10–20% PC) is added to many processed foods in small amounts for the purpose of maintaining texture consistency.

Phosphatidyl choline has been used in connection with the following conditions (refer to the individual health concern for complete information):

Rating	Health Concerns
★★☆	**High homocysteine** (page 235) **Liver cirrhosis** (page 290) **Neural tube defects** (page 63) (prevention) **Tardive dyskinesia** (page 425)
★☆☆	**Alzheimer's disease** (page 19) **Bipolar disorder** (page 61) **Gallbladder attacks** (page 193) **Hepatitis** (page 220) **High cholesterol** (page 223)

Lactase

Who is likely to be deficient?

Although choline deficiencies have been artificially induced in people, little is known about human deficiency in the real world.

How much is usually taken?

Small amounts of choline are present in many **B-complex** (page 603) and **multivitamin** (page 559) supplements.

Are there any side effects or interactions?

With several grams of choline per day, some people will experience abdominal discomfort, **diarrhea** (page 163), or nausea. Supplementing choline in large amounts (over 1,000 mg per day) can lead to a fishy body odor. PC does not have this effect. **Depression** (page 145) has been reported as a side effect in people taking large amounts of choline, such as 9 grams per day.

The body uses both PC and **pantothenic acid** (page 568) to form acetylcholine.

LIPASE

What is it?

Lipase is an **enzyme** (page 506) that is used by the body to break down dietary fats into an absorbable form.

When lipase levels are insufficient to break down dietary fats, greasy, light-colored stools ensue; this condition is called steatorrhea.

Where is it found?

Most of the body's lipase is manufactured in the pancreas, although some of it is secreted in the saliva, as well. Pancreatin contains lipase along with two other groups of **enzymes** (page 506): proteases and amylase.

Lipase has been used in connection with the following conditions (refer to the individual health concern for complete information):

Rating	Health Concerns
★★★	**Cystic fibrosis** (page 143)
★★☆	**Indigestion** (page 260) (for pancreatic insufficiency only)
★☆☆	**Celiac disease** (page 102) **Crohn's disease** (page 141)

Who is likely to be deficient?

People with pancreatic insufficiency and **cystic fibrosis** (page 143) frequently require supplemental lipase and other enzymes. In addition, those with **celiac disease** (page 102)[1] or **Crohn's disease** (page 141)[2] and perhaps some people suffering from **indigestion** (page 260)[3] may be deficient in **pancreatic enzymes** (page 506) including lipase.

How much is usually taken?

Products that contain lipase also usually contain other **enzymes** (page 506) that help digest carbohydrates and protein. In the U.S., pancreatin, which contains lipase, amylase, and proteases, is rated against a government standard. For example, "9X pancreatin" is nine times stronger than the government standard. Each "X" contains 25 USP units of amylase, 2 USP units of lipase, and 25 USP units of proteolytic enzymes. Taking 1.5 grams of 9X pancreatin (or a higher amount at lower potencies) with each meal can help people with pancreatic insufficiency digest food.

Are there any side effects or interactions?

Lipase does not generally cause any side effects at the amounts listed above.

LIVER EXTRACTS

What are they?

Extracts of beef (bovine) liver are a rich natural source of many **vitamins and minerals** (page 559), including **iron** (page 540).

Liver extracts provide the most absorbable form of iron—heme iron—and other nutrients critical in building blood, including **vitamin B$_{12}$** (page 601) and **folic acid** (page 520). Liver extracts can contain as much as 3–4 mg of heme iron per gram. In addition to its use as a source of iron, liver extracts are also used by some healthcare practitioners to support liver function and boost energy levels. Liver extracts have been tested in people with chronic liver disease. However, no clear benefit has been demonstrated.[1, 2]

Where are they found?

Liver extracts are available as nutritional supplements in capsules and tablets.

Liver extracts have been used in connection with the following conditions (refer to it for complete information):

Rating	Health Concerns
★★★	**Iron-deficiency anemia** (page 278)

Who is likely to be deficient?

As it is not an essential nutrient, no deficiency state exists.

How much is usually taken?

The recommended amount depends on the concentration, method of preparation, and quality of the liver extract.

Are there any side effects or interactions?

No side effects or adverse reactions have been reported. Liver extracts should not be used by people suffering from iron-storage disorders, such as hemochromatosis.

As the liver is a major filtering organ for many potentially toxic environmental chemicals, some doctors are concerned that consumption of liver extracts may result in increased intake of these chemicals.

LUTEIN

What is it?

Lutein is an **antioxidant** (page 467) in the **carotenoid** (page 488) family (a group of naturally occurring fat-soluble pigments found in plants). Lutein is the primary carotenoid present in the central area of the retina called the macula.

Lutein may act as a filter to protect the macula from potentially damaging forms of light. Consequently, lutein appears to be associated with protection from age-related **macular degeneration** (page 303) (the leading cause of blindness in older adults).

Where is it found?

Spinach, kale, collard greens, romaine lettuce, leeks, peas, and egg yolks are good sources of lutein.

Lutein has been used in connection with the following conditions (refer to the individual health concern for complete information):

Rating	Health Concerns
★★☆	**Macular degeneration** (page 303) **Cataracts** (page 101)

Who is likely to be deficient?

While a deficiency has not been identified, people who eat more lutein-containing foods appear to be at lower risk of **macular degeneration** (page 303). One study found that adults with the highest dietary intake of lutein had a 57% decreased risk of macular degeneration compared with those people with the lowest intake, and of the **carotenoids** (page 488), lutein and zeaxanthin are most strongly associated with this protection.[1] In a preliminary study, a similar link was suggested between low dietary lutein and increased risk of **cataracts** (page 101).[2]

How much is usually taken?

People showing protection from **macular degeneration** (page 303) have been reported to have eaten about 6 mg of lutein per day from food. Lutein, in supplemental form, should be taken with fat-containing food to improve absorption.[3]

Are there any side effects or interactions?

No adverse effects from lutein have been reported.

Lutein functions together with zeaxanthin, another **antioxidant** (page 467) found in the same foods and supplements as lutein.

LYCOPENE

What is it?

Lycopene, found primarily in tomatoes, is a member of the **carotenoid** (page 488) family—which includes **beta-carotene** (page 469) and similar compounds found naturally in food—and has potent **antioxidant** (page 467) capabilities.

A study conducted by Harvard researchers examined the relationship between carotenoids and the risk of prostate **cancer** (page 87).[1] Of the carotenoids studied, only lycopene was clearly linked to protection. The men who had the greatest amounts of lycopene in their diet (6.5 mg per day or more) showed a 21% decreased risk of **prostate cancer** (page 371) compared with those eating the least. This report suggests that lycopene may be an important tool in the prevention of prostate cancer. This study also reported that those who ate more than ten servings per week of tomato-based foods had a 35% decreased risk of prostate cancer compared with those eating less than 1.5 weekly servings. When the researchers looked at only advanced prostate cancer, the high lycopene eaters had an 86% decreased risk (although this did not reach statistical significance due to the small number of cases).

Contrary to popular opinion, research suggests that there is no preferential concentration of lycopene in prostate tissue.[2] Although prostate cancer patients have been reported to have low levels of lycopene in the blood,[3] and lycopene appears to be a potent inhibitor of human **cancer** (page 87) cells in test-tubes,[4] evidence is conflicting concerning whether an increased intake of tomato products is protective against prostate cancer. Some studies, like the one discussed above, have reported that high consumption of tomatoes and tomato products reduces risk of prostate cancer.[5, 6] Other studies, however, are inconclusive,[7] and some have found no protective association.[8, 9, 10, 11, 12]

There is some evidence that lycopene may be helpful in the treatment of prostate cancer. In a preliminary trial, 26 men with prostate cancer were randomly assigned to receive lycopene (15 mg twice a day) or no lycopene for three weeks before undergoing prostate surgery. Prostate tissue was then obtained during surgery and examined. Compared with the unsupplemented men, those receiving lycopene were found to have significantly less aggressive growth of cancer cells.[13] In addition, a case report has been published of a 62-year-old man with advanced prostate cancer who experienced a regression of his tumor after starting 10 mg of lycopene per day and 300 mg of **saw palmetto** (page 743) three times per day. As saw palmetto has not been previously associated with improvements in prostate cancer, the authors of the report attributed the response to the lycopene.[14] Long-term controlled studies are needed to confirm these promising initial reports.

There is no evidence that tomato intake has any effect on **benign prostatic hyperplasia** (page 58) (BPH).

Another study found that for the 25% of people with the greatest tomato intake, the risk for cancers of the gastrointestinal tract was 30–60% lower, compared with those who ate fewer tomatoes. These reduced risks were statistically significant.[15] A study of women found that the 75% who ate the least amount of tomatoes had between 3.5 and 4.7 times the risk for pre-cancerous changes of the cervix (cervical intraepithelial neoplasia).[16] Other researchers have also reported evidence suggesting that high dietary lycopene may be linked to protection from **cervical dysplasia** (page 3).[17] While preliminary evidence also links dietary lycopene with protection from **breast cancer** (page 65),[18] another study did not find this link.[19]

In a review of 72 studies,[20] one researcher reported 57 associations between tomato intake or blood lycopene levels and decreased risk of cancer. Of these associations, 35 were statistically significant. The benefit was strongest for prostate, **lung** (page 298), and stomach cancers, although protective associations were also found for cancers of the pancreas, **colon** (page 134), rectum, esophagus, oral cavity, breast, and cervix. Because the data were from observational studies, a cause-and-effect relationship cannot be firmly established. However, the consistently lower risk of cancer associated with higher consumption of lycopene-containing tomatoes, provides a strong foundation for further research on lycopene.

In Europe, researchers have found a statistically significant association between high dietary lycopene and a 48% lower risk of **heart disease** (page 98).[21] Lycopene supplementation has also boosted **immune function** (page 255) in the elderly. In that trial, 15 mg of lycopene per day increased natural killer cell activity by 28% in 12 weeks.[22]

Where is it found?

Tomatoes and tomato-containing foods are high in lycopene. In the Harvard study, the only tomato-based food that did not correlate with protection was tomato juice. In an unblinded, controlled trial, lycopene supplementation, but not tomato juice, effectively increased the body's lycopene stores.[23] These studies suggest that the lycopene present in tomato juice is poorly absorbed. However, other research indicates that significant amounts of lycopene from tomato juice can, in fact, be absorbed.[24] Other foods that contain lycopene include watermelon, pink grapefruit, and guava.

Lycopene

Lycopene has been used in connection with the following conditions (refer to the individual health concern for complete information):

Rating	Health Concerns
★★☆	**Asthma** (page 32), exercise-induced **Preeclampsia** (page 361) **Prostate cancer** (page 371)
★☆☆	**Atherosclerosis** (page 38) (prevention only) **Cancer risk reduction** (page 87) **Immune function** (page 255) **Macular degeneration** (page 303)

Who is likely to be deficient?

This is unknown, but people who do not eat diets high in tomatoes or tomato products are likely to consume less than optimal amounts.

How much is usually taken?

The ideal intake of lycopene is currently unknown; however, the men in the Harvard study with the greatest protection against **cancer** (page 87) consumed at least 6.5 mg per day.

Are there any side effects or interactions?

No adverse effects have been reported with the use of lycopene.

LYSINE

What is it?

Lysine is an essential **amino acid** (page 465) needed for growth and to help maintain nitrogen balance in the body. (Essential amino acids cannot be made in the body and must be supplied by the diet or **supplements** [page 559].)

Lysine appears to help the body absorb and conserve **calcium** (page 483).[1] Lysine has many functions in the body because it is incorporated into many proteins, which are used by the body for a variety of purposes. Lysine interferes with replication of **herpes viruses** (page 200) and is therefore often prescribed by doctors to people with **cold sores** (page 119) or genital herpes. A review of the research trials investigating the effects of lysine on people with cold sores shows that most, though not all, trials support the use of lysine.[2]

Where is it found?

Brewer's yeast (page 480), legumes, dairy, fish, and meat all contain significant amounts of lysine.

Lysine has been used in connection with the following conditions (refer to the individual health concern for complete information):

Rating	Health Concerns
★★★	**Cold sores** (page 119) (recurrence prevention)
★★☆	**Genital Herpes** (page 200)
★☆☆	**Shingles** (page 401)

Who is likely to be deficient?

Most people, including vegans (vegetarians who also avoid dairy and eggs), consume adequate amounts of lysine. However, vegans whose diets contain large amounts of grains and only minimal amounts of beans could become deficient in lysine. **Athletes** (page 43) involved in frequent vigorous exercise have increased need for essential **amino acids** (page 465), although most diets meet these increased needs. The essential amino acid requirements of **burn** (page 85) patients may exceed the amount of lysine in the diet.

How much is usually taken?

Most people do not require lysine supplementation. Doctors often suggest that people with recurrent **herpes simplex** (page 119) infections take 1,000–3,000 mg of lysine per day.

Are there any side effects or interactions?

In animals, high amounts of lysine have been linked to increased risk of **gallstones** (page 193)[3] and **elevated cholesterol** (page 223).[4] At supplemental amounts, no consistent problems have been reported in humans, though abdominal cramps and transient **diarrhea** (page 163) have occasionally been reported at very high (15–40 grams per day) intakes.[5]

Lysine supplementation increases the absorption of **calcium** (page 483) and may reduce its excretion.[6] As a result, some researchers believe that lysine may eventually be shown to have a role in the prevention and treatment of **osteoporosis** (page 333).[7]

Lysine works with other essential **amino acids** (page 465) to maintain growth, lean body mass, and the body's store of nitrogen.

MAGNESIUM

What is it?

Magnesium is an essential mineral to the human body. It is needed for bone, protein, and fatty acid formation, making new cells, activating **B vitamins** (page 603), relaxing muscles, clotting blood, and forming adenosine triphosphate (ATP; the energy the body runs on). The secretion and action of insulin also require magnesium.

Magnesium also acts in a way related to **calcium** (page 483) channel blocker drugs. This effect may be responsible for the fact that under certain circumstances magnesium has been found to potentially improve vision in people with glaucoma.[1] Similarly, this action might account for magnesium's ability to **lower blood pressure** (page 246).[2]

Since magnesium has so many different actions in the body, the exact reasons for some of its clinical effects are difficult to determine. For example, magnesium has reduced hyperactivity in children in preliminary research.[3] Other research suggests that some children with attention deficit-hyperactivity disorder (ADHD) have lowered levels of magnesium. In a preliminary but controlled trial, 50 ADHD children with low magnesium (as determined by red blood cell, hair, and serum levels of magnesium) were given 200 mg of magnesium per day for six months.[4] Compared with 25 other magnesium-deficient ADHD children, those given magnesium supplementation had a significant decrease in hyperactive behavior.

Magnesium levels have been reported to be low in those with **chronic fatigue syndrome** (page 111) (CFS),[5] and magnesium injections have been reported to improve symptoms.[6] Oral magnesium supplementation has also improved symptoms in those people with CFS who had low magnesium levels in another report, although magnesium injections were sometimes necessary.[7] However, other research reports no evidence of magnesium deficiency in people with CFS.[8, 9] The reason for this discrepancy remains unclear. People with CFS considering magnesium supplementation should have their magnesium status checked beforehand by a doctor. Only people with magnesium deficiency appear to benefit from this therapy.

People with **diabetes** (page 152) tend to have lower magnesium levels compared with those who have normal glucose tolerance.[10] Supplementation with magnesium overcomes this problem[11] and may help some diabetics improve glucose tolerance.

Magnesium may be beneficial for bladder problems in women, especially common disturbances in bladder control and the sense of "urgency." A double-blind trial found that women who took 350 mg of magnesium hydroxide (providing 147 mg elemental magnesium) twice daily for four weeks had better bladder control and fewer symptoms than women who took a placebo.[12]

Magnesium supplementation may reduce dehydration of red blood cells in **sickle cell anemia** (page 403) patients. Administration of 540 mg per day of magnesium pidolate to sickle cell anemia patients was seen after six months, to reverse some of the characteristic red blood cell abnormalities and to dramatically reduce the number of painful days for these patients.[13] This preliminary trial was not blinded, so placebo effect could not be ruled out. Magnesium pidolate is also an unusual form of magnesium. It is unknown whether other forms of magnesium would produce similar results.

Where is it found?

Nuts and grains are good sources of magnesium. Beans, dark green vegetables, fish, and meat also contain significant amounts.

Magnesium has been used in connection with the following conditions (refer to the individual health concern for complete information):

Rating	Health Concerns
★★★	**Cardiac arrhythmia** (page 93) **Congestive heart failure** (page 134) **Diabetes** (page 152) **Dysmenorrhea** (page 171) **Gestational hypertension** (page 202) **Kidney stones** (page 284) (citrate in combination with **potassium** (page 572) citrate) **Migraine headaches** (page 314) **Mitral valve prolapse** (page 319)
★★☆	**ADHD** (page 55) **Anemia** (page 25) (for thalassemia) **Angina** (page 27) **Asthma** (page 32) **Celiac disease** (page 102) (for deficiency only) **Heart attack** (page 212) (IV magnesium immediately following a myocardial infarction) **High blood pressure** (page 246) (for people taking potassium-depleting diuretics) **Osteoporosis** (page 333) **Premenstrual syndrome** (page 368) Urinary urgency (women)

Magnesium

Rating	Health Concerns
★☆☆	**Alcohol withdrawal support** (page 12)
	Anxiety (page 30)
	Athletic performance (page 43)
	Autism (page 63)
	Chronic fatigue syndrome (page 111)
	Chronic obstructive pulmonary disease (page 114) (COPD)
	Cluster headache (page 117) (intravenous)
	Fibromyalgia (page 191)
	Glaucoma (page 205)
	Heart attack (page 212) (oral magnesium)
	High cholesterol (page 223)
	Hypoglycemia (page 251)
	Insomnia (page 270)
	Insulin resistance syndrome (page 273) (Syndrome X)
	Intermittent claudication (page 276)
	Multiple sclerosis (page 323)
	Preeclampsia (page 361)
	Raynaud's disease (page 382)
	Retinopathy (page 385)
	Sickle cell anemia (page 403)
	Stroke (page 419)

Magnesium *(side tab)*

Who is likely to be deficient?

Magnesium deficiency is common in people taking "**potassium** (page 572)-depleting" prescription diuretics. Taking too many laxatives can also lead to deficiency. **Alcoholism** (page 12), severe **burns** (page 85), **diabetes** (page 152), and **heart failure** (page 134) are other potential causes of deficiency. In a study of urban African-American people (predominantly female), the overall prevalence of magnesium deficiency was 20%. People with a history of alcoholism were six times more likely to have magnesium deficiency than were people without such a history.[14] The low magnesium status seen in alcoholics with **liver cirrhosis** (page 290) contributes to the development of **hypertension** (page 246) in these people.[15]

Almost two-thirds of people in intensive care hospital units have been found to be magnesium deficient.[16] Deficiency may also occur in people with chronic **diarrhea** (page 163), pancreatitis, and other conditions associated with **malabsorption** (page 304).

Fatigue, **abnormal heart rhythms** (page 93), muscle weakness and spasm, **depression** (page 145), loss of appetite, listlessness, and **potassium** (page 572) depletion can all result from a magnesium deficiency. People with these symptoms should be evaluated by a doctor before taking magnesium supplements.

As previously mentioned, magnesium levels have been found to be low in people with **chronic fatigue syndrome** (page 111).

Deficiencies of magnesium that are serious enough to cause symptoms should be treated by medical doctors, as they might require intravenous administration of magnesium.[17]

How much is usually taken?

Most people don't consume enough magnesium in their diets. Many nutritionally oriented doctors recommend 250–350 mg per day of supplemental magnesium for adults.

Are there any side effects or interactions?

Comments in this section are limited to effects from taking oral magnesium. Side effects from intravenous use of magnesium are not discussed.

Taking too much magnesium often leads to **diarrhea** (page 163). For some people this can happen with amounts as low as 350–500 mg per day. More serious problems can develop with excessive magnesium intake from magnesium-containing laxatives. However, the amounts of magnesium found in nutritional supplements are unlikely to cause such problems. People with kidney disease should not take magnesium supplements without consulting a doctor.

Vitamin B₆ (page 600) increases the amount of magnesium that can enter cells. As a result, these two nutrients are often taken together. Magnesium may compete for absorption with other minerals, particularly **calcium** (page 483). Taking a **multimineral supplement** (page 559) avoids this potential problem.

MALIC ACID

What is it?

Malic acid is a naturally occurring compound that plays a role in the complex process of deriving adenosine triphosphate (ATP; the energy currency that runs the body) from food.

Although uncontrolled research had suggested that the combination of 1,200–2,400 mg per day of malic acid and 300–600 mg of **magnesium** (page 551) for eight weeks reduced symptoms of **fibromyalgia** (page

191),[1] double-blind evidence has shown that malic acid plus magnesium fails to help people with this condition.[2]

Where is it found?
Malic acid is found in a wide variety of fruits and vegetables, but the richest source is apples, which is why malic acid is sometimes referred to as "apple acid."

Malic acid has been used in connection with the following conditions (refer to the individual health concern for complete information):

Rating	Health Concerns
★☆☆	Fibromyalgia (page 191)

Who is likely to be deficient?
A deficiency in humans is unlikely, since the body can produce malic acid.

How much is usually taken?
Healthy people do not need to take malic acid as a supplement. Research has been conducted with 1,200–2,400 mg of malic acid in combination with 300–600 mg of elemental **magnesium** (page 551).

Are there any side effects or interactions?
Current research does not indicate any adverse effects from the use of malic acid in moderate amounts.

MANGANESE

What is it?
Manganese is an essential trace mineral needed for healthy skin, bone, and cartilage formation, as well as glucose tolerance. It also helps activate superoxide dismutase (SOD)—an important **antioxidant enzyme** (page 467).

Where is it found?
Nuts and seeds, wheat germ, wheat bran, leafy green vegetables, beet tops, tea, and pineapple are all good sources of manganese.

Manganese has been used in connection with the following conditions (refer to the individual health concern for complete information):

Rating	Health Concerns
★★☆	Tardive dyskinesia (page 425)
★☆☆	Diabetes (page 152)
	Hypoglycemia (page 251)
	Osgood-Schlatter disease (page 327)
	Osteoporosis (page 333)
	Sprains and strains (page 412)

Who is likely to be deficient?
Many people consume less than the 2–5 mg of manganese currently considered safe and adequate. Nonetheless, clear deficiencies are rare. People with **osteoporosis** (page 333) sometimes have low blood levels of manganese, suggestive of deficiency.[1]

How much is usually taken?
Whether most people would benefit from manganese supplementation remains unclear. While there is no recommended dietary allowance, the National Research Council's "estimated safe and adequate daily dietary intake" is 2–5 mg.[2] The Institute of Medicine recommends that intake of manganese from food, water and dietary supplements should not exceed the tolerable daily upper limit of 11 mg per day. In contrast, the 5–15 mg often found in high-potency **multivitamin-mineral supplements** (page 559) is generally considered to be a reasonable level by many doctors, though many manufacturers are likely to reformulate their products to contain no more than 11 mg per daily amount.

Are there any side effects or interactions?
Amounts found in supplements (5–20 mg) have not been linked with any toxicity. Excessive intake of manganese rarely lead to psychiatric symptoms. However, most reports of manganese toxicity in otherwise healthy people have been in those people who chronically inhaled manganese dust at their jobs e.g., miners or alloy plant workers. Other sources of manganese intoxication are now recognized, including total parenteral nutrition (TPN) in patients who are being fed intravenously[3, 4, 5] and pesticides containing manganese in agricultural workers who have been exposed.[6]

Preliminary research suggests that people with **cir-**

rhosis (page 290)[7] or cholestasis (blocked bile flow from the gall bladder)[8] may not be able to properly excrete manganese. Until more is known, these people should not supplement manganese. Manganese supplementation (3–5 mg per day) has caused severe **hypoglycemia** (page 251) (low blood sugar) in a person with insulin-dependent **diabetes** (page 152).[9] People with diabetes who want to take manganese should consult their doctor.

Several minerals, such as **calcium** (page 483) and **iron** (page 540), and possibly **zinc** (page 614), reduce the absorption of manganese.[10] Of these interactions, the link to iron may be the most important. In one study, women with high iron status had relatively poor absorption of manganese.[11] In another report of manganese/iron interactions in women, increased intake of "non-heme iron"—the kind of iron found in most supplements—decreased manganese status.[12] These interactions suggest that taking multi-minerals that include manganese may protect against manganese deficiencies that might otherwise be triggered by taking isolated mineral supplements, particularly iron.

MEDIUM CHAIN TRIGLYCERIDES

What are they?
Medium-chain triglycerides (MCT) are a class of fatty acids. Their chemical composition is of a shorter length than the long-chain fatty acids present in most other fats and oils, which accounts for their name. They are also different from other fats in that they have a slightly lower calorie content[1] and they are more rapidly absorbed and burned as energy, resembling carbohydrate more than fat.[2]

MCT have been shown to increase calorie burning compared with other fats.[3, 4] However, researchers estimate that half of the calories in the diet would have to be eaten as MCT for significant **weight loss** (page 446) to occur.[5] Obese women on a calorie-restricted diet using MCT for 24% of total calories, experienced no greater weight loss after three months, than when regular fat was used.[6] Whether MCT would help people lose weight on a normal diet has not been adequately studied.

Since MCT is more rapidly used for energy than other fats, some **athletes** (page 43) have been inter-

ested in its use, especially during prolonged endurance exercise.[7] However, no effect on carbohydrate sparing or endurance exercise performance has been shown, with moderate amounts of MCT (30–45 grams).[8, 9] Trials using very large amounts (about 85 grams) have produced conflicting results. One study found increased performance when MCT was added to a 10% carbohydrate solution,[10] and another study actually reported decreased performance, probably due to gastrointestinal distress, in athletes using MCT.[11]

Because some short-term studies have shown that MCT lowers blood glucose levels, a group of researchers investigated the use of MCT to treat people with type 2 (adult onset or non-insulin-dependent) **diabetes** (page 152) mellitus.[12] In nonhospitalized people with diabetes who consumed MCT for an average of 17.5% of their total calorie intake for 30 days, MCT did not improve diabetic control by most measures.[13]

Where are they found?
Medium chain triglycerides are found in coconut oil, palm kernel oil, and butter. MCT are also available as a supplement.

Medium chain triglycerides have been used in connection with the following conditions (refer to the individual health concern for complete information):

Rating	Health Concerns
★☆☆	**Athletic performance** (page 43) **Diabetes** (page 152)

Who is likely to be deficient?
Most people consume adequate amounts of fat in their diets and many people consume excessive amounts, so extra fat intake as medium chain triglycerides is unnecessary.

How much is usually taken?
The best amount of medium chain triglycerides to take is currently unknown. Athletes are not likely to benefit from less than 50 grams during **exercise** (page 43). Larger amounts may possibly help some, but may also impair performance if not combined with carbohydrate.

Are there any side effects or interactions?
Consuming medium chain triglycerides on an empty stomach can lead to **gastrointestinal upset** (page 260). Anyone with **cirrhosis** (page 290) or other liver prob-

lems should check with a doctor before using MCT. Two reports suggest that MCT may raise serum **cholesterol** (page 223) and/or **triglycerides** (page 235).[14, 15] MCT is actually the preferred fatty acid source for cirrhotic patients, but only when used intermittently.[16]

MELATONIN

What is it?

Melatonin is a natural hormone that regulates the human biological clock.

Double-blind research with young adults has shown that melatonin facilitates **sleep** (page 270).[1] Another study of healthy, young adults reported that melatonin significantly shortened the time needed to go to sleep, reduced the number of night awakenings, and improved sleep quality.[2] Other researchers reported the time needed to get to sleep was reduced with melatonin.[3]

Melatonin is also helpful in relieving symptoms of **jet lag** (page 283). One double-blind trial, involving a sample of international flight crew members taking either melatonin or a placebo for three days before and five days after an international flight, found that melatonin significantly reduced symptoms of jet lag and resulted in a quicker recovery of preflight energy levels and alertness.[4]

Less than 1 mg of melatonin has lowered pressure within the eyes of healthy people,[5] but studies have not yet been published on the effects of using melatonin with people who have **glaucoma** (page 205).

Melatonin might help some people suffering from **depression** (page 145). A small double-blind study suggested that supplementation with small amounts of melatonin (0.125 mg taken twice per day) may reduce **winter depression** (page 397).[6] People with major depressive disorders sometimes have sleep disturbances. Melatonin has been shown to be effective at improving the quality of sleep of people with major depression.[7] However, because of the possibility that melatonin could exacerbate depression, it should only be used for this purpose, under a doctor's supervision.

When some people take melatonin to treat sleep disorders, chronic **tension headaches** (page 428) are relieved.[8] Melatonin has also relieved **cluster headaches** (page 117) in double-blind research.[9] Some researchers have suggested that melatonin's role in regulating core body temperature may be responsible for preventing cluster headaches,[10] which have been reported to be triggered by increased body heat.[11]

Melatonin also regulates **immunity** (page 255). One group of doctors reported two successfully treated cases of sarcoidosis that it attributed to melatonin's immune-modulating effect.[12] Also, because of its effects on the immune system, melatonin has been given to people with **cancer** (page 87) in many research trials. Low blood levels of melatonin are associated with an increased risk of uterine cancer.[13] Melatonin has significantly reduced the level of prostate specific antigen (PSA, a marker for cancer) in **prostate cancer** (page 371) patients.[14] Melatonin inhibits **breast cancer** (page 65) cells in test tubes[15] and has put some women with breast cancer into remission in preliminary research.[16] Melatonin supplementation has improved disease-free survival in people with melanoma[17] and increased survival in people with brain cancer[18] and **lung cancer** (page 298).[19] Melatonin exerts anti-inflammatory activity that may be responsible for its anticancer properties.[20]

In a double-blind trial, people who had difficulty sleeping as a result of **tinnitus** (page 430) were better able to sleep if given 3 mg melatonin per night for one month rather than a placebo.[21] Although melatonin did not reduce overall symptom scores for tinnitus, people in this trial with higher symptom scores did appear to obtain some benefit.

Melatonin supplementation may be helpful in treating **epilepsy** (page 183); 5–10 mg of melatonin taken at bedtime reduced the frequency of seizures and improved sleep in a group of children with epilepsy in a small, preliminary trial.[22] However, in a group of children suffering from neurological disorders, 1–5 mg of melatonin per night led to an increase in the rate of seizures.[23] Children with a seizure disorder called "myoclonus" were reported to have been cured by supplementing with 3–5 mg of melatonin per day in a preliminary trial.[24] Until more is known, children with neurological conditions should take melatonin only under medical supervision.

Melatonin may be useful in the treatment of **fibromyalgia** (page 191). In a small, uncontrolled preliminary study, 3 mg of melatonin at bedtime was found to reduce tender points associated with this disorder. **Pain** (page 338) and fatigue improved only slightly.[25]

Children with Angelman's syndrome (a rare, genetic disorder characterized by severe mental retardation, seizures, and sleep disturbances) may benefit from low amounts of melatonin. In an uncontrolled study, children with Angelman's Syndrome who took 0.3 mg of melatonin one-half to one hour before bedtime had significant improvement in nighttime sleep patterns and a reduction in movement disturbances during sleep.[26]

Animal studies indicate that melatonin secretion may regulate cardiovascular activity,[27, 28] blood pressure,[29] and blood flow to the brain.[30] In healthy young men, oral administration of 1 mg of melatonin significantly reduced blood pressure and levels of stress hormones within 90 minutes.[31] To date, no clinical trials in humans have tested the efficacy of melatonin for **hypertension** (page 246).

Where is it found?
Melatonin is produced by the pineal gland, located within the brain. Levels of melatonin in the body fluctuate with the cycles of night and day. The highest melatonin levels are found at night. Melatonin is present in foods only in trace amounts.

Melatonin has been used in connection with the following conditions (refer to the individual health concern for complete information):

Rating	Health Concerns
★★☆	Angelman's syndrome (sleep disturbances only) **Cluster headaches** (page 117) **Colon cancer** (page 123) **Depression** (page 145) **Insomnia** (page 270) **Jet lag** (page 283) **Schizophrenia** (page 393) (for sleep disturbances only) **Tardive dyskinesia** (page 425) **Tinnitus** (page 430) (**insomnia** [page 270]-associated)
★☆☆	**Age-related cognitive decline** (page 8) **Breast cancer** (page 65) **Epilepsy** (page 183) **Fibromyalgia** (page 191) **Glaucoma** (page 205) **Lung cancer** (page 298) **Migraine headaches** (page 316) Myoclonus **Prostate cancer** (page 371) Sarcoidosis

Who is likely to be deficient?
Although elderly people often have difficulty sleeping[32] and melatonin supplements have been shown to improve sleep in the elderly,[33] melatonin secretion does not appear to decline in healthy older adults to a significant degree, despite many preliminary reports to the contrary.[34] Most of these preliminary studies failed to verify that older subjects were healthy and not using drugs that suppress melatonin secretion (e.g., aspirin, ibuprofen, beta-blockers). Routine replacement of melatonin in elderly persons is, therefore, not recommended.

Adults with **insomnia** (page 270) have been shown to have lower melatonin levels.[35] Frequent travelers and shift workers are also likely to benefit from melatonin for the resynchronization of their sleep schedules,[36] though a melatonin "deficiency" as such does not exist for these people. Patients with **heart disease** (page 98) have been reported to have low melatonin levels, but whether this abnormality increases the risk of heart disease or whether heart disease leads to the low melatonin level is not yet known.[37] People with **schizophrenia** (page 393) were found to have low melatonin output and experienced significantly improved sleep following melatonin replacement supplementation.[38]

How much is usually taken?
Normally, the body secretes melatonin for several hours per night—an effect best duplicated with time-release supplements. Studies using timed-release melatonin for **insomnia** (page 270) have reported good results.[39] Many doctors suggest 1–3 mg of melatonin taken one to two hours before bedtime. Studies with people suffering from sarcoidosis or **cancer** (page 87) have used very high amounts of melatonin—typically 20 mg per night. Such levels should never be taken without the supervision of a doctor. Melatonin should not be taken during the day.

Are there any side effects or interactions?
Melatonin is associated with few side effects. However, morning grogginess, undesired drowsiness, sleepwalking, and disorientation have been reported. Researchers have hypothesized that certain people should not use melatonin supplements, including **pregnant** (page 363) or breast-feeding women, people with **depression** (page 145) or **schizophrenia** (page 393), and those with autoimmune disease, including **lupus** (page 421), at least until more is known.[40, 41]

In one study, administration of 3 mg per day of melatonin for three months resulted in a marked decline in sperm counts and a decline in sperm quality in two of eight healthy young men.[42] In one of these two men, sperm count and quality became normal after melatonin was discontinued. Although this was a small study, it raises the possibility that long-term use of melatonin could lead to infertility.

In a group of children suffering from neurological disorders, 1–5 mg of melatonin per night led to an increase in the rate of seizures despite the fact that sleep improved.[43] Until more is known, children with neurological conditions should take melatonin only under medical supervision.

Many other side effects have been attributed to melatonin supplementation, including inhibition of sex drive, severe headaches, abdominal cramps, and formation of rudimentary breasts in men.[44, 45] However, these associations have not been supported by solid evidence.[46, 47, 48, 49] Since none of these claims have been well documented or independently confirmed, these problems may not have been due to melatonin.

Though most research reports that melatonin improves the quality of sleep, at least one trial has found that four of fifteen men given melatonin had their sleep patterns disturbed by supplemental melatonin.[50]

One case of painful gynecomastia (enlarged breasts) has been reported involving a 56-year-old man who had been suffering from amyotrophic lateral sclerosis (Lou Gehrig's disease), and was taking 1–2 mg melatonin per day for one and a half years.[51] As the signs and symptoms disappeared after melatonin was discontinued, the authors of the report suspected that melatonin caused this side effect.

According to a preliminary report, blood levels of melatonin may be elevated in women with **fibromyalgia** (page 191).[52] Data in this report did not indicate toxicity from melatonin, nor did the report suggest that melatonin causes or exacerbates the symptoms of fibromyalgia. It *did* suggest there is no current rationale for melatonin supplementation in people with fibromyalgia.

One-time oral administration of 1 mg of melatonin to post-**menopausal** (page 311) women reduced glucose tolerance and insulin sensitivity when tested 45 minutes after administration.[53] This finding suggests that people with **diabetes** (page 152) should use melatonin with caution and only under the supervision of a doctor.

Special United Kingdom considerations

Melatonin is either not available or may require a prescription. People should check with their physicians.

METHIONINE

What is it?

Methionine is one of the essential **amino acids** (page 465) (building blocks of protein), meaning that it cannot be produced by the body, and must be provided by the diet. It supplies **sulfur** (page 590) and other compounds required by the body for normal metabolism and growth. Methionine also belongs to a group of compounds called lipotropics, or chemicals that help the liver process fats (lipids). Others in this group include **choline** (page 546), **inositol** (page 537), and **betaine** (page 472) (trimethylglycine).

People with **AIDS** (page 239) have low levels of methionine. Some researchers suggest this may explain some aspects of the disease process,[1, 2, 3] especially the deterioration that occurs in the nervous system that can cause symptoms, including **dementia** (page 19).[4, 5] A preliminary study has suggested that methionine (6 grams per day) may improve memory recall in people with AIDS-related nervous system degeneration.[6]

Other preliminary studies have suggested that methionine (5 grams per day) may help treat some symptoms of **Parkinson's disease** (page 345).[7] However, another form of methionine, S-adenosylmethionine (**SAMe** [page 583]) may worsen the symptoms of Parkinson's disease and should be avoided until more is known.[8, 9, 10, 11, 12]

Methionine (2 grams per day) in combination with several **antioxidants** (page 467), reduced **pain** (page 338) and recurrences of attacks of pancreatitis in a small but well-controlled trial.[13]

Where is it found?

Meat, fish, and dairy are all good sources of methionine. Vegetarians can obtain methionine from whole grains, but beans are a relatively poor source of this **amino acid** (page 465).

Methionine has been used in connection with the following conditions (refer to the individual health concern for complete information):

Rating	Health Concerns
★★☆	**Pancreatitis** (page 341)
	Parkinson's disease (page 345)
★☆☆	**HIV support** (page 239)
	Liver support

Methionine

Who is likely to be deficient?

Most people consume plenty of methionine through a typical diet. Lower intakes during **pregnancy** (page 363) have been associated with **neural tube defects** (page 63) in newborns, but the significance of this is not yet clear.[14]

How much is usually taken?

Amino acid (page 465) requirements vary according to body weight. However, average-size adults require approximately 800–1,000 mg of methionine per day—an amount easily obtained or even exceeded by most Western diets.

Are there any side effects or interactions?

Animal studies suggest that diets high in methionine, in the presence of B-vitamin deficiencies, may increase the risk for **atherosclerosis** (page 38) (hardening of the arteries) by increasing blood levels of **cholesterol** (page 223) and a compound called **homocysteine** (page 235).[15] This idea has not yet been tested in humans. Excessive methionine intake, together with inadequate intake of **folic acid** (page 520), **vitamin B$_6$** (page 600), and **vitamin B$_{12}$** (page 601), can increase the conversion of methionine to homocysteine—a substance linked to **heart disease** (page 98) and **stroke** (page 419). Even in the absence of a deficiency of **folic acid** (page 520), **B$_6$** (page 600), or **B$_{12}$** (page 601), megadoses of methionine (7 grams per day) have been found to cause elevations in blood levels of homocysteine.[16] Whether such an increase would create a significant hazard for humans taking supplemental methionine has not been established. Supplementation of up to 2 grams of methionine daily for long periods of time has not been reported to cause any serious side effects.[17]

METHOXYISOFLAVONE

What is it?

Methoxyisoflavone is a member of the family of **flavonoids (isoflavones)** (page 516). In a U.S. patent, the developers of this substance claim, based on preliminary animal research, that it possesses muscle-building and bone-building (anabolic) effects without the side effects seen with either androgenic (male) hormones or estrogenic (female) hormones.[1]

Where is it found?

Several substances similar to methoxyisoflavone are found in many plants and some foods, including soybeans. Whether methoxyisoflavone itself is found in nature is unknown.

Methoxyisoflavone has been used in connection with the following conditions (refer to the individual health concern for complete information):

Rating	Health Concerns
★☆☆	Athletic performance (page 43)

Who is likely to be deficient?

Methoxyisoflavone is not an essential nutrient, so no deficiencies are possible.

How much is usually taken?

Manufacturers of methoxyisoflavone recommend 200 to 400 mg twice a day.

Are there any side effects or interactions?

Hormones with anabolic effects on muscle often have side effects that include **acne** (page 4), male-pattern baldness, prostate enlargement, and lower high-density lipoprotein (HDL; "good") **cholesterol** (page 223). Whether methoxyisoflavone can cause these side effects has not been investigated.

METHYLSULFONYLMETHANE

What is it?

Methylsulfonylmethane (MSM) is a naturally occurring, organic, **sulfur** (page 590)-containing compound related to another sulfur-containing substance, dimethyl sulfoxide (**DMSO** [page 508]). MSM is found in small amounts throughout nature and has been detected in small amounts in the blood and urine of humans.[1]

Animal studies have shown that sulfur from oral supplements of MSM is incorporated into body proteins.[2] Animal studies have also reported that joints affected by **osteoarthritis** (OA [page 328]) have lower sulfur content,[3] and mice with arthritis given MSM, experience less joint deterioration.[4] According to a preliminary report, a double-blind trial in people with OA found that MSM, in the amount of 2,250 mg per day, reduced **pain** (page 338) after six weeks.[5]

Where is it found?

A precursor of MSM is formed initially by ocean plankton and released into the atmosphere, where it interacts with ozone and sunlight and returns to earth as MSM in rainfall. MSM can be taken up by plants and incorporated into their structure, but no measurement of the MSM content of foods has been done. Supplements containing MSM are available.

MSM has been used in connection with the following conditions (refer to the individual health concern for complete information):

Rating	Health Concerns
★☆☆	Osteoarthritis (page 328)

Who is likely to be deficient?

Although MSM is present in food, it is not an essential nutrient, so deficiency is not likely.

How much is usually taken?

Some authorities report anecdotally that 250–500 mg per day has beneficial effects on a variety of health problems.[6] However, the only controlled trial using MSM used over 2000 mg per day to treat **osteoarthritis** (page 328). More research is needed before reliable recommendations for MSM supplementation can be made.

Are there any side effects or interactions?

According to some anecdotal reports, MSM has been used in human research for many years in amounts above 2000 mg per day with no significant adverse effects.[7] However, **diarrhea** (page 163), skin rash, headache, and fatigue may be experienced in less than 20% of people, according to other anecdotal reports. Detectable levels of MSM in the brain of a person taking MSM supplements have been reported,[8] but the significance of this finding, if any, is unclear.

MOLYBDENUM

What is it?

Molybdenum is an essential trace mineral needed for the proper function of certain enzyme-dependent processes, including the metabolism of **iron** (page 540).

Preliminary evidence indicates that molybdenum, through its involvement in detoxifying sulfites, might reduce the risk of sulfite-reactive **asthma** (page 32) attacks.[1] However, a physician should be involved in the evaluation and treatment of sulfite sensitivity.

Where is it found?

The amount of molybdenum in plant foods varies significantly and is dependent upon the mineral content of the soil. The best sources of this mineral are beans, dark green leafy vegetables, and grains. Hard tap water can also supply molybdenum to the diet. Molybdeum is also available as a supplement.

Molybdenum has been used in connection with the following condition (refer to the individual health concern for complete information):

Rating	Health Concerns
★☆☆	Asthma (page 32)

Who is likely to be deficient?

Although molybdenum is an essential mineral, no deficiencies have been reported in humans.

How much is usually taken?

No recommended dietary allowance (RDA) has been established for molybdenum. The estimated range recommended by the Food and Nutrition Board as safe and adequate is 75–250 mcg per day for adults.

Are there any side effects or interactions?

Molybdenum is needed to convert purine to uric acid, and excessive intake could, in rare cases, increase uric acid levels and potentially trigger **gout** (page 208). Molybdenum interferes with the absorption of copper; long-term supplementation with molybdenum could, in theory, result in copper deficiency. Molybdenum has been reported to cause psychosis in a patient taking 300 to 800 mcg per day for 18 days. This report is as yet unsubstantiated by any other human or animal research.[2]

MULTIPLE VITAMIN-MINERAL SUPPLEMENTS

What do they do?

Multiple vitamin-mineral (MVM) supplements, sometimes known as multivitamin-mineral supplements, contain a variable number of essential and/or non-essential nutrients. Their primary purpose is to provide a convenient way to take a variety of supplemental nutrients from a single product, in order to prevent vitamin or mineral deficiencies, as well as to achieve higher intakes of nutrients believed to be of benefit above typical dietary levels.

Many MVMs contain at least 100% of the Daily Value (DV) or the U.S. Recommended Dietary Allowance (USRDA) of all vitamins that have been assigned these recommended values. Mineral levels may be lower, or in the case of high potency MVMs, most or all mineral levels may also be at 100% of DV or USRDA. Micronutrients that should be included in a complete MVM are **vitamin A** (page 595) (or **beta-carotene** [page 469]), **vitamin B-complex** (page 603) (**thiamine** [page 597], **riboflavin** [page 598], **niacin** [page 598] and/or **niacinamide** [page 598], **vitamin B₆** [page 600], **folic acid (folate)** [page 520], **vitamin B₁₂** [page 601], **pantothenic acid** [page 568], and **biotin** [page 473]), **vitamin C** (page 604), **vitamin D** (page 607), and **vitamin E** (page 609), and the minerals **calcium** (page 483), **magnesium** (page 551), **zinc** (page 614), **iodine** (page 538), **selenium** (page 584), **copper** (page 499), **manganese** (page 553), **chromium** (page 493), **molybdenum** (page 559), and possibly **iron** (page 540). Some MVMs also contain vitamin K, but people taking the medication warfarin (Coumadin) should consult their doctor before taking vitamin K supplements. **Phosphorus** (page 570) is another essential dietary mineral, but is so abundant in the diet that it does not need to be included in an MVM formula. The only exception is for elderly people, whose diets tend to be lower in phosphorus. Calcium interferes with phosphorus absorption, so older people who are taking a calcium supplement might benefit from taking additional phosphorus.[1]

Potassium (page 572) is an unusual case, as adequate amounts of potassium cannot, by law, be sold in nonprescription products. Thus potassium, when included in an MVM formula, represents only a trivial amount. MVMs may contain **iron** (page 540), but these should be taken only by people who have been diagnosed as having, or being at high risk of, **iron deficiency** (page 278), or who have a history of frequent iron deficiency.

Some nutrients may be beneficial at levels above what is possible to obtain from diet alone, and an MVM formula can provide these levels as well. Nutri-ents that may be useful to most people in larger amounts include **vitamin C** (page 604), **folic acid** (page 520), and **calcium** (page 483). **Vitamin E** (page 609) has long been thought to protect against **heart disease** (page 98) beginning at 100 IU per day, but more recent research has cast doubt on the value of vitamin E for heart-disease prevention.[2] Large amounts of **vitamin B₁** (page 597), **vitamin B₂** (page 598), **vitamin B₃** (page 598), and **pantothenic acid** (page 568) are often included in MVM formulas. Some people claim to experience improvements in mood, energy, and/or overall well-being when taking higher-than-RDA amounts of **B vitamins** (page 603). While there is not a great deal of scientific research to support those observations, one double-blind study of healthy volunteers found that an MVM supplement significantly reduced anxiety and perceived stress levels, and possibly improved energy and the ability to concentrate.[3]

The importance of including the nonessential nutrient **beta-carotene** (page 469) in MVMs remains speculative. The synthetic beta-carotene found in most MVMs clearly does not prevent **cancer** (page 87) and may increase the risk of **lung cancer** (page 298) in smokers. Therefore, the inclusion of synthetic beta-carotene in MVM formulas is of questionable value, and it should be avoided by smokers. This concern was validated by the results of a large study in which male smokers who supplemented with synthetic beta-carotene had an 18% increase in incidence of lung cancer, compared with those given a placebo.[4] On the other hand, because beta-carotene can be converted to **vitamin A** (page 595) without causing vitamin A toxicity, some manufacturers use beta-carotene as a source of vitamin A. In contrast to synthetic beta-carotene, however, natural beta-carotene and several other **carotenoids** (page 488) may be helpful in preventing certain diseases, including some cancers.[5, 6, 7] Increasingly, natural beta-carotene and several other carotenoids are found in higher quality MVMs.

Another class of non-essential nutrients is the **flavonoids** (page 516), which have **antioxidant** (page 467) and other properties and have been reported by some,[8] though not all,[9] researchers to be linked with a reduced risk of **heart disease** (page 98). MVM supplements also frequently include other nutrients of uncertain benefit in the small amounts supplied, such as **choline** (page 546), **inositol** (page 537), and various **amino acids** (page 465).

Preliminary and double-blind trials have shown that

women who use an MVM containing **folic acid** (page 520), beginning three months before becoming pregnant and continuing through the first three months of **pregnancy** (page 363),[10, 11] have a significantly lower risk of having babies with **neural tube defects** (page 63) (e.g., spina bifida) and other congenital defects.

In one double-blind trial, schoolchildren received, for three months, a daily low-potency vitamin-mineral tablet containing 50% of the USRDA for most essential vitamins and the minerals.[12] The subjects were "working class," primarily Hispanic, children, aged 6 to 12 years. Dramatic gains in certain measures of IQ were observed in about 20% of the supplemented children. These gains may have been due to the correction of specific nutrient deficiencies (for example, iron) found in these children. However, it was not possible in this study to identify which nutrients caused the increases in IQ.

What about "one-per-day" multiples?

One-per-day multiples are primarily **B-complex** (page 603) vitamins, with both **vitamin A** (page 595) and **vitamin D** (page 607) included either at high or low potency, depending on the supplement. The rest of the formula tends to be low potency. It does not take much of some of the minerals—for example, **copper** (page 499), **zinc** (page 614), and **iron** (page 540)—to offer 100% or more of what people normally require, so these minerals may appear at reasonable levels in a one-per-day MVM.

One-per-day MVMs usually do not provide sufficient amounts of many nutrient supplements shown to benefit people eating a Western diet, such as **vitamin E** (page 609), **calcium** (page 483), **magnesium** (page 551), and **vitamin C** (page 604). One-per-day MVMs should therefore not be viewed as a way to "cover all bases" in the way that high-potency MVMs, requiring three or more pills per day, are viewed.

How much is usually taken?

The following table shows the USRDA for nutrients as well as suggested optimum amounts of each vitamin and mineral that should be present in a daily MVM supplement for healthy people. Some people may want to take larger amounts because of specific health concerns. They should read the individual nutrient sections to learn about safe upper ranges of supplementation.

Nutrient	Daily Value (includes diet)	Suggested Daily Optimum in an MVM Supplement
Biotin (page 473)	300 mcg	300 mcg
Calcium (page 483)	1,000 mg	800–1,000 mg
Chromium (page 493)	120 mg	120–200 mcg
Copper (page 499)	2 mg	1–3 mg
Folate (page 520)	400 mcg	400 mcg
Iodine (page 538)	150 mcg	150 mcg
Iron (page 540)	18 mg	People should avoid iron supplements unless they have been diagnosed with having, or being at high risk of, **iron deficiency** (page 278).
Magnesium (page 551)	400 mg	250–400 mg
Manganese (page 553)	2 mg	2–5 mg
Molybdenum (page 559)	75 mcg	75 mcg
Niacin (page 598)	20 mg	20 mg
Pantothenic acid (page 568)	10 mg	10 mg
Riboflavin (page 598)	1.7 mg	1.7 mg
Selenium (page 584)	70 mcg	100–200 mcg
Thiamine (page 597)	1.5 mg	1.5 mg
Vitamin A (page 595)	5,000 IU	5,000 IU (as natural beta-carotene)
Vitamin B$_6$ (page 600)	2 mg	10 mg
Vitamin B$_{12}$ (page 601)	6 mcg	50 mcg
Vitamin C (page 604)	60 mg	100–200 mg
Vitamin D (page 607)	400 IU	400 IU
Vitamin E (page 609)	30 IU	30–400 IU
Vitamin K (page 612)	80 mcg	80 mcg
Zinc (page 614)	15 mg	15–25 mg

Multiple Vitamin-Mineral Supplements

Because one-per-day formulas typically do not contain even the minimum recommended amounts of some of the nutrients listed here, multiples requiring several capsules or tablets per day are preferable. With two- to six-per-day multiples, intake should be spread out at two or three meals each day, instead of taking them all at one sitting. The amount of vitamins and minerals can be easily increased or decreased by taking more or fewer of the multiple.

Which is better—capsule or tablet?

Multiples are available as a powder inside a hard-shell pull-apart capsule, as a liquid inside a soft-gelatin capsule, or as a tablet.

Most multiples have all the ingredients mixed together. Occasionally the **B vitamins** (page 603) react with the rest of the ingredients in the capsule or tablet. This reaction, which is sped up in the presence of moisture or heat, can cause the B vitamins to "bleed" through the tablet or capsule, discoloring it and also making the multiple smell. While the multiple is still safe and effective, the smell is off-putting and usually not very well tolerated. Liquid multiples in a soft-gel capsule—or tablets or capsules that are kept dry and cool—do not have this problem.

Capsules are usually not as large as tablets, and thus some people find capsules easier to swallow.

Some people prefer vegetarian multiples. While some capsules are made from vegetarian sources, most come from animal gelatin. Vegetarians need to carefully read the label to ensure they are getting a vegetarian product.

One concern people have with tablets is whether they will break down sufficiently to allow the nutrients to be absorbed. Properly made tablets and capsules will dissolve readily in the stomach.

What about timed-release?

Some multiples are in timed-release form. The theory is that releasing vitamins and minerals slowly into the body over a period of time is better than releasing all of the nutrients at once. Except for work done on **vitamin C** (page 604)—some of which showed timed-release C was better absorbed than non-timed-release—research on this question has been lacking. It is possible that some nutrients, especially minerals, will be poorly absorbed from timed-release multiples. Also, some doctors have concerns about the safety of ingesting the chemicals that are used in tablets or capsules to make them timed-release.

What about nutrient interactions?

Another area of controversy is whether all of the nutrients in a multiple would be better utilized if they were taken separately. While certain nutrients compete with each other for absorption, this is also the case when the nutrients are supplied in food. For example, **magnesium** (page 551), **zinc** (page 614), and **calcium** (page 483) compete; **copper** (page 499) and zinc also compete. However, the body is designed to cope with this competition, which should not be a problem if multiples are spread out over the day.

What about chewables?

Unfortunately, multiples do not taste very good. In order to make chewable multiples palatable, whether for children or adults, some compromises must be made. First, bad-tasting ingredients must be reduced or eliminated. Second, the rest of the ingredients must be masked with a sweetener.

Unless an artificial sweetener like aspartame (NutraSweet) or saccharin is used, the only sweeteners available are sugars. Generally, consuming sugar is undesirable, and not having it in a chewable dietary supplement would be preferable. Xylitol, a natural sugar rarely used in chewables because it is relatively expensive, would be an ideal choice since it does not cause tooth decay or other known problems.

Some chewables, such as **vitamin C** (page 604), contain more sugar than any other ingredient. In such products, the sweetener should be listed as the first ingredient, but often is not. Care needs to be exercised when reading labels about chewable vitamins. If it tastes sweet, it contains sugar or a synthetic sweetener. In addition, chewable vitamin C products should contain buffered vitamin C, rather than the acidic form, ascorbic acid, in order to avoid damaging dental enamel.

When is the best time to take a multiple?

The best time to take vitamins or minerals is with meals. Multiples taken between meals sometimes cause **stomach upset** (page 260) and are likely not to be as well absorbed.

N-ACETYL CYSTEINE

What is it?

N-acetyl cysteine (NAC) is an altered form of the **amino acid cysteine** (page 502), which is commonly found in food and synthesized by the body.

NAC helps break down mucus. Double-blind research has found that NAC supplements improved symptoms and prevented recurrences in people with chronic **bronchitis** (page 80).[1, 2, 3] NAC may also protect lung tissue through its **antioxidant** (page 467) activity.[4]

NAC helps the body synthesize **glutathione** (page 531), an important antioxidant. In animals, the antioxidant activity of NAC protects the liver from the adverse effects of exposure to several toxic chemicals. NAC also protects the body from acetaminophen toxicity and is used at very high levels in hospitals for patients with acetaminophen poisoning. It has also been shown to be effective at treating liver failure from causes other than acetaminophen poisoning (e.g., **hepatitis** [page 220], and other drug toxicity)[5] and at preventing kidney damage caused by injections of iopromide, a contrast medium used in people scheduled to undergo computerized tomography (CT) imaging.[6]

Supplementation with NAC has been shown to reduce the proliferation of certain cells lining the colon and may reduce the risk of **colon cancer** (page 123) in people with recurrent polyps in the colon.[7]

There have been several case reports of oral NAC producing dramatic improvements in Unverricht-Lundborg disease, an inherited degenerative disorder involving seizures and progressive disability.[8, 9] One study used 3 grams of NAC per day.

Oral supplementation with NAC has been used successfully in two cases to treat a rare syndrome that complicates kidney dialysis.[10] This condition, known as pseudoporphyria, has no other known treatment. Controlled clinical trials are needed to confirm these preliminary observations.

People undergoing a certain cardiac procedure (coronary angiography) are at risk of developing kidney damage from the injected dye that is used to visualize the coronary arteries. In a double-blind study, oral administration of NAC reduced by 86% the incidence of kidney damage in people undergoing this procedure.[11] The amount of NAC used in that study was 400 mg twice a day, on the day before and the day of the procedure.[12] Other studies have shown that NAC is protective only when a low dose of dye is used.

Where is it found?

Cysteine (page 502), the **amino acid** (page 465) from which NAC is derived, is found in most high-protein foods. NAC is not found in the diet.

N-acetyl cysteine has been used in connection with the following conditions (refer to the individual health concern for complete information):

Rating	Health Concerns
★★★	Acetaminophen poisoning **Bronchitis** (page 80) (chronic) **Chronic obstructive pulmonary disease** (page 114) (COPD)
★★☆	**Angina pectoris** (page 27) **Gastritis** (page 195) **Heart Attack** (page 212) (IV immediately following a myocardial infarction) **HIV support** (page 239) Prevention of kidney damage during coronary angiography Unverricht-Lundborg Disease
★☆☆	Pseudoporphyria

Who is likely to be deficient?

Deficiencies of NAC have not been defined and may not exist. Deficiencies of the related **amino acid** (page 465) **cysteine** (page 502) have been reported in **HIV-infected** (page 239) patients.[13]

How much is usually taken?

Healthy people do not need to supplement NAC. Optimal levels of supplementation remain unknown, though much of the research uses 250–1,500 mg per day.

Are there any side effects or interactions?

One study reported that 19% of people taking NAC orally experienced nausea, vomiting, headache, dry mouth, dizziness, or abdominal pain.[14] These symptoms have not been consistently reported by other researchers, however.

Although a great deal of research has shown that NAC has **antioxidant** (page 467) activity, one small study found that daily amounts of 1.2 grams or more could lead to *increased* oxidative stress.[15] Extremely large amounts of **cysteine** (page 502), the **amino acid** (page 465) from which NAC is derived, may be toxic to nerve cells in rats.

NAC may increase urinary zinc excretion.[16] Therefore, supplemental **zinc** (page 614) and **copper** (page 499) should be added when supplementing with NAC for extended periods.

N - A c e t y l   C y s t e i n e

N-ACETYL-GLUCOSAMINE

What is it?

N-acetyl-glucosamine (NAG) is a form of glucosamine, one of the building blocks of joint tissue and other connective tissues. NAG differs from **glucosamine sulfate** (page 528) and glucosamine hydrochloride; instead of a sulfur or chloride molecule, NAG has a larger, more complex molecule attached to it. As a result, NAG is an entirely different molecule than either glucosamine sulfate or hydrochloride, and it also appears to be handled by the body differently.

Over the years, numerous researchers have repeatedly demonstrated in animal and test tube studies that NAG is inferior to other forms of glucosamine in terms of absorption and utilization.[1, 2, 3, 4, 5, 6, 7] However, an animal study demonstrated that NAG was able to enhance the manufacture of cartilage in damaged joints.[8] A recent human study compared the absorption of NAG to a long chain of NAG molecules (POLY-Nag).[9] Results showed that orally ingested NAG and POLY-Nag are absorbed and increase the blood levels of NAG, with both forms yielding similar results. In addition, there was some conversion of both molecules to glucosamine. However, the degree of conversion still resulted in lower levels of blood glucosamine levels compared to glucosamine sulfate and glucosamine hydrochloride, which are both absorbed extremely well.[10, 11] Furthermore, unlike glucosamine sulfate, there have been no human clinical studies utilizing NAG to treat arthritis or other health problems.

Where is it found?

NAG is available primarily in tablets and capsules.

Who is likely to be deficient?

As NAG is not an essential nutrient, no deficiency states have been reported.

How much is usually taken?

Most manufacturers recommend supplementation with 1,500 mg daily.

Are there any side effects or interactions?

No significant side effects or interactions have yet been reported in studies on NAG.

NADH

What is it?

NADH (nicotinamide adenine dinucleotide) is the active coenzyme form of **vitamin B_3** (page 598). It plays an essential role in the energy production of every human cell.

In the brain, increased NADH concentrations may result in improved production of essential neurotransmitters.[1] Large preliminary studies using oral or injected NADH to treat **Parkinson's disease** (page 345) showed reductions in physical disability and in the need for medication;[2, 3] however, a small, double-blind, short-term trial using injections of NADH found no significant effects.[4] A small, uncontrolled study showed that oral NADH improved mental function in people with **Alzheimer's disease** (page 19).[5] Preliminary research suggests that NADH may also help people with **depression** (page 145)[6] or **chronic fatigue syndrome** (page 111).[7] These promising results come from research conducted by the developer of the oral NADH supplement and require independent confirmation.

Where is it found?

NADH is found in the muscle tissue of fish and poultry and cattle, as well as in food products made with yeast. However, it is not known whether the NADH from these sources can be efficiently absorbed or utilized by the body. It is also available as a nutritional supplement.

NADH has been used in connection with the following conditions (refer to the individual health concern for complete information):

Rating	Health Concerns
★★☆	**Chronic fatigue syndrome** (page 111) **Parkinson's disease** (page 345)
★☆☆	**Alzheimer's disease** (page 19) **Depression** (page 145)

Who is likely to be deficient?

NADH deficiency is known to occur only in the presence of **vitamin B_3** (page 598) deficiency, which is rare in Western society except in some **alcoholics** (page 12).

Which form of NADH is best?

NADH appears to be a chemically unstable molecule that decomposes rapidly. For this reason, techniques have been developed to stabilize the NADH sold in tablet form. At the present time, it is not known which commercially available NADH products are most effective.

How much is usually taken?

Researchers have used 10 mg per day, taken with water only, on an empty stomach.

Are there any side effects or interactions?

Clinical studies of NADH using oral or intravenous administration have reported no side effects with up to one year or more of use. Longer-term use has not been evaluated.

OCTACOSANOL

What is it?

Octacosanol is a waxy substance naturally present in some plant oils and is the primary component of the sugar cane extract called policosanol.

Octacosanol-containing wheat germ oil was investigated decades ago as an **exercise performance** (page 43)–promoting (ergogenic) agent. These preliminary studies found that octacosanol had promising effects on endurance, reaction time, and other measures of exercise capacity.[1] In another trial, 1,000 mcg per day of octacosanol for eight weeks was found to improve grip strength and visual reaction time, but it had no effect on chest strength, auditory reaction time, or endurance.[2]

Where is it found?

Octacosanol is a waxy substance found in vegetable oils and sugar cane *(Saccharum officinarum)*. Another compound, called policosanol, contains a large amount of octacosanol, along with several similar compounds.

Octacosanol has been used in connection with the following conditions (refer to the individual health concern for complete information):

Rating	Health Concerns
★☆☆	**Athletic performance** (page 43)

Who is likely to be deficient?

Because octacosanol is not an essential bodily constituent, deficiencies do not occur.

How much is usually taken?

When octacosanol is taken as part of policosanol, 5–10 mg of policosanol is taken twice each day with meals. For exercise performance, 1 mg per day of octacosanol has been used.

Are there any side effects or interactions?

Long-term trials in humans using amounts up to 20 mg per day have not shown any negative effects.[3]

ORNITHINE

What is it?

Ornithine, an **amino acid** (page 465), is manufactured by the body when another amino acid, **arginine** (page 467), is metabolized during the production of urea (a constituent of urine).

Animal research has suggested that ornithine, along with arginine, may promote muscle-building activity in the body by increasing levels of growth-promoting (anabolic) hormones such as insulin and growth hormone. However, most human research does not support these claims at reasonable intake levels.[1, 2, 3] One study that did demonstrate increased growth hormone with oral ornithine used very high amounts (an average of 13 grams per day) and reported many gastrointestinal side effects.[4] One controlled study reported greater increases in lean body mass and strength after five weeks of intensive strength training in **athletes** (page 43) taking 1 gram per day each of arginine and ornithine compared with a group doing the exercise but taking a placebo.[5] These findings require independent confirmation.

In clinical studies on people hospitalized for surgery, generalized **infections** (page 265), **cancer** (page 87), trauma, or **burns** (page 85), supplementation with ornithine alpha-ketoglutarate (OKG) has been reported to produce several beneficial effects.[6] A double-blind trial evaluated the effects of OKG supplementation in elderly people recovering from acute illnesses.[7] Those who took 10 grams of OKG per day for two months had marked improvement in appetite, weight gain, and quality of life compared with those taking the placebo. They also had shorter recovery periods and required

O r n i t h i n e

fewer home visits by physicians and nurses and needed fewer medications.

Ornithine aspartate has been shown to be beneficial in people with brain abnormalities (hepatic encephalopathy) due to **liver cirrhosis** (page 290). In a double-blind trial, people with cirrhosis and hepatic encephalopathy received either 18 grams per day of L-ornithine-L-aspartate or a placebo for two weeks.[8] Those taking the ornithine had significant improvements in liver function and blood tests compared with those taking the placebo.

Preliminary[9] and controlled[10] studies of people with severe burns showed that supplementation with 10–30 grams of ornithine alpha-ketoglutarate per day significantly improved **wound healing** (page 319) and decreased the length of hospital stays.

Where is it found?

As with **amino acids** (page 465) in general, ornithine is predominantly found in meat, fish, dairy, and eggs. Western diets typically provide 5 grams per day. The body also produces ornithine.

Ornithine has been used in connection with the following conditions (refer to the individual health concern for complete information):

Rating	Health Concerns
★★☆	**Liver cirrhosis** (page 290) (hepatic encephalopathy) (L-ornithine-L-aspartate) Recovery from illness (ornithine alpha-ketoglutarate)
★☆☆	**Athletic performance** (page 43) (for body composition and strength)

Who is likely to be deficient?

Since ornithine is produced by the body, a deficiency of this nonessential **amino acid** (page 465) is unlikely, though depletion can occur during growth or **pregnancy** (page 363), and after severe trauma or malnutrition.[11]

How much is usually taken?

Most people would not benefit from ornithine supplementation. In human research involving ornithine, 5–10 grams are typically used per day, sometimes combined with **arginine** (page 467).

Are there any side effects or interactions?

No side effects have been reported with the use of ornithine, except for gastrointestinal distress with intakes over 10 grams per day.

The presence of **arginine** (page 467) is needed to produce ornithine in the body, so higher levels of this **amino acid** (page 465) should increase ornithine production.

ORNITHINE ALPHA-KETOGLUTARATE

What is it?

The amino acids **ornithine** (page 565) and **glutamine** (page 530) are combined to form ornithine alpha-ketoglutarate (OKG).

OKG has been shown to improve protein retention, **wound repair** (page 319), and **immune function** (page 255) in hospitalized patients partly by increasing levels of growth-promoting (anabolic) hormones such as insulin and growth hormone.[1] In a large, well-controlled trial,[2] nonhospitalized elderly people benefited from 10 grams per day of OKG as they recovered from various illnesses or surgery, showing improved appetite, weight gain, muscle growth, reduced need for medical care, and improved quality of life. No studies on muscle growth in athletes using OKG have been published.

Where is it found?

Although the **amino acids** (page 465) that comprise OKG are present in protein foods such as meat and poultry and fish, the OKG compound is found only in supplements.

OKG has been used in connection with the following condition (refer to the individual health concern for complete information):

Rating	Health Concerns
★★☆	**Wound healing** (page 319)

Who is likely to be deficient?

A deficiency of OKG has not been reported.

How much is usually taken?

Optimal levels remain unknown, though 10 grams per day has been used in clinical trials.

Are there any side effects or interactions?

No side effects have been reported with the use of OKG.

No clear interactions between OKG and other nutrients have been established.

PABA

What is it?

Para-aminobenzoic acid (PABA) is a compound that is an essential nutrient for microorganisms and some animals, but has not been shown to be essential for people. PABA is considered by some to be a member of the **vitamin B-complex** (page 603), though its actions differ widely from other B vitamins.

PABA has been reported to enhance the effects of cortisone.[1] It may also prevent or even reverse accumulation of abnormal fibrous tissue.

The most well-known property of PABA is as an effective sunscreen, when used topically. Oral PABA supplementation has not been shown to possess any sunscreening properties.[2]

An isolated trial published in 1942 reported that 12 of 16 **infertile women** (page 187) were able to become **pregnant** (page 363) after supplementing with 100 mg of PABA taken four times per day for three to seven months.[3] The effect of PABA on fertility has not been studied in modern research.

Researchers have attempted to discover whether large amounts of PABA would be helpful in various connective tissue disorders. Although preliminary studies have reported that PABA (12 grams per day) was helpful to people with scleroderma,[4, 5, 6] a double-blind trial found that supplementation with PABA did not lead to improvement.[7]

Older published reports of uncontrolled investigations suggest that PABA may be helpful in a variety of conditions, including dermatomyositis,[8] Peyronie's disease (accumulation of abnormal fibrous tissue in the penis),[9] pemphigus (a severe blistering disease),[10] and **vitiligo** (page 443) (a disorder in which patches of skin lose their pigmentation).[11] However, PABA was reported to cause vitiligo in one report.[12]

Older preliminary reports found that PABA darkened gray hair in a minority of elderly (but not younger) people.[13] In these trials, between 200 and 600 mg of PABA was taken per day for several months, in some cases accompanied by other **B vitamins** (page 603). However, at least one other study found that

PABA did not darken gray hair.[14] Therefore, the evidence supporting the use of PABA as a way to return gray hair to its original color remains very weak.

Where is it found?

PABA is found in grains and foods of animal origin.

PABA has been used in connection with the following conditions (refer to the individual health concern for complete information):

Rating	Health Concerns
★☆☆	**Dermatitis herpetiformis** (page 151)
	Dermatomyositis
	Infertility (female) (page 187)
	Pemphigus
	Peyronie's disease
	Scleroderma
	Vitiligo (page 443)

Who is likely to be deficient?

Deficiencies of PABA have not been described in humans, and most nutritionists do not consider it an essential nutrient.

Which form of PABA is best?

PABA is available as a nutritional supplement, but because it is mildly acidic, it can cause stomach irritation when taken in large amounts. The potassium salt of PABA, called Potaba, which is available by prescription, tends to be better tolerated.

How much is usually taken?

Small amounts of PABA are present in some **B-complex vitamins** (page 603) and **multivitamin formulas** (page 559). The amount of PABA used in the studies described above ranged from 300 mg to 12 grams per day. Anyone taking more than 400 mg of PABA per day should consult a physician.

Are there any side effects or interactions?

No serious side effects have been reported with 300–400 mg per day. Larger amounts (such as 8 grams per day or more) may cause **low blood sugar** (page 251), rash, fever, and (on rare occasions) liver damage.[15] One report exists of **vitiligo** (page 443) appearing after ingestion of large amounts of PABA[16] and use of amounts over 20 grams per day in small children has resulted in deaths.[17] There is also a report of a death from toxic **hepatitis** (page 220) in a person with **lupus** (page

421), who took as much as 48 grams per day for six days, followed by 8 grams per day for seven months.[18]

No interactions between PABA and other nutrients have been reported. However, PABA interferes with sulfa drugs (a class of antibiotics) and therefore should not be taken when these medications are being used.

PANTOTHENIC ACID

What is it?

Pantothenic acid, also called vitamin B_5, is a water-soluble vitamin involved in the Kreb's cycle of energy production and is needed to make the neurotransmitter acetylcholine. It is also essential in producing, transporting, and releasing energy from fats. Synthesis of cholesterol (needed to manufacture **vitamin D** (page 607) and steroid hormones) depends on pantothenic acid. Pantothenic acid also activates the adrenal glands.[1] Pantethine—a byproduct of pantothenic acid—has been reported to lower blood levels of **cholesterol** (page 223) and **triglycerides** (page 235).

Where is it found?

Liver, yeast, and salmon have high concentrations of pantothenic acid, but most other foods, including vegetables, dairy, eggs, grains, and meat, also provide some pantothenic acid.

Pantothenic acid or pantethine have been used in connection with the following conditions (refer to the individual health concern for complete information):

Rating	Health Concerns
★★★	**High cholesterol** (page 223) (pantethine) **High triglycerides** (page 235) (pantethine)
★★☆	**Rheumatoid arthritis** (page 387) (pantothenic acid)
★☆☆	**Acne** (page 4) (pantothenic acid) **Lupus** (page 421)

Who is likely to be deficient?

Pantothenic acid deficiencies may occur in people with **alcoholism** (page 12) but are generally believed to be rare.

How much is usually taken?

Most people do not need to supplement with pantothenic acid. However, the 10–25 mg found in many multivitamin (page 559) supplements might improve pantothenic acid status. So-called primitive human diets provided greater amounts of this nutrient than is found in modern diets. Most cholesterol researchers using pantethine have given people 300 mg three times per day (total 900 mg).

Are there any side effects or interactions?

No serious side effects have been reported, even at intakes of up to 10,000 mg (10 grams) per day. Very large amounts of pantothenic acid (several grams per day) can cause **diarrhea** (page 163).

Pantothenic acid works together with **vitamin B_1** (page 597), **vitamin B_2** (page 598), and **vitamin B_3** (page 598) to help make the fuel our bodies run on—ATP.

There is one report of a 76-year-old woman who developed a life-threatening condition (eosinophilic pleuropericardial effusion) while taking 300 mg of pantothenic acid per day and 10 mg of biotin per day.[2] However, it is not clear whether the vitamins caused the problem.

PHENYLALANINE

What are they?

L-phenylalanine (LPA) serves as a building block for the various proteins that are produced in the body. LPA can be converted to **L-tyrosine** (page 544) (another **amino acid** [page 465]) and subsequently to L-dopa, norepinephrine, and epinephrine. LPA can also be converted (through a separate pathway) to phenylethylamine, a substance that occurs naturally in the brain and appears to elevate mood.

D-phenylalanine (DPA) is not normally found in the body and cannot be converted to L-tyrosine, L-dopa, or norepinephrine. As a result, DPA is converted primarily to phenylethylamine (the potential mood elevator). DPA also appears to influence certain chemicals in the brain that relate to **pain** (page 338) sensation.

DLPA is a mixture of LPA and its mirror image DPA. DLPA (or the D- or L-form alone) has been used to treat **depression** (page 145).[1, 2] DPA may be helpful for some people with **Parkinson's disease** (page 345)[3] and has been used to treat chronic pain—including pain from **osteoarthritis** (page 328) and **rheumatoid arthritis** (page 387)—with both positive[4] and negative[5] results. No research has evaluated the effectiveness of DLPA on rheumatoid arthritis.

Where are they found?

LPA is found in most foods that contain protein. DPA does not normally occur in food. However, when phenylalanine is synthesized in the laboratory, half appears in the L-form and the other half in the D-form. These two compounds can also be synthesized individually, but it is more expensive to do so. The combination supplement (DLPA) is often used because of the lower cost and because both components exert different health-enhancing effects.

Phenylalanine has been used in connection with the following conditions (refer to the individual health concern for complete information):

Rating	Health Concerns
★★☆	**Depression** (page 145) (DPA, LPA, DLPA) **Low back pain** (page 293) (DPA) **Pain** (page 328) (DPA) **Parkinson's disease** (page 345) (DPA) **Vitiligo** (page 443) (LPA)
★☆☆	**Alcohol withdrawal support** (page 12) (DLPA) **Osteoarthritis** (page 328) (DPA) **Rheumatoid arthritis** (page 387) (DPA)

Who is likely to be deficient?

People whose diets are very low in protein may develop a deficiency of LPA, although this is believed to be very uncommon. However, one does not necessarily have to be deficient in LPA in order to benefit from a DLPA supplement.

How much is usually taken?

DLPA has been used in amounts ranging from 75–1,500 mg per day. This compound can have powerful effects on mood and on the nervous system, and therefore DLPA should be taken only under medical supervision. LPA has been used in amounts up to 3.5 grams per day. For best results, phenylalanine should be taken between meals, because the protein present in food can interfere with the uptake of phenylalanine into the brain, potentially reducing its effect.

Are there any side effects or interactions?

The maximum amount of DLPA that is safe is unknown. However, consistent toxicity in healthy people has not been reported with 1,500 mg per day or less of DLPA, except for occasional nausea, **heartburn** (page 260), or transient headaches.

When 100 mg of LPA per 2.2 pounds body weight or more was given to animals, a variety of complex problems occurred, leading two researchers to have concerns about potential toxicity of high amounts in humans.[6] While these concerns were directed at LPA specifically, they are likely to be equally applicable to DLPA. Although no serious adverse effects have been reported in humans taking phenylalanine, amounts greater than 1,500 mg per day should be supervised by a doctor.

People with **phenylketonuria** (page 354) must not supplement with phenylalanine.

Some research suggests that people with **tardive dyskinesia** (page 425) may process phenylalanine abnormally. Until more is known, it makes sense for people with this condition to avoid phenylalanine supplementation.

LPA competes with several other **amino acids** (page 465) for uptake into the body and the brain. Therefore, for best results, phenylalanine should be taken between meals, or away from protein-containing foods. People taking prescription or over-the-counter medications should consult a physician before taking DLPA.

PHOSPHATIDYLSERINE

What is it?

Phosphatidylserine (PS) belongs to a special category of fat-soluble substances called phospholipids, which are essential components of cell membranes. PS is found in high concentrations in the brain.

According to double-blind studies, PS may help preserve, or even improve, some aspects of mental functioning in the elderly when taken in the amount of 300 mg per day for three to six months.[1, 2]

In patients with early **Alzheimer's disease** (page 19), placebo-controlled[3] and double-blind studies have shown mild benefits from PS supplementation when used in the amount of 300 mg per day for three to twelve weeks.[4, 5] In one double-blind study, the improvement on standardized tests of mental functioning averaged approximately 15%.[6] Continued improvement has been reported up to three months beyond the end of the supplementation period.[7]

PS is not a cure for Alzheimer's disease. While it may reduce symptoms in the short term, at best PS probably slows the rate of deterioration rather than halting the progression altogether. For example, in a six-month trial, benefits began to fade after the fourth month.[8] PS affects the levels of neurotransmitters in the brain related to mood. In a preliminary trial, elderly women suffering from **depression** (page 145) who were given 300 mg of PS per day for 30 days experienced, on average, a 70% reduction in the severity of their depression.[9]

Where is it found?
PS is found in only trace amounts in a typical diet. Very small amounts are present in **lecithin** (page 546). The body manufactures PS from phospholipid building blocks. PS research has used material derived from a bovine source. Currently, PS that is commercially available is derived from soy.

Phosphatidylserine has been used in connection with the following conditions (refer to the individual health concern for complete information):

Rating	Health Concerns
★★★	**Age-related cognitive decline (ARCD)** (page 8)
★☆☆	**Alzheimer's disease** (page 19) **Depression** (page 145) **Parkinson's disease** (page 345)

Who is likely to be deficient?
PS is not an essential nutrient, and therefore dietary deficiencies do not occur. Adults age 50 and older, especially those with **age-related cognitive decline** (page 8), may not synthesize enough PS, and appear most likely to benefit from supplemental PS.

Which form is best?
Most research has been conducted with PS derived from bovine (cow) brain tissue. Due to concerns about the possibility of humans contracting infectious diseases (such as Creutzfeld-Jakob or "mad cow" disease), bovine PS is not available in the United States. The soy- and bovine-derived PS, however, are not structurally identical.[10] Doctors and researchers have debated whether the structural differences could be important,[11, 12] but so far only a few trials have studied the effects of soy-based PS.

Preliminary animal research shows that the soy-derived PS does have effects on brain function similar to effects from the bovine source.[13, 14, 15] An isolated unpublished double-blind human study used soy-derived PS in an evaluation of memory and mood benefits in non-demented, non-depressed elderly people with impaired memories and accompanying **depression** (page 145).[16] In this three-month study, 300 mg per day of PS was not significantly more effective than a placebo. In a double-blind study, soy-derived PS was administered in the amount of 300 or 600 mg per day for 12 weeks to people with **age-related memory impairment** (page 8). Compared with the placebo, soy-derived PS had no effect on memory or on other measures of cognitive function.[17] While additional research needs to be done, currently available evidence suggests that soy-derived PS is not an effective treatment for age-related cognitive decline.

How much is usually taken?
Positive effects on mental function have been achieved using 200–500 mg per day of bovine PS; most studies used 300 mg per day.

Are there any side effects or interactions?
No significant side effects associated with PS have been reported.

PHOSPHORUS

What is it?
Phosphorus is an essential mineral that is usually found in nature combined with oxygen as phosphate. Most of the phosphate in the human body is in bone, but phosphate-containing molecules (phospholipids) are also important components of cell membranes and lipoprotein particles, such as HDL and LDL ("good" and "bad" cholesterols, respectively). Small amounts of phosphate play important roles in numerous biochemical reactions throughout the body.

The role of phosphate-containing molecules in aerobic exercise reactions has suggested that phosphate loading might enhance **athletic performance** (page 43), though controlled research has produced inconsistent results.[1, 2]

Where is it found?
Phosphorus is highest in protein-rich foods and cereal grains. In addition, phosphorus additives are used in many soft drinks and packaged foods. Phosphorus is

not often present in supplements except for certain **calcium** (page 483) supplements, such as bone meal.

Phosphorus has been used in connection with the following condition (refer to the individual health concern for complete information):

Rating	Health Concerns
★★☆	**Osteoporosis** (page 333) (for elderly people taking calcium supplements)
★☆☆	**Athletic performance** (page 43)

Who is likely to be deficient?
Phosphorus deficiency is uncommon, because dietary intake is usually adequate.[3] Chronic alcoholics may become deficient in phosphorus.[4] and people taking large amounts of aluminum-containing antacids[5]

One study has shown that taking calcium can interfere with the absorption of phosphorus, which, like calcium, is important for bone health.[6]. Although most western diets contain ample or even excessive amounts of phosphorus, older people who supplement with large amounts of calcium may be at risk of developing phosphorus deficiency. For this reason, the authors of this study recommend that, for elderly people, at least some of the supplemental calcium be taken in the form of tricalcium phosphate or some other phosphorus-containing preparation.

How much is usually taken?
Phosphorus supplements are unnecessary. Most multiple vitamin-mineral supplements do not contain phosphorus for this reason.

Are there any side effects or interactions?
People with severe kidney disease must avoid excessive phosphorus. High phosphorus intake may impair absorption of **iron** (page 540), **copper** (page 499), and **zinc** (page 614).[7] Based primarily on animal studies, some authorities have suggested that excess intake of phosphate is hazardous to normal calcium and bone metabolism,[8] but this idea has been challenged.[9] Phosphoric acid–containing soft drinks have been implicated in elevated **kidney stone** (page 284) risk,[10, 11] but not all studies have found this relationship.[12]

Ingestion of excessive amounts of aluminum-containing antacids (such as Di-Gel, Riopan, Maalox, or Mylanta) can cause phosphorus deficiency.

POLICOSANOL

What is it?
Policosanol is a mixture of long-chain alcohols (waxes), including **octacosanol** (page 565), extracted from natural sources.

Where is it found?
The long-chain alcohols found in policosanol are present in many foods of plant origin. Supplemental policosanol is typically extracted from sugar cane or beeswax.

Policosanol has been used in connection with the following condition (refer to the individual health concern for complete information):

Rating	Health Concerns
★★★	**High cholesterol** (page 223)
	Intermittent claudication (page 276)
★★☆	**High triglycerides** (page 235)

Who is likely to be deficient?
Policosanol is not an essential nutrient, so no deficiencies are possible.

How much is usually taken?
Most studies have used 5 to 10 mg of policosanol taken twice per day.

Are there any side effects or interactions?
When policosanol is combined with aspirin, an increased blood-thinning effect occurs.[1] This suggests that policosanol should not be taken with blood-thinning drugs without the supervision of a doctor.

POLLEN

What is it?
Pollen, a substance collected from the flowers of various plants, contains carbohydrates, fat, protein, and some vitamins and minerals.[1]

A proprietary rye pollen extract (Cernilton) has been shown to have anti-inflammatory properties,[2] to relax

Pollen

the muscles that surround the urethra,[3] and to inhibit growth of prostate cells.[4] This rye pollen extract has been reported to improve symptoms of chronic **prostatitis** (page 377) in uncontrolled trials,[5, 6, 7] including a trial in which three tablets daily significantly reduced symptoms in 78% of people with uncomplicated prostatitis. However, only one of eighteen people with complications (such as scar tissue and calcifications) improved.[8]

Preliminary[9, 10, 11] and double-blind[12, 13, 14] trials have demonstrated that a proprietary rye pollen extract is effective at reducing the symptoms of benign prostatic hyperplasia.

A preliminary report from the Ukraine on the use of flower pollen in humans with **rheumatoid arthritis** (page 387) suggested positive effects on related disorders of the liver, gallbladder, stomach, and intestine.[15] Pollen extracts have been used orally to desensitize people to plants to which they are **allergic** (page 14).[16, 17, 18, 19, 20] For example, in a double-blind study, people with **hay fever** (page 211) allergies to grass pollen were asked to place drops of liquid grass pollen extract under their tongues daily for three weeks, using a gradually increasing concentration. After the three-week period, pollen was given twice per week at a "maintenance" level. During the next allergy season they had significantly fewer severe hay fever symptoms than a group given placebo drops.[21]

Melbrosia, a mixture of flower pollen, fermented bee pollen, and **royal jelly** (page 582), was reported to help relieve **menopausal** (page 311) symptoms in about one-third of women in an uncontrolled survey in Denmark.[22] This result agrees with an earlier, controlled study that found melbrosia (amount not stated) was more effective than a placebo for menopausal symptoms, including headache, urinary incontinence, vaginal dryness, and low vitality.[23] According to animal studies, melbrosia does not work by causing estrogen-like effects in body tissues.[24] Whether royal jelly alone might have similar effects on menopausal symptoms is unknown.

Where is it found?

Most noncultivated plants produce pollen. Commercial pollen is collected from bees returning to their hives (bee pollen) or may be directly harvested with machines (flower pollen). It is not clear which plants produce the most effective pollens. Some of the most common pollens used are timothy grass, corn, rye, and pine.

Pollen has been used in connection with the following conditions (refer to the individual health concern for complete information):

Rating	Health Concerns
★★★	**Benign prostatic hyperplasia** (page 58) (rye)
★★☆	**Prostatitis** (page 377) (rye)

Who is likely to be deficient?

Since pollen is not an essential bodily constituent, deficiencies do not occur.

How much is usually taken?

The optimal intake of pollen is unknown. Some doctors recommend using 500 mg two to three times per day. Research on the proprietary rye pollen extract has used three to six tablets, or four capsules, per day.

Are there any side effects or interactions?

Many people have **allergies** (page 14) to inhaled pollen. Allergic reactions to ingested pollen (some of them quite serious) have also been reported.[25, 26, 27] Otherwise, no significant adverse effects have been reported.

POTASSIUM

What is it?

Potassium is an essential mineral needed to regulate water balance, levels of acidity, **blood pressure** (page 246), and neuromuscular function. This mineral also plays a critical role in the transmission of electrical impulses in the heart.

People with low blood levels of potassium who are undergoing heart surgery are at an increased risk of developing **heart arrhythmias** (page 93) and an increased need for cardiopulmonary resuscitation.[1] Potassium is also required for carbohydrate and protein metabolism.

Where is it found?

Most fruits are excellent sources of potassium. Beans, milk, and vegetables contain significant amounts of potassium.

Pollen

Potassium has been used in connection with the following conditions (refer to the individual health concern for complete information):

Rating	Health Concerns
★★★	**High blood pressure** (page 246) (for people *not* taking potassium-sparing diuretics) **Kidney stones** (page 284) (citrate in combination with **magnesium** [page 551] citrate)
★★☆	**Cardiac arrhythmia** (page 93) **Congestive heart failure** (page 134) **Premenstrual syndrome** (page 368) **Stroke** (page 419)

Who is likely to be deficient?

So-called primitive diets provided much greater levels of potassium than modern diets, which may provide too little. Gross deficiencies, however, are rare except in cases of prolonged vomiting, **diarrhea** (page 163), or use of "potassium-depleting" diuretic drugs. People taking one of these drugs are often advised by their doctor to take supplemental potassium. Prescription amounts of potassium provide more than the amounts sold over the counter but not more than the amount found in several pieces of fruit.

How much is usually taken?

The best way to obtain extra potassium is to eat several pieces of fruit per day, as well as liberal amounts of vegetables. The amount of potassium found in the diet ranges from about 2.5 grams to about 5.8 grams per day. The amount allowed in supplements—99 mg per tablet or capsule—is very low, considering that one banana can contain 500 mg. One should not attempt to achieve higher potassium levels by taking large numbers of potassium pills. This concentrated form of potassium can irritate the stomach—a problem not encountered with the potassium in food.

Are there any side effects or interactions?

High potassium intake (several hundred milligrams at one time in tablet form) can produce stomach irritation. People using potassium-sparing drugs should avoid using potassium chloride-containing products, such as Morton Salt Substitute, No Salt, Lite Salt, and others and should not take potassium supplements, except under the supervision of a doctor. Even eating several pieces of fruit each day can sometimes cause problems for people taking potassium-sparing drugs, due to the high potassium content of fruit.

Potassium and sodium work together in the body to maintain muscle tone, blood pressure, water balance, and other functions. Many researchers believe that part of the **blood pressure** (page 246) problem caused by too much salt (which contains sodium) is made worse by too little dietary potassium.

People with kidney failure should not take potassium supplements, except under careful medical supervision.

PREGNENOLONE

What is it?

Pregnenolone serves as a precursor to other hormones, including dehydroepiandrosterone (**DHEA** [page 503]) and **progesterone** (page 577).[1]

The functions of pregnenolone in the body are not well known. It has been suggested the role of pregnenolone in the body is to serve as a "mother steroid" (precursor hormone). Aside from that role, it has no known functions in the body.

Many effects of pregnenolone on the nervous system have been studied. Rat studies indicate powerful memory-enhancing effects,[2] far beyond that of other neuroactive substances.[3, 4] In healthy men aged 20 to 30, administration of pregnenolone (1 mg daily) was found to improve **sleep** (page 270) quality and decrease intermittent wakefulness.[5]

It has been suggested this hormone may play a role in the neuroendocrine response to stress. In a study of airplane pilots subjected to stress, administration of pregnenolone (25 mg twice daily) improved performance without causing adverse side effects.[6] In a study of the stress response in rats, an increase in **anxiety** (page 30) was observed following administration of pregnenolone. The researchers suggested this was a beneficial response during a stressful period and was initiated through the nervous system.[7]

In a study of rats subjected to spinal cord injury, administration of pregnenolone in combination with the anti-inflammatory medication indomethacin (Indocin) and an immune-modulating substance (bacterial lipopolysaccharide) promoted recovery of nerve function. The effect was more pronounced with combination therapy than with any one of these substances given singly or in combinations of two.

Pregnenolone has not been studied in humans with spinal cord injuries.[8]

Pregnenolone appears to exhibit an antagonistic effect on the calming receptors in the brain (gamma-amino butyric acid [**GABA** (page 524)] receptors), resulting in an excitatory effect. It is possible this alteration in nervous system transmission could contribute to seizure activity.[9, 10]

Steroid hormones are known to affect mood and behavior via effects on the nervous system. In people with either current **depression** (page 145) or a history of depression, pregnenolone in the cerebrospinal fluid (the fluid that bathes the brain) was significantly lower, than levels in healthy people. In addition, it was found that patients with active depression had lower levels of pregnenolone compared with those with a prior history of depression.[11]

In a double-blind study of elderly women with wrinkles, daily application of a 0.5% pregnenolone acetate cream improved the visible wrinkling of the skin. When the treatment was discontinued, the benefit was not maintained. Because the results were only temporary, it is suggested the beneficial effect of the cream was due to improved hydration of the skin.[12]

Researchers have reported on the use of pregnenolone in a variety of rheumatologic diseases. In a study of pregnenolone therapy (intramuscular injection, 50–600 mg daily) for **rheumatoid arthritis** (page 387), six of eleven people experienced moderate to marked improvement in symptoms of joint pain and joint mobility. The symptom improvement was apparent two to four days after therapy was initiated. In a study of 13 adults with **osteoarthritis** (page 328), pregnenolone therapy reduced the **pain** (page 338) and improved the range of motion in seven of the study participants. Pain recurred when therapy was discontinued. In a person who suffered from gouty arthritis that was unresponsive to conventional medications, pregnenolone therapy resulted in a dramatic response within three days of initiating therapy. This patient received 300 mg daily of pregnenolone (by intramuscular injection) for four weeks, followed by 200 mg weekly of pregnenolone as a maintenance amount. This study of pregnenolone therapy in rheumatologic diseases also reports a substantial benefit in patients with **systemic lupus erythematosus** (page 421) (SLE), **psoriasis** (page 379), and scleroderma. Of the 59 people reported in this paper, the only adverse effect was redness or pain at the site of injection. No systemic adverse effects were reported.[13]

Where is it found?

The cells of both the adrenal gland and the central nervous system synthesize pregnenolone. Human studies show there are much higher concentrations of pregnenolone in the nervous tissue, than in the bloodstream.[14] Animal studies indicate the concentration of pregnenolone in the brain is ten-fold higher than that of other stress-related hormones (including **DHEA** [page 503]).[15] Pregnenolone is present in the blood as both free pregnenolone and a more stable form, pregnenolone-sulfate.

Who is likely to be deficient?

Since it is not an essential nutrient, pregnenolone is not associated with a deficiency state.

How much is usually taken?

Pregnenolone is generally available in amounts of 10 to 30 mg. It is not known what an appropriate intake is for humans or whether the benefits of taking this hormone outweigh the risks.

Are there any side effects or interactions?

Due to its antagonistic effects on the **GABA** (page 524) receptor in the central nervous system, supplementation with pregnenolone could cause problems in people with a history of seizures. Pregnenolone supplementation may increase the levels of **progesterone** (page 577) and **DHEA** (page 503) in the body and possibly the levels of other hormones (testosterone and estradiol). In theory, pregnenolone could cause disturbances in the endocrine system, which may manifest as changes in the menstrual cycle or the development or aggravation of hormone sensitive diseases (including **breast** [page 65] and **prostate cancer** [page 371]). The side effects and interactions with other therapies are currently unknown.

PROANTHOCYANIDINS

What are they?

Proanthocyanidins—also called "OPCs" for oligomeric procyanidins or "PCOs" for procyanidolic oligomers—are a class of nutrients belonging to the **flavonoid** (page 516) family.

Proanthocyanidins have **antioxidant** (page 467) activity and they play a role in the stabilization of collagen and maintenance of elastin—two critical proteins in

Pregnenolone (side tab)

connective tissue that support organs, joints, blood vessels, and muscle.[1, 2] Possibly because of their effects on blood vessels, proanthocyanidins have been reported in double-blind research to reduce the duration of **edema** (page 180) after face-lift surgery from 15.8 to 11.4 days.[3] In preliminary research, proanthocyanidins were reported to have anti-mutagenic activity (i.e., to prevent chromosomal mutations).[4]

Proanthocyanidins have been shown to strengthen capillaries in double-blind research using as little as 100 mg per day.[5] In another double-blind trial, French researchers reported that women with **chronic venous insufficiency** (page 116) had reduced symptoms using 150 mg per day.[6] In another French double-blind trial, supplementation with 100 mg taken three times per day, resulted in benefits within four weeks.[7]

Proanthocyanidins (200 mg per day for five weeks) have improved aspects of vision (**visual performance in the dark** (page 326) and after exposure to glare) in healthy people.[8, 9] A product that is high in proanthocyanidins has been shown to prevent and reverse abnormal blood clotting in smokers.[10]

Where are they found?

Proanthocyanidins can be found in many plants, most notably pine bark, grape seed, and grape skin. However, **bilberry** (page 634), **cranberry** (page 664), black currant, **green tea** (page 686), black tea, and other plants also contain these **flavonoids** (page 516). Nutritional supplements containing proanthocyanidins extracts from various plant sources are available, alone or in combination with other nutrients, in herbal extracts, capsules, and tablets.

Proanthocyanidins have been used in connection with the following conditions (refer to the individual health concern for complete information):

Rating	Health Concerns
★★★	**Chronic venous insufficiency** (page 116)
★★☆	**Capillary fragility** (page 93) **Retinopathy** (page 385)
★☆☆	**Pancreatic insufficiency** (page 341) **Varicose Veins** (page 440)

Who is likely to be deficient?

Flavonoids (page 516) and proanthocyanidins are not classified as essential nutrients because their absence does not induce a deficiency state. However, proantho-

cyanidins may have many health benefits, and anyone not eating the various plants that contain them would not derive these benefits.

How much is usually taken?

Flavonoids (page 516) (proanthocyanidins and others) are a significant source of **antioxidants** (page 467) in the average diet. Proanthocyanidins at 50–100 mg per day is considered a reasonable supplemental level by some doctors, but optimal levels remain unknown.

Are there any side effects or interactions?

Flavonoids (page 516), in general, and proanthocyanidins, specifically, have not been associated with any consistent side effects. As they are water-soluble nutrients, excess intake is simply excreted in the urine.

PROBIOTICS

What are they?

Probiotic bacteria favorably alter the intestinal microflora balance, inhibit the growth of harmful bacteria, promote good digestion, boost **immune function** (page 255), and increase resistance to **infection** (page 265).[1, 2] People with flourishing intestinal colonies of beneficial bacteria are better equipped to fight the growth of disease-causing bacteria.[3, 4] Lactobacilli and bifidobacteria maintain a healthy balance of intestinal flora by producing organic compounds—such as lactic acid, hydrogen peroxide, and acetic acid—that increase the acidity of the intestine and inhibit the reproduction of many harmful bacteria.[5, 6] Probiotic bacteria also produce substances called bacteriocins, which act as natural antibiotics to kill undesirable microorganisms.[7]

Immune function (page 255) tends to decline with age. Twice daily supplementation with *Bifidobacterium lactis* (a particular strain of bifidobacteria) in milk was found in a double-blind trial to significantly enhance various aspects of immune function in a group of healthy elderly people.[8] Benefits were apparent after only six weeks of supplementation. Yogurt has been purported to support immune function, due to its inclusion of lactic-acid bacteria.[9] While *B. lactis* is a different organism than that found in yogurt, effects on immunity may be similar.

Regular ingestion of probiotic bacteria may help prevent **vaginal yeast infection** (page 454).[10, 11] A review of the research concluded that both topical and oral use

Probiotics

of acidophilus can prevent yeast infection caused by candida overgrowth.[12]

Diarrhea (page 163) flushes intestinal microorganisms out of the gastrointestinal tract, leaving the body vulnerable to opportunistic **infections** (page 265). Replenishing the beneficial bacteria with probiotic supplements can help prevent new infections. The incidence of "traveler's diarrhea," caused by pathogenic bacteria in drinking water or undercooked foods, can be reduced by the preventive use of probiotics.[13]

Most people associate lactobacilli with *L. acidophilus*, the most popular species in this group of probiotic bacteria. However, research shows that other *Lactobacillus* species may be beneficial as well. For example, *L. rhamnosus* and *L. plantarum* appear to be protective intestinal bacteria. They are involved in the production of several "gut nutrients," such as short-chain fatty acids, and the **amino acids** (page 465), **arginine** (page 467), **cysteine** (page 502), and **glutamine** (page 530).[14] These beneficial bacteria may also help remove toxins from the gut and exert a beneficial effect on **cholesterol levels** (page 223).[15]

In a double-blind trial, administration of a preparation containing *L. plantarum* to people with acute pancreatitis reduced the number of complications severe enough to require surgery.[16]

One probiotic, *Saccharomyces boulardii,* has prevented diarrhea in several human trials.[17] Double-blind research studying critically ill patients found this strain of yeast to prevent diarrhea when 500 mg is taken four times per day.[18]

Probiotics are important in recolonizing the intestine during and after antibiotic use. Probiotic supplements replenish the beneficial bacteria, preventing up to 50% of infections occurring after antibiotic use.[19]

Probiotics also promote healthy **digestion** (page 260). **Enzymes** (page 506) secreted by probiotic bacteria aid digestion. Acidophilus is a source of **lactase** (page 545), the enzyme needed to digest milk sugar, which is lacking in **lactose-intolerant** (page 288) people.[20]

Fructo-oligosaccharides (page 522) (FOS) are naturally occurring carbohydrates that cannot be digested or absorbed by humans. They support the growth of bifidobacteria, one of the beneficial bacterial strains.[21] Due to this effect, some doctors recommend that patients taking bifidobacteria also supplement with FOS. Several trials have used 8 grams per day. However, a review of the research has suggested that 4 grams per day appears to be enough to significantly increase the amount of bifidobacteria in the gut.[22]

Where are they found?

Beneficial bacteria present in fermented dairy foods—namely live culture yogurt—have been used as a folk remedy for hundreds, if not thousands, of years. Yogurt is the traditional source of beneficial bacteria. However, different brands of yogurt can vary greatly in their bacteria strain and potency. Some (particularly frozen) yogurts do not contain any live bacteria. Supplements in powder, liquid extract, capsule, or tablet form containing beneficial bacteria are other sources of probiotics.

Probiotics have been used in connection with the following conditions (refer to the individual health concern for complete information):

Rating	Health Concerns
★★★	**Diarrhea** (page 163) **Tooth decay** (page 431) (*Lactobacillus* GG) **Vaginitis** (page 438) **Yeast infection** (page 454)
★★☆	**Canker sores** (page 90) **Colic** (page 121) (*Bifidobacterium lactis* and *Streptococcus thermophilus*) **Crohn's disease** (page 141) (*Saccharomyces boulardii*) **Eczema** (page 177) **Food allergies** (page 14) **HIV support** (page 239) (*Saccharomyces boulardii*) **Immune function** (page 255) **Infection** (page 265) Pancreatitis (acute) (*Lactobacillus plantarum*) **Ulcerative colitis** (page 433)
★☆☆	**Chronic candidiasis** (page 109)

Who is likely to be deficient?

People using antibiotics, eating a poor diet, or suffering from **diarrhea** (page 163) are more likely to have depleted colonies of friendly bacteria.

How much is usually taken?

The amount of probiotics necessary to replenish the intestine varies according to the extent of microbial depletion and the presence of harmful bacteria. One to two billion colony forming units (CFUs) per day of acidophilus is considered to be the minimum amount for the healthy maintenance of intestinal microflora. Some *Saccharomyces boulardii* research has used 500 mg taken four times per day.

Are there any side effects or interactions?

There are at least nine case reports of severe, invasive (internal) fungal **infections** (page 265) developing in people treated with the yeast organism *Saccharomyces boulardii*. All of these people were debilitated or had impaired **immune function** (page 255) prior to receiving *Saccharomyces boulardii*.[23, 24] No such adverse reactions have been reported with other probiotic supplements or in people with normal immune systems.

Acidophilus and bifidobacteria may manufacture **B vitamins** (page 603), including **niacin** (page 598), **folic acid** (page 520), **biotin** (page 473), and **vitamin B$_6$** (page 600).

PROGESTERONE

What is it?

Progesterone is a hormone from a corpus luteum, formed by the cyclical rupture of an ovarian follicle. Progesterone is necessary for proper uterine and breast development and function.

Natural progesterone and synthetic progestins are structurally different and have differing effects in the body. Progestins are recommended by doctors if estrogen is prescribed during or after **menopause** (page 311), because prolonged estrogen replacement therapy without the addition of progestins (or large amounts of natural progesterone), increases the risk of uterine cancer.[1] However, women who have had a hysterectomy—and therefore no longer have a uterus—are typically prescribed estrogens without progestins. Although natural progesterone is considered by some doctors to be safer and more effective for a variety of health problems, researchers have studied the effects of supplemental natural progesterone much less than the effects of synthetic progestins.

Preliminary evidence suggests that progesterone plays a role in bone metabolism and could help reduce the risk of osteoporosis.[2] An uncontrolled study, using topically applied natural progesterone cream in combination with diet, exercise, and **vitamin** (page 559) and **calcium** (page 483) supplementation, reported consistent gains in bone density over a three-year period in postmenopausal women. However, no comparison was made to a similar program without progesterone.[3]

One trial found that adding natural progesterone to estrogen therapy had no better effect on bone mass than estrogen therapy alone[4] and another trial reported that progesterone applied topically over a one-year period had no effect on bone loss.[5] In a more recent double-blind study, progesterone had a modest bone-sparing (protective) effect in post-menopausal women.[6]

Some doctors have observed that progesterone administered vaginally, rectally, or topically (to the skin) can relieve the symptoms of **premenstrual syndrome** (page 368) (PMS).[7] However, most well-controlled studies have not found natural progesterone to be effective against PMS.[8]

One double-blind study found that topical administration of natural progesterone led to a reduction in hot flashes in 83% of women, compared with improvement in only 19% of those given a placebo.[9] Synthetic progestins have also been reported to reduce symptoms of **menopause** (page 311).[10]

Some studies have linked synthetic progestins to increased risk of **breast cancer** (page 65).[11] In contrast, topical progesterone has produced changes in breast tissue that may have a **cancer prevention** (page 87) effect.[12, 13] Other researchers, however, have reported essentially opposite effects, suggesting that natural progesterone may increase proliferation of breast cells.[14]

Looked at as a whole, the research remains incomplete and inconsistent. In one trial, (natural) progesterone deficiency was linked with an increased risk, but only when the breast cancer was diagnosed before menopause.[15] Such a finding fits with the idea that natural progesterone might be protective. This position is further strengthened by a preliminary trial showing that a raised level of progesterone in the blood at the time of breast cancer surgery is associated with an improved prognosis for premenopausal women with operable breast cancer.[16] However, most breast cancer begins postmenopausally, and one trial found that progesterone *deficiency* was associated with a large (though statistically nonsignificant) *decreased* risk of postmenopausal breast cancer.[17] If duplicated by future research, this finding would not suggest protection, nor even necessarily safety.

A recent report found that long-term topical use of natural progesterone on the breast neither increased nor decreased the risk of women eventually being diagnosed with breast cancer.[18] In this trial, some women were also taking oral synthetic progesterone-like drugs. Remarkably, women using this combination experienced a 50% decreased risk of eventually being diagnosed with breast cancer. More research is needed to understand the effects of both synthetic and natural progesterone in both pre- and postmenopausal women.

Synthetic progestins have been linked to effects that might increase the risk of **heart disease** (page 98).[19] However, vaginally applied natural progesterone has been reported to significantly enhance the benefits of estrogen replacement therapy on heart function in women with **coronary artery disease** (page 38).[20] More research is needed to evaluate the effects of natural progesterone on heart disease.

Although the differences in the chemical structure of natural progesterone and synthetic progestins are slight, their effects in the body differ considerably and the two forms should not be considered interchangeable. Synthetic progestins may be useful for **endometriosis** (page 182) and **menorrhagia** (page 314) (prolonged or profuse menstrual flow) because of their specific effects on progesterone receptors in the brain and on the glandular response of the uterine lining. However, these same effects may be detrimental for women with **PMS** (page 368), and may be associated with *increased* symptoms, such as **depression** (page 145), headaches, and **water retention** (page 180). Thus, natural progesterone may be preferable to synthetic progestins for PMS.[21]

Where is it found?

Progesterone is produced in the female body in the ovaries. Progesterone production is high during the luteal phase (second portion) of the menstrual cycle and low during the follicular phase (first portion), as well as being low before puberty and after menopause.

Supplemental sources of progesterone are available in oral and cream forms, as well as lozenges, suppositories, and injectable forms. "Natural" progesterone refers to the molecule that is identical in chemical structure to the progesterone produced in the body, even if the molecule is synthesized in a laboratory.

Progestins are found in oral contraceptive pills and are used in conventional hormone replacement therapy.

Wild yam (page 759) contains precursors to progesterone (such as diosgenin) that can be converted through a chemical process in the laboratory into progesterone—the exact same molecule made in the human body. However, contrary to popular claims, the diosgenin in wild yams cannot be converted into progesterone in the body.[22, 23] Women who require progesterone should consult their physician and not rely on wild yam or other herbs.

Pregnenolone (page 573), another hormone produced by the body, is converted by the body into progesterone. However, it is not clear what effect supplementing with pregnenolone will have on progesterone production in the body.

Progesterone has been used in connection with the following conditions (refer to the individual health concern for complete information):

Rating	Health Concerns
★★☆	**Amenorrhea** (page 22) **Menopause** (page 311) **Osteoporosis** (page 333)
★☆☆	**Dysmenorrhea** (page 171) (topical cream) **Heart disease** (page 98) **Premenstrual syndrome** (page 368)

Who is likely to be deficient?

Postmenopausal women have reduced production of progesterone. While this "deficiency" is normal, progesterone, including the natural forms of progesterone, has been found to relieve **menopausal** (page 311) symptoms when used in combination with estrogen replacement therapy.[24]

How much is usually taken?

The proper amount of progesterone for a woman should be determined in consultation with a doctor. Some research with the natural, oral form of progesterone has used 200 mg per day.[25] Progesterone is used in much lower amounts—such as 20–70 mg per day—by most doctors who prescribe topical natural progesterone. However, the ability of skin-applied progesterone to achieve effective levels in the body is the source of considerable debate.[26] Although progesterone is a natural substance, oral progesterone supplements are available by prescription only. High-dose topical progesterone cream is also treated like a drug and requires a prescription. A few creams containing lower amounts of progesterone are sold without prescription.

Are there any side effects or interactions?

Progesterone is a hormone and, as such, concerns about its inappropriate use have been raised. A physician should be consulted before using this hormone as a supplement. Few side effects have been associated with topical progesterone creams but can include skin reactions. Effects of natural progesterone on **breast cancer** (page 65) risk remain unclear. Research has suggested both increased and reduced risk.

Synthetic progestins have many well-known side effects, including the increase of LDL ("bad") **cholesterol** (page 223) and the decrease of HDL ("good") cholesterol. Other side effects reported with synthetic progestins include **bloating** (page 137), breast soreness,

depression (page 145), and mood swings. Natural progesterone has been shown to have no adverse effect on HDL **cholesterol** (page 223) levels.[27] Overall, natural progesterone is considerably safer than progestins and is therefore preferred by many doctors in situations where either would be effective.[28]

PROPOLIS

What is it?

Propolis is the resinous substance collected by bees from the leaf buds and bark of trees, especially poplar and conifer trees. Bees use the propolis along with beeswax to construct their hives.

Propolis has antibiotic activities that help the hive block out viruses, bacteria, and other organisms. Commercial preparations of propolis appear to retain these antibiotic properties, according to test tube studies.[1, 2] Test tube and animal studies have also shown that propolis exerts some **antioxidant** (page 467),[3] liver protecting,[4] anti-inflammatory,[5, 6, 7] and anticancer properties.[8]

Propolis contains protein, **amino acids** (page 465), vitamins, minerals, and **flavonoids** (page 516).[9, 10, 11] For this reason, some people use propolis as a general nutritional supplement, although it would take large amounts of propolis to supply meaningful amounts of these nutrients. Propolis may stimulate the body's **immune system** (page 255), according to preliminary human studies,[12, 13] and a controlled trial found propolis-containing mouthwash effective in healing surgical **wounds** (page 319) in the mouth.[14] In test tube studies propolis has shown considerable activity against bacteria and yeast associated with **dental cavities** (page 431), **gingivitis** (page 203), and **periodontal disease** (page 203),[15, 16] but one human study showed that propolis was no better than a placebo in inhibiting dental plaque formation.[17]

Propolis extracts may be helpful in protecting against and shortening the duration of the **common cold** (page 129).[18] A preliminary human study reported propolis extract (amount not stated) reduced upper respiratory infections in children.[19] In one small double-blind study of 50 people with the common cold, the group taking propolis extract (amount not stated) became symptom-free more quickly when compared with the placebo group.[20]

The antimicrobial properties of propolis may also help protect against **parasitic infections** (page 343) in the gastrointestinal tract. One preliminary study of children and adults with giardiasis (a common intestinal parasite infection) showed a 52% success rate of parasite elimination in children and a 60% rate in adults in those given propolis extract (amount not stated).[21] However, these results are not as impressive as those achieved with conventional drugs used against giardiasis, so propolis should not be used alone for this condition without first consulting a physician about available medical treatment.

Topical applications of propolis-containing ointments and creams are showing promise in the treatment of certain health conditions. A controlled study found that men and women with recurrent **genital herpes** (page 200) simplex virus infections (HSV type 2) who applied an ointment containing propolis to their lesions experienced significantly faster healing compared with either a topical antiviral medication or placebo.[22] In a small double-blind study, women with inflammation of the cervix (cervicitis) due to infection experienced significant healing after applying a vaginal dressing containing 5% propolis for ten days.[23] Anti-inflammatory effects from topical application of propolis extract have been noted in one animal study,[24] and a preliminary controlled study found that people with **rheumatoid arthritis** (page 387) treated with topical propolis extract had greater improvements in symptoms compared with placebo.[25]

Where is it found?

Propolis is available in liquid extract form as well as in capsules and tablets. Topical creams and sprays containing propolis are also available, but whether they closely resemble topical propolis products used in research is unclear.

Propolis has been used in connection with the following conditions (refer to the individual health concern for complete information):

Rating	Health Concerns
★★☆	Cervicitis (topical use) **Common cold** (page 129) **Genital Herpes** (page 200) (topical use) **Infertility (female)** (page 187) (in women with endometriosis) **Parasites** (page 343) **Rheumatoid arthritis** (page 387) (topical)
★☆☆	**Cold Sores** (page 119) (topical) **Dental caries** (page 431) (topical) **Periodontal disease** (page 203) (topical)

Propolis

Propolis

Who is likely to be deficient?

Propolis is not an essential nutrient and no deficiency states have been reported.

How much is usually taken?

Most manufacturers recommend 500 mg of oral propolis products once or twice daily. For topical applications, follow label instructions.

Are there any side effects or interactions?

Propolis is generally nontoxic, though allergic reactions have been reported.[26] These reactions are typically limited to skin rashes;[27] however, as with other bee products (e.g., **pollen** [page 571] and **royal jelly** [page 582]), more severe allergic reactions are possible. People who are allergic to bee pollen, honey, or conifer and poplar trees should not use propolis unless tested first by an allergy specialist. As the effects of propolis during pregnancy and breast-feeding have not been sufficiently evaluated, women should not use it during these times unless directed to do so by a physician.

PYRUVATE

What is it?

Pyruvate (the buffered form of pyruvic acid) is a product created in the body during the metabolism of carbohydrates and protein.

Pyruvate may aid **weight loss** (page 446) efforts.[1] A clinical trial found that supplementation with 22–44 grams per day of pyruvate, when compared with placebo, enhanced weight loss and resulted in a greater reduction of body fat in overweight adults consuming a low-fat diet.[2] Three controlled studies combining 6–10 grams per day of pyruvate with an exercise program, reported similar effects on weight loss and body fat.[3, 4, 5] Animal studies suggest that pyruvate supplementation leads to weight loss by increasing the resting metabolic rate.[6] A few clinical trials also indicated that pyruvate supplements may improve **exercise endurance** (page 43),[7, 8] though weight-lifting capacity did not improve.[9]

Preliminary research indicates that pyruvate functions as an **antioxidant** (page 467), inhibiting the production of harmful free radicals.[10, 11, 12] Preliminary research with animals suggests that, due to its antioxidant function, pyruvate may inhibit the growth of **cancerous** (page 87) tumors.[13] However, this effect has not been confirmed in human studies.

Where is it found?

Pyruvate is formed in the body as a byproduct of the normal metabolism of carbohydrates and protein and is present in several foods, including red apples, cheese, dark beer, and red wine. Dietary supplements of pyruvate are also available.

Pyruvate has been used in connection with the following conditions (refer to the individual health concern for complete information):

Rating	Health Concerns
★★★	**Weight loss and obesity** (page 446)
★★☆	**Athletic performance** (page 43) (for exercise performance)
★☆☆	**Athletic performance** (page 43) (for improving body composition with strength training in untrained people only)

Who is likely to be deficient?

Because it is not an essential nutrient, pyruvate is not associated with a deficiency state.

How much is usually taken?

Most human research with pyruvate and **weight loss** (page 446) has used at least 30 grams per day. However, such large amounts may not be necessary. In a six-week double-blind trial, as little as 6 grams per day of pyruvate in combination with exercise, led to greater weight loss and loss of body fat, compared with a placebo plus exercise.[14]

Are there any side effects or interactions?

High intakes of pyruvate can trigger **gastrointestinal upset** (page 195), such as gas, bloating, and **diarrhea** (page 163). One preliminary study in exercising women found 10 grams per day of pyruvate reduced blood levels of HDL (the "good" cholesterol) after one month.[15]

QUERCETIN

What is it?

Quercetin belongs to a class of water-soluble plant pigments called **flavonoids** (page 516).

Quercetin acts as an antihistamine and has anti-inflammatory properties. As an **antioxidant** (page

467), it protects LDL **cholesterol** (page 223) ("bad" cholesterol) from becoming damaged. A variety of evidence indicates that quercetin possesses potent antioxidant properties. Cardiologists believe that damage to LDL cholesterol is an underlying cause of **heart disease** (page 98). Quercetin blocks an **enzyme** (page 506) that leads to accumulation of sorbitol, which has been linked to nerve, eye, and kidney damage in those with **diabetes** (page 152). However, no human research has demonstrated these actions of quercetin in people with diabetes patients.

Quercetin is considered a phytoestrogen (i.e., a plant substance with similar functions as that of estrogen). Some phytoestrogens are believed also to have antiestrogenic effects that might lead to reduced risks of certain **cancers** (page 87). Quercetin was found to have this antiestrogenic activity by inhibiting **breast cancer** (page 65) cells in a test tube.[1]

In a double-blind trial, 67% of people taking quercetin had an improvement of **prostatitis** (page 377) symptoms, compared with a 20% response rate in the placebo group.[2]

Where is it found?
Quercetin can be found in onions, apples, **green tea** (page 686), and black tea. Smaller amounts are found in leafy green vegetables and beans.

Quercetin has been used in connection with the following conditions (refer to the individual health concern for complete information):

Rating	Health Concerns
★★★	**Prostatitis** (page 377) (nonbacterial prostatitis, prostadynia)
★☆☆	**Allergies** (page 14) **Asthma** (page 32) **Atherosclerosis** (page 38) **Capillary fragility** (page 93) **Childhood diseases** (page 105) **Cataracts** (page 101) **Diabetes** (page 152) **Edema (water retention)** (page 180) **Gout** (page 208) **Hay fever** (page 211) **Peptic ulcer** (page 349) **Retinopathy** (page 385)

Who is likely to be deficient?
No clear deficiency of quercetin has been established.

How much is usually taken?
Some doctors recommend 200–500 mg of quercetin taken two to three times per day. Optimal intake remains unknown.

Are there any side effects or interactions?
No clear toxicity has been identified. Early quercetin research suggested that large amounts of quercetin could cause cancer in animals.[3] Most,[4, 5, 6] but not all,[7] current research finds quercetin to be safe or actually linked to protection from **cancer** (page 87).

Quercetin has been shown to cause chromosomal mutations in certain bacteria in test tube studies.[8] Although the significance of this finding for humans is not clear, some doctors are concerned about the possibility that **birth defects** (page 63) could occur in the offspring of people supplementing with quercetin at the time of conception or during **pregnancy** (page 363).

Since **flavonoids** (page 516) help protect and enhance **vitamin C** (page 604), quercetin is often taken with vitamin C.

RESVERATROL

What is it?
Resveratrol, a compound found primarily in red wine, is a naturally occurring **antioxidant** (page 467).

In test tube and animal studies, resveratrol decreased the "stickiness" of blood platelets and helped blood vessels remain open and flexible.[1, 2, 3] A series of laboratory experiments suggested that resveratrol inhibits the development of **cancer** (page 87) in animals and prevents the progression of cancer.[4] In other animal studies, resveratrol was shown to be an effective anti-inflammatory agent.[5] However, human research is still needed in all of these areas.

Where is it found?
Resveratrol is present in a wide variety of plants—of the edible plants, mainly in grapes and peanuts.[6] Wine is the primary dietary source of resveratrol. Red wine contains much greater amounts of resveratrol than does white wine, since resveratrol is concentrated in the grape skin and the manufacturing process of red wine includes prolonged contact with grape skins. Resveratrol is also available as a dietary supplement.

Resveratrol

Resveratrol has been used in connection with the following conditions (refer to the individual health concern for complete information):

Rating	Health Concerns
★☆☆	Atherosclerosis (page 38)

Who is likely to be deficient?
Since it is not an essential nutrient, resveratrol is not associated with a deficiency state.

How much is usually taken?
An 8-ounce glass of red wine provides approximately 640 mcg of resveratrol, while a handful of peanuts provides about 73 mcg of resveratrol. Resveratrol supplements (often found in combination with grape extracts or other **antioxidants** [page 467]) are generally taken in the amount of 200–600 mcg per day. This is far less than the amount used in animal studies to prevent **cancer** (page 87): equivalent to more than 500 *mg* (500,000 mcg) per day for an average-sized human. Therefore, one should not assume that the small amounts found in supplements or food would necessarily be protective. The optimal level of intake is not known.

While a moderate intake of red wine may protect against **heart disease** (page 98), the optimal amount required to produce this effect is still unknown. Due to the risks involved with drinking alcohol, drinking red wine cannot be recommended as a means of preventing heart disease until more information is known.

Are there any side effects or interactions?
No side effects have been reported with the use of resveratrol.

RIBOSE

What is it?
Ribose is a type of sugar normally made in the body from glucose. Ribose plays important roles in the synthesis of RNA, DNA, and the energy-containing substance adenosine triphosphate (ATP).

According to preliminary animal and human research, ribose supplementation speeds up regeneration of ATP in muscle cells of the heart or elsewhere in the body when those cells have been deprived of oxygen.[1, 2, 3, 4]

Where is it found?
Ribose is present in small amounts in many foods of plant or animal origin.

Ribose has been used in connection with the following conditions (refer to the individual health concern for complete information):

Rating	Health Concerns
★★☆	Angina (page 27)
★☆☆	Athletic performance (page 43)

Who is likely to be deficient?
Ribose is not an essential nutrient, therefore deficiencies do not occur.

How much is usually taken?
Sports supplement manufacturers recommend 1 to 10 grams per day of ribose.

Are there any side effects or interactions?
No known side effects have been reported from the use of ribose when consumed in amounts of less than 10 grams per day. Larger amounts may cause gastrointestinal distress such as diarrhea,[5] and may lower glucose levels,[6] although it is not known whether symptoms of hypoglycemia might result.

ROYAL JELLY

What is it?
Royal jelly is a thick, milky substance produced by worker bees to feed the queen bee. The worker bees mix honey and bee pollen with enzymes in the glands of their throats to produce royal jelly.

Royal jelly is believed to be a potentially useful supplement because of the queen bee's superior size, strength, stamina, and longevity compared to other bees, but these effects have not been studied in humans. Royal jelly contains all of the B vitamins, including high concentrations of **pantothenic acid** (page 568) (vitamin B_5) and **pyridoxine** (page 600) (vitamin B_6).[1] Other nutritional qualities of royal jelly are similar to those of pollen.[2]

Test tube studies suggest royal jelly may have some cancer-preventive properties.[3] Animal studies have found that royal jelly has some **cholesterol-lowering** (page 223),[4] **immune-stimulating** (page 223),[5] anti-inflammatory, and **wound-healing** (page 319) properties.[6]

Scientific investigation into the health-promoting properties of royal jelly in humans has been limited to its ability to lower blood cholesterol levels. There have been ten human studies published, seven of which were double-blind.[7] Of these seven double-blind studies, only three studies utilized an oral preparation of royal jelly;[8, 9, 10] an injectable form was used in the other four.[11, 12, 13] A detailed analysis of the oral double-blind studies concluded there were many shortcomings in the design of the research, but royal jelly in amounts of 50–100 mg per day reduced total cholesterol levels by about 14% in people with moderately high cholesterol levels.[14]

Melbrosia, a mixture of royal jelly, flower **pollen** (page 571), and fermented bee pollen, was reported to help relieve **menopausal** (page 311) symptoms in about one-third of women in a preliminary study in Denmark.[15] This result agrees with an earlier, controlled study that found melbrosia (amount not stated) was more effective than placebo for menopausal symptoms, including headache, urinary incontinence, vaginal dryness, and low vitality.[16] According to animal studies, melbrosia does not work by causing estrogen-like effects in body tissues.[17] Whether royal jelly alone might have similar effects on menopausal symptoms is unknown.

Where is it found?
Royal jelly is available in liquid form (usually in glass vials), tablets, and capsules.

Royal jelly has been used in connection with the following condition (refer to it for complete information):

Rating	Health Concerns
★★☆	High cholesterol (page 223)

Who is likely to be deficient?
Because royal jelly is not an essential nutrient, deficiencies do not occur.

How much is usually taken?
Royal jelly in the amount of 50–100 mg per day has been used in most of the studies on **cholesterol** (page 223) lowering.

Are there any side effects or interactions?
Allergic reactions are the most common side effect. Allergic reactions from oral intake of royal jelly can range from very mild (e.g., mild gastrointestinal upset) to more severe reactions, including **asthma** (page 32), anaphylaxis (shock), intestinal bleeding, and even death in people who are extremely allergic to bee products.[18, 19, 20] People who are allergic to bee pollen, honey, or conifer and poplar trees should not use royal jelly orally. Topical use of royal jelly has been reported to cause skin irritations in some people.[21]

SAMe

What is it?
S-adenosyl-l-methionine (SAMe) is an important biological agent in the human body, participating in over 40 essential biochemical reactions.

SAMe participates in detoxification reactions and in the manufacture of brain chemicals, **antioxidants** (page 467), joint tissue structures, and many other important components.[1, 2]

SAMe appears to raise levels of dopamine, an important neurotransmitter in mood regulation,[3] and higher SAMe levels in the brain are associated with successful drug treatment of **depression** (page 145).[4] Oral SAMe has been demonstrated to be an effective treatment for depression in some,[5, 6, 7, 8] though not all,[9] double-blind studies. While it does not seem to be as powerful as full amounts of antidepressant medications[10] or **St. John's wort** (page 747), its effects are felt more rapidly, often within one week.[11]

SAMe possesses anti-inflammatory, pain-relieving, and tissue-healing properties that may help protect the health of joints.[12, 13] Several double-blind studies have shown that SAMe is useful for people with **osteoarthritis** (page 328), reducing **pain** (page 338), stiffness, and swelling better than placebos and equal to drugs such as ibuprofen and naproxen.[14, 15, 16, 17, 18, 19, 20, 21]

Intravenous SAMe given to **fibromyalgia** (page 191) patients reduced pain and depression in two double-blind studies,[22, 23] but in a short (ten-day) trial no benefit was seen.[24] Oral SAMe was tested in one double-blind study and significant beneficial effects were noticed, such as reduced pain, fatigue, and stiffness, and improved mood.[25]

Oral and intravenous treatment with SAMe replenishes important substances in damaged livers and im-

SAMe

proves the flow of bile.[26, 27] Preliminary research has indicated that SAMe may be helpful in a variety of liver conditions, including cholestasis, Gilbert's syndrome, alcoholic liver injury, and **cirrhosis** (page 290).[28, 29, 30] In alcoholic cirrhosis, damage to the liver prevents the natural formation of SAMe from the amino acid **methionine** (page 557). In a double-blind trial, people with cirrhosis of the liver due to alcoholism who took SAMe for two years had a 47% lower rate of death or need for liver transplantation, compared with those who received a placebo.[31] However, the improvement did not quite achieve statistical significance. In people with less severe cirrhosis, the results were more impressive and were also statistically significant.

Preliminary research also suggests oral SAMe may increase sperm activity in **infertile men** (page 304)[32] and may be helpful in the treatment of **migraine headaches** (page 316).[33] One double-blind study found injections of SAMe significantly more helpful than placebo injections for reducing the symptoms of post-concussion syndrome.[34]

Where is it found?

SAMe is not abundant in the diet, though its precursor, the **amino acid** (page 465) **methionine** (page 557) is plentiful in many protein foods. It is not known whether increasing one's intake of methionine will increase the body's production of SAMe. Supplements of SAMe have been available in the U.S. since 1997.

SAMe has been used in connection with the following conditions (refer to the individual health concern for complete information):

Rating	Health Concerns
★★★	**Liver cirrhosis** (page 290) **Osteoarthritis** (page 328)
★★☆	**Depression** (page 145) **Fibromyalgia** (page 191) **Hepatitis** (page 220) (for liver cholestasis) **Pregnancy and postpartum support** (page 363) (for cholestasis only)
★☆☆	**Bipolar disorder** (page 61) **Infertility (male)** (page 304) **Migraine headaches** (page 316) Post-concussion syndrome

Who is likely to be deficient?

SAMe is normally produced in the liver from the **amino acid** (page 465) **methionine** (page 557) which is abundant in most diets. **Folic acid** (page 520) and **vitamin B$_{12}$** (page 601) are necessary for the synthesis of SAMe, and deficiencies of these vitamins results in low concentrations of SAMe in the central nervous system.[35] Low blood or central nervous system levels of SAMe have been detected in people with **cirrhosis of the liver** (page 290),[36] **coronary heart disease** (page 38),[37] **Alzheimer's disease** (page 19), and **depression** (page 145).[38]

How much is usually taken?

Healthy people do not need to take this supplement. Researchers working with people suffering from a variety of conditions have been using these amounts of SAMe: **depression** (page 145), 1,600 mg per day; **osteoarthritis** (page 328), 800–1,200 mg per day; **fibromyalgia** (page 191), 800 mg per day; liver disorders, 1,200 mg per day; and **migraine** (page 316), 800 mg per day.

Are there any side effects or interactions?

Clinical trials in thousands of people for up to two years have demonstrated that SAMe is very well tolerated, much better than the medications with which it has often been compared.[39, 40] Occasional **gastrointestinal upset** (page 195) may be experienced by some people. Researchers treating people with **bipolar disorder** (page 61) (manic depression) have reported that SAMe could cause them to switch from depression to a manic episode.[41, 42]

SELENIUM

What is it?

Selenium is an essential trace mineral.

Selenium activates an **antioxidant** (page 467) enzyme called glutathione peroxidase, which may help protect the body from **cancer** (page 87). Yeast-derived forms of selenium have induced "apoptosis" (programmed cell death) in cancer cells in test tubes and in animals.[1, 2, 3] A double-blind trial that included over 1,300 people found those given 200 mcg of yeast-based selenium per day for 4.5 years had a 50% drop in the cancer death rate compared with the placebo group.[4] In that same study, however, selenium supplementation was associated with a significant increase in the risk of developing one type of skin cancer (squamous cell carcinoma).[5] Another study found that men consuming the most dietary selenium (assessed indirectly by measuring toenail selenium levels) developed 65% fewer cases of advanced **prostate cancer** (page 371) than did men with the lowest levels of selenium intake.[6]

Selenium is also essential for healthy **immune functioning** (page 371). Selenium supplementation has reduced the incidence of viral **hepatitis** (page 220) in selenium-deficient populations, presumably by enhancing immune function.[7] Even in a non-deficient population of elderly people, selenium supplementation has been found to stimulate the activity of white blood cells—primary components of the immune system.[8] Selenium is also needed to activate thyroid hormones.

In a placebo-controlled study, supplementation with 200 mcg per day of selenium for three months reduced anti-thyroid antibody levels (indicating a reduction in disease activity) in people with autoimmune thyroiditis (inflammation of the thyroid gland).[9]

In a double-blind trial, selenium supplementation of **infertile men** (page 305) improved the motility of sperm cells and increased the chance of conception.[10]

Where is it found?

Brazil nuts are the best source of selenium. Yeast, whole grains, and seafood are also good sources. Animal studies have found that selenium from yeast is better absorbed than selenium in the form of selenite.[11]

Selenium has been used in connection with the following conditions (refer to the individual health concern for complete information):

Rating	Health Concerns
★★☆	**Asthma** (page 32)
	Atherosclerosis (page 38)
	Colon cancer (page 134) (reduces risk)
	Depression (page 145)
	Dermatitis herpetiformis (page 151)
	Heart attack (page 212)
	HIV support (page 239)
	Immune function (page 255) (for elderly people)
	Infections (page 265) (to prevent hospital-acquired infections in very low birth weight infants)
	Infertility (male) (page 305)
	Lung cancer (page 298) (reduces risk)
	Lymphedema (page 180)
	Pancreatic insufficiency (page 341)
	Phenylketonuria (page 354) (if deficient)
	Prostate cancer (page 371) (reduces risk)
	Rheumatoid arthritis (page 387)
	Thyroiditis (autoimmune)
★☆☆	**Cardiac arrhythmia** (page 93)
	Cardiomyopathy (page 95) (only for Keshan's cardiomyopathy)
	Childhood diseases (page 105)
	Diabetic retinopathy (page 385) (in combination with **vitamin A** [page 595], **vitamin C** [page 604], and **vitamin E** [page 609])
	Down's syndrome (page 169)
	Halitosis (page 209) (if gum disease)
	Hepatitis (page 220)
	Hypothyroidism (page 252) (if deficient)
	Liver cirrhosis (page 290)
	Macular degeneration (page 303)
	Osgood-Schlatter disease (page 327)
	Pap smear (abnormal) (page 3)
	Pre- and post-surgery health (page 357)
	Retinopathy (page 385) (combined with **vitamin A** [page 595], **vitamin C** [page 604], and **vitamin E** [page 609])

Who is likely to be deficient?

While most people probably don't take in enough selenium, gross deficiencies are rare in Western countries. Soils in some areas are selenium-deficient and people who eat foods grown primarily on selenium-poor soils are at risk for deficiency. People with **AIDS** (page 239) have been reported to be depleted in selenium.[12] Similarly, limited research has reported an association between **heart disease** (page 98) and depleted levels of selenium.[13] People who are deficient in selenium have an increased risk of developing certain types of **rheumatoid arthritis** (page 387).[14]

How much is usually taken?

While the Recommended Dietary Allowance for most adults is 55 mcg per day, an adult intake of 100–200 mcg of selenium per day is recommended by many doctors.

Are there any side effects or interactions?

Selenium is safe at the level people typically supplement (100–200 mcg); however, taking more than 900 mcg of selenium per day has been reported to cause adverse effects in some people.[15] Selenium toxicity can result in loss of fingernails, skin rash, and changes in the nervous system. In the presence of **iodine** (page 538)-deficiency-induced **goiter** (page 206), selenium supplementation has been reported to exacerbate low thyroid function.[16] Although most research suggests that selenium prevents cancer, one study found an increased risk of a type of skin cancer (squamous cell carcinoma)

Selenium

in people taking selenium supplements.[17] The National Academy of Sciences recommends that selenium intake not exceed 400 mcg per day, unless the higher intake is monitored by a healthcare professional.[18]

Selenium enhances the **antioxidant** (page 467) effect of **vitamin E** (page 609).

SILICA HYDRIDE

What is it?
Silica hydride is a colloidal mineral compound containing silicon, oxygen, and hydrogen. According to the developers of this supplement, silica hydride contains a large number of loosely bound electrons that are available to help neutralize potentially dangerous free radicals.[1, 2] Test tube studies have demonstrated that silica hydride does neutralize free radicals and preserves the health of cells exposed to these radicals. However, whether silica hydride can be absorbed from the gastrointestinal tract and whether it will affect the health of animals or humans has not been adequately tested.

A preliminary study attempted to measure health-promoting properties of silica hydride with a computerized analysis of blood, urine, and saliva samples called Biological Terrain Assessment (BTA). BTA testing indicated some potentially positive effects of silica hydride in healthy people, but no effects in people with diagnosed health problems.[3] BTA has not been proven to be a reliable method for evaluating health or disease,[4] so even this marginally promising report should be regarded tentatively.

Another claim made is that the electrons in silica hydride can help promote the body's production of the energy-containing substance adenosine triphosphate (ATP). While test tube studies have demonstrated that some preliminary steps in energy production are facilitated by silica hydride,[5] no evidence exists that this will increase ATP production in the body.

Where is it found?
Since silica hydride is not essential, a recommended intake has not been established. Whether it is present in food or water is unknown. Supplements contain 200 to 250 mg per capsule.

Who is likely to be deficient?
Silica hydride is not an essential nutrient, so no deficiencies are possible.

How much is usually taken?
Since silica hydride is not essential, a recommended intake has not been established. Whether it is present in food or water is unknown. Supplements contain 200 to 250 mg per capsule.

Are there any side effects or interactions?
Due to the lack of published scientific research on silica hydride in animals or humans, side effects and interactions are unknown.

SILICON

What is it?
Silicon is a trace mineral.

The functions of silicon are not well understood, although silicon probably plays a role in making and maintaining connective tissue. Silicon is present in areas of bone that are undergoing mineralization, which indicates this mineral might be important for normal bone function; however, evidence for this has not been confirmed in humans.[1]

Where is it found?
Good dietary sources for silicon include whole-grain breads and cereals, root vegetables, and beer. A form of silicon called silicates is added to some processed foods.

Silicon has been used in connection with the following condition (refer to the individual health concern for complete information):

Rating	Health Concerns
★☆☆	**Osteoporosis** (page 333) **Sprains and strains** (page 412)

Who is likely to be deficient?
Silicon is not an essential mineral. Deficiencies have not been reported.

How much is usually taken?
Because silicon has not been established as essential, a recommended intake has not been established. The average diet is estimated to provide 5–20 mg of silicon per day—an amount that appears adequate. When used as a supplement, common amounts range from 1 to 2 mg per day.

Are there any side effects or interactions?

A high dietary intake of silicon is not associated with any toxic effects. Inhalation of large amounts of silicon (in an industrial setting) can cause the respiratory disease silicosis.

SOY

What is it?

Soy, a staple food in many Asian countries, contains valuable constituents, including protein, isoflavones, saponins, and phytosterols. Soy protein provides essential **amino acids** (page 465). When eaten with rice, soy provides protein comparable with that found in animal products. Soy is low in fat and cholesterol-free.

The isoflavones in soy, primarily genistein and daidzein, have been well researched by scientists for their **antioxidant** (page 467) and phytoestrogenic properties.[1] Saponins enhance **immune function** (page 255) and bind to cholesterol to limit its absorption in the intestine. Phytosterols and other components of soy have been reported to lower **cholesterol levels** (page 223).

The soy isoflavone genistein has been reported to inhibit angiogenesis,[2] the growth of new blood vessels that, when abnormal, can contribute to the development of **cancer** (page 87). Soy isoflavones have also been shown to inhibit 5 alpha-reductase,[3] the **enzyme** (page 506) that activates testosterone in the prostate gland and other tissues. 5 Alpha-reductase inhibition represents a potentially effective therapeutic approach to **benign prostate enlargement** (page 58) and male pattern baldness.

Isoflavones may reduce the risk of hormone-dependent cancers, such as **breast** (page 65) and **prostate cancer** (page 371), as well as other cancers. One study of soy research found that 65% of 26 animal-based cancer studies showed a protective effect of soy or soy isoflavones.[4] Human research also suggests a protective role of soy against cancer,[5, 6] but the data are currently insufficient to form any solid conclusions.[7]

A review of 38 different studies revealed that soy consumption reduced **cholesterol** (page 223) levels in 89% of the studies. A meta-analysis of these studies indicated that eating soy resulted, on average, in a cholesterol reduction of 23 mg per deciliter.[8] Exactly how soy lowers cholesterol remains in debate,[9] though isoflavones appear to be one key component.[10]

The mild estrogenic activity of soy isoflavones may ease **menopause** (page 311) symptoms for some women, without creating estrogen-related problems. In one double-blind trial, supplementation with 60 grams of soy protein per day for 12 weeks led to a 45% decrease in the number of hot flashes, compared with a 30% reduction in the placebo group, a statistically significant difference.[11] In addition, soy may help regulate hormone levels in premenopausal women.[12]

Soy may also be beneficial in preventing **osteoporosis** (page 333). Isoflavones from soy have protected against bone loss in animal studies.[13] In a double-blind study of postmenopausal women, supplementation with 40 grams of soy protein powder per day (containing 90 mg of isoflavones per day) protected against bone mineral loss in the spine.[14] Although the use of soy in the prevention of osteoporosis looks hopeful, no long-term human studies have examined the effects of soy or soy-derived isoflavones on bone density or fracture risk.

Where is it found?

Relatively large amounts of isoflavones are present in whole soybeans, roasted soy nuts, tofu, tempeh, soy milk, meat substitutes, soy flour, and some soy protein isolates. In addition, the isoflavones present in soy are available as supplements, in capsules or tablets.

Soy has been used in connection with the following conditions (refer to the individual health concern for complete information):

Rating	Health Concerns
★★★	**High cholesterol** (page 223) **Menopause** (page 311)
★★☆	**High blood pressure** (page 246) **Osteoporosis** (page 333)
★☆☆	**Vaginitis** (page 438)

Who is likely to be deficient?

Although deficiencies do not occur, people who do not consume soy foods will not gain the benefits of soy.

How much is usually taken?

The ideal intake of soy is not known. Researchers suggest the equivalent of one serving of soy foods per day supports good health, and the benefits increase as soy intake increases.[15] Societies in which large amounts of

Soy

soy are consumed ingest between 50 and 100 mg per day of soy isoflavones. The **cholesterol** (page 223)-lowering effects of soy have been observed at amounts as low as 20 grams of soy protein per day, if it replaces animal protein in the diet.[16]

Are there any side effects or interactions?

Soy products and cooked soybeans are safe at a wide range of intakes. However, a small percentage of people have **allergies** (page 14) to soybeans and thus should avoid soy products.

Soy isoflavones have been reported to reduce thyroid function in some people.[17] A preliminary trial of soy supplementation among healthy Japanese, found that 30 grams (about one ounce) per day of soybeans for three months, led to a slight reduction in the hormone that stimulates the thyroid gland.[18] Some participants complained of malaise, **constipation** (page 137), sleepiness, and even **goiter** (page 206). These symptoms resolved within a month of discontinuing soy supplements. However, a variety of soy products have been shown to either cause an *increase* in thyroid function[19] or produce no change in thyroid function.[20] The clinical importance of interactions between soy and thyroid function remains unclear. However, in infants with congenital **hypothyroidism** (page 252), soy formula must not be added, nor removed from the diet, without consultation with a physician, because ingestion of soy may interfere with the absorption of thyroid medication.[21]

Most research, including animal studies, report **anticancer** (page 87) effects of soy extracts,[22] though occasional animal studies have reported cancer-enhancing effects.[23] The findings of several recent studies suggest that consuming soy might, under some circumstances, *increase* the risk of **breast cancer** (page 65). When ovaries have been removed from animals—a situation related to the condition of women who have had a total hysterectomy—dietary genistein has been reported to *increase* the proliferation of breast cancer cells.[24] When pregnant rats were given genistein injections, their female offspring were reported to be at *greater* risk of breast cancer.[25] Although **premenopausal** (page 311) women have shown decreases in estrogen levels in response to soy,[26, 27] pro-estrogenic effects have also been reported.[28] When pre-menopausal women were given soy isoflavones, an increase in breast secretions resulted—an effect thought to *elevate* the risk of breast cancer.[29] In yet another trial, healthy breast cells from women previously given soy supplements containing isoflavones showed an *increase* in proliferation rates—an effect that might also increase the risk of breast cancer.[30]

Of 154 healthy postmenopausal women who received 150 mg of soy isoflavones per day for five years, 3.9% developed an abnormal proliferation of the tissue that lines the uterus (endometrial hyperplasia). In contrast, none of 144 women who received a placebo developed uterine hyperplasia.[31] Although no case of uterine cancer was diagnosed during the study, endometrial hyperplasia is a potential forerunner of uterine cancer. The amount of isoflavones used in this study is two to three times as much as that used in many other studies. Nevertheless, the possibility exists that long-term use of isoflavones could cause uterine hyperplasia, and women taking isoflavones should be monitored appropriately by their doctor.

Soy contains a compound called phytic acid, which can interfere with mineral absorption.

SPLEEN EXTRACTS

What are they?

Spleen extracts are extracts derived from the spleens of beef (bovine) sources. The spleen is a fist-sized, spongy, dark purple organ that lies in the upper left abdomen behind the lower ribs. Weighing about 7 ounces, the spleen is the largest mass of lymphatic tissue in the body. The spleen produces white blood cells, engulfs and destroys bacteria and cellular debris, and destroys worn-out red blood cells and platelets.

A series of case reports in the early 1930s demonstrated that orally administered bovine spleen extracts were able to raise white-blood-cell counts in individuals with extremely low counts, as well as to benefit patients with malaria and typhoid fever.[1, 2, 3] However, there does not appear to be any more recent studies with these sorts of preparations. Most of the recent research with spleen extracts has focused on the use of injectable preparations or isolated spleen proteins, such as tuftsin and splenopentin.[4, 5, 6, 7] Although these preparations have been shown to enhance **immune function** (page 255), it is not known whether the same benefits can be obtained with oral preparations.

Where are they found?

Spleen extracts are available as nutritional supplements in capsules and tablets.

Spleen extracts have been used in connection with the following condition (refer to the individual health concern for complete information):

Rating	Health Concerns
★★☆	Cancer chemotherapy, adverse effects
★☆☆	Low white-blood-cell count

Who is likely to be deficient?

As spleen extract is not an essential nutrient, no deficiency state exists.

How much is usually taken?

The recommended amount depends on the concentration, method of preparation, and quality of the extract. Follow the manufacturer's recommendation on the label.

Are there any side effects or interactions?

No side effects or adverse effects have been reported with the use of oral spleen preparations.

STRONTIUM

What is it?

Strontium is a mineral that is not classified as essential for the human body.

There is research that strontium has been shown to promote strong, **osteoporosis** (page 333)-resistant bones,[1] lessen the risk of dental cavities,[2] and reduce the **pain** (page 338) of bone lesions that occasionally develop in association with certain **cancers** (page 87).[3] The type of strontium used as a supplement is not the radioactive type.

Where is it found?

Strontium is widely distributed throughout nature. Strontium levels in the soil determine how much strontium will be in the foods grown in particular areas. Areas with strontium-rich soils also tend to have higher levels of strontium in the drinking water.

Strontium has been used in connection with the following conditions (refer to the individual health concern for complete information):

Rating	Health Concerns
★☆☆	**Dental cavities** (page 431) **Osteoporosis** (page 333)

Who is likely to be deficient?

Strontium is not an essential mineral, so deficiencies are not seen with this mineral.

How much is usually taken?

No recommended intake levels have been established for strontium, since it is not considered essential for humans. However, preliminary research in humans suggests that 600–1,700 mg of strontium, taken as a supplement in the form of strontium salts, may increase bone mass in the vertebrae of people with **osteoporosis** (page 333).[4]

Are there any side effects or interactions?

No consistent toxicities from strontium supplements have been reported.

SULFORAPHANE

What is it?

Sulforaphane is a compound that was identified in broccoli sprouts by scientists at the Johns Hopkins University School of Medicine in Baltimore, MD.[1]

These researchers were investigating the **anticancer** (page 87) compounds present in broccoli when they discovered that broccoli sprouts contain anywhere from 30 to 50 times the concentration of protective chemicals that are found in mature broccoli plants.[2] Sulforaphane is one of a class of chemicals called isothiocyanates. Sulforaphane and other isothiocyanates are **antioxidants** (page 467) and potent stimulators of natural detoxifying enzymes in the body. These compounds are believed to be responsible for the lowered risk of cancer that is associated with the consumption of broccoli and other cruciferous vegetables, such ascauliflower, cabbage, andkale.[3, 4, 5, 6, 7, 8, 9]

Feeding sulforaphane-rich broccoli-sprout extracts to laboratory rats exposed to a carcinogen dramatically reduced the frequency, size, and number of the rats' tumors.[10, 11, 12] Human studies with sulforaphane and other cruciferous-vegetable components have shown that these compounds stimulate the body's production of detoxification enzymes and exert antioxidant effects.[13, 14, 15]

Preliminary studies suggest that in order to cut the risk of cancer in half, the average person would need to eat about two pounds of broccoli or similar vegetables per week. Since the concentration of sulforaphane is much higher in broccoli sprouts than in mature broccoli, the same reduction in risk theoretically might be had with a weekly intake of just over an ounce of sprouts.

Where is it found?
Sulforaphane is found in highest concentrations in broccoli sprouts, but it is also found in mature broccoli and other cruciferous vegetables, such as cauliflower, cabbage, and kale.

Sulforaphane has been used in connection with the following conditions (refer to the individual health concern for complete information):

Rating	Health Concerns
★☆☆	**Cancer** (page 87) (risk reduction)

Who is likely to be deficient?
Sulforaphane is not an essential nutrient, and thus no deficiency state exists.

How much is usually taken?
The optimal level of intake is not known, but some doctors recommend 200 to 400 mcg of sulforaphane daily from broccoli-sprout extracts.

Are there any side effects or interactions?
No side effects or drug interactions have been reported, although sulforaphane and dietary consumption of cruciferous vegetables does interact with drug detoxifying **enzymes** (page 506).[16] People taking prescription drugs should therefore consult a doctor before taking sulforaphane or broccoli-sprout extracts.

SULFUR

What is it?
Sulfur is a mineral needed for the manufacture of many proteins, including those forming hair, muscles,

and skin. Sulfur contributes to fat digestion and absorption, because it is needed to make bile acids. Sulfur is also a constituent of bones, teeth, and collagen (the protein in connective tissue). As a component of insulin, sulfur is needed to regulate blood sugar. Sulfur is present in **methylsulfonylmethane (MSM)** (page 558), a naturally-occurring substance available as a supplement.

Where is it found?
Most dietary sulfur is consumed as part of certain **amino acids** (page 465) in protein-rich foods. Meat and poultry, organ meats, fish, eggs, beans, and dairy products are all good sources of sulfur-containing amino acids. Sulfur also occurs in **garlic** (page 679) and onions and may be partially responsible for the health benefits associated with these items.[1]

Most of the body's sulfur is found in the sulfur-containing amino acids **methionine** (page 557), cystine, and **cysteine** (page 502). **Vitamin B$_1$** (page 597), **biotin** (page 473), and **pantothenic acid** (page 568) contain small amounts of sulfur.

Who is likely to be deficient?
Deficiencies of sulfur have not been documented, although a protein-deficient diet could theoretically lead to a deficiency of sulfur. Low levels of cystine, and therefore possibly sulfur, were reported many years ago in people with arthritis, but this association is far from proven.[2]

How much is usually taken?
No recommended intake levels have been established for sulfur. Since most Western diets are high in protein, the majority of diets probably supply enough sulfur.

Are there any side effects or interactions?
No side effects have been reported with the use of sulfur.

TAURINE

What is it?
Taurine is an **amino acid** (page 465)-like compound and a component of bile acids, which are used to help absorb fats and fat-soluble **vitamins** (page 559). Taurine also helps regulate the heart beat, maintain cell membrane stability, and prevent brain cell over-activity.

Where is it found?

Taurine is found mostly in meat and fish. Except for infants, the human body is able to make taurine from **cysteine** (page 502)—another **amino acid** (page 465).

Taurine has been used in connection with the following conditions (refer to the individual health concern for complete information):

Rating	Health Concerns
★★★	**Congestive heart failure** (page 134)
★★☆	**Cystic fibrosis** (page 143)
	Iron-deficiency anemia (page 278)
	Liver support
	Pre- and post-surgery health (page 357)
★☆☆	**Cardiomyopathy** (page 95)
	Diabetes (page 152)
	Epilepsy (page 183)
	High blood pressure (page 246)

Who is likely to be deficient?

Most people, including vegans (vegetarians who eat no dairy or eggs), do not need taurine supplements. While infants require taurine, the amount in either human milk or formula is adequate. People with **diabetes** (page 152) have been reported to have lower blood levels of taurine than non-diabetics.[1]

How much is usually taken?

For the treatment of various medical conditions, doctors typically recommend 1.5 grams to as much as 6 grams or more per day.

Are there any side effects or interactions?

Taurine has not been reported to cause any severe adverse effects.

THYMUS EXTRACTS

What are they?

Thymus extracts are extracts derived from the thymus glands usually of young calves (bovine). The thymus is one of our major **immune system** (page 255) glands. It is composed of two soft pinkish-gray lobes lying in bib-like fashion just below the thyroid gland and above the heart. To a large extent, the health of the thymus determines the health of the immune system. The thymus is responsible for many immune system functions, including the production of T lymphocytes, a type of white blood cell responsible for "cell-mediated immunity." Cell-mediated immunity refers to immune mechanisms not controlled or mediated by antibodies. Cell-mediated immunity is extremely important in the resistance to infection by certain bacteria, yeast (including *Candida albicans*), fungi, **parasites** (page 343), and viruses (including **herpes simplex** [page 119], Epstein-Barr, and the viruses that cause **hepatitis** [page 220]). Cell-mediated immunity is also critical in protecting against the development of **cancer** (page 87), **allergies** (page 14), and autoimmune disorders such as **rheumatoid arthritis** (page 387). The thymus gland also releases several hormones, such as thymosin, thymopoeitin, and serum thymic factor, that regulate many immune functions.

The oral calf thymus extract that has been studied scientifically is specially prepared to concentrate small protein-like molecules (polypeptides). This extract (known as Thymomodulin) has been shown effective in preventing recurrent upper respiratory tract infections.

Preliminary studies suggest that Thymomodulin may also be helpful in (1) improving one of the T-cell defects in patients with human immunodeficiency virus infection (**HIV** [page 239]—the virus that causes AIDS); (2) treating acute and chronic **hepatitis** (page 220) B infections; (3) restoring the number of peripheral white blood cells in **cancer** (page 87) patients undergoing chemotherapy or radiation; and (4) relieving **allergies** (page 14), including **asthma** (page 32), **hay fever** (page 211), and food allergies, in children.[1, 2] The effectiveness of Thymomodulin in these conditions may be the result of improved thymus gland activity, or it may be due to the presence of hormones or other biologically active substances in the extract.

The ability of Thymomodulin to improve **immune function** (page 255) and reduce the number of recurrent **infections** (page 265) has been shown in double-blind studies of children and adults with a history of recurrent respiratory-tract infections.[3, 4, 5, 6, 7] Thymomodulin has also been shown in a double-blind study to improve immune function in cases of exercise-induced immune suppression. In addition, preliminary studies have shown the extract to improve immune function in people with **diabetes** (page 152) and in elderly people.[8, 9, 10, 11] (Extreme **exercise** (page 43), diabetes, and aging are all associated with suppression of immune function.)

Preliminary studies in patients with acute or chronic hepatitis suggest that supplementation with Thymomodulin may be helpful.[12, 13] However, additional studies are needed to confirm these findings.

Thymus Extracts

In a preliminary study in patients with early HIV infection, Thymomodulin improved several measures of immune function, including an increase in the number of T-helper cells, one of the goals in the treatment of HIV infection.[14] Thymomodulin (given orally or by injection) has been used in **cancer** (page 87) patients to counteract the decline in white-blood-cell levels that can result from chemotherapy or radiation.[15, 16, 17, 18, 19, 20] In test tube studies, Thymomodulin and other thymus extracts have been shown to exert a number of effects on white blood cells (e.g., increasing both the bone marrow production and functional activity of white blood cells).[21, 22] However, it is not yet known if this effect can be achieved with the use of oral thymus extracts.

The oral administration of Thymomodulin has been shown in preliminary and double-blind clinical trials to improve the symptoms and course of **hay fever** (page 211), allergic **rhinitis** (page 407), **asthma** (page 32), **eczema** (page 177), and food **allergies** (page 14) (in conjunction with an allergy elimination diet).[23, 24, 25, 26, 27, 28, 29, 30] Presumably, this clinical improvement results from restoring proper control over **immune function** (page 255).

Thymomodulin given by injection has also been shown to be helpful in the treatment of diseases of the heart muscle (idiopathic myocarditis and idiopathic dilated **cardiomyopathy** [page 95]).[31, 32] It is not known whether oral thymus extracts can achieve these same benefits.

Where are they found?

Thymus extracts (from bovine sources) are found in capsules and tablets as a dietary supplement. Thymomodulin is not available in the United States, and it is unknown whether any of the thymus extracts that are available have the same effects as Thymomodulin.

Thymus extracts have been used in connection with the following conditions (refer to the individual health concern for complete information):

Rating	Health Concerns
★★★	**Bronchitis** (page 80)
★★☆	**Allergies** (page 14)
	Hay fever (page 211)
	Hepatitis (page 220)
	Immune function (page 255)
	Recurrent upper respiratory tract infections
★☆☆	**Asthma** (page 32)
	HIV infection (page 239)

Who is likely to be deficient?

Since it is not an essential nutrient, no deficiency state exists.

How much is usually taken?

A number of different thymus preparations are commercially available. However, whether any of them have the same effects as Thymomodulin, which is not available in the United States, is still unknown. The recommended amount of thymus extract varies according to the type of preparation.

Are there any side effects or interactions?

No side effects or adverse reactions have been reported with the use of thymus preparations.

THYROID EXTRACTS

What are they?

Thyroid extracts are thyroid extracts derived from the thyroid glands of usually bovine (beef) sources.

The hormones of the thyroid gland regulate metabolism in every cell of the body. The medical treatment of underactive thyroid (**hypothyroidism** [page 252]) usually involves a prescription of synthetic thyroid hormones (thyroxine and/or triiodothyronine) or thyroid extract (desiccated thyroid). The difference between prescription thyroid extract and the thyroid extracts sold as nutritional supplements is the latter are required by the U.S. Food and Drug Administration to be free of the known active thyroid hormones (thyroxine and triiodothyronine). The use of hormone-free thyroid preparations has not been evaluated in scientific studies, but some doctors believe these products may provide nutritional support to the thyroid gland or contain other compounds with possible hormonal activity.

Where are they found?

Thyroid extracts are available as nutritional supplements in capsules and tablets.

Thyroid extracts have been used in connection with the following conditions (refer to the individual health concern for complete information):

Rating	Health Concerns
★☆☆	**Hypothyroidism** (page 252)

Who is likely to be deficient?

As thyroid extract is not an essential nutrient, therefore, no deficiency state exists.

How much is usually taken?

The recommended intake depends on the concentration, method of preparation, and quality of the thyroid extract. Follow the manufacturer's recommendation on the label.

Are there any side effects or interactions?

No side effects or adverse reactions have been reported. However, people taking prescription thyroid hormones should consult their doctor before using non-prescription thyroid extracts.

TOCOTRIENOLS

What are they?

Tocotrienols are members of the **vitamin E** (page 609) family. Like vitamin E, tocotrienols are potent **antioxidants** (page 467) against lipid peroxidation (the damaging of fats by oxidation).[1, 2]

Human studies indicate that, in addition to their antioxidant activity, tocotrienols have other important functions, especially in maintaining a healthy cardiovascular system.[3] Test tube and animal studies indicate a possible role for tocotrienols in protecting against **cancer** (page 87) (particularly **breast** [page 65] and skin cancer).

Like vitamin E, tocotrienols may offer protection against hardening of the arteries (**atherosclerosis** [page 38]) by preventing oxidative damage to LDL **cholesterol** (page 223) (oxidation of LDL cholesterol is believed to be one of the triggering factors for atherosclerosis).[4] In a double-blind study in patients with severe atherosclerosis of the carotid artery—the main artery supplying blood to the head—tocotrienol administration (200 mg per day) reduced the level of lipid peroxides in the blood. Moreover, in a small sample of patients receiving tocotrienols for 12 months, the size of atherosclerotic plaques became smaller. In contrast, none of the patients receiving the placebo showed an improvement in their atherosclerosis.[5]

Although tocotrienols inhibited **cholesterol** (page 223) synthesis in test tube studies,[6, 7] human studies have produced conflicting results. In a preliminary study, supplementation with 200 mg of gamma-tocotrienol reduced total cholesterol levels significantly—by 13% in four weeks.[8] In a double-blind study, 200 mg of tocotrienols per day produced a significant 15% drop in total cholesterol and an 8% reduction in LDL levels. There were no changes in these levels in the placebo group.[9] However, another double-blind study showed that 200 mg of tocotrienols per day failed to lower cholesterol levels.[10] In the most recent double-blind study, a group of men with slightly elevated cholesterol levels given 140 mg of tocotrienols and about 120 IU mg of **vitamin E** (page 609) daily demonstrated no changes in total cholesterol, LDL cholesterol, or HDL cholesterol levels after four weeks of supplementation.[11]

Test tube studies indicate that tocotrienols exert some **anticancer** (page 87 effects, especially against skin and **breast cancer** (page 65).[12, 13, 14, 15, 16] These results still need confirmation in human studies, however.

Where are they found?

Tocotrienols are found primarily in the oil fraction of rice bran, palm fruit, barley, and wheat germ. Supplemental sources of tocotrienols are derived from rice bran oil and palm oil distillates. Tocotrienol supplements are available in capsules and tablets.

Tocotrienols have been used in connection with the following conditions (refer to the individual health concern for complete information):

Rating	Health Concerns
★★★	**Atherosclerosis** (page 38)
★★☆	**High Cholesterol** (page 223)
★☆☆	**Stroke** (page 419)

Who is likely to be deficient?

As it is not an essential nutrient, no deficiency state exists.

How much is usually taken?

The typical recommendation is 140 to 360 mg per day. Most studies have used 200 mg daily.

Are there any side effects or interactions?

No significant adverse effects have been reported with tocotrienols.[17]

Tocotrienols

VANADIUM

What is it?

Vanadium is an ultra-trace mineral found in the human diet and the human body. It is essential for some animals. Deficiency symptoms in these animals include growth retardation, bone deformities, and infertility. However, vanadium has not been proven to be an essential mineral for humans.

Vanadium may play a role in building bones and teeth.

Vanadyl sulfate, a form of this mineral, may improve glucose control in people with type 2 (adult-onset or non-insulin-dependent) **diabetes** (page 152) mellitus, according to a study of eight people with diabetes who supplemented with 100 mg of the mineral daily for four weeks.[1] However, the researchers of this study caution that the long-term safety of such large amounts of vanadium remains unknown. Many doctors expect future research to show that amounts this high will likely prove to be unsafe. Moreover, in a preliminary report, vanadium did not help people with type 1 (childhood-onset or insulin-dependent) diabetes.[2]

Where is it found?

Vanadium is found in very small amounts in a wide variety of foods, including seafood, cereals, mushrooms, parsley, corn, soy, and gelatin.

Vanadium has been used in connection with the following condition

Rating	Health Concerns
★☆☆	**Diabetes** (page 152)

Who is likely to be deficient?

Deficiencies of vanadium have not been reported in humans, and it is not known whether this mineral is essential for humans.

How much is usually taken?

As yet, research indicates that most people would not benefit from vanadium supplementation. Optimal intake of vanadium is unknown. If vanadium turns out to be essential for humans, the estimated requirement would probably be less than 10 mcg per day. An average diet provides 15–30 mcg per day.

Are there any side effects or interactions?

Information about vanadium toxicity is limited. Workers exposed to vanadium dust can develop toxic effects. High blood levels have been linked to **manic-depressive** (page 61) mental disorders, but the meaning of this remains uncertain.[3] Vanadium sometimes inhibits, but at other times stimulates, **cancer** (page 87) growth in animals. However, the effect in humans remains unknown.[4]

Vanadium is not known to interact with other nutrients.

VINPOCETINE

What is it?

Vinpocetine is a chemical substance synthesized from vincamine, a natural constituent found in the leaves of *Vinca minor* (lesser periwinkle).

Vinpocetine appears to have antioxidant,[1] blood flow enhancing,[2, 3, 4, 5] and other effects that may be beneficial to brain function.[6, 7, 8, 9, 10] Research, primarily in Europe, has investigated these possible benefits in people with memory disorders (dementias) and people who have suffered strokes.

Where is it found?

Vinpocetine is synthesized from vincamine, a constituent of the leaves of *Vinca minor* (lesser periwinkle)

Vinpocetine has been used in connection with the following condition (refer to the individual health concern for complete information):

Rating	Health Concerns
★★★	**Age-related cognitive decline** (page 8)
★★☆	**Stroke** (page 419) (intravenous vinpocetine only) **Vertigo** (page 441)
★☆☆	**Alzheimer's disease** (page 19) Memory **Retinopathy** (page 385) Urinary incontinence

Who is likely to be deficient?

Vinpocetine is not an essential nutrient, so no deficiencies are possible.

How much is usually taken?

Research has typically used 30 to 60 mg per day of vinpocetine. Taking vinpocetine with food appears to dramatically improve its absorption.[11]

Are there any side effects or interactions?

Studies on vinpocetine report no serious side effects with amounts up to 60 mg per day.[12] Vinpocetine has blood-thinning effects,[13] which suggests that people with bleeding disorders or who are taking anticoagulant or other blood-thinning medications should consult a doctor before taking vinpocetine. However, one study found no such interaction between vinpocetine and the anticoagulant drug warfarin.[14]

VITAMIN A

See also: Beta-carotene (page 469)

What is it?

Vitamin A is a fat-soluble vitamin with four major functions in the body: (1) It helps cells reproduce normally—a process called differentiation (cells that have not properly differentiated are more likely to undergo pre-cancerous changes). (2) It is required for vision; vitamin A maintains healthy cells in various structures of the eye and is required for the transduction of light into nerve signals in the retina. (3) It is required for normal growth and development of the embryo and fetus, influencing genes that determine the sequential development of organs in embryonic development. (4) It may be required for normal reproductive function, with influences on the function and development of sperm, ovaries and placenta.

For some people, water-soluble forms of vitamin A supplements appear to be better absorbed than fat-soluble vitamin A.

Where is it found?

Liver, dairy products, and **cod liver oil** (page 514) are good sources of vitamin A. Vitamin A is also available in supplement form.

Vitamin A has been used in connection with the following conditions (refer to the individual health concern for complete information):

Rating	Health Concerns
★★★	**Anemia** (page 25) (for deficiency)
	Childhood diseases (page 105)
	Cystic fibrosis (page 143)
	Infection (page 265)
	Leukoplakia (page 289)
	Measles (page 307) (for deficiency)
	Night blindness (page 326)
★★☆	**Bronchitis** (page 80)
	Celiac disease (page 102) (for deficiency only)
	Heart attack (page 212)
	Immune function (page 255)
	Iron-deficiency anemia (page 278) (as an adjunct to supplemental iron)
	Measles (page 307) (for severe cases)
	Menorrhagia (page 314) (heavy menstruation)
	Peptic ulcer (page 349)
	Retinitis pigmentosa
	Sprains and strains (page 412) (for deficiency only)
	Wound healing (page 319)
★☆☆	**Acne** (page 4)
	Alcohol withdrawal support (page 12)
	Conjunctivitis/blepharitis (page 136)
	Crohn's disease (page 141)
	Diabetic retinopathy (page 385) (in combination with **selenium** [page 584], **vitamin C** [page 604], and **vitamin E** [page 609])
	Diarrhea (page 152)
	Gastritis (page 195)
	Goiter (page 206)
	HIV support (page 239)
	Hypothyroidism (page 252)
	Lung cancer (page 298)
	Pap smear (abnormal) (page 3)
	Pre- and post-surgery health (page 357)
	Premenstrual syndrome (page 368) (see dosage warnings)
	Retinopathy (page 385) (in combination with **selenium** [page 584], **vitamin C** [page 604], and **vitamin E** [page 609])
	Sickle cell anemia (page 403)
	Urinary tract infection (page 436)
	Vaginitis (page 438)

Who is likely to be deficient?

People who limit their consumption of liver, dairy foods, and **beta-carotene** (page 469)-containing vegetables can develop a vitamin A deficiency. Extremely low birth weight babies (2.2 pounds or less) are at high

Vitamin A

Vitamin A

risk of being born with a deficiency, and vitamin A shots given to these infants have been reported in double-blind research to reduce the risk of lung disease.[1] The earliest deficiency sign is poor **night vision** (page 326). Deficiency symptoms can also include dry skin, increased risk of **infections** (page 265), and metaplasia (a precancerous condition). Severe deficiencies causing blindness are extremely rare in Western societies.

Less severe deficiencies are more likely to occur with a variety of conditions causing **malabsorption** (page 304). A high incidence of vitamin A deficiency in people infected with **HIV** (page 239) has also been reported. People with **hypothyroidism** (page 252) have an impaired ability to convert **beta-carotene** (page 469) to vitamin A.[2, 3] For this reason, some doctors suggest taking supplemental vitamin A (perhaps 5,000–10,000 IU per day) if they are not consuming adequate amounts in their diet.

Very old people with type 2 **diabetes** (page 152) have shown a significant age-related decline in blood levels of vitamin A, irrespective of their dietary intake.[4]

How much is usually taken?

For most people, up to 25,000 IU (7,500 mcg) of vitamin A per day is considered safe. However, people over age 65 and those with liver disease should probably not supplement with more than 15,000 IU per day, unless supervised by a doctor. In women who could become **pregnant** (page 363), the maximum safe intake is being re-evaluated. However, less than 10,000 IU (3,000 mcg) per day is generally accepted as safe. There is concern that larger intakes could cause **birth defects** (page 63). Whether the average person would benefit from vitamin A supplementation remains unclear.

Are there any side effects or interactions?

Since a 1995 report from the *New England Journal of Medicine,*[5] women who are or could become **pregnant** (page 363) have been told by doctors to take less than 10,000 IU (3,000 mcg) per day of vitamin A to avoid the risk of **birth defects** (page 63). A recent report studied several hundred women exposed to 10,000–300,000 IU (median exposure of 50,000 IU) per day.[6] Three major malformations occurred in this study, but all could have happened in the absence of vitamin A supplementation. Surprisingly, no congenital malformations happened in any of the 120 infants ex-

posed to maternal intakes of vitamin A that exceeded 50,000 IU per day. In fact, the high-exposure group had a 50% decreased risk for malformations compared with infants not exposed to vitamin A. The authors noted that some previous studies found no link between vitamin A and birth defects, and argued the studies that did find such a link suffered from various weaknesses. A closer look at the recent study reveals a 32% higher than expected risk of birth defects in infants exposed to 10,000–40,000 IU of vitamin A per day, but paradoxically a 37% decreased risk for those exposed to even higher levels. This suggests that both "higher" and "lower" risks may have been due to chance.

Excessive dietary intake of vitamin A has been associated with birth defects in humans in fewer than 20 reported cases over the past 30 years.[7, 8] Presently, the level at which vitamin A supplementation may cause birth defects is not known, though combined human and animal data suggest that 30,000 IU per day should be considered safe.[9] Women who are or who could become pregnant should consult with a doctor before supplementing with more than 10,000 IU per day.

Vitamin A supplements can both help and hurt children. Many people have heard that vitamin A supplements support **immune function** (page 255) and prevent **infections** (page 265). This is true under some circumstances. However, vitamin A can also *increase* the risk of infections, according to the findings of a double-blind trial.[10] In a study of African children between six months and five years old, a 44% reduction in the risk of severe **diarrhea** (page 163) was seen in those children given four 100,000–200,000 IU applications of vitamin A (the lower amount for those less than a year old) during an eight-month period. On further investigation, the researchers discovered that the reduction in diarrhea occurred only in children who were very malnourished. For children who were not starving, vitamin A supplementation actually *increased* the risk of diarrhea compared with the placebo group. The vitamin A-supplemented children also had a 67% *increased* risk of coughing and rapid breathing, signs of further lung infection, although this problem did not appear in children infected with AIDS. These findings should be of concern to American parents, whose children are not usually infected with AIDS or severely malnourished. Such relatively healthy children fared poorly in the African trial in terms of both the risk of diarrhea and the risk of continued lung problems. Vitamin A provided no benefit to the well-nourished kids. Therefore, it makes sense to *not* give vitamin A supplements to children unless there is a special reason to do so, such as the presence of a condition causing **malabsorption** (page 304) (e.g., **celiac disease** [page 102]).

In a study of people with retinitis pigmentosa (a degenerative condition of the eye), participants received 15,000 IU of vitamin A per day for 12 years with no signs of adverse effects or toxicity.[11] For other adults, intake above 25,000 IU (7,500 mcg) per day can—in rare cases—cause headaches, dry skin, hair loss, fatigue, bone problems, and liver damage.[12] At higher levels (for example 100,000 IU per day) these problems become more common.

A controlled clinical trial showed that people who took 25,000 IU of vitamin A per day for a median of 3.8 years had an 11% increase in **triglycerides** (page 235), a 3% increase in total **cholesterol** (page 223) and a 1% decrease in HDL cholesterol compared to those who did not take vitamin A.[13] Although the significance of these findings is not clear, people at risk for **cardiovascular disease** (page 98) should use caution when considering long-term vitamin A supplementation.

One study found that increasing the intake of vitamin A in the diet was associated with bone loss and risk of hip fracture, possibly due to a vitamin A-induced stimulation of cells that break down bone.[14] In this study, a vitamin A intake greater than 5,000 IU per day, when compared to a lower intake, was associated with a reduction in bone mineral density that approximately doubles the risk of hip fracture. **Beta-carotene** (page 469) (which can be used by the body to make vitamin A) has not been linked to reduced bone mass. Until more is known, people concerned about **osteoporosis** (page 333) may consider taking beta-carotene supplements rather than supplementing with vitamin A.

Data from test tube, animal, and human studies show that excessive vitamin A intake can accelerate bone loss and inhibit formation of new bone, increasing the risk of osteoporosis.[15] In humans, small studies have found these effects at about 85,000–125,000 IU per day.[16, 17]

Taking vitamin A and **iron** (page 540) together helps overcome **iron deficiency** (page 278) more effectively than iron supplementation alone.[18] Supplementation with **zinc** (page 614), iron, or the combination has been found to improve vitamin A status among children at high risk for deficiency of the three nutrients.[19]

VITAMIN B₁

What is it?
Vitamin B₁ is is a water-soluble vitamin needed to process carbohydrates, fat, and protein. Every cell of the body requires vitamin B₁ to form the fuel the body runs on—adenosine triphosphate (ATP). Nerve cells require vitamin B₁ in order to function normally.

Where is it found?
Wheat germ, whole wheat, peas, beans, enriched flour, fish, peanuts, and meat are all good sources of vitamin B₁.

Vitamin B₁ has been used in connection with the following conditions (refer to the individual health concern for complete information):

Rating	Health Concerns
★★★	**Anemia** (page 25) (for genetic thiamine-responsive anemia)
★★☆	**Alzheimer's disease** (page 19) **Canker sores** (page 90) Childhood intelligence (for deficiency) **Diabetes** (page 152) Dialysis (for encephalopathy and neurologic damage; take only under medical supervision) **Hepatitis** (page 220) **Low back pain** (page 293) (in combination with **vitamin B₆** [page 600] and **vitamin B₁₂** [page 601])
★☆☆	**Cardiomyopathy** (page 95) (only for wet beri beri) **Dysmenorrhea** (page 171) (painful menstruation) **Fibromyalgia** (page 191) **HIV support** (page 239) **Multiple sclerosis** (page 323) **Pre- and post-surgery health** (page 357)

Who is likely to be deficient?
A decline in vitamin B₁ levels occurs with age, irrespective of medical condition.[1] Deficiency is most commonly found in **alcoholics** (page 12), people with **malabsorption** (page 304) conditions, and those eating a very poor diet. It is also common in children with congenital heart disease.[2] People with **chronic fatigue syndrome** (page 111) may also be deficient in vitamin

Vitamin B₁

B_1.[3, 4] Individuals undergoing regular kidney dialysis may develop severe vitamin B_1 deficiency, which can result in potentially fatal complications.[5] Persons receiving dialysis should discuss the need for vitamin B_1 supplementation with their physician.

How much is usually taken?

While the ideal intake is uncertain, one study reported the healthiest people consumed more than 9 mg per day.[6] The amount found in many **multivitamin** (page 559) supplements (20–25 mg) is more than adequate for most people.

Vitamin B_1 is nontoxic, even in very high amounts.

Are there any side effects or interactions?

Vitamin B_1 works hand in hand with **vitamin B_2** (page 598) and **vitamin B_3** (page 598). Therefore, nutritionists usually suggest that vitamin B_1 be taken as part of a **B-complex** (page 603) vitamin or other **multivitamin supplement** (page 559).

VITAMIN B₂

What is it?

Vitamin B_2 is a water-soluble vitamin needed to process **amino acids** (page 465) and fats, activate **vitamin B_6** (page 600) and **folic acid** (page 520), and help convert carbohydrates into the fuel the body runs on—adenosine triphosphate (ATP). Under some conditions, vitamin B_2 can act as an **antioxidant** (page 467).

Where is it found?

Dairy products, eggs, and meat contain significant amounts of vitamin B_2. Leafy green vegetables, whole grains, and enriched grains contain some vitamin B_2.

Vitamin B₂ has been used in connection with the following conditions (refer to the individual health concern for complete information):

Rating	Health Concerns
★★★	**Anemia** (page 25) (if deficient) **Migraine headaches** (page 316)
★★☆	**Canker sores** (page 90) **Cataracts** (page 101) **Parkinson's disease** (page 345)
★☆☆	**Preeclampsia** (page 361) **Sickle cell anemia** (page 403)

Who is likely to be deficient?

Vitamin B_2 deficiency can occur in **alcoholics** (page 12). Also, a deficiency may be more likely in people with **cataracts** (page 101)[1, 2] or **sickle cell anemia** (page 403).[3] In developing countries, vitamin B_2 deficiency has been found to be a risk factor for the development of **preeclampsia** (page 361) in **pregnant** (page 363) women.[4] People with **chronic fatigue syndrome** (page 111) may be deficient in vitamin B_2.[5]

How much is usually taken?

The ideal level of intake is not known. The amounts found in many **multivitamin** (page 559) supplements (20–25 mg) are more than adequate for most people.

Are there any side effects or interactions?

At supplemental and dietary levels, vitamin B_2 is nontoxic.

Vitamin B_2 works with **vitamin B_1** (page 597), **vitamin B_3** (page 598), and **vitamin B_6** (page 600). For that reason, vitamin B_2 is often taken as part of a **B-complex** (page 603) supplement.

VITAMIN B₃ (NIACIN, NIACINAMIDE)

What is it?

The body uses the water-soluble vitamin B_3 in the process of releasing energy from carbohydrates. It is needed to form fat from carbohydrates and to process alcohol. The niacin form of vitamin B_3 also regulates **cholesterol** (page 223), though niacinamide does not.

Vitamin B_3 comes in two basic forms—niacin (also called nicotinic acid) and niacinamide (also called nicotinamide). A variation on niacin, called inositol hexaniacinate, is also available in supplements. Since it has not been linked with any of the usual niacin toxicity in scientific research, some doctors recommend inositol hexaniacinate for people who need large amounts of niacin.

Where is it found?

The best food sources of vitamin B_3 are peanuts, **brewer's yeast** (page 480), fish, and meat. Some vitamin B_3 is also found in whole grains.

Vitamin B$_3$ has been used in connection with the following conditions (refer to the individual health concern for complete information):

Rating	Health Concerns
★★★	**Acne** (page 4) (topical niacinamide) **High cholesterol** (page 223) **High triglycerides** (page 235) (niacin) **Intermittent claudication** (page 276) (niacin–inositol hexaniacinate) **Osteoarthritis** (page 328) (niacinamide)
★★☆	**Dysmenorrhea** (page 171) (painful menstruation) (niacin) **High cholesterol** (page 223) (inositol hexaniacinate) **High triglycerides** (page 235) (inositol hexaniacinate) **Peripheral vascular disease** (page 352) (inositol hexaniacinate) **Raynaud's disease** (page 382) (niacin–inositol hexaniacinate) **Schizophrenia** (page 393)
★☆☆	**Alcohol withdrawal support** (page 12) (niacinamide) **Anxiety** (page 30) (niacinamide) **Cataracts** (page 101) (niacinamide) **Dermatitis herpetiformis** (page 151) (nicotinamide, when combined with tetracycline) **Diabetes** (page 152) (niacinamide) **HIV support** (page 239) **Hypoglycemia** (page 251) (niacinamide) **Hypothyroidism** (page 252) (niacin) **Multiple sclerosis** (page 323) (niacin) **Photosensitivity** (page 356) (niacinamide) **Tardive dyskinesia** (page 425) (niacin or niacinamide)

Who is likely to be deficient?

Pellagra, the disease caused by a vitamin B$_3$ deficiency, is rare in Western societies. Symptoms include loss of appetite, skin rash, **diarrhea** (page 163), mental changes, beefy tongue, and digestive and emotional disturbance.

How much is usually taken?

In part because it is added to white flour, most people generally get enough vitamin B$_3$ from their diets to prevent a deficiency. However, 10–25 mg of the vitamin can be taken as part of a **B-complex** (page 603) or **multivitamin** (page 559) supplement. Larger amounts are used for the treatment of various health conditions.

Are there any side effects or interactions?

Niacinamide is almost always safe to take, though rare liver problems have occurred at amounts in excess of 1,000 mg per day. Niacin, in amounts as low as 50–100 mg, may cause flushing, headache, and **stomachache** (page 260) in some people. Doctors sometimes prescribe very high amounts of niacin (as much as 3,000 mg per day or more) for certain health problems. These large amounts can cause liver damage, **diabetes** (page 152), **gastritis** (page 195), damage to eyes, and elevated blood levels of uric acid (which can cause **gout** [page 208]). Symptoms caused by niacin supplements, such as flushing, have been reduced with sustained-release (also called "time-release") niacin products. However, sustained-release forms of niacin have caused significant liver toxicity and, rarely, liver failure.[1, 2, 3, 4, 5] One partial time-release (intermediate-release) niacin product has demonstrated clinical efficacy without flushing, and also without the liver function abnormalities typically associated with sustained-release niacin formulations.[6] However, this form of niacin is available by prescription only.

In a controlled clinical trial, 1,000 mg or more per day of niacin raised blood levels of **homocysteine** (page 234), a substance associated with increased risk of **heart disease** (page 98).[7] Since other actions of niacin lower heart disease risk,[8, 9] the importance of this finding is unclear. Nonetheless, for all of the reasons discussed above, large amounts of niacin should never be taken without consulting a doctor.

The inositol hexaniacinate form of niacin has not been linked with the side effects associated with niacin supplementation. In a group of people being treated alternatively with niacin and inositol hexaniacinate for skin problems, niacin supplementation (50–100 mg per day) was associated with numerous side effects, including skin flushing, nausea, vomiting and agitation.[10] In contrast, people taking inositol hexaniacinate experienced no complaints whatsoever, even at amounts two to five times higher than the previously used amounts of niacin. However, the amount of research studying the safety of inositol hexaniacinate remains quite limited. Therefore, people taking this supplement in large amounts (2,000 mg or more per day) should be under the care of a doctor.

Vitamin B$_3$ works with **vitamin B$_1$** (page 597) and **vitamin B$_2$** (page 598) to release energy from carbohydrates. Therefore, these vitamins are often taken together in a **B-complex** (page 603) or **multivitamin** (page 559) supplement (although most B$_3$ research uses niacin or niacinamide alone).

Vitamin B$_3$ (Niacin, Niacinamide)

VITAMIN B₆

What is it?

Vitamin B₆ is the master vitamin for processing **amino acids** (page 465)—the building blocks of all proteins and some hormones. Vitamin B₆ helps to make and take apart many amino acids and is also needed to make the hormones, serotonin, **melatonin** (page 555), and dopamine.

Vitamin B₆ aids in the formation of several neurotransmitters and is therefore an essential nutrient in the regulation of mental processes and possibly mood.

In combination with **folic acid** (page 520) and **vitamin B₁₂** (page 601), vitamin B₆ lowers **homocysteine** (page 234) levels—an amino acid linked to **heart disease** (page 98) and **stroke** (page 419), and possibly other diseases as well, such as **osteoporosis** (page 333), and **Alzheimer's disease** (page 19).

A rare, but severe, form of childhood **epilepsy** (page 183) results from an inborn error in the metabolism of vitamin B₆. Children with this form of epilepsy have an abnormal dependence on vitamin B₆ and are usually mentally retarded. Seizure activity is reversible with intravenous injections of vitamin B₆, which must be administered by a doctor.[1]

In some,[2, 3] but not all,[4] studies, vitamin B₆ supplements improved glucose tolerance in women with **diabetes** (page 152) caused by **pregnancy** (page 363).

Where is it found?

Potatoes, bananas, raisin bran cereal, lentils, liver, turkey, and tuna are all good sources of vitamin B₆.

Vitamin B₆ has been used in connection with the following conditions (refer to the individual health concern for complete information):

Rating	Health Concerns
★★★	**Anemia** (page 25) (if deficient and for genetic vitamin B₆-responsive anemia) **Autism** (page 63) **Depression** (page 145) (in women taking oral contraceptives) **High homocysteine** (page 234) (in combination with **folic acid** [page 520] and **vitamin B₁₂** [page 601]) **Morning sickness** (page 320) **Premenstrual syndrome** (page 368)
★★☆	**Age-related cognitive decline** (page 8) **Asthma** (page 32) **Canker sores** (page 90) **Carpal tunnel syndrome** (page 99) Childhood intelligence (for deficiency) **Depression** (page 145) (associated with **premenstrual syndrome** [page 368]) **Diabetes** (page 152) (gestational only) **Low back pain** (page 293) (in combination with **vitamin B₁** [page 597] and **vitamin B₁₂** [page 601]) **MSG sensitivity** (page 322) **Pregnancy and postpartum support** (page 363) (if homocysteine [page 234] levels are elevated) **Schizophrenia** (page 393) **Vertigo** (page 441)
★☆☆	**Acne** (page 4) **Alcohol withdrawal support** (page 12) **Alzheimer's disease** (page 19) (in combination with **iron** [page 540] and **coenzyme Q₁₀** [page 496]) **Amenorrhea** (page 22) **Atherosclerosis** (page 38) **Attention deficit disorder** (page 55) **Celiac disease** (page 102) **Eating disorders** (page 174) (for bulimia) **Epilepsy** (page 183) **Fibrocystic breast disease** (page 189) **Heart attack** (page 212) **HIV support** (page 239) **Hypoglycemia** (page 251) **Kidney stones** (page 284) **Osgood-Schlatter disease** (page 327) (in combination with **manganese** [page 553] and **zinc** [page 614]) **Osteoporosis** (page 333) (to lower **homocysteine** [page 234]) **Parkinson's disease** (page 345) (with Sinemet or Eldepryl) **Photosensitivity** (page 356) **Preeclampsia** (page 361) **Pre- and post-surgery health** (page 357) **Seborrheic dermatitis** (page 400) **Sickle cell anemia** (page 403) **Stroke** (page 419) **Tardive dyskinesia** (page 425)

Who is likely to be deficient?

Vitamin B₆ deficiencies are thought to be very rare. Vitamin B₆ deficiency can cause impaired **immunity** (page 225), skin lesions, and mental confusion. A marginal deficiency sometimes occurs in **alcoholics** (page 12), patients with kidney failure, and women using oral contraceptives. Some doctors believe that most diets do not provide optimal amounts of this vitamin. People with kidney failure have an increased risk of vitamin B_6 deficiency.[5] Vitamin B_6 has also been reported to be deficient in some people with **chronic fatigue syndrome** (page 111).[6]

How much is usually taken?

The most common supplemental intake is 10–25 mg per day. However, high amounts (100–200 mg per day or even more) may be recommended for certain conditions.

Are there any side effects or interactions?

Vitamin B_6 is usually safe, at intakes up to 200 mg per day in adults.[7] However, neurological side effects can sometimes occur at that level.[8] Levels higher than 200 mg are more likely to cause such problems. Vitamin B_6 toxicity can damage sensory nerves, leading to numbness in the hands and feet as well as difficulty walking. The National Academy of Sciences performed an analysis of vitamin B_6 studies. They determined the safe upper limit for long-term use is 100 mg per day. However, under supervision of a healthcare professional, up to 200 mg per day of vitamin B_6 can be safely taken by most men and nonpregnant women for limited periods of time. **Pregnant** (page 363) and breast-feeding women should not take more than 100 mg of vitamin B_6 per day without a doctor's supervision.

Since vitamin B_6 increases the bioavailability of **magnesium** (page 551), these nutrients are sometimes taken together.

VITAMIN B₁₂

What is it?

Vitamin B_{12} is is a water-soluble vitamin needed for normal nerve cell activity, DNA replication, and production of the mood-affecting substance **SAMe** (page 583) (S-adenosyl-L-methionine). Vitamin B_{12} acts with **folic acid** (page 520) and **vitamin B_6** (page 600) to control homocysteine levels. An excess of **homocysteine** (page 234) is associated with an increased risk of **heart disease** (page 98), **stroke** (page 419), and potentially other diseases such as **osteoporosis** (page 333) and **Alzheimer's disease** (page 19).

Vitamin B_{12} deficiency causes fatigue. Years ago, a small, double-blind trial reported that even some people who are *not* deficient in this vitamin had increased energy after vitamin B_{12} injections, compared with the effect of placebo injections.[1] In recent years, however, the relationship between B_{12} injections and the energy level of people who are not vitamin B_{12}-deficient has been rarely studied. In a preliminary trial, 2,500–5,000 mcg of vitamin B_{12}, given by injection every two to three days, led to improvement in 50–80% of a group of people with **chronic fatigue syndrome** (page 111) (CFS), with most improvement appearing after several weeks of vitamin B_{12} shots.[2] The ability of vitamin B_{12} injections to help people with CFS remains unproven, however. People with CFS interested in considering a trial of vitamin B_{12} injections should consult a doctor. Oral or sublingual (administered under the tongue) B_{12} supplements are unlikely to obtain the same results as injectable B_{12}, because the body's ability to absorb large amounts is relatively poor.

Where is it found?

Vitamin B_{12} is found in all foods of animal origin, including dairy, eggs, meat, poultry, and fish. According to one report, small, inconsistent amounts occur in seaweed (including nori and chlorella) and tempeh.[3] Many researchers and healthcare professionals believe that people cannot rely on vegetarian sources to provide predictably sufficient quantities of vitamin B_{12}. However, another study found substantial amounts of vitamin B_{12} in nori (at least 55 mcg per 100 grams of dry weight).[4]

Vitamin B₁₂ has been used in connection with the following conditions (refer to the individual health concern for complete information):

Rating	Health Concerns
★★★	**Anemia** (page 25) (if deficient)
	Depression (page 145) (in people with vitamin B_{12} deficiency)
	High homocysteine (page 234) (combination with **folic acid** [page 520] and **vitamin B_6** [page 600])
	Pernicious anemia (Vitamin B_{12} deficiency)

Vitamin B₁₂

Vitamin B₁₂

Rating	Health Concerns
★★☆	**Age-related cognitive decline** (page 8) (in people with vitamin B₁₂ deficiency) **Anemia** (page 25) (for thalassemia if deficient) **Bell's palsy** (page 57) **Canker sores** (page 90) (for deficiency only) **Chronic fatigue syndrome** (page 111) Cyanide poisoning **Cystic fibrosis** (page 143) (in people with vitamin B₁₂ deficiency) **Indigestion** (page 260) (for people with the combination of low vitamin B₁₂ levels, delayed gastric emptying, and *Helicobacter pylori* infection) **Infertility (male)** (page 305) **Low back pain** (page 293) (in combination with **vitamin B₁** [page 597] and **vitamin B₆** [page 600]) **Migraine headaches** (page 316) **Sickle cell anemia** (page 403) (for sickle cell patients with B₁₂ deficiency)
★☆☆	**Alzheimer's disease** (page 19) **Asthma** (page 32) **Atherosclerosis** (page 38) **Bipolar disorder** (page 61) **Bursitis** (page 87) **Crohn's disease** (page 141) **Dermatitis herpetiformis** (page 151) (in people with vitamin B₁₂ deficiency) **Diabetes** (page 152) **Down's syndrome** (page 169) **Heart attack** (page 212) **Hepatitis** (page 220) **HIV support** (page 239) **Hives** (page 245) **Immune function** (page 255) **Insomnia** (page 270) **Lung cancer** (page 298) (reduces risk) **Osteoporosis** (page 333) (to lower homocysteine) **Pain** (page 338) **Phenylketonuria** (page 354) (in people with vitamin B₁₂ deficiency) **Pre- and post-surgery health** (page 357) **Preeclampsia** (page 361) **Retinopathy** (page 385) (associated with childhood **diabetes** [page 152]) **Schizophrenia** (page 393) **Seborrheic dermatitis** (page 400) (injection) **Shingles (herpes zoster)/postherpetic neuralgia** (page 401) (injection) **Stroke** (page 419) **Tinnitus** (page 430) (injection) **Vitiligo** (page 443)

Who is likely to be deficient?

Vegans (vegetarians who also avoid dairy and eggs) frequently become deficient, though the process often takes many years. People with **malabsorption** (page 303) conditions, including those with tapeworm infestation and those with bacterial overgrowth in the intestines, often suffer from vitamin B₁₂ deficiency. Malabsorption of vitamin B₁₂ can also result from pancreatic disease, the effects of gastrointestinal surgery, or various prescription drugs.[5]

Pernicious anemia is a special form of vitamin B₁₂ malabsorption due to impaired ability of certain cells in the stomach to make intrinsic factor—a substance needed for normal absorption of vitamin B₁₂. By definition, all people with pernicious anemia are vitamin B₁₂-deficient. They require either vitamin B₁₂ injections or oral supplementation with very high levels (1000 mcg per day) of vitamin B₁₂.

Older people with urinary incontinence[6] and hearing loss[7] have been reported to be at increased risk of B₁₂ deficiency.

Infection (page 265) with *Helicobacter pylori*, a common cause of **gastritis** (page 195) and **ulcers** (page 349), has been shown to cause or contribute to adult vitamin B₁₂ deficiency. *H. pylori* has this effect by damaging cells in the stomach that make intrinsic factor—a substance needed for normal absorption of vitamin B₁₂. In one trial, *H. pylori* was detected in 56% of people with anemia due to vitamin B₁₂ deficiency. Successful eradication of *H. pylori* led to improved blood levels of B₁₂ in 40% of those infected.[8] Other studies have also suggested a link between *H. pylori* infection and vitamin B₁₂ deficiency.[9, 10] Elimination of *H. pylori* infection does not always improve vitamin B₁₂ status. People with *H. pylori* infections should have vitamin B₁₂ status monitored.

In a preliminary report, 47% of people with **tinnitus** (page 430) and related disorders were found to have vitamin B₁₂ deficiencies that may be helped by supplementation.[11]

HIV (page 239)-infected patients often have low blood levels of vitamin B₁₂.[12]

A disproportionate amount of people with psychiatric disorders are deficient in B₁₂.[13] Significant vitamin B₁₂ deficiency is associated with a doubled risk of severe **depression** (page 145), according to a study of physically disabled older women.[14]

A preliminary study found that **postmenopausal** (page 311) women who were in the lowest one-fifth of vitamin B₁₂ consumption had an increased risk of developing **breast cancer** (page 65).[15]

Although blood levels of vitamin B_{12} may be higher in **alcoholics** (page 12), actual body stores of vitamin B_{12} in the tissues (e.g., the liver) of alcoholics is frequently deficient.[16, 17]

Low blood levels of vitamin B_{12} are sometimes seen in **pregnant** (page 363) women; however, this does not always indicate a vitamin B_{12} deficiency.[18] The help of a healthcare professional is needed to determine when a true vitamin B_{12} deficiency exists in pregnant women with low blood levels of the vitamin.

Hydroxocobalamin (a form of vitamin B_{12}) has been recognized for more than 40 years as an effective antidote to cyanide poisoning. It is currently being used in France for that purpose. Because of its safety, hydroxocobalamin is considered by some researchers to be an ideal treatment for cyanide poisoning.[19]

How much is usually taken?

Most people do not require vitamin B_{12} supplements. However, vegans should supplement with at least 2 to 3 mcg per day.

People with pernicious anemia are often treated with injections of vitamin B_{12}. However, oral administration of 1,000 mcg per day can be used reliably as an alternative to vitamin B_{12} injections.[20, 21, 22, 23, 24]

Absorption of vitamin B_{12} is reduced with increasing age. Some research suggests that elderly people may benefit from 10 to 25 mcg per day of vitamin B_{12}.[25, 26, 27]

When vitamin B_{12} is used for therapeutic purposes *other than correcting a deficiency*, injections are usually necessary to achieve results.

Sublingual forms of vitamin B_{12} are available,[28] but there is no proof (nor is there any reason to expect) that they offer any advantage to oral supplements (i.e. a sublingual preparation is eventually swallowed).

Are there any side effects or interactions?

Oral vitamin B_{12} supplements are not generally associated with any side effects.

Although quite rare, serious **allergic reactions** (page 14) to *injections* of vitamin B_{12} (sometimes even life-threatening) have been reported.[29, 30] Whether these reactions are to the vitamin itself, or to preservatives or other substances in the injectable vitamin B_{12} solution, remains somewhat unclear. Most, but not all, injectable vitamin B_{12} contains preservatives.

If a person is deficient in vitamin B_{12} and takes 1,000 mcg or more of **folic acid** (page 520) per day, the folic acid supplementation can improve the anemia caused by vitamin B_{12} deficiency. The effect of folic acid on vitamin B_{12} deficiency-induced anemia is not a folic acid toxicity. Rather, the folic acid supplementation is acting to correct one of the problems caused by B_{12} deficiency. The other problems caused by a lack of vitamin B_{12} (mostly neurological) do *not* improve with folic acid supplements, and can become irreversible if vitamin B_{12} is not provided to someone who is vitamin B_{12} deficient.

Some doctors are unaware that vitamin B_{12} deficiencies often occur *without* anemia—even in people who do not take folic acid supplements. This lack of knowledge can delay diagnosis and treatment of people with vitamin B_{12} deficiencies. This can lead to permanent injury. When such a delayed diagnosis occurs in someone who inadvertently erased the anemia of vitamin B_{12} deficiency by taking folic acid supplements, the folic acid supplementation is often blamed for the missed diagnosis. This problem is rare and should not occur in people whose doctors understand that a lack of anemia does not rule out a vitamin B_{12} deficiency. Anyone supplementing 1,000 mcg or more per day of folic acid should be initially evaluated by a doctor before the folic acid can obscure a proper diagnosis of a possible B_{12} deficiency.

VITAMIN B-COMPLEX

The vitamin B-complex refers to all of the known essential water-soluble vitamins except for **vitamin C** (page 604). These include **thiamine** (page 597) (vitamin B_1), **riboflavin** (page 598) (vitamin B_2), **niacin** (page 598) (vitamin B_3), **pantothenic acid** (page 568) (vitamin B_5), pyridoxine (**vitamin B_6** [page 600]), **biotin** (page 473), **folic acid** (page 520), and the cobalamins (**vitamin B_{12}** [page 601]).

"Vitamin B" was once thought to be a single nutrient that existed in extracts of rice, liver, or yeast. Researchers later discovered these extracts contained several vitamins, which were given distinguishing numbers. Unfortunately, this has led to an erroneous belief among non-scientists that these vitamins have a special relationship to each other. Further adding to confusion has been the "unofficial" designation of other substances as members of the B-complex, such as **choline** (page 546), **inositol** (page 537), and para-aminobenzoic acid (**PABA** [page 567]), even though they are not essential vitamins.

Each member of the B-complex has a unique structure and performs unique functions in the human body. Vitamins B$_1$, B$_2$, B$_3$, and biotin participate in different aspects of energy production, vitamin B$_6$ is essential for **amino acid** (page 465) metabolism, and vitamin B$_{12}$ and folic acid facilitate steps required for cell division. Each of these vitamins has many additional functions. However, contrary to popular belief, no functions require all B-complex vitamins simultaneously.

Human requirements for members of the B-complex vary considerably—from 3 mcg per day for vitamin B$_{12}$ to 18 mg per day for vitamin B$_3$ in adult males, for example. Therefore, taking equal amounts of each one— as provided in many B-complex supplements—makes little sense. Furthermore, there is little evidence supporting the use of megadoses of B-complex vitamins to combat everyday stress, boost energy, or control food cravings, unless a person has a deficiency of one or more of them. Again, contrary to popular belief, there is no evidence indicating people should take all B vitamins to avoid an imbalance when one or more individual B vitamin is taken for a specific health condition.

Most **multivitamin-mineral** (page 559) products contain the B-complex along with the rest of the essential vitamins and minerals. Since they are more complete than B-complex vitamins alone, multiple vitamin-mineral supplements are recommended to improve overall micronutrient intake and prevent deficiencies.

Are there any side effects or interactions?

Vitamin B-complex includes several different components, each of which has the potential to interact with drugs. It is recommended that you discuss the use of vitamin B-complex and your current medication(s) with your doctor or pharmacist.

VITAMIN C

What is it?

Vitamin C is a water-soluble vitamin that has a number of biological functions.

Acting as an **antioxidant** (page 467), one of vitamin C's important functions is to protect LDL **cholesterol**

(page 223) from oxidative damage. (Only when LDL is damaged does cholesterol appear to lead to **heart disease** (page 98), and vitamin C may be one of the most important antioxidant protectors of LDL.)[1] Vitamin C may also protect against heart disease by reducing the stiffness of arteries and the tendency of platelets to clump together.[2]

The antioxidant properties of vitamin C are thought to protect smokers, as well as people exposed to second-hand smoke, from the harmful effects of free radicals. A controlled trial demonstrated the ability of 3 grams of vitamin C, taken by nonsmokers two hours prior to being exposed to cigarette smoke, to reduce the free radical damage and LDL cholesterol oxidation associated with exposure to cigarette smoke.[3] The smoke-induced decline in total antioxidant defense was also diminished. These beneficial effects were not observed in nonsmokers under normal conditions (no free radical exposure).

Vitamin C is needed to make collagen, the "glue" that strengthens many parts of the body, such as muscles and blood vessels. Vitamin C also plays important roles in **wound healing** (page 319) and as a natural antihistamine. This vitamin also aids in the formation of liver bile and helps to fight viruses and to detoxify alcohol and other substances.

Recently, researchers have shown that vitamin C improves nitric oxide activity.[4] Nitric oxide is needed for the dilation of blood vessels, potentially important in lowering **blood pressure** (page 246) and preventing spasms of arteries in the heart that might otherwise lead to **heart attacks** (page 212). Vitamin C has reversed dysfunction of cells lining blood vessels.[5] The normalization of the functioning of these cells may be linked to prevention of heart disease.

Evidence indicates that vitamin C levels in the eye decrease with age[6] and that supplementing with vitamin C prevents this decrease,[7] possibly leading to a lower risk of developing **cataracts** (page 101).[8, 9] Healthy people have been reported in some, but not all, studies[10] to be more likely to take vitamin C and **vitamin E** (page 609) supplements than are people with cataracts.[11]

Vitamin C has been reported to reduce activity of the **enzyme** (page 506), aldose reductase, in people.[12] Aldose reductase is the enzyme responsible for accumulation of sorbitol in eyes, nerves, and kidneys of people with **diabetes** (page 152). This accumulation is believed to be responsible for deterioration of these parts of the body associated with diabetes. Therefore, interference with the activity of aldose reductase theoretically helps protect people with diabetes.

Vitamin C may help protect the body against accumulation or retention of the toxic mineral, lead. In one preliminary study, people with higher blood levels of vitamin C had much lower risk of having excessive blood levels of lead.[13] In a controlled trial, male smokers with moderate to high levels of lead received supplements of 1,000 mg per day of vitamin C, 200 mg per day of vitamin C, or a placebo.[14] Only those people taking 1,000 mg per day of vitamin C experienced a drop in the blood lead levels, but the reduction in this group was dramatic.

People with recurrent boils (furunculosis) may have defects in white blood cell function that are correctable with vitamin C supplementation. A preliminary study of people with recurrent boils and defective white blood cell function, found that 1 gram of vitamin C taken daily for four to six weeks, resulted in normalization of white blood cell function.[15] Ten of twelve people receiving vitamin C became symptom-free within one month and remained so for periods of one to three years without additional supplementation. The other two people required long-term vitamin C supplementation to prevent recurrences.

A double-blind trial found that 500 mg of vitamin C per day for one year reduced the risk of developing reflex sympathetic dystrophy (a painful nerve condition of the extremities), after a wrist fracture.[16]

In a small, preliminary trial, vitamin C (500 mg twice daily) combined with rutoside (500 mg twice daily), a derivative of the **flavonoid** (page 516), rutin, produced marked improvement in three women with progressive pigmented purpura (PPP), a mild skin condition.[17] Although not a serious medical condition, cosmetic concerns lead people with PPP to seek treatment with a variety of drugs. The vitamin C/rutoside combination represents a promising, non-toxic alternative to these drug treatments, but larger, controlled trials are needed to confirm these preliminary results.

Where is it found?

Broccoli, red peppers, currants, Brussels sprouts, parsley, potatoes, citrus fruit, and strawberries are good sources of vitamin C.

Vitamin C has been used in connection with the following conditions (refer to the individual health concern for complete information)**:**

Rating	Health Concerns
★★★	**Anemia** (page 25) (if deficient)
	Athletic performance (page 43) (if deficient, or to reduce pain and speed up muscle strength recovery after intense exercise)
	Bronchitis (page 80)
	Bruising (page 84) (for deficiency)
	Burns (page 85) (in combination with **vitamin E** [page 609] for prevention of sunburn only)
	Capillary fragility (page 93)
	Common cold/sore throat (page 129)
	Gingivitis (page 203) (periodontal disease) (for deficiency only)
	Glaucoma (page 205)
	Heart attack (page 212) (for deficiency)
	High cholesterol (page 223) (protection of LDL cholesterol)
	Infection (page 265)
	Infertility (male) (page 305) (for sperm agglutination)
	Reflex sympathetic dystrophy (prevention)
	Scurvy
	Wound healing (page 319)
★★☆	**Asthma** (page 32)
	Atherosclerosis (page 38)
	Athletic performance (page 43) (for exercise recovery)
	Autism (page 63)
	Cataracts (page 101)
	Childhood intelligence (for deficiency)
	Cold sores (page 119)
	Diabetes (page 152)
	Dysmenorrhea (page 171) (plus **vitamin B₃** [page 598] [niacin] and rutin)
	Endometriosis (page 182) (in combination with **vitamin E** [page 609])
	Gastritis (page 195)
	Gingivitis (page 203) (periodontal disease) (in combination with flavonoids)
	Immune function (page 255)
	Infertility (female) (page 187)
	Influenza (page 269)
	Iron-deficiency anemia (page 278) (as an adjunct to supplemental iron)
	Lead toxicity
	Pancreatic insufficiency (page 341)
	Parkinson's disease (page 345) (in combination with **Vitamin E** [page 609])
	Pre- and post-surgery health (page 357) (if deficient)
	Preeclampsia (page 361) (in combination with **vitamin E** [page 609]; for high risk only)
	Schizophrenia (page 393)
	Skin ulcers (page 409)
	Sprains and strains (page 412)

Vitamin C

Rating	Health Concerns
★☆☆	**Age-related cognitive decline** (page 8)
	Alcohol withdrawal support (page 12)
	Amenorrhea (page 22)
	Anemia (page 25) (for thalassemia if deficient)
	Bipolar disorder/manic depression (page 61)
	Boils (recurrent furunculosis)
	Childhood diseases (page 105)
	Chronic obstructive pulmonary disease (page 114) (COPD)
	Colon cancer (page 123) (reduces risk)
	Diabetic retinopathy (page 385) (in combination with **selenium** [page 584], **vitamin A** [page 595], and **vitamin E** [page 609])
	Ear infections (recurrent) (page 383)
	Eczema (page 177)
	Gallstones (page 193)
	Gout (page 208)
	Halitosis (page 209) (if gum disease and deficient)
	Hay fever (page 211)
	Heart attack (page 212) (for those not deficient)
	Hepatitis (page 220)
	High blood pressure (page 246)
	HIV support (page 239) (oral and topical)
	Hives (page 245)
	Hypoglycemia (page 251)
	Leukoplakia (page 289)
	Low back pain (page 293)
	Macular degeneration (page 303)
	Menopause (page 311)
	Menorrhagia (page 314) (heavy menstruation)
	Morning sickness (page 320)
	Peptic ulcer (page 349)
	Progressive pigmented purpura (in combination with rutoside)
	Prostatitis (page 377) (acute bacterial prostatitis, chronic bacterial prostatitis)
	Retinopathy (page 385) (in combination with **selenium** [page 584], **vitamin A** [page 595], and **vitamin E** [page 609])
	Sickle cell anemia (page 403)
	Sinusitis (page 407)
	Tardive dyskinesia (page 425)
	Urinary tract infection (page 436)
	Vitiligo (page 443)

Who is likely to be deficient?

Although scurvy (severe vitamin C deficiency) is uncommon in Western societies, many doctors believe that most people consume less than optimal amounts. Fatigue, easy **bruising** (page 84), and bleeding gums are early signs of vitamin C deficiency that occur long before frank scurvy develops. Smokers have low levels of vitamin C and require a higher daily intake to maintain normal vitamin C levels. Women with **preeclampsia** (page 361) have been found to have lower blood levels of vitamin C than women without the condition.[18] Women who have lower blood levels of vitamin C have an increased risk of **gallstones** (page 193).[19]

People with kidney failure have an increased risk of vitamin C deficiency.[20] However, people with kidney failure should take vitamin C only under the supervision of a doctor.

How much is usually taken?

The recommended dietary allowance (RDA) for vitamin C in nonsmoking adults is 75 mg per day for women and 90 mg per day for men. For smokers, the RDAs are 110 mg per day for women and 125 mg per day for men. Most clinical vitamin C studies have investigated the effects of a broad range of higher vitamin C intakes (100–1,000 mg per day or more), often not looking for (or finding) the "optimal" intake within that range. In terms of **heart disease** (page 98) prevention, as little as 100–200 mg of vitamin C appears to be adequate.[21] Although some doctors recommend 500–1,000 mg per day or more, additional research is needed to determine whether these larger amounts are necessary. Some vitamin C experts propose that adequate intake be considered 200 mg per day because of evidence that the cells of the human body do not take up any more vitamin C when larger daily amounts are used.[22]

Some scientists have recommended that healthy people take multi-gram amounts of vitamin C for the prevention of illness. However, little or no research supports this point of view and it remains controversial. Supplementing more results in an excretion level virtually identical to intake, meaning that consuming more vitamin C does not increase the amount that remains in the body.[23] On the basis of extensive analysis of published vitamin C studies, researchers at the Linus Pauling Institute at Oregon State University have called for the RDA to be increased, but only to 120 mg.[24] This same report reveals that ". . . 90–100 mg vitamin C per day is required for optimum reduction of chronic disease risk in nonsmoking men and women." Thus, the multiple gram amounts of vitamin C taken by many healthy people may be superfluous.

The studies that ascertained approximately 120–200 mg daily of vitamin C is correct for prevention purposes in healthy people have typically not investigated whether people suffering from various diseases can benefit from larger amounts. In the case of the **common cold** (page 129), a review of published trials found that amounts of 2 grams per day in children appear to be more effective than 1 gram per day in adults, suggesting that large intakes of vitamin C may be more effective than smaller amounts, at least for this condition.[25]

Are there any side effects or interactions?

Some people develop **diarrhea** (page 163) after as little as a few grams of vitamin C per day, while others are not bothered by ten times this amount. Strong scientific evidence to define and defend an upper tolerable limit for vitamin C is not available. A review of the available research concluded that high intakes (2–4 grams per day) are well-tolerated by healthy people.[26] However, intake of large amounts of vitamin C can deplete the body of **copper** (page 499)[27, 28]—an essential nutrient. People should be sure to maintain adequate copper intake at higher intakes of vitamin C. Copper is found in many **multivitamin-mineral** (page 559) supplements. Vitamin C increases the absorption of **iron** (page 540) and should be avoided by people with iron overload diseases (e.g., hemochromatosis, hemosiderosis). Vitamin C helps recycle the **antioxidant** (page 467), **vitamin E** (page 609).

It is widely (and mistakenly) believed that mothers who consume large amounts of vitamin C during **pregnancy** (page 363) are at risk of giving birth to an infant with a higher-than-normal requirement for the vitamin. The concern is that the infant could suffer "rebound scurvy," a vitamin C deficiency caused by not having this increased need met. Even some medical textbooks have subscribed to this theory.[29] In fact, however, the concept of "rebound scurvy" in infants is supported by extremely weak evidence.[30] Since the publication in 1965 of the report upon which this mistaken notion is based, millions of women have consumed high amounts of vitamin C during pregnancy and not a single new case of rebound scurvy has been reported.[31]

A preliminary study found that people who took 500 mg per day of vitamin C supplements for one year had a greater increase in wall thickness of the carotid arteries (vessels in the neck that supply blood to the brain) than those who did not take vitamin C.[32] Thickness of carotid artery walls is an indicator of progression of **atherosclerosis** (page 38). Currently, no evidence supports a cause-and-effect relationship for the outcome reported in this study. The vast preponderance of research suggests either a protective or therapeutic effect of vitamin C for **heart disease** (page 98), or no effect at all.

People with the following conditions should consult their doctor before supplementing with vitamin C: glucose-6-phosphate dehydrogenase deficiency, iron overload (hemosiderosis or hemochromatosis), history of kidney stones, or kidney failure.

It has been suggested that people who form calcium oxalate **kidney stones** (page 284) should avoid vitamin C supplements, because vitamin C can be converted into oxalate and increase urinary oxalate.[33, 34] Initially, these concerns were questioned because of potential errors in the laboratory measurement of oxalate.[35, 36] However, using newer methodology that rules out this problem, recent evidence shows that as little as 1 gram of vitamin C per day can increase the urinary oxalate levels in some people, even those without a history of kidney stones.[37, 38] In one case, 8 grams per day of vitamin C led to dramatic increases in urinary oxalate excretion and kidney stone crystal formation causing bloody urine.[39] People with a history of kidney stones should consult a doctor before taking large amounts (1 gram or more per day) of supplemental vitamin C.

Despite possible therapeutic effects of vitamin C in people with **diabetes** (page 152) at lower intakes, one case of *increased* blood sugar levels was reported after taking 4.5 grams per day.[40]

VITAMIN D

What is it?

The fat-soluble vitamin D's most important role is maintaining blood levels of **calcium** (page 483), which it accomplishes by increasing absorption of calcium from food and reducing urinary calcium loss. Both effects keep calcium in the body and therefore spare the calcium that is stored in bones. When necessary, vitamin D transfers calcium from the bone into the bloodstream, which does not benefit bones. Although the overall effect of vitamin D on the bones is complicated, some vitamin D is necessary for healthy bones and teeth.

Vitamin D

Vitamin D plays a role in **immunity** (page 255) and blood cell formation and also helps cells "differentiate"—a process that may reduce the risk of **cancer** (page 87). From animal and human studies, researchers have hypothesized that vitamin D may protect people from **multiple sclerosis** (page 323),[1] autoimmune arthritis, and juvenile **diabetes** (page 152).[2]

Vitamin D is also needed for adequate blood levels of insulin.[3] Vitamin D receptors have been found in the pancreas where insulin is made, and preliminary evidence suggests that supplementation may increase insulin secretion for some people with adult-onset (type 2) **diabetes** (page 152).[4]

Where is it found?

Cod liver oil (page 514) is an excellent dietary source of vitamin D, as are vitamin D-fortified foods. Traces of vitamin D are found in egg yolks and butter. However, the majority of vitamin D in the body is created during a chemical reaction that starts with sunlight exposure to the skin. Cholecalciferol (vitamin D$_3$) is the animal form of this vitamin.

Vitamin D has been used in connection with the following conditions (refer to the individual health concern for complete information):

Rating	Health Concerns
★★★	**Crohn's disease** (page 141)
	Cystic fibrosis (page 143)
	Osteoporosis (page 333)
	Rickets/osteomalacia (page 392)
★★☆	**Burns** (page 85) (severe)
	Cancer (prostate) (page 371)
	Celiac disease (page 102) (for deficiency only)
	Depression (page 145)
	Hypertension (page 246) (for deficiency only)
	Seasonal affective disorder (page 397)
★☆☆	**Alcohol withdrawal support** (page 12)
	Amenorrhea (page 22) (calcium for preventing bone loss)
	Breast cancer (page 65) (reduces risk)
	Cardiac arrhythmia (page 93)
	Colon cancer (page 123) (reduces risk)
	Diabetes (page 152)
	Migraine headaches (page 316)
	Multiple sclerosis (page 323)
	Parkinson's disease (page 345)
	Vitiligo (page 443) (topical calcipotriol only)

Who is likely to be deficient?

In adults, vitamin D deficiency may result in a softening of the bones known as **osteomalacia** (page 392). This condition is treated with vitamin D, sometimes in combination with **calcium** (page 483) supplements. Osteomalacia should be diagnosed, and its treatment monitored, by a doctor. In people of any age, vitamin D deficiency causes abnormal bone formation. It occurs more commonly following winter, owing to restricted sunlight exposure during that season. Living in an area with a lot of atmospheric pollution, which can block the sun's ultraviolet rays, also appears to increase the risk of vitamin D deficiency.[5]

Vitamin D deficiency is more common in strict vegetarians (who avoid vitamin D-fortified dairy foods), dark-skinned people,[6] alcoholics, and people with liver or kidney disease. People with liver and kidney disease can make vitamin D but cannot activate it.

Vitamin D deficiency is more common in people suffering from intestinal **malabsorption** (page 304), which may have occurred following previous intestinal surgeries, or from **celiac disease** (page 102).[7] People with insufficient pancreatic function (e.g., those with pancreatitis or **cystic fibrosis** [page 143]) tend to be deficient in vitamin D. Vitamin D deficiency is also common in individuals with hyperthyroidism (Graves' disease), particularly women.[8]

In children, vitamin D deficiency is called **rickets** (page 392) and causes a bowing of bones not seen in adults with vitamin D deficiency. Vitamin D deficiency is common among people with hyperparathyroidism, a condition in which the parathyroid gland is overactive. In a study of 124 people with mild hyperparathyroidism, vitamin D levels were below normal in 7% of them and suboptimal in 53% of them.[9] Vitamin D deficiency is also common in men with advanced **prostate cancer** (page 371). In one study, 44% of 16 men with advanced prostate cancer had decreased blood levels of vitamin D.[10]

One in seven adults has been reported to be deficient in vitamin D.[11] In one study, 42% of hospitalized patients under age 65 were reported to be vitamin D deficient.[12] In this same study, 37% of the people were found to be deficient in vitamin D, despite the fact they were eating the currently recommended amount of this nutrient. Vitamin D deficiency is particularly common among the elderly. Age-related decline in vitamin D status may be due to reduced absorption, transport, or liver metabolism of vitamin D.[13]

Vitamin D

How much is usually taken?

People who get plenty of sun exposure do not require supplemental vitamin D, since sunlight increases vitamin D synthesis when it strikes bare skin. Although the recommended dietary allowance for vitamin D is 200 IU per day for adults, there is some evidence that elderly people need 800 to 1,000 IU per day for maximum effects on preserving bone density and preventing fractures.[14, 15, 16, 17] Sun-deprived people should take no less than 600 IU per day and ideally around 1,000 IU per day.[18]

Are there any side effects or interactions?

People with hyperparathyroidism should not take vitamin D without consulting a physician. People with sarcoidosis should not supplement with vitamin D, unless a doctor has determined that their **calcium** (page 483) levels are not elevated. Too much vitamin D taken for long periods of time may lead to headaches, **weight loss** (page 446), and **kidney stones** (page 284). Rarely, excessive vitamin D may even lead to deafness, blindness, increased thirst, increased urination, **diarrhea** (page 163), irritability, children's failure to gain weight, or death.

Most people take 400 IU per day, a safe amount for adults. Some researchers believe that amounts up to 10,000 IU per day are safe for the average healthy adult, although adverse effects may occur even at lower levels among people with hypersensitivity to vitamin D (e.g. hyperparathyroidism).[19] In fact, of all published cases of vitamin D toxicity for which a vitamin D amount is known, only one occurred at a level of intake under 40,000 IU per day.[20] Nevertheless, people wishing to take more than 1,000 IU per day for long periods of time should consult a physician. People should remember the total daily intake of vitamin D includes vitamin D from fortified milk and other fortified foods, **cod liver oil** (page 514), supplements that contain vitamin D, and sunlight. People who receive adequate sunlight exposure do not need as much vitamin D in their diet as do people who receive minimal sunlight exposure.

Vitamin D increases both **calcium** (page 483) and phosphorus absorption and has also been reported to increase absorption of aluminum. Increased blood levels of calcium (which may be a marker for vitamin D status) have been linked to **heart disease** (page 98).[21] Some,[22] but not all,[23] research suggests that vitamin D may slightly raise blood levels of **cholesterol** (page 333) in humans.

VITAMIN E

What is it?

Vitamin E is an **antioxidant** (page 467) that protects cell membranes and other fat-soluble parts of the body, such as low-density lipoprotein (LDL; "bad" cholesterol) **cholesterol** (page 333), from damage.

Only when LDL is damaged does cholesterol appear to lead to **heart disease** (page 98), and vitamin E is an important antioxidant protector of LDL.[1] Several studies,[2, 3] including two double-blind trials,[4, 5] have reported that 400 to 800 IU of natural vitamin E per day reduces the risk of heart attacks. Other recent double-blind trials have found either limited benefit[6] or no benefit at all from supplementation with synthetic vitamin E.[7] One of the negative trials used 400 IU of natural vitamin E[8]—a similar amount and form to previous successful trials. In attempting to make sense of these apparently inconsistent findings, the following is clear: less than 400 IU of synthetic vitamin E, even when taken for years, does not protect against heart disease. Whether 400 to 800 IU of natural vitamin E is, or is not, protective remains unclear.

Vitamin E also plays some role in the body's ability to process glucose. Some, but not all, trials suggest that vitamin E supplementation may eventually prove to be helpful in the prevention and treatment of **diabetes** (page 152).

In the last ten years, the functions of vitamin E in the cell have been further clarified. In addition to its antioxidant functions, vitamin E is now known to act through other mechanisms, including direct effects on inflammation, blood cell regulation, connective tissue growth, and genetic control of cell division.[9]

Where is it found?

Wheat germ oil, nuts and seeds, whole grains, egg yolks, and leafy green vegetables all contain vitamin E. Certain vegetable oils should contain significant amounts of vitamin E. However, many of the vegetable oils sold in supermarkets have had the vitamin E removed in processing. The high amounts found in supplements, often 100 to 800 IU per day, are not obtainable from eating food.

Vitamin E

Vitamin E has been used in connection with the following conditions (refer to the individual health concern for complete information):

Rating	Health Concerns
★★★	**Anemia** (page 25) (if deficient)
	Burns (page 85) (in combination with **vitamin C** [page 604] for prevention of sunburn only)
	Epilepsy (page 183) (for children)
	Immune function (page 255) (for elderly people)
	Intermittent claudication (page 276)
	Rheumatoid arthritis (page 387)
	Tardive dyskinesia (page 425)
★★☆	**Alzheimer's disease** (page 19)
	Anemia (page 25) (injections for thalassemia, orally for glucose-6-phosphate dehydrogenase deficiency [G6PD] anemia and anemia caused by kidney dialysis)
	Angina (page 27)
	Atherosclerosis (page 38)
	Athletic performance (page 43) (for exercise recovery and high-altitude exercise performance only)
	Bronchitis (page 80)
	Cold sores (page 119)
	Dermatitis herpetiformis (page 151)
	Diabetes (page 152) (for glucose tolerance and prevention of diabetic retinopathy)
	Down's syndrome (page 169)
	Dysmenorrhea (page 171)
	Endometriosis (page 182) (in combination with **vitamin C** [page 604])
	Hay fever (page 211)
	Heart attack (page 212) (at 400 to 800 IU of natural vitamin E)
	High blood pressure (page 246)
	Leukoplakia (page 289)
	Lung cancer (page 298) (reduces risk)
	Osteoarthritis (page 328)
	Pancreatic insufficiency (page 341)
	Parkinson's disease (page 345) (in combination with **vitamin C** [page 604])
	Preeclampsia (page 361) (in combination with **vitamin C** [page 604; for high risk only)
	Premenstrual syndrome (page 368)
	Prostate cancer (page 371) (reduces risk)
	Radiation therapy (side-effect prevention in people with cancer of the oral cavity)
	Retinopathy (page 385) (diabetic retinopathy and retrolental fibroplasia)
	Skin ulcers (page 409) (oral vitamin E)
	Wound healing (page 319)
	Yellow nail syndrome (page 456)
★☆☆	**Abnormal pap smear** (page 3)
	Age-related cognitive decline (page 8) (ARCD)
	Alcohol withdrawal support (page 12)
	Burns (minor) (page 85) (topical)
	Cataracts (page 101)
	Childhood diseases (page 105)
	Colon cancer (page 123) (reduces risk)
	Cystic fibrosis (page 143)
	Dupuytren's contracture (page 171)
	Epilepsy (page 183) (for adults)
	Fibrocystic breast disease (page 189)
	Fibromyalgia (page 191)
	Goiter (page 206)
	Halitosis (page 209) (if gum disease and deficient)
	Hepatitis (page 220)
	High cholesterol (page 223)
	HIV support (page 239)
	Hypoglycemia (page 251)
	Infertility (female) (page 187)
	Infertility (male) (page 305)
	Insulin resistance syndrome (page 273) (Syndrome X)
	Kidney stones (page 284) (prevention)
	Liver cirrhosis (page 290)
	Lupus (page 421)
	Macular degeneration (page 303)
	Menopause (page 311)
	Menorrhagia (heavy menstruation) (page 314)
	Osgood-Schlatter disease (page 327)
	Photosensitivity (page 356)
	Pre- and post-surgery health (page 357)
	Restless legs syndrome (page 384)
	Retinopathy (page 385) (abetalipoproteinemia)
	Retinopathy (page 385) (in combination with **selenium** [page 584], **vitamin A** [page 595], and **vitamin C** [page 604])
	Shingles (page 401)
	Sickle cell anemia (page 403)
	Skin ulcers (page 409) (topical vitamin E)
	Sprains and strains (page 412) (for exercise-related muscle strain)
	Stroke (page 419)
	Vaginitis (page 438)

Who is likely to be deficient?

Severe vitamin E deficiencies are rare. People with a genetic defect in a vitamin E transfer protein called thrombotic thrombocytopenic purpura (TTP) have severe vitamin E deficiency, characterized by low blood and tissue levels of vitamin E and progressive nerve abnormalities.[10, 11]

Low vitamin E status has been associated with an

increased risk of **rheumatoid arthritis** (page 387)[12] and major **depression** (page 145).[13] Women with **preeclampsia** (page 361) have been found to have lower blood levels of vitamin E than women without the condition.[14]

Very old people with type 2 **diabetes** (page 152) have shown a significant age-related decline in blood levels of vitamin E, irrespective of their dietary intake.[15]

Which form is best?

The names of all types of vitamin E begin with either "d" or "dl," which refer to differences in chemical structure. The "d" form is natural (also known as RRR-alpha tocopherol) and "dl" is synthetic (more correctly known as all-rac-alpha tocopherol). The natural form is more active and better absorbed. Little is known about how the "unnatural" "l" portion of the synthetic "dl" form affects the body, though no clear toxicity has been discovered.

In theory, when a vitamin E supplement is labeled "400 IU" it should have the same level of activity regardless of its source. This is purportedly achieved by using more synthetic vitamin E to reach the same potency as a lesser amount of natural vitamin E. For example, 100 IU of vitamin E requires about 67 mg of the natural form but closer to 100 mg of the synthetic. However, a recent review of the scientific evidence suggests that natural vitamin E probably has greater activity in the body than indicated on the label.[16] Natural vitamin E may be as much as twice as bioavailable as synthetic vitamin E, not 1.36 times as is generally accepted.[17] Many doctors advise people to use only the natural, the "d" form, of vitamin E.

After the "d" or "dl" designation, often the Greek letter "alpha" appears, which also describes the structure. Synthetic "dl" vitamin E is found only in the alpha form—as in "dl-alpha tocopherol." Natural vitamin E may be found either as alpha—as in "d-alpha tocopherol"—or in combination with beta, gamma, and delta, labeled "mixed"—as in mixed natural tocopherols.

Little is known about the importance of the beta and delta forms of vitamin E, but a debate has arisen concerning gamma tocopherol. In a test tube study, gamma tocopherol was found to be more effective than alpha tocopherol in protecting against certain specific types of oxidative damage.[18] In addition, some research has shown that supplementation with large amounts of alpha tocopherol (such as 1,200 IU per day) increases the breakdown, and decreases blood levels, of gamma tocopherol.[19]

Human trials with vitamin E have almost always been done with the alpha (not gamma) form. Historically the synthetic "dl" form was used in most trials, but some trials are now using the natural form. The issue of alpha vs. gamma form requires more research before it can be fully understood.

Almost all vitamin E research shows that, when positive results are obtained, hundreds of units per day are required—an amount easily obtained with supplements but impossible with food. Therefore, switching to food sources, as suggested by some researchers, is impractical. On the other hand, the vitamin E occurring naturally in food contains gamma tocopherol and other tocopherols. Thus, it possibly may turn out to be more effective than the vitamin E taken in supplement form. Additional research is needed in this area.

Vitamin E forms are listed as either plain "tocopherol" or tocopheryl followed by the name of what is attached to it, as in "tocopheryl acetate." The two forms are not greatly different. However, plain tocopherol may be absorbed a little better, while tocopheryl attached forms have a slightly better shelf life. Both forms are active when taken by mouth. However, the skin utilizes the tocopheryl forms very slowly,[20, 21] so those planning to apply vitamin E to the skin should buy plain tocopherol. In health food stores, the most common forms of vitamin E are d-alpha tocopherol and d-alpha tocopheryl acetate or succinate. Both of these d (natural) alpha forms are frequently recommended by doctors. Although the succinate form is slightly weaker than the acetate form, more milligrams of the succinate form are added to supplements to compensate for this small difference in potency. Therefore, 400 IU of either form should have equivalent potency.

How much is usually taken?

The recommended dietary allowance for vitamin E is low, just 15 mg or approximately 22 International Units (IU) per day. The most commonly recommended amount of supplemental vitamin E for adults is 400 to 800 IU per day. However, some leading researchers suggest taking only 100 to 200 IU per day, since trials that have explored the long-term effects of different supplemental levels suggest no further benefit beyond that amount. In addition, research reporting positive effects with 400 to 800 IU per day has not investigated the ef-

Vitamin E

fects of lower intakes.[22] For **tardive dyskinesia** (page 425), the best results have been achieved from 1,600 IU per day,[23] a large amount that should be supervised by a healthcare practitioner.

Are there any side effects or interactions?

Vitamin E toxicity is very rare and supplements are widely considered to be safe. The National Academy of Sciences has established the daily tolerable upper intake level for adults to be 1,000 mg of vitamin E, which is equivalent to 1,500 IU of natural vitamin E or 1,100 IU of synthetic vitamin E.[24]

In a double-blind study of healthy elderly people, supplementation with 200 IU of vitamin E per day for 15 months had no effect in the incidence of respiratory infections, but increased the severity of those infections that did occur.[25] For elderly individuals, the risks and benefits of taking this vitamin should be assessed with the help of a doctor or nutritionist.

In contrast to trials suggesting vitamin E improves glucose tolerance in people with **diabetes** (page 152), one trial reported that 600 IU per day of vitamin E led to impairment in glucose tolerance in obese people with diabetes.[26] The reason for the discrepancy between reports is not known.

In a double-blind study of people with established **heart disease** (page 98) or **diabetes** (page 152), participants who took 400 IU of vitamin E per day for an average of 4.5 years developed **heart failure** (page 134) significantly more often than did those taking a placebo.[27] Hospitalizations for heart failure occurred in 5.8% of those in the vitamin E group, compared with 4.2% of those in the placebo group, a 38.1% increase. Considering that some other studies have shown a beneficial effect of vitamin E against heart disease, the results of this study are difficult to interpret. Nevertheless, individuals with heart disease or diabetes should consult their doctor before taking vitamin E.

A review of 19 clinical trials of vitamin E supplementation concluded that long-term use of large amounts of vitamin E (400 IU per day or more) was associated with a small (4%) but statistically significant increase in risk of death.[28] Long-term use of less than 400 IU per day was associated with a small and statistically nonsignificant reduction in death rates. This research has been criticized because many of the studies on which it was based used a combination of nutritional supplements, not just vitamin E. For example, the adverse ef-

fects reported in some of the studies may have been due to the use of large amounts of zinc or synthetic beta-carotene, and may have had nothing to do with vitamin E. It is also possible that long-term use of large amounts of pure alpha-tocopherol may lead to a deficiency of gamma-tocopherol, with potential negative consequences. For that reason, some doctors recommend that people who need to take large amounts of vitamin E take at least part of it in the form of mixed tocopherols.

Patients on kidney dialysis who are given injections of **iron** (page 540) frequently experience "oxidative stress." This is because iron is a pro-oxidant, meaning that it interacts with oxygen molecules in ways that may damage tissues. These adverse effects of iron therapy may be counteracted by supplementation with vitamin E.[29]

A diet high in unsaturated fat increases vitamin E requirements. Vitamin E and **selenium** (page 584) work together to protect fat-soluble parts of the body.

VITAMIN K

What is it?

Vitamin K is needed for proper bone formation and blood clotting. In both cases, vitamin K does this by helping the body transport **calcium** (page 483). Vitamin K is used by doctors when treating an overdose of the drug warfarin. Also, doctors prescribe vitamin K to prevent excessive bleeding in people taking warfarin but requiring surgery.

There is preliminary evidence that vitamin K_2 (menadione), not vitamin K_1 (phylloquinone; phytonadione), may improve a group of blood disorders known as myelodysplastic syndromes (MDS).[1] These syndromes carry a significantly increased risk of progression to acute myeloid leukemia. Large-scale trials of vitamin K_2 for MDS are needed to confirm these promising early results.

Where is it found?

Leafy green vegetables, such as spinach, kale, collards, and broccoli, are the best sources of vitamin K. The greener the plant, the higher the vitamin K content.[2] Other significant dietary sources of vitamin K include soybean oil, olive oil, cottonseed oil, and canola oil.[3]

Vitamin K has been used in connection with the following conditions (refer to the individual health concern for complete information):

Rating	Health Concerns
★★☆	**Celiac disease** (page 102) (for deficiency only) **Crohn's disease** (page 141) **Cystic fibrosis** (page 143) **Osteoporosis** (page 333)
★☆☆	Acute myeloid leukemia (vitamin K₂ only) **Morning sickness** (page 320) Myelodysplastic syndromes (vitamin K₂ only) **Phenylketonuria** (page 354) (if deficient)

Who is likely to be deficient?

A vitamin K deficiency, which causes uncontrolled bleeding, is rare, except in people with certain **malabsorption diseases** (page 304). However, there are reports of severe vitamin K deficiency developing in hospitalized patients who had poor food intake and were receiving antibiotics.[4] All newborn infants receive vitamin K to prevent deficiencies that sometimes develop in breast-fed infants.

How much is usually taken?

The recommended dietary allowance for vitamin K is about 1 mcg per 2.2 pounds of body weight per day or about 65 to 80 mcg per day for most adults.[5] This level of intake may be achieved by consuming adequate amounts of leafy green vegetables. However, studies have shown that many men and women aged 18 to 44 years ingest less than the recommended amount of vitamin K.[6, 7]

Are there any side effects or interactions?

Allergic reactions to vitamin K injections have been reported on rare occasions.[8]

Vitamin K facilitates the effects of **calcium** (page 483) in building bone and proper blood clotting.

WHEY PROTEIN

What is it?

Whey protein is a mixture of some of the proteins naturally found in milk. The major proteins found in whey protein include beta-lactoglobulin and alpha-lactalbumin. Whey protein has one of the highest protein digestibility-corrected amino acid scores (PDCAAS; a measure of protein bioavailability) and is more rapidly digested than other proteins, such as casein (another milk protein).[1]

Alpha-lactalbumin is a whey protein high in the **amino acid tryptophan** (page 465), which the body uses to make the neurotransmitter serotonin. A double-blind study found that supplementing the diet with alpha-lactalbumin helped improve scores on a memory test in people who were vulnerable to experiencing problems with stress.[2] The researchers speculated that the alpha-lactalbumin raised brain serotonin levels in these subjects, which may have improved their tolerance to stress.

Where is it found?

During the process of making milk into cheese, whey protein is separated from the milk. This whey protein is then incorporated into ice cream, bread, canned soup, infant formulas, and other food products. Supplements containing whey protein are also available.

Whey protein has been used in connection with the following conditions (refer to the individual health concern for complete information):

Rating	Health Concerns
★★☆	**Athletic performance** (page 43)
★☆☆	**Cancer** (page 87) **Hepatitis** (page 220) **HIV infection** (page 239) **Immune function** (page 255) **Osteoporosis** (page 333) **Stress** (page 415) **Weight loss and obesity** (page 446)

Who is likely to be deficient?

People who do not include dairy foods in their diets do not consume whey protein. However, the amino acids in whey protein are available from other sources, and a deficiency of these amino acids is unlikely.

People who do not include dairy foods in their diets do not consume whey protein. However, the **amino acids** (page 465) in whey protein are available from other sources, and a deficiency of these amino acids is unlikely. In fact, most Americans consume too much, rather than too little, protein.

Whey Protein

Whey Protein

How much is usually taken?
Some benefits of whey protein have been demonstrated with as little as 20 grams per day. For **athletes in training** (page 43) a commonly used amount is 25 grams of whey protein per day, and shouldn't exceed 1.2 grams per 2.2 pounds body weight. Most clinical research has used similar amounts of whey protein.

Are there any side effects or interactions?
People who are **allergic to dairy products** (page 14) could react to whey protein and should, therefore, avoid it.[3] As with protein in general, long-term, excessive intake may be associated with deteriorating kidney function and possibly **osteoporosis** (page 333). However, neither kidney nor bone problems have been directly associated with consumption of whey protein, and the other dietary sources of protein typically contribute more protein to the diet than does whey protein. The possibility that certain proteins in milk may contribute to the development of diabetes in children is controversial. But since whey proteins include some of the same milk proteins, people who are avoiding milk because of concerns about the risk of diabetes should not consume whey protein either.

XYLITOL

What is it?
Xylitol is the alcohol form of xylose, which is used as a sweetener in chewing gums and other dietetic products. Xylitol has less effect on blood sugar or insulin levels compared with sucrose,[1] so it may be a useful sugar substitute for **diabetics** (page 152).[2] In addition, xylitol inhibits the growth of several types of bacteria, including those that cause **tooth decay** (page 431) and **ear infections** (page 383).[3, 4, 5, 6]

Where is it found?
Xylitol occurs naturally in straw, corncobs, fruit, vegetables, cereals, mushrooms, and some seaweeds. For use in food manufacturing, xylitol is extracted from birch wood chips. Xylitol may be found in many foods labeled as "sugar-free," including hard candies, cookies, chewing gums, soft drinks, and throat lozenges.

Xylitol has been used in connection with the following conditions (refer to the individual health concern for complete information):

Rating	Health Concerns
★★★	**Ear infections** (page 383) **Tooth decay** (page 431)

Who is likely to be deficient?
Xylitol is not an essential nutrient; therefore, no deficiencies are possible.

How much is usually taken?
For prevention of dental caries (cavities), 7 to 20 grams per day are given, divided into several doses in candies or chewing gum. For prevention of ear infections, 1.7 to 2.0 grams are given fives times per day in gum, lozenges, or syrup.

Are there any side effects or interactions?
Xylitol is recognized as a safe food additive by the U.S. government.[7] Large amounts (30 to 40 grams) taken all at once can produce diarrhea and intestinal gas.

ZINC

What is it?
Zinc is an essential mineral that is a component of more than 300 **enzymes** (page 506) needed to **repair wounds** (page 319), maintain fertility in adults and growth in children, synthesize protein, help cells reproduce, preserve vision, boost **immunity** (page 255), and protect against **free radicals** (page 467), among other functions.

In double-blind trials, zinc lozenges have reduced the duration of **colds** (page 129) in adults,[1, 2, 3] but have been ineffective in children.[4] The ability of zinc to shorten colds may be due to a direct, localized antiviral action in the throat. For the alleviation of cold symptoms, lozenges providing 13–25 mg of zinc, in the form of zinc gluconate, zinc gluconate-glycine, or zinc acetate, are used, typically every two hours while awake, but only for several days. The best effect is obtained when lozenges are used at the first sign of a cold.

Lozenges containing zinc gluconate, zinc gluconate-glycine, or zinc acetate have been effective, whereas most other forms of zinc and lozenges flavored with citric acid,[5] tartaric acid, sorbitol, or mannitol, have been ineffective.[6] Trials using forms other than zinc gluconate, zinc gluconate-glycine, or zinc acetate have failed, as have trials that use insufficient amounts of zinc.[7] Therefore, until more is known, people should only use zinc gluconate, zinc gluconate-glycine, or zinc acetate.

Zinc reduces the body's ability to utilize the essential mineral **copper** (page 499). (For healthy people, this interference is circumvented by supplementing with copper, along with zinc.) The ability to interfere with copper makes zinc an important therapeutic tool for people with **Wilson's disease** (page 453)—a genetic condition that causes copper overload.

Zinc supplementation in children in developing countries is associated with improvements in stunted growth, increased weight gain in underweight children, and substantial reductions in the rates of **diarrhea** (page 163) and pneumonia, the two leading causes of death in these settings.[8, 9, 10] Whether such supplementation would help people in better nourished populations remains unclear.

A small, preliminary trial has found zinc sulfate to be effective for contact dermatitis (a skin rash caused by contact with an **allergen** (page 14) or irritant).[11] Participants with active skin rashes took approximately 23 mg of zinc (in the form of zinc sulfate) three times daily, for one month. 73% of those taking the zinc sulfate had complete resolution of their skin rashes, while the remaining participants had a 50–75% improvement. Further trials are needed to confirm these preliminary findings, however.

Where is it found?
Good sources of zinc include oysters, meat, eggs, seafood, black-eyed peas, tofu, and wheat germ.

Zinc has been used in connection with the following conditions (refer to the individual health concern for complete information):

Rating	Health Concerns
★★★	**Acne** (page 4)
	Acrodermatitis enteropathica (page 7)
	Childhood intelligence (for deficiency)
	Common cold/sore throat (page 129) (as lozenges)
	Down's syndrome (page 169)
	Infertility (male) (page 305) (for deficiency)
	Night blindness (page 326) (for deficiency)
	Wilson's disease (page 453)
	Wound healing (page 319) (oral and topical)
★★☆	**Anemia** (page 25) (for thalassemia if deficient)
	Anorexia nervosa (page 174)
	Attention deficit–hyperactivity disorder (page 55)
	Birth defects prevention (page 63)
	Canker sores (page 90) (for deficiency only)
	Celiac disease (page 102) (for deficiency)
	Cold sores (page 119) (topical)
	Common cold (page 129) (as nasal spray)
	Crohn's disease (page 141)
	Diabetes (page 152) (preferably for those with a documented deficiency)
	Genital herpes (page 200)
	Gingivitis (page 203) (zinc plus **bloodroot** [page 641] toothpaste)
	Halitosis (page 209) (zinc chloride rinse or toothpaste)
	Hepatitis C (page 220) (zinc-L-carnosine)
	HIV support (page 239)
	Immune function (page 255) (for elderly people)
	Infection (page 265)
	Liver cirrhosis (page 290) (for deficiency)
	Macular degeneration (page 303)
	Peptic ulcer (page 349)
	Pregnancy support (page 363)
	Rheumatoid arthritis (page 387)
	Sickle cell anemia (page 403)
	Skin ulcers (page 409) (oral and topical zinc)
	Sprains and strains (page 412) (if deficient)
	Tinnitus (page 430) (for deficiency only)
	Warts (page 445)
★☆☆	**Amenorrhea** (page 22)
	Athletic performance (page 43)
	Benign prostatic hyperplasia (page 58) (BPH)
	Contact dermatitis
	Cystic fibrosis (page 143)
	Dermatitis herpetiformis (page 151) (for deficiency)
	Diarrhea (page 163)
	Ear infections (recurrent) (page 383)
	Gastritis (page 195)
	Gestational hypertension (page 202)
	Goiter (page 206)
	Hypoglycemia (page 251)
	Hypothyroidism (page 252)
	Immune function (page 255) (for non-elderly people)
	Insulin resistance syndrome (page 273) (Syndrome X)
	Osgood-Schlatter Disease (page 327)
	Osteoarthritis (page 328) (in combination with **boswellia** [page 644], **ashwagandha** [page 629], and **turmeric** [page 753])
	Osteoporosis (page 333)
	Pre- and post-surgery health (page 357)
	Preeclampsia (page 361)
	Prostatitis (page 377) (CBP, NBP)

Zinc

Who is likely to be deficient?

Zinc deficiencies are quite common in people living in poor countries. Phytate, a substance found in unleavened bread (pita, matzos, and some crackers) significantly reduces absorption of zinc, increasing the chance of zinc deficiency. However, phytate-induced deficiency of zinc appears to be a significant problem only for people already consuming marginally low amounts of zinc.

Even in developed countries, low-income **pregnant** (page 363) women and pregnant teenagers are at risk for marginal zinc deficiencies. Supplementing with 25–30 mg per day improves pregnancy outcome in these groups.[12, 13]

People with **liver cirrhosis** (page 290) appear to be commonly deficient in zinc.[14] This deficiency may be due to cirrhosis-related zinc **malabsorption** (page 304).[15]

People with Down's syndrome are also commonly deficient in zinc.[16] Giving zinc supplements to children with Down's syndrome has been reported to improve impaired immunity[17] and thyroid function,[18] though optimal intake of zinc for people with Down's syndrome remains unclear.

Children with alopecia areata (patchy areas of hair loss) have been reported to be deficient in zinc.[19, 20]

The average diet frequently provides less than the Recommended Dietary Allowance for zinc, particularly in vegetarians. To what extent (if any) these small deficits in zinc intake create clinical problems remains unclear. Nonetheless, a low-potency supplement (15 mg per day) can fill in dietary gaps. Zinc deficiencies are more common in **alcoholics** (page 12) and people with **sickle cell anemia** (page 403), **malabsorption** (page 304) problems, and chronic kidney disease.[21]

How much is usually taken?

Moderate intake of zinc, approximately 15 mg daily, is adequate to prevent deficiencies. Higher levels (up to 50 mg taken three times per day) are reserved for people with certain health conditions, under the supervision of a doctor. For the alleviation of **cold** (page 129) symptoms, lozenges providing 13–25 mg of zinc in the form zinc gluconate, zinc gluconate-glycine, or zinc acetate are generally used frequently but only for several days.

Are there any side effects or interactions?

Zinc intake in excess of 300 mg per day has been reported to impair **immune function** (page 255).[22] Some people report that zinc lozenges lead to stomach ache, nausea, mouth irritation, and a bad taste. One source reports that gastrointestinal upset, metallic taste in the mouth, blood in the urine, and lethargy can occur from chronic oral zinc supplementation over 150 mg per day,[23] but those claims are unsubstantiated. In topical form, zinc has no known side effects when used as recommended. However, using zinc nasal spray has been reported to cause severe or complete loss of smell function in at least ten people. In some of those cases, the loss of smell was long-lasting or permanent.[24]

Preliminary research had suggested that people with **Alzheimer's disease** (page 19) should avoid zinc supplements.[25] More recently, preliminary evidence in four patients actually showed improved mental function with zinc supplementation.[26] In a convincing review of zinc/Alzheimer's disease research, perhaps the most respected zinc researcher in the world concluded that zinc does not cause or exacerbate Alzheimer's disease symptoms.[27]

Zinc inhibits **copper** (page 499) absorption. Copper deficiency can result in anemia, lower levels of HDL ("good") **cholesterol** (page 223), or **cardiac arrhythmias** (page 93).[28, 29, 30] Copper intake should be increased if zinc supplementation continues for more than a few days (except for people with **Wilson's disease** [page 453]).[31] Some sources recommend a 10 to 1 ratio of zinc to copper. Evidence suggests that no more that 2 mg of copper per day is needed to prevent zinc-induced copper deficiency. Many zinc supplements include copper in the formulation to prevent zinc-induced copper deficiency. Zinc-induced copper deficiency has been reported to cause reversible anemia and suppression of bone marrow.[32]

Marginal zinc deficiency may be a contributing factor in some cases of anemia. In a study of women with normocytic anemia (i.e., their red blood cells were of normal size) and low total iron-binding capacity (a blood test often used to assess the cause of anemia), combined **iron** (page 540) and zinc supplementation significantly improved the anemia, whereas iron or zinc supplemented alone had only slight effects.[33] Supplementation with zinc, or zinc and iron together, has been found to improve **vitamin A** (page 595) status among children at high risk for deficiency of the three nutrients.[34]

Zinc competes for absorption with **copper** (page 499), **iron** (page 540),[35, 36] **calcium** (page 483),[37] and **magnesium** (page 551).[38] A **multimineral** (page 559) supplement will help prevent mineral imbalances that can result from taking high amounts of zinc for extended periods of time.

N-acetyl cysteine (page 562) (NAC) may increase urinary excretion of zinc.[39] Long-term users of NAC may consider adding supplements of zinc and copper.

Zinc

PART THREE
Herbs

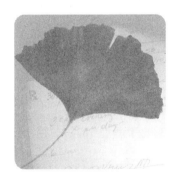

UNDERSTANDING HERBAL TERMINOLOGY

There are many words used to describe herbs and their actions on the body. The following is a guide to understanding these unique terms.

Adaptogen
A substance that invigorates or strengthens the system (also called a tonic).

Alterative
A substance that produces a gradual, beneficial change in the body.

Alkaloid
Heterogeneous group of alkaline, organic, compounds containing nitrogen and usually oxygen; generally colorless and bitter-tasting; especially found in seed plants.

Analgesic
A substance that reduces or relieves pain.

Anodyne
A pain relieving agent, less potent than an anesthetic or narcotic.

Antihelmintic, anthelmintic
A substance that expels or destroys intestinal worms (also called a vermifuge).

Antihydrotic
A substance that reduces or suppresses perspiration.

Antipyretic
An agent that reduces or prevents fever (also called a febrifuge).

Antispasmodic
An agent that relieves spasms or cramps.

Aperient
A mild and gentle-acting laxative.

Aperitif
An agent that stimulates the appetite.

Aphrodisiac
A substance that increases sexual desire or potency.

Aromatic
A substance with a strong, volatile, fragrant aroma; often with stimulant properties.

Astringent
An agent that contracts or shrinks tissues; it is used to decrease secretions or control bleeding.

Bitter tonic
A substance with an acrid, astringent or disagreeable taste that stimulates flow of saliva and gastric juices.

Bolus
A suppository poultice used for vaginal or rectal application; made by mixing powdered herb material in melted cocoa butter or similar base and hand-forming suppositories as the matrix cools.

Calmative
An agent with mild sedative or hypnotic properties.

Carminative
a substance that stops the formation of intestinal gas and helps expel gas that has already formed.

Catarrh
Inflammation of a mucous membrane, especially of the respiratory tract.

Cathartic
A powerful agent used to relieve severe constipation (also called a purgative).

Cholegogue
An agent that stimulates secretion and release of bile.

Choleretic

An agent that stimulates the formation of bile.

Concentration

The amount of material in a solution in relationship to the amount of solvent; expressed as the ratio. For example:

- 1:5 concentration means that 5 parts of an extract contains the equivalent of one part of the raw herb;
- 4:1 concentration means that 1 part of an extract contains the equivalent of 4 parts of the raw herb.

Counterirritant

An agent that causes a distracting irritation intended to relieve another irritation.

Decoction

Extract of a crude drug made by boiling or simmering (cooking) herbs in water; stronger than a tea or infusion.

Demulcent

An oily or mucilaginous substance that soothes irritated tissue, especially mucous membranes.

Diaphoretic

An agent, taken internally to promote sweating (also called sudorific).

Diuretic

An agent that promotes urine production and flow.

Emetic

A substance that induces vomiting.

Emmenogogue

An agent, taken internally, to promote menstrual flow.

Emollient

An externally applied agent that softens or soothes skin.

Essential oil

Any of a class of volatile oils that impart the characteristic odors of plants; used especially in perfumes, food flavorings and aromatherapy; also called volatile oil.

Expectorant

An agent that increases bronchial secretions and facilitates their expulsion through coughing, spitting or sneezing.

Extract

A concentrate, made by steeping raw plant material(s) in solvent (alcohol and/or water), after which the solvent is allowed to evaporate.

Febrifuge

An agent that reduces fever (also called an antipyretic).

Flatulence

Gas in the stomach or intestines.

Fluid extract

A liquid extract of raw plant material(s), usually of a concentration ratio of 1 part raw herb to 1 part solvent (1:1).

Fomentation

Application of a warm and moist cloth, soaked in an infusion or decoction, as treatment.

Galactogogue

An agent that increases secretion of milk (synonym for lactagogue).

Galenical

Herb and other vegetable drugs as distinguished from mineral or chemical remedies; crude drugs and the tinctures, decoctions, and other preparations made from them, as distinguished from the alkaloids and other active principles.

Glycoside

Esters containing a sugar component (glycol) and a nonsugar (aglycone) component attached via oxygen or nitrogen bond; hydrolysis of a glycoside yields one or more sugars.

Hemostatic

An agent used to stop internal bleeding.

Herb

Plant or part of a plant used for medicinal, taste or aromatic purposes.

Humectant

A substance used to obtain a moistening effect.

Hygroscopic

A substance that readily attracts and retains water.

Infusion

Tea made by steeping herb(s) in hot water.

Lactagogue

An agent that increases secretion of milk (synonym for galactogogue).

Laxative

A substance that promotes bowel movements.

Maceration

A process of softening tissues by soaking in liquid.

Mucilage

A gelatinous substance, containing proteins and polysaccharides, that soothes inflammation.

Mucilaginous

An agent characterized by a gummy or gelatinous consistency.

Nervine

An agent that calms nervousness, tension, or excitement.

Oleoresin

A homogenous mixture of resin(s) and volatile oil(s).

Pharmacognosy

The study of the biochemistry and pharmacology of plant drugs, herbs, and spices.

Phlogistic

Referring to inflammation or fever.

Poultice

A soft, moist mass applied to the skin to provide heat and moisture.

Purgative

A powerful agent used to relieve severe constipation (also called a cathartic).

Raw herb

The form of the plant, or plant parts, unchanged by processing other than separation of parts, drying or grinding.

Resin

Any of several solid or semi-solid, flammable, natural organic substances soluble in organic solvents and not water; commonly formed in plant secretions; complex chemical mixtures of acrid resins, resin alcohols, resinol, tannols, esters, and resenes.

Rubefacient

An agent, applied to the skin, causing a local irritation and redness; for relief of internal pain.

Salve

An herbal preparation mixed in oil and thickened with bees wax applied to the skin.

Saponin

Any of several surfactant glycosides that produce a soapy lather; found in plants.

Sedative

A substance that reduces nervous tension; usually stronger than a calmative.

Sialogogue

An agent that stimulates secretion of saliva.

Solid extract

An extract of plant material(s) made by removing the solvent from a fluid extract.

Soporific

A substance that induces sleep.

Stimulant

An agent that excites or quickens a process or activity of the body.

Stomachic

An agent that gives strength and tone to the stomach or stimulates the appetite by promoting digestive secretions.

Styptic

A substance that stops external bleeding (usually an astringent).

Sudorific

An agent, taken internally, to promote sweating (also called diaphoretic).

Tannin

A complex mixture of polyphenols; gives a color reaction to iron-containing substances.

Terpene

Any of several isomeric hydrocarbons; most volatile oils consist primarily of terpenes.

Tincture

A solution prepared by steeping or soaking (maceration) plant materials in alcohol and water.

Tonic

A substance that invigorates or strengthens the system (also called adaptogen); tonics often act as stimulants or aleratives.

Vermifuge

A substance that expels or destroys intestinal worms (also called antihelmintic or anthelmintic).

Volatile oil

An odorous plant oil that evaporates readily; also called essential oil.

Vulnerary

A substance used in the treatment or healing of wounds.

Herbs are listed by common names; if you don't find what you're looking for, look in the index.

AHCC

Common name: Active Hexose Correlated Compound
Botanical name: *Basidiomycetes*

Parts used and where grown

AHCC™ is a newly developed "functional food" made through the hybridization of several kinds of mushrooms belonging to the Basidiomycetes family, including shiitake (Lentinula edodes), cultured in a liquid medium. The mushroom's sources and details of methods of preparation have not been fully disclosed.

AHCC has been used in connection with the following conditions (refer to the individual health concern for complete information):

Rating	Health Concerns
★★☆	Cancer

Historical or traditional use (may or may not be supported by scientific studies)

AHCC was not used in traditional medicine. The mushrooms of the type from which AHCC is made were historically used as tonics and for chronic infections, anemia, and a variety of other conditions.[1]

Active constituents

AHCC consists of polysaccharides, particularly low molecular weight alpha-1,3-glucans, amino acids, and minerals.

How much is usually taken?

Studies have typically administered 3 grams per day orally.

Are there any side effects or interactions?

In the studies in which AHCC was given to people with cancer, no side effects or drug interactions were observed. However, thorough studies establishing its safety have not been conducted. There are no reports that AHCC is contraindicated in any condition. Use in pregnancy and lactation have not been studied.

ALDER BUCKTHORN

Common name: Frangula
Botanical name: *Rhamnus frangula*

Parts used and where grown

Alder buckthorn is a tall shrub native to northern Europe. The bark of alder buckthorn is removed, cut into small pieces, and dried for one year before being used medicinally. Fresh bark has an emetic or vomit-inducing property and is therefore not used.

Alder Buckthorn has been used in connection with the following conditions (refer to the individual health concern for complete information):

Rating	Health Concerns
★★☆	Constipation (page 137)

Historical or traditional use (may or may not be supported by scientific studies)

Alder buckthorn has been used as a cathartic laxative in northern and central Europe, including England, for centuries.[1] Despite its decline in importance when the similar shrub *Rhamnus purshiana* or **Cascara sagrada** (page 652) was discovered in America,[2] alder buckthorn is still used, particularly in Europe.

Active constituents

Alder buckthorn is high in anthraquinone glycosides. Resins, tannins, and lipids make up the bulk of the bark's other ingredients. Anthraquinone glycosides have a cathartic action, inducing the large intestine to increase its muscular contraction (peristalsis) and increasing water movement from the cells of the colon into the feces, resulting in strong, soft bowel movements.[3] It takes six to ten hours for alder buckthorn to act after taking it by mouth.

How much is usually taken?

Only the dried form of alder buckthorn should be used. Capsules providing 20 to 30 mg of anthraquinone glycosides (calculated as glucofrangulin A) per day can be used; however, the smallest amount necessary to maintain regular bowel movements should be used.[4] As a tincture, 5 ml once at bedtime is generally taken. Alder buckthorn is usually taken at bedtime to induce a bowel movement by morning. It is important to drink

AHCC

eight six-ounce glasses of water throughout the day while taking alder buckthorn, and to consume plenty of fresh fruits and vegetables. Alder buckthorn should be taken for a maximum of eight to ten days consecutively or else it can lead to dependence on it to have a bowel movement.[5] Some people take **peppermint tea** (page 726) or capsules with alder buckthorn to prevent griping, an unpleasant sensation of strong contractions in the colon sometimes induced by the herb.

Are there any side effects or interactions?

Alder buckthorn may turn the urine dark yellow or red, but this is harmless. Women who are pregnant or breast-feeding and children under the age of 12 should not use alder buckthorn without the advice of a physician. Those with an intestinal obstruction, **Crohn's disease** (page 141) or any other acute inflammatory problem in the intestines, **diarrhea** (page 163), appendicitis, or abdominal pain should not use this herb.[6] Use or abuse of alder buckthorn for more than ten days consecutively may cause a loss of electrolytes (especially the mineral potassium) or may weaken the colon. Long-term use can also cause kidney damage.[7]

ALFALFA

Common name: Lucerne
Botanical name: *Medicago sativa*

Parts used and where grown

Alfalfa, also known as lucerne, is a member of the pea family and is native to western Asia and the eastern Mediterranean region. Alfalfa sprouts have become a popular food. Alfalfa herbal supplements primarily use the dried leaves of the plant. The heat-treated seeds of the plant have also been used.

Alfalfa has been used in connection with the following conditions (refer to the individual health concern for complete information):

Rating	Health Concerns
★★☆	**Menopause** (page 311) (in combination with sage [page 740])
★☆☆	**High cholesterol** (page 223) **Menopause** (page 311) Poor appetite

Historical or traditional use (may or may not be supported by scientific studies)

Many years ago, traditional Chinese physicians used young alfalfa leaves to treat disorders of the digestive tract.[1] Similarly, the Ayurvedic physicians of India prescribed the leaves and flowering tops for poor digestion. Alfalfa was also considered therapeutic for water retention and arthritis. North American Indians recommended alfalfa to treat jaundice and to encourage blood clotting.

Although conspicuously absent from many classic textbooks on herbal medicine, alfalfa did find a home in the texts of the Eclectic physicians (19th-century physicians in the United States who used herbal therapies) as a tonic for **indigestion** (page 260), dyspepsia, anemia, loss of appetite, and poor assimilation of nutrients.[2] These physicians also recommended the alfalfa plant to stimulate lactation in nursing mothers, and the seeds were made into a poultice for the treatment of boils and insect bites.

Active constituents

While the medicinal benefits of alfalfa are poorly understood, the constituents in alfalfa have been extensively studied. The leaves contain approximately 2–3% saponins.[3] Animal studies suggest that these constituents block absorption of **cholesterol** (page 223) and prevent the formation of atherosclerotic plaques.[4] One small human trial found that 120 grams per day of heat-treated alfalfa seeds for eight weeks led to a modest reduction in cholesterol.[5] However, consuming the large amounts of alfalfa seeds (80–120 grams per day) needed to supply high amounts of these saponins may potentially cause damage to red blood cells in the body.[6] Herbalists also claim that alfalfa may be helpful for people with **diabetes** (page 152). But while high amounts of a water extract of the leaves led to increased insulin release in animal studies, there is no evidence that alfalfa would be useful for the treatment of diabetes in humans.[7]

Alfalfa leaves also contain flavones, isoflavones, sterols, and coumarin derivatives. The isoflavones are thought to be responsible for the estrogen-like effects seen in animal studies.[8] Although this has not been confirmed with human trials, alfalfa is sometimes used to treat **menopause** (page 311) symptoms.

Alfalfa contains protein and **vitamin A** (page 595), **vitamin B₁** (page 597), **vitamin B₆** (page 600), **vitamin C** (page 604), **vitamin E** (page 609), and **vitamin K** (page 612). Nutrient analysis demonstrates the presence of **calcium** (page 483), **potassium** (page 572), **iron** (page 540), and **zinc** (page 614).

Alfalfa

How much is usually taken?

Dried alfalfa leaf is available as a bulk herb, and in tablets or capsules. It is also available in liquid extracts. No therapeutic amount of alfalfa has been established for humans. Some herbalists recommend 500–1,000 mg of the dried leaf per day or 1–2 ml of tincture three times per day.[9]

Are there any side effects or interactions?

Use of the dried leaves of alfalfa in the amounts listed above is usually safe. There have been isolated reports of people who are allergic to alfalfa. Ingestion of very large amounts (the equivalent of several servings) of the seed and/or sprouts has been linked to the onset of **systemic lupus erythematosus** (page 421) (SLE) in animal studies.[10] It has also been linked to the reactivation of SLE in people consuming alfalfa tablets.[11] SLE is an autoimmune illness characterized by inflamed joints and a high risk of damage to kidneys and other organs. The chemical responsible for this effect is believed to be canavanine.

ALOE

Botanical names: *Aloe vera, Aloe barbadensis*

Parts used and where grown

The aloe plant originally came from Africa. The leaves, which are long, green, fleshy, and have spikes along the edges, are used medicinally. The fresh leaf gel and latex are used for many purposes. Aloe latex is the sticky residue left over after the liquid from cut aloe leaves has evaporated.

Aloe has been used in connection with the following conditions (refer to the individual health concern for complete information):

Rating	Health Concerns
★★★	**Constipation** (page 137)
★★☆	**Burns (minor)** (page 85)
	Canker sores (page 90)
	Diabetes (page 152)
	Genital herpes (page 200) (topical)
	Psoriasis (page 379)
	Seborrheic dermatitis (page 400) (topical)
	Skin ulcers (page 409)
	Ulcerative colitis (page 433)
	Wound healing (page 319) (topical)
★☆☆	**Crohn's disease** (page 141)
	Gastroesophageal reflux disease (page 198) (GERD)

Historical or traditional use (may or may not be supported by scientific studies)

Aloe has been historically used for many of the same conditions for which it is used today—particularly **constipation** (page 137) and minor **cuts** (page 319) and **burns** (page 85). In India, it has been used by herbalists to treat intestinal **infections** (page 265), suppressed menses, and **colic** (page 121).

Active constituents

The constituents of aloe latex responsible for its laxative effects are known as anthraquinone glycosides. These molecules are split by the normal bacteria in the large intestines to form other molecules (aglycones), which exert the laxative action. Since aloe is such a powerful laxative, other plant laxatives such as senna or **cascara** (page 652) are often recommended first.

Topically, it is not yet clear which constituents are responsible for the **wound healing** (page 319) properties of aloe.[1] Test tube studies suggest polysaccharides, such as acemannon, help promote skin healing by antiinflammatory, antimicrobial, and immune-stimulating actions. Aloe's effects on the skin may also be enhanced by its high concentration of **amino acids** (page 465), as well as **vitamin E** (page 609), **vitamin C** (page 604), **zinc** (page 614), and essential fatty acids.

Aloe has been used to treat minor **burns** (page 85).[2] Stabilized aloe gel is applied to the affected area of skin three to five times per day. Older case studies reported that aloe gel applied topically could help heal radiation burns,[3] and a small clinical trial found it more effective than a topical petroleum jelly in treating burns.[4] However, a large, modern, placebo-controlled trial did not find aloe effective for treating minor burns.[5]

Two small controlled human trials have found that aloe, either alone or in combination with the oral hypoglycemic drug, glibenclamide, effectively lowers blood sugar in people with type 2 (non-insulin-dependent) **diabetes** (page 152).[6, 7]

An aloe extract in a cream has been shown effective in a double-blind, controlled trial in people with **psoriasis** (page 379).[8]

Alfalfa

How much is usually taken?

For **constipation** (page 137), a single 50–200 mg capsule of aloe latex can be taken each day for a maximum of ten days.

For minor **burns** (page 85), the stabilized aloe gel is applied topically to the affected area of skin three to five times per day. Treatment of more serious burns should only be done under the supervision of a healthcare professional. For internal use of aloe gel, two tablespoons (30 ml) three times per day is used by some people for **inflammatory bowel** (page 269) conditions, such as **Crohn's disease** (page 141) and **ulcerative colitis** (page 433) (see precautions below). For type 2 **diabetes** (page 152), clinical trials have used one tablespoon (15 ml) of aloe juice, twice daily. Treatment of diabetes with aloe should only be done under the supervision of a qualified healthcare professional.

Are there any side effects or interactions?

Except in the rare person who is allergic to aloe, topical application of the gel is generally safe. For any **burn** (page 85) that blisters significantly or is otherwise severe, medical attention is absolutely essential. In some severe burns and **wounds** (page 319), aloe gel may actually impede healing.[9]

The latex form of aloe should not be used by anyone with inflammatory intestinal diseases, such as **Crohn's disease** (page 141), **ulcerative colitis** (page 433), or appendicitis. It should also not be used by children, or by women during **pregnancy** (page 363) or **breast-feeding** (page 74).[10]

In people with constipation, aloe latex should not be used for more than ten consecutive days as it may lead to dependency and fluid loss. Extensive fluid loss may lead to depletion of important electrolytes in the body such as **potassium** (page 572).[11]

AMERICAN GINSENG

Botanical name: *Panax quinquefolius*

Parts used and where grown

Like its more familiar cousin **Asian ginseng** (page 630) *(Panax ginseng)*, the root of American ginseng is used medicinally. The plant grows wild in shady forests of the northern and central United States, as well as in parts of Canada. It is cultivated in the United States, China, and France.

American ginseng has been used in connection with the following conditions (refer to the individual health concern for complete information):

Rating	Health Concerns
★★☆	**Diabetes** (page 152)
★☆☆	**Athletic performance** (page 43) **Infection** (page 265) Stress

Historical or traditional use (may or may not be supported by scientific studies)

Many Native American tribes used American ginseng. Medicinal applications ranged from digestive disorders to sexual problems.[1] The Chinese began to use American ginseng after it was imported during the 1700s.[2] The traditional applications of American ginseng in China are significantly different from those for *Panax ginseng* (Asian ginseng).[3]

Active constituents

American ginseng contains ginsenosides, which are thought to fight fatigue and stress by supporting the adrenal glands and the use of oxygen by exercising muscles.[4] The type and ratio of ginsenosides are somewhat different in American and Asian ginseng. The extent to which this affects their medicinal properties is unclear. A recent preliminary trial with healthy volunteers found no benefit in exercise performance after one week of taking American ginseng.[5]

In a small pilot study, 3 grams of American ginseng was found to lower the rise in blood sugar following the consumption of a drink high in glucose by people with type 2 **diabetes** (page 152).[6] The study found no difference in blood sugar lowering effect if the herb was taken either 40 minutes before the drink or at the same time. A follow-up to this study found that increasing the amount of American ginseng to either 6 or 9 grams did not increase the effect on blood sugar following the high-glucose drink in people with type 2 diabetes.[7] This study also found that American ginseng was equally effective in controlling the rise in blood sugar if it was given up to two hours before or together with the drink.

How much is usually taken?

Standardized extracts of American ginseng, unlike Asian ginseng, are not available. However, dried root powder, 1–3 grams per day in capsule or tablet form, can be used.[8] Some herbalists also recommend 3–5 ml of tincture three times per day.

Are there any side effects or interactions?
Occasional cases of **insomnia** (page 270) or agitation have been reported with the use of American ginseng. These conditions are more likely, however, when caffeine-containing foods and beverages are also being consumed.[9]

AMERICAN SCULLCAP

Common name: Scullcap
Botanical name: *Scutellaria lateriflora*

Parts used and where grown
Scullcap is a member of the mint family. *Scutellaria lateriflora* grows in eastern North America and is most commonly used in United States and European herbal products containing scullcap. The aboveground (aerial) part of the plant is used in herbal preparations. It is not interchangeable with **Chinese scullcap** (page 658).

Scullcap has been used in connection with the following conditions (refer to the individual health concern for complete information):

Rating	Health Concerns
★☆☆	**Anxiety** (page 30) **Insomnia** (page 270) **Pain** (page 338)

Historical or traditional use (may or may not be supported by scientific studies)
As is the case in modern herbal medicine, scullcap was used historically as a sedative for people with nervous tension and **insomnia** (page 270). It was, and continues to be, commonly combined with **valerian** (page 756) for insomnia.[1] It was also used by herbalists as a remedy for **epilepsy** (page 183) and nerve **pain** (page 338).

Active constituents
Few studies have been completed on the constituents of American scullcap. One of its constituents, scutellarian, has been reportedly shown to have mild sedative and antispasmodic actions in animal studies.[2] Human trials have not yet been conducted to confirm the use of scullcap for **anxiety** (page 30) or insomnia.

How much is usually taken?
Scullcap tea can be made by pouring 1 cup (250 ml) of boiling water over 1–2 teaspoons (5–10 grams) of the dried herb and steeping for 10 to 15 minutes. This tea may be drunk three times per day.[3] Alternatively, tincture made from fresh scullcap, ⅓–¾ teaspoon (2–4 ml) three times per day, may be taken.

Are there any side effects or interactions?
Use of scullcap in the amounts listed above is generally safe. However, scullcap use during **pregnancy** (page 363) and breast-feeding should be avoided due to limited information about its safety. Cases of liver damage have been reported in association with the intake of scullcap. However, on closer examination, it appears these scullcap products actually contained germander (*Teucrium chamaedrys*), an herb known to cause liver damage.[4]

One case report exists of a 28-year-old man who died of liver failure after taking unspecified amounts of scullcap, pau d'arco, and zinc.[5] It appears likely that this, too, may have been a case of adulteration of scullcap with germander.[6]

ANDROGRAPHIS

Common names: Chiretta, chuan xin lian, kalmegh, kirata
Botanical name: *Andrographis paniculata*

Parts used and where grown
Andrographis originated in the plains of India, and it also grows in China. The leaves and flowers are used medicinally.

Andrographis has been used in connection with the following conditions (refer to the individual health concern for complete information):

Rating	Health Concerns
★★★	**Common cold** (page 129) **Immune function** (page 255) **Infection** (page 265)
★★☆	Dysentery
★☆☆	**HIV infection** (page 239) **Indigestion** (page 260) **Viral hepatitis** (page 220)

American Ginseng

Historical or traditional use (may or may not be supported by scientific studies)

Andrographis has long been used in traditional Indian and Chinese herbal medicine. The most common reported uses were for digestive problems (as is the case with most non-toxic bitter herbs such as andrographis), snakebite, and **infections** (page 265) ranging from malaria to dysentery.[1, 2] Interestingly, some of these uses have been validated by modern scientific research. Although the roots were sometimes used in traditional medicine, the leaves and flowers are now more commonly used.

Active constituents

The major constituents in andrographis are diterpene lactones known as andrographolides. These bitter constituents are believed to have **immune-stimulating** (page 255), anti-inflammatory, fertility-decreasing, liver-protective, and bile secretion-stimulating actions.[3] Though some older studies suggested andrographis was antibacterial, modern research has been unable to confirm this finding.[4]

Several double-blind clinical trials have found that andrographis can help reduce symptom severity in people with **common colds** (page 129).[5, 6, 7, 8, 9] Though the earliest clinical trial among these showed modest benefits, later studies have tended to be more supportive. Standardized andrographis extract combined with **eleuthero** (page 672) (Siberian ginseng), known as Kan jang, has also been shown in a double-blind clinical trial to reduce symptoms of the common cold.[10]

A preliminary uncontrolled study using isolated andrographolide found that while it tended to decrease viral load and increase CD4 lymphocyte levels in people with **HIV infection** (page 239), at the amount used, the preparation led to side effects, including headache, fatigue, a bitter/metallic taste in the mouth, and elevated liver enzymes (which returned to normal after the medication was stopped).[11] It is unknown whether the andrographolides used in this study directly killed HIV or had an immune-strengthening effect.

Andrographis has proven helpful in combination with antibiotics for people with dysentery, a severe form of **diarrhea** (page 163).[12] It has also shown preliminary benefit for people with chronic viral **hepatitis** (page 220).[13]

How much is usually taken?

Andrographis is generally available as capsules with dried herb or as standardized extracts (containing 11.2 mg andrographolides per 200 mg of extract). For dried herb,

500–3,000 mg are taken three times per day. In clinical trials, 100 mg of a standardized extract were taken two times per day to treat the **common cold** (page 129).[14] For **indigestion** (page 260), andrographis may be taken as a tea. Use 1 teaspoon (5 grams) of the herb for each cup (250 ml) of hot water. Allow the mixture to stand for 10–15 minutes before drinking (sip before meals).

Are there any side effects or interactions?

Some people develop intestinal upset when taking andrographis. If this occurs, reduce the amount taken or take it with meals. Headache, fatigue, a bitter/metallic taste, and elevated liver enzymes were reported in one trial with HIV-infected people taking high doses of isolated andrographolides.[15] This has not been reported in people using whole andrographis or standardized extracts at the amounts recommended above. As with all bitter herbs, andrographis may aggravate **ulcers** (page 349) and **heartburn** (page 260). The safety of andrographis during **pregnancy** (page 363) and breast-feeding is unknown.

ANISE

Botanical name: *Pimpinella anisum*

Parts used and where grown

The seeds of this aromatic plant are used as both medicine and as a cooking spice. Anise comes from Eurasia but is now grown in gardens all over the world.

Anise has been used in connection with the following conditions (refer to the individual health concern for complete information):

Rating	Health Concerns
★☆☆	Adjunct to cathartic laxatives
	Breast-feeding support (page 74)
	Bronchitis (page 80)
	Chronic Obstructive Pulmonary Disease (page 114) (COPD)
	Cough (page 139)
	Indigestion and gas (page 260)
	Parasites (page 343)

Historical or traditional use (may or may not be supported by scientific studies)

Anise has been an important flavoring in European cooking since time immemorial. Its oil has also been used as an anthelmintic—a drug used to remove intestinal **parasites** (page 343)—though it is not considered the strongest plant in this regard.[1] Anise has also been used for centuries in European herbalism to treat **coughs** (page 139) and **indigestion** (page 260).[2]

Active constituents

The active constituents in anise, particularly the terpenoid anethole, are contained in its volatile oil. The volatile oil gives the plant a delightful flavor and has been combined with other less pleasant tasting medicinal herbs to offset their taste. The oil is also antispasmodic, helping to relieve **intestinal gas** (page 260) and spasmodic **coughs** (page 139).[3] Anise has been combined with cathartic laxatives to help reduce the spasmodic cramping they can cause.[4] It may also have modest antiparasitic actions and has been recommended by some practitioners to treat mild intestinal **parasite** (page 343) infections.[5] Anethole has been documented to have phytoestrogen activity in test tubes and animals;[6] the relevance of this to humans is unknown. No clinical trials have been conducted to support any of these uses, though anise is approved for use by the German Commission E for relieving coughs and indigestion.[7]

How much is usually taken?

Three grams (½ tsp) of the seeds can be used three times per day to treat indigestion. To make a tea, boil 2 to 3 grams (½ tsp) of crushed seeds in 250 ml (1 cup) of water for ten to fifteen minutes, keeping the pot covered. Three cups of this tea can be drunk per day. It has been recommended to combine approximately 0.5 ml anise volatile oil with 4 oz (120 ml) tincture of anise and then take 10 to 30 drops (½ to 1.5 ml) of this mixture three times daily for coughs.[8] The volatile oil can also be inhaled (by placing it in a vaporizer or in a steaming bowl of water) to help relieve a cough.[9]

Are there any side effects or interactions?

There are no known adverse effects from anise other than occasional allergic reactions of the skin with topical use and of the respiratory or gastrointestinal tract with internal use. It is frequently used to alleviate cough in children because of its gentleness and pleasant taste.[10] The safety of using anise during **pregnancy** (page 363) and **breast-feeding** (page 74) is unknown, though it is very likely safe and has traditionally been used to support breast-feeding in some cultures.[11]

ARTICHOKE

Botanical name: *Cynara scolymus*

Parts used and where grown

This large thistle-like plant is native to the regions of southern Europe, North Africa, and the Canary Islands. The leaves of the plant are used medicinally. However, the roots and the immature flower heads may also contain beneficial compounds.[1]

Artichoke has been used in connection with the following conditions (refer to the individual health concern for complete information):

Rating	Health Concerns
★★★	**Indigestion** (page 260) and lack of appetite (digestive aid)
★★☆	**High cholesterol** (page 223)
★☆☆	**Irritable bowel syndrome** (page 280)

Historical or traditional use (may or may not be supported by scientific studies)

The artichoke is one of the world's oldest medicinal plants. The ancient Egyptians placed great value on the plant—it is clearly seen in drawings involving fertility and sacrifice. Moreover, this plant was used by the ancient Greeks and Romans as a digestive aid. In 16th century Europe, the artichoke was favored as a food by royalty.[2]

Active constituents

Artichoke leaves contain a wide number of active constituents, including cynarin, 1,3 dicaffeoylquinic acid, 3-caffeoylquinic acid, and scolymoside.[3] The choleretic (bile stimulating) action of the plant has been well documented in a controlled trial involving a small sample of healthy volunteers.[4] After the administration of 1.92 grams of standardized artichoke extract directly into the duodenum, liver bile flow increased significantly. This choleretic effect has led to the popular use of artichoke extract in Europe for the treatment of mild indigestion—particularly following a meal high in fat. In an uncontrolled clinical trial with 553 people suffering from non-specific digestive disorders (including indigestion), 320–640 mg of a standardized artichoke extract taken three times per day was found to reduce nausea, abdominal pain, **constipation** (page 137), and flatulence in over 70% of the study participants.[5]

The standardized extract has also been used to treat **high cholesterol** (page 223) and **triglycerides** (page 235). In one preliminary trial[6] and one controlled trial,[7] use of a standardized artichoke extract was found to lower cholesterol and triglycerides significantly when taken in amounts ranging from 900 to 1,920 mg per day. One preliminary trial failed to find any effect.[8]

While scientists are not certain how artichoke leaves lower cholesterol, test tube studies have suggested that the action may be due to an inhibition of cholesterol synthesis and/or the increased elimination of cholesterol because of the plant's choleretic action.[9] In test tube studies, the **flavonoids** (page 516) from the artichoke (e.g., luteolin) have been shown to prevent LDL-cholesterol oxidation—an effect that may reduce risk of **atherosclerosis** (page 38).[10]

How much is usually taken?

The suggested adult amount of the standardized leaf extract is 300–640 mg three times daily for a minimum of six weeks.[11] Alternatively, if a standardized extract is not available, the amount of the crude, dried leaves is 1–4 grams, three times a day.[12]

Are there any side effects or interactions?

At the recommended amount and according to the German Commission E Monograph,[13] there are no known side effects or drug interactions. The use of artichoke is not recommended for those who are allergic to artichokes and other members of the Compositae (e.g., daisy) family. In addition, those who have any obstruction of the bile duct (e.g., as a result of **gallstones** [page 193]) should not employ this plant therapeutically. The plant's safety during **pregnancy** (page 363) and breast-feeding has not been established.

ASHWAGANDHA

Botanical name: *Withania somniferum*

Parts used and where grown

Ashwagandha, which belongs to the pepper family, is found in India and Africa. The roots of ashwagandha are used medicinally.

Ashwagandha has been used in connection with the following conditions (refer to the individual health concern for complete information):

Rating	Health Concerns
★★☆	**Immune function** (page 255)
★☆☆	**Osteoarthritis** (page 328)
	Stress

Historical or traditional use (may or may not be supported by scientific studies)

The health applications for ashwagandha in traditional Indian and Ayurvedic medicine are extensive. Of particular note is its use against tumors, inflammation (including arthritis), and a wide range of infectious diseases.[1] The shoots and seeds are also used as food and to thicken milk in India. Traditional uses of ashwagandha among tribal peoples in Africa include fevers and inflammatory conditions.[2] Ashwagandha is frequently a constituent of Ayurvedic formulas, including a relatively common one known as shilajit.

Active constituents

The constituents believed to be active in ashwagandha have been extensively studied.[3] Compounds known as withanolides are believed to account for the multiple medicinal applications of ashwagandha.[4] These molecules are steroidal and bear a resemblance, both in their action and appearance, to the active constituents of **Asian ginseng** (page 630) (*Panax ginseng*) known as ginsenosides. Indeed, ashwagandha has been called "Indian ginseng" by some. Ashwagandha and its withanolides have been extensively researched in a variety of animal studies examining effects on **immune function** (page 255), inflammation, and even **cancer** (page 87). Ashwagandha stimulates the activation of immune system cells, such as lymphocytes.[5] It has also been shown to inhibit inflammation[6] and improve memory in animal experiments.[7] Taken together, these actions may support the traditional reputation of ashwagandha as a tonic or adaptogen[8]—an herb with multiple, nonspecific actions that counteract the effects of stress and generally promote wellness.

How much is usually taken?

Some experts recommend 3–6 grams of the dried root, taken each day in capsule or tea form.[9] To prepare a tea, ¾–1¼ teaspoons (3–6 grams) of ashwagandha root are boiled for 15 minutes and cooled; 3 cups (750 ml) may be drunk daily. Alternatively, tincture ½–¾ teaspoon (2–4 ml) three times per day, is sometimes recommended.

Ashwagandha

Are there any side effects or interactions?

No significant side effects have been reported with ashwagandha. The herb has been used safely by children in India. Its safety during **pregnancy** (page 363) and breastfeeding is unknown.

ASIAN GINSENG

Common names: Korean ginseng, Chinese ginseng
Botanical name: *Panax ginseng*

Parts used and where grown

Asian ginseng is a member of the *Araliaceae* family, which also includes the closely related **American ginseng** (page 625) *(Panax quinquefolius)* and less similar Siberian ginseng *(Eleutherococcus senticosus),* also known as **eleuthero** (page 672). Asian ginseng commonly grows on mountain slopes and is usually harvested in the fall. The root is used, preferably from plants older than six years of age.

Asian ginseng has been used in connection with the following conditions (refer to the individual health concern for complete information):

Rating	Health Concerns
★★★	**Erectile dysfunction** (page 185)
★★☆	**Athletic performance** (page 43) **Diabetes** (page 152) **Epilepsy** (page 183) (in combination with **bupleurum** [page 647], peony root, pinellia root, cassia bark, **ginger** [page 680] root, jujube fruit, **Chinese scullcap** [page 658] root, and **licorice** [page 702] root) **Immune function** (page 255) **Infertility (male)** (page 304)
★☆☆	Aerobic capacity **Chronic fatigue syndrome** (page 111) **Common cold/sore throat** (page 129) **HIV support** (page 239) **Infection** (page 265) **Influenza** (page 270) **Lung cancer** (page 298) **Menopause** (page 311) Stress

Historical or traditional use (may or may not be supported by scientific studies)

Asian ginseng has been a part of Chinese medicine for over 2,000 years. The first reference to the use of Asian ginseng dates to the 1st century A.D. Ginseng is commonly used by elderly people in the Orient to improve mental and physical vitality.

Active constituents

Ginseng's actions in the body are thought to be due to a complex interplay of constituents. The primary group are the ginsenosides, which are believed to counter the effects of stress and enhance intellectual and physical performance. Thirteen ginsenosides have been identified in Asian ginseng. Two of them, ginsenosides Rg1 and Rb1, have been closely studied.[1] Other constituents include the panaxans, which may help lower blood sugar, and the polysaccharides (complex sugar molecules), which are thought to support **immune function** (page 255).[2, 3]

Long-term intake of Asian ginseng may be linked to a reduced risk of some forms of **cancer** (page 87).[4, 5] A double-blind trial found that 200 mg of Asian ginseng per day improved blood sugar levels in people with type 2 (non-insulin-dependent) **diabetes** (page 152).[6] Human trials have mostly failed to confirm the purported benefit of Asian ginseng for the enhancement of **athletic performance** (page 43).[7, 8] One preliminary trial suggests it may help those in poor physical condition to tolerate exercise better.[9] In combination with some vitamins and minerals, 80 mg of ginseng per day was found to effectively reduce fatigue in a double-blind trial.[10] Another double-blind trial also found it helpful for relief of fatigue and, possibly, stress.[11] Although there are no human clinical trials, adaptogenic herbs such as Asian ginseng may be useful for people with **chronic fatigue syndrome** (page 111). This may be because these herbs are thought to have an immunomodulating effect and also help support the normal function of the hypothalamic-pituitary-adrenal axis, the hormonal stress system of the body.[12]

Asian ginseng may also prove useful for **male infertility** (page 304). A double-blind trial with a large group of infertile men found that 4 grams of Asian ginseng per day for three months led to an improvement in sperm count and sperm motility.[13]

Asian ginseng may also help men with **erectile dysfunction** (page 185). A double-blind trial in Korea found that 1,800 mg per day of Asian ginseng extract for three months helped improve libido and the ability to maintain an erection in men with erectile dysfunction.[14] This finding was confirmed in another double-blind study, in which 900 mg three times a day was given for eight weeks.[15]

How much is usually taken?

The most researched form of ginseng, standardized herbal extracts, supply approximately 5–7% ginsenosides.[16] Ginseng root extracts are sometimes recommended at 200–500 mg per day. Non-standardized extracts require a higher intake, generally 1–4 grams per day for tablets or 2–3 ml for dried root tincture three times per day. Ginseng is traditionally used for two to three weeks continuously, followed by a one- to two-week "rest" period before resuming.

Are there any side effects or interactions?

Used in the recommended amounts, ginseng is generally safe. In rare instances, it may cause over-stimulation and possibly **insomnia** (page 270).[17] Consuming caffeine with ginseng increases the risk of over-stimulation and gastrointestinal upset. People with uncontrolled **high blood pressure** (page 246) should use ginseng cautiously. Long-term use of ginseng may cause menstrual abnormalities and breast tenderness in some women. Ginseng is not recommended for **pregnant** (page 363) or **breast-feeding** (page 74) women.

ASTRAGALUS

Common name: Huang qi
Botanical name: *Astragalus membranaceus*

Parts used and where grown

Astragalus is native to northern China and the elevated regions of the Chinese provinces, Yunnan and Sichuan. The portion of the plant used medicinally is the four- to seven-year-old dried root, collected in the spring. While over 2,000 types of astragalus exist worldwide, the Chinese version has been extensively tested, both chemically and pharmacologically.[1]

Astragalus has been used in connection with the following conditions (refer to the individual health concern for complete information):

Rating	Health Concerns
★☆☆	**Common cold/sore throat** (page 129)
	Heart attack (page 212)
	Hepatitis (page 220)
	Immune function (page 255)
	Infection (page 265)
	Systemic lupus erythematosus (page 421)

Historical or traditional use (may or may not be supported by scientific studies)

Shen Nung, the founder of Chinese herbal medicine, classified astragalus as a superior herb in his classical treatise *Shen Nung Pen Tsao Ching* (circa A.D. 100). The Chinese name *huang qi* translates as "yellow leader," referring to the yellow color of the root and its status as one of the most important tonic herbs. Traditional Chinese Medicine used this herb for night sweats, deficiency of chi (e.g., fatigue, weakness, and loss of appetite), and **diarrhea** (page 163).[2]

Active constituents

Astragalus contains numerous components, including **flavonoids** (page 516), polysaccharides, triterpene glycosides (e.g., astragalosides I–VII), **amino acids** (page 465), and trace minerals.[3] Several preliminary clinical trials in China have suggested that astragalus can benefit **immune function** (page 255) and improve survival in some people with **cancer** (page 87).[4] Given the poor quality of these trials, it is difficult to know how useful astragalus really was. One Chinese trial also found that astragalus could decrease overactive immune function in people with **systemic lupus erythematosus** (page 421) (SLE), an autoimmune disease.[5] Further trials are needed, however, to know if astragalus is safe for people with SLE, or any other autoimmune disease.

A double-blind trial found that, in people undergoing dialysis for kidney failure, intravenous astragalus improved one facet of immune function compared to the immune function of untreated people.[6] Further study is needed to determine if astragalus can help prevent **infections** (page 265) in people undergoing dialysis. Early clinical trials in China suggest astragalus root might also benefit people with chronic viral **hepatitis** (page 220), though it may take one to two months to see results.[7]

In preliminary trials in China, astragalus has been used after people suffer **heart attacks** (page 212).[8] More research is needed to determine whether astragalus is truly beneficial in this situation.

How much is usually taken?

Textbooks on Chinese herbs recommend taking 9–15 grams of the crude herb per day in decoction form.[9] A decoction is made by boiling the root in water for a few minutes and then brewing the tea. Alternatively, 3–5 ml of tincture three times per day, are sometimes recommended.

Astragalus

Are there any side effects or interactions?

Astragalus has no known side effects when used as recommended.

BACOPA

Common names: Brahmi, water hyssop
Botanical name: *Bacopa monniera*

Parts used and where grown

Bacopa is native to India, where it grows in marshy areas. In the West, bacopa is a familiar water plant used in aquariums. Most parts of the plant have been used traditionally, but modern preparations are extracts of the stem and leaves.

Bacopa has been used in connection with the following conditions (refer to the individual health concern for complete information):

Rating	Health Concerns
★☆☆	**Alzheimer's disease** (page 19)
	Anxiety (page 30)
	ARCD (page 8)
	Epilepsy (page 183)

Historical or traditional use (may or may not be supported by scientific studies)

Since at least the sixth century A.D., bacopa (Brahmi) has been used in Ayurvedic medicine (the traditional medicine of India) as a diuretic and as a tonic for the nervous system and the heart. Specific uses include the treatment of asthma, insanity, and epilepsy.[1]

Active constituents

The leaves of bacopa contain saponins, including the bacosides,[2, 3, 4] which are thought responsible for the therapeutic properties of the herb. In animal studies, both purified bacosides and extracts of bacopa standardized for bacosides have been found to enhance several aspects of mental function and learning ability.[5, 6, 7] Additional brain effects of bacopa demonstrated in animal research include reduction of both anxiety and depression.[8, 9] Biochemically, these nervous-system effects have been attributed to an enhancement of the effects of the neurotransmitters acetylcholine and,[10, 11] possibly, serotonin or GABA (gamma aminobutyric acid).[12, 13]

Bacopa extracts also appear to have significant antioxidant activity in the brain,[14] and other effects that may help protect brain cells.[15]

Animal research has also reported that bacopa extracts can relax the muscles that control the blood vessels, the intestine, and the airways of the respiratory system,[16, 17, 18, 19] and can help both prevent and heal ulcers in the stomach.[20]

Traditional herbal references recommend 5 to 10 grams per day of the powdered herb.[21] Human research has used 300 to 450 mg per day of an extract standardized to contain 55% bacosides.

Bacopa appears to be well tolerated when taken in typical amounts,[22] although one double-blind study reported significantly more symptoms of dry mouth, nausea, and muscle fatigue in participants taking bacopa.[23]

BARBERRY

Botanical name: *Berberis vulgaris*

Parts used and where grown

The root and stem bark contain the medicinally active components of barberry. The barberry bush also produces small red berries. Although this particular species is native to Europe, it now also grows throughout North America. A closely related species, **Oregon grape** (page 721) *(Berberis aquifolium)*, is native to North America.

Barberry has been used in connection with the following conditions (refer to the individual health concern for complete information):

Rating	Health Concerns
★☆☆	**Chronic candidiasis** (page 109)
	Diarrhea (page 163) (berberine)
	Indigestion (page 260)
	Infection (page 265)
	Parasites (page 343)
	Psoriasis (page 379)
	Vaginitis (page 438)

Historical or traditional use (may or may not be supported by scientific studies)

Traditionally, in European and American herbalism, barberry was used to treat a large number of conditions, particularly **infections** (page 265) and stomach problems.[1] It has also been used internally to treat skin conditions.

Active constituents

The alkaloid, berberine, receives the most research and widest acclaim as the active component of barberry and its relatives. Berberine is also a key constituent of **goldenseal** (page 683) *(Hydrastis canadensis).* Berberine and its related constituents (such as oxyacanthine) are antibacterial[2] and have been shown to kill amoebae in a test tube study.[3] Berberine inhibits bacteria from attaching to human cells, which helps prevent **infection** (page 265).[4] This compound treats **diarrhea** (page 163) caused by bacteria, such as *E. coli.*[5] Berberine also stimulates some **immune system cells** (page 255) to function better.[6] Berbamine is another alkaloid found in barberry. It may help reduce inflammation[7] and is an **antioxidant** (page 467).[8]

The bitter compounds in barberry, including the alkaloids mentioned above, stimulate digestive function following meals.

How much is usually taken?

For digestive conditions, barberry is often combined with other bitter herbs, such as **gentian** (page 680), in tincture form. Such mixtures are taken 15 to 20 minutes before a meal, usually 2–5 ml each time. As a tincture, 2–3 ml of barberry can be taken three times per day. Standardized extracts containing 5–10% alkaloids, with a total of approximately 500 mg of berberine taken each day, are preferable for preventing **infections** (page 265). Standardized extracts of **goldenseal** (page 683) are a more common source of berberine, since goldenseal contains a higher concentration of berberine than barberry. An ointment made from a 10% extract of barberry can be applied topically three times per day for **psoriasis** (page 379). A tea/infusion can be prepared using 2 grams of the herb in a cup of boiling water. This can be repeated two to three times daily.[9]

Are there any side effects or interactions?

Berberine has been reported to interfere with normal liver function in infants, raising a concern that it might worsen jaundice.[10] For this reason, berberine-containing plants, including barberry, goldenseal, and Oregon grape should be used with caution during **pregnancy** (page 363) and breast-feeding. Strong standardized extracts may cause stomach upset and should be used for

no more than two weeks continuously. Other symptoms of excessive berberine intake include lethargy, nose bleed, skin and eye irritation, and kidney irritation.[11]

BASIL

Common names: Common basil, sweet basil
Botanical name: *Ocimum basilicum*

Parts used and where grown

The leaves of basil and its many close relatives are used as medicine. The seeds are also used medicinally in India and Southeast Asia. Though it originates on the shores of the Mediterranean Sea and the Middle East, common basil now grows in gardens all over the world. Three important relatives with similar properties are *Ocimum canum* (hairy basil), *O. gratissimum* (basil), and *O. sanctum* (holy basil).

Basil has been used in connection with the following conditions (refer to the individual health concern for complete information):

Rating	Health Concerns
★★☆	**Constipation** (page 137) **Diabetes** (page 152)
★☆☆	**Indigestion** (page 260)

Historical or traditional use (may or may not be supported by scientific studies)

Basil has been a culinary herb in Europe and Central Asia since before the written word.[1] In India the seeds were used for **diarrhea** (page 163), mucous discharges, **constipation** (page 137), and as a general demulcent (soothes mucous membranes);[2] the leaves were used for **indigestion** (page 260) and skin diseases. In traditional Thai herbalism, the plant is used for **coughs** (page 139), skin diseases, and intestinal problems. The seed is used as a bulk-forming laxative and diuretic.[3]

Active constituents

Basil contains a strong-scented volatile oil composed primarily of terpenoids, particularly eugenol, thymol, and estragole. Basil also has what are known as chemotypes, minor variations among plants that contain significantly different mixes of constituents. The exact components of basil oil vary widely, being affected not only by these chemotypes but also by factors such as the time of day of harvest.[4] This may account for some of the variability in scientific research and reports of medicinal efficacy of basil from culture to culture.

Preliminary studies on holy basil and hairy basil have shown that the leaf and seed may help people with type 2 **diabetes** (page 152) control their blood sugar levels.[5, 6, 7] While the action-mechanism of the leaf is not understood, the seed may work by providing dietary **fiber** (page 512), which helps prevent rapid blood sugar elevations after meals. In addition, the seed has been found to relieve **constipation** (page 137) by acting as a bulk-forming laxative in one uncontrolled human study.[8] A similar study showed the seeds useful in elderly people who experienced constipation after undergoing major surgery.[9]

The volatile oil of basil has shown antibacterial, antifungal, and antiviral activity in test tube studies.[10] It is also believed to act as a carminative, relieving **intestinal gas** (page 260), and as a mild diuretic, though these actions have yet to be definitively proven.[11]

How much is usually taken?
A tea can be made by steeping 1 teaspoon of basil leaves in one cup of water for ten minutes. Three cups of this tea can be drunk per day. Capsules of basil can be taken in the amount of 2.5 grams per day. The volatile oil can be taken internally in the amount of 2 to 5 drops three times per day.[12]

Are there any side effects or interactions?
Although concerns have been raised about the possible cancer-causing effects of estragole, a component found in variable amounts in basil volatile oil, small amounts of basil would not seem to pose a significant threat.[13] However, because some herbal books suggest that estragole may be potentially carcinogenic and has been thought to stimulate uterine contractions, some herbal experts feel it may be best for **pregnant** (page 363) or **breast-feeding** (page 74) women to avoid use of the herb, especially the volatile oil.[14] People with serious kidney or liver damage should not use basil volatile oil internally, as they could theoretically have trouble eliminating it from their bodies. However, use of basil as a seasoning in food is unlikely to be of concern.

BILBERRY

Botanical name: *Vaccinium myrtillus*

Parts used and where grown
A close relative of American **blueberry** (page 641), bilberry grows in northern Europe, Canada, and the United States. The ripe berries are primarily used in modern herbal extracts.

Bilberry has been used in connection with the following conditions (refer to the individual health concern for complete information):

Rating	Health Concerns
★★☆	**Diabetes** (page 152)
	Retinopathy (page 385)
★☆☆	**Atherosclerosis** (page 38)
	Cataracts (page 101)
	Diarrhea (page 163)
	Macular degeneration (page 303)
	Night blindness (page 326)

Historical or traditional use (may or may not be supported by scientific studies)
The dried berries and leaves of bilberry have been recommended for a wide variety of conditions, including scurvy, **urinary tract infections** (page 436), **kidney stones** (page 284), and **diabetes** (page 152). Perhaps the most sound historical application is the use of the dried berries to treat **diarrhea** (page 163). Modern research of bilberry was partly based on its use by British World War II pilots, who noticed that their night vision improved when they ate bilberry jam prior to night bombing raids.[1]

Active constituents
Anthocyanosides, the **flavonoid** (page 516) complex in bilberries, speed the regeneration of rhodopsin, the purple pigment that is used by the rods in the eye for night vision.[2] While earlier trials suggested that taking bilberry could benefit people with **night blindness** (page 326),[3, 4] more recent trials with healthy volunteers have found no effect of bilberry on night vision.[5, 6] Preliminary human trials conducted in Europe show that bilberry may prevent **cataracts** (page 101),[7] and may even help to treat people with mild retinopathies (such as **macular degeneration** [page 303] and diabetic

Basil

retinopathy [page 385]).[8, 9] Anthocyanosides are potent **antioxidants** (page 467).[10] They support normal formation of connective tissue and strengthen capillaries in the body. Anthocyanosides may also improve capillary and venous blood flow. Bilberry may also prevent blood vessel thickening due to **diabetes** (page 152).[11]

Bilberry protects cholesterol from oxidizing in test tubes.[12] While this action is thought to help prevent **atherosclerosis** (page 38), no human trials have studied whether bilberry may be useful in the regard.

How much is usually taken?
Bilberry herbal extract in capsules or tablets standardized to provide 25% anthocyanosides are typically recommended at 240–600 mg per day.[13] Herbalists have traditionally recommended taking 1–2 ml two times per day in tincture form, or 20–60 grams of the fruit daily.

Are there any side effects or interactions?
In recommended amounts, no side effects have been reported with bilberry extract.

BITTER MELON

Botanical name: *Momordica charantia*

Parts used and where grown
Bitter melon grows in tropical areas, including parts of East Africa, Asia, the Caribbean, and South America, where it is used as a food as well as a medicine. The fruit of this plant lives up to its name—it tastes bitter. Although the seeds, leaves, and vines of bitter melon have all been used, the fruit is the safest and most prevalent part of the plant used medicinally.

Bitter melon has been used in connection with the following conditions (refer to the individual health concern for complete information):

Rating	Health Concerns
★★☆	Diabetes (page 152)
★☆☆	Indigestion (page 260)

Historical or traditional use (may or may not be supported by scientific studies)
Being a relatively common food item, bitter melon was traditionally used for an array of conditions by people in tropical regions. Numerous **infections** (page 265), **can-**

cer (page 87), and **diabetes** (page 152) were among the most common conditions it has been purported to improve.[1] The leaves and fruit have both been used in the Western world to make teas and beer or to season soups.

Active constituents
At least three different groups of constituents in bitter melon have been reported to have blood-sugar lowering actions of potential benefit in **diabetes** (page 152) mellitus. These include a mixture of steroidal saponins known as charantin, insulin-like peptides, and alkaloids. It is still unclear which of these is most effective, or if all three work together. Some clinical trials have confirmed the benefit of bitter melon for people with diabetes.[2]

In traditional herbal medicine, bitter melon—like other bitter-tasting herbs—is thought to stimulate digestive function and improve appetite. This has yet to be tested in human studies.

How much is usually taken?
For those with a taste or tolerance for bitter flavor, a small melon can be eaten as food, or up to 3 1/3 ounces (100 ml) of a decoction or 2 ounces (60 ml) of fresh juice can be drunk per day.[3] Though still bitter, tinctures of bitter melon (1 teaspoon [5 ml] two to three times per day) are also sometimes used. The amounts recommended would be appropriate for people with **diabetes** (page 152).

Are there any side effects or interactions?
Ingestion of excessive amounts of bitter melon juice (several times more than the amount recommended above) can cause abdominal pain and **diarrhea** (page 163).[4] Excessive ingestion of the seeds had been associated with headache, fever, and coma. Bitter melon is not recommended for **pregnant** (page 363) women. People with **hypoglycemia** (page 251) (low blood sugar) should not take bitter melon, because it may trigger or worsen the problem. This effect has been reported in two young children and one adult patient with **diabetes** (page 152).

BITTER ORANGE

Common names: Seville orange, zhi shi, chongcao
Botanical name: *Citrus X aurantium*

Parts used and where grown
The dried outer peel of the fruit of bitter orange, with the white pulp layer removed, is used medicinally. The

leaves are also commonly used in many folk traditions. The bitter orange tree is indigenous to eastern Africa, Arabia, and Syria, and cultivated in Spain, Italy, and North America.

Bitter orange has been used in connection with the following conditions (refer to the individual health concern for complete information):

Rating	Health Concerns
★★☆	**Indigestion** (page 260) Loss of appetite
★☆☆	**Insomnia** (page 270) **Weight loss** (page 446)

Historical or traditional use (may or may not be supported by scientific studies)

Bitter orange is used similarly in a wide variety of traditions. In Mexico and South America the leaf is used as a tonic, as a laxative, as a sedative for insomnia, and to calm frazzled nerves.[1, 2] The peel of the fruit is used for stomach aches and high blood pressure.[3, 4] The Basque people in Europe use the leaves for stomach aches, insomnia, and palpitations and the bitter orange peel as an anti-spasmodic.[5] In traditional Chinese medicine, the peel of the immature fruit is used for indigestion, abdominal pain, constipation, and dysenteric diarrhea. Where the patient is weak, the milder, mature fruit is used similarly.[6] Bitter orange continues to be widely used for insomnia and indigestion in many parts of the world.[7]

Active constituents

Bitter orange has a complex chemical makeup, though it is perhaps most known for the volatile oil in the peel. The familiar oily residue that appears after peeling citrus fruit, including bitter orange, is this volatile oil. It gives bitter orange its strong odor and flavor, and accounts for many of its medicinal effects. Besides the volatile oil, the peel contains flavones, the alkaloids synephrine, octopamine, and N-methyltyramine, and carotenoids.[8, 9]

How much is usually taken?

Usually 1 to 2 grams of dried peel is simmered for 10 to 15 minutes in a cup of water; three cups are drunk daily. As a tincture, 2 to 3 ml (with a weight-to-volume ratio ranging from 1:1 to 1:5) is often recommended

for use three times per day.[10] The purified volatile oil is generally avoided for reasons discussed in the side effects section.

Are there any side effects or interactions?

Bitter orange oil may possibly cause light sensitivity (photosensitivity), especially in fair-skinned individuals.[11] Generally this occurs only if the oil is applied directly to the skin and then exposed to bright light; in rare cases it has also been known to occur in people who have taken bitter orange internally. The oil should not be applied topically and anyone who uses it internally should avoid bright light, including tanning booths.

Internal use of the volatile oil of bitter orange is also potentially unsafe and should not be undertaken without expert guidance. Large amounts of orange peel have caused intestinal colic, convulsions, and death in children.[12] The amounts recommended above for internal use should not be exceeded.

One text on Chinese medicine cautions against the use of bitter orange in pregnancy.[13] This concern is not raised in any other reference, and the American Herbal Products Association classifies the herb as "class 1," an herb that can be safely consumed during pregnancy when used appropriately.[14]

Decoctions of bitter orange substantially increased blood levels of cyclosporine in pigs, causing toxicity.[15] Bitter orange also inhibited human cytochrome P450 3A (CYP3A) in the test tube.[16] This is an enzyme that helps the liver get rid of numerous toxins, and strongly affects metabolism of certain drugs. Bitter orange might, therefore, interact with drugs that are metabolized by CYP3A. To be on the safe side, bitter orange should not be combined with prescription medications, unless someone is under the care of an experienced natural medicine clinician.

BLACKBERRY

Common names: Dewberry, European blackberry
Botanical name: *Rubus fructicosus*

Parts used and where grown

Blackberries grow in wet areas across the United States and Europe. Several species of blackberry exist: *Rubus fructicosus* is the most common European species and

Rubus canadensis is a common North American species. While the leaves are used most frequently for medicinal preparations, the root is sometimes used as well.

Blackberry has been used in connection with the following conditions (refer to the individual health concern for complete information):

Rating	Health Concerns
★☆☆	**Common cold/sore throat** (page 129)
	Diarrhea (page 163)

Historical or traditional use (may or may not be supported by scientific studies)

Since ancient Greek physicians prescribed blackberry for **gout** (page 208), the leaves, roots, and even berries have been used as herbal medicines.[1] The most common uses were for treating **diarrhea** (page 163), **sore throats** (page 129), and **wounds** (page 319). These are similar to the uses of its close cousin, the **red raspberry** (page 735) *(Rubus idaeus),* and a somewhat more distant relative, the **blueberry** (page 641) *(Vaccinium corymbosum).*

Active constituents

The presence of large amounts of tannins give blackberry leaves and roots an astringent effect that may be useful for treating **diarrhea** (page 163).[2] These same constituents may also be helpful for soothing **sore throats** (page 129).

How much is usually taken?

The German Commission E monograph recommends 4.5 grams of blackberry leaf per day.[3] Blackberry tea is prepared by adding 1.5 grams of leaves or powdered root to 250 ml of boiling water and allowing it to steep for 10 to 15 minutes. Three cups per day should be drunk. Alternatively, one may use 3–4 ml of tincture three times each day.

Are there any side effects or interactions?

Tannins can cause nausea and even vomiting in people with sensitive stomachs. People with chronic gastrointestinal problems might be particularly at risk for such reactions. Taking blackberry leaf or root preparations with food may reduce risk of gastrointestinal problems in some people.

BLACK COHOSH

Botanical name: *Cimicifuga racemosa*

Parts used and where grown

Black cohosh is a shrub-like plant native to the eastern deciduous forests of North America, ranging from southern Ontario to Georgia, north to Wisconsin and west to Arkansas. The dried root and rhizome are used medicinally.[1] When harvested from the wild, the root is black in color. Cohosh, an Algonquin Indian word meaning "rough," refers to the plants gnarly root structure.[2]

Black cohosh has been used in connection with the following conditions (refer to the individual health concern for complete information):

Rating	Health Concerns
★★★	**Menopause** (page 311)
★☆☆	**Dysmenorrhea** (page 171) (painful menstruation)
	Osteoporosis (page 333)
	Premenstrual syndrome (page 368)

Historical or traditional use (may or may not be supported by scientific studies)

Native Americans valued the herb and used it for many conditions, ranging from gynecological problems to rattlesnake bites. Some 19th century American physicians used black cohosh for fever, menstrual cramps, arthritis, and **insomnia** (page 270).[3]

Active constituents

Black cohosh contains several ingredients, including triterpene glycosides (e.g., acetin and 27-deoxyactein) and isoflavones (e.g., formononetin). Other constituents include aromatic acids, tannins, resins, fatty acids, starches, and sugars. As a woman approaches **menopause** (page 311), the signals between the ovaries and pituitary gland diminish, slowing down estrogen production and increasing luteinizing hormone (LH) secretions. Hot flashes can result from these hormonal changes. Earlier animal studies[4, 5] and a human clinical trial[6] suggested that black cohosh had some estrogen activity in the body and also decreased LH secretions. However, more recent animal studies[7] and a clinical trial[8] have found no estrogen activity for black cohosh extracts. Further clinical trials are needed to determine whether black cohosh has significant estrogenic actions in the body.

Small German clinical trials support the usefulness of black cohosh for women with hot flashes associated with menopause.[9, 10] A review of eight clinical trials found black cohosh to be both safe and effective for symptomatic relief of menopausal hot flashes.[11] Other symptoms which improved included night sweats, **insomnia** (page 270), nervousness, and irritability. A clinical trial compared the effects of 40 mg versus 130 mg of black cohosh in menopausal women with complaints of hot flashes.[12] While hot flashes were reduced equally at both amounts, there was no evidence of any estrogenic effect in any of the women. Although further trials are needed, this trial suggests that black cohosh is best reserved only for the symptomatic treatment of hot flashes associated with menopause and is not thought to be a substitute for hormone replacement therapy in menopausal and postmenopausal women.

A recent study suggests black cohosh may protect animals from **osteoporosis** (page 333).[13] Human studies have not confirmed this action.

How much is usually taken?

Black cohosh can be taken in several forms, including crude, dried root or rhizome (300–2,000 mg per day), or as a solid, dry powdered extract (250 mg three times per day). Standardized extracts of the herb are available. The recommended amount is 20–40 mg twice per day.[14] The best researched extract provides 1 mg of deoxyactein per 20 mg of extract. Tinctures can be taken at 2–4 ml three times per day.[15] Black cohosh can be taken for up to six months, and then it should be discontinued.[16]

Are there any side effects or interactions?

Black cohosh should not be used by **pregnant** (page 363) or **breast-feeding women** (page 74).[17] Very large amounts (over several grams daily) of this herb may cause abdominal pain, nausea, headaches, and dizziness. There is one case report of a woman developing autoimmune hepatitis while using black cohosh.[18] A cause–effect relationship is in doubt, however, because the hepatitis did not resolve after black cohosh was discontinued. A few cases have also been reported in which severe liver failure was attributed to the use of black cohosh.[19] While a cause–effect relationship is difficult to prove, and while such a side effect appears to

be rare, people taking black cohosh should be alert to signs of possible liver disease, such as nausea, loss of appetite, fatigue, and tan-colored urine. Black cohosh is not a substitute for hormone replacement therapy during **menopause** (page 311).

BLACK HOREHOUND

Botanical name: *Ballota nigra*

Parts used and where grown

This European mint family (Lamiaceae) plant now grows in North America and on other continents as well. The leaf and flower are used medicinally. This plant should not be confused with **white horehound** (page 691), which acts differently.

Black horehound has been used in connection with the following conditions (refer to the individual health concern for complete information):

Rating	Health Concerns
★☆☆	**Motion sickness** (page 322)
	Nausea

Historical or traditional use (may or may not be supported by scientific studies)

Black horehound has primarily been used in European traditional herbalism to relieve nausea, **anxiety** (page 30), or the combination of these conditions.[1] It was also used as a mild expectorant and to help normalize menstruation.

Active constituents

Phenylpropanoids—flavonoids and compounds found in the volatile oil of black horehound—are believed to be the plant's major active constituents.[2, 3] A recent test tube study found black horehound phenylpropanoids to have both **antioxidant** (page 467) properties and a sedating effect on overactive nerve cells.[4] Although no human studies have been conducted with black horehound, the herb is believed to be useful for treating nausea associated **motion sickness** (page 322) due to a possible effect on the central nervous system.[5]

How much is usually taken?

Black horehound is traditionally used as a tea or tincture. Approximately 2 teaspoons of the leaves are added to 1 cup hot water and allowed to steep for 10 to 15 minutes.[6] One cup is drunk three times per day. If a tincture is preferred, 1 to 2 ml may be taken three times per day. Black horehound is rarely used alone, and is frequently combined with **meadowsweet** (page 709), **chamomile** (page 656), or **ginger** (page 680) for relief of nausea.

Are there any side effects or interactions?

There are no reports of adverse effects from use of black horehound when taken in the amounts listed above. Black horehound was traditionally used to treat **nausea during pregnancy** (page 363), though no scientific evaluation of the safety or efficacy of this practice has been conducted. Some sources report that black horehound could induce miscarriage when taken in large amounts.[7] Consult with a doctor who is trained in botanical medicine before using horehound during pregnancy.

BLADDERWRACK

Botanical name: *Fucus vesiculosus*

Parts used and where grown

Bladderwrack is a type of brown algae (seaweed) that grows on the northern Atlantic and Pacific coasts of the United States and on the northern Atlantic coast and Baltic coast of Europe. The main stem of bladderwrack, known as the thallus, is used medicinally. The thallus has tough, air-filled pods or bladders to help the algae float—thus the name bladderwrack. Although bladderwrack is sometimes called kelp, that name is not specific to this species and should be avoided.

Bladderwrack has been used in connection with the following conditions (refer to the individual health concern for complete information):

Rating	Health Concerns
★☆☆	**Constipation** (page 137)
	Diarrhea (page 163)
	Gastritis (page 195)
	Gastroesophageal Reflux Disease (page 198) (GERD)
	Heartburn (page 260)
	Hypothyroidism (page 252)
	Indigestion (page 260)
	Iodine deficiency
	Wound healing (page 319) (topical)

Historical or traditional use (may or may not be supported by scientific studies)

Bladderwrack's mucilaginous thallus has long been used to soothe irritated and inflamed tissues in the body.[1] It was also historically used as a bulk-forming laxative.[2] People living near oceans or seas have a historically low rate of **hypothyroidism** (page 252), due, in part, to ingestion of iodine-rich food, such as seafood and seaweeds like bladderwrack. It has also been used to counter **obesity** (page 446), possibly due to its reputation for stimulating the thyroid gland. Clinical research in this area has failed to confirm that seaweeds like bladderwrack help with weight loss,[3] though more specific research is warranted.

Active constituents

There are three major active constituents in bladderwrack: **iodine** (page 538), alginic acid, and fucoidan.

The amount of iodine in bladderwrack is highly variable,[4] probably as a result of different amounts of iodine in the water where it grows. A reasonable portion of bladderwrack may contain the U.S. adult recommended dietary allowance (RDA) of iodine (150 mcg). The RDA amount of iodine is believed to be necessary for maintenance of normal thyroid function in adults (infants and children need proportionally less). Thus, in people with insufficient iodine in their diet, bladderwrack may serve as a supplemental source of iodine. Either **hypothyroidism** (page 252) or **goiter** (page 206) due to insufficient intake of iodine may possibly improve with bladderwrack supplementation, though human studies have not confirmed this.

Alginic acid is a type of dietary **fiber** (page 512) that can be used to help relieve **constipation** (page 137) and **diarrhea** (page 163). However, human studies have not been done on how effective bladderwrack is for either of these conditions. An over-the-counter antacid, Gaviscon, containing magnesium carbonate and sodium alginate (the sodium salt of alginic acid), has been shown to effectively relieve the symptoms of **heartburn** (page 260) compared to other antacids in a double-blind study.[5] However, bladderwrack has not been studied for use in people with heartburn. Bladderwrack might also help indigestion, though again clinical trials have not been conducted. Calcium alginate (the calcium salt of alginic acid) has shown promise as an agent to speed **wound healing** (page 319) in animal studies[6] but has not been demonstrated to be effective in humans.

Alginic acid has also been shown to inhibit **HIV** (page 239) in the test tube.[7] However, this effect has

Bladderwrack

not been studied in humans. Alginic acid may help lower LDL ("bad") **cholesterol** (page 223) levels, according to animal studies.[8] No human trials have studied this effect of bladderwrack. It is widely used in food and pharmaceuticals as a thickener and gelling agent.[9]

Fucoidan is another type of dietary fiber in bladderwrack that contains numerous sulfur groups. According to test tube and animal studies, this appears to give fucoidan several properties, such as lowering LDL cholesterol levels,[10] lowering blood glucose levels,[11] anti-inflammatory activity,[12] possible anticoagulant effects,[13] and antibacterial[14] and anti-HIV activity.[15] Though it has not been definitively proven, fucoidan is thought to prevent bacteria and viruses from binding to human cells, a necessary step in starting an **infection** (page 265), as opposed to killing the microbes directly.[16, 17] To date, no human clinical trials have been done with fucoidan or bladderwrack to support their use for any of these conditions.

How much is usually taken?

For short-term use (a few days) to relieve **constipation** (page 137), powdered bladderwrack can be taken in the amount of 1 teaspoon three times per day along with at least 8 oz of water each time.[18] For **thyroid problems** (page 252), **gastritis** (page 195), or **heartburn** (page 260), 5 to 10 grams of dried bladderwrack in capsules three times per day has been recommended. Alternately, bladderwrack may be eaten whole or made into a tea using 1 teaspoon per cup of hot water, allowing each cup to sit at least 10 minutes before drinking. Three cups per day of tea can be drunk. No more than 150 mcg **iodine** (page 538) should be consumed from all sources, including bladderwrack, per day.[19] However, most bladderwrack products do not give any indication of their iodine content. Therefore, anyone considering taking bladderwrack should first consult a physician trained in nutrition and herbal medicine.

Are there any side effects or interactions?

Bladderwrack is generally safe, though there are three potential problems with its consumption: **acne** (page 4), thyroid dysfunction, and heavy-metal contamination. Iodine in any form—including from bladderwrack and other seaweeds—can cause or aggravate acne in some people.[20] Excessive iodine ingestion can cause either hypothyroidism or hyperthyroidism and should be avoided.[21, 22] Bladderwrack and other seaweeds that grow in heavy-metal-contaminated waters may contain high levels of these toxins (particularly arsenic and

lead), leading to nerve damage,[23] kidney damage,[24] or other problems. Only bladderwrack known to have been harvested from clean water or labeled to indicate the absence of heavy metals or other contaminants should be consumed. The safety of using bladderwrack during **pregnancy** (page 363) and **breast-feeding** (page 74) is unknown. People who are allergic to iodine may need to avoid bladderwrack.

BLESSED THISTLE

Botanical name: *Cnicus benedictus*

Parts used and where grown

Although native to Europe and Asia, blessed thistle is now cultivated in many areas of the world, including the United States. The leaves, stems, and flowers are all used in herbal preparations.

Blessed thistle has been used in connection with the following conditions (refer to the individual health concern for complete information):

Rating	Health Concerns
★☆☆	**Indigestion and heartburn** (page 260) Poor appetite

Historical or traditional use (may or may not be supported by scientific studies)

Folk medicine used blessed thistle tea for digestive problems, including gas, **constipation** (page 137), and stomach upset. This herb was also used—like its well-known relative, **milk thistle** (page 710)[1]—for liver and gallbladder diseases.

Active constituents

The sesquiterpene lactones, such as cnicin, provide the main beneficial effects of blessed thistle in the treatment of **indigestion** (page 260). The bitterness of these compounds stimulates digestive activity, including the flow of saliva and secretion of gastric juice, which leads to improved appetite and digestion.[2] Some pharmacological evidence suggests that blessed thistle may also have anti-inflammatory properties.[3]

How much is usually taken?

The German Commission E monograph recommends 4–6 grams of blessed thistle per day.[4] Alternatively, tincture (½ teaspoon [2 ml] three times per day) may be used. Approximately ½ teaspoon (2 grams) of the dried herb can also be added to 1 cup (250 ml) of boiling water and steeped 10 to 15 minutes to make a tea. Three cups can be drunk each day.

Are there any side effects or interactions?
Blessed thistle is generally safe and is not associated with side effects. Anyone with **allergies** (page 14) to plants in the daisy family should use blessed thistle cautiously.

BLOODROOT

Botanical name: *Sanguinaria canadensis*

Parts used and where grown
Bloodroot grows primarily in North America and in India. The rhizomes and root of the plant contain an orange-red latex.

Bloodroot has been used in connection with the following conditions (refer to the individual health concern for complete information):

Rating	Health Concerns
★★☆	**Gingivitis** (page 203) (periodontal disease)
★☆☆	**Cough** (page 139) **Halitosis** (page 209) (rinse)

Historical or traditional use (may or may not be supported by scientific studies)
Native Americans employed bloodroot extensively in ritual and medicine. The dye was used as a body paint.[1] **Sore throats** (page 129), **cough** (page 139), rheumatic pains, and various types of **cancer** (page 87) were all treated with bloodroot.

Active constituents
Alkaloids—principally sanguinarine—constitute the primary active compounds in bloodroot. These are sometimes used in toothpaste and other oral hygiene products because they inhibit the growth of oral bacteria.[2, 3] Not all trials have found sanguinaria-containing dental products helpful for gum disease, however.[4]

How much is usually taken?
Sanguinarine-containing toothpastes and mouth rinses should be used according to manufacturer's directions.

Bloodroot tincture is sometimes included in **cough** (page 139)-relieving formulas, and 10 drops or less may be taken three times per day.[5] However, bloodroot is rarely used alone for this purpose.

Are there any side effects or interactions?
Although previous studies have suggested the long-term use of dental products containing sanguinarine is safe,[6] a recent report suggests that use of dental preparations containing blood root may be associated with **leukoplakia** (page 289)—a condition characterized by white spots or patches in the mouth that is thought to be precancerous.[7] Only small amounts of bloodroot should be taken internally, since amounts as small as 1 ml (approximately 20–30 drops) of tincture or 1 gram (approximately 1/30th ounce) can cause nausea and vomiting.[8, 9]

Long-term use or overdose of bloodroot can also cause stomach pain, **diarrhea** (page 163), visual changes, paralysis, fainting, and collapse.[10] Long-term oral intake of sanguinarine-contaminated cooking oils has been linked in India to **glaucoma** (page 205), **edema** (page 180), **heart disease** (page 98), miscarriage, and diarrhea.[11] The sanguinarine in these cases came from plants other than bloodroot. Nevertheless, bloodroot should not be used long term. The plant is unsafe for use in children and should not be used by **pregnant** (page 363) or lactating women.

Recently the practice of applying ointments containing bloodroot, such as the so-called "black salve," has been promoted for treatment of skin and other types of **cancer** (page 87).[12] These ointments have never been tested in clinical studies, so their efficacy for treating cancer is unknown. They can cause severe **pain** (page 338), **burns** (page 85), and damage to healthy skin. It is imperative to seek professional diagnosis and treatment for all forms of cancer.

BLUEBERRY

Botanical name: *Vaccinium* spp.

Parts used and where grown
Blueberry is closely related to the European **bilberry** (page 634) *(Vaccinium myrtillus)*. Several species of blueberries exist—including *V. pallidum* and *V. corymbosum*—and grow throughout the United States. Blueberry leaves are the primary part of the plant used medicinally. However, the berries are occasionally used.

Blueberry has been used in connection with the following conditions (refer to the individual health concern for complete information):

Rating	Health Concerns
★☆☆	**Common cold/sore throat** (page 129)
	Diarrhea (page 163)
	Urinary tract infection (page 436)

Historical or traditional use (may or may not be supported by scientific studies)

According to traditional herbal textbooks, a tea made from blueberry leaves was considered helpful in **diabetes** (page 152), **urinary tract infections** (page 436), and poor appetite.[1] The berries were a prized commodity among the indigenous peoples of North America.

Active constituents

Tannins make up as much as 10% of blueberry leaves. The astringent nature of tannins likely accounts for the usefulness of blueberry leaf in treating **diarrhea** (page 163).[2] The astringent effect may also be soothing for **sore throats** (page 129).[3] **Bilberry** (page 634), blueberry's European cousin, is used primarily for maintaining blood vessels, particularly those in the eyes. Some preliminary evidence indicates that anthocyanosides, the bioflavonoid complex common to bilberry and blueberry may help people with **diabetes** (page 152), particularly if they have damage to the retina (**retinopathy** [page 385]). However, these studies are primarily based on a standardized extract from bilberry fruit.[4]

How much is usually taken?

A tea is prepared by combining 1 cup (250 ml) boiling water and 1–2 teaspoons (5–10 grams) of dried leaves and steeping for 15 minutes. As many as 6 cups (1,500 ml) each day may be taken for diarrhea and 3 cups (750 ml) each day for diabetes. Alternatively, 1 teaspoon (5 ml) of tincture can also be used three times per day.

Are there any side effects or interactions?

If the tea does not significantly reduce diarrhea within two to three days, consult with a healthcare practitioner. Fresh (but not dried) berries tend to be laxative and should be avoided in cases of **diarrhea** (page 163).[5]

BLUE COHOSH

Botanical name: *Caulophyllum thalictroides*

Parts used and where grown

Blue cohosh grows throughout North America. The roots of this flower are used medicinally. Blue cohosh is not related to **black cohosh** (page 637) *(Cimicifuga racemosa)*. However, both herbs are primarily used to treat women's health problems.

Blue cohosh has been used in connection with the following conditions (refer to the individual health concern for complete information):

Rating	Health Concerns
★☆☆	**Amenorrhea** (page 22) (lack of menstruation)
	Dysmenorrhea (page 171) (painful menstruation)

Historical or traditional use (may or may not be supported by scientific studies)

Native Americans are believed to have used blue cohosh flowers to induce labor and menstruation.[1] Blue cohosh is a traditional remedy for lack of menstruation. It is considered an emmenagogue (agent that stimulates menstrual flow) and a uterine tonic. No clinical trials have validated this traditional use. It has also been used traditionally to treat painful periods (**dysmenorrhea** [page 171]). Early-20th-century physicians in the United States who treated with natural remedies (known as Eclectic physicians) used blue cohosh for these same purposes and also to treat kidney infections, arthritis, and other ailments.

Active constituents

A saponin from blue cohosh called caulosaponin is believed to stimulate uterine contractions.[2] Several other alkaloids may be active in this herb. However, current research about the active constituents of blue cohosh is insufficient.

How much is usually taken?

Blue cohosh is generally taken as a tincture and should be limited to no more than 1–2 ml taken three times per day. The whole herb (300–1,000 mg per day) is sometimes used. Blue cohosh is generally used in combination with other herbs.

Blueberry

Are there any side effects or interactions?

Large amounts of blue cohosh can cause nausea, headaches, and **high blood pressure** (page 246). Blue cohosh should only be used under medical supervision and in limited amounts. Using blue cohosh during **pregnancy** (page 363) has been brought into question by reports of an infant developing a stroke and another infant being born with **congestive heart failure** (page 134).[3, 4] Safety studies need to be completed to determine whether blue cohosh is safe to use during pregnancy.

BLUE FLAG

Botanical name: *Iris versicolor*

Parts used and where grown

The rhizome, or underground stem, of the blue flag (indicating its showy blue flowers) is used medicinally. Blue flag and closely related species (particularly *Iris missouriensis,* western blue flag) grow across North America.

Blue flag has been used in connection with the following conditions (refer to the individual health concern for complete information):

Rating	Health Concerns
★☆☆	Impetigo (topical)

Historical or traditional use (may or may not be supported by scientific studies)

Based on Native American traditions, Eclectic physicians (19th century doctors who relied on herbs) and herbalists used blue flag for a number of conditions. Of note was its use as a nonspecific **immune enhancer** (page 255), as a laxative, and to detoxify the intestinal tract.[1] Topical application of fresh, sliced rhizomes to the sores of impetigo (a common bacterial skin infection in children) has been recommended by herbalists.[2] Traditional herbalists have used blue flag to treat poor digestion characterized by fat malabsorption.

Active constituents

The resinous fraction of blue flag contains numerous phenolic glycosides. Traditional herbal texts suggest these constituents stimulate the parasympathetic nervous system, leading to production of bile, saliva, and sweat.[3] However, modern clinical trials have not confirmed these effects for blue flag.

How much is usually taken?

Herbalists sometimes recommend up to 10 drops of tincture of the dried rhizome be taken three times per day.[4] The tea form is unlikely to be effective, since the active compounds in blue flag are not water soluble.

Are there any side effects or interactions?

Blue flag can cause nausea, vomiting, and loose stools if too much is taken.[5] People should not exceed the recommended amount given above. Fresh rhizome should only be applied topically and never taken internally, since it can irritate the mouth[6] and is much more likely to cause nausea and **diarrhea** (page 163). Blue flag should only be taken on the advice of a physician or herbalist trained in its use. Blue flag is unsafe for use during **pregnancy** (page 363) or breast-feeding. People should not give blue flag to children.

BOLDO

Botanical name: *Peumus boldus*

Parts used and where grown

Boldo is an evergreen shrub or small tree that is native to Chile and is naturalized to the Mediterranean region of Europe. The leaves are used medicinally.[1]

Boldo has been used in connection with the following conditions (refer to the individual health concern for complete information):

Rating	Health Concerns
★☆☆	**Indigestion and heartburn** (page 260)

Historical or traditional use (may or may not be supported by scientific studies)

Boldo has a long history of use by the indigenous people of Chile, as a liver tonic and in the treatment of **gallstones** (page 193).

Active constituents

Boldo contains several types of primary constituents, including volatile oils (e.g., ascaridole, eucalyptol), **flavonoids** (page 516), and alkaloids. Boldine, which constitutes about one-fourth of the total number of alkaloids present, is the major alkaloid.[2] Scientists believe that boldine is responsible for the plant's choloretic (bile stimulating) and diuretic actions.[3] In conjunction with other herbs, such as **cascara** (page 652), rhubarb, and **gentian** (page 680), boldo has been reported to improve appetite.[4] Ascaridole, a compound found in the volatile oil of the plant, has been used as an anti-parasitic agent but is no longer recommended due its to toxic side effects.[5]

How much is usually taken?

Tinctures that are free of ascaridoles are sometimes recommended. People may take 1 ml of tincture three times per day. Volatile oil of boldo is not recommended due to its high ascaridole content.[6, 7] The dried leaf can be used as an infusion at 3 grams per day.

Are there any side effects or interactions?

The German Commission E monograph[8] suggests that only an ascaridole-free preparation should be used internally. Boldo contains terpene-4-ol, an ingredient similar to that found in **juniper** (page 698), and should be avoided by people with kidney disease, as it could cause kidney irritation.[9] In addition, the herb should not be taken during **pregnancy** (page 363) or breast-feeding. It should also be avoided by people who have obstruction of the liver bile duct, or severe liver disease.[10] Excessive use of the herb over long time periods (more than three to four weeks continuously) is not recommended.

BONESET

Botanical name: *Eupatorium perfoliatum*

Parts used and where grown

Boneset belongs to the same botanical family as **echinacea** (page 669) and daisy *(Asteraceae)*. It grows primarily in North America. Boneset's leaves and flowering tops are used medicinally.

Boneset has been used in connection with the following conditions (refer to the individual health concern for complete information):

Rating	Health Concerns
★☆☆	**Common cold/sore throat** (page 129) **Influenza** (page 269)

Historical or traditional use (may or may not be supported by scientific studies)

Native Americans used boneset as a treatment for a wide range of infectious and fever-related conditions. Europeans eventually adopted the use of the plant, and extended its traditional uses to include malaria.[1]

Active constituents

Boneset contains sesquiterpene lactones, such as euperfolin, euperfolitin, and eufoliatin, as well as polysaccharides and **flavonoids** (page 516). In a test tube study, a particular polysaccharide in boneset was found to stimulate **immune cell function** (page 255).[2] This may partially explain its use to treat minor viral infections, such as **colds** (page 129) and the **flu** (page 269). Boneset also triggers sweating by raising body temperature, potentially of benefit for colds and flu as well.[3]

How much is usually taken?

Traditionally, boneset is taken as a tea or tincture. To prepare a tea, boiling water is added to ¼–½ teaspoon (1–2 grams) of the herb and allowed to steep, covered, for ten to fifteen minutes. Three cups (750 ml) a day may be taken (the tea is quite bitter). Tincture, ¼–¾ teaspoon (1–4 ml) three times per day, is also often taken.[4]

Are there any side effects or interactions?

A small number of people experience nausea and/or vomiting when using boneset. The fresh plant, however, is more likely to cause this than the dried herb. Although potentially liver-damaging chemicals, called pyrrolizidine alkaloids, are found in some plants similar to boneset, the levels in boneset are minimal. There are no known reports of liver damage from taking boneset. Nevertheless, patients with liver disease should avoid boneset, and no one should take it consistently for longer than six months. Boneset is not recommended during **pregnancy** (page 363) or breast-feeding. Boneset should not be used when a high fever (over 102 degrees F) is present.

BOSWELLIA

Common name: Salai guggal
Botanical name: *Boswellia serrata*

Parts used and where grown

Boswellia is a moderate to large branching tree found in the dry hilly areas of India. When the tree trunk is tapped, a gummy oleoresin is exuded. A purified extract of this resin is used in modern herbal preparations.

Boswellia has been used in connection with the following conditions (refer to the individual health concern for complete information):

Rating	Health Concerns
★★★	**Osteoarthritis** (page 328)
★★☆	**Asthma** (page 32) **Rheumatoid arthritis** (page 387) **Ulcerative colitis** (page 433)
★☆☆	**Bursitis** (page 87)

Historical or traditional use (may or may not be supported by scientific studies)

In the ancient Ayurvedic medical texts of India, the gummy exudate from boswellia is grouped with other gum resins and referred to collectively as guggals. Historically, the guggals were recommended by Ayurvedic physicians for a variety of conditions, including **osteoarthritis** (page 328), **rheumatoid arthritis** (page 387), **diarrhea** (page 163), dysentery, pulmonary disease, and ringworm.

Active constituents

The gum oleoresin consists of essential oils, gum, and terpenoids. The terpenoid portion contains the boswellic acids that have been shown to be the active constituents in boswellia.[1] Today, extracts are typically standardized to contain 37.5–65% boswellic acids.

Studies have shown that boswellic acids have an anti-inflammatory action[2]—much like the conventional nonsteroidal anti-inflammatory drugs (NSAIDs) used for inflammatory conditions. Boswellia inhibits pro-inflammatory mediators in the body, such as leukotrienes.[3] As opposed to NSAIDs, long-term use of boswellia does not appear to cause irritation or ulceration of the stomach. One small, controlled, double-blind trial has shown that boswellia extract may be helpful for **ulcerative colitis** (page 433).[4]

How much is usually taken?

The standardized extract of the gum oleoresin of boswellia is recommended by many doctors. For **rheumatoid arthritis** (page 387) or **osteoarthritis** (page 328), 150 mg of boswellic acids are taken three times per day.[5] As an example, if an extract contains 37.5% boswellic acids, 400 mg of the extract would be

taken three times daily. Treatment with boswellia generally lasts eight to twelve weeks. In the one clinical trial to date, people with **ulcerative colitis** (page 433) used 550 mg of boswellia extract three times per day.

Are there any side effects or interactions?

Boswellia is generally safe when used as directed. Rare side effects can include **diarrhea** (page 163), skin rash, and nausea. Any inflammatory joint condition should be closely monitored by a physician.

BUCHU

Botanical names: *Barosma betulina, Agathosma betulina, Agathosma crenultata*

Parts used and where grown

Buchu is a low shrub native to the Cape region of South Africa. The dried leaves are harvested during the flowering season. The oil can be obtained by steam distillation of the leaves. The two primary species of buchu used commercially are *Agathosma betulina* (syn. *Barosma betulina)* and *Agathosma crenulata* (syn. *Barosma crenultata).*

Buchu has been used in connection with the following conditions (refer to the individual health concern for complete information):

Rating	Health Concerns
★☆☆	**Urinary tract infections and inflammation** (page 436)

Historical or traditional use (may or may not be supported by scientific studies)

Buchu leaf preparations have a long history of use in traditional herbal medicine as a urinary tract disinfectant and diuretic.[1] Buchu was used by herbalists to treat **urinary tract infections** (page 436) and inflammation, as well as inflammation of the prostate. In Europe, it was also used to treat **gout** (page 208).[2] The original use of buchu by the native peoples of southern Africa is unclear because buchu is a general term for aromatic plants.[3] It appears to have been applied topically, possibly as an insect repellant, and also used internally for stomach problems, rheumatism and bladder problems.

Active constituents

The leaves of buchu contain 1.0–3.5% volatile oils as well as flavonoids.[4] The urinary tract antiseptic actions of buchu are thought to be due to the volatile oils. The primary volatile oil component thought to have anti-bacterial action is the monoterpene disophenol. However, one test tube study using buchu oil found no significant antibacterial effect.[5]

How much is usually taken?

The German Commission E Monograph concludes there is insufficient evidence to support the modern use of buchu for the treatment of urinary tract infections or inflammation.[6] However, some traditional herbal practitioners continue to recommend the herb for these conditions. Traditional recommendations for the herb include the use of 1–2 grams of the dried leaf taken three times daily in capsules or in a tea.[7] Tinctures can be used at 2–4 ml three times per day.

Are there any side effects or interactions?

Buchu may cause gastrointestinal irritation and should only be taken with meals. Also, it should not be used by **pregnant** (page 363) or breast-feeding women.

BUCKTHORN

Botanical name: *Rhamnus catharticus*

Parts used and where grown

Buckthorn is a tall shrub native to northern Europe. The dried berries and dried bark are used medicinally. The bark is allowed to dry for up to a year before being used, which reduces the potential of buckthorn to cause vomiting.

Buckthorn has been used in connection with the following conditions (refer to the individual health concern for complete information):

Rating	Health Concerns
★★☆	**Constipation** (page 137)

Historical or traditional use (may or may not be supported by scientific studies)

Buckthorn has been used as a cathartic laxative in northern and central Europe, including England, for centuries.[1] While its importance declined when the similar shrub *Rhamnus purshiana* or **Cascara sagrada** (page 652) was discovered in America,[2] buckthorn is still used, particularly in Europe.

Active constituents

Buckthorn bark and berries are high in anthraquinone glycosides. Resins, tannins, and lipids make up the bulk of the bark's other ingredients. Buckthorn berries also contain flavonoids. Anthraquinone glycosides have a cathartic action, inducing the large intestine to increase its muscular contraction (peristalsis) and increasing water movement from the cells of the colon into the feces, resulting in strong, soft bowel movement.[3] It takes six to ten hours for buckthorn to act after taking it by mouth.

How much is usually taken?

Only the dried form of buckthorn berries and bark should be used. Capsules providing 20 to 30 mg of anthraquinone glycosides (calculated as glucofrangulin A) per day can be used; however, the smallest amount necessary to maintain regular bowel movements should be used.[4] As a tincture, 5 ml once at bedtime is generally taken. Usually buckthorn is taken at bedtime, so it will have time to act and by morning a bowel movement is induced. It is important to drink eight six-ounce glasses of water throughout the day while taking buckthorn, and to consume plenty of fresh fruits and vegetables. Buckthorn should be taken for a maximum of eight to ten days consecutively or else it can lead to dependence on it to have a bowel movement.[5] Some people take peppermint tea or capsules with buckthorn to prevent griping, an unpleasant sensation of strong contractions in the colon sometimes induced by buckthorn.

Are there any side effects or interactions?

Buckthorn may turn the urine dark yellow or red, but this is harmless. Women who are pregnant or breast-feeding and children under the age of 12 should not use buckthorn without the advice of a physician. Those with an intestinal obstruction, **Crohn's disease** (page 141) or any other acute inflammatory problem in the intestines, **diarrhea** (page 163), appendicitis, or abdominal pain should not use this herb.[6] Use or abuse of buckthorn for more than ten days consecutively may cause a loss of electrolytes (especially the mineral potassium) or may weaken the colon. Long-term use can also cause kidney damage.[7]

Buchu

BUGLEWEED

Botanical name: *Lycopus virginicus*

Parts used and where grown
The leaves and flowers of this plant from the mint family are used medicinally. Both bugleweed and its European cousin, gypsywort *(Lycopus europaeus)*, grow in very wet areas.

Bugleweed has been used in connection with the following conditions (refer to the individual health concern for complete information):

Rating	Health Concerns
★☆☆	Breast pain
	Hyperthyroidism

Historical or traditional use (may or may not be supported by scientific studies)
The modern applications of bugleweed, unlike many medicinal plants, do not match its traditional use. Historically, bugleweed and related species were used to treat coughs and as a sedative.[1] Today, the main use of this herb is for treating mild hyperthyroidism.

Active constituents
Lithospermic acid and other organic acids are believed to be responsible for bugleweed's activity. These acids decrease levels of several hormones in the body, particularly thyroid-stimulating hormones[2] and the thyroid hormone thyroxine (T4).[3] Bugleweed inhibits the binding of antibodies to the thyroid gland.[4] These antibodies can cause the most common form of hyperthyroidism, Graves' disease. All these actions may help explain bugleweed's benefit in people with mildly overactive thyroids.

How much is usually taken?
The German Commission E monograph recommends 1–2 grams of the whole herb per day.[5] Intake of tincture should be limited to 1–2 ml three times a day. Bugleweed is often combined with other herbs used to treat mildly overactive thyroid function, including **lemon balm** (page 701) *(Melissa officinalis)* and gromwell *(Lithospermum ruderale)*.

Are there any side effects or interactions?
Excessive intake of bugleweed by people with thyroid disease or use by healthy people may cause a potentially harmful decrease in thyroid function. Thyroid disease is dangerous and should only be treated under the supervision of a healthcare professional. However, long-term use of bugleweed is considered safe for people with hyperthyroidism.[6] Bugleweed should not be taken by people with **hypothyroidism** (page 252). Bugleweed should also not be used during **pregnancy** (page 363) and breast-feeding.[7]

BUPLEURUM

Common names: Thorowax, saiko, hare's ear, chai hu
Botanical names: *Bupleurum chinense, Bupleurum falcatum*

Parts used and where grown
These Asian plants are part of the *Apiaceae (Umbelliferae)* family, and resemble dill or fennel. However, bupleurum has long thin leaves rather than the lacy appearance of fennel and dill leaves. The Chinese name for bupleurum, *chai hu*, means "kindling of the barbarians." The origin of this name is unclear. The roots of the plant are used in herbal medicine.

Bupleurum has been used in connection with the following conditions (refer to the individual health concern for complete information):

Rating	Health Concerns
★★☆	**Epilepsy** (page 183)
	Hepatitis (page 220) (viral)
	Irritable bowel syndrome (page 280) (Chinese herbal combination formula containing **wormwood** [page 762], **ginger** [page 680], bupleurum, **schisandra** [page 744], dan shen, and other extracts)
	Liver cirrhosis (page 290)
★☆☆	**HIV/AIDS** (page 239)

Historical or traditional use (may or may not be supported by scientific studies)
Bupleurum has been used in Traditional Chinese Medicine for thousands of years to help relieve numerous conditions. Most particularly, **infections** (page 265) with fever, liver problems, **indigestion** (page 260), **hemorrhoids** (page 219), and uterine prolapse.[1]

Bupleurum is a key ingredient in the formula known as sho-saiko-to. This is a Japanese kampo or traditional herbal medicine formula based on the traditional Chinese formula xiao-chai-hu-tang. In English, it has been called minor bupleurum formula. Bupleurum makes up 16% of the formula for sho-saiko-to (see below for the complete contents of the formula). Results reported for sho-saiko-to cannot be attributed solely to bupleurum because the other herbs in the formula also contribute.[2]

Sho-saiko-to (xao-chai-hu-tang or minor bupleurum formula) contains the following:

- *Bupleurum falcatum* (thorowax) root, 16%
- *Paeonia lactiflora* (peony) root, 16%
- *Pinellia ternata* (ban xia) rhizome, 14%
- *Cinnamomum cassia* (cassia) bark, 11%
- *Zingiber officinale* (page 680) (ginger) rhizome, 11%
- *Zizyphus jujuba* (jujube) fruit, 11%
- *Panax ginseng* (page 630) (Asian ginseng) root, 8%
- *Scutellaria baicalensis* (page 658) (Chinese scullcap) root, 8%
- *Glycyrrhiza uralensis* (page 702) (licorice, gan cao) rhizome, 5%

Active constituents

Bupleurum contains constituents known as saikosaponins that appear to account for much of the medicinal activity of the plant. Test tube studies have shown that the sho-saiko-to combination can increase production of various chemicals (known as cytokines) that immune cells use to signal one another.[3] Test tube studies have also found that saikosaponins can inhibit growth of liver cancer cells,[4] and are anti-inflammatory.[5, 6]

Human trials, only one double-blind, have shown that the bupleurum-containing formula sho-saiko-to may help reduce symptoms and blood liver enzyme levels in children and adults with chronic active viral **hepatitis** (page 220).[7, 8, 9, 10] Most of these studies were in people with hepatitis B infection, though one preliminary human trial has also shown a benefit in people with hepatitis C.[11] Sho-saiko-to was also found, in a large, preliminary (but not double-blind), study to decrease the risk of people with chronic viral hepatitis developing liver cancer.[12]

Sho-saiko-to has also been used to reduce symptoms of and possibly decrease the severity of **liver cirrhosis** (page 290), though clinical studies on this condition are generally lacking. One randomized trial (it was unclear if this trial was double-blind) found that sho-saiko-to could reduce the rate of liver cancer in people with liver cirrhosis.[13]

Several uncontrolled trials in Japan have shown that sho-saiko-to or very similar traditional Japanese and Chinese herbal formulas (all containing bupleurum) can reduce seizure frequency and/or severity in people with **epilepsy** (page 183) that does not respond to anti-seizure medications.[14, 15, 16, 17] However, double-blind trials are still needed to determine the importance of these findings.

Sho-saiko-to has been found to inhibit human immunodeficiency virus (**HIV** [page 239]) in the test tube.[18] Yet, it is unclear to what degree bupleurum or saikosaponins contributed to this effect. Sho-saiko-to also increased the efficacy of the standard anti-HIV drug lamivudine in the test tube.[19] Human data are lacking on the benefit of sho-saiko-to or bupleurum in people with HIV infection or acquired immunodeficiency syndrome (AIDS).

How much is usually taken?

Generally 500–2,000 mg bupleurum dry root are taken three times daily in capsules.[20] Traditionally, and in some clinical studies, bupleurum was prepared as a tea in which the root is decocted or cooked for hours before use. Some people take 1–4 grams per cup of water, three times daily. Sho-saiko-to formula is typically given in capsules (1.8–2.5 grams) three times per day. The amount given to children should be proportionally reduced based on individual weight and height as compared to adults.[21]

Are there any side effects or interactions?

Bupleurum and sho-saiko-to taken as a tea can upset the stomach, an effect that tends to be lessened by taking them with food or in capsules. Bupleurum and sho-saiko-to are not recommended during **pregnancy** (page 363) and breast-feeding.

Sho-saiko-to has been used alone and with interferon to treat **hepatitis** (page 220). Eighty or more cases of drug-induced pneumonitis (inflammation of the lungs) have been associated with the use of sho-saiko-to alone or with interferon.[22, 23, 24, 25, 26] Until more is known, sho-saiko-to should not be combined with interferon.

BURDOCK

Botanical name: *Arctium lappa*

Parts used and where grown

Burdock is native to Asia and Europe. The root is the primary source of many herbal preparations. The root becomes very soft with chewing and tastes sweet, with a mucilaginous (sticky) texture.

Burdock has been used in connection with the following conditions (refer to the individual health concern for complete information):

Rating	Health Concerns
★☆☆	**Acne rosacea** (page 4)
	Acne vulgaris (page 6)
	Menopause (page 311)
	Psoriasis (page 379)
	Rheumatoid arthritis (page 387)

Historical or traditional use (may or may not be supported by scientific studies)

In traditional herbal texts, burdock root is described as a "blood purifier" or "alterative"[1] and was believed to clear the bloodstream of toxins. It was used both internally and externally for **eczema** (page 177) and **psoriasis** (page 379), as well as to treat painful joints and as a diuretic. In Traditional Chinese Medicine, burdock root in combination with other herbs is used to treat **sore throats** (page 129), tonsillitis, **colds** (page 129), and even **measles** (page 307).[2] In Japan, it is eaten as a vegetable.

Burdock root has recently become popular as part of a tea to treat **cancer** (page 87). To date, however, research is insufficient to promote burdock for this application.[3]

Active constituents

Burdock root contains high amounts of inulin and mucilage. This may explain its soothing effects on the gastrointestinal tract. Bitter constituents in the root may also explain the traditional use of burdock to improve digestion. Additionally, burdock has been shown to reduce liver damage in animal studies.[4] This has not been confirmed in human studies, however. It also contains polyacetylenes that have demonstrated anti-microbial activity.[5] Even though test tube and animal studies have indicated some anti-tumor activity in burdock root, these results have not been duplicated in human studies.[6] Several animal and test tubes studies have also suggested an anti-inflammatory effect of unknown compounds in burdock root or seeds, including an ability to inhibit the potent inflammation-causing chemical platelet activating factor.[7, 8]

How much is usually taken?

Traditional herbalists recommend 2–4 ml of burdock root tincture per day.[9] For the dried root preparation in capsule form, some herbalists recommend 1–2 grams three times per day. Many herbal preparations combine burdock root with other alterative "blood cleansing" herbs, such as **yellow dock** (page 763), **red clover** (page 735), or **cleavers** (page 660).

Are there any side effects or interactions?

Burdock root contains approximately 50% inulin,[10] a fiber widely distributed in fruits, vegetables and plants. Inulin is classified as a food ingredient (not as an additive) and is considered to be safe to eat.[11] In fact, inulin is a significant part of the daily diet of most of the world's population.[12] However, there is a report of a 39-year-old man having a life-threatening allergic reaction after consuming high amounts of inulin from multiple sources.[13] Allergy to inulin in this individual was confirmed by laboratory tests. Such sensitivities are exceedingly rare. Moreover, this man did not take burdock. Nevertheless, people with a confirmed sensitivity to inulin should avoid burdock. There is one published case report of a severe allergic reaction, apparently due to burdock itself.[14]

BUTCHER'S BROOM

Botanical name: *Ruscus aculeatus*

Parts used and where grown

Butcher's broom is a spiny, small-leafed evergreen bush native to the Mediterranean region and northwest Europe. It is a member of the lily family and is similar, in many ways, to asparagus. The roots and young stems of butcher's broom are used medicinally.

Butcher's broom has been used in connection with the following conditions (refer to the individual health concern for complete information):

Rating	Health Concerns
★★★	**Chronic venous insufficiency** (page 116)
★☆☆	**Atherosclerosis** (page 38)
	Varicose veins (page 440)

Historical or traditional use (may or may not be supported by scientific studies)

Butcher's broom is so named because the mature branches were bundled and used as brooms by butchers. The young shoots were sometimes eaten as food. Ancient physicians used the roots as a diuretic in the treatment of urinary problems.[1]

Active constituents

Steroidal saponins are thought to be responsible for the medicinal actions of butcher's broom.[2] These constituents are reported to improve the strength and tone of the veins and act as mild diuretics. They may also lead to constriction of the veins, which helps blood return from the extremities.[3, 4] Butcher's broom extracts also exert a mild anti-inflammatory effect.

Clinical trials, one double-blind, have confirmed the benefit of a combination of **vitamin C** (page 604), **flavonoids** (page 516), and butcher's broom for treatment of **chronic venous insufficiency** (page 116) (CVI).[5, 6] In a comparison study, a product combining butcher's broom extract, the flavonoid hesperidin, and vitamin C was more effective than a synthetic flavonoid product for treating CVI.[7] A double-blind study, in which Butcher's broom alone was used, has confirmed the beneficial effect of this herb in the treatment of CVI.[8]

How much is usually taken?

Encapsulated butcher's broom extracts, in the amount of 1,000 mg three times per day, can be used for **chronic venous insufficiency** (page 116). These extracts are often combined with vitamin C and/or flavonoids. Standardized extracts (9–11% ruscogenins) can be taken in the amount of 100 mg three times per day.

Are there any side effects or interactions?

Side effects are rarely seen if butcher's broom is used as directed above. However, in certain cases, butcher's broom can cause nausea.[9]

CALENDULA

Common name: Marigold
Botanical name: *Calendula officinalis*

Parts used and where grown

Calendula grows as a common garden plant throughout North America and Europe. The golden-orange or yellow flowers of calendula have been used as medicine for centuries.

Calendula has been used in connection with the following conditions (refer to the individual health concern for complete information):

Rating	Health Concerns
★★☆	**Dermatitis** (page 151) (radiation-induced)
★☆☆	**Breast-feeding support** (page 74) (topical for sore nipples)
	Burns (minor, including sunburn) (page 85)
	Conjunctivitis/blepharitis (page 136)
	Eczema (page 117)
	Peptic ulcer (page 349)
	Ulcerative colitis (page 433)
	Wound healing (page 319) (topical)

Historical or traditional use (may or may not be supported by scientific studies)

Calendula flowers were historically considered beneficial for reducing inflammation, **wound healing** (page 319), and as an antiseptic. Calendula was used to treat various skin diseases, ranging from skin ulcerations to **eczema** (page 117).[1] Internally, the soothing effects of calendula have been used for **stomach ulcers** (page 349) and inflammation. Traditionally, a sterile tea was topically applied in cases of **conjunctivitis** (page 136).

Active constituents

Flavonoids (page 516), found in high amounts in calendula, are thought to account for much of its anti-inflammatory activity.[2] Other potentially important constituents include the triterpene saponins[3] and **carotenoids** (page 488).

Investigations into anticancer and antiviral actions of calendula are continuing. At this time, insufficient evidence exists to recommend the use of calendula for **cancer** (page 87). Nevertheless, test tube studies have found antiviral activity for calendula.[4, 5] The constituents responsible for these actions are not clear, however, and the relevance of these actions for human health care has not been established.

How much is usually taken?

A tea of calendula can be made by pouring 1 cup (250 ml) of boiling water over 1–2 teaspoons (5–10 grams) of the flowers; the tea is then steeped, covered for ten to fifteen minutes, strained, and drunk.[6] At least 3 cups of tea are recommended per day. Tincture is similarly used three times a day, at ¼–½ teaspoon (1–2 ml) each time. The tincture can be taken in water or tea. In addition, prepared ointments can be used topically for skin problems, although wet dressings made by dipping a cloth into the cooled tea are also effective. Topical treatment for eye conditions is not recommended, as absolute sterility must be maintained.

Are there any side effects or interactions?
Side effects are rare with the use of calendula. Some people may experience a skin rash with topical use and should be tested to see if they are allergic to the herb.

CARAWAY

Botanical name: *Carum carvi*

Parts used and where grown
Caraway is a biennial that is widely cultivated throughout the world, and is native to Europe, Asia, and North Africa. The dried ripe fruit or seeds are used medicinally.[1]

Caraway has been used in connection with the following conditions (refer to the individual health concern for complete information):

Rating	Health Concerns
★★★	**Irritable bowel syndrome** (page 280) (combination with **peppermint** (page 726) oil)
★★☆	**Gingivitis** (page 203) (periodontal disease) (as mouthwash, in combination with **sage** [page 740], **peppermint** [page 726] oil, menthol, **chamomile** [page 656] tincture, expressed juice from **echinacea** [page 669], **myrrh** [page 713] tincture, and clove oil) **Indigestion** (page 260)
★☆☆	**Colic** (page 121)

Historical or traditional use (may or may not be supported by scientific studies)
The use of caraway as a medicinal agent has remained unchanged for centuries. Its use as a digestive aid was first mentioned in the Egyptian *Eberus Papyrus* about 1500 B.C.[2] In Shakespeare's *Henry IV,* the character Falstaff is invited to have a serving of baked apples and caraway to aid the digestion and relieve gas.[3] Nine-

teenth-century American Eclectic physicians (doctors who recommended herbs), such as Harvey Felter, pointed out the seeds not only promote digestion but also ease the symptoms of children suffering from digestive **colic** (page 121).[4]

Active constituents
Caraway contains 3–7% volatile oil, with the main components divided into carvone (50–60%) and limonene (40%).[5] The fruit also contains approximately 10% fixed oil along with 20% carbohydrate and 20% protein. Caraway belongs to a class of herbs called carminatives, which are plants helpful in easing gastrointestinal discomfort, including gas. The volatile oils derived from this group of plants may help alleviate bowel spasm.[6]

There are no human clinical trials on caraway as a single entity. However, it has been used with success in combination with enteric-coated **peppermint oil** (page 726) in the treatment of **irritable bowel syndrome** (page 280) (IBS).[7, 8] People using this combination reported experiencing less pain and noted an overall improvement in their bowel symptoms compared to those who took a comparable placebo. A combination of caraway with the other carminative herbs anise and **fennel** (page 676) has shown to be helpful in dealing with conditions of flatulence and mild abdominal cramping, especially in children.[9]

How much is usually taken?
Use approximately ¼–½ teaspoon (0.5–2 grams) of powdered caraway fruit to make tea; drink it three times a day. Tinctures of the extracted herb (0.5–4 ml) are sometimes used three times per day. The enteric-coated volatile oil (0.05–0.2 ml) can be taken three times daily (usually in combination with enteric-coated **peppermint** (page 726) oil) for **irritable bowel syndrome** (page 280).[10]

Are there any side effects or interactions?
Caraway is generally safe for internal use. However, the purified volatile oil should not be used by children under two years of age, as oil from caraway and other herbs in the *Umbelliferae* family can be irritating to the skin and mucous membranes.[11] Large amounts of the oil (several times higher than the dosages listed above) may be potentially abortifacient and neurotoxic and should be avoided, especially by **pregnant** (page 363) women.

Carob

CAROB

Common names: St. John's bread, locust bean
Botanical name: *Ceratonia siliqua*

Parts used and where grown

Carob is originally from the Mediterranean region and the western part of Asia. Today it is grown mostly in Mediterranean countries. The gum from carob seeds is called locust bean gum. The dried, powdered pods of the plant are used in herbal medicine.

Carob has been used in connection with the following conditions (refer to the individual health concern for complete information):

Rating	Health Concerns
★★☆	Diarrhea (page 163)

Historical or traditional use (may or may not be supported by scientific studies)

Carob has long been eaten as food. John the Baptist is said to have eaten it, and thus it is sometimes called St. John's bread. Powdered carob pods have been used to treat **diarrhea** (page 163) for centuries.

Active constituents

The main constituents of carob are sugars and tannins. Carob tannins have an astringent effect in the gastrointestinal tract making them useful for treating **diarrhea** (page 163). They may also bind to (and thereby inactivate) toxins and inhibit growth of bacteria. The sugars make carob gummy and able to act as a thickener to absorb water—another action that may help decrease diarrhea. A double-blind clinical trial found carob useful for treating diarrhea in infants.[1] A less rigorous trial showed it did not help adults with traveler's diarrhea.[2]

How much is usually taken?

Some trials have used up to 15 grams of carob powder for treating **diarrhea** (page 163) in children.[3] Adults should take at least 20 grams a day for treating diarrhea. The powder can be mixed in applesauce or with sweet potatoes. Carob should be taken with plenty of water. Please note that infant diarrhea must be monitored by a healthcare professional and that proper hydration with a high electrolyte fluid is critical during acute diarrhea.

Are there any side effects or interactions?

Carob is generally safe. Only rarely have allergic reactions been reported.

CASCARA

Common names: Cascara sagrada, sacred bark
Botanical names: *Cascara sagrada*, *Rhamnus purshiani cortex*

Parts used and where grown

Cascara is a small to medium-size tree native to the provinces and states of the Pacific coast, including British Columbia, Washington, Oregon, and northern California. The bark of the tree is removed, cut into small pieces, and dried for one year before being used medicinally. Fresh cascara bark has an emetic or vomit-inducing property and therefore is not used.

Cascara has been used in connection with the following conditions (refer to the individual health concern for complete information):

Rating	Health Concerns
★★★	Constipation (page 137)

Historical or traditional use (may or may not be supported by scientific studies)

Northern California Indians introduced this herb, which they called sacred bark, to 16th century Spanish explorers. As it is much milder in its laxative action than the herb buckthorn, cascara became popular in Europe as a treatment for **constipation** (page 137). Cascara has been an approved treatment for constipation in the U.S. Pharmacopoeia since 1890.[1]

Active constituents

Cascara bark is high in hydroxyanthraquinone glycosides called cascarosides. Resins, tannins, and lipids make up the bulk of the other bark ingredients. Cascarosides have a cathartic action that induces the large intestine to increase its muscular contraction (peristalsis), resulting in bowel movement.[2]

How much is usually taken?

Only the dried form of cascara should be used. Capsules providing 20–30 mg of cascarosides per day can be used. However, the smallest amount necessary to maintain soft stool should be used.[3] As a tincture, ¼–1 teaspoon (1–5 ml) per day is generally taken. It is important to drink eight 6-ounce (180 ml) glasses of water throughout the day while using cascara. Cascara should be taken consecutively for no longer than eight to ten days.[4]

Are there any side effects or interactions?

Women who are **pregnant** (page 363) or breast-feeding, and children under the age of 12 should not use cascara without the advice of a physician. People with an intestinal obstruction, **Crohn's disease** (page 141), appendicitis or abdominal pain should not employ this herb.[5] Long-term use or abuse of cascara may result in weakened bowel function. It may also cause a loss of electrolytes (especially the mineral **potassium** [page 572]). Loss of potassium can lead to abnormalities of heart function and may augment the action of digitalis-like medications with fatal consequences.

CATNIP

Botanical name: *Nepeta cataria*

Parts used and where grown

Catnip is a whitish-gray plant with a minty odor. The flowers are white with crimson dots. The catnip plant grows in North America and Europe. The leaves and flowers are used as medicine.

Catnip has been used in connection with the following conditions (refer to the individual health concern for complete information):

Rating	Health Concerns
★☆☆	**Cough** (page 139)
	Insomnia (page 270)

Historical or traditional use (may or may not be supported by scientific studies)

Catnip is famous for inducing a delirious, stimulated state in felines. Throughout history, this herb has been used in humans to produce a sedative effect.[1] Several other conditions (including **cancer** [page 87], toothache, corns, and **hives** [page 245]) have been treated with catnip by traditional herbalists.

Active constituents

The volatile oil in catnip contains the monoterpene, nepetalactone, which is similar to the valepotriates found in **valerian** (page 756), a more commonly used herbal sedative.[2] Human trials are lacking to prove the effectiveness of catnip for treating **insomnia** (page 270). It has been used traditionally to reduce gas and act as a digestive aid.[3]

How much is usually taken?

A catnip tea can be made by adding 1 cup (250 ml) of boiling water to 1–2 teaspoons (5–10 grams) of the herb; cover, then steep for ten to fifteen minutes. Drink 2–3 cups per day.[4] For children with **coughs** (page 139), 1 teaspoon (5 ml) of tincture three times per day can be used. Adults may take twice this amount.

Are there any side effects or interactions?

No common side effects have been associated with the use of catnip. Since catnip (particularly the volatile oil) may act to promote uterine contractions, it should not be used during **pregnancy** (page 363).

CAT'S CLAW

Common name: Uña de gato
Botanical name: *Uncaria tomentosa*

Parts used and where grown

Cat's claw grows in the rain forests of the Andes Mountains in South America, particularly in Peru. The two species of the plant used most commonly are *U. tomentosa*, which makes up most of the cat's claw imported to the U.S., and *U. guianensis*, which is more widely used in Europe. In South America, both species are used interchangeably. The root bark is used as medicine.

Cat's claw has been used in connection with the following conditions (refer to the individual health concern for complete information):

Rating	Health Concerns
★★★	**Osteoarthritis** (page 328)
★☆☆	**HIV support** (page 239)
	Immune function (page 255)
	Rheumatoid arthritis (page 387)

Historical or traditional use (may or may not be supported by scientific studies)

Cat's claw has been reportedly used by indigenous peoples in the Andes to treat inflammation, rheumatism, gastric ulcers, tumors, dysentery, and as birth control.[1] Cat's claw is popular in South American folk medicine for treating intestinal complaints, gastric ulcers, arthritis, and to promote **wound healing** (page 319).

Active constituents

According to test tube studies, oxyindole alkaloids in cat's claw stimulate **immune function** (page 255).[2] Alkaloids and glycosides in cat's claw have also demonstrated anti-inflammatory and antioxidant activity.[3, 4]

Although clinical trials are lacking, cat's claw has become very popular in North America and is sometimes recommended for people with **cancer** (page 87) or **HIV** (page 239) infection. A cigarette smoker who took a freeze-dried extract of cat's claw root bark for one month showed a sharp decrease in one urinary cancer marker.[5] This finding, however, does little to support the use of the herb in persons with cancer and points toward the need for actual clinical studies to determine its effectiveness.

Cat's claw has been used traditionally for **osteoarthritis** (page 328) and **rheumatoid arthritis** (page 387). In a double-blind trial, 100 mg per day of a freeze-dried preparation of cat's claw taken for four weeks was significantly more effective than a placebo at relieving pain and improving the overall condition.[6]

How much is usually taken?

In a study of patients with **osteoarthritis** (page 328), 100 mg per day of a freeze-dried preparation was used. Cat's claw tea is prepared from ¼ teaspoon (1 gram) of root bark by adding 1 cup (250 ml) of water and boiling for ten to fifteen minutes. Cool, strain and drink one cup three times per day. Alternatively, ¼–½ teaspoon (1–2 ml) of tincture can be taken up to two times per day, or 20–60 mg of a dry standardized extract can be taken once per day.[7]

Are there any side effects or interactions?

Although no serious adverse effects have been reported for cat's claw, there is little known about its safety because most reports have been based on anecdotal evidence. Cat's claw should be used with caution in people with autoimmune illness, **multiple sclerosis** (page 323), and tuberculosis. Until proven safe, cat's claw should not be taken by **pregnant** (page 363) or **breastfeeding** (page 74) women.

CAYENNE

Botanical names: *Capsicum annuum, Capsicum frutescens*

Parts used and where grown

Originally from South America, the cayenne plant is now used worldwide as a food and spice. Cayenne is very closely related to bell peppers, jalapeños, paprika, and other similar peppers. The fruit is used medicinally.

Cayenne has been used in connection with the following conditions (refer to the individual health concern for complete information):

Rating	Health Concerns
★★★	**Diabetes** (page 152) (topical for neuropathy) Neurogenic bladder (administered by urologist) **Osteoarthritis** (page 328) (topical, for pain only) **Pain** (page 338) (topical use only) **Psoriasis** (page 379) (topical) **Shingles (herpes zoster)/postherpetic neuralgia** (page 401) (topical, for pain only)
★★☆	**Cluster headaches** (page 117) **Indigestion and heartburn** (page 260) Itching (anal; pruritus ani) **Obesity** (page 446) **Rheumatoid arthritis** (page 387) (topical)
★☆☆	**Bursitis** (page 87) **Low back pain** (page 293) (topical) **Migraine headaches** (page 316)

Historical or traditional use (may or may not be supported by scientific studies)

The potent, hot fruit of cayenne has been used as medicine for centuries. It was considered helpful by herbalists for various conditions of the gastrointestinal tract, including stomach aches, cramping pains, and gas. Cayenne was frequently used to treat diseases of the circulatory system. It is still traditionally used in herbal medicine as a circulatory tonic (a substance believed to improve circulation). Rubbed on the skin, cayenne is a traditional, as well as modern, remedy for rheumatic pains and arthritis due to what is termed a counterirritant effect. A counterirritant is something that causes irritation to a tissue to which it is applied, thus distracting from the original irritation (such as joint pain in the case of arthritis).

Active constituents

Cayenne contains a resinous and pungent substance known as capsaicin. Topical application of capsaicin relieves pain and itching by acting on sensory nerves.[1] Capsaicin temporarily depletes "substance P", a chemical in nerves that transmits pain sensations. Without substance P, pain signals can no longer be sent. The effect is temporary. Numerous double-blind trials have proven topically applied capsaicin creams are helpful for a range of conditions, including nerve pain in **diabetes** (page 152) (diabetic neuropathy),[2, 3] post-surgical pain,[4, 5, 6] **psoriasis** (page 379),[7] muscle pain due to **fibromyalgia** (page 191),[8] nerve pain after **shingles** (page 401) (postherpetic neuralgia),[9, 10] **osteoarthritis** (page 328) pain,[11, 12] and **rheumatoid arthritis** (page 387) pain.[13]

With the aid of a healthcare professional, capsaicin administered via the nose may also be a potentially useful therapy for **cluster headaches** (page 117). This is supported by a double-blind trial.[14] Weaker scientific support exists for the use of capsaicin for **migraines** (page 316).[15]

Injecting capsaicin directly into the urinary bladder has reduced symptoms of one type of bladder dysfunction (neurogenic hyperreflexic bladder)[16] that results from spinal cord and other nerve injuries. Capsaicin is not known to help other bladder conditions, such as chronic bladder pain. The placing of cayenne or capsaicin products into the bladder has only been performed in clinical experiments and should only be done by a urologist.

Modest reductions in appetite have been found in healthy Japanese women and white men when they consumed 10 grams of cayenne pepper along with meals in a double-blind trial.[17] A similar trial found that cayenne could increase metabolism of dietary fats in Japanese women.[18] These trials suggest cayenne may help in the treatment of **obesity** (page 446).

In a double-blind study of people with dyspepsia (**heartburn** [page 260]), supplementation with 833 mg of cayenne powder in capsules, three times per day before meals, reduced heartburn symptoms by 48%, compared with a placebo. However, two of 15 individuals receiving cayenne discontinued it because of abdominal pain.[19]

How much is usually taken?
Topical creams containing 0.025% to 75% capsaicin are generally used.[20] People often apply the cream to the affected area three or four times per day. A burning sensation may occur the first several times the cream is applied. However, this should gradually decrease with each use. The hands must be carefully and thoroughly washed after use, or gloves should be worn, to prevent the cream from accidentally reaching the eyes, nose, or mouth, which would cause a burning sensation. Do not apply the cream to areas of broken skin. For internal use, cayenne tincture (0.3–1 ml) can be taken three times per day. An infusion can be made by pouring 1 cup (250 ml) of boiling water onto ½–1 teaspoon (2.5 to 5 grams) of cayenne powder and let set for 10 minutes. A teaspoon of this infusion can be mixed with water and taken three to four times daily. In the treatment of heartburn, researchers have used 833 mg of cayenne powder in capsule form, taken three times per day before meals.[21]

Are there any side effects or interactions?
Besides causing a mild burning during the first few applications (or severe burning if accidentally placed in sensitive areas, such as the eyes), side effects are few with the use of capsaicin cream.[22] As with anything applied to the skin, some people may have an allergic reaction to the cream, so the first application should be to a very small area of skin. Do not attempt to use capsaicin cream intra-nasally for headache treatment without professional guidance.

When consumed as food—one pepper per day for many years—cayenne may increase the risk of stomach cancer, according to one study.[23] A different human study found that people who ate the most cayenne actually had lower rates of stomach cancer.[24] Overall, the current scientific evidence is contradictory. Thus, the relationship between cayenne consumption and increased risk of stomach cancer remains unclear.[25] Oral intake of even 1 ml of tincture three times per day can cause burning in the mouth and throat, and can cause the nose to run and eyes to water. People with **ulcers** (page 349), **heartburn** (page 260), or **gastritis** (page 195) should use any cayenne-containing product cautiously as it may worsen their condition.

CENTAURY

Botanical name: *Centaurium minus*

Parts used and where grown
This small grassland plant is native to Eurasia. The leaves, stems, and flowers of centaury are used medicinally.

Centaury has been used in connection with the following conditions (refer to the individual health concern for complete information):

Rating	Health Concerns
★☆☆	**Hypochlorhydria** (page 260) (low stomach acid) **Indigestion** (page 260) Loss of appetite

Historical or traditional use (may or may not be supported by scientific studies)

Centaury is one of the mainstays of European folk herbalism as a tonic for the digestive tract.[1] It was also used as a general tonic for people who had fevers.

Active constituents

Centaury contains bitter glycosides that stimulate secretion of stomach acid and digestive enzymes as well as activity of the entire digestive tract.[2] Centaury is recommended by the German Commission E for people with poor appetite and **indigestion** (page 260).[3] One preliminary animal study showed the herb had anti-inflammatory and fever-lowering effects.[4]

How much is usually taken?

Centaury is generally taken prior to a meal. A tea is made by adding 1 to 2 teaspoons of the herb to one cup of hot water and allowing it to steep for 15 minutes.[5] The tea should be sipped slowly. The bitter taste can be covered up by adding **ginger** (page 680) tea. Alternately, capsules can be used in the amount of 1 to 2 grams three times per day before a meal.[6]

Are there any side effects or interactions?

Centaury could theoretically worsen the conditions of **peptic ulcer disease** (page 349), elevated stomach acid levels, **heartburn** (page 260), **gastroesophageal reflux disease** (page 198), **diarrhea** (page 152), or acute inflammation of the intestinal tract, such as **Crohn's disease** (page 141), and should be avoided in such cases. Centaury is otherwise safe.[7] The safety of centaury in **pregnancy** (page 363) and **breast-feeding** (page 74) is unknown.

CHAMOMILE

Botanical name: *Matricaria recutita*

Parts used and where grown

Chamomile, a member of the daisy family, is native to Europe and western Asia. German chamomile is the most commonly used. The dried and fresh flowers are used medicinally.

Chamomile has been used in connection with the following conditions (refer to the individual health concern for complete information):

Rating	Health Concerns
★★☆	**Colic** (page 121) **Eczema** (page 177) **Gingivitis** (page 203) (periodontal disease) (as mouthwash, in combination with **sage** [page 740], **peppermint** [page 726] oil, menthol, expressed juice from **echinacea** [page 669], **myrrh** [page 713] tincture, and **caraway** [page 651] oil) **Wound healing** (page 319)
★☆☆	**Anxiety** (page 30) **Canker sores** (page 90) **Conjunctivitis/blepharitis** (page 136) **Crohn's disease** (page 141) **Diarrhea** (page 163) **Gastritis** (page 195) **Gingivitis** (page 203) (periodontal disease) **Indigestion and heartburn** (page 260) **Insomnia** (page 270) **Irritable bowel syndrome** (page 280) **Peptic ulcer** (page 349) **Ulcerative colitis** (page 433)

Historical or traditional use (may or may not be supported by scientific studies)

Chamomile has been used for centuries in Europe as a medicinal plant, mostly for gastrointestinal complaints. This practice continues today.

Active constituents

The flowers of chamomile contain 1–2% volatile oils including alpha-bisabolol, alpha-bisabolol oxides A & B, and matricin (usually converted to chamazulene).[1] Other active constituents include the **flavonoids** (page 516) apigenin, luteolin, and **quercetin** (page 580). These active ingredients contribute to chamomile's

Centaury

anti-inflammatory, antispasmodic, and smooth-muscle relaxing action, particularly in the gastrointestinal tract.[2, 3, 4, 5]

Topical applications of chamomile have been shown to be moderately effective in the treatment of **eczema** (page 177).[6, 7] One double-blind trial found it to be about 60% as effective as 0.25% hydrocortisone cream.[8] Topical use of chamomile ointment was also found to successfully treat mild stasis ulcers bed sores in elderly bedridden patients.[9]

How much is usually taken?

Chamomile is often taken three to four times daily between meals[10] as a tea. Common alternatives are to use 2–3 grams of the herb in tablet or capsule form or 4–6 ml of tincture three times per day between meals. Standardized extracts containing 1% apigenin and 0.5% volatile oils may also be used. One to two capsules containing 300–400 mg of extract may be taken three times daily. Topical creams or ointments can be applied to the affected area three to four times daily.

Are there any side effects or interactions?

Though rare, allergic reactions to chamomile have been reported.[11] These reactions have included bronchial constriction with internal use and allergic skin reactions with topical use.[12] While reports of such side effects are uncommon, people with allergies to plants of the Asteraceae family (ragweed, aster, and chrysanthemums), as well as mugwort pollen should avoid using chamomile.[13] Chamomile is usually considered to be safe during **pregnancy** (page 363) or breast-feeding. However, there is one case report in which a pregnant woman who took chamomile as an enema had an allergic reaction that led to the death of her newborn.[14]

CHAPARRAL

Common names: Creosote bush, greasewood
Botanical name: *Larrea tridentata*

Parts used and where grown

Chaparral takes its name from the area in which it grows, the desert regions of the southwestern United States and northern Mexico known as the chaparral ecosystem. The leaves and stems of this ancient plant are used as medicine.

Chaparral has been used in connection with the following conditions (refer to the individual health concern for complete information):

Rating	Health Concerns
★☆☆	**Cold sores** (page 119)
	Indigestion and heartburn (page 260)
	Infection (page 265)
	Intestinal cramps (topical)
	Parasites (page 343)
	Rheumatoid arthritis (page 387) (topical)
	Wound healing (page 319) (topical)

Historical or traditional use (may or may not be supported by scientific studies)

Chaparral has been used for thousands of years by Native Americans for a variety of purposes. It has been employed primarily in tea form to help with cramping pains, joint pains, and allergic problems, as well as to eliminate **parasites** (page 343).[1, 2] Externally it has been applied to reduce inflammation and pain, and to promote healing of **minor wounds** (page 319).[3]

Active constituents

The major lignan in chaparral, known as nordihydroguaiaretic acid (NDGA) is a potent antioxidant and was thought by some scientists to be a potential cancer treatment. In a rat study, NDGA and a leaf extract of a South American subspecies of chaparral were found to exert an antitumor effect.[4] However, one report suggests that NDGA may stimulate further growth of tumors in cancer patients.[5] Clinical trials, therefore, are still needed to establish whether chaparral is a safe and effective treatment for people with cancer.

Other reported effects for chaparral include anti-inflammatory properties[6, 7] as well as antimicrobial actions in test tubes.[8] These actions have note been established in human clinical trials

How much is usually taken?

A tea can be prepared by steeping 1 teaspoon (approximately 5 grams) of leaves and flowers in 1 cup (250 ml) of hot water for ten to fifteen minutes.[9] People should drink three cups per day for a maximum of two weeks unless under the care of a physician expert in the use of botanical medicines. Alternatively, 0.5–1 ml of tincture can be taken three times per day.[10] Topically, cloths can be soaked in oil preparations or tea of chaparral and applied several times per day (with heat if helpful) over

Chaparral

the affected area. Capsules of chaparral should be avoided.

Are there any side effects or interactions?

There have been sporadic reports of people developing liver or kidney problems after taking chaparral, particularly in capsules.[11] Almost all of these cases involved either the use of capsules or excessive amounts of tea. Some of these cases were people with established liver disease prior to using the herb. Tea and tincture of chaparral have an extremely strong taste considered disagreeable by most people, which restricts the amount they can tolerate before feeling nauseous. Capsules bypass this protective mechanism and should therefore be avoided. Since human studies have shown that large amounts of chaparral tea and injections of NDGA in people with **cancer** (page 87) do not cause liver or kidney problems,[12] it is likely the cases of toxicity represented individual reactions.[13]

Special United Kingdom considerations

Chaparral is either not available or may require a prescription. People should check with a qualified herbalist.

CHICKWEED

Botanical name: *Stellaria media*

Parts used and where grown

The small, green chickweed plant originated in Europe, but now grows across the United States. The leaves, stems, and flowers are used medicinally.

Chickweed has been used in connection with the following conditions (refer to the individual health concern for complete information):

Rating	Health Concerns
★☆☆	**Eczema** (page 177) Insect stings and bites

Historical or traditional use (may or may not be supported by scientific studies)

Chickweed was reportedly used at times for food.[1] It enjoys a reputation in folk medicine for treating a wide spectrum of conditions, ranging from **asthma** (page 32) and **indigestion** (page 260) to skin diseases such as **eczema** (page 177) and **psoriasis** (page 379). It is

sometimes used to alleviate itching secondary to insect bites.

Active constituents

The active constituents in chickweed are largely unknown. It contains relatively high amounts of vitamins (e.g., **vitamin C** [page 604]) and **flavonoids** (page 516), which may partly explain its effectiveness as a topical treatment for skin irritations and itching. Although some older information suggests a possible benefit for chickweed in rheumatic conditions, this has not been validated in clinical trials.[2]

How much is usually taken?

Although formerly used as a tea, chickweed is mainly used today as a cream applied liberally several times each day to rashes and inflammatory skin conditions (e.g., **eczema** [page 177]) to ease itching and inflammation.[3] As a tincture, ¼–1 teaspoon (1–5 ml) per day can be taken three times per day. Two teaspoonfuls (10 grams) of the dried herb may also be drunk as a tea three times daily.

Are there any side effects or interactions?

No side effects with chickweed have been reported.

CHINESE SCULLCAP

Common name: Baikal scullcap
Botanical name: *Scutellaria baicalensis*

Parts used and where grown

Scutellaria baicalensis, a mint family member, is grown in China and Russia. The root of this plant is used in traditional Chinese herbal medicines and has been the focus of most scientific studies on scullcap. **American scullcap** (page 626) and Chinese scullcap are not interchangeable.

Chinese scullcap has been used in connection with the following conditions (refer to the individual health concern for complete information):

Rating	Health Concerns
★★☆	**Epilepsy** (page 183) (in combination with **bupleurum** [page 647], peony root, pinellia root, cassia bark, **ginger** [page 680] root, jujube fruit, **Asian ginseng** [page 630] root, and **licorice** [page 702] root)

Chaparral

Rating	Health Concerns
★☆☆	**Bronchitis** (page 80) **Hepatitis** (page 220) **HIV support** (page 239) (in combination with **bupleurum** [page 647], peony root, pinellia root, cassia bark, **ginger** [page 680] root, jujube fruit, **Asian ginseng** [page 630] root, Asian scullcap root, and **licorice** [page 702] root)

Historical or traditional use (may or may not be supported by scientific studies)

Chinese scullcap is typically used in herbal combinations in Traditional Chinese Medicine to treat inflammatory skin conditions, **allergies** (page 14), **high cholesterol** (page 223) and **triglycerides** (page 235).[1]

Active constituents

The root of Chinese scullcap contains the **flavonoid** (page 516) baicalin that has been shown in test tube studies to have protective actions on the liver. Anti-allergy actions and the inhibition of bacteria and viruses in test tube studies have also been documented with Chinese scullcap.[2] Some preliminary Chinese human trials, generally of low quality, suggest that Chinese scullcap may help people with acute lung, intestinal, and liver infections, as well as **hay fever** (page 211).[3] More extensive clinical research is needed to clearly demonstrate Chinese scullcap's effectiveness for these conditions.

How much is usually taken?

In traditional Chinese herbal medicine, Chinese scullcap is typically recommended as a tea made from 3–9 grams of the dried root.[4] Fluid extract, 1–4 ml three times per day, is also used.[5]

Are there any side effects or interactions?

Use of Chinese scullcap in the amounts listed above appears to be safe. The safety of Chinese scullcap during **pregnancy** (page 363) and breast-feeding is unknown and should be avoided during these times.

CINNAMON

Botanical name: *Cinnamomum zeylanicum*

Parts used and where grown

Most people are familiar with the sweet but pungent taste of the oil, powder, or sticks of bark from the cinnamon tree. Cinnamon trees grow in a number of tropical areas, including parts of India, China, Madagascar, Brazil, and the Caribbean.

Cinnamon has been used in connection with the following conditions (refer to the individual health concern for complete information):

Rating	Health Concerns
★★☆	**Diabetes** (page 152)
★☆☆	**Colic** (page 121) **Indigestion and heartburn** (page 260) **Menorrhagia** (page 314) (heavy menstruation) Poor appetite **Yeast infection** (page 454)

Historical or traditional use (may or may not be supported by scientific studies)

Cinnamon is an ancient herbal medicine mentioned in Chinese texts as long ago as 4,000 years. It has a broad range of historical uses in different cultures, including the treatment of **diarrhea** (page 163), rheumatism, and certain menstrual disorders.[1]

Active constituents

Various terpenoids found in the volatile oil are believed to account for cinnamon's medicinal effects. Important among these compounds are eugenol and cinnamaldehyde. Both cinnamaldehyde and cinnamon oil vapors are potent anti-fungal compounds.[2] Preliminary human evidence confirms this effect in a clinical trial with **AIDS** (page 239) patients suffering from oral candida (thrush) infections that improved with topical application of cinnamon oil.[3] Antibacterial actions have also been demonstrated for cinnamon.[4] The diterpenes in the volatile oil have shown anti-allergic activity[5] as well. In addition, water extracts may help reduce ulcers.[6] Test tube studies also show that cinnamon can augment the action of insulin.[7] However, use of cinnamon to improve the action of insulin in people with **diabetes** (page 152) has yet to be proven in clinical trials.

How much is usually taken?

The German Commission E monograph suggests ½–¾ teaspoon (2–4 grams) of the powder per day.[8] A tea can be prepared from the powdered herb by boiling ½ teaspoon (2–3 grams) of the powder for ten to fifteen minutes, cooling, and then drinking. No more than a few

Cinnamon

drops of volatile oil should be used and only for a few days at a time. A tincture (½ teaspoon or 2–3 ml) may also be taken three times per day.

Are there any side effects or interactions?

Some people develop bronchial constriction or skin rash after exposure to cinnamon.[9] Therefore, only small amounts should be used initially in people who have not previously had contact with cinnamon, and anyone with a known allergy should avoid it. Chronic use of the concentrated oil may cause inflammation in the mouth. According to the German Commission E monograph, cinnamon is not recommended for use by **pregnant** (page 363) women.[10]

CLEAVERS

Common names: Bedstraw, goose grass
Botanical name: *Galium aparine*

Parts used and where grown

Cleavers grow in wet areas of Britain, Europe, Asia, and North America. Small prickles grow on the leaves of cleavers, causing it to have a sticky feeling and giving it its name. The leaves and flowers of cleavers are used medicinally.

Cleavers has been used in connection with the following conditions (refer to the individual health concern for complete information):

Rating	Health Concerns
★☆☆	**Edema** (page 180)

Historical or traditional use (may or may not be supported by scientific studies)

Cleavers is one of numerous plants considered in ancient times to act as a diuretic.[1] It was therefore used to relieve **edema** (page 180) and to promote urine formation during bladder infections. It has also been used by people with lymph swellings, jaundice, and wounds.

Active constituents

Galiosin, an anthraquinone glycoside, other glycosides, tannins, and **flavonoids** (page 516) may be the major constituents of cleavers. Little research has been conducted on this plant, but preliminary lab experiments suggest it may have antispasmodic activity.[2]

How much is usually taken?

Cleavers tincture and tea are most widely recommended by herbal practitioners. Tincture (½–1 teaspoon or 3–5 ml) can be taken three times per day. Tea is made by steeping 2–3 teaspoons (10–15 grams) of the herb in 1 cup (250 ml) of hot water for ten to fifteen minutes. People can drink three or more cups per day.

Are there any side effects or interactions?

Cleavers has no known side effects and is thought to be safe for use by children and **pregnant** (page 363) or nursing women.

COLEUS

Common name: Makandi
Botanical name: *Coleus forskohlii*

Parts used and where grown

This attractive, perennial member of the mint *(Lamiaceae)* family originated in the lower elevations of India. It is now grown around the world as an ornamental plant. The root is used medicinally.

Coleus has been used in connection with the following conditions (refer to the individual health concern for complete information):

Rating	Health Concerns
★★☆	**Asthma** (page 32) (forskolin)
	Glaucoma (page 205) (forskolin)
★☆☆	**Cardiomyopathy** (page 95) (forskolin)
	Congestive heart failure (page 134)
	Hypertension (page 246) (forskolin)
	Obesity (page 446)
	Psoriasis (page 379)

Historical or traditional use (may or may not be supported by scientific studies)

As recorded in ancient Sanskrit texts, coleus was used in Ayurvedic medicine[1] to treat heart and lung diseases, intestinal spasms, **insomnia** (page 270), and convulsions.

Active constituents

Forskolin, a chemical found in coleus, activates the enzyme adenylate cyclase.[2] This enzyme is a turnkey compound that initiates a cascade of critical events within every cell of the body. Adenylate cyclase and the chemicals it activates comprise a "second messenger" system that is responsible for carrying out the complex and powerful effects of hormones in the body. Stimulation of the second messenger system by forskolin leads to blood vessel dilation,[3] inhibition of allergic reactions,[4] and an increase in thyroid hormone secretion.[5] Forskolin has other properties as well, including inhibition of the pro-inflammatory substance known as platelet-activating factor (PAF)[6] and inhibition of the spread of cancer cells.[7]

Studies in healthy humans, including at least one double-blind trial, have shown that direct application of an ophthalmic preparation of forskolin to the eyes lowers eye pressure,[8, 9] thus reducing the risk of **glaucoma** (page 205). Direct application of the whole herb to the eyes has not been studied and is not recommended.

Forskolin may help dilate blood vessels and improve the forcefulness with which the heart pumps blood. A preliminary trial found that forskolin reduced **blood pressure** (page 246) and improved heart function in people with **cardiomyopathy** (page 95).[10] It is unknown if oral coleus extracts would have the same effect. A small double-blind trial found that inhaled forskolin could decrease lung spasms in **asthmatics** (page 32).[11] It is unclear if oral ingestion of coleus extracts will provide similar benefits.

How much is usually taken?
Coleus extracts standardized to 10% to 18% forskolin are available. While some doctors expert in herbal medicine recommend 50–100 mg two to three times per day of standardized coleus extract, these amounts are extrapolations and have yet to be confirmed by direct clinical research.[12] Most studies have used injected forskolin, so it is unclear if oral ingestion of coleus extracts will provide similar benefits in the amounts recommended above. Until ophthalmic preparations of coleus or forskolin are available, people with glaucoma should consult with a skilled healthcare practitioner to obtain a sterile fluid extract for use in the eyes.

Are there any side effects or interactions?
Few adverse effects of coleus have been reported. It should be avoided in people with **ulcers** (page 349), because it may increase stomach acid levels. Direct application to the eyes may cause transitory tearing, burning, and itching. The safety of coleus in **pregnancy** (page 363) and breast-feeding is unknown.

COLTSFOOT

Botanical name: *Tussilago farfara*

Parts used and where grown
The flowers, leaves, and roots of coltsfoot have been used as herbal medicines. However, the roots are generally avoided now. Coltsfoot originates in Eurasia and North Africa, and now also grows throughout damp areas of North America.

Coltsfoot has been used in connection with the following conditions (refer to the individual health concern for complete information):

Rating	Health Concerns
★☆☆	**Cough** (page 139)
	Sore throat (page 129)

Historical or traditional use (may or may not be supported by scientific studies)
Coltsfoot historically has been used by herbalists to alleviate **coughs** (page 139) due to all manner of conditions. It was considered particularly useful for people with chronic coughs, such as those due to emphysema or silicosis.[1] Coltsfoot leaf was originally approved for the treatment of **sore throats** (page 129) in the German Commission E monograph[2] but has since been banned in Germany for internal use.[3]

Active constituents
Mucilage, bitter glycosides, and tannins are considered the major constituents of coltsfoot.[4] These are thought to give the herb anti-inflammatory and antitussive (cough prevention and treatment) activity.[5] Coltsfoot also contains pyrrolizidine alkaloids, potentially toxic constituents.

How much is usually taken?
Internal use of coltsfoot root is not recommended due to the potential liver toxicity of its pyrrolizidine alkaloids. Tea of coltsfoot leaf or flower is made by steeping 1–2 teaspoons (5–10 grams) in 1 cup (250 ml) hot water for ten to twenty minutes.[6] People can drink three cups (750 ml) daily. Alternatively, ½–1 teaspoon (2–4 ml) of tincture of the leaf or flower can be taken three times per day. Some practitioners of herbal medicine have recommended having hot coltsfoot tea ready in a thermos to drink for morning coughs due to em-

physema.[7] People should not use coltsfoot for more than one month consecutively unless on the advice of a doctor. Also, preparations guaranteed to be pyrrolizidine-free can be used indefinitely and are preferable.

Are there any side effects or interactions?

Coltsfoot contains potentially liver-damaging pyrrolizidine alkaloids, with much higher levels appearing in the root than in the leaves or the flowers. Animal studies using amounts of coltsfoot hundreds of times higher than those used as medicine have shown these alkaloids can cause cancer in animals.[8] A single case of an infant who developed liver disease and died after the mother drank tea containing coltsfoot during pregnancy has been reported.[9] This eventually led to the banning of coltsfoot in Germany in 1992.

Coltsfoot should not be taken during **pregnancy** (page 363) or breast-feeding.[10] Otherwise, coltsfoot is generally safe.[11]

Coltsfoot should be differentiated from the plant called western coltsfoot *(Petastites frigidus),* because western coltsfoot can contain higher amounts of pyrrolizidine alkaloids. Use of western coltsfoot is not recommended.

COMFREY

Common names: Knitbone, boneset
Botanical name: *Symphytum officinale*

Parts used and where grown

The leaf and root of comfrey have been employed medicinally for centuries. Originally from Europe and western Asia, it is now also grown in North America.

Comfrey has been used in connection with the following conditions (refer to the individual health concern for complete information):

Rating	Health Concerns
★☆☆	Broken bones (topical)
	Bruises (page 84) (topical)
	Chronic skin ulcer (topical)
	Conjunctivitis/blepharitis (page 136) (topical eye application)
	Cough (page 139)
	Peptic ulcer (page 349)
	Sprains (page 412) (topical)
	Thrombophlebitis (topical)
	Wound healing (page 319) (topical)

Historical or traditional use (may or may not be supported by scientific studies)

Comfrey has a long history of use as a topical agent for treating **wounds** (page 319), skin ulcers, thrombophlebitis, **bruises** (page 84), and **sprains and strains** (page 412).[1, 2] Comfrey was used by herbalists to promote more rapid repair of broken bones, hence the common names boneset and knitbone. Topically, comfrey was also used to treat minor skin irritations and inflammation. It has also been used as a wash or topical application for eye irritations and for treating **conjunctivitis** (page 136). Internally, it was used to treat gastrointestinal problems, such as stomach **ulcers** (page 349) and **inflammatory bowel disease** (page 269), and lung problems.

Active constituents

Mucilage and allantoin are considered the major constituents in comfrey responsible for the herbs soothing and anti-inflammatory actions.[3]

How much is usually taken?

Fresh, peeled root or dried root, approximately 3.5 ounces (100 grams), is simmered in 1 pint (500 ml) of water for ten to fifteen minutes to prepare comfrey for topical use.[4] Cloth or gauze is soaked in this liquid, then applied to the skin for at least 15 minutes. Fresh leaves can be ground up lightly and applied directly to the skin. Alternatively, creams or ointments made from root or leaf can be applied. All topical preparations should be applied several times per day.

Due to variations in pyrrolizidine alkaloid content, root preparations are unsafe for internal use unless they are guaranteed pyrrolizidine-free. Although comfrey root tea has been used traditionally, the danger of its pyrrolizidine alkaloids is significant. Therefore, comfrey root and young leaf preparations should not be taken internally.

Are there any side effects or interactions?

Comfrey contains potentially dangerous compounds known as pyrrolizidine alkaloids. The roots contain higher levels of these compounds and mature leaves contain very little, if any, of these alkaloids.[5, 6] Fresh young leaves contain higher amounts (up to 16 times more than mature leaves) and should be avoided.[7] Other related forms, such as Russian comfrey *(Symphytum uplandicum)* and prickly comfrey *(S. asperum),* are sometimes available or mistakenly sold as regular comfrey but contain higher levels of these alkaloids.[8] Several

Coltsfoot

cases of people who developed liver disease or other serious problems from taking capsules or tea of comfrey have been reported over the years.[9]

Most comfrey products do not list their pyrrolizidine alkaloid content on the label. Therefore, it is best to avoid internal use of products made from comfrey root or young leaves altogether.

Special United Kingdom considerations

Comfrey for internal use is only available as an herbal tea, unless prescribed by a Medicinal Herbalist. People should consult with a qualified herbalist for other forms of this herb.

CORDYCEPS

Common names: Caterpillar fungus, deer fungus parasite, chongcao
Botanical name: *Cordyceps* spp.

Parts used and where grown

Cordyceps sinensis in its sexual stage is the primary form used.[1] However, more than ten related species (in sexual and asexual stages) as well as artificially cultured mycelium are today used as substitutes in commercial preparations. *C. sinensis*, *C. ophioglossoides*, *C. capita*, and *C. militaris* are the most common species in commerce.

Cordyceps has been used in connection with the following conditions (refer to the individual health concern for complete information):

Rating	Health Concerns
★★☆	**Chronic hepatitis B** (page 220) Kidney disease
★☆☆	**Immune function** (page 255) Liver disease

Historical or traditional use (may or may not be supported by scientific studies)

In ancient China, cordyceps was used in the Emperor's palace and was considered to have ginseng-like properties.[2] It was used to strengthen the body after exhaustion or long-term illness, and for impotence, neurasthenia, and backache. It was also used to cure opium addiction.

Active constituents

Cordyceps contains a wide variety of potentially important constituents, including polysaccharides, ophiocordin (an antibiotic compound), cordycepin, cordypyridones, nucleosides, bioxanthracenes, sterols, alkenoic acids, and exo-polymers.[3, 4, 5, 6, 7, 8, 9]

Many studies on the medicinal effects of cordyceps do not give a clear picture of its actions because many of the studies (1) are in animals or test tubes; (2) use different species, preparations, and intake levels; (3) inject cordyceps and/or its constituents rather than administering them orally; or (4) are not available in English and, therefore, cannot be reviewed for accuracy and design.

There are some clinical trials supporting the efficacy of cordyceps, particularly for liver, kidney, and immune problems. A number of studies indicate that cordyceps may have a anti-cancer, anti-metastatic, immuno-enhancing, and antioxidant effects.[10, 11, 12, 13, 14]

How much is usually taken?

The recommended intake of cordyceps is 3 to 9 grams taken twice daily as a liquid extract, as food, or as powdered extract.[15]

Are there any side effects or interactions?

There are insufficient studies on the safety of cordyceps. However, it has a long history of use as a food and is generally considered safe.[16] There is no information available about safety in pregnancy, lactation, or use in children.

There are two reported cases of lead poisoning associated with the use of apparently contaminated cordyceps powder.[17] Cordyceps should only be purchased from companies that test to exclude heavy metal contamination.

CORYDALIS

Common name: Yan hu so
Botanical names: *Corydalis turtschaninovii*, *Corydalis yanhusuo*

Parts used and where grown

Corydalis is an herb native to the Chinese province of Zhejiang. The portion of the plant that is used medicinally is the tuberous rhizome.[1]

Corydalis

Corydalis has been used in connection with the following conditions (refer to the individual health concern for complete information):

Rating	Health Concerns
★★☆	**Insomnia** (page 270) **Pain** (page 338) (nerve)
★☆☆	**Dysmenorrhea** (page 171) (painful menstruation) **Heart arrhythmia** (page 93) **Peptic ulcer** (page 349)

Historical or traditional use (may or may not be supported by scientific studies)

In Traditional Chinese Medicine, corydalis is said to invigorate the blood, move qi (energy that travels through the body), and alleviate **pain** (page 338), including menstrual, abdominal, and hernial.[2]

Active constituents

Scientists have isolated a number of alkaloids from the tuber of corydalis, including corydaline, tetrahydropalmatine (THP), dl-Tetrahydropalmatine (dl-THP), protopine, tetrahydrocoptisine, tetrahydrocolumbamine, and corybulbine.[3] Of the full range of 20 alkaloids found in the plant, THP is considered to be the most potent. In laboratory research, it has been shown to exhibit a wide number of pharmacological actions on the central nervous system, including analgesic and sedative effects.[4] dl-THP has been found to exhibit a tranquilizing action in mice. Scientists have suggested that dl-THP blocks certain receptor sites (e.g., dopamine) in the brain to cause sedation.[5]

In addition to its central nervous system effects, studies in the laboratory have shown the alkaloids from corydalis also have cardiovascular actions. For example, dl-THP has been shown to both decrease the stickiness of platelets and protect against **stroke** (page 419),[6] as well as lower **blood pressure** (page 246) and heart rate in animal studies.[7] Additionally, it seems to exert an anti-arrhythmic action on the heart. This was found in a small double-blind clinical trial with patients suffering from a specific type of **heart arrhythmia** (page 93) (e.g., supra-ventricular premature beat or SVPB).[8] People taking 300–600 mg of dl-THP per day in tablet form, had a significantly greater improvement than those taking placebo pills.

Other human clinical trials on dl-THP have shown the ability to fall asleep was improved in people suffering from **insomnia** (page 270) after taking 100–200 mg of dl-THP at bedtime. No drug hangover symptoms such as morning grogginess, dizziness or **vertigo** (page 441) were reported by people taking the alkaloid extract.[9]

Reports from Chinese researchers also note that 75 mg of THP daily was effective in reducing nerve pain in 78% of the patients tested.[10] Painful menstruation (**dysmenorrhea** [page 171]), abdominal pain after childbirth, and headache have also been reported to be successfully treated with THP.[11]

Extracts of the herb may also be useful in the treatment of **stomach ulcers** (page 349). In a large sample of patients with stomach and intestinal ulcers or chronic inflammation of the stomach lining, a 90–120 mg extract of the herb per day (equal to 5–10 grams of the crude herb) was found to improve healing and symptoms in 76% of the patients.[12]

How much is usually taken?

For an analgesic or sedative effect, the crude, dried rhizome is usually recommended at 5–10 grams per day.[13] Alternatively, one can take 10–20 ml per day of a 1:2 extract.[14]

Are there any side effects or interactions?

Corydalis should not be taken by **pregnant** (page 363) or nursing women.[15] There have been several reports in Western journals of THP toxicity, including acute **hepatitis** (page 220).[16, 17, 18] In addition, people taking corydalis can experience **vertigo** (page 441), fatigue, and nausea.[19]

CRANBERRY

Botanical name: *Vaccinium macrocarpon*

Parts used and where grown

Cranberry is a member of the same family as **bilberry** (page 634) and blueberry. It is from North America and grows in bogs. The ripe fruit is used medicinally.

Cranberry has been used in connection with the following conditions (refer to the individual health concern for complete information):

Rating	Health Concerns
★★☆	**Urinary tract infection** (page 436) prevention

Corydalis

Historical or traditional use (may or may not be supported by scientific studies)

In traditional North American herbalism, cranberry has been used to prevent **kidney stones** (page 284) and "bladder gravel" as well as to remove toxins from the blood. Cranberry has long been recommended by herbalists as well as doctors to help prevent **urinary tract infections** (page 436) (UTIs).

Active constituents

In test tube studies, cranberry prevents *E. coli,* the most common bacterial cause of UTIs, from adhering to the cells lining the wall of the bladder. This anti-adherence action is thought to reduce the ability of the bacteria to cause a UTI.[1, 2] The **proanthocyanidins** (page 574) in the berry have exhibited this anti-adherence action.[3] Cranberry has been shown to reduce bacteria levels in the urinary bladders of older women significantly better than placebo, an action that may help to prevent UTIs.[4] A small double-blind trial with younger women ages 18–45 years with a history of recurrent **urinary tract infections** (page 436), found that daily treatment with an encapsulated cranberry concentrate (400 mg twice per day) for three months significantly reduced the recurrence of urinary tract infections compared to women taking a placebo.[5] Other preliminary trials in humans suggest cranberry may help people with urostomies and enterocystoplasties to keep their urine clear of mucus buildup and possibly reduce the risk of UTIs.[6] However, one trial found that cranberry did not reduce the risk of UTIs in children with neurogenic bladder disease (a condition that does not allow for proper flow of urine from the bladder) who were receiving daily catheterization.[7]

How much is usually taken?

One capsule of concentrated cranberry juice extract (400 mg) can be taken two times per day.[8] Several 16-ounce (500 ml) glasses of high-quality unsweetened cranberry juice from concentrate each day approximate the effect of the cranberry extract. Cranberry tincture, ½–1 teaspoon (3–5 ml) three times per day, can also be taken.

Are there any side effects or interactions?

Cranberry concentrate has not been reported to cause side effects and has no known contraindications to use during **pregnancy** (page 363) and **breast-feeding** (page 74). According to one report, supplementation with an unspecified number of cranberry tablets for seven days increased the urinary excretion of oxalate by 43%, suggesting that long term use of cranberry supplements might increase the risk of developing a **kidney stone** (page 284).[9] On the other hand, in the same study, urinary excretion of magnesium and potassium (which are inhibitors of stone formation) also increased. Until more is known, individuals with a personal or family history of calcium-oxalate kidney stones should consult a doctor before using cranberry supplements for long periods of time (e.g., more than a week). Cranberry should not be used as a substitute for antibiotics during an acute **urinary tract infection** (page 436), except under medical supervision.

CRANESBILL

Botanical name: *Geranium maculatum*

Parts used and where grown

Cranesbill originated in North America and is sometimes grown ornamentally in a variety of flower colors. The root is primarily used in herbal medicine, but the above-ground part of the plant has also been used traditionally by herbalists.

Cranesbill has been used in connection with the following conditions (refer to the individual health concern for complete information):

Rating	Health Concerns
★☆☆	**Canker sores** (page 90)
	Crohn's disease (page 141)
	Diarrhea (page 163)
	Menorrhagia (page 314)

Historical or traditional use (may or may not be supported by scientific studies)

The Blackfoot Indians of North America used the root of cranesbill and closely related plants to stop bleeding.[1] Cranesbill has also been used by other indigenous tribes of North America to treat **diarrhea** (page 163).

Active constituents

Cranesbill is high in tannins, which may account for its anti-diarrheal activity.[2] Little scientific research exists to clarify cranesbill's constituents and actions.

Cranesbill

How much is usually taken?

A tea can be prepared by boiling 1–2 teaspoons (5–10 grams) of the root for ten to fifteen minutes in 2 cups (500 ml) of water.[3] People can drink three (750 ml) or more cups per day. Cranesbill tincture (approximately ½ teaspoon or 3 ml) three times per day is also commonly used, although generally in combination with other herbs, for **diarrhea** (page 163). Dried, powdered cranesbill root is sometimes used in an herbal combination to treat **Crohn's disease** (page 141); however, there are no scientific studies to support this combination.

Are there any side effects or interactions?

Cranesbill tea should not be used for more than two to three consecutive weeks. Due to the high tannin content, some people may develop an upset stomach after using cranesbill.

DAMIANA

Botanical name: *Turnera diffusa*

Parts used and where grown

The leaves of damiana were originally used as medicine by the indigenous cultures of Central America, particularly Mexico. Today the plant is found in hot, humid climates, including Mexico and parts of Texas, the Caribbean, and southern Africa.

Damiana has been used in connection with the following conditions (refer to the individual health concern for complete information):

Rating	Health Concerns
★☆☆	**Depression** (page 145)
	Erectile dysfunction (page 185)

Historical or traditional use (may or may not be supported by scientific studies)

Damiana has been hailed as an aphrodisiac since ancient times, particularly by the native peoples of Mexico.[1] Other folk uses have included **asthma** (page 32), **bronchitis** (page 80), neurosis, and various sexual disorders.[2] It has also been promoted as a euphoria-inducing substance.

Active constituents

Most research has been done on the volatile oil of damiana, which includes numerous small, fragrant substances called terpenes.[3] As yet, it is unclear if the volatile oil is truly the main active constituent of damiana. Damiana extracts have been shown, in a test tube, to weakly bind to **progesterone** (page 577) receptors.[4] Thus, damiana may be a potentially useful herb for some female health problems. However, no human studies have investigated this possibility and it is not a primary traditional use.

How much is usually taken?

To make a tea, add 1 cup (250 ml) boiling water to ¼ teaspoon (1 gram) of dried leaves and allow to steep for ten to fifteen minutes. People can drink three cups (750 ml) per day. To use in tincture form, take ½–¾ teaspoon (2–3 ml) three times daily. Tablets or capsules (400–800 mg three times per day) may also be used. Damiana is commonly used in herbal combinations. However, the authors of the German Commission E monographs do not feel that traditional use of this herb is justified by modern research.[5]

Are there any side effects or interactions?

The leaves have a minor laxative effect and may cause loosening of the stools at higher amounts. Until more is known about damiana's effects on the female hormonal system, it should be avoided during **pregnancy** (page 363).[6]

DANDELION

Botanical name: *Taraxacum officinale*

Parts used and where grown

Closely related to chicory, dandelion is a common plant worldwide and the bane of those looking for the perfect lawn. The plant grows to a height of about 12 inches, producing spatula-like leaves and yellow flowers that bloom year-round. Upon maturation, the flower turns into the characteristic puffball containing seeds that are dispersed in the wind. Dandelion is grown commercially in the United States and Europe. The leaves and root are used in herbal supplements.

Dandelion has been used in connection with the following conditions (refer to the individual health concern for complete information):

Rating	Health Concerns
★☆☆	**Constipation** (page 137) (root) **Edema (water retention)** (page 180) (leaves) **Indigestion and heartburn** (page 260) (leaves and root) Liver support (root) **Pregnancy and postpartum support** (page 363) (leaves and root)

Historical or traditional use (may or may not be supported by scientific studies)

Dandelion is commonly used as a food. The leaves are used in salads and teas, while the roots are sometimes used as a coffee substitute. Dandelion leaves and roots have been used for hundreds of years to treat liver, gallbladder, kidney, and joint problems. In some traditions, dandelion is considered a blood purifier and is used for conditions as varied as **eczema** (page 177) and **cancer** (page 87). As is the case today, dandelion leaves have also been used historically to treat **water retention** (page 180).

Active constituents

The primary constituents responsible for dandelion's action on the digestive system and liver are the bitter principles. Previously referred to as taraxacin, these constituents are sesquiterpene lactones of the eudesmanolide and germacranolide type, and are unique to dandelion.[1] Dandelion is also a rich source of vitamins and minerals. The leaves have a high content of **vitamin A** (page 595) as well as moderate amounts of **vitamin D** (page 607), **vitamin C** (page 604), various **B vitamins** (page 603), **iron** (page 540), **silicon** (page 586), **magnesium** (page 551), **zinc** (page 614), and **manganese** (page 553).[2]

An animal study found that at high amounts (2 grams per 2.2 pounds [1 kg] of body weight), the leaves possess diuretic effects comparable to the prescription diuretic furosemide (Lasix).[3] However, to date, these results have not been demonstrated in human clinical trials. Since **edema** (page 180), or water retention, may be a sign of a more serious disease, people should seek the guidance of a physician before using dandelion leaves for either of these conditions.

The bitter compounds in the leaves and root help stimulate digestion and are mild laxatives.[4] These bitter principles also increase bile production in the gallbladder and bile flow from the liver.[5] For this reason dandelion is recommended by some herbalists for people with sluggish liver function due to alcohol abuse or poor diet. The increase in bile flow may help improve fat (including cholesterol) metabolism in the body.

How much is usually taken?

As a general liver/gallbladder tonic and to stimulate digestion, ½–1 teaspoon (3–5 grams) of the dried root or 1–2 teaspoons (5–10 ml) of a tincture made from the root can be used three times per day.[6] Some experts recommend the alcohol-based tincture because the bitter principles are more soluble in alcohol.[7]

As a mild diuretic or appetite stimulant, 1–2 teaspoons (4–10 grams) of dried leaves can be added to a 1 cup (250 ml) of boiling water and drunk as a decoction.[8] Or, 1–2 teaspoons (5–10 ml) of fresh juice or ½–1 teaspoon (2–5 ml) of tincture made from the leaves can be used three times per day. Fresh dandelion leaves can be eaten as part of a salad.

Are there any side effects or interactions?

Dandelion leaf and root should not be used by people with **gallstones** (page 193) without the supervision of a healthcare practitioner.[9] People with an obstruction of the bile ducts should not take dandelion. In cases of stomach **ulcer** (page 349) or **gastritis** (page 195), dandelion should be used cautiously, as it may cause overproduction of stomach acid. Those experiencing fluid or water retention should consult a doctor before taking dandelion leaves. The milky latex in the stem and leaves of fresh dandelion may cause an allergic rash in some people.

Dandelion root contains approximately 40% inulin,[10] a fiber widely distributed in fruits, vegetables and plants. Inulin is classified as a food ingredient (not as an additive) and is considered to be safe to eat.[11] In fact, inulin is a significant part of the daily diet of most of the world's population.[12] However, there is a report of a 39-year old man having a life-threatening allergic reaction after consuming high amounts of inulin from multiple sources.[13] Allergy to inulin in this individual was confirmed by laboratory tests. Such sensitivities are exceedingly rare. Moreover, this man did not take dandelion. Nevertheless, people with a confirmed sensitivity to inulin should avoid dandelion.

Dandelion

DEVIL'S CLAW

Botanical name: *Harpagophytum procumbens*

Parts used and where grown

Devil's claw is a native plant of southern Africa, especially the Kalahari desert, Namibia and the island of Madagascar. The name devil's claw is derived from the herb's unusual fruits, which are covered with numerous small claw-like appendages. The secondary storage roots, or tubers, of the plant are used in herbal supplements.[1]

Devil's claw has been used in connection with the following conditions (refer to the individual health concern for complete information):

Rating	Health Concerns
★★☆	**Osteoarthritis** (page 328) **Rheumatoid arthritis** (page 387)
★☆☆	**Indigestion** (page 260) **Low back pain** (page 293)

Historical or traditional use (may or may not be supported by scientific studies)

Numerous tribes native to southern Africa have used devil's claw for a wide variety of conditions, ranging from gastrointestinal difficulties to arthritic conditions.[2] Devil's claw has been widely used in Europe as a treatment for arthritis.

Active constituents

The devil's claw tuber contains three important constituents belonging to the iridoid glycoside family: harpagoside, harpagide, and procumbide. The secondary tubers of the herb contain twice as much harpagoside as the primary tubers and are the chief source of devil's claw used medicinally.[3] Harpagoside and other iridoid glycosides found in the plant may be responsible for the herb's anti-inflammatory and analgesic actions. However, research has not entirely supported the use of devil's claw in alleviating arthritic pain symptoms.[4, 5] In one trial it was found to reduce pain associated with **osteoarthritis** (page 328) as effectively as the slow-acting analgesic/cartilage-protective drug diacerhein.[6] One double-blind study reported that devil's claw (600 or 1200 mg per day) was helpful in reducing **low back pain** (page 293).[7]

Devil's claw is also considered by herbalists to be a potent bitter. Bitter principles, like the iridoid glycosides found in devil's claw, can be used in combination with carminative (gas-relieving) herbs by people with **indigestion** (page 260), but not **heartburn** (page 260).

How much is usually taken?

As a digestive stimulant, 1.5–2 grams per day of the powdered secondary tuber are used.[8] For tincture, the recommended amount is 1–2 ml three times daily. For **osteoarthritis** (page 328) and **rheumatoid arthritis** (page 387), 4.5–10 grams of powder are used per day. Alternatively, standardized extracts, 1,200–2,500 mg per day, may be taken.

Are there any side effects or interactions?

Since devil's claw promotes the secretion of stomach acid, anyone with gastric or duodenal **ulcers** (page 349), **heartburn** (page 260), **gastritis** (page 195), or excessive stomach acid should not use the herb. Additionally, people with **gallstones** (page 193) should consult a physician before taking devil's claw.[9]

DONG QUAI

Common names: Dang-gui, Chinese angelica
Botanical name: *Angelica sinensis*

Parts used and where grown

Dong quai is a member of the celery family. Greenish-white flowers bloom from May to August, and the plant is typically found growing in damp mountain ravines, meadows, river banks, and coastal areas. The root is used in herbal medicine.

Dong quai has been used in connection with the following conditions (refer to the individual health concern for complete information):

Rating	Health Concerns
★☆☆	Anemia (due to dialysis) **Dysmenorrhea** (page 171) (painful menstruation) **Menopause** (page 311) **Premenstrual syndrome** (page 368)

Historical or traditional use (may or may not be supported by scientific studies)

Also known as dang-gui in Traditional Chinese Medicine (TCM), dong quai is sometimes referred to as the female ginseng. In Traditional Chinese Medicine, dong quai is often included in herbal combinations for abnormal menstruation, suppressed menstrual flow, **dysmenorrhea** (page 171) (painful menstruation), and uterine bleeding. It is not used in TCM for treating symptoms associated with **menopause** (page 311), such as hot flashes. It is also used in TCM for both men and women with **cardiovascular disease** (page 98), including **high blood pressure** (page 246) and problems with peripheral circulation.[1]

Active constituents

Traditionally, dong quai is believed to have a balancing or "adaptogenic" effect on the female hormonal system. Contrary to the opinion of some authors, dong quai does not qualify as a phytoestrogen and does not appear to have any hormone-like actions in the body. This is partially supported by a double-blind trial with **menopausal** (page 311) women that found no estrogenic activity for the herb.[2] In Traditional Chinese Medicine, dong quai is rarely used alone and is typically used in combination with herbs such as peony and ligusticum for conditions such as menstrual cramps.[3]

Dong quai has been traditionally used as a way to promote formation of red blood cells, an effect partially supported in a case study of a man with kidney failure who had a significant improvement in anemia due to dialysis while drinking a tea composed of dong quai and peony.[4] No clinical trials have examined dong quai alone for this purpose, or for the treatment of other forms of anemia.

How much is usually taken?

The powdered root can be used in capsules or tablets.[5] Women may take 3–4 grams daily in three divided applications. Alternatively, 3–5 ml of tincture may be taken three times per day.

Are there any side effects or interactions?

Dong quai may cause some fair-skinned people to become more sensitive to sunlight. People using it on a regular basis should limit prolonged exposure to the sun or other sources of ultraviolet radiation. Dong quai is not recommended for **pregnant** (page 363) or breastfeeding women.[6]

ECHINACEA

Common name: Purple coneflower
Botanical names: *Echinacea purpurea, Echinacea angustifolia, Echinacea pallida*

Parts used and where grown

Echinacea is a wildflower native to North America. While echinacea continues to grow and is harvested from the wild, the majority used for herbal supplements comes from cultivated plants. The root and/or the above-ground part of the plant during the flowering growth phase are used in herbal medicine.

Echinacea has been used in connection with the following conditions (refer to the individual health concern for complete information):

Rating	Health Concerns
★★★	**Common cold/sore throat** (page 129) (for symptoms; effective only for adults)
★★☆	**Gingivitis** (page 203) (periodontal disease) (as mouthwash, in combination with **sage** [page 740], **peppermint** [page 726] oil, menthol, **chamomile** [page 656] tincture, **myrrh** [page 713] tincture, clove oil, and **caraway oil** [page 651]) **Immune function** (page 255) **Infection** (page 265) **Influenza** (page 269)
★☆☆	**Bronchitis** (page 80) **Canker sores** (page 90) **Chronic candidiasis** (page 109) **Cold sores** (page 119) **Ear infections (recurrent)** (page 383) **Gingivitis (periodontal disease)** (page 203) **HIV support** (page 239) **Pap smear (abnormal)** (page 3) **Vaginitis** (page 438) **Wound healing** (page 319) (topical) **Yeast infection** (page 454)

Historical or traditional use (may or may not be supported by scientific studies)

Echinacea was used by Native Americans for a variety of conditions, including venomous bites and other external wounds. It was introduced into U.S. medical practice in 1887 and was touted for use in conditions ranging from **colds** (page 129) to syphilis. Modern research started in the 1930s in Germany.

Echinacea

Active constituents

Echinacea is thought to support the **immune system** (page 255) by activating white blood cells.[1] Three major groups of constituents may work together to increase the production and activity of white blood cells (lymphocytes and macrophages), including alkylamides/polyacetylenes, caffeic acid derivatives, and polysaccharides. More studies are needed to determine if and how echinacea stimulates the immune system in humans.

Echinacea may also increase production of interferon, an important part of the body's response to viral infections.[2] Several double-blind studies have confirmed the benefit of echinacea for treating **colds** (page 129) and **flu** (page 269).[3, 4, 5, 6, 7] Recent studies have suggested that echinacea may not be effective for the *prevention* of colds and flu and should be reserved for use at the onset of these conditions.[8, 9] In terms of other types of infections, research in Germany using injectable forms or an oral preparation of the herb along with a medicated cream (econazole nitrate) reduced the recurrence of vaginal **yeast infections** (page 454) as compared to women given the cream alone.[10]

How much is usually taken?

At the onset of a cold or flu, 3–4 ml of echinacea in a liquid preparation or 300 mg of a powdered form in capsule or tablet, can be taken every two hours for the first day of illness, then three times per day for a total of 7 to 10 days.[11]

Are there any side effects or interactions?

Echinacea is rarely associated with side effects when taken orally.[12] According to the German Commission E monograph, people should not take echinacea if they have an autoimmune illness, such as **lupus** (page 421), or other progressive diseases, such as tuberculosis, **multiple sclerosis** (page 323), or **HIV** (page 239) infection. However, the concern about echinacea use for those with autoimmune illness is not based on clinical research and some herbalists question the potential connection. Those who are allergic to flowers of the daisy family should not take echinacea. Cases of allergic responses to echinacea (e.g., wheezing, skin rash, **diarrhea** [page 163]) have been reported in medical literature.[13] In the first study to look at echinacea's possible effect on fetal development and pregnancy outcome, women taking echinacea during **pregnancy** (page 363) were found to have no greater incidence of miscarriage or **birth defects** (page 63) than women not taking the herb.[14]

Echinacea root contains approximately 20% inulin,[15] a fiber widely distributed in fruits, vegetables, and plants. Inulin is classified as a food ingredient (not as an additive) and is considered safe to eat.[16] In fact, inulin is a significant part of the daily diet of most of the world's population.[17] However, there is a report of a 39-year-old man having a life-threatening allergic reaction after consuming high amounts of inulin from multiple sources.[18] Allergy to inulin in this individual was confirmed by laboratory tests. Such sensitivities are exceedingly rare. Moreover, this man did not take echinacea. Nevertheless, people with a confirmed sensitivity to inulin should avoid echinacea.

ELDERBERRY

Common names: European elderberry (black elderberry), North American elderberry
Botanical name: *Sambucus nigra*

Parts used and where grown

Numerous species of elder or elderberry grow in Europe and North America. Only those with blue/black berries are medicinal. The flowers and berries are both used. Species with red berries are not medicinal.

Elderberry has been used in connection with the following conditions (refer to the individual health concern for complete information):

Rating	Health Concerns
★★☆	**Influenza** (page 269)
★☆☆	**Cold sores** (page 119)
	Common cold/sore throat (page 129)
	Infection (page 265)
	Inflammation

Historical or traditional use (may or may not be supported by scientific studies)

Elderberries have long been used as food, particularly in the dried form. Elderberry wine, pie, and lemonade are some of the popular ways to prepare this plant as food. The leaves were touted by European herbalists to be pain relieving and to promote healing of injuries when applied as a poultice.[1] Native American herbalists used the plant for **infections** (page 265), **coughs** (page 139), and skin conditions.

Active constituents

Flavonoids (page 516), including **quercetin** (page 580), are believed to account for the therapeutic actions of the elderberry flowers and berries. These flavonoids include anthocyanins that are powerful **antioxidants** (page 467) and protect cells against damage according to test tube studies.[2] According to laboratory research, an extract from the leaves, combined with **St. John's wort** (page 747) and soapwort, inhibits the **influenza** (page 269) virus and **herpes simplex** (page 119) virus.[3] The effect on influenza of a syrup made from the berries of the black elderberry has been studied in a small double-blind trial.[4] People receiving an elderberry extract (2 tablespoons [30 ml] per day for children, 4 tablespoons [60 ml] per day for adults) appeared to recover faster than did those receiving a placebo. Animal studies have shown the flowers to have anti-inflammatory properties.[5] These actions have not been verified in human clinical trials.

How much is usually taken?

A syrup of black elderberry extract (1 teaspoon–1 tablespoon [5–15 ml] for children, 2 teaspoons–2 tablespoons [10–30 ml] for adults) can be taken twice daily. A tea made from ½–1 teaspoon (3–5 grams) of the dried flowers steeped in 1 cup (250 ml) boiling water for ten to fifteen minutes may be drunk three times per day.[6]

Are there any side effects or interactions?

The safe internal use of elderberry is limited to the use of the dried flowers or syrups made from the ripe berries.[7] The roots, stems, leaves, and unripe berries may contain poisonous constituents that can cause nausea, vomiting, and **diarrhea** (page 163).[8] Preparations containing any of these parts of the elder plant should be avoided.

ELECAMPANE

Common name: Inula
Botanical name: *Inula helenium*

Parts used and where grown

Elecampane is indigenous to Europe and Asia and is now grown in the United States. The dried roots and rhizomes (branching part of the root) are collected in fall or early winter and used in herbal preparations.

Elecampane has been used in connection with the following conditions (refer to the individual health concern for complete information):

Rating	Health Concerns
★☆☆	**Asthma** (page 32)
	Bronchitis (page 80)
	Chronic obstructive pulmonary disease (page 114) (COPD)
	Cough (page 139)
	Indigestion (page 260)

Historical or traditional use (may or may not be supported by scientific studies)

Traditionally, herbalists have used elecampane to treat **coughs** (page 139), particularly those associated with **bronchitis** (page 80), **asthma** (page 32), and whooping cough.[1] The herb has also been used historically to treat poor digestion and general complaints of the intestinal tract.

Active constituents

Elecampane root and rhizome contain approximately 1–4% volatile oils.[2] Most of these volatile oils are composed of sesquiterpene lactones, including alantolactone. Elecampane is also very high in inulin (44%)[3] and mucilage. Most herbal texts attribute the actions of elecampane to alantolactone.[4] The antitussive (cough prevention and treatment) and carminative (soothing effect on the intestinal tract) effects of elecampane, however, may possibly be due to the inulin and mucilage content. Isolated alantolactone has been used to treat **parasites** (page 343) (e.g., roundworm, threadworm, hookworm, whipworm). This use is only by prescription and is not approved in all European countries.[5]

How much is usually taken?

The German Commission E Monograph states the historical application of elecampane has not been adequately proven to recommend its use.[6] This is partially based on the potential side effects listed below. For traditional use, elecampane is typically recommended as a tea. Boiling water is poured over ¼ teaspoon (1 gram) of the ground root and rhizome, left to steep for ten to fifteen minutes, then strained. One cup of this preparation is taken three to four times daily. Some texts recommend ½ to 1 teaspoon (3–5 ml) of a tincture three times daily.[7]

Are there any side effects or interactions?

The inulin in elecampane root is widely distributed in fruits, vegetables and plants. It is classified as a food ingredient (not as an additive) and is considered safe to eat.[8] In fact, inulin is a significant part of the daily diet of most of the world's population.[9] However, there is a report of a 39-year-old man having a life-threatening allergic reaction after consuming high amounts of inulin from multiple sources.[10] Allergy to inulin in this individual was confirmed by laboratory tests. Such sensitivities are extremely rare. Moreover, this man did not take elecampane. Nevertheless, people with a confirmed sensitivity to inulin should avoid elecampane.

Alantolactone can be an irritant to the intestinal tract and, along with other sesquiterpene lactones in elecampane, may cause localized irritation in the mouth. Amounts several times higher than those stated above may cause vomiting, **diarrhea** (page 163), spasms, and signs of paralysis.[11] If these symptoms occur, people should contact their local poison control center. **Pregnant** (page 363) or nursing women should not use elecampane.

ELEUTHERO

Common names: Siberian ginseng, ci wu jia, touch-me-not, devil's shrub
Botanical names: *Eleutherococcus senticosus, Acanthopanax senticosus*

Parts used and where grown
Eleuthero belongs to the Araliaceae family and is a distant relative of **Asian ginseng** (page 630) *(Panax ginseng)*. Also known commonly as touch-me-not and devil's shrub, eleuthero has been most frequently nicknamed Siberian ginseng in this country. Eleuthero is native to the Taiga region of the Far East (southeastern part of Russia, northern China, Korea, and Japan). The root and the rhizomes (underground stem) are used medicinally.

Eleuthero has been used in connection with the following conditions (refer to the individual health concern for complete information):

Rating	Health Concerns
★★☆	**Athletic performance** (page 43)
	Fatigue
	Immune function (page 255)
	Stress

★☆☆	**Breast cancer** (page 65)
	Chronic fatigue syndrome (page 111)
	Common cold/sore throat (page 129)
	Diabetes (page 152)
	HIV support (page 239)
	Infection (page 265)
	Influenza (page 269)

Historical or traditional use (may or may not be supported by scientific studies)
Although not as popular as **Asian ginseng** (page 630), eleuthero use dates back 2,000 years, according to Chinese medicine records. Referred to as ci wu jia in Chinese medicine, it was used to prevent respiratory tract infections, **colds** (page 129) and **flu** (page 269). It was also believed to provide energy and vitality. In Russia, eleuthero was originally used by people in the Siberian Taiga region to increase performance and quality of life and to decrease **infections** (page 265).

In more modern times, eleuthero has been used to increase stamina and endurance in Soviet Olympic athletes. Russian explorers, divers, sailors, and miners also used eleuthero to prevent stress-related illness. After the Chernobyl accident, many Russian and Ukrainian citizens were given eleuthero to counteract the effects of radiation.

Active constituents
The constituents in eleuthero that have been most studied are the eleutherosides.[1] Seven primary eleutherosides have been identified, with most of the research attention focusing on eleutherosides B and E.[2] Eleuthero also contains complex polysaccharides (complex sugar molecules).[3] These constituents may play a critical role in eleuthero's ability to support **immune function** (page 255).

Eleuthero is an "adaptogen" (an agent that helps the body adapt to stress). It is thought to help support adrenal gland function when the body is challenged by stress.[4]

Eleuthero has been shown to enhance mental acuity and physical endurance without the letdown that comes with caffeinated products.[5] Research has shown that eleuthero improves the use of oxygen by the exercising muscle.[6] This means that a person is able to maintain aerobic **exercise** (page 43) longer and recover from workouts more quickly. Preliminary research from Russia indicates it may be effective for this purpose.[7] Other trials have been inconclusive[8] or have shown no beneficial effect.[9]

Eleuthero may also support the body by helping the liver detoxify harmful toxins. It has shown a protective action in animal studies against chemicals such as ethanol, sodium barbital, tetanus toxoid, and chemotherapeutic agents.[10] According to a test tube study eleuthero also helps protect the body during radiation exposure.[11] Preliminary research in Russia has suggested that eleuthero may help alleviate side effects and help the bone marrow recover more quickly in people undergoing chemotherapy and radiation therapy for **cancer** (page 87).[12]

Eleuthero may be useful as a preventive measure during the **cold** (page 129) and **flu** (page 269) season. However, it has not yet been specifically studied for this purpose. Preliminary evidence also suggests that eleuthero may prove valuable in the long-term management of various diseases of the immune system, including **HIV** (page 239) infection and **chronic fatigue syndrome** (page 111). Healthy people taking 2 teaspoons (10 ml) of tincture three times daily have been shown to have increased numbers of the immune cells (T4 lymphocytes) that have been found to decrease during HIV-infection and AIDS.[13] Further human clinical trials are needed to confirm that eleuthero may be helpful for this disease.

How much is usually taken?
Dried, powdered root and rhizomes, 2–3 grams per day, are commonly used.[14] Alternatively, 300–400 mg per day of concentrated solid extract standardized on eleutherosides B and E can be used, as can alcohol-based extracts, 8–10 ml in two to three divided dosages. Historically, eleuthero is taken continuously for six to eight weeks, followed by a one- to two-week break before resuming.

Are there any side effects or interactions?
Reported side effects have been minimal with use of eleuthero.[15] Mild, transient **diarrhea** (page 163) has been reported in a very small number of users. Eleuthero may cause **insomnia** (page 270) in some people if taken too close to bedtime. Eleuthero is not recommended for people with uncontrolled **high blood pressure** (page 246). There are no known reasons to avoid eleuthero during **pregnancy** (page 363) and breast-feeding. However, pregnant or breast-feeding women should be aware that some products may be adulterated with herbs that should *not* be taken in pregnancy, such as **Asian ginseng** (page 630). Only eleuthero from a trusted source should be used.

In one case report, a person taking eleuthero with digoxin developed dangerously high serum digoxin levels.[16] Although a clear relationship could not be established, it is wise for someone taking digoxin to seek the advise of a doctor before taking eleuthero.

EUCALYPTUS

Botanical name: *Eucalyptus globulus*

Parts used and where grown
Eucalyptus is an evergreen tree native to Australia but is cultivated worldwide. The plant's leaves—and the oil that is steam-distilled from them—are used medicinally.[1]

Eucalyptus has been used in connection with the following conditions (refer to the individual health concern for complete information):

Rating	Health Concerns
★★☆	Insect repellant (topical)
★☆☆	**Athletic performance** (page 43) (topical) **Bronchitis** (page 80) **Chronic obstructive pulmonary disease** (page 114) (COPD) **Common cold** (page 129) **Cough** (page 139) **Genital herpes** (page 200) (topical) **Infection** (page 265) **Low back pain** (page 293) Rheumatism (topical use) **Rheumatoid arthritis** (page 387) (oil, topical) **Sinus congestion** (page 405) **Sinusitis** (page 407)

Historical or traditional use (may or may not be supported by scientific studies)
Eucalyptus was first used by Australian aborigines, who not only chewed the roots for water in the dry outback but used the leaves as a remedy for fevers. In the 1800s, crew members of an Australian freighter developed high fevers, but were able to successfully cure their condition using eucalyptus tea. Thus, eucalyptus became well known throughout Europe and the Mediterranean as the Australian fever tree. Early 19th century Eclectic physicians in the United States not only used eucalyptus oil to sterilize instruments and wounds, but recommended a steam inhalation of the vapor of its oil to help

treat **asthma** (page 32), **bronchitis** (page 80), whooping cough, and emphysema.[2]

Active constituents

The major constituent in eucalyptus leaves is a volatile oil known as eucalyptol (1,8-cineol). In order to provide an effective expectorant and antiseptic action, the leaf oil should contain approximately 70–85% eucalyptol.[3] Eucalyptus oil is said to function in a fashion similar to that of menthol by acting on receptors in the nasal mucosa, leading to a reduction in symptoms such as **nasal congestion** (page 405).[4] In test tube studies, eucalyptus species have been shown to possess antibacterial actions against such organisms as *Bacillus subtilis*,[5] as well as several strains of *Streptococcus*.[6] These actions have not been researched in human clinical trials.

Peppermint (page 726) (10 grams) and eucalyptus oil (5 grams) in combination, applied topically to the forehead and temples for three minutes with a small sponge, have been shown to be helpful as a muscle relaxant (but not for pain relief) in people with tension headaches.[7] A eucalyptus oil extract containing 50% p-methane-3,8-diol (PMD) as the active ingredient has been shown to be effective in protecting human volunteers from various types of biting insects.[8] On human forearms, it was determined that the eucalyptus extract was nearly as effective as a 20% solution of diethyltoluamine (used in many insect repellents) in repelling bites of the *Anopheles* mosquito (the insect that spreads malaria) for up to five hours. The eucalyptus extract was also effective at repelling flies (94%) and midges (100%) for up to six hours.

A preliminary study suggests the combination of eucalyptus and menthol as a nasal inhalant is helpful in cases of mild to moderate snoring.[9] Also, in a double-blind trial, a eucalyptus-based rub was found helpful for warming muscles in athletes.[10] This further suggests eucalyptus may help relieve minor muscle soreness when applied topically, though studies are needed to confirm this possibility.

How much is usually taken?

Eucalyptus oil (0.05–0.2 ml per day) can be taken internally by adults.[11] It should always be diluted in warm water before consuming. For local applications, 30 ml of the oil can be mixed in 500 ml of lukewarm water and applied topically as an insect repellent or used over the temporal areas of the forehead for tension headaches. As an inhalant, add a few drops of eucalyptus oil to hot water or a vaporizer. Deeply inhale the

steam vapor. For eucalyptus leaf preparations, an infusion of 2–3 grams of the chopped leaves may be boiled in 150 ml of water and taken two times per day. Eucalyptus oil needs to be used very cautiously since as little as 3.5 ml of the oil taken internally has proven fatal.[12] It is best for people to discuss internal use with a qualified healthcare professional.

> **Warning:** Eucalyptus oil needs to be used very cautiously since as little as 3.5 ml of the oil taken internally has proven fatal. It is best for individuals to discuss internal use with a qualified healthcare professional.

Are there any side effects or interactions?

Side effects from the internal use of eucalyptus can include nausea, vomiting, and **diarrhea** (page 163). Eucalyptus oil should not be used by infants and children under the age of two, especially near the face and nose, due to the risk of airway spasm and possible cessation of breathing.[13] The oil may aggravate bronchial spasms in people with **asthma** (page 32) and should not be taken internally by those with severe liver diseases and inflammatory disorders of the gastrointestinal tract and kidney.[14, 15] Whole-body application of eucalyptus oil (double-distilled, containing 80–85% cineole oil) resulted in severe nervous system toxicity in a six year old girl.[16] Parents are advised to use topical eucalyptus oil in moderation with children.

Although there are no known reports of drug interactions, the German Commission E monograph suggests that because eucalyptus oil may activate certain enzyme systems in the liver, it may potentially weaken or shorten the action of some medications, including pentobarbital, aminopyrine, and amphetamine.[17, 18] Eucalyptus should not be used in large amounts by people with low blood pressure as it may cause a further drop in blood pressure.[19] The safety of eucalyptus oil has not been established in **pregnant** (page 363) or nursing women.

EYEBRIGHT

Botanical name: *Euphrasia officinalis*

Parts used and where grown

In the wild, European eyebright grows in meadows, pastures, and grassy places in Bulgaria, Hungary, and the former Yugoslavia. Eyebright is also grown commercially in Europe. The plant flowers in late summer and autumn. The whole herb is used in herbal medicine.

Eyebright has been used in connection with the following conditions (refer to the individual health concern for complete information):

Rating	Health Concerns
★☆☆	**Conjunctivitis/blepharitis** (page 136) Irritated eyes

Historical or traditional use (may or may not be supported by scientific studies)

Eyebright was and continues to be used by herbalists primarily as a poultice for the topical treatment of eye inflammations, including **conjunctivitis/blepharitis** (page 136) and sties. Traditionally, a compress made from a decoction of eyebright is used to give relief from redness, swelling, and visual disturbances due to eye **infections** (page 265).[1] A tea is sometimes given internally along with the topical treatment. It has also been used for the treatment of eye fatigue and other disturbances of vision. In addition, herbalists have recommended eyebright for problems of the respiratory tract, including **sinus infections** (page 407), **coughs** (page 139), and **sore throat** (page 129).[2] None of the traditional uses of eyebright have been studied in clinical research.

Active constituents

While there are many chemicals that may be active in eyebright, none of them has been proven to have any effect on eye inflammation or irritation. Some herbal texts suggest that the astringent actions of eyebright may reduce eye irritation while others suggest that eyebright may also have antibacterial actions topically. To date, there are no clinical studies to support or refute these proposed actions.

How much is usually taken?

Traditional herbal texts recommend a compress made with 1 tablespoon (15 grams) of the dried herb combined with 2 cups (500 ml) of water and boiled for ten minutes.[3] The undiluted liquid is used as a compress after cooling. The German Commission E monograph does not support this application, due to possible impurities in non-pharmaceutical preparations.[4] Consult with a physician knowledgeable in the use of herbs before applying eyebright to the eyes.

Internally, two to three cups per day of eyebright tea is sometimes recommended. Dried herb, ½–¾ teaspoon (2–4 grams) three times per day, may also be taken. The tincture is typically taken in ½–1¼ teaspoons (2–6 ml) three times per day.

Are there any side effects or interactions?

Due to limited information on the active constituents in eyebright and the need for sterility in substances used topically in the eyes, the traditional use of eyebright as a topical compress currently cannot be recommended without professional support. Used internally at the amounts listed above, eyebright is generally safe. However, its safety during **pregnancy** (page 363) and breastfeeding has not been proven.

FALSE UNICORN

Botanical name: *Chamaelirium luteum*

Parts used and where grown

False unicorn is native to Mississippi and continues to grow primarily in the southern part of the United States. The roots of false unicorn are most commonly used in herbal medicine.

False unicorn has been used in connection with the following conditions (refer to the individual health concern for complete information):

Rating	Health Concerns
★☆☆	**Dysmenorrhea** (page 171) (painful menstruation)

Historical or traditional use (may or may not be supported by scientific studies)

The medicinal use of false unicorn root is based in traditional Native American herbalism. It was recommended for many women's health conditions, including **dysmenorrhea** (page 171) (painful menstruation) and other irregularities of menstruation, as well as to prevent miscarriages.[1] False unicorn was also used as a remedy for **morning sickness** (page 320).

Active constituents

Steroidal saponins are generally credited with providing false unicorn root's activity.[2] However, modern investigations have not confirmed this, and no research exists about the medical applications of this herb.

How much is usually taken?
False unicorn root tincture, ½–1 teaspoon (2–5 ml) three times per day, is sometimes recommended .[3] The dried root, ¼–½ teaspoon (1–2 grams) three times per day, is also used.

Are there any side effects or interactions?
No adverse effects have been reported with the use of false unicorn. Although false unicorn has been used historically for nausea and vomiting of pregnancy and to prevent miscarriages, its actions as a possible uterine tonic make its use during **pregnancy** (page 363) potentially unsafe.

FENNEL

Botanical name: *Foeniculum vulgare*

Parts used and where grown
The fennel plant came originally from Europe, where it is still grown. Fennel is also cultivated in many parts of North America, Asia, and Egypt. Fennel seeds are used in herbal medicine.

Fennel has been used in connection with the following conditions (refer to the individual health concern for complete information):

Rating	Health Concerns
★★☆	**Colic** (page 121) (in combination with **chamomile** [page 656], **vervain** [page 756], **licorice** [page 702] and **lemon balm** [page 701])
	Colic (page 121) (fennel seed oil)
	Indigestion and heartburn (page 260)
★☆☆	**Irritable bowel syndrome** (page 280)

Historical or traditional use (may or may not be supported by scientific studies)
According to the Greek legend of Prometheus, fennel was thought to have bestowed immortality.[1] Fennel seeds are a common cooking spice, particularly for use with fish. After meals, they are used in several cultures to prevent gas and upset stomach.[2] Fennel has also been used as a remedy for **cough** (page 139) and **colic** (page 121) in infants.

Active constituents
The major constituents, which include the terpenoid anethole, are found in the volatile oil. Anethole and other terpenoids inhibit spasms in smooth muscles,[3] such as those in the intestinal tract, and this is thought to contribute to fennel's use as a carminative (gas-relieving and gastrointestinal tract cramp-relieving agent). Related compounds to anethole may have mild estrogenic actions, although this has not been proven in humans. Fennel is also thought to possess diuretic (increase in urine production), choleretic (increase in production of bile), pain-reducing, fever-reducing, and anti-microbial actions.[4] Fennel was formerly an official drug in the United States and was listed as being used for **indigestion** (page 260).[5]

How much is usually taken?
The German Commission E monograph recommends 1–1½ teaspoons (5–7 grams) of seeds per day.[6] To make a tea, boil ½ teaspoon (2–3 grams) of crushed seeds per 1 cup (250 ml) of water for ten to fifteen minutes, keeping the pot covered during the process. Cool, strain, and then drink three cups (750 ml) per day. As a tincture, 1–2 teaspoons (5–10 ml) can be taken three times per day between meals.

Are there any side effects or interactions?
No significant adverse effects have been reported. However, in rare cases fennel can cause allergic reactions of the skin and respiratory tract.[7] Anyone with an estrogen-dependent **cancer** (page 87) (e.g., some **breast cancer** (page 65) patients) should avoid fennel in large quantities until the significance of its estrogen-like activity is clarified.

FENUGREEK

Botanical name: *Trigonella foenum-graecum*

Parts used and where grown
Although originally from southeastern Europe and western Asia, fenugreek grows today in many parts of the world, including India, northern Africa, and the United States. The seeds of fenugreek are used medicinally.

Fenugreek has been used in connection with the following conditions (refer to the individual health concern for complete information):

Rating	Health Concerns
★★★	Diabetes (page 152) High cholesterol (page 223)
★★☆	Atherosclerosis (page 38) High triglycerides (page 235)
★☆☆	Constipation (page 137)

Historical or traditional use (may or may not be supported by scientific studies)

A wide range of uses were found for fenugreek in ancient times. Medicinally it was used for the treatment of **wounds** (page 319), abscesses, arthritis, **bronchitis** (page 80), and digestive problems. Traditional Chinese herbalists used it for kidney problems and conditions affecting the male reproductive tract.[1] Fenugreek was, and remains, a food and a spice commonly eaten in many parts of the world.

Active constituents

Fenugreek seeds contain alkaloids (mainly trigonelline) and protein high in **lysine** (page 550) and L-tryptophan. Its steroidal saponins (diosgenin, yamogenin, tigogenin, and neotigogenin) and mucilaginous **fiber** (page 512) are thought to account for many of the beneficial effects of fenugreek. The steroidal saponins are thought to inhibit cholesterol absorption and synthesis,[2] while the fiber may help lower blood sugar levels.[3] One human study found that fenugreek can help lower **cholesterol** (page 223) and blood sugar levels in people with moderate **atherosclerosis** (page 38) and non-insulin-dependent (type 2) **diabetes** (page 152).[4] Preliminary and double-blind trials have found that fenugreek helps improve blood sugar control in patients with insulin-dependent (type 1) and non-insulin-dependent (type 2) diabetes.[5, 6, 7] Double-blind trials have shown that fenugreek lowers elevated cholesterol and **triglyceride** (page 235) levels in the blood,[8, 9] This has also been found in a controlled clinical trial with diabetic patients with elevated cholesterol.[10] Generally, fenugreek does not lower HDL ("good") cholesterol levels.

How much is usually taken?

Due to the somewhat bitter taste of fenugreek seeds, de-bitterized seeds or encapsulated products are pre-ferred. The German Commission E monograph recommends a daily intake of 6 grams.[11] The typical range of intake for **diabetes** (page 152) or **cholesterol** (page 223)-lowering is 5–30 grams with each meal or 15–90 grams all at once with one meal. As a tincture, 3–4 ml of fenugreek can be taken up to three times per day.

Are there any side effects or interactions?

Use of more than 100 grams of fenugreek seeds daily can cause intestinal upset and nausea. Otherwise, fenugreek is extremely safe. Due to the potential uterine stimulating properties of fenugreek, which may cause miscarriages, fenugreek should not be used during **pregnancy** (page 363).[12]

FEVERFEW

Botanical name: *Tanacetum parthenium*

Parts used and where grown

Feverfew grows widely across Europe and North America. The leaves are used in herbal medicine.

Feverfew has been used in connection with the following conditions (refer to the individual health concern for complete information):

Rating	Health Concerns
★★★	Migraine headaches (page 316)

Historical or traditional use (may or may not be supported by scientific studies)

Feverfew was mentioned in Greek medical literature as a remedy for inflammation and for menstrual discomforts. Traditional herbalists in Great Britain used it to treat fevers, rheumatism, and other aches and pains.

Active constituents

Feverfew contains a range of compounds known as sesquiterpene lactones. Over 85% of these are a compound called parthenolide. In test tube studies, parthenolide prevents excessive clumping of platelets and inhibits the release of certain chemicals, including serotonin and some inflammatory mediators.[1, 2] Feverfew's parthenolide content was originally thought to account for the anti-migraine action of this herb, but this has been a matter of recent debate.[3]

According to three double-blind trials with migraine patients, feverfew reduces the severity, duration, and frequency of **migraine headaches** (page 316).[4, 5, 6] These successful studies employed dried, powdered leaves. One negative study used an alcohol extract suggesting the dried leaf preparation is superior.[7]

How much is usually taken?

Feverfew leaf products with at least 0.2% parthenolide content are generally used. Standardized leaf extracts may contain up to 0.7% parthenolide. Herbal products in capsules or tablets providing at least 250 mcg of parthenolide per day may be taken.[8] It may take four to six weeks before benefits are noticed. Feverfew is useful for decreasing the severity and incidence of migraines. However, it is not an effective treatment for an acute migraine attack.

Are there any side effects or interactions?

Taken as recommended, standardized feverfew causes minimal side effects. Minor side effects include gastrointestinal upset and nervousness. Chewing feverfew leaves has been reported to cause **canker sores** (page 90).[9] Feverfew is not recommended during **pregnancy** (page 363) or breast-feeding and should not be used by children under the age of two years.

FO-TI

Common name: He-shou-wu
Botanical name: *Polygonum multiflorum*

Parts used and where grown

Fo-ti is a plant native to China, where it continues to be widely grown. It also grows extensively in Japan and Taiwan. The unprocessed root is sometimes used medicinally. However, once it has been boiled in a special liquid made from black beans, it is considered a superior and rather different medicine according to Traditional Chinese Medicine. The unprocessed root is sometimes called white fo-ti and the processed root red fo-ti. According to Chinese herbal medicine, the unprocessed root is used to relax the bowels and detoxify the blood, and the processed root is used to strengthen the blood, invigorate the kidneys and liver, and serve as a tonic to increase overall vitality.

Fo-ti has been used in connection with the following conditions (refer to the individual health concern for complete information):

Rating	Health Concerns
★☆☆	**Constipation** (page 137) **High cholesterol** (page 223) **Immune function** (page 255)

Historical or traditional use (may or may not be supported by scientific studies)

The Chinese common name for fo-ti, he-shou-wu, was the name of a Tang dynasty man whose infertility was supposedly cured by fo-ti. In addition, his long life was attributed to the tonic properties of this herb.[1] Since then, Traditional Chinese Medicine has used fo-ti to treat premature aging, weakness, vaginal discharges, numerous infectious diseases, **angina pectoris** (page 27), and **erectile dysfunction** (page 185).

Active constituents

The major constituents of fo-ti are anthraquinones, phospholipids (e.g., lecithin), tannins, and tetrahydroxystilbene glucoside. The processed root has been used to lower cholesterol levels in Traditional Chinese Medicine. According to animal research, it helps to decrease fat deposits in the blood and possibly prevent **atherosclerosis** (page 38).[2, 3] However, human clinical trials are lacking to support this use. Test tube studies have suggested fo-ti's ability to stimulate **immune function** (page 255), increase red blood cell formation, and exert an antibacterial action.[4] None of these effects has been studied in humans. The unprocessed roots have a mild laxative action.

How much is usually taken?

The typical recommended intake is 1–1½ teaspoons (4–8 grams) per day.[5] A tea can be made from processed roots by boiling ½–1 teaspoons (3–5 grams) in 1 cup (250 ml) of water for ten to fifteen minutes. Three or more cups are suggested each day. Five fo-ti tablets (500 mg each) can be taken three times per day.

Are there any side effects or interactions?

The unprocessed roots may cause mild **diarrhea** (page 163).[6] Some people who are sensitive to fo-ti may develop a skin rash. Taking more than 15 grams of processed root powder may cause numbness in the arms or legs.

GARLIC

Botanical name: *Allium sativum*

Parts used and where grown

Garlic has been used since time immemorial as a culinary spice and medicinal herb. Garlic has been cultivated in the Middle East for more than 5,000 years and has been an important part of Traditional Chinese Medicine. The region with the largest commercial garlic production is central California. China is also a supplier of commercial garlic. The bulb is used medicinally.

Garlic has been used in connection with the following conditions (refer to the individual health concern for complete information):

Rating	Health Concerns
★★★	**Atherosclerosis** (page 38)
★★☆	**BPH** (page 58) (Kastamonu Garlic) **Breast-feeding support** (page 74) **Colon cancer** (page 123) (reduces risk of stomach, esophageal, and colon cancers) **Common cold** (page 129) **High blood pressure** (page 246) **High cholesterol** (page 223) **High triglycerides** (page 235) **Intermittent claudication** (page 276) **Warts** (page 445) (topical application)
★☆☆	**Athlete's foot** (page 42) **Chronic candidiasis** (page 109) **Ear infections (recurrent)** (page 383) **HIV support** (page 239) **Infection** (page 265) **Parasites** (page 343) **Peptic ulcer** (page 349) **Sickle cell anemia** (page 403)

Historical or traditional use (may or may not be supported by scientific studies)

Garlic is mentioned in the Bible and the Talmud. Hippocrates, Galen, Pliny the Elder, and Dioscorides all mention the use of garlic for many conditions, including **parasites** (page 343), respiratory problems, poor digestion, and low energy. Its use in China was first mentioned in A.D. 510. Louis Pasteur studied the antibacterial action of garlic in 1858.

Active constituents

The sulfur compound allicin, produced by crushing or chewing fresh garlic or by taking powdered garlic products with allicin potential, in turn produces other sulfur compounds: ajoene, allyl sulfides, and vinyldithiins.[1] Aged garlic products lack allicin, but may have activity due to the presence of S-allylcysteine.

Many publications have shown that garlic supports the cardiovascular system. While earlier trials suggest it may mildly lower **cholesterol** (page 223) and **triglyceride** (page 235) levels in the blood,[2, 3, 4] more recent trials found garlic to have minimal success in lowering cholesterol and triglycerides.[5, 6, 7] Garlic also inhibits platelet stickiness (aggregation) and increases fibrinolysis,[8] which results in a slowing of blood coagulation. It is mildly **antihypertensive** (page 246)[9] and has **antioxidant** (page 467) activity.[10]

Garlic's cardiovascular protective effects were illustrated in a four-year clinical trial on people 50–80 years old with **atherosclerosis** (page 38).[11] It was found that consumption of 900 mg of a standardized garlic supplement reduced arterial plaque formation by 5–18%. The benefits were most notable in women.

In test tube studies garlic has been found to have antibacterial, antiviral, and antifungal activity.[12] However, these actions are less clear in humans and do not suggest that garlic is a substitute for antibiotics or antifungal medications.

Human population studies suggest that eating garlic regularly reduces the risk of esophageal, stomach, and **colon cancer** (page 123).[13, 14] This may be partly due to garlic's ability to reduce the formation of carcinogenic compounds.

How much is usually taken?

People who wish to consume garlic and have no aversion to its odor can chew from one to two whole cloves of raw garlic daily. For those who prefer it with less odor, enteric-coated tablets or capsules with approximately 1.3% allin are available. Clinical trials have used 600–900 mg (delivering approximately 5,000–6,000 mcg of allicin potential) per day in two or three divided amounts.[15, 16] Aged-garlic extracts have been studied in amounts ranging from 2.4–7.2 grams per day.

Are there any side effects or interactions?

Many people enjoy eating garlic. However, some people who are sensitive to it may experience **heartburn** (page 260) and flatulence. Because of garlic's anti-clotting properties, people taking anticoagulant drugs should check with their doctor before taking garlic.[17] Those scheduled for surgery should inform their surgeon if they are taking garlic supplements. Garlic appears to be safe during **pregnancy** (page 363) and breast-feeding. In fact, two studies have shown that babies like breast milk better from mothers who eat garlic.[18, 19]

GENTIAN

Botanical name: *Gentiana lutea*

Parts used and where grown
Gentian originally comes from meadows in Europe and Turkey. However, it is now also cultivated in North America. The root is used in herbal medicine.

Gentian has been used in connection with the following conditions (refer to the individual health concern for complete information):

Rating	Health Concerns
★☆☆	**Indigestion** (page 260)
	Poor appetite
	Sinusitis (page 407) (in combination with primrose flowers, sorrel herb, elder flowers, and European **vervain** [page 756])

Historical or traditional use (may or may not be supported by scientific studies)
Gentian root and other highly bitter plants have been used for centuries by herbalists in Europe as digestive aids (the well-known Swedish bitters often contain gentian). Other folk uses included topical application on skin tumors, decreasing fevers, and treatment of **diarrhea** (page 163).[1]

Active constituents
Gentian contains bitter substances such as the glycosides gentiopicrin and amarogentin. The bitter taste of these can be detected even when diluted 50,000 times.[2] Besides stimulating secretion of saliva in the mouth and hydrochloric acid in the stomach, gentiopicrin may protect the liver.[3] Gentian is used to treat poor appetite and **indigestion** (page 260).[4] An open study shows that gentian tincture inhibits the feeling of fullness after eating, suggesting it could improve poor appetite.[5]

How much is usually taken?
Tincture can be taken 20 minutes before each meal, for a total of ¼–½ teaspoon (1–3 ml) daily. Alternatively, whole root, ½–¾ teaspoon (2–4 grams) per day, can be used. Since capsules of the herb bypass the taste buds, they may not have the same effect as other dosage methods.

Are there any side effects or interactions?
Gentian should not be used by people suffering from excessive stomach acid, **heartburn** (page 260), **peptic ulcer disease** (page 349), or **gastritis** (page 195).[6]

GINGER

Botanical name: *Zingiber officinale*

Parts used and where grown
Ginger is a perennial plant that grows in India, China, Mexico, and several other countries. The rhizome (underground stem) is used as both a spice and in herbal medicine.

Ginger has been used in connection with the following conditions (refer to the individual health concern for complete information):

Rating	Health Concerns
★★★	**Motion sickness** (page 322)
	Osteoarthritis (page 328)
★★☆	**Epilepsy** (page 183) (in combination with **bupleurum** [page 647], peony root, pinellia root, cassia bark, jujube fruit, **Asian ginseng** [page 630] root, **Chinese scullcap** [page 658] root, and **licorice** [page 702] root)
	Indigestion (page 260)
	Irritable bowel syndrome (page 280) (Chinese herbal combination formula containing **wormwood** [page 762], ginger, **bupleurum** [page 647], **schisandra** [page 744], dan shen, and other extracts)
	Morning sickness (page 320)
	Nausea and vomiting following **surgery** (page 357)
	Nausea following chemotherapy
	Pre- and post-surgery health (page 357)
	Vertigo (page 441)
★☆☆	**Atherosclerosis** (page 38)
	Hay fever (page 211) (Sho-seiryu-to: contains **licorice** [page 702], cassia bark, **schisandra** [page 744], ma huang [ephedra], ginger, peony root, pinellia, and asiasarum root)
	HIV support (page 239) (in combination with **bupleurum** [page 647], peony root, pinellia root, cassia bark, ginger root, jujube fruit, **Asian ginseng** [page 630] root, **Chinese scullcap** [page 658] root, and **licorice** [page 702] root)
	Low back pain (page 293)
	Migraine headaches (page 316)
	Rheumatoid arthritis (page 387)

Historical or traditional use (may or may not be supported by scientific studies)

Traditional Chinese Medicine has recommended ginger for over 2,500 years. It is used for abdominal bloating, **coughing** (page 139), vomiting, **diarrhea** (page 163), and rheumatism. Ginger is commonly used in the Ayurvedic and Tibb systems of medicine for the treatment of inflammatory joint diseases, such as arthritis and rheumatism.

Active constituents

The dried rhizome of ginger contains approximately 1–4% volatile oils. These are the medically active constituents of ginger and are also responsible for ginger's characteristic odor and taste. The aromatic constituents include zingiberene and bisabolene, while the pungent constituents are known as gingerols and shogaols.[1] The pungent constituents are credited with the anti-nausea and anti-vomiting effects of ginger.

In humans, ginger is thought to act directly on the gastrointestinal system to reduce nausea.[2] Ginger has been shown to reduce the symptoms of **motion sickness** (page 322) associated with travel by boat and, to a lesser extent, car.[3, 4, 5] Two double-blind clinical trials have found that ginger may reduce nausea due to anesthesia following surgery,[6, 7] although one trial could not confirm this benefit.[8] A preliminary trial has suggested ginger may be helpful for preventing chemotherapy-induced nausea.[9]

While ginger is a popular remedy for **nausea of pregnancy** (page 320), it has only been clinically studied for very severe nausea and vomiting known as hyperemesis gravidarum.[10] This condition is life threatening and should only be treated by a qualified healthcare professional. Because ginger contains some compounds that cause chromosomal mutation in the test tube, some doctors are concerned about the safety of using ginger during pregnancy. However, the available clinical research, combined with the fact that ginger is widely used in the diet of certain cultures, suggests that prudent use of ginger for morning sickness is safe in amounts up to 1 gram per day.

Ginger is considered a tonic for the digestive tract, stimulating digestion and toning the intestinal muscles.[11] This action eases the transport of substances through the digestive tract, lessening irritation to the intestinal walls.[12] Ginger may protect the stomach from the damaging effect of alcohol and non-steroidal anti-inflammatory drugs (NSAIDs, such as ibuprofen) and may help prevent **ulcers** (page 349).[13]

Ginger also supports **cardiovascular health** (page 98). Ginger may make blood platelets less sticky and less likely to aggregate.[14, 15] However, not all human research has confirmed this.[16, 17]

How much is usually taken?

For prevention or treatment of motion sickness, 500 mg of dried ginger powder can be taken one-half to one hour before travel, and then 500 mg every two to four hours as necessary. Children below the age of six should use one-half the adult amount. For the treatment of nausea associated with **pregnancy** (page 320), women can take up to 1 gram daily,[18] but should only use ginger for symptomatic relief of nausea and not on an ongoing basis. Ginger may potentially be used for nausea associated with anesthesia or chemotherapy, but only under the supervision of a physician.

Are there any side effects or interactions?

Side effects due to ginger are rare when used as recommended. However, some people sensitive to the taste may experience **heartburn** (page 260). People with a history of **gallstones** (page 193) should consult a doctor before using ginger.[19] Short-term use of ginger for nausea and vomiting during **pregnancy** (page 320) appears to pose no safety problems. However, long-term use during pregnancy is not recommended. A doctor should be informed if ginger is used before surgery as the herb may increase bleeding.

GINKGO BILOBA

Common name: Maidenhair tree
Botanical name: *Ginkgo biloba*

Parts used and where grown

Ginkgo biloba is the world's oldest living species of tree. Individual trees live as long as 1,000 years. Ginkgo grows most predominantly in the southern and eastern United States, southern France, China, and Korea. The leaves of the tree are used in modern herbal medicine.

Ginkgo biloba has been used in connection with the following conditions (refer to the individual health concern for complete information):

Rating	Health Concerns
★★★	**Age-related cognitive decline** (page 8) (ARCD)
	Alzheimer's disease (page 19) (early-stage)
	Glaucoma (page 205) (normal tension glaucoma)
	Intermittent claudication (page 276)

Ginkgo Biloba

Rating	Health Concerns
★★☆	Altitude sickness (prevention)
	Depression (page 145) (for elderly people)
	Erectile dysfunction (page 185) (of vascular origin)
	Macular degeneration (page 303)
	Schizophrenia (page 393) (in combination with haloperidol)
	Vertigo (page 441)
	Vitiligo (page 443)
★☆☆	**Asthma** (page 32)
	Atherosclerosis (page 38)
	Deafness, acute cochlear
	Diabetes (page 152)
	Memory enhancement (in healthy adults)
	Ménière's disease (page 308)
	Migraine headaches (page 316)
	Multiple sclerosis (page 323) (injections)
	Premenstrual syndrome (page 368)
	Raynaud's disease (page 382)
	Retinopathy (page 385)
	Tinnitus (page 430)

Historical or traditional use (may or may not be supported by scientific studies)

Medicinal use of ginkgo can be traced back almost 5,000 years in Chinese herbal medicine. The nuts of the tree were most commonly recommended and used to treat respiratory tract ailments. The use of the leaves is a modern development originating in Europe.

Active constituents

The medical benefits of *Ginkgo biloba* extract (GBE) are attributed primarily to two groups of active constituents: the ginkgo flavone glycosides and the terpene lactones. Ginkgo flavone glycosides, which typically make up approximately 24% of the extract, are primarily responsible for GBE's **antioxidant** (page 467) activity and may mildly inhibit platelet aggregation (stickiness). These two actions may help GBE prevent circulatory diseases, such as **atherosclerosis** (page 38), and support the brain and central nervous system.[1] In addition to the cardiovascular system, GBE's antioxidant action may also extend to the brain and retina of the eye.[2] Preliminary trials have suggested potential benefit for people with **macular degeneration** (page 303)[3] and **diabetic retinopathy** (page 385).[4] The terpene lactones found in GBE, known as ginkgolides and bilobalide, typically make up approximately 6% of the extract. They are associated with increasing circulation to the brain and other parts of the body and may exert a protective action on nerve cells.[5] GBE regulates the tone and elasticity of blood vessels,[6] making circulation more efficient.[7]

Ginkgo is also well-known for its effect on memory and thinking (cognitive function). It may enhance cognitive performance in healthy older adults,[8] in people with **age-related cognitive decline** (page 8), and in people with **Alzheimer's disease** (page 19).

How much is usually taken?

Most clinical trials have used between 120 and 240 mg of GBE (standardized to contain 6% terpene lactones and 24% flavone glycosides) per day, generally divided into two or three portions.[9] The higher amount (240 mg per day) has been used in some people with mild-to-moderate **Alzheimer's disease** (page 19), **age-related cognitive decline** (page 8), **intermittent claudication** (page 276), and resistant **depression** (page 145). GBE may need to be taken for eight to twelve weeks before desired actions such as cognitive improvement are noticed. Although nonstandardized *Ginkgo biloba* leaf and tinctures are available, there is no well-established amount or use for these forms.

Are there any side effects or interactions?

Excessive bleeding has been reported in a few individuals taking GBE,[10, 11] although a cause/effect relationship was not proven. In addition, two elderly individuals with well-controlled epilepsy developed recurrent seizures within two weeks after starting GBE.[12] Mild headaches lasting for a day or two and mild upset stomach have been reported in a small number of people using GBE.

Ginkgo leaves are known to contain a group of potentially toxic constituents known as alkylphenols. The ginkgo extracts known as EGb 761 and LI 1370 have been shown to conform to the safety limits for these constituents (less that 5 ppm), as set forth by the German Commission E. Other forms of ginkgo may contain higher concentrations of alkylphenols.[13]

One small clinical trial found that ginkgo supplementation for three months increased secretion of insulin by the pancreas, but did not affect blood glucose levels, in healthy young adults.[14] These results suggest that the participants may have developed an insensitivity to insulin, a potential concern because insulin insensitivity may be a precursor to type 2 **diabetes** (page 152). However, this trial does not prove that ginkgo causes insulin insensitivity, nor does it prove that long-term ginkgo supplementation increases the risk for any

Ginkgo Biloba

disease. In addition, the results of this trial are not consistent with other research on ginkgo. Larger and more rigorously designed clinical trials of ginkgo supplementation have found no significant adverse effects after as many as 12 months of supplementation.[15]

People should seek an accurate medical diagnosis prior to self-prescribing GBE. This is especially important for the elderly, whose circulatory conditions can involve serious disease, and for people scheduled for surgery, as GBE may affect bleeding time.

GOLDENSEAL

Botanical name: *Hydrastis canadensis*

Parts used and where grown
Goldenseal is native to eastern North America and is cultivated in Oregon and Washington. It is seriously threatened by over-harvesting in the wild. The dried root and rhizome are used in herbal medicine.

Goldenseal has been used in connection with the following conditions (refer to the individual health concern for complete information):

Rating	Health Concerns
★☆☆	**Canker sores** (page 90)
	Chronic candidiasis (page 109)
	Cold sores (page 119)
	Common cold/sore throat (page 129)
	Conjunctivitis/blepharitis (page 136)
	Diarrhea (page 163) (berberine)
	Gastritis (page 195)
	Indigestion (page 260)
	Infection (page 265)
	Influenza (page 269)
	Pap smear (abnormal) (page 3)
	Parasites (page 343)
	Urinary tract infection (page 436)
	Vaginitis (page 438)

Historical or traditional use (may or may not be supported by scientific studies)
Goldenseal was used by Native Americans as a treatment for irritations and inflammation of the mucous membranes of the respiratory, digestive, and urinary tracts. It was commonly used topically for skin and eye infections and has been used historically as a mouthwash to help heal **canker sores** (page 90). Because of

its anti-microbial activity, goldenseal has a long history of use for infectious **diarrhea** (page 163), upper respiratory tract infections, and vaginal infections. Goldenseal is often recommended by herbalists in combination with **echinacea** (page 669) for the treatment of **colds** (page 129) and **flu** (page 269). Its benefits are most likely limited to helping ease the discomfort of a **sore throat** (page 129) associated with these conditions. Goldenseal was considered a critical remedy for stomach and intestinal problems of all kinds by early 20th century Eclectic physicians (doctors who recommended herbs).[1]

Active constituents
Little research has been done on whole goldenseal root or rhizome, but many studies have evaluated the properties of its two primary alkaloids, berberine and hydrastine. Berberine, the more extensively researched of the two, accounts for 0.5–6.0% of the alkaloids present in goldenseal root and rhizome. However, the effect of goldenseal in the gastrointestinal tract is most likely localized as its alkaloids (particularly berberine) are poorly absorbed into the bloodstream, limiting any systemic antibiotic effects.[2] Goldenseal also has strong astringent properties which may partially explain its historical use for **sore throats** (page 129) and **diarrhea** (page 163). In test tube studies, it has shown a wide spectrum of antibiotic activity against disease-causing organisms, such as *Chlamydia, E. coli, Salmonella typhi,* and *Entamoeba histolytica*.[3] Human trials have used isolated berberine to treat diarrhea and gastroenteritis with good results.[4] The whole root has not been clinically studied.

How much is usually taken?
Powdered goldenseal root and rhizome, 4–6 grams per day in tablet or capsule form, is sometimes recommended.[5] For liquid herbal extracts, use 2–4 ml three times per day. Alternatively, 250–500 mg three times per day of standardized extracts supplying 8–12% alkaloids, are suggested. Continuous use should not exceed three weeks, with a break of at least two weeks between each use.

Due to environmental concerns of overharvesting,[6] many herbalists recommend alternatives to goldenseal, such as **Oregon grape** (page 721) or goldthread.

Are there any side effects or interactions?
Taken as recommended, goldenseal is generally safe. However, as with all alkaloid-containing plants, high

amounts (several times higher than the recommended amount above) may lead to gastrointestinal distress and possible nervous system effects.[7] Goldenseal is not recommended for **pregnant** (page 363) or breast-feeding women. Also, despite some traditional reports, goldenseal is not a substitute for antibiotics.

GOTU KOLA

Botanical name: *Centella asiatica*

Parts used and where grown
This plant grows in a widespread distribution in tropical, swampy areas, including parts of India, Pakistan, Sri Lanka, Madagascar, and South Africa. It also grows in Eastern Europe. The roots and leaves are used medicinally.

Gotu kola has been used in connection with the following conditions (refer to the individual health concern for complete information):

Rating	Health Concerns
★★☆	**Chronic venous insufficiency** (page 116) **Skin ulcers** (page 409) (topical and by intramuscular injection) **Wound healing** (page 319)
★☆☆	**Burns (minor)** (page 85) Scars Scleroderma **Varicose veins** (page 440)

Historical or traditional use (may or may not be supported by scientific studies)
Gotu kola has been important in the medicinal systems of central Asia for centuries. In Sri Lanka, it was purported to prolong life, as the leaves are commonly eaten by elephants. Numerous skin diseases, ranging from poorly healing wounds to leprosy, have been treated with gotu kola. Gotu kola also has a historical reputation for boosting mental activity and for helping a variety of illnesses, such as **high blood pressure** (page 246), rheumatism, fever, and nervous disorders. Some of its common applications in Ayurvedic medicine include **heart disease** (page 98), **water retention** (page 180), hoarseness, **bronchitis** (page 80), and **coughs** (page 139) in children, and as a poultice for many skin conditions.[1]

Active constituents
The primary active constituents of gotu kola are saponins (also called triterpenoids), which include asiaticoside, madecassoside and madasiatic acid.[2] These saponins may prevent excessive scar formation by inhibiting the production of collagen (the material that makes up connective tissue) at the wound site. These constituents are also associated with promoting wound healing. One preliminary trial in humans found that a gotu kola extract improved healing of infected wounds (unless the infection had reached bone).[3] Additionally, a review of French studies suggests that topical gotu kola can improve healing of **burns** (page 85) and **wounds** (page 319).[4] Clinical trials have also shown it can help those with **chronic venous insufficiency** (page 116)[5, 6] Another trial found gotu kola extract helpful for preventing and treating enlarged scars (keloids).[7]

How much is usually taken?
Dried gotu kola leaf can be made into a tea by adding 1–2 teaspoons (5–10 grams) to about ⅔ cup (150 ml) of boiling water and allowing it to steep for ten to fifteen minutes. Three cups (750 ml) are usually suggested per day. Fluid extract (½–1 teaspoon (3–5 ml) per day) or a tincture (2–4 teaspoons (10–20 ml) per day) are sometimes recommended. Standardized extracts containing up to 100% total saponins (triterpenoids), 60 mg once or twice per day, are frequently used in modern herbal medicine.[8]

Are there any side effects or interactions?
Except for the rare person who is allergic to gotu kola, no significant adverse effects are experienced with internal or topical use of this herb.[9]

GREATER CELANDINE

Botanical name: *Chelidonium majus*

Parts used and where grown
Greater celandine grows primarily in Europe and Asia, although it has been introduced in North America. The leaves and small yellow flowers of greater celandine are

used as medicine. Although the roots and rhizomes of the plant have also been used medicinally, most clinical trials have used the above-ground parts of the plant collected at the time of flowering.[1]

Greater celandine has been used in connection with the following conditions (refer to the individual health concern for complete information):

Rating	Health Concerns
★★★	**Indigestion** (page 260)
★☆☆	Biliary dyskinesia Cholecystitis **Warts** (page 445)

Historical or traditional use (may or may not be supported by scientific studies)

European herbal traditions regard greater celandine as a valuable remedy for the topical treatment of **warts** (page 445).[2] It was also a folk remedy for **cancer** (page 87), **gout** (page 208), jaundice, and a variety of skin diseases. The famous French herbalist Maurice Mességué used greater celandine extensively in hand and foot baths and teas for many conditions, particularly those affecting the liver.[3] In eastern Asia it was also valued as a treatment for **peptic ulcer** (page 349).[4]

Active constituents

Greater celandine, like other members of the Papaveraceae (poppy) family, contains alkaloids as its major constituents. These include chelidoxanthine, chelidonine, and coptisine. Greater celandine extracts have been shown to stimulate production of bile and pancreatic digestive enzymes in human studies.[5]

Animal and test tube studies have shown that the alkaloids and whole plant extract can relieve gallbladder spasms and stimulate an under-active gallbladder.[6, 7] Test tube and animal studies have also shown celandine extracts and purified alkaloids to have anti-inflammatory, anti-cancer and antimicrobial properties.[8, 9, 10] They have also shown greater celandine's ability to protect animal livers from toxic substances.[11, 12]

A double-blind trial found that a standardized extract of greater celandine could relieve symptoms of **indigestion** (page 260) (such as abdominal cramping, sensation of fullness, and nausea) significantly better than a placebo.[13] The trial used an extract standardized

to 4 mg of chelidonine per capsule and gave 1–2 tablets three times daily for six weeks. An earlier, preliminary trial also found the same extract reduced symptoms in people with indigestion.[14]

Preliminary reports from Russia and China have reported that a tincture of greater celandine applied topically was useful for **warts** (page 445).[15] However, these results have not yet been confirmed by double-blind clinical trials.

Several reports describe Eastern European clinical trials using semi-synthetic derivatives of greater celandine alkaloids for people with **cancer** (page 87).[16] This injectable product goes by the name Ukrain. The findings on this drug cannot be applied to greater celandine because the alkaloids have been modified from their original form.

How much is usually taken?

One explanation for the variable results obtained from using greater celandine is improperly prepared, dried extracts.[17] Drying extracts quickly at high temperature is necessary to preserve the alkaloids.[18] Extracts standardized to a content of 4 mg chelidonine per capsule are recommended to be taken three times per day.[19] Alternatively, one may mix 1–3 ml tincture into water and sip slowly 10–30 minutes before eating. Topical applications should consist of either concentrated tinctures or the fresh yellow latex. Herbalists and doctors recommend applying fresh latex once per day to warts and allowing it to dry in place.[20]

Are there any side effects or interactions?

Use of fresh plant products may cause stomach upset.[21] Topical use has been associated with intense itching and a rash in one case.[22] Greater celandine should be avoided during **pregnancy** (page 363) and in children under age 12.[23] A recent report of ten women in Germany suffering from acute **hepatitis** (page 220) following supplementation with a standardized extract of greater celandine (dosage was not given) suggest this herb should be avoided by people with hepatitis or impaired liver function. Greater celandine should be used cautiously and under the supervision of a healthcare professional until more is understood about its potential liver toxicity.[24]

Special United Kingdom considerations

Greater celandine is available only by prescription in the United Kingdom.

Greater Celandine

GREEN TEA

Common name: Epigallocatechin gallate (EGCG)
Botanical name: *Camellia sinensis*

Parts used and where grown

All teas (green, black, and oolong) are derived from the same plant, *Camellia sinensis*. The difference is in how the plucked leaves are prepared. Green tea, unlike black and oolong tea, is not fermented, so the active constituents remain unaltered in the herb. The leaves of the tea plant are used both as a social and a medicinal beverage.

Green tea has been used in connection with the following conditions (refer to the individual health concern for complete information):

Rating	Health Concerns
★★☆	**Atherosclerosis** (page 38)
	Cervical dysplasia (page 3) (poly E or (-)-epigallocatechin-3-gallate)
	Colon cancer (page 123) (reduces risk)
	High cholesterol (page 223)
	Leukoplakia (page 289)
	Tooth decay (page 430)
	Weight loss (page 446)
★☆☆	**Breast cancer** (page 65) (risk reduction)
	Crohn's disease (page 141)
	Hemochromatosis (iron overload)
	High triglycerides (page 235)
	Hives (page 246)
	Immune function (page 255)
	Infection (page 265)
	Lung cancer (page 298) (risk reduction)

Historical or traditional use (may or may not be supported by scientific studies)

According to Chinese legend, tea was discovered accidentally by an emperor 4,000 years ago. Since then, Traditional Chinese Medicine has recommended green tea for headaches, body **aches and pains** (page 338), digestion, **depression** (page 145), **immune enhancement** (page 255), detoxification, as an energizer, and to prolong life.

Active constituents

Green tea contains volatile oils, vitamins, minerals, and caffeine, but the primary constituents of interest are the polyphenols, particularly the catechin called epigallo-catechin gallate (EGCG). The polyphenols are believed to be responsible for most of green tea's roles in promoting good health.[1]

Green tea has been shown to mildly lower total **cholesterol** (page 223) levels and improve the cholesterol profile (decreasing LDL "bad" cholesterol and increasing HDL "good" cholesterol) in most,[2, 3, 4, 5] but not all,[6] studies. Green tea may also promote **cardiovascular health** (page 98) by making platelets in the blood less sticky.

Green tea has also been shown to protect against damage to LDL ("bad") cholesterol caused by oxygen.[7] Consumption of green tea increases antioxidant activity in the blood.[8] Oxidative damage to LDL can promote **atherosclerosis** (page 38). While population studies have suggested that consumption of green tea is associated with protection against atherosclerosis,[9] the evidence is still preliminary.

Several animal and test tube studies have demonstrated an anticancer effect of polyphenols from green tea.[10, 11, 12] In one of these studies, a polyphenol called catechin from green tea effectively inhibited metastasis (uncontrolled spread) of melanoma (skin cancer) cells.[13] The polyphenols in green tea have also been associated with reduced risk of several types of **cancer** (page 87) in humans.[14, 15, 16] However, some human studies have found no association between green tea consumption and decreased cancer risk.[17, 18]

In a double-blind trial, people with **leukoplakia** (page 289) (a pre-cancerous oral condition) took 3 grams orally per day of a mixture of whole green tea, green tea polyphenols, and green tea pigments orally, and also painted a mixture of the tea on their lesions three times daily for six months.[19] As compared to the placebo group, those in the green tea group had significant decreases in the pre-cancerous condition.

Compounds in green tea, as well as black tea, may reduce the risk of dental caries.[20] Human volunteers rinsing with an alcohol extract of oolong tea leaves before bed each night for four days had significantly less plaque formation, but similar amounts of plaque-causing bacteria, compared to those with no treatment.[21]

Green tea polyphenols have been shown to stimulate the production of several **immune system** (page 255) cells, and have topical antibacterial properties—even against the bacteria that cause dental plaque.[22, 23, 24]

One study found that intake of 10 cups or more of green tea per day improved blood test results, indicating protection against liver damage.[25] Further studies are needed to determine if taking green tea helps those with liver diseases.

Tea **flavonoids** (page 516) given by capsule reduced fecal odor and favorably altered the gut bacteria in elderly Japanese with feeding tubes living in nursing homes.[26] The study was repeated in bedridden elderly not on feeding tubes, and green tea was again shown to improve their gut bacteria.[27] These studies raise the possibility of using green tea in other settings where gut bacteria are disturbed, such as after taking antibiotics. Further studies are needed to clarify the role of green tea in this respect, however.

High-tannin tea has been shown to reduce the need for blood removal from people with iron overload, or hemochromatosis, in an open study.[28] The tea had to be taken with meals and without lemon or milk to be effective. Tea is believed to help in hemochromatosis by preventing iron absorption.

How much is usually taken?

Much of the research documenting the health benefits of green tea is based on the amount of green tea typically consumed in Asian countries—about 3 cups (750 ml) per day (providing 240–320 mg of polyphenols).[29] However, other research suggests as much as 10 cups (2,500 ml) per day is necessary to obtain noticeable benefits from green tea ingestion.[30, 31] To brew green tea, 1 teaspoon (5 grams) of green tea leaves are combined with 1 cup (250 ml) of boiling water and steeped for three minutes. Decaffeinated tea is recommended to reduce the side effects associated with caffeine, including **anxiety** (page 30) and **insomnia** (page 270). Tablets and capsules containing standardized extracts of polyphenols, particularly EGCG, are available. Some provide up to 97% polyphenol content—which is equivalent to drinking 4 cups (1,000 ml) of tea. Many of these standardized products are decaffeinated.

Are there any side effects or interactions?

Green tea is generally free of side effects. The most common adverse effects reported from consuming large amounts (several cups per day) of green tea are **insomnia** (page 270), **anxiety** (page 30), and other symptoms caused by the caffeine content in the herb.

An extract of green tea taken by healthy women with a meal inhibited the absorption of non-heme iron (e.g., the form of iron in plant foods) by 26%.[32] Frequent use of green tea could, in theory, promote the development of iron deficiency in susceptible individuals.

GUARANÁ

Botanical name: *Paullinia cupana*

Parts used and where grown

Guaraná is an evergreen vine indigenous to the Amazon basin. The vast majority of guaraná is grown in a small area in northern Brazil. Guaraná gum or paste is derived from the seeds and is used in herbal preparations.

Guaraná has been used in connection with the following conditions (refer to the individual health concern for complete information):

Rating	Health Concerns
★☆☆	**Athletic performance** (page 43)
	Fatigue
	Weight loss and obesity (page 446)

Historical or traditional use (may or may not be supported by scientific studies)

The indigenous people of the Amazon rain forest have used crushed guaraná seed as a beverage and a medicine. Guaraná was used to treat **diarrhea** (page 163), decrease fatigue, reduce hunger, and to help arthritis.[1] It also has a history of use in treating hangovers from alcohol abuse and headaches related to menstruation.

Active constituents

Caffeine and the closely related alkaloids theobromine and theophylline make up the primary active constituents in guaraná. Caffeine's effects are well known and include stimulating the central nervous system, increasing metabolic rate, and having a mild diuretic effect.[2] One preliminary trial found no significant actions on thinking or mental function in humans taking guaraná.[3] Guaraná also contains tannins, which act as astringents and may prevent **diarrhea** (page 163). However, this action has not been studied in human clinical trials.

How much is usually taken?

A cup of guaraná, prepared by adding ¼–½ teaspoon (1–2 grams) of crushed seed or resin to 1 cup (250 ml) of water and boiling for ten minutes, can be consumed three times per day.[4] Each cup may provide up to 50 mg of caffeine.

Are there any side effects or interactions?

As with any caffeinated product, guaraná may cause **insomnia** (page 270), trembling, **anxiety** (page 30), palpitations, and urinary frequency.[5] Guaraná should be avoided during **pregnancy** (page 363) and breast-feeding.

GUGGUL

Common names: Gugulipid, gum guggulu
Botanical name: *Commiphora mukul*

Parts used and where grown

The mukul myrrh *(Commiphora mukul)* tree is a small, thorny plant distributed throughout India. Guggul and gum guggulu are the names given to a yellowish resin produced by the stem of the plant. This resin has been used historically and is also the source of modern extracts of guggul.

Guggul has been used in connection with the following conditions (refer to the individual health concern for complete information):

Rating	Health Concerns
★★★	**High triglycerides** (page 235)
★★☆	**Acne vulgaris** (page 6) **Atherosclerosis** (page 38) **High cholesterol** (page 223) **Osteoarthritis** (page 328)
★☆☆	**Obesity** (page 446)

Historical or traditional use (may or may not be supported by scientific studies)

The classical treatise on Ayurvedic medicine, *Sushrita Samhita,* describes the use of guggul for a wide variety of conditions, including rheumatism and **obesity** (page 446). One of its primary indications was a condition known as *medoroga.* This ancient diagnosis is similar to the modern description of **atherosclerosis** (page 38). Standardized guggul extracts are approved in India for lowering elevated serum **cholesterol** (page 223) and **triglyceride** (page 235) levels.

Active constituents

Guggul contains resin, volatile oils, and gum. The extract isolates ketonic steroid compounds known as gug-

gulsterones. These compounds have been shown to provide the cholesterol- and triglyceride-lowering actions noted for guggul.[1] Guggul significantly lowers serum **triglycerides** (page 235) and **cholesterol** (page 223) as well as LDL and VLDL cholesterols (the "bad" cholesterols).[2] At the same time, it raises levels of HDL cholesterol (the "good" cholesterol). As **antioxidants** (page 467), guggulsterones keep LDL cholesterol from oxidizing, an action which protects against **atherosclerosis** (page 38).[3] Guggul has also been shown to reduce the stickiness of platelets—another effect that lowers the risk of coronary artery disease.[4] One double-blind trial found guggul extract similar to the drug clofibrate for lowering cholesterol levels.[5] Other clinical trials in India (using 1,500 mg of extract per day) have confirmed guggul extracts improve lipid levels in humans.[6]

A combination of guggul, phosphate salts, hydroxycitrate, and **tyrosine** (page 544) coupled with exercise has been shown in a double-blind trial to improve mood with a slight tendency to improve weight loss in overweight adults.[7]

One small clinical trial found that guggul *(Commiphora mukul)* compared favorably to tetracycline in the treatment of cystic acne.[8] The amount of guggul extract taken in the trial was 500 mg twice per day.

How much is usually taken?

Daily recommendations for the purified guggul extract are typically based on the amount of guggulsterones in the extract.[9] A common intake of guggulsterones is 25 mg three times per day. Most extracts contain 2.5–5% guggulsterones and can be taken daily for 12 to 24 weeks for lowering **high cholesterol** (page 223) and/or **triglycerides** (page 235).

Are there any side effects or interactions?

Early studies with the crude oleoresin reported numerous side effects, including **diarrhea** (page 163), **anorexia** (page 174), abdominal pain, and skin rash. Modern extracts are more purified, and fewer side effects (e.g., mild abdominal discomfort) have been reported with long-term use. Rash was reported, however, as a fairly common side effect in one recent study.[10] Guggul should be used with caution by people with liver disease and in cases of **inflammatory bowel disease** (page 269) and **diarrhea** (page 163). A physician should be consulted before treating elevated **cholesterol** (page 223) and **triglycerides** (page 235).

GYMNEMA

Common names: Gurmarbooti, gurmar
Botanical name: *Gymnema sylvestre*

Parts used and where grown

Gymnema sylvestre is a woody climbing plant that grows in the tropical forests of central and southern India. The leaves are used in herbal medicine preparations. *G. sylvestre* is known as "periploca of the woods" in English and *meshasringi* (meaning "ram's horn") in Sanskrit. The leaves, when chewed, interfere with the ability to taste sweetness, which explains the Hindi name *gurmar*—"destroyer of sugar."

Gymnema has been used in connection with the following condition (refer to the individual health concern for complete information):

Rating	Health Concerns
★★☆	**Diabetes** (page 152)

Historical or traditional use (may or may not be supported by scientific studies)

Gymnema has been used in India for the treatment of **diabetes** (page 152) for over 2,000 years. The leaves were also used for stomach ailments, **constipation** (page 137), **water retention** (page 180), and liver disease.

Active constituents

The hypoglycemic (blood sugar-lowering) action of gymnema leaves was first documented in the late 1920s.[1] This action is attributed to members of a family of substances called gymnemic acids.[2, 3] Gymnema leaves raise insulin levels, according to research in healthy volunteers.[4] Based on animal studies, this may be due to regeneration of the cells in the pancreas that secrete insulin,[5, 6] or by increasing the flow of insulin from these cells.[7] Other animal research shows that gymnema can also reduce glucose absorption from the intestine,[8] improve uptake of glucose into cells, and prevent adrenal hormones from stimulating the liver to produce glucose, thereby reducing blood sugar levels.[9, 10]

Other animal studies have shown that extracts of gymnema leaves can lower serum **cholesterol** (page 223) and **triglycerides** (page 235) and prevent weight gain,[11, 12, 13, 14] but these effects have not been tested in humans. When placed directly on the tongue, gur-marin, another constituent of the leaves, and gymnemic acid have been shown to block the ability in humans to taste sweets.[15, 16]

How much is usually taken?

Clinical trials with diabetics in India have used 400 mg per day of a water-soluble acidic fraction of the gymnema leaves. The gymnemic acid content of this extract is not clear. A recent preliminary trial in the United States reported promising results in a group of type 1 and type 2 diabetics who took 800 mg per day of an extract standardized for 25% gymnemic acids.[17] Traditionally, 2 to 4 grams per day of the leaf powder is used.

Are there any side effects or interactions?

Used at the amounts suggested, gymnema is generally safe and devoid of side effects. The safety of gymnema during **pregnancy** (page 363) and breast-feeding has not yet been determined. People with **diabetes** (page 152) should only use gymnema to lower blood sugar under the clinical supervision of a healthcare professional. Gymnema cannot be used in place of insulin to control blood sugar by people with either type 1 or type 2 diabetes.

HAWTHORN

Botanical names: *Crataegus laevigata, Crataegus oxyacantha, Crataegus monogyna*

Parts used and where grown

Hawthorn is commonly found in Europe, western Asia, North America, and North Africa. Modern medicinal extracts primarily use the leaves and flowers. Traditional preparations use the fruit.

Hawthorn has been used in connection with the following conditions (refer to the individual health concern for complete information):

Rating	Health Concerns
★★★	**Congestive heart failure** (page 134) (early-stage)
★★☆	**Angina** (page 27) **Cardiomyopathy** (page 95) (if **congestive heart failure** [page 134] is also present)
★☆☆	**Cardiac arrhythmia** (page 93) **Cardiomyopathy** (page 95) (if **congestive heart failure** [page 134] is not present) **Hypertension** (page 246)

Hawthorn

Historical or traditional use (may or may not be supported by scientific studies)

Dioscorides, a Greek herbalist, reportedly used hawthorn in the first century A.D. Although numerous passing mentions are made for a variety of conditions, support for the heart is the main benefit of hawthorn.

Active constituents

The leaves, flowers, and berries of hawthorn contain a variety of bioflavonoids that appear to be primarily responsible for the cardiac actions of the plant. **Flavonoids** (page 516) found in hawthorn include **oligomeric procyanidins** (page 574) (OPCs), vitexin, vitexin 4'-O-rhamnoside, **quercetin** (page 580), and hyperoside. These compounds are often standardized in leaf and flower extracts, which are widely used in Europe.

Hawthorn is thought to exert many beneficial effects on the heart and blood vessels. These include improved coronary artery blood flow and strengthening of the contractions of the heart muscle.[1] Hawthorn may also improve circulation to the extremities by lowering the resistance to blood flow in peripheral blood vessels.[2] The bioflavonoids in hawthorn are potent **antioxidants** (page 467).[3] Hawthorn extracts may mildly lower blood pressure in some people with **high blood pressure** (page 246) but should not be thought of as a substitute for cardiac medications for this condition.

Clinical trials have confirmed that hawthorn leaf and flower extracts are beneficial for people with stage II (early-stage) **congestive heart failure** (page 134).[4, 5, 6, 7, 8] People with congestive heart failure taking 160–900 mg of hawthorn extract per day for eight weeks showed improved quality of life including greater ability to exercise without shortness of breath and exhaustion. Congestive heart failure is a serious medical condition that requires expert management rather than self-treatment. One study has shown that hawthorn leaf and flower extract may also help those with stable **angina** (page 27).[9]

How much is usually taken?

Extracts of the leaves and flowers are most commonly used in modern herbal medicine. Hawthorn extracts standardized for total bioflavonoid content (usually 2.2%) or **oligomeric procyanidins** (page 574) (usually 18.75%) are often suggested. Many doctors recommend 80–300 mg of the herbal extract in capsules or tablets two to three times per day.[10] If traditional berry preparations are used, the recommendation is at least 4–5 grams per day or a tincture of 4–5 ml three times daily. However, this form has not been clinically studied. Hawthorn is slow acting and may take one to two months for maximum effects to be seen. However, it appears to be safe and should be considered a long-term therapy.

Are there any side effects or interactions?

Hawthorn is safe for long-term use. People taking prescription cardiac medications should consult with their doctor before using hawthorn-containing products. Reports of hawthorn interacting with digitalis to augment its effects have not been confirmed in clinical trials. There are no apparent restrictions to use of hawthorn during **pregnancy** (page 363) or breast-feeding.

HOPS

Botanical name: *Humulus lupulus*

Parts used and where grown

The hops plant, *Humulus lupulus,* is a climbing plant native to Europe, Asia, and North America. Hops are the cone-like, fruiting bodies (strobiles) of the plant and are typically harvested from cultivated female plants. Hops are most commonly used as a flavoring agent in beer.

Hops have been used in connection with the following conditions (refer to the individual health concern for complete information):

Rating	Health Concerns
★☆☆	**Anxiety** (page 30)
	Insomnia (page 270)
	Poor appetite

Historical or traditional use (may or may not be supported by scientific studies)

Soothing the stomach and promoting healthy digestion have been the strongest historical use of this herb. Hops tea was also recommended by herbalists as a mild sedative and remedy for **insomnia** (page 270), particularly for those with insomnia resulting from an upset stomach.[1] A pillow filled with hops was sometimes used to

Hawthorn

encourage sleep. Traditionally, hops were also thought by herbalists to have a diuretic effect and to treat sexual neuroses. A poultice of hops was used topically to treat sores and skin injuries and to relieve muscle spasms and nerve pain.[2]

Active constituents

Hops are high in bitter substances. The two primary bitter constituents are known as humulone and lupulone.[3] These are thought to be responsible for the appetite-stimulating properties of hops. Hops also contain about 1–3% volatile oils. Hops have been shown to have mild sedative properties, although the mechanism is unclear.[4] Some herbal preparations for insomnia combine hops with more potent sedative herbs, such as **valerian** (page 756). Hops also contain phytoestrogens that bind estrogen receptors in test tube studies but are thought to have only mild estrogen-like actions.[5]

How much is usually taken?

The German Commission E monograph recommends a single application of 500 mg of dried herb for **anxiety** (page 30) or **insomnia** (page 270).[6] The dried fruits can be made into a tea by pouring 1 cup (250 ml) of boiling water over 1–2 teaspoons (5–10 grams) of the fruit. Steep for ten to fifteen minutes before drinking. Tinctures, ¼–½ teaspoon (1–2 ml) two or three times per day, can also be used. As mentioned above, many herbal preparations use hops in combination with herbal sedatives, including **valerian** (page 756), **passion flower** (page 722), and scullcap.

Are there any side effects or interactions?

Use of hops is generally safe. However, some people have been reported to experience an allergic skin rash after handling the dried flowers. This is most likely due to a pollen sensitivity.[7]

HOREHOUND

Botanical name: *Marrubium vulgare*

Parts used and where grown

Horehound is a perennial plant with small white flowers found growing in the wild throughout Europe and Asia. All parts of the plant are used medicinally.[1]

Horehound has been used in connection with the following conditions (refer to the individual health concern for complete information):

Rating	Health Concerns
★☆☆	**Bronchitis** (page 80)
	Cough (page 139)
	Indigestion (page 260)
	Lack of appetite

Historical or traditional use (may or may not be supported by scientific studies)

Horehound was reportedly first used in ancient Rome by the physician Galen, who recommended it as a therapy for coughs and other respiratory ailments. Like Galen, Nicholas Culpeper, the 17th-century English pharmacist, commented that it was helpful for a **cough** (page 139) and was also useful in helping remove stubborn phlegm from the lung. Similarly, American Eclectic physicians (doctors who recommended herbs) of the 19th century remarked on its value as a medicinal plant not only for coughs and **asthma** (page 32) but also in menstrual complaints.[2]

Active constituents

Horehound contains a number of constituents, including alkaloids, **flavonoids** (page 516), diterpenes (e.g., marrubiin), and trace amount of volatile oils.[3] The major active constituent in horehound is marrubiin, which is thought to be responsible for the expectorant (promotion of coughing up of mucus) action of the herb. In addition, marrubiin contributes to the bitter taste of horehound, an action that increases the flow of saliva and gastric juice, thereby stimulating the appetite.[4] These actions likely explain the long-standing use of horehound as a cough suppressant and expectorant as well as a bitter digestive tonic.

How much is usually taken?

For adults, the German Commission E monograph recommends approximately ¾ teaspoon (4.5 grams) of horehound per day or 2–6 tablespoons (30–90 ml) of the pressed juice.[5] Alternatively, horehound tea can be prepared from approximately ¼–½ teaspoon (1–2 grams) of root boiled in about 7 ounces (200 ml) of water for ten minutes. Three cups (750 ml) of this tea can be drunk per day. Horehound is sometimes found in herbal lozenges that are used for coughs.

Horehound

Are there any side effects or interactions?

Since horehound acts as a bitter and may increase production of stomach acid, people with gastritis or **peptic ulcer** (page 349) disease should use it cautiously. Horehound should not be used during **pregnancy** (page 363), as it may stimulate contractions.

HORSE CHESTNUT

Botanical name: *Aesculus hippocastanum*

Parts used and where grown

The horse chestnut tree is native to Asia and northern Greece, but it is now cultivated in many areas of Europe and North America. The tree produces fruits that are made up of a spiny capsule containing one to three large seeds, known as horse chestnuts. Traditionally, many of the aerial parts of the horse chestnut tree, including the seeds, leaves, and bark, were used in medicinal preparations. Modern extracts of horse chestnut are usually made from the seeds, which are high in the active constituent aescin (also known as escin).

Horse chestnut has been used in connection with the following conditions (refer to the individual health concern for complete information):

Rating	Health Concerns
★★★	**Chronic venous insufficiency** (page 116)
★★☆	**Hemorrhoids** (page 219) **Sprains and strains** (page 412) (topical) **Wound healing** (page 319) (topical)
★☆☆	**Edema (water retention)** (page 180) **Varicose veins** (page 440)

Historical or traditional use (may or may not be supported by scientific studies)

Horse chestnut leaves have been used by herbalists as a **cough** (page 139) remedy and to reduce fevers.[1] The leaves were also believed to reduce pain and inflammation of arthritis and rheumatism. In traditional herbal medicine, poultices of the seeds have been used topically to treat skin ulcers and skin **cancer** (page 87). Other uses include the internal and external application for problems of venous circulation, including **varicose veins** (page 440) and **hemorrhoids** (page 219).

Active constituents

The seeds are the source of a saponin known as aescin, which has been shown to promote circulation through the veins.[2] Aescin fosters normal tone in the walls of the veins, thereby promoting return of blood to the heart. This has made both topical and internal horse chestnut extracts popular in Europe for the treatment of **chronic venous insufficiency** (page 116) and, to a lesser extent, **varicose veins** (page 440). Aescin also possesses anti-inflammatory properties and has been shown to reduce **edema** (page 180) (swelling with fluid) following trauma, particularly following sports injury, surgery, and head injury.[3, 4] A topical aescin preparation is very popular in Europe for the treatment of acute sprains during sporting events. Horse chestnuts also contain **flavonoids** (page 516), sterols, and tannins.

Double-blind and preliminary clinical trials have shown that oral horse chestnut extracts reduce the symptoms of **chronic venous insufficiency** (page 116), including swelling and pain.[5, 6] Those suffering edema after surgery have also found relief from topical application of horse chestnut extracts, according to preliminary studies.[7]

How much is usually taken?

For treatment of **chronic venous insufficiency** (page 116) horse chestnut seed extracts standardized for aescin content (16–20%), 300 mg two to three times per day, are recommended.[8, 9] Tincture, 1–4 ml taken three times per day, can be used though it is questionable whether a significant amount of aescin can be absorbed this way.[10] Gels or creams containing 2% aescin can be applied topically three or four times per day for **hemorrhoids** (page 219), skin ulcers, **varicose veins** (page 440), sports injuries, and trauma of other kinds.

Are there any side effects or interactions?

Internal use of horse chestnut seed extracts standardized for aescin at recommended amounts is generally safe. However, in rare cases oral intake of horse chestnut may cause itching, nausea, and upset stomach.[11] Based on reports of worsening kidney function in people with kidney disease who received intravenous aescin, horse chestnut should be avoided by anyone with kidney disease.[12, 13] People with liver disease should also avoid the use of horse chestnut. There are no known reasons to avoid horse chestnut during **pregnancy** (page 363).[14] Topically, horse chestnut has been associated with rare cases of allergic skin reactions. Circulation disorders and trauma associated with swelling may be the sign of a serious condition. Therefore, a healthcare professional should be consulted before self-treating with horse chestnut.

HORSERADISH

Botanical name: *Cochlearia armoracia*

Parts used and where grown
Horseradish likely originated in Eastern Europe, but today it is cultivated worldwide. The root is used as both food and medicine.

Horseradish has been used in connection with the following conditions (refer to the individual health concern for complete information):

Rating	Health Concerns
★☆☆	**Bronchitis** (page 80)
	Common cold/sore throat (page 129)
	Sinusitis (page 407)
	Urinary tract infection (page 436)

Historical or traditional use (may or may not be supported by scientific studies)
Horseradish, known for its pungent taste, has been used as a medicine and condiment for centuries in Europe. Its name is derived from the common practice of naming a food according to its similarity with another food (horseradish was considered a rough substitute for radishes).

Horseradish was utilized both internally and externally by European herbalists. Applied to the skin, it causes reddening and was used on arthritic joints or irritated nerves. Internally, it was considered to be a diuretic and was used by herbalists to treat **kidney stones** (page 284) or **edema** (page 180). It was also recommended as a digestive stimulant and to treat worms, **coughs** (page 139), and **sore throats** (page 129).[1]

Active constituents
Horseradish contains volatile oils that are similar to those found in mustard. These include glucosinolates (mustard oil glycosides), gluconasturtiin, and sinigrin, which yield allyl isothiocynate when broken down in the stomach. In test tubes, the volatile oils in horseradish have shown antibiotic properties, which may account for its effectiveness in treating throat and upper respiratory tract infections.[2] At levels attainable in human urine after taking the volatile oil of horseradish, the oil has been shown to kill bacteria that can cause **urinary tract infections** (page 436)[3] and one early trial found that horseradish extract may be a useful treatment for people with urinary tract infections.[4] Further studies are still necessary, however, to confirm horseradish's safety and effectiveness in treating urinary tract infections.

How much is usually taken?
The German Commission E monograph suggests an average daily intake of 4 teaspoons (20 grams) of the fresh root for adults.[5] Alternatively, ½–1 teaspoon (3–5 grams) of the freshly grated root can be eaten three times per day. Horseradish tincture is also available and is sometimes taken at ½–¾ teaspoon (2–3 ml) three times daily. The German Commission E also recommends external use of horseradish for respiratory tract congestion as well as minor muscle aches. A poultice can be prepared by grating the fresh root and spreading it on a linen cloth or thin gauze. This is then applied against the skin once or twice per day until a burning sensation is experienced.

Are there any side effects or interactions?
If used in amounts higher than recommended, horseradish can cause stomach upset,[6] vomiting, or excessive sweating. Direct application to the skin or eyes may cause irritation and burning. Horseradish should be avoided by people with **hypothyroidism** (page 252), **gastritis** (page 195), **peptic ulcer disease** (page 349), and kidney disorders. Horseradish should not be used by women during **pregnancy** (page 363) or breast-feeding or by children under four years of age.[7]

HORSETAIL

Common names: Bottlebrush plant, shave grass, scouring rush
Botanical name: *Equisetum arvense*

Parts used and where grown
Horsetail is widely distributed throughout the temperate climate zones of the Northern Hemisphere, including Asia, North America, and Europe.[1] Horsetail is a unique plant with two distinctive types of stems.

Horsetail

One variety of stem grows early in spring and looks like asparagus, except for its brown color and spore-containing cones on top. The mature form of the herb, appearing in summer, has branched, thin, green, sterile stems and looks like a feathery tail.

Horsetail has been used in connection with the following conditions (refer to the individual health concern for complete information):

Rating	Health Concerns
★☆☆	**Brittle nails** (page 79)
	Edema (water retention) (page 180)
	Osteoarthritis (page 328)
	Osteoporosis (page 333)
	Urinary tract infection (page 436)
	Wound healing (page 319) (topical)

Historical or traditional use (may or may not be supported by scientific studies)

Reportedly first recommended by the Roman physician Galen, several cultures have employed horsetail as a folk remedy for kidney and bladder troubles, arthritis, bleeding ulcers, and tuberculosis. In addition, the topical use of horsetail was used traditionally to stop the bleeding of wounds and promote rapid healing. The use of this herb as an abrasive cleanser to scour pots or shave wood illustrates the origin of horsetail's common names—scouring rush and shave grass.[2]

Active constituents

Horsetail is rich in silicic acid and silicates, which provide approximately 2–3% elemental **silicon** (page 586). **Potassium** (page 572), aluminum, and **manganese** (page 553), along with fifteen different types of **flavonoids** (page 516), are also found in this herb. The presence of these flavonoids, as well as saponins, is believed to cause the diuretic effect, while the silicon content is thought to exert a connective tissue-strengthening and anti-arthritic action.[3] Some experts have suggested the element silicon in horsetail is also a vital component for bone and cartilage formation.[4] Anecdotal reports suggest that horsetail may be of some use in the treatment of **brittle nails** (page 79).[5]

How much is usually taken?

The German Commission E monograph suggests up to 6 grams of the herb per day for internal use.[6] A tincture can also be used at 2 teaspoons (10 ml) three times per day. A horsetail tea may be made by boiling 2–4 tea-spoons of the herb in one cup (250 ml) of water for five minutes. Steep the tea for an additional 15 minutes, strain, and drink two or three times daily. The tea can also be used externally as well as internally.

Are there any side effects or interactions?

Horsetail is generally considered safe. The only concern would be that the correct species of horsetail is used. *Equisetum palustre* is another species of horsetail, which contains toxic alkaloids and is a well-known livestock poison. Due to a lack of clear safety information, horsetail should be avoided during **pregnancy** (page 363) and breast-feeding.

The Canadian Health Protection Branch requires supplement manufacturers to document that their products do not contain the enzyme thiaminase, found in crude horsetail, which destroys the B vitamin **thiamine** (page 597). Since alcohol, temperature, and alkalinity neutralize this potentially harmful enzyme, tinctures, fluid extracts, or preparations of the herb subjected to 100°C temperatures during manufacturing are preferred for medicinal use.[7]

HUPERZIA

Common names: Qian ceng ta, huperzine A

Parts used and where grown

Huperzia is a type of moss that grows in China. It is related to club mosses (the *Lycopodiaceae* family) and is known to some botanists as *Lycopodium serratum*. The whole prepared moss was used traditionally. Modern herbal preparations use only the isolated alkaloid known as huperzine A.

Huperzia has been used in connection with the following conditions (refer to the individual health concern for complete information):

Rating	Health Concerns
★★☆	**Alzheimer's disease** (page 19)
	Age-related cognitive decline (page 8)

Historical or traditional use (may or may not be supported by scientific studies)

Huperzia moss tea has been used for centuries in traditional Chinese herbalism for fever, as a diuretic, for blood loss, and for irregular menstruation.[1]

Active constituents

Huperzine A is an alkaloid found in huperzia that has been reported to prevent the breakdown of acetylcholine, an important substance needed by the nervous system to transmit information from cell to cell.[2] Animal research has suggested that huperzine A's ability to preserve acetylcholine may be greater than that of some prescription drugs.[3, 4] Loss of acetylcholine function is a primary feature of several disorders of brain function, including **Alzheimer's disease** (page 19). Huperzine A may also have a protective effect on brain tissue, further increasing its theoretical potential for helping reduce symptoms of some brain disorders.[5, 6]

In a double-blind trial, people with **Alzheimer's disease** (page 19) had significant improvement in memory and cognitive and behavioral functions after taking 200 mcg of huperzine A twice per day for eight weeks.[7] Another double-blind trial using injected huperzine A confirmed a positive effect in people with dementia, including, but not limited to, Alzheimer's disease.[8] Another double-blind trial found that huperzine A (100–150 mcg two to three times per day for four to six weeks) was more effective for improving minor memory loss associated with **age-related cognitive decline** (page 8) than the drug piracetam.[9]

Huperzine A has also been shown to enhance memory in adolescent middle school students. A small controlled trial found that 100 mcg of huperizine A two times per day for four weeks was effective in improving memory and learning performance.[10] Although no side effects were reported in this short trial, long-term safety studies are needed before huperizine A is recommended for adolescents or younger children to improve memory and learning performance.

How much is usually taken?

Human research on huperzine A has used 100–200 mcg taken two to three times per day.[11]

Are there any side effects or interactions?

Medications that prevent acetylcholine breakdown often produce side effects, including nausea, vomiting, excess saliva and tear production, and sweating. However, while dizziness was reported in a few people in one study, no severe side effects have been reported in human trials using huperzine A. Further studies are needed to determine the long-term safety of huperzine A.

HYSSOP

Botanical name: *Hyssopus officinalis*

Parts used and where grown

Hyssop reportedly originated in the area around the Black Sea in central Asia and today is widely cultivated in other arid regions, partly because it thrives even in the most desolate soils. Hyssop's fragrant flowers and leaves are used as medicine.

Hyssop has been used in connection with the following conditions (refer to the individual health concern for complete information):

Rating	Health Concerns
★☆☆	**Asthma** (page 32) **Colic** (page 121) **Common cold** (page 129)/pharyngitis **Cough** (page 139)

Historical or traditional use (may or may not be supported by scientific studies)

The most common uses of hyssop in traditional herbalism have been to relieve chest congestion and **coughs** (page 139), to soothe **sore throats** (page 129), and to act as a mild sedative.[1] Some herbalists consider it stronger for relieving gas or intestinal cramping than for easing a cough.[2] In addition to using hyssop for the above conditions, early 20th century Eclectic physicians (doctors who recommended herbs) in the United States used the herb topically to soothe burned skin.[3]

Active constituents

Due to the presence of volatile oil constituents in hyssop, it may provide relief for mild irritations of the upper respiratory tract that accompany the **common cold** (page 129). The expectorant action of hyssop's volatile oil may partially explain its traditional use for **coughs** (page 139), **asthma** (page 32), and **bronchitis** (page 80).[4] The volatile oils are also thought to contribute to hyssop's carminative actions and use for mild cramping and discomfort in the digestive tract. The German Commission E has not approved hyssop for any medical indication.[5] Test tube studies have found that certain fractions of hyssop (one being a polysaccharide designated as MAR-10) may inhibit the activity of the **human immunodeficiency virus** (page 239)

Hyssop

(HIV).[6, 7] Yet, there have been no studies in humans to determine whether hyssop or any of its constituents are effective in treating HIV infection or AIDS.

How much is usually taken?

Hyssop may be taken as a tea or tincture. The tea is prepared by infusing 2–3 teaspoons of herb in one cup (250 ml) of hot water for ten to fifteen minutes. Three cups can be drunk per day. Alternatively, 1–4 ml of tincture can be taken three times per day.[8] If hyssop is being used to help soothe a **sore throat** (page 129), gargle with the tea or tincture before swallowing. The essential oil should never be used at a level higher than 1–2 drops per day internally, though more can be used topically on unbroken skin. One teaspoon (5 grams) of hyssop herb steeped in 1 cup (250 ml) hot water in a closed vessel for 15–20 minutes, then given in sips from a bottle over a period of 2–3 hours, may help calm **colic** (page 121).

Are there any side effects or interactions?

Tea and tincture of hyssop are unlikely to cause adverse effects.[9] Although, the volatile oil, particularly its constituent pinocamphone, has been reported to cause seizures in laboratory animals as well as in humans when taking more than 10 drops in a day or a child taking 2–3 drops over several days.[10] For this reason, the volatile oil should be used with extreme caution and is not recommended for those with **epilepsy** (page 183) or any other seizure disorder. The herb is not recommended during **pregnancy** (page 363).[11]

IPECAC

Botanical name: *Cephaelis ipecacuanha*

Parts used and where grown

Ipecac grows in the rain forests of Brazil and other parts of South and Central America. It is also cultivated to a small degree in India and Southeast Asia. Ipecac roots are used as medicine.

Ipecac has been used in connection with the following conditions (refer to the individual health concern for complete information):

Rating	Health Concerns
★★★	Poisoning
★★☆	**Intestinal parasites** (page 343)

Historical or traditional use (may or may not be supported by scientific studies)

In traditional herbal medicine, ipecac appears to have been primarily used as an emetic, or an agent that induces vomiting.[1] The herb was reportedly first exported to Europe in 1672.[2] The alkaloids in the plant were identified originally in 1817.

Active constituents

Ipecac's major constituents are the alkaloids emetine and cephaline. The roots also contain tannins and small amounts of anthraquinone glycosides.[3] The alkaloids have several important actions, including activation of brain centers that can induce vomiting, inhibition of the sympathetic nervous system, and inhibition of protein synthesis.[4]

Ipecac syrup is commonly used as a remedy for poisoning, taken following ingestion of toxic but noncaustic substances. In most people, ingestion of adequate amounts leads to vomiting within 30 minutes.[5]

The protein-inhibiting effects of emetine and other alkaloids of ipecac may account for the ability of the plant to inhibit growth of or kill several types of **parasites** (page 343), including ameba, pinworms, and tapeworms.[6, 7] However, the amount of ipecac needed to produce these effects in people are high and can lead to severe side effects. Emetine or its somewhat safer form, dihydroemetine, are reserved for rare cases of people infected with amebas that are not cured by using anti-ameba drugs.[8] Due to the danger involved, ipecac or emetine should never be used without first consulting a physician.

How much is usually taken?

To induce vomiting after ingesting something poisonous (after consulting with poison control centers or emergency services), adults are generally advised to take 15–30 ml of ipecac syrup followed by 3–4 glasses of water.[9] Children age 1–12 years should take 15 ml of ipecac syrup followed by 1–2 glasses of water. Children under age 1 year should be given 5–10 ml syrup followed by one half to 1 glass of water. The poisoned subject should be kept moving and the head kept upright after taking ipecac. It may take up to 30 minutes before vomiting occurs. A second application of 15 ml followed by more water can be used if vomiting does not occur after 30 minutes. If vomiting still does not occur after the second use, it is best to go immediately to the nearest hospital to have the ipecac pumped out of the stomach and obtain further help for the original poisoning. Milk or carbonated drinks should not be substituted for water after taking ipecac, as they might interfere with ipecac's absorption and efficacy. Activated charcoal will also interfere with the absorption and efficacy of ipecac. Charcoal should only be given after ipecac has caused vomiting. Ipecac should never be used to induce vomiting of caustic poisons such as gasoline, acids, or bleach. Ipecac tincture and fluid extract are much stronger than ipecac syrup. Ipecac tincture or fluid extract should never be taken in the amounts listed above for ipecac syrup.

Are there any side effects or interactions?

When used as directed for poisoning, ipecac will cause severe nausea, vomiting, and intestinal cramps. If too much ipecac is ingested, it may cause dizziness, rapid heartbeat, and palpitations. Cases have been reported of people with bulimia who abused ipecac by taking it frequently to induce vomiting and developed severe muscle damage or heart damage, and, in some cases, died.[10, 11] Since emetine is removed from the body slowly, the amounts can build up with repeated use and cause damage later. Ipecac should not be used during **pregnancy** (page 363) or breast-feeding.

IVY LEAF

Botanical name: *Hedera helix*

Parts used and where grown

Ivy is an evergreen climber native to the damp woods of western, central, and southern Europe. The leaf is used medicinally.[1] It should be carefully distinguished from poison ivy found in the Americas.

Ivy has been used in connection with the following conditions (refer to the individual health concern for complete information):

Rating	Health Concerns
★★☆	**Asthma** (page 32) **Bronchitis** (page 80) **Chronic obstructive pulmonary disease** (page 114) (COPD)
★☆☆	**Cough** (page 139) Stretch marks (topical)

Historical or traditional use (may or may not be supported by scientific studies)

Ivy leaves were held in high regard by the ancients. They formed not only the poet's crown but also the wreath of the Greek god of wine, Dionysus. The ancient Greeks believed that binding the forehead with ivy leaves would prevent the effects of inebriation.[2] Greek priests presented a wreath of ivy to newlyweds, and ivy has been traditionally regarded as a symbol of fidelity. Romans regarded ivy as excellent feed for their cattle.[3] Traditional herbalists have used ivy for a wide number of complaints, including **bronchitis** (page 80), whooping cough, arthritis, rheumatism, and dysentery. Decoctions of the herb were applied externally against lice, scabies, and sunburn.[4]

Active constituents

Although ivy's composition has not been subject to detailed scientific investigations, it is known to contain 5–8% saponins.[5] Other constituents in the leaf include an alkaloid called emetine that is similar to one found in the herb **tylophora** (page 754). Although emetine typically induces vomiting, in ivy leaf it seems to increase the secretion of mucus in the lungs. While the emetine content is very low in ivy, this could in part explain its traditional use as an expectorant (a substance that promotes the removal of mucous from the respiratory tract).[6] Animal studies have shown the saponins found in ivy extract prevent the spasm of muscles in the bronchial area.[7]

While very few human clinical trials have been performed on ivy, a controlled trial in a group of children with bronchial **asthma** (page 32) found that 25 drops of ivy leaf extract given twice per day was effective in improving airflow into the lungs after only three days of use.[8] However, the incidence of **cough** (page 139) and shortness of breath symptoms did not change during the short trial period. Ivy leaf is approved by the German Commission E for use against chronic inflammatory bronchial conditions and productive coughs due to its actions as an expectorant.[9] One double-blind human trial found ivy leaf to be as effective as the drug ambroxol for treating the symptoms of chronic bronchitis.[10]

In addition to the use of ivy to treat asthma, clinical reports from Europe suggest that topical cream preparations containing ivy, **horsetail** (page 693), and lady's mantle are beneficial in reducing, although not eliminating, skin stretch marks.[11]

How much is usually taken?

Standardized ivy leaf extract can be taken by itself or in water at 25 drops twice per day as a supportive treatment for children with **asthma** (page 32).[12] At least double this amount may be necessary to benefit adults with asthma. However, ivy is not intended to replace standard medical therapies and should only be used following consultation with a healthcare professional. A similar amount can be used for people with a **cough** (page 139) or **bronchitis** (page 80).

Are there any side effects or interactions?
The 0.3 gram daily tea preparation of the herb, suggested in the German Commission E monographs,[13] is not recommended for pediatric use because the quantities of the saponins it contains are too variable and could induce nausea and vomiting. Since ivy contains small amounts of emetine, it is not recommended during **pregnancy** (page 363), as this specific alkaloid may increase uterine contractions.[14] In addition, the leaf itself can be quite irritating when handled and may cause allergic skin reactions.[15]

JUNIPER

Botanical name: *Juniperus communis*

Parts used and where grown
Juniper, an evergreen tree, grows mainly in the plains regions of Europe as well as in other parts of the world. The medicinal portions of the plant are referred to as berries, but they are actually dark blue-black scales from the cones of the tree. Unlike other pine cones, the juniper cones are fleshy and soft.

Juniper has been used in connection with the following conditions (refer to the individual health concern for complete information):

Rating	Health Concerns
★☆☆	**Edema (water retention)** (page 180) **Indigestion** (page 260) **Urinary tract infection** (page 436)

Historical or traditional use (may or may not be supported by scientific studies)
Aside from being used as the flavoring agent in gin, juniper trees have contributed to the making of everything from soap to perfume.[1] Many conditions have

been treated in traditional herbal medicine with juniper berries, including **gout** (page 208), **warts** (page 445) and skin growths, **cancer** (page 87), **upset stomach** (page 260), and various **urinary tract** (page 436) and kidney diseases.

Active constituents
The volatile oils, particularly terpinen-4-ol, may cause an increase in urine volume.[2] According to some sources, juniper increases urine volume without a loss of electrolytes such as potassium.[3] Juniper contains bitter substances, at least partly accounting for its traditional use in digestive upset and related problems.

How much is usually taken?
The German Commission E monograph suggests ½–2 teaspoons of the dried fruit daily.[4] To make a tea, 1 cup (250 ml) of boiling water is added to 1 teaspoon (5 grams) of juniper berries and allowed to steep for twenty minutes in a tightly covered container. Drink one cup (250 ml) each morning and night. Juniper is often combined with other diuretic and anti-microbial herbs. As a capsule or tablet, 1–2 grams can be taken three times per day, or ¼–½ teaspoon (1–2 ml) of tincture can be taken three times daily.

Are there any side effects or interactions?
Excessive applications (greater than the amounts listed above) may cause kidney irritation. People with either acute or chronic inflammation of the kidneys or kidney failure should not use juniper. Juniper should not be taken for greater than four weeks without first consulting a healthcare professional. One report suggests that people with diabetes should use juniper cautiously as it may raise glucose levels.[5]

Application of the volatile oil directly to skin can cause a rash. **Pregnant** (page 363) women should avoid juniper until further information is available, as it may cause uterine contractions.

KAVA

Botanical name: *Piper methysticum*

Parts used and where grown
Kava is a member of the pepper family and is native to many Pacific Ocean islands. The rhizome (underground stem) is used in modern herbal preparations.

Warning: Kava should be taken only with medical supervision. Kava is not for sale in certain parts of the world.

Historical or traditional use (may or may not be supported by scientific studies)

A nonalcoholic drink made from the root of kava played an important role in social ceremonies in some Pacific islands, including welcoming visiting royalty and at meetings of village elders. Kava was valued both for its mellowing effects and to encourage socializing. It was also noted for initiating a state of contentment, a greater sense of well-being, and enhanced mental acuity, memory, and sensory perception. Kava has also been used traditionally by healers in the Pacific islands to treat **pain** (page 338).

Active constituents

The kava-lactones, sometimes referred to as kava-pyrones, are the most important active constituents in kava extracts. High-quality kava rhizome contains 5.5–8.3% kava-lactones.[1] Medicinal extracts used in Europe contain 30–70% kava-lactones. Kava-lactones are thought to have anti-anxiety, mild analgesic (pain-relieving), muscle-relaxing, and anticonvulsant effects.[2, 3] Some researchers speculate that kava may directly influence the limbic system, the ancient part of the brain associated with emotions and other brain activities.[4] Kava is a unique anti-anxiety alternative because it does not seem to impair reaction time or alertness when used in the amounts recommended below.[5]

Kava has been extensively studied as a treatment for **anxiety** (page 30).[6] The amount often used in clinical trials is 100 mg of an extract (standardized to 70% kava-lactones) three times per day. Double-blind trials, including one that lasted six months, have shown that kava effectively reduces symptoms of anxiety in people with mild to moderate anxiety.[7, 8] One trial found that kava also reduced symptoms of anxiety in menopausal women,[9] and in another study kava enhanced the anti-anxiety effect of hormone replacement therapy.[10] One trial found kava to be just as effective as benzodiazepines (a common class of drugs prescribed for anxiety) in treating mild anxiety over the course of six weeks.[11]

How much is usually taken?

For treatment of mild to moderate anxiety, kava extracts supplying 120–240 mg of kava-lactones per day in two or three divided doses are commonly recommended.[12] Alternatively (although it has not been researched), 1–3 ml of fresh liquid kava tincture can be taken three times per day. Kava should not be taken for more than three months without the advice of a physician, according to the German Commission E monograph.[13]

Are there any side effects or interactions?

In November 2001, German authorities announced that 24 cases of liver disease (including hepatitis, liver failure, and cirrhosis) associated with the use of kava had been reported in Germany; of these, one person died and three required a liver transplant.[14]

Prior to this report, it had been widely believed that kava did not cause any serious side effects. The 1998 edition of the German *Commission E Monographs,* considered to be an authoritative source on herbal medicines, does not mention liver disease in its discussion of kava's side effects.[15] Since that time, four case reports of kava-related liver toxicity have appeared in medical journals.[16, 17, 18, 19] In two of these cases, severe liver failure resulted in the need for a liver transplant. Most, though not all, of the individuals who developed liver damage while taking kava were also taking at least one other medication that has been associated with liver injury.[20] That raises the possibility that these other drugs, rather than kava, may have been responsible for the problem in some cases. It is also conceivable that kava interacts with some of these drugs, thereby increasing their toxicity. However, some of the cases of kava-related liver disease cannot be explained by the concomitant use of other drugs.

The possibility that kava can cause liver damage is supported by a survey of an Aboriginal community in Australia. Although occasional users of kava in this community generally had normal liver function, laboratory evidence of liver injury was quite common among heavy users of the herb.[21] Furthermore, the risk of liver damage was directly related to the amount of kava consumed. It is not clear how relevant these findings are to other communities, since the overall health of the Aborigines who were studied was relatively poor.

It is also unclear whether kava is safe when taken in "normal" amounts. A recent survey of 400 German medical practices revealed that 78% of the kava prescriptions that were written significantly exceeded the recommended amount.[22] However, some of the 24 patients reported to German authorities were not exceeding the manufacturer's recommended level of intake

Kava

when they developed liver disease. In addition, in two of the four published case reports, the amount of kava used was equal to or only slightly higher than the manufacturer's recommendation.[23] Therefore, one cannot assume that the recommended level of intake of kava is safe for all individuals.

Health authorities worldwide are considering or implementing a ban on kava. Until additional information clarifies the extent of the risk involved, it is strongly recommended that all individuals consult their physician before taking kava. In addition, based on the available information, it seems that people with liver disease and those taking medications that have the potential to damage the liver should not take kava.

In recommended amounts, the most common side effect from kava use is mild gastrointestinal disturbances in some people. Kava may temporarily turn the skin yellow, according to some case studies.[24] If this occurs, people should discontinue kava use. In rare cases, an allergic skin reaction, such as a rash, may occur.[25] Enlargement of the pupils has also been reported after long-term use of kava.[26] In the amounts discussed above, kava does not appear to be addictive.

Kava is not recommended for use by **pregnant** (page 363) or breast-feeding women. It should not be taken together with other substances that also act on the central nervous system, such as alcohol, barbiturates, antidepressants, and antipsychotic drugs. One study found that large amounts of a traditional kava preparation did worsen cognitive impairment caused by alcohol consumption.[27] However, at the amounts recommended above, kava does not appear to impair cognitive performance. Kava has also been reported to cause excessive sedation and grogginess when combined with benzodiazepines.[28] One study found it was safe to drive after taking kava at the amounts listed above.[29] However, the German Commission E monograph states that kava, when taken at the recommended levels, may adversely affect a person's ability to safely drive or operate heavy machinery.[30]

Caution: Aside from the reported interactions, kava inhibits a number of the cytochrome P450 enzymes that play a role in the breakdown of many medications.[31] Therefore, kava has the potential to interact with a wide range of medications, even if such interactions have not yet been reported. Individuals taking any medication who wish to use kava should check with their physician or pharmacist to determine whether inhibiting cytochrome P450 could cause an adverse drug interaction.

KUDZU

Common name: Ge-gen
Botanical name: *Pueraria lobata*

Parts used and where grown

Kudzu is a coarse, high-climbing, twining, trailing, perennial vine. The huge root, which can grow to the size of a human, is the source of medicinal preparations used in Traditional Chinese Medicine and modern herbal products. Kudzu grows in most shaded areas in mountains, fields, along roadsides, thickets, and thin forests throughout most of China and the southeastern United States. The root of another Asian species of kudzu, *Pueraria thomsonii,* is also used for herbal products.

Kudzu has been used in connection with the following conditions (refer to the individual health concern for complete information):

Rating	Health Concerns
★☆☆	**Alcohol withdrawal support** (page 12) **Angina** (page 27)

Historical or traditional use (may or may not be supported by scientific studies)

Kudzu root has been known for centuries in Traditional Chinese Medicine as ge-gen. The first written mention of the plant as a medicine is in the ancient herbal text of Shen Nong (circa A.D. 100). In Traditional Chinese Medicine, kudzu root is used in prescriptions for the treatment of wei, or "superficial," syndrome (a disease that manifests just under the surface—mild, but with fever), thirst, headache, and stiff neck with pain due to **high blood pressure** (page 236).[1] It is also recommended for **allergies** (page 14), **migraine headaches** (page 316), and **diarrhea** (page 163). The historical application for drunkenness has become a major focal point of modern research on kudzu. It is also used in modern Chinese medicine as a treatment for **angina pectoris** (page 27).

Active constituents

Kudzu root is high in isoflavones, such as daidzein, as well as isoflavone glycosides, such as daidzin and puerarin. Depending on its growing conditions, the total isoflavone content varies from 1.77–12.0%, with puerarin in the highest concentration, followed by daidzin and daidzein.[2]

A widely publicized 1993 animal study showed that both daidzin and daidzein inhibit the desire for alcohol.[3] The authors concluded the root extract may in fact be useful for reducing the urge for alcohol and as treatment for **alcoholism** (page 12). However, a small controlled clinical trial with alcoholic adults taking 1.2 grams of kudzu two times per day failed to show any effect on decreasing alcohol consumption or cravings.[4]

How much is usually taken?
The 1985 *Chinese Pharmacopoeia* suggests 9–15 grams of kudzu root per day.[5] In China, standardized root extracts (10 mg tablet is equivalent to 1.5 grams of the crude root) are used to treat **angina pectoris** (page 27). Some sources recommend 30–120 mg of the extract two to three times per day.

Are there any side effects or interactions?
At the amounts recommended above, there have been no reports of kudzu toxicity in humans.

LAVENDER

Botanical name: *Lavandula officinalis*

Parts used and where grown
Eastern European countries, particularly Bulgaria, as well as France, Britain, Australia, and Russia grow large quantities of lavender. The fragrant flowers of lavender are used in the preparation of herbal medicines.

Lavender has been used in connection with the following conditions (refer to the individual health concern for complete information):

Rating	Health Concerns
★★☆	**Pregnancy** (page 363) (in bath, for perineal pain after childbirth)
★☆☆	**Indigestion and heartburn** (page 260) **Insomnia** (page 270)

Historical or traditional use (may or may not be supported by scientific studies)
Traditionally, herbalists used lavender for a variety of conditions of the nervous system, including **depression** (page 145) and fatigue.[1] It has also been used for headache and rheumatism. Due to its delightful odor, lavender has found wide application in perfumes and cosmetics throughout history.

Active constituents
The volatile oil (also called essential oil) of lavender contains many constituents, including perillyl alcohol and linalool. The oil is thought to be calming[2] and thus can be helpful in some cases of **insomnia** (page 270). One trial of elderly people with sleeping troubles found that inhaling lavender oil was as effective as some commonly prescribed sleep medications.[3] A large clinical trial found that lavender oil added to a bath was no more effective than a placebo for relieving perineal discomfort immediately after childbirth.[4] However, perineal pain was reduced three to five days afterward. Lavender is recommended by the German Commission E monograph for indigestion and nervous intestinal discomfort.[5]

How much is usually taken?
The German Commission E monograph suggests 1–2 teaspoons (5–10 grams) of the herb be taken as a tea.[6] The tea can be made by steeping 2 teaspoons (10 grams) of leaves in 1 cup (250 ml) of boiling water for fifteen minutes. Three cups (750 ml) can be consumed each day. For internal applications, ½–¾ teaspoon (2–4 ml) of tincture can be taken two or three times per day. Several drops of the oil can be added to a bath or diluted in vegetable oil for topical applications. The concentrated oil is not for internal use, except under medical supervision.

Are there any side effects or interactions?
Internal use of the volatile oil can cause severe nausea. Very small amounts should be used only under the supervision of a healthcare professional. Excessive intake (several times more than listed above) may cause drowsiness.[7] External use in reasonable amounts is safe during **pregnancy** (page 363) and breast-feeding.

LEMON BALM

Common name: Melissa
Botanical name: *Melissa officinalis*

Parts used and where grown
The lemon balm plant originated in southern Europe and is now found throughout the world. The lemony

smell and pretty white flowers of the plant have led to its widespread cultivation in gardens. The leaves, stems, and flowers of lemon balm are used medicinally.

Lemon balm has been used in connection with the following conditions (refer to the individual health concern for complete information):

Rating	Health Concerns
★★★	**Cold sores** (page 119) (topical)
★★☆	**Alzheimer's disease** (page 19) **Colic** (page 121) (in combination with **vervain** [page 756], **licorice** [page 702], and **fennel** [page 676]) **Genital herpes** (page 200) (topical)
★☆☆	Grave's disease (hyperthyroidism) **Indigestion and heartburn** (page 260) **Infection** (page 265) (antiviral) **Insomnia** (page 270) Nerve pain

Historical or traditional use (may or may not be supported by scientific studies)

Charlemagne once ordered lemon balm planted in every monastery garden because of its beauty.[1] It has been used traditionally by herbalists to treat gas, sleeping difficulties, and heart problems. In addition, topical applications to the temples were sometimes used by herbalists for **insomnia** (page 270) or nerve pain.

Active constituents

The terpenes, part of the pleasant smelling volatile oil from lemon balm, are thought to produce this herb's relaxing and gas-relieving (carminative) effects. **Flavonoids** (page 516), phenolic acids, and other compounds appear to be responsible for lemon balm's anti-herpes and thyroid-regulating actions. Test tube studies have found that lemon balm blocks attachment of antibodies to the thyroid cells that cause Grave's disease (hyperthyroidism).[2] The brain's signal to the thyroid (thyroid-stimulating hormone or TSH) is also blocked from further stimulating the excessively active thyroid gland in this disease. However, clinical trials proving lemon balm's effectiveness in treating Grave's disease are lacking.

One small preliminary trial studying sleep quality compared the effect of a combination product containing an extract of lemon balm *(Melissa officinalis)* and an extract of **valerian** (page 756) root with that of the sleeping drug triazolam (Halcion). The effectiveness of the herbal combination was similar to that of Halcion,

as determined by the ability to fall asleep and the quality of sleep.[3] Another trial also found that the same combination of valerian and lemon balm, taken over a two-week period, is effective in improving quality of sleep.[4]

According to double-blind research, topical use of a concentrated lemon balm extract speeds healing time of herpes simplex virus sores (**cold sores** [page 119]) on the mouth.[5, 6]

How much is usually taken?

The German Commission E monograph suggests 1.5–4.5 grams of lemon balm in a tea several times daily.[7] The herb can be steeped for ten to fifteen minutes in 150 ml of boiling water to make the tea. Tincture can also be used at 2–3 ml three times per day. Concentrated extracts, 160–200 mg 30 minutes to one hour before bed, are sometimes recommended for **insomnia** (page 270). Highly concentrated topical extract ointments for herpes can be applied three to four times per day to lesions.

Lemon balm is frequently combined with other medicinal plants. For example, **peppermint** (page 726) and lemon balm together are effective for calming **upset stomach** (page 260). **Valerian** (page 756) is often combined with lemon balm for insomnia. **Bugleweed** (page 647) *(Lycopus virginicus)* and lemon balm have been used together for Graves' disease.

Are there any side effects or interactions?

There is one published report of a severe allergic reaction (anaphylaxis) occurring in a person who took a supplement that contained willow bark.[8] The possibility of allergy to willow bark should be considered by anyone who is allergic to aspirin or other salicylates. As with aspirin, some people may experience stomach upset from taking willow. Although such symptoms are less likely from willow than from aspirin, people with **ulcers** (page 349) and **gastritis** (page 195) should, nevertheless, avoid this herb.[9] Again, as with aspirin, willow should not be used to treat fevers in children since it may cause Reye's syndrome.

LICORICE

Botanical names: *Glycyrrhiza glabra, Glycyrrhiza uralensis*

Parts used and where grown

Originally from central Europe, licorice now grows all across Europe and Asia. The root is used medicinally.

Licorice has been used in connection with the following conditions (refer to the individual health concern for complete information):

Rating	Health Concerns
★★★	**Infection** (page 265) **Peptic ulcer** (page 349) (chewable DGL)
★★☆	**Canker sores** (page 90) (DGL) **Colic** (page 121) (in combination with **vervain** [page 756], **fennel** [page 676], and **lemon balm** [page 701]) **Epilepsy** (page 183) (in combination with **bupleurum** [page 647], peony root, pinellia root, cassia bark, **ginger** [page 680] root, jujube fruit, **Asian ginseng** [page 630] root, and **Chinese scullcap** [page 658] root) **Gastroesophageal reflux disease** (page 198) (GERD) (DGL) **Hepatitis** (page 220) (intravenous glycyrrhizin) **HIV support** (page 239) **Infections** (page 265) (viral)
★☆☆	**Asthma** (page 32) **Chronic fatigue syndrome** (page 111) **Cold sores** (page 119) (topical) **Cough** (page 139) **Crohn's disease** (page 141) **Eczema** (page 177) **Gastritis** (page 195) **Genital herpes** (page 200) (topical) **Hay fever** (page 211) (Sho-seiryu-to: contains licorice, cassia bark, **schisandra** [page 744], ma huang [ephedra], **ginger** [page 680], peony root, pinellia, and asiasarum root) **Hepatitis** (page 220) (oral glycyrrhizin) **Indigestion and heartburn** (page 260) (DGL) Melasma (topical liquirtin) **Menopause** (page 311) **Shingles (herpes zoster)/postherpetic neuralgia** (page 401) (topical gel) **Ulcerative colitis** (page 433)

Historical or traditional use (may or may not be supported by scientific studies)

Licorice has a long and highly varied record of uses. It was and remains one of the most important herbs in Traditional Chinese Medicine. Among its most consistent and important uses are as a demulcent (soothing, coating agent) in the digestive and urinary tracts, to help with **coughs** (page 139), to soothe **sore throats** (page 129), and as a flavoring. It has also been used in Traditional Chinese Medicine to treat conditions ranging from **diabetes** (page 152) to tuberculosis.

Active constituents

The two major constituents of licorice are glycyrrhizin and **flavonoids** (page 516). According to test tube studies, glycyrrhizin has anti-inflammatory actions and may inhibit the breakdown of the cortisol produced by the body.[1, 2] Licorice may also have antiviral properties, although this has not been proven in human pharmacological studies. Licorice flavonoids, as well as the closely related chalcones, help heal digestive tract cells. They are also potent **antioxidants** (page 467) and work to protect liver cells. In test tubes, the flavonoids have been shown to kill *Helicobacter pylori*, the bacteria that causes most **ulcers** (page 349) and stomach inflammation.[3] However, it is unclear whether this action applies to the use of oral licorice for the treatment of ulcers in humans.

An extract of licorice, called liquiritin, has been used as a treatment for melasma, a pigmentation disorder of the skin. In a preliminary trial,[4] topical application of liquiritin cream twice daily for four weeks led to a 70% improvement, compared to only 20% improvement in the placebo group.

A preliminary trial found that while the acid-blocking drug cimetidine (Tagamet) led to quicker symptom relief, chewable deglycyrrhizinated licorice (DGL) tablets were just as effective at healing and maintaining the healing of stomach ulcers.[5] Chewable DGL may also be helpful in treating ulcers of the duodenum, the first part of the small intestine.[6] Capsules of DGL may not work for ulcers, however, as DGL must mix with saliva to be activated.[7] One preliminary human trial has found DGL used as a mouthwash was effective in quickening the healing of **canker sores** (page 90).[8]

How much is usually taken?

There are two types of licorice, "standard" licorice and "de-glycyrrhizinated" licorice (DGL). Each type is suitable for different conditions. The standard licorice containing glycyrrhizin should be used for respiratory infections, **chronic fatigue syndrome** (page 111) or herpes (topical). Licorice root in capsules, 5–6 grams per day, can be used. Concentrated extracts, 250–500 mg three times per day, are another option. Alternatively, a tea can be made by boiling ½ ounce (14 grams) of root in 1 pint (500 ml) of water for fifteen minutes, then drinking two to three cups (500–750 ml) per day. Long-term internal use (more than two to three weeks) of high amounts (over 10 grams per day) of glycyrrhizin-containing products should be attempted only under the supervision of a doctor. Licorice creams or gels can be applied directly to herpes sores three to four times per day.

DGL is prepared without the glycyrrhizin in order to circumvent potential safety problems (see below), and is used for conditions of the digestive tract, such as **ulcers** (page 349). For best results, one 200–300 mg tablet is chewed three times per day before meals and before bed.[9] For **canker sores** (page 90), 200 mg of DGL powder can be mixed with 200 ml warm water, swished in the mouth for three minutes, and then expelled. This may be repeated three or four times per day.

Are there any side effects or interactions?

Licorice products that include glycyrrhizin may increase **blood pressure** (page 246) and cause **water retention** (page 180).[10] Some people are more sensitive to this effect than others. Long-term intake (more than two to three weeks) of products containing more than 1 gram of glycyrrhizin (the amount in approximately 10 grams of root) daily is the usual amount required to cause these effects. Consumption of 7 grams licorice (containing 500 mg glycyrrhizin) per day for seven days has been shown to decrease serum testosterone levels in healthy men by blocking the enzymes needed to synthesize testosterone.[11] However, in another study, a similar amount of licorice had only a small and statistically insignificant effect on testosterone levels.[12] As a result of these possible side effects, long-term intake of high levels of glycyrrhizin is discouraged and should only be undertaken if prescribed by a qualified healthcare professional. Consumption of plenty of fresh fruits and vegetables to increase **potassium** (page 572) intake is recommended to help decrease the chance of side effects. According to the German Commission E monograph, licorice is inadvisable for **pregnant** (page 363) women as well as for people with liver and kidney disorders.[13]

De-glycyrrhizinated licorice extracts do not cause these side effects since they contain no glycyrrhizin.

LIGUSTRUM

Common name: Privet
Botanical name: *Ligustrum lucidum*

Parts used and where grown

This shrub is native to China and eastern Asia and is now grown ornamentally in the United States. The berry of ligustrum is used medicinally.

Ligustrum has been used in connection with the following conditions (refer to the individual health concern for complete information):

Rating	Health Concerns
★☆☆	**Immune function** (page 255) **Infection** (page 265)

Historical or traditional use (may or may not be supported by scientific studies)

Since ancient times, ligustrum berries have been employed as a "yin" tonic in Traditional Chinese Medicine.[1] Ligustrum was used for a wide range of conditions, including premature aging and **ringing in the ears** (page 430).[2]

Active constituents

The major constituent in ligustrum is ligustrin (oleanolic acid). Preliminary studies, mostly conducted in China, suggest that ligustrum stimulates the **immune system** (page 255), decreases inflammation, and protects the liver.[3] Ligustrum is often combined with **astragalus** (page 631) in Traditional Chinese Medicine. Although used for long-term support of the immune system in people with depressed immune function or cancer, more research is needed to demonstrate the optimal length of time to use ligustrum.

How much is usually taken?

Powdered, encapsulated berries, 1–3 teaspoons (5–15 grams) per day, are sometimes recommended.[4] A similar amount of berries can be made into tea by adding ½–1 teaspoon (2–5 grams) of powdered or crushed berries to 1 cup (250 ml) of boiling water and steeping for ten to fifteen minutes. Alternatively, ¾–1 teaspoon (3–5 ml) of tincture three times per day can be taken.

Are there any side effects or interactions?

No adverse effects have been reported.

LINDEN

Common names: Lime blossom, lime flower
Botanical name: *Tilia* spp.

Parts used and where grown

This tree grows in the northern, temperate climates of Europe, Asia, and North America. Many medicinal species of linden exist, with *Tilia cordata* and *Tilia platyphyllos* generally being the most available and studied. Regardless of species, the flowers are used as medicine. Though sometimes called lime flower, linden is not related to the familiar green lime fruit.

Linden has been used in connection with the following conditions (refer to the individual health concern for complete information):

Rating	Health Concerns
★★☆	**Indigestion** (page 260)
★☆☆	**Anxiety** (page 30) **Common cold** (page 129) **Ear infection** (page 383)

Historical or traditional use (may or may not be supported by scientific studies)

Since time immemorial, the fragrant and tasty linden flowers have been used medicinally as a calming agent and to relieve **indigestion** (page 260), the **common cold** (page 129), and griping or colicky pain in the abdomen.[1, 2] Many of these uses have been confirmed or partially confirmed in modern research.

Active constituents

The major active constituents in linden are **flavonoids** (page 516), glycosides, and possibly a volatile oil. One study found that a complex mixture of compounds, primarily flavonoids, reduced anxiety in mice.[3] Although used as a traditional herbal remedy for **anxiety** (page 30), these results have not been confirmed in human clinical trials. Older clinical trials have shown that linden flower tea can help people with mild gallbladder problems (but not gallstones), **upset stomach** (page 260) or dyspepsia, and excessive gas that causes the stomach to push up and put pressure on the heart (also known as the gastrocardiac syndrome.)[4, 5] Linden's reputed antispasmodic action, particularly in the intestines, has been confirmed in at least one human trial.[6]

Linden flowers act as a diaphoretic when consumed as a hot tea. Diaphoretics induce a mild fever, thereby possibly helping promote the immune system's ability to fight **infections** (page 265). The fever usually does not go very high because the diaphoretic also causes sweating, the body's natural way of lowering its temperature. The German Commission E has approved linden flower for the treatment of **colds** (page 129) and cold-related **coughs** (page 139).[7]

How much is usually taken?

A tea of linden is prepared by adding 2–3 teaspoons (5–10 grams) of dried or fresh flowers to a pint (500 ml) of just boiled water. After steeping the flowers in a covered container for ten to fifteen minutes, sip the tea while it is still hot. During an acute problem, several cups can be taken daily for up to one week.[8] For longer term use (three to six months), three cups (750 ml) per day can be used. A tincture or fluid extract of linden, ¾–1 teaspoon (3–5 ml) three times daily, may alternatively be used.

Are there any side effects or interactions?

Statements that overuse of linden can cause heart problems[9] lack scientific merit. Both the German Commission E monograph and the American Herbal Products Association's guide on herbal safety state that linden has no toxic effects.[10, 11] In fact, linden is considered safe for use in children[12] and there are no known reasons to avoid it during **pregnancy** (page 363) and breast-feeding.

LOBELIA

Common name: Indian tobacco
Botanical name: *Lobelia inflata*

Parts used and where grown

Lobelia grows throughout North America. The leaves are primarily used in herbal medicine.

Lobelia has been used in connection with the following conditions (refer to the individual health concern for complete information):

Rating	Health Concerns
★☆☆	**Asthma** (page 32) **Bronchitis** (page 80) **Chronic obstructive pulmonary disease** (page 114) (COPD) **Cough** (page 139) Smoking cessation

Historical or traditional use (may or may not be supported by scientific studies)

Eclectic physicians, early North American doctors who used herbs as their primary medicine, considered lobelia to be one of the most important medicinal plants.[1] It was used by Eclectics to treat **coughs** (page 139) and spasms in the lungs from varying causes, as well as spasms elsewhere in the body, including the intestines and ureters (passages from the kidney to the bladder).[2] Lobelia was also considered a useful pain reliever and in higher amounts was used to induce vomiting in people who had been poisoned.

Active constituents

The alkaloid lobeline is responsible for most of lobelia's actions. Lobeline has been used as a traditional herbal approach to help people stop smoking. Results of human trials using lobeline for smoking cessation have been mixed and generally negative.[3] Preliminary trials suggest lobeline may improve lung function, perhaps by its abilities to reduce bronchial constriction and to thin mucus so that it can be coughed out.[4]

How much is usually taken?

Eclectic physicians generally recommended using a tincture of lobelia made partially or entirely with vinegar instead of alcohol.[5] A vinegar extract is known as an acetract. At most, 1 ml was given three times per day. The absolute maximum amount to take should be that which causes no, or minimal, nausea. Lobelia ointment has also been used topically on the chest to relieve **asthma** (page 32) and **bronchitis** (page 80). People should apply such ointments liberally several times per day.

Are there any side effects or interactions?

Lobelia frequently causes nausea and vomiting when the amount used is too high. Generally, more than 1 ml of tincture or acetract taken at one time will cause nausea and possibly vomiting and should be avoided.[6] Although lobelia has a reputation for being toxic, a thorough review of the medical literature was unable to find any well-documented case of serious problems or death due to lobelia.[7] This may be because a toxic amount cannot be ingested without first causing vomiting. Signs of lobelia poisoning may include weakness, heartburn, weak pulse, difficulty breathing, and collapse.[8] Nevertheless, lobelia should not be used for more than one month consecutively and should be avoided during **pregnancy** (page 363) and breast-feeding.[9] Due to its emetic (vomit-inducing) actions, lobelia should be used cautiously with children under the age of six years.

LOMATIUM

Botanical name: *Lomatium dissectum*

Parts used and where grown

Lomatium is native to western North America. Lomatium is potentially threatened in some parts of its habitat, so it should not be picked from the wild without consulting local experts familiar with the plant. The root of lomatium is used medicinally.

Lomatium has been used in connection with the following conditions (refer to the individual health concern for complete information):

Rating	Health Concerns
★☆☆	**Infection** (page 265)

Historical or traditional use (may or may not be supported by scientific studies)

Native Americans of many tribes reportedly used lomatium root to treat a wide variety of infections, particularly those affecting the lungs.[1] Lomatium was used, particularly in the southwestern United States, during the **influenza** (page 269) pandemic of 1917 with reportedly good results.

Active constituents

According to obscure sources, lomatium is reputed to have antiviral effects. One source suggests the constituents tetronic acids and a glucoside of luteolin may be potentially antiviral.[2] However, little is known about how these compounds act or if other ones might be as important.

How much is usually taken?

Lomatium extracts with the resins removed (often called lomatium isolates), 1–3 ml per day, have been recommended. Lomatium tincture, 1–3 ml three times per day, can also be used, but it may cause a rash in susceptible people. The tincture should not be used unless a very small amount of it is first tested for a reaction. However, even very small amounts can cause a reaction in sensitive people.

Are there any side effects or interactions?

Use of lomatium extracts or tinctures containing the resin (and possibly the coumarins) can, in some people,

Lobelia

cause a whole-body rash.[3] This herb may also lead to nausea in some people. The safety of lomatium during **pregnancy** (page 363) and breast-feeding is unknown and is therefore not recommended.

MAITAKE

Botanical name: *Grifola frondosa*

Parts used and where grown
Maitake is a very large mushroom, which grows deep in the mountains of northeastern Japan, as well as in North America and Europe. Famous for its taste and health benefits, maitake is also known as the "dancing mushroom."[1] Legend holds that those who found the rare mushroom began dancing with joy. Others attribute its name to the way the fruit bodies of the mushroom overlap each other, giving the appearance of dancing butterflies.

Maitake is extremely sensitive to environmental changes, which have presented many challenges to those cultivating this mushroom. However, Japanese farmers have succeeded in producing high-quality organic maitake mushrooms, allowing for wider availability both in Japan and the U.S. The fruiting body and mycelium of maitake are used medicinally.

Maitake has been used in connection with the following conditions (refer to the individual health concern for complete information):

Rating	Health Concerns
★☆☆	**High cholesterol** (page 223) and **high triglyceride** (page 235) levels **HIV support** (page 239) **Immune function** (page 255) **Infection** (page 265)

Historical or traditional use (may or may not be supported by scientific studies)
Historically, maitake has been used as a tonic and adaptogen (a substance that invigorates or strengthens the system). Along with other "medicinal" mushrooms, such as **shiitake** (page 746) and **reishi** (page 737), maitake was used as a food to help promote wellness and vitality.

Active constituents
A common denominator among some mushrooms and some herbs is the presence of complex polysaccharides in their structure. These active constituents help support **immune system function** (page 255) and are sometimes called immunomodulators. The polysaccharides present in maitake have a unique structure and are among the most powerful studied in test tubes to date.[2] The primary polysaccharide, beta-D-glucan, is well absorbed when taken orally and is being studied as a potential tool for prevention and treatment of cancer and as a adjunctive treatment for **HIV infection** (page 239).[3, 4] Animal studies suggest maitake may lower serum cholesterol and triglycerides.[5, 6] However, this research is still preliminary and requires human trials for confirmation.

How much is usually taken?
Maitake can be used as a food or tea and is also available as a capsule or tablet containing the entire fruiting body of the mushroom. For maitake, the fruit body is higher in polysaccharides than the mycelium, which is why it is recommended. Whole-mushroom maitake supplements, 3–7 grams per day, can be taken.[7] Liquid maitake extracts with variable concentrations of polysaccharides are available, and should be taken as directed.

Are there any side effects or interactions?
Used as recommended above, there have been no reports of side effects with maitake.

MALLOW

Common names: High mallow, common mallow
Botanical name: *Malva sylvestris*

Parts used and where grown
Mallow originates from southern Europe and Asia but has spread all over the world as a common weed. Its cousin, the dwarf mallow (*Malva neglecta*), is another Eurasian plant that has spread far and wide. Other similar plants in the same family (*Malvaceae*) are hibiscus and **marshmallow** (page 708). The dried or fresh flowers and leaves of high mallow and dwarf mallow are used as food and medicine.

Mallow has been used in connection with the following conditions (refer to the individual health concern for complete information):

Rating	Health Concerns
★☆☆	**Cough** (page 139) (dry)
	Dermatitis (page 151) (atopic)
	Sore throat (page 129)

Historical or traditional use (may or may not be supported by scientific studies)

Mallow has been used as food and medicine in Europe since the time of ancient Greece and Rome. Traditional herbal medicine continues to regard the plant as a useful anti-inflammatory agent for the respiratory tract, the skin, and the gastrointestinal tract.[1] The esteemed German physician and herbal authority, Rudolf Weiss, MD, recommended mallow primarily for irritations of the mouth and throat, as well as for dry, irritating coughs.[2] He also mentions its use topically for mild cases of **eczema** (page 177).

Active constituents

Like its close relative **marshmallow** (page 708) *(Althea officinalis),* mallow leaves and flowers contain high amounts of mucilage.[3] Mucilage, made up of complex carbohydrates, gives mallow most of its soothing activity, though flavonoids and anthocyanidins may also contribute. In herbal medicine, mallow is classified as a demulcent—a soothing agent that counters irritation and mild inflammation. Both mallow leaf and flower preparations are approved by the German Commission E for relief of **sore throats** (page 129) and dry **coughs** (page 139).[4] Mallow is typically used as a tea or gargle for these indications.

In test tube studies, one carbohydrate in mallow has been shown to inhibit a component of the immune system known as the complement cascade.[5] Excessive activation of the complement cascade has been implicated in chronic inflammation and autoimmune disorders, suggesting that further research on mallow in these areas is warranted. A polysaccharide from the seeds of a related mallow *(Malva verticillata)* stimulated white blood cells known as macrophages in a test tube study.[6] Crude powder of one mallow species showed anticancer effects in another test tube study.[7]

How much is usually taken?

Mallow leaf and flower preparations are most commonly consumed as teas.[8] Boil 2 to 4 teaspoons of the dried leaves or flowers in 150 ml of boiling water for 10 to 15 minutes. One cup of the tea can be drunk three times per day. For topical use, a cloth can be dipped in the hot tea, allowed to cool, and then applied to inflamed skin. Alternatively, a cold infusion can be made, by soaking 6 teaspoons of the dry herb in a quart of cold water overnight, and then applied topically. According to some herbalists, the cold infusion likely extracts the plant's mucilage (a soothing, gelatinous substance) most effectively and may work best for both internal and topical use.

Are there any side effects or interactions?

There are no known adverse effects from mallow when used in the amounts suggested above.

MARSHMALLOW

Botanical name: *Althea officinalis*

Parts used and where grown

The marshmallow plant thrives in wet areas and grows primarily in marshes. Originally from Europe, it now grows in the United States as well. The root and leaves are used medicinally.

Marshmallow has been used in connection with the following conditions (refer to the individual health concern for complete information):

Rating	Health Concerns
★☆☆	**Asthma** (page 32)
	Common cold/sore throat (page 129)
	Cough (page 139)
	Crohn's disease (page 141)
	Diarrhea (page 163)
	Gastritis (page 195)
	Gastroesophageal reflux disease (page 198) (GERD)
	Indigestion (page 260)
	Pap smear (abnormal) (page 3)
	Peptic ulcer (page 349)
	Ulcerative colitis (page 433)

Mallow

Historical or traditional use (may or may not be supported by scientific studies)

Marshmallow (not to be confused with confectionery marshmallows) has long been used by herbalists to treat **coughs** (page 139) and **sore throats** (page 129).[1] Due to its high mucilage content, this plant is soothing to inflamed mucous membranes. Marshmallow is also used by herbalists to soothe chapped skin, chilblains (sores caused by exposure to cold), and minor wounds.

Active constituents

Mucilage, made up of large carbohydrate (sugar) molecules, is thought to be the active constituent in marshmallow. This smooth, slippery substance is believed to soothe and protect irritated mucous membranes. Marshmallow has primarily been used as a traditional herbal soothing agent for conditions of the respiratory and digestive tracts.[2]

How much is usually taken?

The German Commission E monograph suggests 1¼ teaspoon (6 grams) of the root per day.[3] Marshmallow can be made into a hot or cold water tea. Often 2–3 teaspoons (10–15 grams) of the root and/or leaves are used per cup (250 ml) of water. Generally, a full day's amount is steeped overnight when making a cold water tea, 6–9 teaspoons (30–45 grams) per three cups (750 ml) of water, or for fifteen to twenty minutes in hot water. Drink three to five cups (750–1250 ml) a day. Since the plant is so gooey, it does not combine well with other plants. Nevertheless, it can be found in some herbal cough syrups. Herbal extracts in capsules and tablets providing 5–6 grams of marshmallow per day can also be used, or it may be taken as a tincture—1–3 teaspoons (5–15 ml) three times daily.

Are there any side effects or interactions?

Marshmallow is generally safe with only rare allergic reactions reported.

MEADOWSWEET

Botanical name: *Filipendula ulmaria*

Parts used and where grown

Meadowsweet is found in northern and southern Europe, North America, and northern Asia. The flowers and flowering top are primarily used in herbal preparations, although there are some historical references to using the root.

Meadowsweet has been used in connection with the following conditions (refer to the individual health concern for complete information):

Rating	Health Concerns
★☆☆	**Common cold** (page 129)
	Influenza (page 139)
	Osteoarthritis (page 328)
	Rheumatoid arthritis (page 387)

Historical or traditional use (may or may not be supported by scientific studies)

Meadowsweet was used historically by herbalists for a wide variety of conditions, including treating rheumatic complaints of the joints and muscles.[1] Nicholas Culpeper, a 17th-century English pharmacist, mentioned its use to help break fevers and promote sweating during a **cold** (page 129) or **flu** (page 269). Traditional herbal references also indicate its use as a diuretic for people with poor urinary flow. It was also thought to have antacid properties and was used by herbalists to treat stomach complaints, including **heartburn** (page 260).

Active constituents

While the flowers are high in **flavonoids** (page 516), the primary constituents in meadowsweet are the salicylates, including salicin, salicylaldehyde, and methyl salicylate.[2] In the digestive tract, these compounds are oxidized into salicylic acid, a substance that is closely related to aspirin (acetylsalicylic acid). While not as potent as **willow** (page 760), which has a higher salicin content, the salicylates in meadowsweet may give it a mild anti-inflammatory effect and ability to reduce fevers during a **cold** (page 129) or **flu** (page 269). However, this role is only based on historical use and knowledge of the chemistry of meadowsweet's constituents, and to date, no human trials have examined the therapeutic potential of meadowsweet.

How much is usually taken?

The German Commission E monograph recommends 2.5–3.5 grams of the flower or 4–5 grams of the herb—often in a tea or infusion—per day.[3] Unfortunately, to achieve an aspirin-like effect, one would realistically need to consume about 50–60 grams of meadowsweet daily. This means that **willow** (page 760) bark extracts standardized to salicin are a far more practical as a potential herbal substitute for aspirin for minor aches and **pains** (page 338) or mild fevers. Tinctures, 2–4 ml three times per day, may alternatively be used.

Are there any side effects or interactions?

People with sensitivity to aspirin should avoid the use of meadowsweet. It should not be used to lower fevers in children as it may possibly lead to Reye's syndrome.

MILK THISTLE

Common names: Holy thistle, marythistle, St. Mary's thistle, Marian thistle
Botanical names: *Silybum marianum, Carduus marianus*

Parts used and where grown

Milk thistle is commonly found growing wild in a variety of settings, including roadsides. The dried fruit (also called achenes) are used to produce modern herbal extracts.

Milk Thistle has been used in connection with the following conditions (refer to the individual health concern for complete information):

Rating	Health Concerns
★★★	**Alcohol-related** (page 12) liver disease
★★☆	**Hepatitis** (page 220) **Liver cirrhosis** (page 290)
★☆☆	**Gallstones** (page 193)

Historical or traditional use (may or may not be supported by scientific studies)

Medical use of milk thistle can be traced back more than 2,000 years. Nicholas Culpeper, the well-known 17th-century pharmacist, cited its use for opening "obstructions" of the liver and spleen and recommended it for the treatment of jaundice.

Active constituents

The dried fruit of milk thistle contain a **flavonoid** (page 516) complex known as silymarin. This constituent is responsible for the medical benefits of the plant.[1] Silymarin is made up of three parts: silibinin, silidianin, and silicristin. Silibinin is the most active and is largely responsible for the benefits attributed to silymarin.[2]

Milk thistle extract may protect the cells of the liver by blocking the entrance of harmful toxins and helping remove these toxins from the liver cells.[3, 4] As with other bioflavonoids, silymarin is a powerful **antioxidant** (page 467).[5] Silymarin has also been shown to regenerate injured liver cells.[6] Recent studies have shown that silymarin has the ability to block fibrosis, a process that contributes to the eventual development of **cirrhosis** (page 290) in people with inflammatory liver conditions secondary to diseases such as **alcohol abuse** (page 12) or **hepatitis** (page 220).[7]

Milk thistle extract is most commonly recommended to counteract the harmful actions of alcohol on the liver. Double-blind trials indicate that it helps the liver return to a healthy state once a person stops drinking.[8, 9] Some trials suggest it may improve quality of life and even life expectancy in people with liver cirrhosis.[10, 11] However, another trial found no effect in cirrhosis patients.[12] Milk thistle alters bile makeup, thereby potentially reducing risk of **gallstones** (page 193).[13] However, this needs to be verified by human clinical trials. Milk thistle extract has been shown to protect the liver from the potentially damaging effect of drugs used to treat **schizophrenia** (page 393) and other forms of psychosis.[14] However, one trial found that it did not protect the liver from the potentially harmful effects of the drug Cognex (tacrine hydrochloride) used to treat early-stage **Alzheimer's disease** (page 19).[15]

How much is usually taken?

For liver disease and impaired liver function, research suggests the use of 420–600 mg of silymarin per day from an herbal extract of milk thistle standardized to 80% silymarin content.[16] According to research and clinical experience, improvement should be noted in about eight to twelve weeks. For people with chronic liver disease, milk thistle extract may be considered a long-term therapy.

For those who prefer, 12–15 grams of milk thistle dried fruits can be ground and eaten or made into a tea. This should not be considered therapeutic for conditions of the liver, however.

Are there any side effects or interactions?

Milk thistle extract is virtually devoid of any side effects and may be used by most people, including **pregnant** (page 363) and breast-feeding women. In fact, it has been recommended as a treatment for itching due to poor gallbladder function during pregnancy.[17] Since silymarin stimulates liver and gallbladder activity, it may have a mild, transient laxative effect in some people. This will usually cease within two to three days.

There is one case report of a 57-year-old Australian woman experiencing several episodes of nausea, abdominal pain, vomiting and weakness after taking a milk thistle preparation.[18] This case is so atypical, however, that the Adverse Drug Reactions Advisory Committee of Australia questioned whether the product taken might not have contained other herbs or additives that could be responsible for the adverse reaction.

MISTLETOE

Common name: European mistletoe
Botanical name: *Viscum album*

Parts used and where grown
Mistletoe grows as a partial parasite on a variety of trees—particularly pine, apple, plum, poplar, and spruce—across northern Europe and Asia. The young leafy twigs with flowers are used. Mistletoe's white berries are potentially toxic and should be avoided. American mistletoe, various species of *Phoradendron,* are similar but have not been widely studied. They should not be substituted for European mistletoe until more information is available.

Mistletoe has been used in connection with the following conditions (refer to the individual health concern for complete information):

Rating	Health Concerns
★☆☆	**Breast cancer** (page 65)
	Diabetes (page 152)
	High blood pressure (page 246)
	HIV support (page 239)

Historical or traditional use (may or may not be supported by scientific studies)
The ancient Druids of northern Europe and other pagan groups revered mistletoe, particularly when it

infected oak trees (a rare occurrence). Over time, this reverence of mistletoe was translated into the Christian ritual of hanging mistletoe over doorways at Christmas. The custom of kissing under the mistletoe may be a remnant of pagan orgies held before mistletoe altars.[1]

The name mistletoe is said to derive from the Celtic word for "all-heal." This correlates with its historical use for everything from nervous complaints to bleeding to tumors.[2] It is difficult to categorize all of the uses of mistletoe, particularly when one looks at the vast number of uses for this herb in traditional Chinese and Korean medicine. In the early 20th century, Rudolf Steiner created what is known as anthroposophical medicine. This mystical system used a variety of unusual remedies, including special extracts of mistletoe for injection. Steiner helped bring mistletoe into the modern era of scientific research, particularly as a potential treatment for **cancer** (page 87).[3]

Active constituents
Several constituents have been shown to contribute to the medicinal action of mistletoe. Most notable are mistletoe lectins (also called viscotoxins), choline derivatives, alkaloids, polypeptides, and polysaccharides. Human pharmacological studies have found that mistletoe extract given by injection stimulates **immune system function** (page 255).[4, 5, 6] Some test tube and animal studies suggest that certain mistletoe constituents, including the alkaloids, can also kill cancer cells.[7, 8] Numerous clinical trials have found that subcutaneous injections of mistletoe extracts can help people with cancer of various organs, though some have also failed to show any benefit.[9, 10] There is no evidence that people with cancer would benefit from receiving mistletoe orally.

Mistletoe's other uses have been less rigorously studied. Preliminary trials carried out using oral mistletoe have found it can reduce the symptoms of **high blood pressure** (page 246), particularly headaches and dizziness.[11, 12] However, mistletoe has a small (if any) effect on actually lowering blood pressure.[13]

Test tube and animal studies suggest that mistletoe extracts can stimulate insulin secretion from pancreas cells and may improve blood sugar levels in people with **diabetes** (page 152).[14, 15] Given both mistletoe's tradition around the world for helping people with diabetes and these promising preclinical results, human clinical trials are needed to establish mistletoe's potential for this condition.

Mistletoe

How much is usually taken?

Traditionally a cold water extract (cold infusion) is made by soaking 2–4 teaspoons (10–20 grams) of chopped mistletoe in two cups (500 ml) of water overnight.[16] This is taken first thing in the morning and can be sweetened with honey. Another batch is left to steep during the day and drunk at bedtime. Alternately a hot tea can be made by infusing 1 teaspoon (5 grams) of leaves in a cup (250 ml) of just-boiled water for 5–10 minutes. Two cups (500 ml) are consumed per day.[17] A tincture, approximately ⅛ teaspoon (½ ml) three times per day, can also be used.

At least three standardized, injectable extracts have been studied in Europe: Iscador, Helixor, and Eurixor. These products are not designed for self-treatment and are not commercially available in the United States. Iscador is the only fermented extract of the three, and each is standardized in a different way, making comparisons between the extracts difficult. In addition, there are different forms of each extract taken from mistletoe growing on different host trees. Typically, one weekly injection providing 1 mg of mistletoe lectin I per kilogram of body weight is given. People interested in subcutaneous or other injectable forms of mistletoe should consult with a physician.

Are there any side effects or interactions?

In the oral amounts mentioned above, mistletoe is rarely associated with side effects.[18] Two reports, however, have confirmed the danger of ingesting mistletoe leaves and berries in large quantities, particularly when children accidentally eat the berries at Christmas.[19, 20] Many of these exposures involved American mistletoe and not European mistletoe. European mistletoe is less toxic than the American species. If six to twenty berries or four to five leaves are eaten, then activated charcoal or ipecac can be used at home to induce vomiting. Emergency room care is only indicated if more than 20 berries or five leaves are ingested or if symptoms develop at lower levels of exposure. Possible symptoms of overdose are nausea, vomiting, low blood pressure, or dizziness. Injectable forms of mistletoe may cause local redness and pain but otherwise have rarely been associated with serious side effects. There is one case report of a severe allergic reaction to an injected mistletoe preparation.[21] Mistletoe is not recommended for use in children, or for women during **pregnancy** (page 363) or **breastfeeding** (page 74).

MOTHERWORT

Common name: Yi mu cao
Botanical name: *Leonurus cardiaca*

Parts used and where grown

Motherwort came from central Eurasia originally, but has spread to all temperate areas of the world, primarily as a garden plant but also as an escaped weed. A similar plant, *Leonurus heterophyllus,* is used in China. The Chinese name for motherwort is yi mu cao, meaning "benefit mother herb." The leaves and flowers of this mint family plant are used as medicine. In Chinese herbal medicine, the seeds are also employed.

Motherwort has been used in connection with the following conditions (refer to the individual health concern for complete information):

Rating	Health Concerns
★☆☆	**Amenorrhea** (page 22) (lack of menses) **Anxiety** (page 30) **Menopause** (page 311)

Historical or traditional use (may or may not be supported by scientific studies)

The use of motherwort is practically the same in European folk medicine and traditional Chinese herbal medicine. It was widely used to regulate menses and to treat associated conditions.[1] It was also considered a helpful diuretic and heart-strengthening herb by herbalists in both cultures, particularly to alleviate heart palpitations associated with **anxiety** (page 30) attacks.[2] Europeans used motherwort as a sedative as well.[3]

Active constituents

The identities of the active constituents of motherwort are not entirely clear, though they likely include compounds in its volatile oil and the alkaloids. Little research has been done on motherwort in the West. Animal research performed in China suggests that motherwort alkaloids can calm the central nervous system and stimulate the uterus to contract.[4] A report suggests that preliminary human trials have found that Chinese motherwort stimulates uterine contraction after delivery and may alleviate glomerulonephritis (kidney disease secondary to infection).[5] However, insufficient details were provided to assess the quality or results of these studies.

How much is usually taken?

A tea can be prepared by steeping approximately ¾ teaspoon (4.5 grams) of the cut herb in ½–¾ cups (150 ml) of water.[6] Three cups (750 ml) of the tea may be consumed daily. Alternatively, a tincture, ½–¾ teaspoon (2–4 ml) three times per day, can be taken.

Are there any side effects or interactions?

One source suggests that a single application of motherwort extract (concentration not reported) in excess of 3 grams may cause **diarrhea** (page 163), uterine bleeding, and stomach irritation.[7] It should be avoided in **pregnancy** (page 363) as large amounts may cause uterine contraction and potential miscarriage.[8]

MULLEIN

Botanical name: *Verbascum thapsus*

Parts used and where grown

Mullein is native to much of Europe and Asia and is naturalized to North America. There are over 360 species of *Verbascum* with *V. thapsus, V. phlomides,* and *V. densiflorum* mentioned most often in herbal texts. The leaves and flowers are both used medicinally.

Mullein has been used in connection with the following conditions (refer to the individual health concern for complete information):

Rating	Health Concerns
★☆☆	**Asthma** (page 32)
	Bronchitis (page 80)
	Chronic obstructive pulmonary disease (page 114) (COPD)
	Common cold/sore throat (page 129)
	Cough (page 139)
	Ear infections (page 383)

Historical or traditional use (may or may not be supported by scientific studies)

Mullein leaves and flowers are classified in traditional herbal literature as expectorants (promotes the discharge of mucus) and demulcents (soothes irritated

mucous membranes). Historically, mullein has been used by herbalists as a remedy for the respiratory tract, particularly in cases of irritating **coughs** (page 139) with bronchial congestion.[1] Some herbal texts extend the therapeutic use to pneumonia and **asthma** (page 32).[2] Due to its mucilage content, mullein has also been used topically by herbalists as a soothing emollient for inflammatory skin conditions and burns.

Active constituents

Mullein contains approximately 3% mucilage and small amounts of saponins and tannins.[3] The mucilaginous constituents are thought to be responsible for the soothing actions on mucous membranes. The saponins may be responsible for the expectorant actions of mullein.[4] Human clinical trials are lacking to confirm the use of mullien for any condition, however.

How much is usually taken?

A tea of mullein is made by pouring 1 cup (250 ml) of boiling water over 1–2 teaspoons (5–10 grams) of dried leaves or flowers and steeping for ten to fifteen minutes. The tea can be drunk three to four times per day. For the tincture, ¼–¾ teaspoon (1–4 ml) is taken three to four times per day. As a dried product, ½–¾ teaspoon (3–4 grams) is used three times per day.[5] Mullein is sometimes combined with other demulcent or expectorant herbs when used to treat **coughs** (page 139) and bronchial irritation. For **ear infections** (page 383), some doctors apply an oil extract directly in the ear. If the eardrum has ruptured, nothing should be put directly in the ear. Therefore, a qualified healthcare professional should always do an ear examination before mullein oil is placed in the ear.

Are there any side effects or interactions?

Mullein is generally safe except for rare reports of skin irritation. There are no known reasons to avoid its use during **pregnancy** (page 363) or breast-feeding.

MYRRH

Botanical name: *Commiphora molmol*

Parts used and where grown

Myrrh grows as a shrub in desert regions, particularly in northeastern Africa and the Middle East. The resin obtained from the stems is used in medicinal preparations.

Myrrh

Myrrh has been used in connection with the following conditions (refer to the individual health concern for complete information):

Rating	Health Concerns
★★☆	**Gingivitis** (page 203) (periodontal disease) (as mouthwash, in combination with **sage** [page 740], **peppermint** [page 726] oil, menthol, **chamomile** [page 656] tincture, expressed juice from **echinacea** [page 669], clove oil, and **caraway** [page 651] oil) **Parasites** (page 343) (schistosomiasis)
★☆☆	**Canker sores** (page 90) **Cold sores** (page 119) **Common cold/sore throat** (page 129) **Halitosis** (page 209) (rinse) **Infection** (page 265) **Pap smear (abnormal)** (page 3) **Ulcerative colitis** (page 433)

Historical or traditional use (may or may not be supported by scientific studies)

In ancient times, the red-brown resin of myrrh was used to preserve mummies. It was also used as a remedy for numerous infections, including leprosy and syphilis. Myrrh was also recommended by herbalists for relief from **bad breath** (page 209) and for dental conditions.[1] In Traditional Chinese Medicine, it has been used to treat bleeding disorders and **wounds** (page 319).

Active constituents

The three main constituents of myrrh are the resin, the gum, and the volatile oil. All are thought to be important in myrrh's activity as an herbal medicine. The resin has reportedly been shown to kill various microbes and to stimulate macrophages (a type of white blood cell) in test tube studies.[2] Myrrh also has astringent properties and has a soothing effect on inflamed tissues in the mouth and throat. Studies continue on the potential anticancer and pain-relieving actions of myrrh resin.[3, 4] Human clinical trials are lacking to confirm most uses of myrrh.

In a preliminary trial, patients with schistosomiasis (a parasitic infection) were treated with a combination of resin and volatile oil of myrrh, in the amount of 10 mg per 2.2 pounds of body weight per day for three days. The cure rate was 91.7% and, of those who did not respond, 76.5% were cured by a second six-day course of treatment, increasing the overall cure rate to 98.1%.[5]

How much is usually taken?

The German Commission E monograph recommends that persons either dab the undiluted tincture in the mouth or gargle with 5–10 drops of tincture in a glass of water three times daily.[6] In addition, tincture of myrrh, 1–2 ml three times per day, can be taken. The tincture can also be applied topically for **canker sores** (page 90). Due to the gummy nature of the product, a tea cannot be made from myrrh. Capsules, containing up to 1 gram of resin taken three times per day, can be used as well.

Are there any side effects or interactions?

No adverse effects from myrrh usage have been reported.

NETTLE

Botanical name: *Urtica dioica*

Parts used and where grown

Nettle is a leafy plant that is found in most temperate regions of the world. The Latin root of *Urtica* is *uro,* meaning "I burn," indicative of the small stings caused by the little hairs on the leaves of this plant that burn when contact is made with the skin. The root and leaves of nettle are used in herbal medicine.

Nettle has been used in connection with the following conditions (refer to the individual health concern for complete information):

Rating	Health Concerns
★★☆	**Benign prostatic hyperplasia** (page 58) (root extract) **Osteoarthritis** (page 328)
★☆☆	**Hay fever** (page 211) **Pregnancy and postpartum support** (page 363) **Rheumatoid arthritis** (page 387) **Urinary tract infection** (page 436)

Historical or traditional use (may or may not be supported by scientific studies)

Nettle has a long history of use. The tough fibers from the stem have been used to make cloth and cooked nettle leaves were eaten as vegetables. From ancient Greece to the present, nettle has been documented for its tradi-

Myrrh

tional use in treating **coughs** (page 139), tuberculosis, and arthritis and in stimulating hair growth.

Active constituents

There has been a great deal of controversy regarding the identity of nettle's active constituents. Currently, it is thought that polysaccharides (complex sugars) and lectins are probably the active constituents. Test tube studies suggest the leaf has anti-inflammatory actions. This is thought to be caused by nettle preventing the body from making inflammatory chemicals known as prostaglandins.[1] Nettle's root affects hormones and proteins that carry sex hormones (such as testosterone or estrogen) in the human body. This may explain why it helps **benign prostatic hyperplasia** (page 58) (BPH).[2] Although less frequently used alone like **saw palmetto** (page 743) or **pygeum** (page 734), some limited clinical trials suggest benefit of nettle root extract for men with milder forms of BPH.[3]

A preliminary trial reported that capsules made from freeze-dried leaves reduced sneezing and itching in people with **hay fever** (page 211).[4] Further studies are needed to confirm this finding, however.

The historical practice of intentionally applying nettle topically with the intent of causing stings to relieve arthritis has been assessed by a questionnaire in modern times.[5] The results found intentional nettle stings safe, except for a sometimes painful, sometimes numb rash that lasts 6–24 hours. Additional trials are required to determine if this practice is therapeutically effective.

How much is usually taken?

During the **allergy** (page 14) season, two to three 300 mg nettle leaf capsules or tablets or 2–4 ml tincture can be taken three times per day. For **BPH** (page 58), 120 mg of a concentrated root extract in capsules can be taken two times per day.[6] Many products for BPH will combine nettle root with **saw palmetto** (page 743) or **pygeum** (page 734) extracts. Intentional stinging with nettles should only be undertaken after consultation with a physician knowledgeable in botanical medicine.

Are there any side effects or interactions?

Nettle may cause mild gastrointestinal upset in some people. Although allergic reactions to nettle are rare, when contact is made with the skin, fresh nettle can cause a rash secondary to the noted stings.[7] Nettle leaf is considered safe for use in **pregnancy** (page 363) and breast-feeding.

NONI

Common name: Indian mulberry
Botanical name: *Morinda citrifolia*

Parts used and where grown

Native to Polynesia, the noni plant (also known as Indian mulberry) is a small tree that usually grows to a height of ten feet. The fruit, which starts out green and turns yellow, is used medicinally.

Noni has been used in connection with the following conditions (refer to the individual health concern for complete information):

Rating	Health Concerns
★☆☆	**Immune enhancement** (page 255)

Historical or traditional use (may or may not be supported by scientific studies)

Traditional Polynesian healers have used the fruit of the noni plant for just about everything—from a tonic drink to mending broken bones—but it is said that because of its strong, unpleasant odor and bitter taste, a person won't take it until they are too sick and desperate. The bark yields a red dye while the root yields a yellow one. Both colors were used in the ceremonial outfits of Hawaiian chiefs. In the early 1990s, noni juice became heavily marketed in the United States primarily through network marketing companies. However, despite tremendous claims and testimonials, there is little scientific documentation on noni.

Active constituents

The major constituents in noni appear to be polysaccharides and a compound known as damnacanthal.[1, 2, 3] The developer of a commercial noni product claims the alkaloid xeronine is an important constituent, but there has been no confirmation by independent researchers. Animal and test tubes studies show noni to have **immune-enhancing** (page 255) activity, and an earlier animal study seemed to indicate the fruit exerts a mild sedative effect.[4, 5, 6] Specifically, the polysaccharide component has been shown to increase the release of immune-enhancing compounds that activate white blood cells. Also, damnacanthal is thought to be responsible for producing sedative effects in animal studies.

Noni

How much is usually taken?

The usual recommendation is 4 ounces (120 ml) of noni juice 30 minutes before breakfast (effectiveness is thought to be best on an empty stomach). Commercial products are now available that have either eliminated the odor, altered the taste, or made it available as an extract in tablets or capsules to increase palatability. For liquid concentrates the typical recommendation is 2 tablespoons (30 ml) per day. For powdered extracts the typical recommendation is 500 to 1,000 mg daily.

Are there any side effects or interactions?

There have been no commonly reported side effects following the ingestion of noni. Since the use of noni during **pregnancy** (page 363) and breast-feeding has not been adequately studied, it is recommended that it not be used during these times.

OAK

Botanical name: *Quercus* spp.

Parts used and where grown

Oak trees grow throughout North America. Some species of oak grow around the world, including in China and the Middle East. The bark of the oak tree is used medicinally.

Oak has been used in connection with the following conditions (refer to the individual health concern for complete information):

Rating	Health Concerns
★☆☆	**Canker sores** (page 90)
	Crohn's disease (page 141)
	Diarrhea (page 163)
	Eczema (page 177)
	Menorrhagia (page 314)

Historical or traditional use (may or may not be supported by scientific studies)

Oak bark was used traditionally by herbalists to treat **hemorrhoids** (page 219), **varicose veins** (page 440), **diarrhea** (page 163), and **cancer** (page 87). Tannic acid derived from oak trees has a long history of application in tanning hides and making ink.[1]

Active constituents

Tannins are the primary constituents of oak bark.[2] These tannins are potent astringents, akin to those found in **witch hazel** (page 760) *(Hamamelis virginiana)*. Tannins bind liquids, absorb toxins, and soothe inflamed tissues. The oak tannin, known as ellagitannin, inhibits intestinal secretion,[3] which helps resolve **diarrhea** (page 163). The nonirritating, astringent nature of oak has led to its recommendation for treating mild, acute diarrhea in children (along with plenty of electrolyte-containing fluids) in Europe.[4] Astringents such as oak may also help relieve the pain of **sore throats** (page 129) and **canker sores** (page 90).

How much is usually taken?

The German Commission E monograph suggests ¾ teaspoon (3 grams) of the bark per day.[5] For **eczema** (page 177), oak is applied topically by first boiling 1–2 tablespoons (15–30 grams) of the bark for fifteen minutes in 2 cups (500 ml) of water. After cooling, a cloth is dipped into the liquid and applied directly to the rash several times per day. The liquid prepared this way in the morning can be used throughout the day. Unused portions should then be discarded. Up to 5 cups (1250 ml) of this same solution can be taken each day in cases of **diarrhea** (page 163). Alternatively, a tincture of oak, approximately ½ teaspoon (2–3 ml) three times daily, can be used.

Are there any side effects or interactions?

Except for the occasional upset stomach or **constipation** (page 137) reported after drinking the tea, oak bark is rarely associated with side effects. There are no known reasons to avoid oak during **pregnancy** (page 363) or breast-feeding, though oak can cause constipation. It is safe for use in children and infants. The German Commission E monograph warns against people with open sores, **wounds** (page 319), high fever, or **infection** (page 265) bathing in water with oak bark.[6]

OATS

Common name: Wild oats
Botanical name: *Avena sativa*

Parts used and where grown

The common oat used in herbal supplements and foods is derived from cultivated sources. For some herbal supplements, the green or rapidly dried aerial parts of the

Noni

plant are harvested just before reaching full flower. Many herbal texts refer to using the fruits (seeds) or green tops. Although some herb texts discuss oat straw, there is little medicinal action in this part of the plant.

Oats have been used in connection with the following conditions (refer to the individual health concern for complete information):

Rating	Health Concerns
★★★	**High triglycerides** (page 235)
★☆☆	**Anxiety** (page 30) **Eczema** (page 177) Nicotine withdrawal

Historical or traditional use (may or may not be supported by scientific studies)

In folk medicine, oats are used by herbalists to treat nervous exhaustion, **insomnia** (page 270), and "weakness of the nerves." A tea made from oats was thought by herbalists to be useful in rheumatic conditions and to treat **water retention** (page 180). A tincture of the green tops of oats was also used to help with withdrawal from tobacco addiction.[1] Oats were often used in baths to treat insomnia and **anxiety** (page 30) as well as a variety of skin conditions, including **burns** (page 85) and **eczema** (page 177).

Active constituents

The fruits (seeds) contain alkaloids, such as gramine and avenine, and saponins, such as avenacosides A and B.[2] The seeds are also rich in **iron** (page 540), **manganese** (page 553), and **zinc** (page 614). The straw is high in silica. Oat alkaloids are believed to account for the relaxing action of oats, but it should be noted this continues to be debated in Europe. The German Commission E does not approve this herb as a sedative.[3] However, an alcohol-based tincture of the fresh plant has reportedly shown some promise in countering nicotine withdrawal and helping with smoking cessation.[4]

How much is usually taken?

A tea can be made from a heaping tablespoonful (approximately 15 grams) of oats brewed with 1 cup (250 ml) of boiling water. After cooling and straining, the tea can be taken several times a day and shortly before going to bed.[5] As a tincture, oats are often taken at ½–1 teaspoon (3–5 ml) three times per day. Capsules or tablets, 1–4 grams per day, can be taken. A soothing

bath to ease irritated skin can be made by running the bath water through a sock containing several tablespoons of oats, then bathing in the water for several minutes.

Are there any side effects or interactions?

Oats are not associated with any adverse effects.

OLIVE LEAF

Botanical name: *Olea europa*

Parts used and where grown

Olive is a small evergreen tree native to Mediterranean regions. The characteristic green to blue-black fruit of this tree yields a useful, edible oil. Both the oil and the dried green-grayish colored leaves are used medicinally.[1, 2]

Olive leaf has been used in connection with the following conditions (refer to the individual health concern for complete information):

Rating	Health Concerns
★☆☆	**Diabetes** (page 152) **High blood pressure** (page 246) **Infection** (page 265)

Historical or traditional use (may or may not be supported by scientific studies)

The olive tree has been held in high esteem throughout history. Moses reportedly decreed that men who cultivated the leaf be exempt from serving in the army. The oil is symbolic of purity and goodness, while the olive branch represents peace and prosperity. Winners in the Greek Olympic games were crowned with a wreath of olive leaves.[3] Historically, medicinal use of olive leaf has been for treatment of fevers and for the topical treatment of **wounds** (page 319) or **infection** (page 265). As a poultice, it was also used by herbalists to treat skin rashes and boils.[4]

Active constituents

Olive leaf has a wide number of constituents, including oleuropein and several types of **flavonoids** (page 516) (e.g., rutin, apigenin, luteolin).[5] While olive leaf is traditionally associated with a wide number of medicinal claims, few of these have been verified by experimental study. In an animal study oleuropein (when given by injection or in intravenous form) was found to decrease blood pressure (e.g., systolic and diastolic) and dilate the coronary arteries surrounding the heart.[6] This ability to lower blood pressure may justify the traditional use of olive leaf in the treatment of mild to moderate **hypertension** (page 246).[7] However, human studies are needed to clearly establish olive leaf as a potential treatment for high blood pressure.

In addition, a test tube study has revealed that oleuropein inhibits the oxidation of LDL ("bad") cholesterol. LDL oxidation is one part in a series of damaging events that, if left unchecked, can lead to the development of atherosclerosis.[8] This action may provide one clue as to why those consuming a Mediterranean-based diet may lower their risk of developing **atherosclerosis** (page 38).

Oleuropein from olives may also have antibacterial properties. When unheated olives are brined to preserve them, oleuropein is converted into another chemical called elenolic acid. Elenolic acid has shown antibacterial actions against several species of *Lactobacilli* and *Staphylococcus aureus* and *Bacillus subtilus* in a test tube study.[9] Whether or not the oleuropein in the leaf undergoes such a transformation is open to question at this point, raising some question as to its antibacterial effects and potential use for this purpose in humans.

Olive leaf extracts have been employed experimentally to lower elevated blood-sugar levels in animals with diabetes.[10] These results have not been reproduced in human clinical trials and as such, no clear conclusions can be made from this animal study in the treatment of **diabetes** (page 152).

How much is usually taken?
The effective amount of olive leaf for human use is not established. To make a tea, steep 1 teaspoon (5 grams) of dried leaves in 1 cup (250 ml) of hot water for 10–15 minutes.[11] Dried leaf extracts containing 6–15% oleuropein are available commercially, but no standard amount has been established.

Are there any side effects or interactions?
The safety of olive leaf has not been established in **pregnancy** (page 363). Olive leaf can be irritating to the stomach lining and should be taken with meals.[12]

ONION

Botanical name: *Allium cepa*

Parts used and where grown
Like its close cousins **garlic** (page 679), chives, scallions, and leeks, onion is a member of the lily family (Liliaceae). It is native to Eurasia but now grows all over the world, due mostly to people bringing it with them as a staple food wherever they migrated. The French explorer Pere Marquette was saved from starvation in 1624 by eating wild onions near the present site of Chicago—the name of the city is derived from a Native American word for the odor of onions.[1] The bulb of the plant is used medicinally.

Onion has been used in connection with the following conditions (refer to the individual health concern for complete information):

Rating	Health Concerns
★★☆	**Atherosclerosis** (page 38) **Cancer prevention** (page 87) **Diabetes** (page 152) Hyperlipidemia
★☆☆	**Asthma** (page 32) **Cough** (page 139) **Eczema** (page 177) **Hypertension** (page 246) **Infection** (page 265)

Historical or traditional use (may or may not be supported by scientific studies)
Onion has been used as food for many centuries.[2] Onion was also a popular folk remedy, being applied to tumors, made into a syrup for relieving **coughs** (page 139), or prepared in a tincture (using gin) to relieve "dropsy" (heart failure–related edema).[3] It was considered a weaker version of **garlic** (page 679) by many herbal practitioners. Like garlic, onion has a longstanding but unsubstantiated reputation as an aphrodisiac.[4]

Active constituents
Two sets of compounds make up the majority of onion's known active constituents—sulfur compounds, such as allyl propyl disulphide (APDS), and **flavonoids** (page 516), such as **quercetin** (page 580). Each of these groups of compounds has multiple medicinal actions.

The sulfur compounds form a strongly scented oil,

particularly the compound known as thioproanal-s-oxide or lacrimatory factor. It is responsible for the tearing many people suffer while cutting onions.[5] Onion and onion oil constituents have been repeatedly shown to kill various microbes in the test tube.[6, 7] Studies have not been conducted in humans to determine whether onion is a useful antimicrobial agent.

APDS has been shown to block the breakdown of insulin by the liver and possibly to stimulate insulin production by the pancreas, thus increasing the amount of insulin and reducing sugar levels in the blood.[8] Several uncontrolled human studies[9, 10] and at least one double-blind clinical trial[11] have shown that large amounts of onion can lower blood sugar levels in people with **diabetes** (page 152). Onion does not reduce blood sugar levels in healthy nondiabetic people.[12]

Sulfur compounds in onion oil have also been shown to be anti-inflammatory, both by inhibiting formation of thromboxanes and by inhibiting the action of platelet-activating factor (PAF).[13, 14] Not all studies have confirmed that these actions occur in humans.[15] The anti-inflammatory effect is strong enough that subcutaneous onion injections and topical onion applications inhibit skin reactions to intensely inflammatory compounds in people with or without **eczema** (page 177), according to the results of one double-blind study.[16] Human studies have not been performed to determine whether onion would be useful in people with **asthma** (page 32) or **cough** (page 139), though the anti-inflammatory action cited above suggests it might be. These actions, coupled with an ability to reduce the stickiness of platelets[17] and, overall, to decrease the thickness of the blood,[18] have led to interest in onion as a way to prevent or possibly reduce **atherosclerosis** (page 38).

Human studies have proven mixed as to whether onion is helpful for people with atherosclerosis.[19] Intake of quercetin in the diet, primarily from onion, tea, and apples, has been linked to a decreased risk of having a heart attack.[20] High intake of quercetin and other flavonoids from onion and other foods has been shown to decrease risk of atherosclerosis in an epidemiologic study in the United States, although the result was not considered statistically significant.[21] One open clinical trial showed that a crude onion extract could lower blood pressure in some people with **hypertension** (page 246).[22] On the whole, it is unclear whether or not onion supplements, as opposed to onions eaten as food, have a beneficial effect on heart disease.

In a preliminary study of healthy male volunteers, administration of 50 grams of raw or boiled onion prevented the rise in serum cholesterol induced by consumption of a high-fat meal.[23]

The evidence on **cancer prevention** (page 87) with onion suggests a benefit for some but not necessarily for all types of cancer. Onion consumption at a level of at least half an onion a day was associated with a 50% decline in stomach cancer risk in one study.[24] Higher onion intake was also correlated with lower risk of breast cancer in a French epidemiological study.[25] No protective effect against colorectal cancer was seen from higher onion intake.[26]

How much is usually taken?

Most human studies that have shown an effect from onions used at least 25 grams per day and often two to four times that amount.[27, 28] Though some studies have found cooked onions acceptable, several studies suggest that onion constituents are degraded by cooking and that fresh or raw onions are probably most active.[29, 30, 31, 32] If a tincture, syrup, or oil extract is used, 1 tablespoon three times per day may be necessary for several months before effects are noted.[33]

Are there any side effects or interactions?

Most people can eat onion in food without any difficulties. Higher intakes of onion may worsen existing **heartburn** (page 260), though it does not seem to cause heartburn in people who do not already have it.[34] There are also isolated reports of **allergy** (page 14) to onion, including among people with **asthma** (page 32),[35] manifesting as skin rash and red, itchy eyes.

Onion is safe for use in children and, in small amounts in food, during pregnancy (though some pregnant women may have heartburn that onions could exacerbate) and nursing. It is unknown whether larger amounts of onion are safe during pregnancy and nursing. One study did find that baby rats nursing from mothers that were fed onion developed a taste for onion and suffered no ill effects.[36]

OREGANO/WILD MARJORAM

Botanical name: *Origanum vulgare*

Parts used and where grown

Oregano is an aromatic perennial herb that can grow to about two feet in height. It is native to the Mediterean region but is cultivated worldwide. In addition to European oregano, there are several types of related species, including Greek/Turkish oregano *(Origanum onites)* and Mexican oregano *(Lippia graveolens, Lippa palmeri)*. These should not be considered substitutes for true oregano, though they may have similar properties. The leaves as well as the volatile oil of these various species are used medicinally, but must be carefully distinguished as they are quite different.[1]

Oregano has been used in connection with the following conditions (refer to the individual health concern for complete information):

Rating	Health Concerns
★☆☆	**Athlete's foot** (page 42) (oil topically)
	Chronic candidiasis (page 109) (oil internally)
	Indigestion (page 260) (leaf tea)
	Infection (page 265) (oil internally)
	Ringworm (tinea) (oil internally)
	Yeast infection (page 454)

Historical or traditional use (may or may not be supported by scientific studies)

The name *Origanum* is the contraction of two Greek words, *oros* meaning mountain and *ganos* meaning joy. Together the words suggest the beauty that oregano lends to the fields and hilltops on which it grows.[2] Oregano was used extensively by the Greeks for conditions ranging from convulsions to heart failure. Nineteenth-century American Eclectic physicians (doctors who recommended herbal medicines) employed oregano as both a general tonic and to promote menstruation.[3]

Active constituents

This dried herb contains several constituents, including volatile oil (up to 3%), such as carvacrol, thymol, and borneol, plus **flavonoids** (page 516), rosmarinic acid, triterpenoids (e.g., ursolic and oleanolic acid), sterols, and **vitamin A** (page 595) and **vitamin C** (page 604).[4] The thymol and carvacrol contents in oregano are responsible for its antimicrobial and antifungal effects.[5] A test tube study demonstrated that oil of oregano, and carvacrol in particular, inhibited the growth of *Candida albicans* far more effectively than a commonly employed antifungal agent called calcium magnesium caprylate.[6] Clinical studies are still needed to confirm these actions in humans.

In addition to its anti-fungal action, and according to the results of another test tube study from Australia, oregano oil has a strong anti-microbial action against a wide number of bacteria, including *Escherichia coli, Klebsiella pneumoniae, Salmonella enterica,* and *Staphylococcus aureus*.[7] Other test tube studies have shown that oregano from the Mexican *(Lippia)* species was more effective than the prescription medication tinidazol in inhibiting the parasite giardia *(Giardia duodenalis)*.[8] In another test tube study, volatile oils of oregano, **thyme** (page 52), **cinnamon** (page 659), and cumin were individually able to stop the growth of another food-borne pathogen called *Aspergillus parasiticus*. Higher concentrations of these volatile oils were also able to stop the production of aflatoxin, a potent poison from the food mold *Aspergillus*.[9] Together these facts suggest the volatile oils in oregano used during food processing have an important role in preventing the spoilage of food and in reducing the risk of ingesting harmful bacteria, fungi, and **parasites** (page 343). Again, these actions have not yet been confirmed by human clinical trials.

The German Commission E does not approve oregano for any medical indication.[10]

How much is usually taken?

Dried or fresh leaf of oregano can be made into a tea by steeping 1 to 2 teaspoons (5 to 10 grams) in hot water for ten minutes. This tea can be consumed three times a day.[11] The oil (50% or greater dilution) may be applied topically twice a day to areas affected by athlete's foot or other fungal infections. The affected area should be covered by the oil with each application. The safety of the internal use of the oil has not been well studied and should be used with caution or after consulting with a healthcare professional.

Are there any side effects or interactions?

Oregano leaf is very safe. The German Commission E and American Herbal Products Association both state there are no known risks with oregano leaf;[12] neither of these references mentions oregano oil.

Due to the lack of human research and the highly concentrated nature of oregano volatile oil, there is potential for harm from its use; therefore, until its internal use in humans has been proven safe, it should taken with caution if not recommended by a healthcare professional.[13] Volatile oils are generally considered contraindicated in **pregnancy** (page 363) as they likely reach the baby and may cause harm.[14] Topically, the volatile oil of oregano may be moderately irritating to skin and can be a potent mucous membrane irritant. It should not be applied topically to mucous membranes in greater than a 1% concentration.[15] Children less than two years of age and people with damaged or very sensitive skin should not use the oil topically.[16]

OREGON GRAPE

Botanical name: *Berberis aquifolium*

Parts used and where grown
Oregon grape is an evergreen shrub which grows throughout the American northwest. It is somewhat misnamed, as the fruit are not actually grapes. It is, however, grown in Oregon (it is the official state flower). Oregon grape is a close relative of **barberry** (page 632) *(Berberis vulgaris),* and shares many common uses and constituents. The root is used medicinally.

Oregon grape has been used in connection with the following conditions (refer to the individual health concern for complete information):

Rating	Health Concerns
★☆☆	**Chronic candidiasis** (page 109)
	Conjunctivitis/blepharitis (page 136)
	Diarrhea (page 163)
	Infection (page 265)
	Parasites (page 343)
	Poor digestion (page 260)
	Psoriasis (page 379)
	Urinary tract infections (page 436)

Historical or traditional use (may or may not be supported by scientific studies)
Before European colonists arrived, the indigenous peoples of North America treated all manner of complaints with Oregon grape.[1] The berries were used for poor appetite. A tea made from the root was used to treat jaundice, arthritis, **diarrhea** (page 163), fever, and many other health problems.

Active constituents
Alkaloids, including berberine, berbamine, canadine, and hydrastine, may account for the activity of Oregon grape. Isolated berberine has been shown to effectively treat **diarrhea** (page 163) in patients infected with *E. coli.*[2] One of the ways berberine may ease diarrhea is by slowing the transit time in the intestine.[3] Berberine inhibits the ability of bacteria to attach to human cells, which helps prevent **infections** (page 265), particularly in the throat, intestines, and **urinary tract** (page 436).[4] These actions, coupled with berberine's ability to enhance **immune cell function** (page 255),[5] make Oregon grape possibly useful for mild infections although clinical trials are lacking on the whole root.

In one clinical trial, an ointment of Oregon grape was found to be mildly effective for reducing skin irritation, inflammation and itching in people with mild to moderate **psoriasis** (page 379).[6] Whole Oregon grape extracts were shown in one pharmacological study to reduce inflammation (often associated with psoriasis) and stimulate the white blood cells known as macrophages.[7] In this study, isolated alkaloids from Oregon grape did not have these actions. This suggests that something besides alkaloids are important to the properties of Oregon grape responsible for reducing inflammation.

The bitter-tasting compounds as well as the alkaloids in Oregon grape root are thought to stimulate **digestive function** (page 260).

How much is usually taken?
A tea can be prepared by boiling 1–3 teaspoons (5–15 grams) of chopped roots in 2 cups (500 ml) of water for fifteen minutes. After straining and cooling, 3 cups (750 ml) can be taken per day. Tincture, ½–¾ teaspoon (3 ml) three times per day, can be used. Since berberine is not well absorbed, Oregon grape root might not provide adequate amounts of this compound to treat significant systemic **infections** (page 265). A physician should be consulted in the case of infection before attempting to use Oregon grape. An ointment made with 10% Oregon grape extract applied three or more times daily may be useful for **psoriasis** (page 379).

Are there any side effects or interactions?
Oregon grape is thought to be safe in the amounts indicated above. Long-term (more than two to three weeks) internal use is not recommended. Berberine alone has been reported to interfere with normal bilirubin metabolism in infants, raising a concern that it might worsen jaundice.[8] For this reason, berberine-containing plants should be used with caution during **pregnancy** (page 363) and breast-feeding.

Oregon Grape

Passion Flower

PASSION FLOWER

Botanical name: *Passiflora incarnata*

Parts used and where grown

Passion flower is a climbing vine renowned for its beautiful white flowers with purple, blue, or pink calyx crown blooms. The plant is native to North, Central, and South America. While primarily tropical, some of its 400 species can grow in colder climates. The mystery of such a beautiful blossom emerging from an unassuming bud has been compared to the Passion of Christ. This inspired the plant's name, which dates back to the 17th century. The leaves, stems, and flowers are used for medicinal purposes.

Passion flower has been used in connection with the following conditions (refer to the individual health concern for complete information):

Rating	Health Concerns
★★☆	**Anxiety** (page 30)
★☆☆	**Insomnia** (page 270) **Pain** (page 338)

Historical or traditional use (may or may not be supported by scientific studies)

The historical use of passion flower is not dissimilar to its current use as a mild sedative. Medicinal use of the herb did not begin until the late 19th century in the United States. Passion flower was used to treat nervous restlessness and gastrointestinal spasms. In short, the effects of passion flower were believed to be primarily on the nervous system, particularly for **anxiety** (page 30) due to mental worry and overwork.[1]

The effectiveness of passion flower as a treatment for anxiety has been confirmed in a double-blind study. In that study, 45 drops per day of an extract of passion flower taken for four weeks was as effective as 30 mg per day of oxazepam (Serax), a medication used for anxiety.[2]

Active constituents

For many years, plant researchers believed that a group of harman alkaloids were the active constituents in passion flower. Recent studies, however, have pointed to the **flavonoids** (page 516) in passion flower as the primary constituents responsible for its relaxing and anti-anxiety effects.[3] European herbal pharmacopoeias typically recommend passion flower products containing no less than 0.8% total flavonoids. The European literature involving passion flower recommends it primarily for the treatment of mild to moderate **anxiety** (page 30). In this context, it is often combined with **valerian** (page 756), **lemon balm** (page 701), and other herbs with sedative properties.

How much is usually taken?

The recommended intake of the dried herb is 4–8 grams per day.[4] To make a tea, 0.5 to 2.5 grams of the herb can be steeped with boiling water for ten to fifteen minutes and drunk two to three times per day. Alternatively, 5–10 ml of passion flower tincture can be taken three to four times per day.

Are there any side effects or interactions?

Used in the amounts listed above, passion flower is generally safe and has not been found to adversely interact with other sedative drugs. Some practitioners suggest not using passion flower with MAO-inhibiting antidepressant drugs because of concerns that they may interact with the harman alkaloids in passion flower.[5] However, this interaction is theoretical and has not been reported in the medical literature. A single case has been reported of a 34-year-old female who developed severe nausea, vomiting, drowsiness, and heart symptoms following self-administration of passion flower. It is not known for certain if passion flower caused her symptoms.[6] Passion flower has not been proven to be safe during **pregnancy** (page 363) and **breast-feeding** (page 74).

PAU D'ARCO

Common names: Lapacho, taheebo
Botanical names: *Tabebuia avellanedae, Tabebuia impestiginosa*

Parts used and where grown

Various related species of pau d'arco trees grow in rain forests throughout Latin America. The bark is used for medical purposes.

Pau d'arco has been used in connection with the following conditions (refer to the individual health concern for complete information):

Rating	Health Concerns
★☆☆	Infection (page 265) Prostatitis (page 377)

Historical or traditional use (may or may not be supported by scientific studies)

Native peoples in Central and South America reportedly use pau d'arco bark to treat **cancer** (page 87), **lupus** (page 421), infectious diseases, **wounds** (page 319), and many other health conditions.[1] Caribbean folk healers use the leaf of this tree in addition to the bark for the treatment of backache, toothache, sexually transmitted diseases, and as an aphrodisiac.

Active constituents

Lapachol and beta-lapachone (known collectively as naphthaquinones) are two primary active compounds in pau d'arco. According to laboratory tests, both have anti-fungal properties as potent as ketoconazole, a common antifungal drug.[2] However, amounts of these constituents needed to exert an antifungal effect may be toxic to humans. Although these compounds also have anticancer properties according to test tube studies, the effective amount for this effect may also be toxic.[3, 4] Therefore, pau d'arco cannot currently be recommended as a treatment for cancer.

How much is usually taken?

A traditional recommendation is 2–3 teaspoons (10–15 grams) of the inner bark simmered in a pint (500 ml) of water for fifteen minutes three times per day.[5] However, the naphthaquinones believed to give pau d'arco its major effects are very poorly extracted in water, so teas are not usually recommended in modern herbal medicine.[6] Capsules or tablets providing 500–600 mg of powdered bark can be taken three times per day. A tincture, ⅛–¼ teaspoon (0.5–1 ml) three times per day, can also be used.

Are there any side effects or interactions?

High amounts (several grams daily over several days) of lapachol can cause uncontrolled bleeding, nausea, and vomiting.[7] Use of the whole bark is typically safer than isolated lapachol—side effects have included nausea and gastrointestinal upset.[8] **Pregnant** (page 363) or breast-feeding women should avoid use of pau d'arco.

One case report exists of a 28-year-old man who died of liver failure after taking unspecified amounts of pau d'arco, scullcap, and zinc.[9] It appears likely that this may have been a case of adulteration of scullcap with germander.[10]

PENNYROYAL

Common names: European pennyroyal, American pennyroyal, fleabane

Botanical names: *Hedeoma pulegoides, Mentha pulegium*

Parts used and where grown

Two similar plants go by the name pennyroyal, one native to Europe (and therefore called European pennyroyal) and one native to North America (and therefore called American pennyroyal). Both are members of the mint family *(Lamiaceae)* and grow in temperate regions of Europe and the Americas. The flowering tops are used as medicine, but the internal use of the volatile oil should be strictly avoided.

Pennyroyal has been used in connection with the following conditions (refer to the individual health concern for complete information):

Rating	Health Concerns
★☆☆	Anxiety (page 30) Cough (page 139) Insect repellant

Historical or traditional use (may or may not be supported by scientific studies)

Since the time of the ancient Greeks, pennyroyal was considered a useful insect repellant, reflected in modern times by the common name fleabane.[1] The Latin names of both plants also reflect this insect-repelling power—*pulegoides* and *pulegium* both derive from the Latin word for flea. It was also believed to stimulate menstruation. Various folk herb traditions have employed American or European pennyroyal to help relieve **coughs** (page 139), **upset stomachs** (page 260), and **anxiety** (page 30).[2]

Pennyroyal

Active constituents

Like all mint family plants, pennyroyal owes much of its medicinal activity to the presence of a volatile oil. The primary component of this oil is known as pulegone. Pulegone is converted to menthofuran by the body. If large enough amounts of pulegone are consumed, the amount of menthofuran produced can seriously damage the liver and nervous system.[3] Smaller amounts of the volatile oil contained in the whole plant appear to have mild, smooth, muscle-relaxing effects that might help explain the historical use of pennyroyal for **indigestion** (page 260), stomach cramps, and **cough** (page 139).[4] No modern clinical trials have been completed to support these indications, and other herbs with soothing effects on the gastrointestinal tract, such as **chamomile** (page 656) and **peppermint** (page 726), have a much greater history of safety than pennyroyal.

How much is usually taken?

For adults (excluding **pregnant** [page 363] or nursing women, children, and people with liver or kidney disease), a tea of pennyroyal can be prepared by putting 1–2 teaspoons (5–10 grams) of the herb in 1 cup (250 ml) of boiling water and allowing it to steep for 10–15 minutes.[5] Up to 2 cups (500 ml) per day can be drunk. Pennyroyal tincture can be mixed with a skin cream and applied topically to repel insects, though it is unknown whether this is effective due to a lack of scientific study. The tincture and volatile oil are not recommended for internal use.

Are there any side effects or interactions?

Used internally in the amounts stated above, pennyroyal is generally safe, though an occasional person may experience intestinal upset or temporary dizziness.[6] Pulegone and its toxic metabolites, particularly menthofuran, damage the liver and nerves if taken in sufficiently large quantities.[7] If used during **pregnancy** (page 363), pennyroyal may cause fetal death by liver and brain damage as well as promote uterine contractions to expel the fetus.[8] Therefore pregnant or nursing women should absolutely avoid pennyroyal in any form. The traditional use of the herb to induce an abortion has led to many reports of nervous system toxicity in pregnant women. Internal ingestion of pennyroyal volatile oil should be avoided by everyone. People with liver failure or kidney failure, and all children, should avoid pennyroyal. Signs and symptoms of pennyroyal toxicity include severe stomach pain, dizziness, seizures, vomiting, difficulty walking, and coma. Since 1905, 18 cases of injury (with complete recovery in every case) and four deaths related to pennyroyal have been reported in the medical literature.[9] The majority of acute poisonings and deaths reported with pennyroyal have been in cases of women using the oil attempting to induce an abortion.

PEONY

Common names: Moutan (mu dan), red peony (chi shao), white peony (bai shao)

Botanical names: *Paeonia suffruticosa, Paeonia lactiflora, Paeonia veitchii*

Parts used and where grown

Three similar plants are all called peony, and different parts are used in some cases. The bark of the root of *Paeonia suffruticosa* is called moutan or mu dan in China, where it naturally grows. Red peony root comes from wild harvested *Paeonia lactiflora* or *Paeonia veitchii*. White peony root comes from cultivated *Paeonia lactiflora*. The bark, red peony root, and white peony root all have somewhat different properties. Dried versus charred roots also have different properties. The color indicated does not refer to flower color. An important formula used in Chinese and Japanese herbal medicine called shakuyaku-kanzo-to contains white peony root and **licorice** (page 702) root. The roots and flowers of *Paeonia officinalis* have been used in European herbal medicine. However, the German Commission E did not approve this plant for medicinal use.[1]

Peony has been used in connection with the following conditions (refer to the individual health concern for complete information):

Rating	Health Concerns
★★☆	**Chronic viral hepatitis** (page 220)
	Liver cirrhosis (page 290) (shakuyaku-kanzo-to formula)
	Muscle cramps (shakuyaku-kanzo-to formula)
★☆☆	**Atherosclerosis** (page 38) (red peony root)
	Dysmenorrhea (page 171) (painful menses)
	Fever (moutan bark)
	Polycystic ovary syndrome (shakuyaku-kanzo-to)
	Premenstrual syndrome (page 368) (PMS)

Pennyroyal

Historical or traditional use (may or may not be supported by scientific studies)

Peony is an ancient, traditional Chinese herbal medicine.[2] The plant was and is extensively cultivated as an ornamental plant as well. Peony is named for the mythical Greek figure Paeon, who was said to be a student of Aesculapius, the great physician.[3] Paeon used the peony plant (various species also grow in Europe) to heal a wound for the god Pluto. This earned Aesculapius's jealous wrath, but Pluto saved Paeon from death by turning him into a peony plant.

Bai shao or white peony was considered useful for **hypertension** (page 246), chest pain, muscle cramping and spasms, and fever.[4] It was an important remedy for female reproductive conditions ranging from **dysmenorrhea** (page 171) (painful menstruation) to irregular menses.[5] Chi shao or red peony was used for bleeding or lack of blood movement, depending on how it was prepared.[6] Moutan was also considered helpful for problems characterized by bleeding, such as nosebleeds, bleeding wounds, or menorrhagia (excessive menstrual bleeding).[7]

Active constituents

Peony contains a unique glycoside called paeoniflorin. Proanthocyanidins, flavonoids, tannins, polysaccharides, and paeoniflorin are all considered to contribute to the medicinal activity of various forms of peony. Paeoniflorin's major effect seems to be to calm nerves and alleviate spasm. One study has confirmed the efficacy of shakuyaku-kanzo-to (formula with peony and **licorice** [page 702]) for relieving muscle cramps due to **cirrhosis of the liver** (page 290), **diabetes** (page 152), and dialysis.[8] Shakuyaku-kanzo-to is approved by the Japanese Ministry of Health and Welfare for treatment of muscle cramps. Another Japanese formulation known as toki-shakuyaku-san combines peony root with **dong quai** (page 668) and four other herbs and has been found to effectively reduce symptoms of cramping and pain associated with **dysmenorrhea** (page 171) (painful menses).[9]

Paeoniflorin and peony extracts also enhance mental function in animal studies,[10] suggesting a potential benefit for dementia. Human studies have not yet been conducted to confirm this theory.

Red peony root and moutan bark have both shown **antioxidant** (page 467) activity in test tubes, likely due to the presence of paeoniflorin, proanthocyanidins, and

flavonoids.[11] Polysaccharides found in peony bark and root have shown an ability to stimulate immune cells in the test tube.[12, 13]

Animal studies have found that red peony root, alone or in combination with other Chinese herbs, could help prevent liver damage due to various chemical toxins.[14] A crude extract of red peony root was shown in a small, preliminary trial to reduce liver fibrosis in some patients with **chronic viral hepatitis** (page 220).[15] Other case studies published in Chinese have found red peony root helpful for people with viral hepatitis.[16]

Crude red peony root extracts and combinations of these extracts with other Chinese herbs inhibit platelet aggregation, thrombosis, and excessive clotting in the test tube and in animals.[17, 18] A rabbit study found that peony was effective at lowering **cholesterol** (page 223) levels in the aorta.[19] A preliminary human study confirmed that peony could inhibit platelet clumping.[20] This suggests that peony might be helpful for prevention of **atherosclerosis** (page 38). However, clinical studies are needed to confirm this effect.

One uncontrolled clinical trial reported that moutan bark could significantly lower blood pressure in people with **hypertension** (page 246).[21]

Peony shows some weak estrogen-like effects, acting like a very weak anti-estrogen, particularly as part of the formula shakuyaku-kanzo-to. In a preliminary study, this formula was shown to improve fertility in women affected by polycystic ovary syndrome.[22]

How much is usually taken?

White peony capsules are used in the amount of 1.5 to 4 grams three times per day. Red peony and moutan capsules are used in the amount of 1 to 3 grams three times per day.[23] Capsules of shakuyaku-kanzo-to formula are used in the amount of 2.5 grams three times per day.[24]

Are there any side effects or interactions?

If used in the amounts listed above, peony is not associated with side effects. It is not known whether peony is safe for use during pregnancy, though there is an uncontrolled study showing it could safely be used to lower blood pressure in pregnant women.[25]

Shakuyaku-kanzo-to should be taken only while under the care of a healthcare professional trained in herbal medicine.

Peony

PEPPERMINT

Botanical name: *Mentha piperita*

Parts used and where grown

Peppermint is a hybrid of water mint and spearmint and was first cultivated near London in 1750. Peppermint is now cultivated widely, particularly in the U.S. and Europe. The two main cultivated forms are the black mint, which has violet-colored leaves and stems and a relatively high oil content, and the white mint, which has pure green leaves and a milder taste. The leaves are used medicinally.

Peppermint has been used in connection with the following conditions (refer to the individual health concern for complete information):

Rating	Health Concerns
★★★	**Irritable bowel syndrome** (page 280) (combination with **caraway** [page 651] oil)
★★☆	**Gingivitis (periodontal disease)** (page 203) **Indigestion** (page 260) **Irritable bowel syndrome** (page 280) **Shingles** (page 401) (postherpetic neuralgia) (topical) **Tension headache** (page 430) (topical)
★☆☆	**Chronic candidiasis** (page 109) **Colic** (page 121) **Common cold** (page 129) **Gallstones** (page 193) **Low back pain** (page 293) (topical)

Historical or traditional use (may or may not be supported by scientific studies)

Recognized in the early 18th century, the historical use of peppermint is not dramatically different than its use in modern herbal medicine. Classified as a carminative herb, peppermint has been used as a general digestive aid and employed in the treatment of **indigestion** (page 260) and intestinal **colic** (page 121) by herbalists.[1]

Active constituents

Peppermint leaves yield approximately 0.1–1.0% volatile oil which is composed primarily of menthol (29–48%) and menthone (20–31%).[2] Peppermint oil is classified as a carminative (prevents and relieves intestinal gas).[3] It may also relieve spasms in the intestinal tract. Peppermint oil or peppermint tea is often used to treat gas and indigestion.

Three double-blind trials found that enteric-coated peppermint oil reduced the pain associated with intestinal spasms, commonly experienced in **irritable bowel syndrome** (page 280) (IBS).[4, 5, 6] However, another trial found no effect of peppermint on IBS.[7] A double-blind trial found that an enteric-coated combination of peppermint and **caraway** (page 651) oils was superior to a placebo for people with gastrointestinal complaints including IBS.[8] A combination of peppermint, caraway seeds, and two other carminative herbs (**fennel** [page 676] seeds and **wormwood** [page 762]) was reported to be effective for gastrointestinal complaints including IBS in another double-blind study.[9]

A tea of peppermint is a traditional therapy for **colic** (page 121) in infants but has never been investigated in a human trial. Peppermint should be used cautiously in infants (see side effects below).

Peppermint oil's relaxing action also extends to topical use. When applied topically, it acts as an analgesic and reduces pain.[10] A trial of topical peppermint oil applied to the temples of healthy volunteers (with or without **eucalyptus** [page 673] oil) found that peppermint oil had a muscle-relaxing action and it decreased tension.[11] Topical peppermint oil alone reduced pain in people with tension headaches as well.

How much is usually taken?

For internal use, a tea can be made by pouring 1 cup (250 ml) of boiling water over 1 heaped teaspoon (5 grams) of the dried leaves and steeping for five to ten minutes. Three to four cups (750–1000 ml) daily between meals can be taken to relieve stomach and gastrointestinal complaints.[12] Peppermint leaf tablets and capsules, 3–6 grams per day, can be taken. For treatment of **irritable bowel syndrome** (page 280), 1–2 enteric-coated capsules containing 0.2 ml of peppermint oil taken two to three times per day is recommended.

For headaches, a combination of peppermint oil and eucalyptus oil diluted with base oil can be applied to the temples at the onset of the headache and every hour after that or until symptom relief is noted.

Are there any side effects or interactions?

Peppermint tea is generally considered safe for regular consumption. Peppermint oil can cause burning and gastrointestinal upset in some people.[13] It should be avoided by people with chronic **heartburn** (page 260), severe liver damage, inflammation of the gallbladder, or obstruction of bile ducts.[14] People with **gallstones** (page 193) should consult a physician before using peppermint leaf or peppermint oil. Some people using enteric-coated peppermint capsules may experience a burning sensation in the rectum. Rare allergic reactions have been reported with topical use of peppermint oil. Peppermint oil should not be applied to the face—in particular, the nose—of children and infants. Peppermint tea should be used with caution in infants and young children, as they may choke in reaction to the strong menthol. **Chamomile** (page 656) is usually a better choice for this group for treating **colic** (page 121) and mild gastrointestinal complaints.

PERIWINKLE

Common name: Lesser periwinkle
Botanical name: *Vinca minor*

Parts used and where grown
The flower and leaf of lesser periwinkle are used medicinally. Periwinkle is an evergreen shrub that grows in Europe, northwestern Africa, central Asia, and some parts of North America.

Periwinkle has been used in connection with the following conditions (refer to the individual health concern for complete information):

Rating	Health Concerns
★★☆	**Alzheimer's disease** (page 19)
★☆☆	**Canker sores** (page 90)
	Dementia (vascular)
	Dialysis
	Diarrhea (page 163)
	Glaucoma (page 205)
	Hearing loss (presbyacusis)
	Menorrhagia (page 314)
	Stroke (page 419)
	Tinnitus (page 430)

Historical or traditional use (may or may not be supported by scientific studies)
Periwinkle has likely been used for medicine for a long time; its Latin name, *Vinca*, is derived from the Latin word *vincere*, meaning "to overcome." European herbalists have used periwinkle for headaches, vertigo, and poor memory since medieval times.[1] It was also considered a helpful remedy for conditions with a watery or bloody discharge such as **diarrhea** (page 163), bleeding gums, or **menorrhagia** (page 314).[2]

Active constituents
There are two classes of active compounds in lesser periwinkle—alkaloids and tannins. The major alkaloid is known as vincamine. A closely related semisynthetic derivative of vincamine most widely used as medicine is known as ethyl-apovincaminate or vinpocetine. It has vasodilating, blood thinning, and memory-enhancing actions. It has been shown in double-blind studies to help alleviate a type of dementia known as vascular dementia, in which the arteries supplying blood to the brain develop **atherosclerotic** (page 38) plaques.[3, 4, 5] A double-blind study found that vincamine can help people with **Alzheimer's disease** (page 19),[6] while one open study did not.[7] Vinpocetine has also been found to prevent the decline in short-term memory induced by the anti-anxiety benzodiazepine drug flunitrazepam in one preliminary study.[8] Further study is needed to determine whether vinpocetine would be a helpful adjunct to use of benzodiazepines.

One double-blind study found that high amounts of vinpocetine (60 mg per day) could have a beneficial effect on hearing loss due to aging (presbyacusis).[9] A preliminary study concluded that supplementation with ethyl-apovincaminate (a vinca alkaloid) may reduce symptoms of **tinnitus** (page 430) (ringing in the ears) due to impaired blood flow to the inner ear.[10] One review of the use of vinpocetine in people who have suffered **strokes** (page 419) found that the only double-blind study did not show efficacy,[11] though previous uncontrolled studies have suggested there might be a benefit.[12, 13]

Vinpocetine tends to act as a calcium-chelating agent. One uncontrolled study found that use of vinpocetine for 3 to 12 months could eliminate calcium buildup in people undergoing dialysis.[14] Further research is needed to determine whether this could be helpful in other conditions associated with excess calcium, or whether vinpocetine might interfere with calcium's beneficial actions.

One double-blind and one preliminary study have found that brovincamine, a compound closely related to vinpocetine, was helpful in people with chronic **glaucoma** (page 205).[15, 16] Until studies have been conducted using actual vinpocetine, it is unknown whether it would be as effective as brovincamine.

Periwinkle

Crude periwinkle also contains tannins. These make it a mild astringent. It may relieve pain from canker sores or sore throats, according to traditional use. Clinical trials have not been conducted to confirm this.

How much is usually taken?
The amount of vinpocetine used in most studies is 15 mg one to three times per day.[17] Vinpocetine should be taken with food, as it has been shown to be better absorbed with meals than when taken away from meals.[18] It may take three to six weeks before any improvement is noted.[19]

A tincture can be taken in the amount of 1 to 2 ml three times per day.[20] A tea can be made by infusing 1 teaspoon of herb into a cup of water for 10 to 15 minutes; three cups per day should be drunk.[21] Research has not been conducted to determine whether a tincture or a tea provides enough periwinkle compounds to have the same effects as vinpocetine.

Are there any side effects or interactions?
Vinpocetine has been reported to occasionally cause an upset stomach, flushing of the skin, and a skin rash;[22] these effects are mild and rarely cause anyone to stop taking it. The whole periwinkle herb may also cause minor stomach upset. This may be remedied by taking the herb with food. Neither vinpocetine nor periwinkle should be taken during pregnancy or breast-feeding until more information is available. The Commission E of the German government states that some animal studies suggest periwinkle could suppress the immune system.[23] This problem has not been observed to date in studies involving vinpocetine.

PHYLLANTHUS

Common names: Bahupatra, bhuiamla
Botanical name: *Phyllanthus niruri*

Parts used and where grown
Phyllanthus is an herb found in central and southern India. It can grow from 30–60 centimeters in height and blooms with many yellow flowers. Phyllanthus species are also found in other countries, including China (e.g., *Phyllanthus urinaria*), the Philippines, Cuba, Nigeria, and Guam.[1] All parts of the plant are used medicinally.

Phyllanthus has been used in connection with the following conditions (refer to the individual health concern for complete information):

Rating	Health Concerns
★★☆	**Hepatitis** (page 220)
★☆☆	**Pain** (page 338)

Historical or traditional use (may or may not be supported by scientific studies)
Phyllanthus has been used in Ayurvedic medicine for over 2,000 years and has a wide number of traditional uses including internal use for jaundice, gonorrhea, frequent menstruation, and **diabetes** (page 152) and topical use as a poultice for skin ulcers, sores, swelling, and itchiness. The young shoots of the plant are administered in the form of an infusion for the treatment of chronic dysentery.[2]

Active constituents
Phyllanthus primarily contains lignans (e.g., phyllanthine and hypophyllanthine), alkaloids, and **flavonoids** (page 516) (e.g., **quercetin** [page 580]).

Phyllanthus blocks DNA polymerase, the enzyme needed for the **hepatitis** (page 220) B virus to reproduce. In one study, 59% of those infected with chronic viral hepatitis B lost one of the major blood markers of HBV infection (e.g., hepatitis B surface antigen) after using 900 mg of phyllanthus per day for 30 days.[3] While clinical trials on the effectiveness of phyllanthus for HBV have been mixed, the species *P. urinaria* and *P. niruri* seem to work better than *P. amarus*.[4] Clinical trials with hepatitis B patients have used 900–2,700 mg of phyllanthus per day.

How much is usually taken?
Research has used the powdered form of phyllanthus ranging from 900–2,700 mg per day for three months.[5]

Are there any side effects or interactions?
No side effects have been reported using phyllanthus as recommended in the amounts above.

PICRORHIZA

Common names: Kutki, katuka
Botanical name: *Picrorhiza kurroa*

Parts used and where grown

The herb originated in and continues to grow primarily in the Himalayan mountains. The rhizomes or underground stems of picrorhiza are used.

Picrorhiza has been used in connection with the following conditions (refer to the individual health concern for complete information):

Rating	Health Concerns
★★☆	**Asthma** (page 32)
	Vitiligo (page 443)
★☆☆	**Hepatitis (acute viral)** (page 220)
	Indigestion (page 260)
	Infection (page 265)
	Rheumatoid arthritis (page 387)

Historical or traditional use (may or may not be supported by scientific studies)

The bitter rhizomes of picrorhiza have been used for thousands of years in India to treat people with **indigestion** (page 260).[1] It is also used to treat people with **constipation** (page 137) due to insufficient digestive secretion and for fever due to all manner of **infections** (page 265).[2]

Active constituents

The major constituents in picrorhiza are the glycosides picroside I, kutkoside, androsin, and apocynin. They have been shown in animal studies to be antiallergic, to inhibit platelet-activating factor (an important pro-inflammatory molecule),[3] and to decrease joint inflammation.[4] According to test tube and animal studies, picrorhiza has antioxidant actions, particularly in the liver.[5, 6] Picroliv (a commercial mixture containing picroside I and kutkoside) has been shown to have an immunostimulating effect in hamsters, helping to prevent infections.[7] Picrorhiza increases bile production in the liver, according to rat studies.[8] It has also been shown to protect animals from damage by several potent liver toxins, offering protection as good as or better than silymarin (the **flavonoids** [page 516] found in **milk thistle** [page 710]).[9, 10] However, it does not have the amount of human research as silymarin. Picrorhiza has also shown to reduce formation of liver **cancer** (page 87) due to chemical exposures in animal studies.[11]

Human studies on this plant are not prolific. A series of cases of acute viral **hepatitis** (page 220) in India were reportedly treated successfully by a combination of picrorhiza with a variety of minerals.[12] A number of similar reports have appeared in Indian literature over the years. No double-blind clinical trials have yet been published, however.

Two preliminary trials suggest that picrorhiza may improve breathing in asthma patients and reduce the severity of **asthma** (page 32).[13, 14] Although, a follow-up double-blind trial did not confirm these earlier trials.[15]

A preliminary trial conducted in India found a small benefit for people with arthritis (primarily **rheumatoid arthritis** [page 387]).[16]

Picrorhiza in combination with the drug methoxsalen was found in a preliminary trial to hasten recovery in people with **vitiligo** (page 443) faster than those receiving methoxsalen and sun exposure alone.[17]

How much is usually taken?

Between 400 and 1,500 mg of powdered, encapsulated picrorhiza per day has been recommended. One author considers this equivalent to the use of 1–2 ml of fluid extract twice per day.[18] Picrorhiza tastes quite bitter. Combining with **ginger** (page 680) root powder capsules or taking as tea can improve palatability.

Are there any side effects or interactions?

Loose stools and **colic** (page 121) have been reported when unprepared picrorhiza rhizomes are used as medicine. However, extracts in alcohol have shown much less tendency to cause such effects.[19] No other adverse effects have been reported with picrorhiza. Although the use of the herb is not discouraged in India during **pregnancy** (page 363) and breast-feeding, there is little information to determine the safety of the herb during these times.

PLANTAIN

Common names: Broadleaf plantain, lanceleaf plantain, ribwort
Botanical names: *Plantago lanceolata, Plantago major*

Parts used and where grown

These green, weedy plants are native to Europe and Asia, but now grow practically anywhere in the world where there is sufficient water. Plantain should not be confused with the banana-like vegetable of the same name. The leaves of plantain are primarily used as medicine. The seeds of plantain can also be used medicinally, having mild laxative effects similar to the seeds of **psyllium** (page 732), a close relative of plantain.

Plantain has been used in connection with the following conditions (refer to the individual health concern for complete information):

Rating	Health Concerns
★★☆	**Chronic bronchitis** (page 80)
★☆☆	**Burns** (page 85) (topical) **Cough** (page 139) Dermatitis (topical) Insect bites or stings (topical) **Peptic ulcer** (page 349) **Urinary tract infections** (page 436) **Wounds** (page 319) (topical)

Historical or traditional use (may or may not be supported by scientific studies)

Plantain has long been considered by herbalists to be a useful remedy for **cough** (page 139), **wounds** (page 319), inflamed skin or dermatitis, and insect bites.[1] Bruised or crushed leaves have been applied topically to treat insect bites and stings, **eczema** (page 177), and small wounds or cuts. It was considered by herbalists to be a gentle, soothing expectorant, and additionally to have a mild astringent effect said to help remedy **hemorrhoids** (page 219) or **bladder infections** (page 436) with mild amounts of blood in the urine.[2]

Active constituents

The major constituents in plantain are mucilage, iridoid glycosides (particularly aucubin), and tannins. Together these constituents are thought to give plantain mild anti-inflammatory, antimicrobial, antihemorrhagic, and expectorant actions.[3, 4] Plantain is approved by the German Commission E for internal use to ease **coughs** (page 139) and mucous membrane irritation associated with upper respiratory tract infections as well as topical use for skin inflammations.[5] Two Bulgarian clinical trials have suggested that plantain may be effective in the treatment of chronic **bronchitis** (page 80).[6, 7] Insufficient details were provided in these reports to determine the quality of the trials or their findings. Although plantain was thought to possess diuretic properties, one double-blind trial failed to show any diuretic effect for this plant.[8] A preliminary trial found that topical use of a plantain ointment (10% ground plantain in a base of petroleum jelly) was helpful as part of the treatment of people with impetigo and ecthyma, two inflammatory skin disorders.[9] Insufficient details were provided in this report, however, to determine the quality of the study or its findings.

How much is usually taken?

The German Commission E recommends using ¼–½ teaspoon (1–3 grams) of the leaf daily in the form of tea made by steeping the herb in 1 cup (250 ml) of hot water for 10–15 minutes (making three cups (750 ml) per day).[10] The fresh leaves can be applied directly three or four times per day to **minor injuries** (page 319), dermatitis, and insect stings.[11] Syrups or tinctures, approximately ½ teaspoon (2–3 ml) three times per day, can also be used, particularly to treat a **cough** (page 139).[12] Finally, ½–1¼ teaspoons (2–6 grams) of the fresh plant can be juiced and taken in three evenly divided oral administrations throughout the day.[13]

Are there any side effects or interactions?

Plantain is not associated with any common side effects and is thought to be safe for children.[14] There is no information available about its use by **pregnant** (page 363) or nursing women, though topical application appears to be safe. Adulteration of plantain with digitalis leading to dangerous side effects has been reported in Switzerland and the United States.[15] Although rare, it points to the need for consumers to purchase herbs from companies that carefully test their herbal products for adulteration.

PLEURISY ROOT

Botanical name: *Asclepias tuberosa*

Parts used and where grown

As its common name indicates, the root of pleurisy root is used as medicine. This brilliant-orange-flowered herb is native to and continues to grow primarily in the southwestern and midwestern United States. Many plants similar to pleurisy root are known as milkweeds because they produce a milky sap—something pleurisy root does not do.

Plantain

Pleurisy root has been used in connection with the following conditions (refer to the individual health concern for complete information):

Rating	Health Concerns
★☆☆	**Bronchitis** (page 80) Fever Pleurisy Pneumonia

Historical or traditional use (may or may not be supported by scientific studies)

Pleurisy root was used by Native American tribes both internally as a remedy for pulmonary infections and topically to treat wounds.[1] The Eclectic physicians seized upon these ideas and continued to use the plant primarily for lung problems such as pleurisy and pneumonia. It was also used as a diaphoretic (a substance that causes sweating) for all manner of **infections** (page 265).[2] Pleurisy root was an official medicine in the United States Pharmacopoeia from 1820 to 1905.[3]

Active constituents

Insufficient work has been done to identify the active constituents in pleurisy root or its medicinal actions. No human studies have been conducted to determine whether it is effective for any indication. It is still used by herbalists and some physicians trained in herbal medicine as a diaphoretic (promotes sweating), and for lung infections and conditions of the pleura that lines the lungs.[4]

How much is usually taken?

A pleurisy root tea can be made by lightly simmering one teaspoon of the dried, chopped root in one pint of water for 10 to 15 minutes. One cup of this tea can be drunk twice per day.[5] Alternately, 1 to 2 ml of tincture of the fresh root can be used three times per day.[6]

Are there any side effects or interactions?

At the amounts recommended above, pleurisy root generally has no adverse effects. Excessive intake (1 tablespoon or more of the root at one time) can cause intestinal cramping, nausea, vomiting, and **diarrhea** (page 163).[7] Pleurisy root should be avoided by pregnant women as it may stimulate uterine contractions.[8]

PRICKLY ASH

Common names: Toothache tree, American prickly asn
Botanical names: *Zanthoxylum clava-herculis, Zanthoxylum americanum*

Parts used and where grown

The bark and sometimes the berries of these two American trees are used as medicine. There are many other trees in this genus that grow on other continents, including Chinese prickly ash *(Zanthoxylum bungeanum),* which grows in Asia.

Prickly ash has been used in connection with the following conditions (refer to the individual health concern for complete information):

Rating	Health Concerns
★☆☆	**Indigestion** (page 260) Insufficient salivation Rheumatism Toothache

Historical or traditional use (may or may not be supported by scientific studies)

Many eastern Native American tribes valued prickly ash as a remedy for **upset stomach** (page 260), **sore throats** (page 129), aching muscles, skin **infections** (page 265), to stimulate saliva flow, and various other conditions.[1] Eclectic physicians (doctors who recommended herbal medicines) in the United States at the end of the 19th century continued the traditional uses of prickly ash, primarily as a digestive aid, to strengthen the nervous system, and for cholera.[2] The bark was also widely used by herbalists to treat rheumatic conditions.[3] Prickly ash is also considered an alterative in traditional herbalism, meaning it enhances the body's ability to fight against and recover from all manner of difficulties.[4] Chinese prickly ash *(Zanthoxylum simulans)* is used for similar indications as its American relative as well as for killing **parasites** (page 343).[5]

Active constituents

Prickly ash bark contains alkaloids and a volatile oil. The fruit is rich in the volatile oil. Little research has been done specifically on the constituents or actions of American prickly ash. Preliminary Chinese trials have reportedly found that oral use of Chinese prickly ash berries can alleviate pain due to **indigestion** (page 260), gallbladder disease, or ulcers, as well as eliminating **pinworms** (page 343).[6] Herculin, an alkamide in the plant, produces a localized numbing effect on the tongue when consumed.[7] Whether this explains the historical use of prickly ash for toothaches remains to be confirmed in clinical trials.

How much is usually taken?

A tea of prickly ash is made by simmering 1–2 teaspoons (5–10 grams) of the bark for 10–15 minutes. Three cups (750 ml) per day are recommended.[8] Alternatively, a tincture, ½–¾ teaspoon (2–4 ml) three times per day, may also be used.[9] Prickly ash is best taken just before meals. Traditionally, the bark was chewed to relieve tooth pain.[10]

Are there any side effects or interactions?

There are no known side effects from using the amounts of prickly ash noted above. Since it stimulates digestive function, prickly ash should best be avoided in conditions such as **ulcerative colitis** (page 433), **peptic ulcer disease** (page 349), or **gastroesophageal reflux** (page 198). Some herbal experts suggest that prickly ash be avoided by **pregnant** (page 363) women because it may stimulate menstruation and increase risk of a miscarriage.[11]

PSYLLIUM

Common names: Flea seed, ispaghula, spogel
Botanical names: *Plantago ovata*, *Plantago ispaghula*

Parts used and where grown

Psyllium is native to Iran and India and is currently cultivated in these countries. The seeds are primarily used in traditional herbal medicine. Psyllium seed husks are mainly used to treat constipation.

Psyllium has been used in connection with the following conditions (refer to the individual health concern for complete information):

Rating	Health Concerns
★★★	Constipation (page 139) Diabetes (page 152) Diverticular disease (page 168) High cholesterol (page 223) Irritable bowel syndrome (page 280)
★★☆	Atherosclerosis (page 38) Diarrhea (page 163) Hemorrhoids (page 219) High triglycerides (page 238) Ulcerative colitis (page 433) (to maintain remission)
★☆☆	Parkinson's disease (page 345) (for constipation) Weight loss and obesity (page 446)

Historical or traditional use (may or may not be supported by scientific studies)

In addition to its traditional and current use for **constipation** (page 137), psyllium was also used topically by herbalists to treat skin irritations, including poison ivy reactions and insect bites and stings. It has also been used in traditional herbal systems of China and India to treat **diarrhea** (page 163), **hemorrhoids** (page 219), bladder problems, and **high blood pressure** (page 246).

Active constituents

Psyllium is a bulk-forming laxative and is high in both **fiber** (page 512) and mucilage. Psyllium seeds contain 10–30% mucilage. The laxative properties of psyllium are due to the swelling of the husk when it comes in contact with water. This forms a gelatinous mass that keeps feces hydrated and soft, provided it is taken with sufficient water. The resulting bulk stimulates a reflex contraction of the walls of the bowel, followed by emptying.[1]

Psyllium is a common ingredient in over-the-counter bulk laxative products. One preliminary trial found that psyllium seeds relieved **constipation** (page 137) when it was due to lifestyle factors (e.g., inadequate **fiber** [page 512], sedentary lifestyle), but not when an actual disease was the cause.[2] Numerous double-blind trials have found that supplementation with psyllium can lower total **cholesterol** (page 223) and LDL ("bad") cholesterol.[3] However, levels of HDL ("good") cholesterol are not affected by psyllium supplementation.[4] The cholesterol-lowering effect of psyllium has been reported in children,[5] as well as in adults.[6] Psyllium supplementation has also improved blood sugar levels in some people with **diabetes** (page 152).[7, 8, 9] The soluble fiber component of psyllium is believed to account for this effect.

In a double-blind trial, people with **ulcerative colitis** (page 433) had a reduction in symptoms such as bleeding and remained in remission longer when they took 20 grams of ground psyllium seeds twice daily with water compared to the use of the medication mesalamine alone.[10] Also, the combination of the two was slightly more effective than either alone.

How much is usually taken?

The suggested intake of psyllium husks to treat constipation is 1 teaspoon (approximately 5 grams) three times per day. Alternatively, some references suggest taking 2–6 teaspoons (10–30 grams) of the whole seeds per day—typically taken in three even amounts throughout the day.[11] This is stirred into a large glass of water or juice and drunk immediately before it thickens.[12] It is best to follow label instructions on over-the-counter psyllium products for **constipation** (page 137). It is important to maintain a high water intake when using psyllium.

Are there any side effects or interactions?

Using psyllium in recommended amounts is generally safe. People with chronic **constipation** (page 137) should seek the advice of a healthcare professional. Some people with **irritable bowel syndrome** (page 280) feel worse when taking psyllium and may do better with soluble fiber, such as in fruit. People with an obstruction of the bowel or people with **diabetes** (page 152) who have difficulty regulating their blood sugar should not use psyllium.[13] Side effects, such as allergic skin and respiratory reactions to psyllium dust, have largely been limited to people working in factories manufacturing psyllium products.

PUMPKIN

Botanical names: *Cucurbita pepo, Cucurbita maxima*

Parts used and where grown

Pumpkins and other squashes are native to North and Central America, but have since been cultivated around the world. The seeds are primarily used in herbal medicine. The yellow blossoms of pumpkins are also used as medicine in some native traditions.

Pumpkin seeds have been used in connection with the following conditions (refer to the individual health concern for complete information):

Rating	Health Concerns
★★☆	**Benign prostatic hyperplasia (BPH)** (page 58)
★☆☆	**Depression** (page 145) **Kidney stone** (page 284) **Parasites** (page 343)

Historical or traditional use (may or may not be supported by scientific studies)

(may or may not be supported by scientific studies): Native Americans used pumpkin flesh and seeds for food. Their use of the seeds for the treatment of intestinal infections eventually led the United States Pharmacopoeia to list pumpkin seeds as an official medicine for **parasite** (page 343) elimination from 1863 to 1936.[1] Native Americans also commonly used pumpkin seeds to treat a variety of kidney problems. The flowers were used topically to soothe **minor injuries** (page 319).[2] Eclectic physicians (doctors who recommended herbal medicine) at the end of the 19th century used pumpkin seeds to treat **urinary tract** (page 436) problems and **gastritis** (page 195), and to remove tapeworms and roundworms from the intestines.[3]

Active constituents

Pumpkin seeds contain several major groups of active constituents: essential fatty acids, **amino acids** (page 465), phytosterols (e.g., beta-sitosterol) minerals, and vitamins. Other major constituents include mucilaginous carbohydrates and minerals.

Pumpkin seed oil has been used in combination with **saw palmetto** (page 743) in two double-blind trials to effectively reduce symptoms of **benign prostatic hyperplasia** (page 58) (BPH).[4, 5] Only one open label trial evaluated the effectiveness of pumpkin seed oil alone for BPH.[6] Animal studies have shown that pumpkin seed extracts can improve the function of the bladder and urethra. This might partially account for BPH symptom relief.[7]

Curcurbitin is a constituent in pumpkin seeds that has shown anti-parasitic activity in the test tube.[8] Human trials conducted in China have shown pumpkin seeds to be helpful for people with acute schistosomiasis, a severe parasitic disease occurring primarily in

Asia and Africa that is transmitted through snails.[9] Preliminary human research conducted in China and Russia has shown pumpkin seeds may also help resolve tapeworm infestations.[10, 11] The assistance of a physician is required to help diagnose and treat any suspected intestinal **parasite** (page 343) infections.

Due to the purported L-tryptophan content of pumpkin seeds, they have been suggested to help remedy **depression** (page 145).[12] However, research is needed before pumpkin seeds can be considered for this purpose.

Two trials in Thailand have reportedly found that eating pumpkin seeds as a snack can help prevent the most common type of **kidney stone** (page 284).[13, 14] Pumpkin seeds appear to both reduce levels of substances that promote stone formation in the urine and increase levels of substances that inhibit stone formation. The active constituents of pumpkin seeds responsible for this action have not been identified.

How much is usually taken?

Pumpkin seed oil extracts standardized for fatty acid content have been used in BPH trials. Men with BPH have used 160 mg three times per day with meals.[15] Approximately 5–10 grams per day of pumpkin seeds may be needed for kidney stone prevention.[16] As a treatment for parasites, 200–400 grams are ground and taken with milk and honey, followed by castor oil two hours later. This treatment, however, should not be attempted unless under medical supervision.

Are there any side effects or interactions?

Pumpkin seeds may cause an upset stomach, but are otherwise extremely safe. There is no reason to believe pumpkin seeds should be avoided during **pregnancy** (page 363) or breast-feeding as they are commonly consumed as food during these times without any indication of harm.

PYGEUM

Botanical names: *Prunus africanum*, *Pygeum africanum*

Parts used and where grown

Pygeum is an evergreen tree found in the higher elevations of central and southern Africa. The bark is used medicinally. Wild pygeum is environmentally threatened and efforts are being made to grow pygeum on plantations and control harvesting in the wild.

Pygeum has been used in connection with the following conditions (refer to the individual health concern for complete information):

Rating	Health Concerns
★★☆	**Benign prostatic hyperplasia** (page 58) (BPH)
★☆☆	**Prostatitis** (page 377) (CBP, NBP)

Historical or traditional use (may or may not be supported by scientific studies)

The powdered bark was used as a tea for relief of urinary disorders in African herbal medicine. European scientists were so impressed with reports of pygeum's actions, they began laboratory investigations into the active constituents in the bark. This led to the development of the modern lipophilic (fat-soluble) extract used today.

Active constituents

Chemical analysis and pharmacological studies indicate the lipophilic extract of pygeum bark has three categories of active constituents: 1) Phytosterols, including **beta-sitosterol** (page 471), have anti-inflammatory effects by interfering with the formation of hormone-like substances in the body (prostaglandins) that tend to accumulate in the prostate of men with **benign prostatic hyperplasia** (page 58) (BPH); 2) pentacyclic terpenes have an anti-**edema** (page 180), or decongesting, effect; 3) ferulic esters indirectly control testosterone activity in the prostate, which may reduce the risk of BPH.[1] While these effects have been shown in test tube studies, human studies are still needed to confirm these effects in the body. Pygeum alone has been shown in some double-blind trials to help men with BPH by improving urinary flow and other symptoms of BPH.[2, 3] It has also been used successfully in combination with **nettle** (page 714) root to treat BPH.[4] Long-term BPH studies (six months or greater) on pygeum are lacking, however.

How much is usually taken?

The accepted form of pygeum used in Europe for treatment of **BPH** (page 58) is a lipophilic extract standardized to 13% total sterols (typically calculated as beta-sitosterol).[5] Men with mild to moderate BPH sometimes take 50–100 mg two times per day. A double-blind trial found that 100 mg once daily was as effective as 50 mg twice per day.[6] Pygeum should be monitored over at least a six-month period to determine efficacy. Men with BPH who are using pygeum should be supervised by a doctor.

Are there any side effects or interactions?
Side effects from the lipophilic extract of pygeum are rare. In clinical trials, there were reports of mild gastrointestinal upset in some men.

RED CLOVER

Botanical name: *Trifolium pratense*

Parts used and where grown
This plant grows in Europe and North America. The flowering tops are used in botanical medicine. Another plant, white clover, grows in similar areas. Both have white arrow-shaped patterns on their leaves.

Red clover has been used in connection with the following conditions (refer to the individual health concern for complete information):

Rating	Health Concerns
★★☆	**Menopause** (page 311)
	Osteoporosis (page 333)
★☆☆	**Cough** (page 139)
	Eczema (page 177)

Historical or traditional use (may or may not be supported by scientific studies)
Traditional Chinese Medicine and Western folk medicine used this plant as a diuretic, a **cough** (page 139) expectorant (an agent that promotes discharge of mucus from the respiratory passages), and an alterative.[1] Alterative plants were considered beneficial for chronic conditions, particularly those afflicting the skin.

Active constituents
Red clover is known as an alterative agent (i.e., one that produces gradual beneficial changes in the body, usually by improving nutrition; also known as a "blood cleanser"). It is a traditional remedy for **psoriasis** (page 379) and **eczema** (page 177). However, the mechanism of action and constituents responsible for red clover's purported benefit in skin conditions are unknown. Modern research has revealed that red clover also contains high amounts of isoflavones, such as genistein, which have weak estrogen-like properties.[2] Modern re-

search has focused on a red clover extract high in isoflavones as a possible treatment for symptoms associated with **menopause** (page 311) and **cardiovascular health** (page 98) in menopausal women. In a double-blind study, administration of 80 mg of isoflavones per day from red clover reduced the frequency of hot flashes in postmenopausal women. The benefit was noticeable after 4 weeks of treatment and became more pronounced after a total of 12 weeks.[3] Another double-blind trial found that red clover improved cardiovascular function in menopausal women,[4] Various laboratory studies and one case report of a man with prostate cancer suggest red clover isoflavones may help prevent **cancer** (page 87).[5, 6] In another case study, use of red clover by a man with prostate cancer led to noticeable anticancer effects in his prostate after the cancer was surgically removed. Although the isoflavones in red clover may help prevent certain forms of cancer (e.g., **breast** [page 65] and **prostate** [page 371]), further studies are needed before red clover is recommended for cancer patients.

How much is usually taken?
Traditionally, red clover is taken as a tea, by adding 1 cup (250 ml) of boiling water to 2–3 teaspoons (10–15 grams) of dried flowers and steeping, covered, for ten to fifteen minutes.[7] Three cups (750 ml) can be drunk each day. Red clover can also be used in capsule or tablet form, equivalent to 2–4 grams of the dried flowers. Also, ½–¾ teaspoon (2–4 ml) of tincture three times per day may be taken. Standardized extracts providing 40 mg isoflavones per day are available as well.[8]

Are there any side effects or interactions?
Non-fermented red clover is relatively safe. However, fermented red clover may cause bleeding and should be avoided. Red clover supplements should be avoided by **pregnant** (page 363) or breast-feeding women and their safety has not been established in young children and infants.

RED RASPBERRY

Botanical name: *Rubus idaeus*

Parts used and where grown
Raspberry bushes are native to North America and are cultivated in Canada. Although most well known for its delicious berries, raspberry's leaves are used in medicine.

Red raspberry has been used in connection with the following conditions (refer to the individual health concern for complete information):

Rating	Health Concerns
★☆☆	**Common cold/sore throat** (page 129) **Diarrhea** (page 163) **Pregnancy and postpartum support** (page 363)

Historical or traditional use (may or may not be supported by scientific studies)

Raspberry leaves have been used by herbalists to treat **diarrhea** (page 163). In traditional herbalism and midwifery, red raspberry has been connected to female health, including **pregnancy** (page 363). It was considered a remedy for excessive menstrual flow (**menorrhagia** [page 314]) and as a "partus prepartor," or an agent used during pregnancy to help prevent complications.[1]

Active constituents

Raspberry leaves are high in tannins and like its relative, **blackberry** (page 636), may relieve acute **diarrhea** (page 163).[2] The constituents that affect the smooth muscles, such as in the uterus, have not yet been clearly identified. The German Commission E monograph has concluded there is insufficient proof to recommend red raspberry in modern herbal medicine.[3]

How much is usually taken?

Traditionally, raspberry leaf tea is prepared by pouring 1 cup (250 ml) boiling water over 1–2 teaspoons (5–10 grams) of the herb and steeping for ten to fifteen minutes. Up to 6 cups (1500 ml) per day may be necessary for acute problems such as **diarrhea** (page 163) or sore throats due to a **cold** (page 129), while less (two to three cups [500–750 ml]) is used for preventive use during **pregnancy** (page 363). By itself, raspberry is usually not a sufficient treatment for diarrhea. Tincture, ¾–1 teaspoon (4–8 ml) three times per day, may also be taken.

Are there any side effects or interactions?

Raspberry leaf may cause mild loosening of stools and nausea. Otherwise, use of the herb appears to be safe.

RED YEAST RICE

Botanical name: *Monascus purpureus*

Parts used and where grown

This substance, native to China, is a fermentation by-product of cooked non-glutinous rice on which red yeast has been grown.[1] The dried, powdered red yeast rice is used medicinally.

Red yeast rice has been used in connection with the following conditions (refer to the individual health concern for complete information):

Rating	Health Concerns
★★★	**High cholesterol** (page 223)
★★☆	**High triglycerides** (page 235)

Historical or traditional use (may or may not be supported by scientific studies)

Since A.D. 800, red yeast rice has been employed by the Chinese as both a food and a medicinal agent. Its therapeutic benefits as both a promoter of blood circulation and a digestive stimulant were first noted in the traditional Chinese pharmacopoeia, *Ben Cao Gang Mu-Dan Shi Bu Yi,* during the Ming Dynasty (1368–1644).[2] Practitioners of Traditional Chinese Medicine use red yeast rice to treat abdominal pain due to stagnant blood and dysentery, as well as external and internal trauma.[3] In addition to its therapeutic applications, red yeast rice has been used for centuries as a flavor enhancer, a food preservative, and a base for a Taiwanese alcoholic rice-wine beverage.[4, 5]

Active constituents

In addition to rice starch, protein, **fiber** (page 512), sterols, and fatty acids, red yeast rice contains numerous active constituents, including monacolin K, dihydromonacolin, and monacolin I to VI.

Researchers have determined that one of the ingredients in red yeast rice, called monacolin K, inhibits the production of **cholesterol** (page 223) by stopping the action of a key enzyme in the liver (e.g., HMG-CoA reductase) that is responsible for manufacturing cholesterol.[6] The drug lovastatin (Mevacor) acts in a similar

Red Raspberry

fashion to this red yeast rice ingredient. However, the amount per volume of monacolin K in red yeast rice is small (0.2% per 5 mg) when compared to the 20–40 mg of lovastatin available as a prescription drug.[7] This has prompted researchers to suggest that red yeast rice may have other ingredients, such as sterols, that might also contribute to lowering cholesterol.

Along with its evaluation in animal trials,[8] red yeast rice has been clinically investigated as a therapy for reducing **cholesterol** (page 223) in two human trials. In one trial, both men and women taking 1.2 grams (approximately 13.5 mg total monacolins) of a concentrated red yeast rice extract per day for two months had significant decreases in serum cholesterol levels.[9] In addition, people taking red yeast rice had a significant increase in HDL ("good") cholesterol and a decrease in LDL ("bad") cholesterol. Elevated **triglycerides** (page 235) were also found to be lowered.

A double-blind trial at the UCLA School of Medicine determined that red yeast rice in the amount of 2.4 grams per day (approximately 10 mg total monacolins) in capsules significantly decreased total- and LDL-cholesterol levels in a sample of people with elevated cholesterol after 12 weeks of therapy. Triglycerides were also reduced in those taking red yeast rice. However, unlike the original study, HDL values did not increase substantially.[10]

How much is usually taken?
The red yeast rice used in various studies was a proprietary product called Cholestin, which contains ten different monacolins. The amount of Cholestin used in these studies was 1.2–2.4 grams (5–10 mg of monacolins) per day in divided amounts for 8-12 weeks.[11, 12]

Note: Cholestin has been banned in the United States, as a result of a lawsuit alleging patent infringement.

Other red yeast rice products currently on the market differ from Cholestin in their chemical makeup. None contain the full complement of ten monacolin compounds that are present in Cholestin, and some contain a potentially toxic fermentation product called citrinin.[13] Until further information is available, red yeast rice products other than Cholestin cannot be recommended

Are there any side effects or interactions?
The Cholestin brand of red yeast rice has been generally well tolerated with possible temporary mild side effects such as **heartburn** (page 260), gas, and dizziness.[14] This product should not be used by people with liver disorders[15] and its safety during **pregnancy** (page 363) has not been established. As in the case of medications that inhibit HMG-CoA, it is advisable that people using red yeast rice products also supplement 30–60 mg of **coenzyme Q10** (page 496) daily.

There is one case report of muscle weakness and joint pain occurring in a man who was taking red yeast rice.[16] Because the man was also taking several prescription drugs, it was not clear whether the symptoms were caused by red yeast rice. The report should be taken seriously, however, since muscle problems are common side effects of prescription HMG CoA-reductase inhibitors.

REISHI

Common names: Ling chih, ling zhi
Botanical name: *Ganoderma lucidum*

Parts used and where grown
Reishi mushrooms grow wild on decaying logs and tree stumps in the coastal provinces of China. The fruiting body of the mushroom is employed medicinally. Reishi grows in six different colors, but the red variety is most commonly used and commercially cultivated in North America, China, Taiwan, Japan, and Korea.[1]

Reishi has been used in connection with the following conditions (refer to the individual health concern for complete information):

Rating	Health Concerns
★☆☆	Altitude sickness
	Diabetes (page 152)
	Hepatitis (page 220)
	HIV support (page 239)
	Hypertension (page 246)
	Infection (page 265)

Historical or traditional use (may or may not be supported by scientific studies)
Reishi has been used in Traditional Chinese Medicine for at least 2,000 years.[2] The Chinese name *ling zhi* translates as the "herb of spiritual potency" and was highly prized as an elixir of immortality.[3] Its Traditional

Reishi

Chinese Medicine indications include treatment of general fatigue and weakness, **asthma** (page 32), **insomnia** (page 270), and **cough** (page 139).[4]

Active constituents

Reishi contains several major constituents, including sterols, coumarin, mannitol, polysaccharides, and triterpenoids called ganoderic acids. Ganoderic acids may lower **blood pressure** (page 246) as well as decrease LDL ("bad") **cholesterol** (page 223). These specific triterpenoids also help reduce blood platelets from sticking together—an important factor in lowering the risk for **coronary artery disease** (page 38). While human research has been reported that demonstrates some efficacy for the herb in treating altitude sickness and chronic **hepatitis B** (page 220), these uses still need to be confirmed in well-designed human trials.[5] Animal studies and some very preliminary trials in humans suggest reishi may have some beneficial action in people with **diabetes mellitus** (page 152) and **cancer** (page 87).[6] Two controlled clinical trials have investigated the effects of reishi on **high blood pressure** (page 246) in humans and both found it could lower blood pressure significantly compared to a placebo or controls.[7, 8] The people with hypertension in the second study had previously not responded to medications, though these were continued during the study.

How much is usually taken?

Reishi can be taken either as 1.5–9 grams per day of the crude dried mushroom, 1–1.5 grams per day in powdered form, 1 ml per day of tincture, or as a tea.[9]

Are there any side effects or interactions?

Side effects from reishi can include dizziness, dry mouth and throat, nosebleeds, and abdominal upset. These rare effects may develop with continuous use over three to six months.[10] **Pregnant** (page 363) or breast-feeding women should consult a physician before taking reishi.

RHODIOLA

Common name: Golden root, roseroot
Botanical name: *Rhodiola rosea*

Parts used and where grown

There are some 50 species of rhodiola, but it is the fragrant root of the species *Rhodiola rosea* that is used medicinally. *Rhodiola rosea* grows throughout the mountainous regions in the higher latitudes and elevations of the Northern hemisphere.

Rhodiola has been used in connection with the following conditions (refer to the individual health concern for complete information):

Rating	Health Concerns
★★☆	**Athletic performance** (page 43) (to improve endurance) Fatigue Mental performance

Historical or traditional use (may or may not be supported by scientific studies)

Rhodiola has long been used in traditional medicine, primarily in Russia and Scandinavia.[1] The Vikings used rhodiola to enhance physical strength and endurance, and it was commonly used by many Northern peoples to treat fatigue, poor physical endurance, nervous system disorders, and infections, and to enhance fertility. Rhodiola was included in the first Swedish Pharmacopeia, and Dioscorides, the Greek physician, reported on its use in his treatise *De Materia Medica*. In middle Asia, rhodiola was considered a premier treatment for colds and flu during the severe winters that occur there.

Active constituents

Rhodiola contains a number of potentially active compounds, including phenylpropanoids (rosavin, rosin, rosarin),; phenylethanol derivatives (salidroside [also known as rhodioloside], tyrosol); flavonoids (rodiolin, rodionin, rodiosin, acetylrodalgin, tricin); monoterpenes (rosiridol, rosaridin); triterpenes (daucosterol, beta-sitosterol); and phenolic acids (chlorogenic, hydroxycinnamic, and gallic acids). The presence of rosavin distinguishes the species *R. rosea* from other rhodiolas, and many products are standardized to rosavin content to ensure that they contain the proper species.

There are numerous animal and test tube studies showing that rhodiola has both a stimulating and a sedating effect on the central nervous system (depending on intake amount); enhances physical endurance; improves thyroid, thymus, and adrenal function; protects the nervous system, heart, and liver; and has antioxidant and anticancer properties.[2]

How much is usually taken?

Rhodiola has a more stimulating effect at lower amounts, and a more sedating effect at higher amounts. In medical treatment, the usual amounts taken are 200 to 600 mg per day of a standardized extract to at least 3% rosavins and 0.8 to 1% salidroside.[3] The nonstandardized amount would be 1 gram three times daily of the root, the amount for the alcoholic extract (40% alcohol) is 5 to 40 drops two to three times per day (with a weight to volume ratio of 1:1 to 1:5). Rhodiola is usually taken before meals.

Are there any side effects or interactions?

The safety of rhodiola has not been firmly established. However, rhodiola has a history of centuries of folk use and has been the subject of many clinical studies. No side effects or interactions have been reported. Animal studies indicate that rhodiola has a low level of toxicity, and that there is a huge margin of safety at the typical recommended intake amounts.[4] There is no information available about the safety of rhodiola in pregnancy or lactation.

ROOIBOS

Common name: Bushman tea, red bush tea
Botanical name: *Aspalathus linearis*

Parts used and where grown

Rooibos is a nitrogen-fixing shrub native to South Africa. Its leaves are fermented and sun dried for use as a tea.

Rooibos has been used in connection with the following conditions (refer to the individual health concern for complete information):

Rating	Health Concerns
★☆☆	**Allergies** (page 14) Anti-aging Cancer prevention **Indigestion** (page 260)

Historical or traditional use (may or may not be supported by scientific studies)

Rooibos is a pleasant-tasting beverage that has been used traditionally to sooth digestion and relieve stomach cramps, colic, and diarrhea. Rooibos tea has also been used to relieve allergies and eczema, and to slow aging.

Active constituents

Rooibos is completely caffeine free and, unlike black tea *(Camellia sinensis),* does not contain tannins that may interfere with iron absorption. Rooibos is rich in flavonoids, polyphenols, and phenolic acids (including aspalathin, (+)-catechin, isoquercitrin, luteolin, quercetin, rutin, caffeic acid, ferulic acid, and vanillic acid). The polyphenol aspalathin is unique to rooibos. The plant also contains oligosaccharides, polysaccharides, and a variety of minerals, though at levels that are of questionable clinical relevance.[1]

Preliminary studies show that rooibos has antimutagenic and antioxidant properties.[2, 3, 4, 5] It has also shown some ability to prevent radiation damage in animals.[6, 7, 8] This research somewhat supports rooibos's traditional use to slow the aging process, and its modern use as a cancer preventative. Laboratory and animal studies indicate that it affects antibody production and has anti-HIV activity.[9, 10, 11] These studies raise the possibility that the herb could be useful in aiding deficient immune responses in allergies, AIDS, and infections. No clinical trials have yet been published on this herb, however, so its efficacy is still unknown.

How much is usually taken?

A tea can be made by steeping 1 to 4 teaspoons (5 to 20 grams) of rooibos in 1 cup (240 ml) of water for up to ten minutes. Three cups of this tea per day may be drunk, with or without food.[12]

Are there any side effects or interactions?

As rooibos has not been studied scientifically in humans, there is no information available about its safety in pregnancy or lactation or in people with kidney or liver failure. However, it is generally considered a very safe herb, and there are no known side effects, contraindications, or drug interactions.[13]

ROSEMARY

Botanical name: *Rosmarinus officinalis*

Parts used and where grown

Rosemary is a small, fragrant evergreen shrub. The rosemary plant originated in the countries surrounding the

Mediterranean Sea. However, it now grows in North America as well. The leaf is used in herbal medicine.

Rosemary has been used in connection with the following conditions (refer to the individual health concern for complete information):

Rating	Health Concerns
★☆☆	**Atherosclerosis** (page 38)
	Chronic candidiasis (page 109)
	Indigestion (page 260)
	Infection (page 265)
	Rheumatoid arthritis (page 387) (topical)

Historical or traditional use (may or may not be supported by scientific studies)

Throughout history, rosemary was used to preserve meats.[1] It has long played a role in European herbalism and popular folklore. Sprigs of rosemary were considered a love charm, a sign of remembrance, and a way to ward off the plague. Rosemary was used by herbalists as a tonic for the elderly and to help with **indigestion** (page 260).[2] In ancient China, rosemary was used for headaches and topically for baldness.[3]

Active constituents

A number of constituents have shown activity in the test tube. The volatile oil, including eucalyptol (cineole), is considered to have potent antibacterial effects[4] and to relax smooth muscles in the lungs.[5] Rosmarinic acid has **antioxidant** (page 467) activity[6] and another ingredient of rosemary, known as carnosol, inhibits **cancer** (page 87) formation in animal studies.[7] No human studies have confirmed rosemary's use for these conditions.

How much is usually taken?

The German Commission E monograph suggests ¾ to 1¼ tsp (4 to 6 grams) of rosemary leaf per day.[8] A tea can be prepared by adding 2 teaspoons (10 grams) of herb to 1 cup (250 ml) boiling water and allowing it to steep in a covered container for 10 to 15 minutes. This tea can be taken several times per day. Rosemary tincture, ½ to 1 teaspoon (2 to 5 ml) three times per day, may also be used. The concentrated volatile oil should not be taken internally.

Are there any side effects or interactions?

There is no evidence to indicate that intermittent intake of moderate amounts of rosemary poses any threat during breast-feeding. However, internal intake of the herb and oil should be avoided during **pregnancy** (page 363) because the oil may act as an abortifacient (an agent that may induce an abortion).[9]

An extract of rosemary taken with a meal by healthy women inhibited the absorption of non-heme iron (e.g., the form of iron in plant foods) by 15%.[10] Frequent use of rosemary could, in theory, promote the development of iron deficiency in susceptible individuals.

SAGE

Botanical name: *Salvia officinalis*

Parts used and where grown

Sage is a silvery-green shrub with very fragrant leaves. The most commonly cultivated species of sage originally came from the area around the Mediterranean but now also grows in North America. The leaves of this common kitchen herb are used in medicine as well as in cooking.[1]

Sage has been used in connection with the following conditions (refer to the individual health concern for complete information):

Rating	Health Concerns
★★☆	**Alzheimer's disease** (page 19)
	Excessive perspiration
	Gingivitis (page 203) (periodontal disease) (as mouthwash, in combination with **peppermint** [page 726] oil, menthol, **chamomile** [page 656] tincture, expressed juice from **echinacea** [page 669], **myrrh** [page 713] tincture, clove oil, and **caraway** [page 651] oil)
	Indigestion (page 260)
	Menopause (page 311) (in combination with **alfalfa** [page 623])
★☆☆	**Infection** (page 265)
	Menopause (page 311)
	Pregnancy and postpartum support (page 363)
	Sore throat (page 129)

Historical or traditional use (may or may not be supported by scientific studies)

Sage has one of the longest histories of use of any culinary or medicinal herb. It was used by herbalists externally to treat sprains, swelling, ulcers, and bleeding.[2]

Rosemary

Internally, a tea made from sage leaves has had a long history of use to treat **sore throats** (page 129) and **coughs** (page 139)—often used as a gargle. It was also used by herbalists for rheumatism, excessive menstrual bleeding, and to dry up a mother's milk when nursing was stopped. It was particularly noted for strengthening the nervous system, improving memory, and sharpening the senses.[3] Sage was officially listed in the *United States Pharmacopoeia* from 1840 to 1900.

Active constituents

The volatile oil of sage contains the constituents alpha- and beta-thujone, camphor, and cineole.[4] It also contains rosmarinic acid, tannins, and flavonoids. In modern European herbal medicine, a gargle of sage tea is commonly recommended to treat **sore throat** (page 129), inflammations in the mouth, and **gingivitis** (page 203) (inflammation of the gums).[5] Test tube studies have found that sage oil has antibacterial, antifungal, and antiviral activity which may partially explain the effectiveness of sage for these indications.[6]

Sage is also approved in Germany for mild gastrointestinal upset and excessive sweating.[7] An unpublished, preliminary German study with people suffering from excessive perspiration found that either a dry leaf extract or an infusion of the leaf reduced sweating by as much as 50%.[8] A report from the United Kingdom indicates that herbalists there employ sage to treat symptoms of **menopause** (page 311) such as hot flashes.[9]

How much is usually taken?

For treatment of **sore throats** (page 129), inflammation in the mouth, or **gingivitis** (page 203), 3 grams of the chopped leaf can be added to 150 ml of boiling water and strained after 10 minutes.[10] This is then used as a mouthwash or gargle several times daily. Alternatively, one may use 5 ml of fluid extract (1:1) diluted in one glass of water, several times daily. For internal use, the same tea preparation described above may be taken three times per day.

Are there any side effects or interactions?

Concern has been expressed about the internal use of sage due to the presence of thujone.[11] Even when consumed in small amounts for long periods of time, thujone may cause increased heart rate and mental confusion. Very high amounts (several times greater than one receives if taking sage as instructed above), may lead to convulsions. If one takes sage internally, it is best to limit use to the amounts listed above and to

periods of no more than one to two weeks. Extracts of sage made with alcohol are likely to be higher in thujone than those made with water. Sage oil should never be consumed without being first diluted in water. Sage should not be used internally during **pregnancy** (page 363). These concerns do not extend to the use of sage as a gargle or mouth rinse. Sage should be avoided when fever is present.

SANDALWOOD

Botanical name: *Santalum album*

Parts used and where grown

Sandalwood trees grow in India and other parts of Asia. The wood is renowned for carving and also yields the volatile oil used in herbal medicine.

Sandalwood has been used in connection with the following conditions (refer to the individual health concern for complete information):

Rating	Health Concerns
★☆☆	**Infection** (page 265)

Historical or traditional use (may or may not be supported by scientific studies)

Sandalwood oil was used traditionally by herbalists to treat skin diseases, **acne** (page 4), dysentery, gonorrhea, and a number of other conditions.[1] In Traditional Chinese Medicine, sandalwood oil is considered an excellent sedating agent.

Active constituents

The volatile oil contains high amounts of alpha- and beta-santalol. According to a test tube study, these small molecules possess antibacterial properties.[2] This makes it a potential topical treatment for skin infections. Synthetic sandalwood oil does not contain these active ingredients. Internal use of sandalwood is approved by the German Commission E for the supportive treatment of infections of the lower urinary tract (usually the urinary bladder).[3] However, clinical trials are lacking to support this use.

How much is usually taken?

The German Commission E monograph suggests ¼ teaspoon (1–1.5 grams) of the volatile oil for the support-

Sandalwood

ive treatment of **urinary tract infections** (page 436).[4] This should only be done under the supervision of a doctor. Treatment should not exceed six weeks. For external use, a few drops of sandalwood oil are dissolved in 6 ounces (180 ml) of water and applied directly to the infected area of skin several times daily.

Are there any side effects or interactions?
Some people may experience mild skin irritation from topical application of sandalwood oil.[5] People with kidney disease should not use sandalwood internally. Until more is known, sandalwood oil should be avoided for internal use during **pregnancy** (page 363) and breastfeeding. Infants and children should not take sandalwood oil internally.

SARSAPARILLA

Botanical name: *Smilax* spp.

Parts used and where grown
Many different species are called by the general name sarsaparilla. Various species are found in Mexico, South America, and the Caribbean. The root is used in herbal medicine.

Sarsaparilla has been used in connection with the following conditions (refer to the individual health concern for complete information):

Rating	Health Concerns
★☆☆	**Eczema** (page 177)

Historical or traditional use (may or may not be supported by scientific studies)
In Mexico, sarsaparilla was used by herbalists for rheumatism, **cancer** (page 87), skin diseases, and a host of other conditions.[1] At the turn of the 20th century, there were reports of its use by herbalists for the treatment of leprosy.[2] Sarsaparilla also has a tradition of use in various women's health concerns and was rumored to have a **progesterone** (page 577)-like effect. Sarsaparilla was formerly a major flavoring agent in root beer.

Active constituents
Sarsaparilla contains steroidal saponins, such as sarsasapogenin, which may mimic the action of some human

hormones. This property remains undocumented, however. Sarsaparilla also contains phytosterols, such as **beta-sitosterol** (page 471), which may contribute to the anti-inflammatory effect of this herb. Reports have shown anti-inflammatory[3] and liver-protecting[4] effects for this herb. Similar reports on the effect of sarsaparilla on psoriasis occur in early European literature.[5]

How much is usually taken?
Sarsaparilla is often taken in capsules, 2–4 grams three times per day.[6] A tincture, 2–4 ml three times per day, may also be used.

Are there any side effects or interactions?
According to the German Commission E monograph, sarsaparilla may cause stomach irritation and temporary kidney irritation.[7] Sarsaparilla should not be taken during **pregnancy** (page 363) or breast feeding.

SASSAFRAS

Botanical name: *Sassafras albidum*

Parts used and where grown
Sassafras is native to eastern North America. It is a tree that can grow up to 90 feet tall, and it has distinctive three-fingered mitten-shaped leaves, as well as other leaf shapes. The inner bark of the root is used medicinally and in the preparation of beverages.

Sassafras has been used in connection with the following conditions (refer to the individual health concern for complete information):

Rating	Health Concerns
★☆☆	Fever
	Lice (topical oil)
	Rheumatism
	Urinary tract infection (page 436) (as irrigation therapy)

Historical or traditional use (may or may not be supported by scientific studies)
Sassafras was used by Native Americans for many purposes, primarily for infections and gastrointestinal problems.[1] Sassafras was one of the first and largest exports from the New World back to Europe as a beverage

and medicine.[2] Commercially, the pleasant tasting volatile oil was valued as a flavoring agent in root beer and similar beverages. Eclectic physicians in the late 19th and early 20th centuries considered sassafras a useful diaphoretic (a substance that causes sweating) and diuretic plant, primarily for relieving rheumatism and fevers, and as part of the treatment of **urinary tract infections** (page 436).[3]

Active constituents

The volatile oil of sassafras is believed to be the major active constituent of the plant. This oil contains up to 85% of the terpenoid known as safrole.[4] Safrole causes liver cancer when given to laboratory animals in high doses for long periods of time.[5] Sassafras bark, sassafras oil, and safrole are currently prohibited by the U.S. Food and Drug Administration from use as flavorings or food additives. Human studies are lacking to verify the efficacy of sassafras for any condition. However, one case study has been published showing that sassafras acted as a diaphoretic in an otherwise healthy woman.[6] While the amount of sassafras that could potentially cause cancer in humans remains unknown, one cup of strong sassafras tea is reported to contain as much as 200 mg of safrole, an amount that is four times higher than the amount considered potentially hazardous to humans if consumed regularly.[7]

How much is usually taken?

The safety of long-term internal use of sassafras has not been proven. Only guaranteed safrole-free products should be consumed. Note that safrole-containing food products are illegal in the United States and Canada.[8] Some sources suggest a dilute tincture can be used in the amount of 1 to 2 ml three times per day.[9] Volatile oil of sassafras can be applied topically three times per day for lice, but should never be taken internally.[10]

Are there any side effects or interactions?

Safrole causes liver cancer if given to laboratory animals "in high doses and for extended periods of time."[11] This requires metabolism of safrole by the liver into other toxic compounds, though the liver also removes some of these compounds for excretion through the urine.[12, 13] The overall risk of sassafras causing cancer in humans is thought to be low because it is only weakly active and the amounts normally consumed are low.[14] To eliminate the risk, sassafras products that contain safrole should not be consumed.

Safrole and its toxic metabolites do cross the placenta and enter breast milk in laboratory animals, and thus sassafras should be avoided by women who are pregnant or breast-feeding.[15]

SAW PALMETTO

Common name: Sabal
Botanical names: *Serenoa serrulata, Serenoa repens, Sabal serrulata*

Parts used and where grown

Saw palmetto (sometimes referred to as sabal in Europe) is a native of the southeast United States. The berries of the plant are used medicinally.

Saw palmetto has been used in connection with the following conditions (refer to the individual health concern for complete information):

Rating	Health Concerns
★★★	**Benign prostatic hyperplasia (BPH)** (page 58)
★☆☆	**Prostatitis** (page 377) (NBP)

Historical or traditional use (may or may not be supported by scientific studies)

In the early part of the twentieth century, saw palmetto berry tea was commonly recommended by herbalists for a variety of urinary tract ailments in men. Some believed the berry increased sperm production and sex drive in men.

Active constituents

The liposterolic (fat-soluble) extract of saw palmetto provides concentrated amounts of free fatty acids and sterols. One study with a saw palmetto extract suggests that it reduces the amount of dihydrotestosterone (DHT) (an active form of testosterone) binding in the part of the prostate surrounding the urethra (the tube carrying urine from the bladder).[1] Test tube studies also suggest that saw palmetto weakly inhibits the action of 5-alpha-reductase, the enzyme responsible for converting testosterone to DHT.[2] In test tubes, saw palmetto also inhibits the actions of growth factors and inflammatory substances that may contribute to **benign prostatic hyperplasia** (page 58) (BPH). Contrary to some opinions, saw palmetto does not have an estrogen-like effect in men's bodies.

Over the last decade, double-blind clinical trials have proven that 320 mg per day of the liposterolic extract of saw palmetto berries is a safe and effective treatment for the symptoms of **BPH** (page 58). A recent review of studies, published in the *Journal of the American Medical Association,* concluded that saw palmetto extract was as effective as finasteride (Proscar) in the treatment of BPH.[3] The clinical effectiveness of saw palmetto has been shown in trials lasting six months to three years.

A three-year trial in Germany found that taking 160 mg of saw palmetto extract twice daily reduced nighttime urination in 73% of patients and improved urinary flow rates significantly.[4] In a double-blind trial, 160 mg of saw palmetto extract taken twice daily was found to treat BPH as effectively as finasteride (Proscar) without side effects, such as loss of libido.[5]

Saw palmetto extract has also been combined with a **nettle** (page 714) root extract to successfully treat BPH. One trial using a combination of saw palmetto extract (320 mg per day) and nettle root extract (240 mg per day) showed positive actions on symptoms of BPH (e.g. improved urine flow, decreased nighttime urination, etc.) over a one-year treatment period.[6] Another study compared the same combination to finasteride for one year with positive results.[7]

How much is usually taken?

For early-stage **BPH** (page 58), 160 mg per day of liposterolic saw palmetto herbal extract in capsules is taken two times per day. One trial suggested that 320 mg once per day may be equally effective.[8] It may take four to six weeks to see results with BPH. If improvement is noted, the saw palmetto should be used continuously. It is important to work closely with a urologist to determine clinical improvement. Although it has not been tested for efficacy, saw palmetto is occasionally taken as a tea made with 5–6 grams of the powdered dried fruit. Ground, nonstandardized berry preparations (1–2 grams per day) and liquid extracts of whole herb at 5–6 ml per day are also sometimes used but have not been specifically tested.

Are there any side effects or interactions?

No significant side effects have been noted in clinical trials with saw palmetto extracts. However, in rare cases, saw palmetto can cause stomach problems,[9] and one individual who was taking saw palmetto developed severe bleeding during surgery.[10] According to some clinical

trials, saw palmetto extract does not appear to interfere with accurate measuring of prostate-specific antigen (PSA)—a marker for **prostate cancer** (page 371).[11] One test tube study found that saw palmetto did not prevent the release of PSA from prostate cells.[12] Saw palmetto is most effective in managing symptoms of BPH but has not been shown to aggressively shrink the size of the prostate. BPH can only be diagnosed by a physician (preferably a urologist). Use of saw palmetto extract for BPH should only occur after a thorough workup and diagnosis by a doctor. There are no proven uses of saw palmetto for women.

SCHISANDRA

Common name: Wu-wei-zi
Botanical name: *Schisandra chinensis*

Parts used and where grown

Schisandra is a woody vine with numerous clusters of tiny, bright red berries. It is distributed throughout northern and northeast China and the adjacent regions of Russia and Korea.[1] The fully ripe, sun-dried fruit is used medicinally. It is purported to have sour, sweet, salty, hot, and bitter tastes. This unusual combination of flavors is reflected in schisandra's Chinese name wu-wei-zi, meaning "five taste fruit."

Schisandra has been used in connection with the following conditions (refer to the individual health concern for complete information):

Rating	Health Concerns
★★☆	**Irritable bowel syndrome** (page 280) (Chinese herbal combination formula containing **wormwood** [page 762], **ginger** [page 680], **bupleurum** [page 647], schisandra, dan shen, and other extracts)
★☆☆	**Common cold/sore throat** (page 129) Fatigue **Hay fever** (page 211) (Sho-seiryu-to: contains **licorice** [page 702], cassia bark, schisandra, ma huang [ephedra], **ginger** [page 680], peony root, pinellia, and asiasarum root) **Hepatitis** (page 220) **Infection** (page 265) Liver support Stress

Historical or traditional use (may or may not be supported by scientific studies)

A classical treatise on Chinese herbal medicine, *Shen Nung Pen Tsao Ching*, describes schisandra as a high-grade herbal drug useful for a wide variety of medical conditions—especially as a kidney tonic and lung astringent. In addition, other textbooks on Traditional Chinese Medicine note that schisandra is useful for **coughs** (page 139), night sweats, **insomnia** (page 270), thirst, and physical exhaustion.[2] Adaptogenic herbs, like schisandra, have been used in Traditional Chinese Medicine to improve the ability of the body to respond to stress.

Active constituents

The major constituents in schisandra are lignans (schizandrin, deoxyschizandrin, gomisins, and pregomisin) found in the seeds of the fruit. Modern Chinese research suggests these lignans have a protective effect on the liver and an immunomodulating effect. Two human trials completed in China (one double-blind and the other preliminary) have shown that schisandra may help people with chronic viral **hepatitis** (page 220).[3, 4] Schisandra lignans appear to protect the liver by activating the enzymes in liver cells that produce **glutathione** (page 531), an important **antioxidant** (page 467) substance.[5]

Schisandra fruit may also have an adaptogenic action, much like the herb **Asian ginseng** (page 630), but with weaker effects. Laboratory work suggests that schisandra may improve work performance, build strength, and help to reduce fatigue.[6]

How much is usually taken?

Use of schisandra fruit ranges from 1.5–15 grams per day.[7] The tincture, 2–4 ml three times per day, can also be used.

Are there any side effects or interactions?

Side effects involving schisandra are uncommon but may include abdominal upset, decreased appetite, and skin rash.[8]

SENNA

Botanical names: *Cassia senna, Cassia angustifolia*

Parts used and where grown

The senna shrub grows in India, Pakistan, and China. The leaves and pods are used medicinally.

Senna has been used in connection with the following conditions (refer to the individual health concern for complete information):

Rating	Health Concerns
★★★	**Constipation** (page 137)
★★☆	Bowel Surgery (preparation for)

Historical or traditional use (may or may not be supported by scientific studies)

People in northern Africa and southwestern Asia have used senna as a laxative for centuries. It was considered a "cleansing" herb because of its cathartic effect. In addition, the leaves were sometimes made into a paste and applied to various skin diseases. Ringworm and **acne** (page 4) were both treated in this way.

Active constituents

Senna contains hydroxyanthracene glycosides known as sennosides. These glycosides stimulate colon activity and thus have a laxative effect. Also, these glycosides increase fluid secretion by the colon, with the effect of softening the stool and increasing its bulk.[1] Double-blind trials have confirmed the benefit of senna in treating **constipation** (page 137).[2, 3] Constipation induced by drugs such as the anti-**diarrhea** (page 163) medicine loperamide (Imodium) has also been shown to be improved by senna in a clinical trial.[4]

A double-blind trial showed that senna was more effective as a preparatory agent for bowel surgery than the commonly used polyethylene glycol (PEG).[5] Patients scheduled to undergo bowel surgery received either 120 mg of senna in a glass of water or 118 mg of PEG in about 2–3 quarts of water the night before surgery. Surgeons rated the efficacy of senna at clearing the bowels at 70%, compared to 58% efficacy for PEG. Supplementation with senna for this purpose should always be supervised by the surgeon.

How much is usually taken?

People using over-the-counter senna products should carefully follow label instructions. An extract in capsules or tablets providing 20–60 mg of sennosides per day is sometimes recommended.[6] This can be continued for a maximum of ten days. Use beyond ten days is strongly discouraged. If constipation is not alleviated within ten days, people should seek the help of a healthcare professional.

Are there any side effects or interactions?

Some people may develop a dependency on senna for normal bowel movements. Therefore, senna must not be used for more than ten consecutive days. Chronic senna use can also cause loss of fluids, low **potassium** (page 572) levels and **diarrhea** (page 163), all of which can lead to dehydration and potentially negative effects on the heart and muscles. The safety of senna during **pregnancy** (page 363) and breast-feeding is controversial. Most guidelines suggest avoiding senna during the first trimester of pregnancy.[7, 8] It is best to consult a physician. Senna is not recommended for children under the age of ten years. People with **Crohn's disease** (page 141), **ulcerative colitis** (page 433), appendicitis, intestinal obstructions, and abdominal pain should not supplement with senna.[9]

SHIITAKE

Common name: Hua gu
Botanical name: *Lentinus edodes*

Parts used and where grown

Wild shiitake mushrooms are native to Japan, China, and other Asian countries and typically grow on fallen broadleaf trees. Shiitake is now widely cultivated throughout the world, including the United States. The fruiting body is used medicinally.

Shiitake has been used in connection with the following conditions (refer to the individual health concern for complete information):

Rating	Health Concerns
★☆☆	**Hepatitis** (page 220)
	HIV support (page 239)
	Infection (page 265)
	Prostate cancer (page 371)

Historical or traditional use (may or may not be supported by scientific studies)

(may or may not be supported by scientific studies): Shiitake has been revered in Japan and China as both a food and medicinal herb for thousands of years. Wu Ri, a physician from the Chinese Ming Dynasty era (A.D. 1368–1644), wrote extensively about this mushroom,

noting its ability to increase energy, cure **colds** (page 129), and eliminate worms.[1]

Active constituents

Shiitake contains proteins, fats, carbohydrates, soluble **fiber** (page 512), vitamins, and minerals. In addition, shiitake's key ingredient—found in the fruiting body—is a polysaccharide called lentinan. Commercial preparations employ the powdered mycelium of the mushroom before the cap and stem grow. This preparation is called lentinus edodes mycelium extract (LEM). LEM is rich in polysaccharides and lignans.

One preliminary trial suggested that oral shiitake may be useful for people with **hepatitis B** (page 220).[2] A highly purified, intravenous form of lentinan is used in Japan and has been reported to increase survival in people with recurrent stomach **cancer** (page 87), particularly when used in combination with chemotherapy.[3] Similar findings have been found in one small clinical trial with people suffering from pancreatic cancer.[4] Case reports from Japan suggest that intravenous lentinan may be helpful in treating people with **HIV** (page 239) infection.[5] However, large-scale clinical trials to confirm this action have not yet been performed.

Oral supplementation of lentinan from shiitake has been shown to significantly reduce the recurrence rate of genital warts (condyloma acuminata). A preliminary trial involving a group of men and women with genital warts found that those who took 12.5 mg of lentinan twice a day for two months after laser surgery had significantly fewer recurrences (10.53% recurrence rate) compared to those who only had the laser surgery (47.06% recurrence rate).[6]

How much is usually taken?

The traditional intake of the whole, dried shiitake mushroom is 6–16 grams per day.[7] The mushroom is typically eaten in soups or taken as a decoction (i.e., boiled for 10–20 minutes, cooled, strained, and drunk). Recommended intake of LEM is 1–3 grams two to three times per day. Purified lentinan is considered a drug in Japan and is not currently available as an herbal supplement in North America.

Are there any side effects or interactions?

Shiitake has an excellent record of safety but has been known to induce temporary **diarrhea** (page 163) and abdominal bloating when used in high amounts (above 15–20 grams per day). Its safety during **pregnancy** (page 363) and breast feeding has not yet been established.

SLIPPERY ELM

Botanical names: *Ulmus rubra, Ulmus fulva*

Parts used and where grown

The slippery elm tree is native to North America, where it still grows primarily. The inner bark of the tree is the main part used for medicinal preparations.

Slippery elm has been used in connection with the following conditions (refer to the individual health concern for complete information):

Rating	Health Concerns
★☆☆	**Common cold/sore throat** (page 129)
	Cough (page 139)
	Crohn's disease (page 141)
	Gastritis (page 195)
	Gastroesophageal reflux disease (page 198) (GERD)
	Heartburn (page 260) (symptom relief)

Historical or traditional use (may or may not be supported by scientific studies)

Native Americans found innumerable medicinal and other uses for this tree. Canoes, baskets, and other household goods were made from the tree and its bark. Slippery elm was also used internally for conditions such as **sore throats** (page 129) and **diarrhea** (page 163).[1] As a poultice, it was considered a remedy for many inflammatory skin conditions.

Active constituents

The mucilage of slippery elm, found in the inner bark, gives it the soothing effect for which it is known.[2] In people with **heartburn** (page 260), the mucilage appears to act as a barrier against the damaging effects of acid on the esophagus. It may also have an anti-inflammatory effect locally in the stomach and intestines. This soothing effect may also extend to the throat. Clinical research, verifying these effects in humans has not been conducted.

How much is usually taken?

The dried inner bark in capsules or tablets, 800–1,000 mg three to four time per day, may be used. A tea can also be made by boiling ½–2 grams of the bark in 200 ml of water for ten to fifteen minutes, then cooled before drinking. Three to four cups a day can be used.[3]

Tincture, 5 ml three times per day, can be taken as well. Slippery elm is also an ingredient of some sore throat and cough lozenges.

Are there any side effects or interactions?

Slippery elm is quite safe. There are no known reasons to avoid its use during **pregnancy** (page 363) or breast feeding. However, because it is so mucilaginous, it may interfere with the absorption of medicine taken at the same time.

ST. JOHN'S WORT

Common name: Klamath weed
Botanical name: *Hypericum perforatum*

Parts used and where grown

St. John's wort is found in Europe and the United States. It is especially abundant in northern California and southern Oregon. The above-ground (aerial) parts of the plant are gathered during the flowering season.

St. John's wort has been used in connection with the following conditions (refer to the individual health concern for complete information):

Rating	Health Concerns
★★☆	**Depression** (page 145)
	Eczema (topical application) (page 177)
	Seasonal affective disorder (page 397)
	Somatoform disorders
★☆☆	**Anxiety** (page 30)
	Cold sores (page 90)
	Ear infections (recurrent) (page 383)
	HIV support (page 239)
	Infection (page 265)
	Menopause (page 311)
	Ulcerative colitis (page 433)
	Wound healing (page 319)

Historical or traditional use (may or may not be supported by scientific studies)

In ancient Greece, St. John's wort was used to treat many ailments, including sciatica and poisonous reptile bites. In Europe, St. John's wort was used by herbalists for the topical treatment of **wounds** (page 319) and **burns** (page 85). It is also a folk remedy for kidney and lung ailments as well as for **depression** (page 145).

St. John's Wort

Active constituents

The major constituents in St. John's wort include hypericin and other dianthrones, **flavonoids** (page 516), xanthones, and hyperforin.[1] While it was previously thought the antidepressant actions of St. John's wort were due to hypericin and the inhibition of the enzyme monoamine oxidase,[2] current research has challenged this belief, focusing on other constituents, such as hyperforin, and flavonoids.[3, 4, 5] Test tube studies suggest that St. John's wort extracts may exert their antidepressant actions by inhibiting the reuptake of the neurotransmitters serotonin, norepinephrine, and dopamine.[6] This action is possibly due to the constituent hyperforin.[7] St. John's wort is able to act as an antidepressant, by making more of these neurotransmitters available to the brain.

How much is usually taken?

The standard recommendation for mild to moderate depression is 500–1,050 mg of St. John's wort extract per day.[8, 9, 10] Results may be noted as early as two weeks. Length of use should be discussed with a healthcare professional. For more severe depression, higher intakes may be used, under the supervision of a healthcare professional.

Are there any side effects or interactions?

St. John's wort has a low incidence of side effects compared to prescription antidepressants. An adverse events profile of St. John's wort found that, of 14 controlled clinical trials, seven reported no adverse reactions, two had no information, and five reported a total of seven mild reactions.[11] Adverse effects reported included stomach upset, fatigue, itching, sleep disturbance, and skin rash. The rate of adverse reactions was always similar to that of the placebo. Additionally, in seven trials comparing St. John's wort with other antidepressants, the adverse reaction rate for St. John's wort was consistently lower than that of the antidepressant drugs with which it was compared.

St. John's wort can make the skin more sensitive to sunlight.[12] Therefore, fair-skinned people should be alert for any rashes or burns following exposure to the sun. Three cases of severe blistering and burns were reported in people taking St. John's wort internally or applying it topically and then being exposed to sunlight.[13] There is a case report of a woman experiencing neuropathy (nerve injury and pain) in sun-exposed skin areas after taking 500 mg of whole St. John's wort for four weeks.[14] Although St. John's wort has photosensi-

tizing properties, the severity of this reaction is not typical for people taking the herb.

People with a history of manic-depressive illness (**bipolar disorder** [page 61]) or a less severe condition known as hypomania, should avoid use of St. John's wort as it may trigger a manic episode.[15, 16, 17, 18]

There is a single case report in which ingestion of St. John's wort appeared to cause **high blood pressure** (page 246) in a 56-year-old man. The blood pressure returned to normal when the herb was discontinued.[19]

Caution: It is likely that there are many drug interactions with St. John's wort that have not yet been identified. St. John's wort stimulates a drug-metabolizing enzyme (cytochrome P450 3A4) that metabolizes at least 50% of the drugs on the market.[20] Consequently, St. John's wort could potentially interfere with a large number of medications. Individuals taking any medication should, therefore, consult with a physician before taking St. John's wort.

STEVIA

Common name: Sweetleaf
Botanical name: *Stevia rebaudiana*

Parts used and where grown

The stevia plant originally came from the rain forests of Brazil and Paraguay. It is now grown in those areas, as well as in Japan, Korea, Thailand, and China. It is most widely used as a non-sugar sweetener in food and drink, particularly because it does not appear to have any calories or affect on blood sugar like most natural sweeteners (like sugar or honey). The leaf is used in herbal preparations.

Historical or traditional use (may or may not be supported by scientific studies)

The native peoples in South America used stevia primarily as a sweetener, a practice adopted by European colonists. The indigenous tribes also used stevia to treat **diabetes** (page 152).[1] During World War II, stevia was grown in England as a sugar substitute. The greatest use of stevia as a sweetener today can be found in Japan.

Active constituents

Various glycosides, particularly stevioside, give stevia its sweetness. Stevioside is between 100 and 200 times sweeter than sugar. Early reports suggested that stevia might reduce blood sugar (and therefore potentially help with **diabetes** [page 152]),[2] although this has not been confirmed in all reports.[3]

How much is usually taken?
Less than 1 gram per day can be used effectively as a sweetener. Usually, the powdered herb is added directly to tea or to food.

Are there any side effects or interactions?
Extensive reviews of human and animal data indicate stevia to be safe.[4] Stevia accounts for nearly 40% of the sweetener market in Japan and is commonly used in various parts of South America.[5]

SUMA

Common name: Para todo
Botanical names: *Pfaffia paniculata, Hebanthe paniculata*

Parts used and where grown
Suma is a large shrubby vine native to the rain forests of the Amazon and other tropical regions of Latin America, including Brazil, Ecuador, Panama, Peru, and Venezuela.[1] The root of the plant is used medicinally.

Historical or traditional use (may or may not be supported by scientific studies)
Although suma is claimed as an ancient Brazilian folk remedy, no confirmation of that statement is found in the modern literature on medicinal plants. Advocates have claimed suma is an immune enhancer, an adaptogen (helps combat stress), and that it possesses anticancer activities. Test tube studies do indicate possible anti-tumor activity of suma constituents called pfaffosides. Suma has been marketed as Brazilian ginseng, though it is not an adaptogen (a substance that invigorates or strengthens the system) and is not related to **Asian ginseng** (page 630) or **American ginseng** (page 625). In light of the lack of known traditional use, and of modern research confirming health benefits, use of suma is not recommended for any condition at this time.[2]

Active constituents
Suma root contains several major constituents, including the nortriterpene pfaffic acid, six pfaffic acid

saponins (pfaffosides A–F), pterosterone, ecdysterone, and ecdysteroid glycosides.[3, 4] Although widespread claims are made for this herb for the treatment of **chronic fatigue** (page 111), stress, **menopausal symptoms** (page 311), and **diabetes** (page 152), they are not supported by current human clinical research. What little research has been done focuses on the plant's anti-tumor, anti-inflammatory, and aphrodisiac effects and has been completed only in test tubes or with animals.[5, 6, 7, 8]

How much is usually taken?
Suma root, 500 to 1,000 mg two to three times per day, can be used.[9]

Are there any side effects or interactions?
Very little is known about the adverse effects of this herb. Saponins, such as the pfaffosides found in this plant, can cause nausea when taken in excessive quantities. Occupational inhalation of suma dust has been known to trigger **asthma** (page 32).[10] The safety of this plant has not been established for use during **pregnancy** (page 363) or breast-feeding.

SUNDEW

Botanical names: *Drosera rotundifolia, Drosera ramentacea, Drosera intermedia, Drosera anglica*

Parts used and where grown
These carnivorous plants have their primary origins in East Africa and Madagascar but are cultivated throughout the world. The main species originally used in cough preparations in Germany, *D. rotundifolia, D. intermedia,* and *D. anglica,* are now rarely used currently due to threat of extinction. Instead, *D. ramentacea* and other *Drosera* species from Australia are employed. Herbal medicine preparations are made primarily from the roots, flowers, and fruit-like capsules.[1]

Sundew has been used in connection with the following conditions (refer to the individual health concern for complete information):

Rating	Health Concerns
★☆☆	**Coughs** (page 139) (particularly dry and irritating)

Historical or traditional use (may or may not be supported by scientific studies)

The historical use of sundew is similar to its use in modern herbal medicine. In 1685, Johann Schroder wrote in his book, *The Apothecary or a Treasure Chest of Valuable Medicines,* that sundew was a beneficial herb that "cures lung ailments and cures coughs." Sundew tea was specifically recommended in Europe by herbalists for dry **coughs** (page 139), **bronchitis** (page 80), whooping cough, **asthma** (page 32), and "bronchial cramps."[2]

Active constituents

Naphthaquinones are believed to give sundew the antispasmodic (or relief from coughing spasms) effect that has made it such a popular **cough** (page 139) remedy in Europe.[3] These naphthaquinones include plumbagin, ramentone, ramentaceon, and biramentaceone. Pharmacological studies show a clear antispasmodic effect in the respiratory tract.[4] One naphthaquinone was found in an animal study to be comparable to codeine in its ability to suppress the impulse to cough. This finding has not been repeated in human studies, however. Based on this effect, sundew is often referred to as an herbal antitussive (a substance capable of preventing or relieving coughing). Human trials have shown its value either alone or in combination with other herbs for the treatment of coughs associated with **bronchitis** (page 80), pharyngitis, laryngitis, and even whooping cough.[5]

How much is usually taken?

Adults and children older than 12 years of age may take ½–¾ teaspoons (3 grams) per day.[6] To prepare tea, boiling water is poured over ¼–½ teaspoon (1 to 2 grams) of finely cut sundew root and above-ground parts, then strained after steeping for ten minutes. One cup (250 ml) may be taken three to four times daily. In Europe, liquid preparations of sundew are often combined with **thyme** (page 752), another antitussive, in cough syrups for adults and children. A tincture of sundew, ⅛–¼ teaspoon (0.5 to 1.0 ml) three times per day, is also sometimes used.

Are there any side effects or interactions?

At the amounts listed above, sundew is thought to be safe.[7] Higher levels may lead to gastrointestinal irritation in some people. **Pregnant** (page 363) and breastfeeding women should avoid use of sundew.

SWEET ANNIE

Common names: Qinghao, sweet wormwood
Botanical name: *Artemisia annua*

Parts used and where grown

This inconspicuous herb originated in Europe and Asia and has since spread to North America. It is now a common weed around the world. The above ground parts of the plant are used medicinally.

Sweet Annie has been used in connection with the following conditions (refer to the individual health concern for complete information):

Rating	Health Concerns
★★☆	Malaria (isolated artemisinin, an experimental drug)
★☆☆	Fever **Infectious diarrhea** (page 163) **Intestinal parasites** (page 343)

Historical or traditional use (may or may not be supported by scientific studies)

Ancient Chinese medical texts dating from around 150 B.C. suggest the use of sweet Annie for people with **hemorrhoids** (page 219).[1] Other writings from A.D. 340 are the first known to mention sweet Annie as a treatment for people with fevers.[2] It has been used ever since for a variety of infections in Traditional Chinese Medicine.

Active constituents

Artemisinin, called qinghaosu in China where it was first discovered, is thought to account for the antimalarial activity of the plant.[3, 4] This compound is a sesquiterpene lactone and is believed to cause damage to the organisms that cause malaria inside the red blood cells they infect. Preliminary and double-blind trials, have shown that injections or oral use of artemisinin or similar compounds rapidly and effectively cure people with malaria.[5] A human trial has also found that artemisinin reduced mortality due to malaria by 50% compared with treatment with a standard quinoline anti-malarial drug.[6] Artemisinin-based drugs have not been studied for prevention of malaria. Test tube studies suggest artemisinin can kill other **parasites** (page 343) and bacteria,[7] possibly supporting the traditional notion of using it for parasitic infections of the gastrointestinal tract.

How much is usually taken?

Artemisinin-based drugs are not readily available in the United States or Europe and are still considered experimental. Sweet Annie cannot be substituted for artemisinin as a drug and cannot be used to treat people with malaria, a potentially lethal disease requiring immediate treatment. Traditionally, 3 grams of the powdered herb was taken each day.[8]

Are there any side effects or interactions?

No serious adverse effects have been seen in clinical trials with artemisinin.[9] The use of the whole herb as well as artemisinin may cause upset stomach, loose stools, abdominal pain, and occasional fever.

TEA TREE

Common name: Tea tree oil
Botanical name: *Melaleuca alternifolia*

Parts used and where grown

The tea tree grows in Australia and Asia. This tall evergreen tree has a white, spongy bark. The oil from the leaves is used medicinally.

Tea tree has been used in connection with the following conditions (refer to the individual health concern for complete information):

Rating	Health Concerns
★★★	**Acne** (page 4) (topical)
★★☆	**Athlete's foot** (page 42) (topical) Toenail fungal infection (topical)
★☆☆	**Chronic candidiasis** (page 109) (topical) **Halitosis** (page 209) (tea tree oil rinse or toothpaste) **HIV support** (page 239) **Infection** (page 265) (topical) **Vaginitis** (page 438) (topical) **Wound healing** (page 319) (oil, topical) **Yeast infection** (page 454) (topical)

Historical or traditional use (may or may not be supported by scientific studies)

Australian Aborigines used the leaves to treat cuts and skin infections. They would crush the leaves and apply them to the affected area. Captain James Cook and his crew named the tree "tea tree," using its leaves as a substitute for tea as well as to flavor beer. Australian soldiers participating in World War I were given tea tree oil as a disinfectant, leading to a high demand for its production.

Active constituents

The oil contains numerous chemicals known as terpenoids. Australian standards were established for the amount of one particular compound, terpinen-4-ol, which must make up at least 30% and preferably 40–50% of the oil for it to be medically useful. Another compound, cineole, should make up less than 15% and preferably 2.5% of the oil. The oil kills fungus and bacteria, including those resistant to some antibiotics.[1, 2] For common **acne** (page 4), a double-blind trial compared the topical use of 5% tea tree oil to 5% benzoyl peroxide.[3] Although the tea tree oil was slower and less potent in its action, it had far fewer side effects and was thus considered more effective overall.

A double-blind trial found that a 10% tea tree oil cream was as effective as anti-fungal medicine at improving *symptoms* associated with **athlete's foot** (page 42), though it was not more effective than a placebo for eliminating the fungal infection.[4] A double-blind trial found 100% tea tree oil applied topically was as effective as the anti-fungal medicine clotrimazole (Lotrimin, Mycelex) for people with fungus affecting the toe nails, a condition known as onychomycosis.[5] In another double-blind trial with toenail fungus sufferers, a combination of 5% tea tree oil and 2% butenafine (Mentax), a synthetic anti-fungal drug, in a cream proved more effective than an unspecified concentration of tea tree oil in cream alone.[6] The results are not entirely surprising, as the tea tree product alone was probably not at a sufficiently high enough concentration to be effective.

A preliminary trial found that rinsing the mouth with 1 tablespoon (15 ml) tea tree oil solution four times daily effectively treated thrush (oral yeast infections) in **AIDS** (page 239) patients.[7] Solutions containing no more than 5% should be used orally and should never be swallowed.

A concern for hospital staff and patients is the spread of the bacteria *Staphylococcus aureus*—sometimes referred to as a "staph infection." One small clinical trial found that use of a 4% tea tree oil nasal ointment as well as a 5% tea tree oil body wash was slightly more effective than standard drugs used to prevent the spread of the bacteria.[8]

How much is usually taken?

Oil at a strength of 70–100% should be applied moderately at least twice per day to the affected areas of skin or nail.[9] For topical treatment of **acne** (page 4), the oil is used at a dilution of 5–15%. Concentrations as strong as 40% may be used—with extreme caution and qualified advice—as vaginal douches. For thrush in immune-compromised adults, tea tree oil diluted to 5% or less is used in the amount of 1 tablespoon (15 ml) four times daily (as a mouth rinse). Tea tree oil should never be swallowed.

Are there any side effects or interactions?

While tea tree oil can be applied to minor cuts and scrapes, use caution for more extensive areas of broken skin or areas affected by rashes not due to fungus. The oil may burn if it gets into the eyes, nose, mouth, or other tender areas. Some people have allergic reactions, including rashes and itching, when applying tea tree oil.[10] For this reason, only a small amount should be applied when first using it. Tea tree oil should never be swallowed, as it may cause nerve damage and other problems.

THYME

Botanical name: *Thymus vulgaris*

Parts used and where grown

This fragrant plant is indigenous to the Mediterranean region of Europe and is extensively cultivated in the United States. The dried or partially dried leaves and flowering tops are used medicinally.

Thyme has been used in connection with the following conditions (refer to the individual health concern for complete information):

Rating	Health Concerns
★☆☆	**Bronchitis** (page 80)
	Chronic candidiasis (page 109)
	Cough (page 139)
	Halitosis (page 209) (oil of thyme rinse)
	Indigestion (page 260)
	Infection (page 265)
	Whooping cough

Historical or traditional use (may or may not be supported by scientific studies)

Other than its use as a spice, thyme has a long history of use in Europe for the treatment of dry, spasmodic **coughs** (page 139) as well as **bronchitis** (page 80).[1] Its antispasmodic actions have made it a common traditional recommendation for whooping cough. Thyme has also been used to ease an irritated gastrointestinal tract. The oil has been used to treat topical fungal infections and is also used in toothpastes to prevent **gingivitis** (page 203).

Active constituents

Many constituents in thyme team up to provide its antitussive (preventing and treating a cough), antispasmodic, and expectorant (thinning the mucus to allow for coughing out) actions. The primary constituents are the volatile oils, which include the phenols, thymol and carvacol.[2] These are complemented by the actions of **flavonoids** (page 516). Thyme, either alone or in combination with herbs such as **sundew** (page 749), continues to be one of the most commonly recommended herbs in Europe for the treatment of dry, spasmodic coughs as well as whooping cough.[3] Due to the low toxicity of the herb, it has become a favorite for treating coughs in small children.

How much is usually taken?

The German Commission E monograph recommends a cup (250 ml) of tea made from ¼–½ teaspoon (1–2 grams) of the herb taken several times daily as needed for a **cough** (page 139).[4] A fluid extract, ¼–¾ teaspoon (1–4 ml) three times per day, can also be used. Another alternative is to use a tincture, ⅓–1 teaspoon (2–6 ml) three times per day.

Are there any side effects or interactions?

Used as indicated above, thyme herbal preparations are generally safe. However, a spasmodic cough, particularly in a young child, may be dangerous and a healthcare professional should be consulted before deciding on the proper course of treatment. The use of thyme by **pregnant** (page 363) or breast-feeding women is considered to be safe. Thyme oil should be reserved for topical use, as internally it may lead to dizziness, vomiting, and breathing difficulties.[5] Some people may be sensitive to use of thyme oil topically on the skin or as a mouth rinse.

TURMERIC

Botanical name: *Curcuma longa*

Parts used and where grown

The vast majority of turmeric comes from India. Turmeric is one of the key ingredients in many curries, giving them color and flavor. The root and rhizome (underground stem) are used medicinally.

Turmeric has been used in connection with the following conditions (refer to the individual health concern for complete information):

Rating	Health Concerns
★★☆	**Indigestion** (page 260) **Rheumatoid arthritis** (page 387)
★☆☆	Anterior uveitis (chronic) **Atherosclerosis** (page 38) **Bursitis** (page 87) **Genital herpes** (page 200) (topical) **HIV support** (page 239) Inflammation **Low back pain** (page 293) **Osteoarthritis** (page 38) (in combination with **boswellia** [page 644], **ashwagandha** [page 629], and **zinc** [page 614]) **Pre- and post-surgery health** (page 357)

Historical or traditional use (may or may not be supported by scientific studies)

In Ayurvedic medicine, turmeric was prescribed for treatment of many conditions, including poor vision, rheumatic pains, and **coughs** (page 139), and to increase milk production. Native peoples of the Pacific sprinkled the dust on their shoulders during ceremonial dances and used it for numerous medical problems ranging from **constipation** (page 137) to skin diseases. Turmeric was used for numerous intestinal infections and ailments in Southeast Asia.

Active constituents

The active constituent is known as curcumin. It has been shown to have a wide range of therapeutic actions. First, it protects against free radical damage because it is a strong **antioxidant** (page 467).[1, 2] Second, it reduces inflammation by lowering histamine levels

and possibly by increasing production of natural cortisone by the adrenal glands.[3] Third, it protects the liver from a number of toxic compounds.[4] Fourth, it has been shown to reduce platelets from clumping together, which in turn improves circulation and may help protect against **atherosclerosis** (page 38).[5] There are also test-tube and animal studies showing a **cancer** (page 87)-preventing action of curcumin. In one of these studies, curcumin effectively inhibited metastasis (uncontrolled spread) of melanoma (skin cancer) cells.[6] This may be due to its antioxidant activity in the body. Curcumin inhibits **HIV** (page 239) in test tubes, though human trials are needed to determine if it has any usefulness for treating humans with this condition.[7]

A preliminary trial in people with **rheumatoid arthritis** (page 387) found curcumin to be somewhat useful for reducing inflammation and symptoms such as pain and stiffness.[8] A separate double-blind trial found that curcumin was superior to placebo or phenylbutazone (an NSAID) for alleviating post-surgical inflammation.[9]

While a double-blind trial has found turmeric helpful for people with **indigestion** (page 260),[10] results in people with stomach or intestinal **ulcers** (page 349) have not shown it to be superior to a placebo and have demonstrated it to be less effective than antacids.[11, 12]

Preliminary research indicates a possible benefit of oral curcumin supplementation (375 mg of turmeric extract with 95% curcuminoids three times daily for 12 weeks) for chronic anterior uveitis (inflammation of the iris and middle coat of the eyeball).[13]

How much is usually taken?

Turmeric extracts standardized at 90 to 95% curcumin can be taken in the amount of 250 to 500 mg three times per day.[14] Tincture, 0.5–1.5 ml three times per day, is sometimes recommended.

Are there any side effects or interactions?

Used in the recommended amounts, turmeric is generally safe. It has been used in large quantities as a condiment with no adverse reactions. Some herbal books recommend not taking high amounts of turmeric during **pregnancy** (page 363) as it may cause uterine contractions and people with **gallstones** (page 193) or obstruction of bile passages should consult their healthcare practitioner before using turmeric.[15, 16]

Turmeric

TYLOPHORA

Common name: Indian ipecac
Botanical names: *Tylophora indica, Tylophora asthmatica*

Parts used and where grown

Tylophora is a perennial climbing plant native to the plains, forests, and hills of southern and eastern India. The portions of the plant used medicinally are the leaves and root.[1]

Tylophora has been used in connection with the following conditions (refer to the individual health concern for complete information):

Rating	Health Concerns
★★☆	**Asthma** (page 32)
★☆☆	**Diarrhea** (page 163) **Hay fever** (page 211)

Historical or traditional use (may or may not be supported by scientific studies)

This plant has been traditionally used as a folk remedy in certain regions of India for the treatment of bronchial **asthma** (page 32), **bronchitis** (page 80), rheumatism, and dermatitis. In the latter half of the 19th century, it was called Indian ipecacuahna, as the roots of the plant have often been employed as an effective substitute for ipecac. The use to induce vomiting led to tylophora's inclusion in the Bengal Pharmacopoeia of 1884.[2]

Active constituents

The major constituent in tylophora is the alkaloid tylophorine. Laboratory research has shown this isolated plant extract exerts a strong anti-inflammatory action.[3] Test tube studies suggest that tylophorine is able to interfere with the action of mast cells, which are key components in the process of inflammation.[4] These actions seem to support tylophora's traditional use as an anti-asthmatic and antiallergic medication by Ayurvedic practitioners.

These historical and laboratory findings have been supported by several human clinical trials using differing preparations of tylophora, including the crude leaf, tincture, and capsule. One clinical trial with **asthma** (page 32) sufferers, found that tylophora leaf (150 mg of the leaf by weight) chewed and swallowed daily in the early morning for six days led to moderate to complete relief of their asthma symptoms.[5] In a follow-up trial with asthma patients, an alcoholic extract of crude tylophora leaves in 1 gram of glucose had comparable effects to that of chewing the crude leaf.[6] Another trial found similar success in reducing asthma symptoms using a tylophora leaf powder (350 mg per day.)[7] However, the tylophora was not as effective as a standard asthma drug combination. One double-blind trial failed to show any effect on asthma for tylophora.[8]

How much is usually taken?

Tylophora leaf—200 to 400 mg of the dried leaf per day or 1 to 2 ml of tincture per day—can be used to treat **asthma** (page 32).[9]

Are there any side effects or interactions?

Patients using tylophora may experience temporary nausea and vomiting, soreness of the mouth, and loss of taste for salt, particularly with the fresh leaf and tincture.[10, 11, 12] The herb's safety for use during **pregnancy** (page 363) and breast-feeding has not been established. People with asthma should be closely monitored by a qualified healthcare professional.

USNEA

Common name: Old man's beard
Botanical name: *Usnea barbata*

Parts used and where grown

Usnea, also known as old man's beard, is not a plant but a lichen—a symbiotic relationship between an algae and a fungus. The entire lichen is used medicinally. Usnea looks like long, fuzzy strings hanging from trees in the forests of North America and Europe, where it grows.

Usnea has been used in connection with the following conditions (refer to the individual health concern for complete information):

Rating	Health Concerns
★☆☆	**Common cold/sore throat** (page 129) **Cough** (page 139) **Infection** (page 265) **Pap smear (abnormal)** (page 3)

Tylophora

Historical or traditional use (may or may not be supported by scientific studies)

Due to its bitter taste, usnea stimulates digestion and was historically used by herbalists to treat **indigestion** (page 260). It was also reportedly used over 3,000 years ago in ancient Egypt, Greece, and China to treat unspecified infections.[1]

Active constituents

Usnic acid gives usnea its bitter taste and also acts as an antibiotic in test tube studies.[2] Test tube studies have suggested an anti-**cancer** (page 87) activity for usnic acid. However, this action has not been sufficient to warrant further investigation in humans.[3] Usnea also contains mucilage, which may be helpful in easing irritating **coughs** (page 139). Again, this has not been studied in humans.

How much is usually taken?

Usnea, 100 mg three times per day, can be taken in capsules.[4] Tincture, 3–4 ml three times per day, can also be used.

Are there any side effects or interactions?

There are no known side effects of usnea. It is considered safe for use in children. The safety of usnea during **pregnancy** (page 363) and breast-feeding has not been established.

UVA URSI

Common name: Bearberry
Botanical name: *Arctostaphylos uva-ursi*

Parts used and where grown

The uva ursi plant is found in colder, northern climates. It has red flowers and red berries, which bears like to eat. The leaf is used medicinally.

Uva ursi has been used in connection with the following conditions (refer to the individual health concern for complete information):

Rating	Health Concerns
★☆☆	Urinary tract infection (page 436)

Historical or traditional use (may or may not be supported by scientific studies)

The leaves and berries were used by numerous indigenous people from northern latitudes. Combined with tobacco, Native Americans sometimes smoked uva ursi. It was also used as a beverage tea in some places in Russia. The berries were considered beneficial as a **weight-loss** (page 446) aid. It was found in wide use for **infections** (page 265) of all parts of the body because of its astringent, or "drying," action.

Active constituents

The glycoside arbutin is the main active constituent in uva ursi and comprises up to 10% of the plant by weight. Hydroquinone derived from arbutin and *methyl*arbutin is a powerful anti-bacterial agent and is thought to be responsible for uva ursi's ability to treat **urinary tract infections** (page 436). It is believed to be most effective as a urinary tract antiseptic agent if the urine is alkaline.[1] No human trials have been published confirming the effectiveness of uva ursi in people with urinary tract infections.

How much is usually taken?

The German Commission E monograph suggests ½–¾ teaspoon (3 grams) of uva ursi steeped in about 5 ounces (150 ml) of boiling water and drunk as an infusion three to four times daily.[2] For alcohol-based tinctures, 1 teaspoon (5 ml) three times per day can be used. Standardized extracts in capsules or tablets (containing 20% arbutin), 700–1,000 mg three times per day, can also be taken. Use of uva ursi should be limited to no more than 14 days. To ensure alkaline urine, about 1½ teaspoons (6–8 grams) of sodium bicarbonate (baking soda) mixed in a glass of water can be taken. Baking soda should also not be taken for more than 14 days. People with **high blood pressure** (page 246) should not take baking soda. Uva ursi should not be used to treat an **infection** (page 265) without first consulting a physician.

Are there any side effects or interactions?

Due to the high tannin content in uva ursi, some people may experience cramping, nausea, or vomiting. It is also not recommended for long-term use. Uva ursi should not be taken by **pregnant** (page 363) or breast-feeding women and should be used in young children only with the guidance of a healthcare professional.

VALERIAN

Botanical name: *Valeriana officinalis*

Parts used and where grown

Although valerian grows wild all over Europe, most of the valerian used for medicinal extracts is cultivated. The root is used in herbal medicine preparations.

Valerian has been used in connection with the following conditions (refer to the individual health concern for complete information):

Rating	Health Concerns
★★★	**Insomnia** (page 270)
★★☆	**Anxiety** (page 30) (in combination with passion flower)
★☆☆	**Pain** (page 338)

Historical or traditional use (may or may not be supported by scientific studies)

The Greek physician Dioscorides reportedly recommended valerian for a host of medical issues, including digestive problems, nausea, liver problems, and even urinary tract disorders. Use of valerian for **insomnia** (page 270) and nervous conditions has been common for many centuries. By the 18th century, it was an accepted sedative and was also used for nervous disorders associated with a restless digestive tract.

Active constituents

Valerian root contains many different constituents, including volatile oils that appear to contribute to the sedating properties of the herb. Central nervous system sedation is regulated by receptors in the brain known as GABA-A receptors. According to test tube studies, valerian may weakly bind to these receptors to exert a sedating action.[1] This might explain why valerian may help some people deal with stress more effectively.[2]

Double-blind trials have found that valerian is an effective treatment for people with mild to moderately severe insomnia.[3, 4] Generally, valerian makes sleep more restful as well as making the transition to sleep easier, but does not tend to increase total time slept, according to these studies. Two trials have also found that a combination with **lemon balm** (page 701) is effective in improving quality of sleep and in treating **insomnia** (page 270).[5, 6]

How much is usually taken?

For **insomnia** (page 270), some doctors suggest 300–500 mg of a concentrated valerian root herbal extract (standardized to at least 0.5% volatile oils) in capsules or tablets 30 to 60 minutes before bedtime.[7] Non-standardized dried root products, 1.5 to 2 grams 30 to 60 minutes before bedtime, may also be used. As an alcohol-based tincture, 5 ml can be taken before bedtime. Combination products with **lemon balm** (page 701), **hops** (page 690), **passion flower** (page 722), and scullcap can also be used.

Are there any side effects or interactions?

Research suggests that valerian does not impair one's ability to drive or operate machinery.[8] There is one case reported of a man experiencing severe cardiac symptoms that may have been due to withdrawing from valerian. This man abruptly discontinued taking valerian, after having used 5–20 times the recommended amount "for many years."[9] However, when taken at recommended amounts, valerian supplementation does not lead to addiction or dependence. In the case of an 18-year old college student who tried to kill herself by ingesting approximately 20,000 mg of valerian root (approximately 40–50 times the recommended amount), the only symptoms reported were fatigue, abdominal pain, and a mild tremor of the hands and feet.[10] Valerian does not appear to impair reaction time, alertness, or concentration the morning after use.[11] There are no known reasons to avoid valerian during **pregnancy** (page 363) or breast-feeding.

VERVAIN

Botanical name: *Verbena officinalis*

Parts used and where grown

The most commonly used species is European vervain *(Verbena officinalis)*, though blue vervain *(V. hastata)* and *V. macdougalii*, among others, are probably interchangeable. *V. officinalis* is native to Europe, Asia, and Africa and has spread to North America. Other medicinal species are native to North America. The leaf and flower are used in herbal medicine.

Valerian

Vervain has been used in connection with the following conditions (refer to the individual health concern for complete information):

Rating	Health Concerns
★★☆	**Colic** (page 121) (in combination with **chamomile** [page 656], **licorice** [page 702], **fennel** [page 676], and **lemon balm** [page 701])
★☆☆	**Depression** (page 145) **Dysmenorrhea** (page 171) (painful menstruation) **Indigestion** (page 260) **Sinusitis** (page 407) (in combination with **gentian** [page 680] root, primrose flowers, sorrel herb, and elder flowers)

Historical or traditional use (may or may not be supported by scientific studies)

Due to its bitter taste, herbalists used vervain to improve digestion. Vervain was also used to treat people with **depression** (page 145) and spastic pains in the gastrointestinal tract, as a mild diaphoretic (to induce sweating and promote mild fevers), and for all manner of female reproductive system problems when associated with melancholy or anxiety.[1] Early 20th century Eclectic physicians (doctors who recommended herbal medicines) in the United States felt vervain might be helpful for mild **digestive problems** (page 260).[2] Vervain also has a reputation as a traditional remedy for stimulating production of breast milk.[3]

Active constituents

The active constituents of vervain have not been thoroughly demonstrated. Glycosides, such as verbenalin and aucubin, and a volatile oil may all contribute to its activity.[4] No human studies have documented the use of this herb for any condition.

How much is usually taken?

A tea of vervain leaves and flowers is prepared by adding 1–2 teaspoons (2–4 grams) to a pint (500 ml) of hot water which is left to steep, covered, for 10–15 minutes.[5] Three cups (750 ml) per day are typically recommended by doctors. The taste of the tea is fairly disagreeable, therefore, most people prefer a tincture. Tincture, 1–2 teaspoons (5–10 ml) three times per day, is also suggested.[6]

Are there any side effects or interactions?

No adverse effects of vervain have been reported. Vervain should be avoided during **pregnancy** (page 363).[7] Although, traditionally, its use was during the last two weeks of pregnancy to facilitate labor. Vervain should be used during pregnancy only under the guidance of a healthcare professional experienced in herbal medicine.

VITEX

Common names: Chaste tree, monk's pepper
Botanical name: *Vitex agnus-castus*

Parts used and where grown

Vitex grows in Mediterranean countries and central Asia. The dried fruit, which has a pepper-like aroma and flavor, is used in herbal medicine preparations.

Vitex has been used in connection with the following conditions (refer to the individual health concern for complete information):

Rating	Health Concerns
★★★	**Premenstrual syndrome** (page 368)
★★☆	**Female infertility** (page 187) **Fibrocystic breast disease** (page 189)
★☆☆	**Acne** (page 6) (associated with menstrual cycle) **Amenorrhea** (page 22) **Dysmenorrhea** (page 171) **Endometriosis** (page 182) **Menorrhagia** (page 314) (heavy menstruation) **Pregnancy and postpartum support** (page 363)

Historical or traditional use (may or may not be supported by scientific studies)

Hippocrates, Dioscorides, and Theophrastus mention the use of vitex for a wide variety of conditions, including hemorrhage following childbirth and assisting with the "passing of afterbirth." Decoctions of the fruit and plant were also used in sitz baths for diseases of the uterus. In addition, vitex was believed to suppress libido and inspire chastity, which explains one of its common names, chaste tree.

Active constituents

Vitex contains several different constituents, including flavonoids, iridoid glycosides, and terpenoids. The

Vitex

whole fruit extract, rather than one of its individual constituents, appears to be necessary for the medicinal activity of vitex.[1] Vitex does not contain hormones. The benefits of vitex stem from its actions upon the pituitary gland—specifically on the production of a hormone called luteinizing hormone (LH). This indirectly increases **progesterone** (page 577) production and helps regulate the menstrual cycle. Vitex also keeps prolactin secretion in check.[2, 3] The ability to decrease mildly elevated prolactin levels may benefit some **infertile women** (page 187) as well as some women with breast tenderness associated with **premenstrual syndrome** (page 368) (PMS).

A controlled clinical trial found that women taking 20 mg per day of a concentrated vitex extract for three menstrual cycles had a significant reduction in symptoms of PMS, including irritability, mood swings, headache, and breast tenderness.[4] Another double-blind trial found that women taking vitex had slightly greater relief from symptoms of PMS, including breast tenderness, cramping, and headaches, than those taking **vitamin B₆** (page 600).[5] These trials support the findings of preliminary vitex trials for women with PMS.[6, 7] Vitex (32.4 mg per day), in combination with some homeopathic remedies, has also been found in a double-blind trial to successfully treat breast tenderness (also called mastalgia).[8]

A review of other trials and case reports suggests there is at least preliminary support that vitex should be considered for women with irregular periods, infertility, and mildly elevated prolactin levels.[9] Double-blind trials have confirmed the effectiveness of vitex at lowering mildly elevated prolactin levels in women.[10] According to one small trial, **acne** (page 6) associated with PMS, may also be reduced using vitex.[11]

How much is usually taken?

The German Commission E monograph recommends a daily intake—30–40 mg of the dried herb—in capsules or in liquid preparations.[12] Vitex is typically taken once in the morning with liquid for several months consecutively.

With its emphasis on long-term balancing of a woman's hormonal system, vitex is not a fast-acting herb and is unlikely to give immediate relief to the discomfort associated with PMS. For **premenstrual syndrome** (page 368), frequent or heavy periods, vitex can be used continuously for four to six months. **Infertile women** (page 187) with **amenorrhea** (page 22) (lack of menstruation) can remain on vitex for 12 to 18 months, unless **pregnancy** (page 363) occurs during treatment.

Are there any side effects or interactions?

Side effects may include minor stomach upset and a mild skin rash with itching. Vitex is not recommended for use during **pregnancy** (page 363) and should not be used concurrently with hormone therapy (e.g., estrogen, **progesterone** [page 577]).

WILD CHERRY

Botanical name: *Prunus serotina*

Parts used and where grown

Although native to North America, wild cherry trees now grow in many other countries. The bark of the wild cherry tree is used for medicinal preparations.

Wild cherry has been used in connection with the following conditions (refer to the individual health concern for complete information):

Rating	Health Concerns
★☆☆	**Chronic obstructive pulmonary disease** (page 114) (COPD) **Cough** (page 139)

Historical or traditional use (may or may not be supported by scientific studies)

Wild cherry syrup has been used traditionally by herbalists to treat **coughs** (page 139) and other lung problems. It has also been used to treat **diarrhea** (page 163) and to relieve pain.[1]

Active constituents

Wild cherry bark contains cyanogenic glycosides, particularly prunasin. These glycosides, once broken apart in the body, act to relieve choughs by quelling spasms in the smooth muscles lining bronchioles.[2] Although wild cherry is a commonly used ingredient in cough syrups, there are no published clinical trials in humans to support its use for this indication.

How much is usually taken?

Wild cherry tincture or syrup, 2–4 ml three to four times per day, is sometimes recommended for coughs.[3]

Are there any side effects or interactions?

Very large amounts (several times the recommended amount above) of wild cherry pose the theoretical risk

Vitex

of causing cyanide poisoning, due to hydrocyanic acid.[4] However, this has not been reported in clinical practice. The safety of wild cherry during **pregnancy** (page 363) has also not been established.

WILD INDIGO

Botanical name: *Baptisia tinctoria*

Parts used and where grown
The plant is native to the midwestern United States and continues to grow primarily in this region. The root of wild indigo is used medicinally.

Wild indigo has been used in connection with the following conditions (refer to the individual health concern for complete information):

Rating	Health Concerns
★☆☆	**Common cold/sore throat** (page 129)
	Infection (page 265)
	Influenza (page 269)

Historical or traditional use (may or may not be supported by scientific studies)
Historically, the root of wild indigo was used to make blue dye. It was also used by European herbalists to treat **ulcers** (page 349) and several types of infections, including those affecting the mouth and gums, lymph nodes, and throat.[1]

Active constituents
According to test tube experiments, the polysaccharides and proteins in wild indigo are believed to stimulate the **immune system** (page 255).[2] This might account for its role against the **common cold** (page 129) and **flu** (page 269). Wild indigo is rarely used alone and is a part of a popular European product for colds and flu that combines the herb with **echinacea** (page 669) and thuja.[3] The root also contains alkaloids, which may contribute to its medicinal actions.

How much is usually taken?
Wild indigo is generally used in combination with herbs such as **echinacea** (page 669) and thuja. A tincture, 1–2 ml three times per day, is sometimes used. When taking the whole herb, 500–1,000 mg is taken as a tea three times daily.[4]

Are there any side effects or interactions?
Higher intakes (over 30 grams per day) of wild indigo can cause nausea and vomiting.[5] Long-term use (more than two to three weeks) is not recommended. The safety of wild indigo during **pregnancy** (page 363) and breast-feeding has only been established in a product combining it with echinacea and thuja. Used according to the manufacturer's recommendations, the combination delivers 90 mg of wild indigo per day.

WILD YAM

Botanical name: *Dioscorea villosa*

Parts used and where grown
Wild yam plants are found across the midwestern and eastern United States, Latin America (especially Mexico), and Asia. Several different species exist. All of which possess similar constituents and properties. The root is used medicinally.

Wild yam has been used in connection with the following conditions (refer to the individual health concern for complete information):

Rating	Health Concerns
★☆☆	**High cholesterol** (page 223)
	Menopause (page 311)

Historical or traditional use (may or may not be supported by scientific studies)
Wild yam has been used by herbalists as an expectorant for people with **coughs** (page 139). It was also used for **gastrointestinal upset** (page 195), nerve pain, and **morning sickness** (page 320).[1] Eventually, it was discovered that the saponins from wild yam could be converted industrially into cortisone, estrogens, and **progesterone** (page 577)-like compounds. Wild yam and other plants with similar constituents continue to be a source for these drugs.

Active constituents
The steroidal saponins (such as diosgenin) account for some of the activity of wild yam. Another compound, dioscoretine, has been shown in animal studies to lower blood sugar levels.[2] An extract of wild yam was also found in a clinical trial to have **antioxidant** (page 467) properties and raised HDL, the "good," **cholesterol** (page 223) in elderly adults.[3]

Wild Yam

Contrary to popular claims, wild yam roots do not contain and are not converted into **progesterone** (page 577) or dehydroepiandrosterone (**DHEA** [page 503]) in the body.[4, 5] Pharmaceutical progesterone is made from wild yam using a chemical conversion process. This can lead to confusion—while wild yam can be a source of progesterone, it cannot be used without this pharmaceutical conversion, which cannot be duplicated by the body. Women who require progesterone should consult with their physician and not rely on wild yam supplements.

How much is usually taken?
Up to 2–3 ml of wild yam tincture can be taken three to four times per day. Alternatively, 1 gram of dried, powdered root can be taken three times each day.[6]

Are there any side effects or interactions?
Some people may experience nausea or vomiting when taking large amounts of wild yam (several times the amounts listed above). The safety of wild yam during **pregnancy** (page 363) and breast feeding has not been established.

WILLOW

Common name: Willow bark
Botanical name: *Salix alba*

Parts used and where grown
The willow tree grows primarily in central and southern Europe, although it is also found in North America. The bark is used to make herbal extracts.

Willow has been used in connection with the following conditions (refer to the individual health concern for complete information):

Rating	Health Concerns
★★☆	**Low back pain** (page 293) **Osteoarthritis** (page 328)
★☆☆	**Bursitis** (page 87) Fever **Pain** (page 338) **Rheumatoid arthritis** (page 387)

Historical or traditional use (may or may not be supported by scientific studies)
Willow bark was used traditionally by herbalists for fever, headache, **pain** (page 338), and rheumatic complaints.[1] In the late 19th century, the constituent sali-cylic acid was isolated from willow bark and went on to become the model for the development of aspirin (acetylsalicylic acid).[2]

Active constituents
The glycoside salicin, from which the body can split off salicylic acid, is thought to be the source of the anti-inflammatory and pain-relieving actions of willow.[3] The analgesic actions of willow are typically slow to develop but may last longer than the effects of standard aspirin products. One trial has found that a combination herbal product including 100 mg willow bark taken for two months improved functioning via pain relief in people with **osteoarthritis** (page 328).[4] Another trial found that 1360 mg of willow bark extract per day (delivering 240 mg of salicin) for two weeks was somewhat effective in treating pain associated with knee and/or hip osteoarthritis.[5] Use of high amounts of willow bark extract may also help people with low back pain. One four-week trial found 240 mg of salicin from a willow extract was effective in reducing exacerbations of low back pain.[6]

How much is usually taken?
Willow extracts standardized for salicin content are available. The commonly recommended intake of salicin has been 60–120 mg per day.[7] However, newer studies suggest a higher salicin intake of 240 mg per day may be more effective for treating pain.[8] A willow tea can be prepared from ¼–½ teaspoon (1–2 grams) of bark boiled in about 7 ounces (200 ml) of water for ten minutes. Five or more cups (1250 ml) of this tea can be drunk per day. Tincture, 1–1½ teaspoons (5–8 ml) three times per day, is also occasionally used.

Are there any side effects or interactions?
As with aspirin, some people may experience stomach upset from taking willow. Although such symptoms are less likely from willow than from aspirin, people with **ulcers** (page 349) and **gastritis** (page 195) should, nevertheless, avoid this herb.[9] Again, as with aspirin, willow should not be used to treat fevers in children since it may cause Reye's syndrome.

WITCH HAZEL

Botanical name: *Hamamelis virginiana*

Parts used and where grown
Although native to North America, witch hazel now also grows in Europe. The leaves and bark of the tree are used in herbal medicine.

Witch hazel has been used in connection with the following conditions (refer to the individual health concern for complete information):

Rating	Health Concerns
★★☆	**Cold sores** (page 119) (topical) **Eczema** (page 177) (topical) **Hemorrhoids** (page 219) (topical)
★☆☆	**Canker sores** (page 90) **Crohn's disease** (page 141) **Menorrhagia** (page 314) **Skin ulcers** (page 409) (topical) **Varicose veins** (page 440) **Wound healing** (page 319) (topical)

Historical or traditional use (may or may not be supported by scientific studies)

Native Americans used poultices of witch hazel leaves and bark to treat **hemorrhoids** (page 219), **wounds** (page 319), painful tumors, insect bites, and skin ulcers.[1]

Active constituents

Tannins and volatile oils are the main active constituents in witch hazel. These constituents contribute to the strong astringent effect of witch hazel. Pharmacological studies have suggested that witch hazel strengthens veins and is anti-inflammatory.[2, 3] Topical creams are currently used in Europe to treat inflammatory skin conditions, such as **eczema** (page 177). One double-blind trial found that a topical witch hazel ointment (applied four times per day) was as effective as the topical anti-inflammatory drug bufexamac for people with eczema.[4] However, another trial found that witch hazel was no better than a placebo when compared to hydrocortisone for people with eczema.[5] Witch hazel is approved in Germany for relief of local mouth inflammations such as **canker sores** (page 90).

How much is usually taken?

A tea of witch hazel can be made by steeping 2–3 grams of the leaves or bark in 150 ml of boiled water for 10 to 15 minutes.[6] The tea can be drunk two to three times daily between meals. A tincture, 2–4 ml three times per day, is also occasionally used.

In combination with warm, moist compresses, witch hazel extracts can be applied liberally at least twice each day (in the morning and at bedtime) on **hemorrhoids** (page 219). For other skin problems, ointment or cream can be applied three or four times a day, or as needed.[7]

Are there any side effects or interactions?

With internal use, witch hazel may cause stomach irritation and cramping.[8] In particular, it should not be taken internally in combination with medications, supplements or herbs containing alkaloids, as the tannins in witch hazel may interfere with absorption.

There are no known restrictions to the internal use of witch hazel during **pregnancy** (page 363) or breastfeeding.[9]

WOOD BETONY

Common name: Betony, lousewort
Botanical name: *Stachys officinalis*

Parts used and where grown

Native to Europe, wood betony is now planted in many parts of the world with temperate climates. The primary portions of the plant that are used as medicine are the leaves and flowers, though historically the root has also been used. There are many similar species originating from Eurasia, including *Stachys sieboldii* (Chinese artichoke, kan lu) and *S. atherocalyx* (hedge nettle).

Wood betony has been used in connection with the following conditions (refer to the individual health concern for complete information):

Rating	Health Concerns
★☆☆	**Anxiety** (page 30) **Gastritis** (page 195) **Shingles** (page 401) **Sinusitis** (page 407) **Stress** (page 415)

Historical or traditional use (may or may not be supported by scientific studies)

Wood betony was used in European folk herbalism as a remedy for respiratory tract inflammation, **heartburn** (page 260), urinary tract inflammation, **varicose veins** (page 440), **intestinal worm infestations** (page 343), and failure to thrive.[1] It was considered a calming remedy and was used for headaches as well as some forms of neuralgia, including **shingles** (page 401).[2]

Active constituents

The active constituents of wood betony have not been clearly identified. The tannins, alkaloids, glycosides, and volatile oil found in this plant and its cousins may all contribute to its activity. Almost no research has been conducted on wood betony. Some Russian research in humans apparently suggests it may promote lactation, though the details of these studies are not readily available.[3, 4]

How much is usually taken?

A tea of wood betony can be made by steeping 1 to 2 tsp dried leaf and flower in a cup of water for 15 minutes. One or two cups of this tea can be drunk per day.[5] Though generally better between meals, it can be taken with food for convenience or if there is any gastrointestinal upset.

Are there any side effects or interactions?

There are no known adverse effects from use of wood betony other than occasional mild gastrointestinal upset. Its safety in **pregnancy** (page 363) and breast-feeding is generally unknown, though as noted above it has been studied in Russia as a way to increase lactation.

WORMWOOD

Botanical name: *Artemisia absinthium*

Parts used and where grown

The wormwood shrub grows wild in Europe, North Africa, and western Asia. It is now cultivated in North America as well. The leaves and flowers, and the oil obtained from them, are all used in herbal medicine.

Wormwood has been used in connection with the following conditions (refer to the individual health concern for complete information):

Rating	Health Concerns
★★☆	**Irritable bowel syndrome** (page 280) (in combination with **ginger** [page 680], **bupleurum** [page 647], **schisandra** [page 744], dan shen, and other extracts)
★☆☆	Gallbladder inflammation **Indigestion** (page 260) **Parasites** (page 343) Poor appetite

Historical or traditional use (may or may not be supported by scientific studies)

Wormwood is perhaps best known because of the use of its oil to prepare certain alcoholic beverages, most notably vermouth and absinthe. Absinthe, popular in the 19th century in Europe, caused several cases of brain damage and even death and was banned in most places in the early 20th century.[1] Wormwood oil continues to be used as a flavoring agent for foods, although in much smaller amounts than were found in absinthe.

As a traditional medicine, wormwood was used by herbalists as a bitter to improve digestion, to fight worm infestations, and to stimulate menstruation.[2] It was also regarded as a useful remedy for liver and gallbladder problems.

Active constituents

The aromatic oil of wormwood contains the toxins thujone and isothujone. Very little of this oil is present in ordinary wormwood teas or tinctures.[3] Also existent in the plant are strong bitter agents known as absinthin and anabsinthin. These stimulate digestive and gallbladder function.[4] Modern herbal medicine rarely uses wormwood alone. It is typically combined with herbs such as **peppermint** (page 726) or **caraway** (page 651) to treat **heartburn** (page 260) and even **irritable bowel syndrome** (page 280). Clinical trials are lacking to support the use of wormwood for any indication, however.

How much is usually taken?

A wormwood tea can be made by adding ½ to 1 teaspoon (2.5 to 5 grams) of the herb to 1 cup (250 ml) of boiling water, then steeping for ten to fifteen minutes.[5] Many doctors recommend drinking three cups (750 ml) each day. Tincture, 10–20 drops in water, can be taken ten to fifteen minutes before each meal.[6] Either preparation should not be used consecutively for more than four weeks.[7]

Are there any side effects or interactions?

Longer-term use (over four weeks) or intake of amounts higher than those recommended can cause nausea, vomiting, **insomnia** (page 270), restlessness, vertigo, tremors, and seizures.[8] Thujone-containing oil or alcoholic beverages (absinthe) made with the oil is strictly inadvisable—the oil is addictive and may cause brain damage, seizures, and even death.[9] Short-term use (two to four weeks) of a wormwood tea or tincture has not resulted in any reports of significant side effects. One study found there were no side effects when using less than 1 ml tincture three times per day for as long as nine months to promote digestive function.[10] Nevertheless, consult with a healthcare professional knowledgeable in herbal medicine before taking wormwood. Wormwood is not recommended during **pregnancy** (page 363) and breast-feeding.[11]

YARROW

Botanical name: *Achillea millefolium*

Parts used and where grown

This prolific plant grows in Europe, North America, and Asia. A number of species are used as garden ornamentals. The flowering tops of yarrow are used in herbal medicine.

Yarrow has been used in connection with the following conditions (refer to the individual health concern for complete information):

Rating	Health Concerns
★☆☆	**Amenorrhea** (page 22)
	Colic (page 121)
	Common cold/sore throat (page 129)
	Crohn's disease (page 141)
	Indigestion and heartburn (page 260)
	Inflammation
	Pap smear (abnormal) (page 3)
	Premenstrual syndrome (page 368)
	Ulcerative colitis (page 433)

Historical or traditional use (may or may not be supported by scientific studies)

Traditional herbal medicine has used yarrow in three broad categories.[1] First, it was used to help stop minor bleeding and to treat **wounds** (page 319). Second, it was used to treat inflammation in a number of conditions, especially in the intestinal and female reproductive tracts. Third, it was utilized as a mild sedative. Some or all of these historical uses occurred in Europe, China, and India. The ancient Chinese fortune-telling system known as the I Ching first used dried yarrow stems, then later replaced them with coins.[2]

Active constituents

A number of chemicals may contribute to yarrow's actions. The volatile oil, which is rich in sesquiterpene lactones, and alkamides has been found to have anti-inflammatory properties in test tube studies.[3, 4] Animal studies have shown this herb can reduce smooth muscle spasms, which might further explain its usefulness in gastrointestinal conditions.[5] The alkaloid obtained from yarrow, known as achilletin, reportedly stops bleeding in animals.[6] No human clinical studies have confirmed the traditional uses of yarrow.

How much is usually taken?

The German Commission E monograph suggests approximately 1 teaspoon (4.5 grams) of yarrow daily or 3 teaspoons (15 ml) of the fresh pressed juice.[7] A tea can be prepared by steeping 1–2 teaspoons (5–10 grams) of yarrow in 1 cup (250 ml) boiling water for ten to fifteen minutes. Three cups (750 ml) a day can be taken. A tincture, ½–¾ teaspoon (3–4 ml) three times per day, can be taken. The tea, or cloths dipped in the tea, can be used topically as needed for minor skin injuries.

Are there any side effects or interactions?

People who take yarrow may occasionally develop an allergy or rash.[8] Yarrow might increase sensitivity to sunlight. Yarrow should not be used to treat large, deep, or infected **wounds** (page 319), all of which require medical attention. Yarrow is not recommended during **pregnancy** (page 363) or breast-feeding.[9]

YELLOW DOCK

Botanical name: *Rumex crispus*

Parts used and where grown

Yellow dock is found in many places throughout North America. The root of the plant is used in herbal medicine.

Yellow dock has been used in connection with the following conditions (refer to the individual health concern for complete information):

Rating	Health Concerns
★☆☆	**Poor digestion** (page 260)
	Skin conditions

Historical or traditional use (may or may not be supported by scientific studies)

Yellow dock has a long history of use as an alterative. Alterative herbs have nonspecific effects on the gastrointestinal tract and the liver. As a result, they are thought to treat skin conditions attributed to toxic metabolites from **poor digestion** (page 260) and poor liver function.

Active constituents

Yellow dock contains relatively small amounts of anthraquinone glycosides, which may contribute to its mild laxative effect.[1] It is also thought to stimulate bile production. It is often used as a digestive bitter for people with poor digestion. No human studies have been done on its use as medicine.

How much is usually taken?

A tincture of yellow dock, ¼– ½ teaspoon (1–2 ml) three times per day, can be used.[2] Alternatively, a tea can be made by boiling 1–2 teaspoons (5–10 grams) of root in 2 cups (500 ml) of water for ten minutes. Three cups (750 ml) may be drunk each day.

Are there any side effects or interactions?

Aside from mild **diarrhea** (page 163) or loose stools in some people, yellow dock is rarely associated with side effects.[3]

YOHIMBE

Botanical name: *Pausinystalia yohimbe*

Parts used and where grown

Yohimbe is a tall evergreen forest tree native to southwestern Nigeria, Cameroon, Gabon, and the Congo. The bark of this African tree is used medicinally. There are concerns, however, that the tree may be endangered due to over-harvesting for use as medicine.

Yohimbe has been used in connection with the following conditions (refer to the individual health concern for complete information):

Rating	Health Concerns
★★★	**Erectile dysfunction** (page 185)
★★☆	**Weight loss** (page 446)
★☆☆	**Depression** (page 145)

Historical or traditional use (may or may not be supported by scientific studies)

Historically, yohimbe bark was used in western Africa for fevers, leprosy, and **coughs** (page 139).[1] It has also been used to dilate pupils, for **heart disease** (page 98), and as a local anesthetic. It has a more recent history of use as an aphrodisiac and a hallucinogen.

Active constituents

The alkaloid known as yohimbine is the primary active constituent in yohimbe, although similar alkaloids may also play a role. Yohimbine blocks alpha-2 adrenergic receptors, part of the sympathetic nervous system.[2] It also dilates blood vessels. Yohimbine inhibits monoamine oxidase (MAO) and therefore may theoretically be of benefit in depressive disorders. However, it does not have the clinical research of other herbs used for **depression** (page 145), such as **St. John's wort** (page 747).

Yohimbine has been shown in double-blind trials to help treat men with **erectile dysfunction** (page 185).[3, 4] Although, negative studies have also been reported.[5, 6]

How much is usually taken?

Standardized yohimbe products are available. A safe daily amount of yohimbine from any product is 15–30 mg.[7] Yohimbine should be used under the supervision of a physician. Traditionally, a tincture of the bark, 5–10 drops three times per day, has been used.

Are there any side effects or interactions?

Patients with kidney disease, **peptic ulcer** (page 349) or **pregnant** (page 363) or breast-feeding women should not use yohimbe.[8] Standard amounts may occasionally cause dizziness, nausea, **insomnia** (page 270), **anxiety** (page 30), increased **blood pressure** (page 246), and rapid heart beat,[9] though all of these are rare.[10] Using more than 40 mg of yohimbine per day can cause dangerous side effects, including loss of muscle function, chills, and vertigo. Some people will also experience hallucinations when taking higher amounts of yohimbine.[11] Taking 200 mg yohimbine in one case led to only a brief episode of hypertension, palpitations, and anxiety.[12] People with post-traumatic stress disorder[13] and panic disorder[14] should avoid yohimbe as it may worsen their condition.

Foods with high amounts of tyramine (such as cheese, red wine, and liver) should not be eaten while a person is taking yohimbe, as they may theoretically cause severe high blood pressure and other problems. Similarly, yohimbe should only be combined with other antidepressant drugs under the supervision of a physician, though at least one study suggests it may benefit those who are not responding to serotonin reuptake inhibitors such as fluoxetine (Prozac).[15]

Special United Kingdom considerations

Yohimbe may be prescribed by a doctor or dispensed under the supervision of a pharmacist.

Index

About Healthnotes

Healthnotes, Inc. (HNI) is the premier provider of reliable, easy-to-use health, food, and lifestyle information for Web sites and interactive touch-screen kiosks. Used by leading supermarkets, pharmacies, and health food stores in the United States, Canada, and the United Kingdom, Healthnotes Retail Solutions empower consumers to make educated decisions and drive product sales—online and in-store. HNI also generates Web applications that are licensed to e-commerce and health-related Internet sites worldwide. On the Web: www.healthnotes.com.

Overseen by Chief Medical Editor Alan R. Gaby, M.D., the Healthnotes interdisciplinary writing team includes experts from the fields of medicine, pharmacy, nursing, naturopathy, public health, and chiropractic. We regularly update our knowledge base, annually reviewing thousands of articles published in more than 600 peer-reviewed medical journals to ensure that consumers receive fully referenced, up-to-date health information based on the latest scientific and medical research.

Alan R. Gaby, M.D., *Chief Medical Editor*

An expert in nutritional therapies, Chief Medical Editor Alan R. Gaby is a former professor at Bastyr University of Natural Health Sciences, where he served as the Endowed Professor of Nutrition. He is past president of the American Holistic Medical Association and gave expert testimony to the White House Commission on Complementary and Alternative Medicine on the cost-effectiveness of nutritional supplements. He has authored *Preventing and Reversing Osteoporosis* (Prima Lifestyles, 1995) and *B_6: The Natural Healer* (Keats, 1987) and coauthored *The Patient's Book of Natural Healing* (Prima, 1999), *The Natural Pharmacy* (Three Rivers Press, 2006), and the *A–Z Guide to Drug-Herb-Vitamin Interactions* (Three Rivers Press, 2006). Dr. Gaby has conducted nutritional seminars for physicians and has collected more than 30,000 scientific papers related to the field of nutritional and natural medicine.

Also Available From Healthnotes

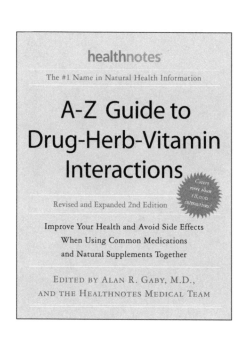

A–Z Guide to Drug-Herb-Vitamin Interactions

0-307-33664-6
$22.95 paper (Canada: $32.95)

Written by a team of experts from the fields of medicine, pharmacy, naturopathy, and public health, the *A–Z Guide to Drug-Herb-Vitamin Interactions* covers the ways in which common prescription and over-the-counter drugs interact with herbs, vitamins, and foods, including potential nutrient depletions, interference with drug actions, reduction of drug side effects, and interference with drug absorption (bioavailability). Learn how some herbs and vitamins help drugs work better, discover why certain drugs and supplements should never be taken together, and find out which drug side effects can be reduced by taking the right vitamin or herb.

Healthnotes reliable health, food, and lifestyle information is available throughout the United States and United Kingdom. Ask your local pharmacy, supermarket, or health food store if they offer Healthnotes in-store or online.

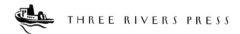 THREE RIVERS PRESS   *Available from Three Rivers Press wherever books are sold*